GLOBAL CLIMATE CHANGE AND HUMAN HEALTH

GLOBAL CLIMATE CHANGE AND HUMAN HEALTH

FROM SCIENCE TO PRACTICE

Second Edition

Edited by

Jay Lemery, MD

University of Colorado, Anschutz Medical Campus
Aurora, CO

Kim Knowlton, DrPH

Columbia University, Mailman School of Public Health
New York, NY

Cecilia Sorensen, MD

University of Colorado, Anschutz Medical Campus
Aurora, CO

JB **JOSSEY-BASS**™

A Wiley Brand

Registered Office
John Wiley & Sons, Inc., 111 River Street, Hoboken, NJ 07030, USA

Editorial Office
111 River Street, Hoboken, NJ 07030, USA

For details of our global editorial offices, customer services, and more information about Wiley products visit us at www.wiley.com.

Wiley also publishes its books in a variety of electronic formats and by print-on-demand. Some content that appears in standard print versions of this book may not be available in other formats.

Library of Congress Cataloging-in-Publication Data

Names: Luber, George, editor. | Lemery, Jay, editor. | Knowlton, Kim,
    editor. | Sorensen, Cecilia, editor.
Title: Global climate change and human health : from science to practice /
    edited by George Luber, Jay Lemery, Kim Knowlton, Cecilia Sorensen.
Description: Second edition. | San Francisco : Jossey-Bass, 2020. |
    Includes bibliographical references and index.
Identifiers: LCCN 2020028113 (print) | LCCN 2020028114 (ebook) | ISBN
    9781119667957 (paperback) | ISBN 9781119670018 (Adobe PDF) | ISBN
    9781119669999 (epub)
Subjects: MESH: Climate Change | Environmental Health | Global Health
Classification: LCC RA793 (print) | LCC RA793 (ebook) | NLM WA 30.2 |
    DDC 615.9/02—dc23
LC record available at https://lccn.loc.gov/2020028113
LC ebook record available at https://lccn.loc.gov/2020028114

Cover Design: Wiley
Cover Image: © Usman Ahmad/EyeEm/Getty Images, Ratnakorn Piyasirisorost/Getty Images, Mitch Diamond/Getty Images, Rehman Asad/Getty Images, Marco Bottigelli/Getty Images

Set in size of 10.5/14 and Warnock Pro by SPi Global, Chennai

SKY10058714_102723

JL: In loving memory of two of the world's most formidable mentors: Dean Jack Blackburn and Mr. Jim Westhall. Here's some evidence that you are indeed still changing the world!

KK: With love and gratitude to my parents, Stewart Knowlton and Nadine Wolfe, for their kindness and encouraging hours of scientific discovery under the big willow tree; and to my loving husband, Allen, for his patience and for asking the best questions.

CS: To future generations—may you enjoy the beauty of this wondrous planet. To my mentors for their inspiration and determination; and of course to Zach—for all the love, encouragement, and laughs.

CONTENTS

Jay Lemery, Kim Knowlton, Cecilia Sorensen, and Hanna Linstadt

Christopher K. Uejio, James D. Tamerius, Yoonjung Ahn, and Elaina Gonsoroski

Mark E. Keim

Xiangmei (May) Wu and Rupa Basu

Chapter 31   The Global Energy Transition and Public Health in a

Hanna Linstadt, Cecilia J. Sorensen and Morgan D. Bazilian

Carolyn Sotka

The *Nurses Climate Challenge*: A Model for Health Professional

Shanda Demorest

Recently, we took a field trip with a group of public health and medical students to the National Science Foundation Ice Core Facility in Lakewood, Colorado. The students were taking one of the nation's first medical school courses in climate change and health, and it was time to get out of the classroom to see science in action. We weren't quite sure what to expect as, essentially, we were going to visit a warehouse full of ancient ice.

It was May, but we were told to bring our deep winter gear—down jackets, hats, and gloves. The room was built for Arctic winter, set at 40° below, the singular temperature where Fahrenheit is the same as Celsius. After a short film explaining the process of ice core science, we were introduced to the star of the show: there, in all its cryogenic glory, a recumbent ice tube containing the atmospheric carbon record of the last several thousand years. The staff was masterful in recounting a science narrative explaining how the project was conceived, data obtained, and conclusions rendered.

The students were mesmerized. We witnessed a cascade of "ah-ha!" moments, the Holy Grail for any educator where the abstract notions, numbers, and equations all come together in a spark of enlightenment for the learner. For us, that day was more than a lesson in science, it was a lesson in the power of science communication—our highest aspiration as we bring you the most up-to-date expert climate and health science in this second edition.

Much has changed since we published our first edition in 2015.

We can be thankful that the science of climate change has advanced remarkably, while simultaneously, economically viable green technologies have emerged at an unprecedented rate. Despite public acceptance around climate science globally, we've seen a backlash against science-backed climate policy and intransigence toward policy action, especially in the United States. Understanding public opinion and perceptions around climate change and science, which can shape or hinder smart policy, has become a science unto itself, and we explore that in this book.

New challenges have emerged that are rewriting climate narratives. We now must incorporate the profound impact of the recent pandemic into our work and understand how they are related. Do the public health remedies for both coincide? Although we have yet to fully digest this experience, what is clear is that COVID-19 shows us how fragile our interconnections are and how rapidly we can mobilize resources—both human action and financial resources—to address a common threat. It also offers a palpable admonishment of our custodianship of the commons and the limitations of current governance—both national and international—to implement policy. Yet there is no doubt the COVID-19 crisis presents an opportunity for us to upgrade our operating system, to think about public health resilience, energy policy, and global governance.

Despite the rapidly changing events, the goal of this textbook remains the same: to serve as a resource for public health and clinical medicine practitioners, students, and learners. We crafted this book to be a comprehensive source on climate and health issues, authored by the experts who demonstrate mastery of the many complex facets of this topic. We added innovative pedagogical elements, expanded clinical correlations from the first edition, led each chapter with key concepts; included a glossary, and are again supporting educators with materials in the form of electronic teaching slides with accompanying multiple choice and essay questions.

New to this second edition are updates to the core climate and health science topics, issues of health equity, novel perspectives from clinical medicine and allied health professions, and an expansive discussion on the dizzying aspects of global governance. We have likewise recruited experts to share science on the unique vulnerabilities that women suffer from climate change as well as the interrelated topics of ecosystem services and loss of biodiversity.

It is our sober assessment that when it comes to protecting our health from climate change, we are not keeping pace. It's easy to look at the table of contents and feel pessimistic. Yet there is much for which to be hopeful. Since the publication of our last edition, medical societies have banded together in action and joined thousands of public entities in divesting from fossil fuels, major medical journals have prioritized climate-related topics, graduate schools of public health and medicine have launched dedicated climate and health curricula, and energetic grassroots student groups have emerged across campuses. Perhaps most telling is that public opinions are slowly changing.

One thing is certain: the science will advance, and in that regard, we feel fortunate to have this platform to share with you. May our next edition reflect the health implications from shifts in grassroots perceptions, the maturation of clean technologies in the marketplace, and the efficacy of smart policies enacted.

We believe this is the grand health challenge of our times. For us, there is no better outlet for our intellectual and creative energies than to present the work of our accomplished authors to you.

Jay Lemery
Kim Knowlton
Cecilia Sorensen

My career in medicine and public health has brought me to sub-Saharan Africa and southeast Asia, as well as the American southwest. I've responded to outbreaks of hepatitis E in Chad, Ebola in West Africa, and most recently on the frontlines of coronavirus disease 2019 (COVID-19) in New York City.

Despite being different outbreaks in different places, the one constant similarity in all was how public health crises always disproportionately affect already marginalized and vulnerable communities.

For a long time, we've known that we were susceptible to a global pandemic. In recent decades, outbreaks of SARS (severe acute respiratory syndrome coronavirus 2) and MERS (Middle East respiratory syndrome) alerted us to the possible implications of global spread. The 2014–2016 West Africa Ebola outbreak further highlighted how a public health threat anywhere represents a threat everywhere. In the aftermath of all of these outbreaks, lessons learned documents formed the basis for adaptations and change. Yet despite all this, when COVID-19 rapidly spread around the world in 2020, we found ourselves unprepared.

Along with the recent rise of nationalism and antimigrant rhetoric, there has been increasing critique of the globalist mindset—this idea that the people and nations of the world are inextricably linked. As countries have gradually receded and focused inward, they've taken apart and undermined much of the preparedness done to prevent and respond to a global public health threat.

The Social Injustice of the Pandemic

In that sense, it's not the COVID-19 pandemic that was surprising. It's how poorly we managed it. Throughout history, epidemics arise on the margins of our society, the disease taking root among the most vulnerable. It was Virchow who noted that *medicine is a social science and politics is nothing else but medicine on a large scale* (Virchow 1985). The mortality rate from COVID-19 is highest among the elderly, communities of color, and those with preexisting health conditions and is likely to be devastating for the poorest and in the developing world.

Climate Justice

Unfortunately, we know this is a harbinger of things to come. The pandemic experience foreshadows the health impacts from climate change, compounding every year with extreme weather patterns, sea level rise, food and water insecurity, and many other drivers articulated in this textbook. As the authors consistently point out in each of these chapters, it's the most marginalized and vulnerable who will suffer the most—through geography, age, socioeconomic status, and medical comorbidities. The public health policy response to the COVID-19 pandemic has pitted individual rights against collective action. I am too sanguine to think that apolitical unity would be a default societal response in these times; however, we do have powerful tools to lead and to continue to shape the policy narrative.

We can lead on the incredible successes of data-driven public health responses. Even before John Snow's eureka moment at the Broad Street pump, the world has benefited from global health initiatives proven to be a sound investment. No better example exists than the global campaign against smallpox, which was finally eradicated in 1980. Smallpox had long been humanity's greatest scourge. In the late 1700s, smallpox was so feared that even the first president of the United States—George Washington, himself a smallpox survivor—described it as a "greater threat than. . .the Sword of the Enemy." For the unparalleled commitment to smallpox eradication, the United States saves the total of all its historic contributions to ending smallpox every 26 days because it does not have to vaccinate or treat the disease (Center for Global Development n.d.).

The worldwide response to the HIV/AIDS pandemic recognized that supporting global health initiatives not only has a humanitarian impact. PEPFAR (President's Emergency Plan for AIDS Relief) was established in 2003 by President George W. Bush to increase access to HIV/AIDS treatment around the world. Since its inception, this program has greatly reduced HIV/AIDS-related morbidity and mortality by providing treatment to millions of men, women, and children worldwide. Subsequently, we have also seen the profound strategic national and international benefits by preventing social unrest and political instability in the countries most affected by HIV/AIDS in the developing world.

To date, many in the developed world have equated emergency preparedness with individual preparedness. But none of us has the individual ability to affect our sick neighbors' risk of disease spread or to roll out widespread testing for evidence of infection. Collective action is a precondition for managing any public health crisis, be it from a pandemic or global environmental change—and these actions are not necessarily rooted in protecting the individual as much as protecting the most vulnerable in our communities.

Leading

Yet because the pandemic has upended many of our assumptions—not only about public health but also governance, economic models, and social policies—you readers have an unprecedented opportunity to lead on this issue. And the rhetoric you choose does not have to be steeped in dour consequences—we have a lot to be excited about and to give the public a positive reason for change. We can lead on solutions.

Technology is giving us better ways tools to decarbonize while reducing the cost of energy. *Wright's law*—a model that predicts plummeting costs as new technology comes to scale—has proven true for wind, solar, and battery power. In many instances these technologies are now cheaper than oil and gas, ushering a future of cheap and abundant clean energy. As we think about how to reinvigorate our economy from the pandemic, such opportunities afford us a synergistic benefit in both job creation for a growing market and reduced greenhouse gas emissions.

The reputation of science has taken some bruising in recent years. But when it comes to illness or injury, everyone wants the best science working for themselves and their loved ones. Therein lies our ability to affect public risk assessment and to advance an evidence-based approach toward risk and opportunity.

I conclude by sharing with you a moment from my time on the frontlines of Ebola in West Africa. I had seen so many succumb to this disease and I felt like I hadn't made a difference. Yet one day, while being treated for Ebola myself in a hospital in New York City, I received a call from someone far away. She heard I was sick and called to thank me for caring for her family and to wish me well. I recognized then that I had indeed made an impact. Because over and over she thanked me. She believed if I hadn't been there to take care of her and her family none of them would have survived this disease.

In caring for others I had created a community of people across the world who cared about me because I had cared about them.

If we are to successfully tackle the public health and climate challenges in coming years, we will need collective action. Action based on creating a worldwide community that cares about others. If the COVID-19 pandemic taught us anything, it's that in times of global crisis we need global solidarity.

This book is a framework for the actions and decisions we need to foster this global community of caring. But it is only by operationalizing our voices, our advocacy, and our passion that we will create the collective response necessary to confront the public health and climate crises that undoubtedly lie in front of us.

References

Center for Global Development. n.d. *Case 1: Eradicating Smallpox.* https://www.cgdev.org/page/case-1-eradicating-smallpox

Virchow, R. 1985. "The Charity Physician (1848)." In *Collected Essays on Public Health and Epidemiology*, edited by L. J. Rather. Canton, MA: Science History Publications.

ACKNOWLEDGEMENTS

We would like to acknowledge the incredible efforts from our editorial team! We are grateful for their superb contributions to this second edition.

Beth Gillespie, MD, associate editor for pedagogical elements

Elaine Reno, MD, associate editor for supporting education materials, who led a team of motivated and talented editorial assistants: Ian Liu, William Mundo, Jessica Phan, Gavriel Roda, and Alessandra Santiago

Caitlin Rublee, MD, assistant editor for Clinical Correlates

Jay Lemery, MD, is professor of emergency medicine at the University of Colorado School of Medicine, chief of the Section of Wilderness and Environmental Medicine, and professor in the Department of Environmental and Occupational Health at the Colorado School of Public Health. He is a past-president of the Wilderness Medical Society.

In 2015 Dr. Lemery coedited the first edition of *Global Climate Change and Human Health: From Science to Practice*, and in 2017 he coauthored *Enviromedics: The Impact of Climate Change on Human Health*. He was a technical contributor to the *Fourth National Climate Assessment* (2018) produced by thirteen federal agencies, and from 2011 to 2016, he was a consultant for the Climate and Health Program at the Centers for Disease Control and Prevention.

Dr. Lemery graduated as an Echols Scholar from the University of Virginia and has a medical degree from the Geisel School of Medicine at Dartmouth. He also holds academic appointments at the Harvard School of Public Health (FXB Center), where he is a contributing editor for its journal, *Health and Human Rights*. Dr. Lemery sits on the National Academy of Medicine's Roundtable on Environmental Health Sciences, Research, and Medicine and is currently the medical director for the National Science Foundation's Polar Research program.

* * *

Kim Knowlton, DrPH, MS, is assistant professor of environmental health sciences at the Mailman School of Public Health, Columbia University; and past chair of the Climate Change Topic Committee of the American Public Health Association's Environment Section. She served as co-convening lead author for the human health chapter of the U.S. Third National Climate Assessment; as a member of the 2nd and the 4th New York City Panel on Climate Change and participated in the Intergovernmental Panel on Climate Change's 2007 Fourth and 2013 Fifth Assessment Reports. She is a health scientist specializing in the human health impacts of climate change, particularly air pollution and extreme heat.

Her work with the New York Climate and Health Project 2001–2007 described some of the first downscaled global-to-regional climate-air quality/heat-health effect modeling results in the United States and served as a foundation for her collaboration with climate, atmospheric chemistry, and land use modelers. She also serves as senior scientist and deputy director of the Science Center at the Natural Resources Defense Council in New York, where she works to help communities in the United States and partners in India adapt to our changed climate, connect the dots between climate and health for multiple audiences, and put science in the service of advocacy to protect people and the planet.

* * *

Cecilia Sorensen, MD, is an emergency medicine physician-investigator in the area of climate change and health at the University of Colorado School of Medicine and the Colorado School of Public Health. Following residency training at Denver Health in Denver, Colorado, she became the inaugural Living Closer Foundation Fellow in Climate and Health Science Policy, based at the University of Colorado School of Medicine and the National Institute of Environmental Health Sciences.

Dr. Sorensen has a broad range of expertise at the intersection of human health, environmental health, and social justice. Her recent work has spanned domestic as well as international emergent health issues related to climate change, including heat stress and worker health in Guatemala, wildfires and health care utilization in the United States, the emergence of Zika virus in Ecuador following the earthquake of 2016, climate change and women's health in India, and mortality following hurricane Maria in Puerto Rico.

Translating this research into policy to order to build resilience in vulnerable communities is the focus of her work. To this end, she has served as a health author for the U.S. Fourth National Climate Assessment and serves as a technical advisor for the annual Lancet Climate and Health U.S. Policy Brief. Additionally, she is a founding member of the Colorado Chapter of Physicians for Social Responsibility, a member of the Colorado Consortium for Climate Change, a scientific advisor for the Citizens Climate Lobby and the course director for the nation's first medical school course on climate change and human health.

Salma M. Abdalla, MBBS, MPH, School of Public Health, Boston University, Boston, Massachusetts

Yoonjung Ahn, MS, Florida State University, Tallahassee, Florida

Micaela Y. Arthur, MPH, Washington, DC

Louise Aubin, MES, Public Health, Health Services, Region of Peel, Mississauga, Ontario

John M. Balbus, MD, MPH, National Institute of Environmental Health Sciences, Bethesda, Maryland

Satchit Balsari, MD, MPH, Department of Emergency Medicine, Beth Israel Deaconess Medical Center, Boston, Massachusetts

Rupa Basu, PhD, OEHHA/CalEPA, Oakland, California

Morgan D. Bazilian, PhD, Payne Institute, Colorado School of Mines, Golden, Colorado

Charles B. Beard, PhD, Centers for Disease Control and Prevention, Fort Collins, Colorado

Peter Berry, PhD, Health Canada, Ottawa, Ontario8

Alison Blaiklock, MBChB, MPHTM, FNZCPHM, University of Otago, Wellington, New Zealand

Ellen Bloomer, MSc, Global Public Health, Public Health England, London, United Kingdom

Andrea Buchwald, PhD, Colorado School of Public Health, Aurora, Colorado

Emilie J. Calvello Hynes, MD, MPH, University of Colorado School of Medicine, Aurora, Colorado

Stuart Capstick, PhD, School of Psychology, University of Cardiff, Cardiff, United Kingdom

Elizabeth J. Carlton, PhD, Colorado School of Public Health, University of Colorado, Anschutz Campus, Aurora, Colorado

Amit Chandra, MD, MSc, Arlington, Virginia

Amy Collins, MD, Wellesley, Massachusetts

Adam Corner, PhD, Climate Outreach, Oxford, United Kingdom

Allison Crimmins, MS, MPP, Washington, DC

Tracy A. Cushing, MD, University of Colorado School of Medicine, Aurora, Colorado

Miranda Dally, MS, University of Colorado, Anschutz Medical Campus, Aurora, Colorado

Shanda Demorest, DNP, RN, PHN, LaCrescent, Minnesota

Caleb Dresser, MD, Department of Emergency Medicine, Beth Israel Deaconess Medical Center, Boston, Massachusetts

Kristie L. Ebi, PhD, MPH, Departments of Global Health and of Environmental and Occupational Health Sciences, University of Washington, Seattle, Washington

Abdulrahman M. El-Sayed, MD, DPhil, Department of Public Health, Wayne State University, Detroit, Michigan

Kenneth L. Gage, PhD, Centers for Disease Control and Prevention, Fort Collins Colorado

Sandro Galea, MD, MPH, DrPH, School of Public Health, Boston University, Boston, Massachusetts

Jada F. Garofalo, Centers for Disease Control and Prevention, Fort Collins Colorado

Elaina Gonsoroski, Florida State University, Tallahassee, Florida

Mark R. Hafen, PhD, University of South Florida, School of Public Affairs, Tampa, Florida

Micah Hahn, PhD, MPH, Anchorage, Alaska

Sherilee L. Harper, PhD, School of Public Health, University of Alberta, Edmonton, AB

Jeremy J. Hess, MD, MPH, Center for Health and the Global Environment, University of Washington, Seattle, Washington

Rhys Jones, MBChB, MPH, FNZCPHM, University of Auckland, Auckland, New Zealand

Kristopher B. Karnauskas, PhD, University of Colorado, Boulder, Colorado

Mark Keim, MD, MBA, DisasterDoc LLC, Lawrenceville, Georgia

Amber S. Khan, Division of Environmental Health Sciences, School of Public Health, Berkeley, California

Kim Knowlton, DrPH, Columbia University Mailman School of Public Health, New York, New York

Randall Kramer, PhD, Nicholas School of the Environment and The Global Health Institute, Duke University, Durham, North Carolina

Joleah Lamb, PhD, University of California, Irvine, Irvine, California

Jay Lemery, MD, University of Colorado School of Medicine, Aurora, Colorado

Vijay S. Limaye, PhD, Natural Resources Defense Council, New York, New York

Hanna Linstadt, MD, University of Colorado School of Medicine, Aurora, Colorado

Cecilia Martinez, PhD, Center for Earth, Energy and Democracy, Minneapolis, Minnesota

Sara Mason, MS, Nicholas Institute for Environmental Policy Solutions, Duke University, Durham, North Carolina

Yuta Masuda, PhD, The Nature Conservancy, Arlington, Virginia

J. S. Metcalf, PhD, Brain Chemistry Labs, Jackson, Wyoming

Virginia Murray, FFPH, FRCP, FFOM, Global Disaster Risk Reduction, Public Health England, London, United Kingdom

Lee S. Newman, MD, MA, Center for Health, Work & Environment, University of Colorado, Anschutz Medical Campus, Aurora, Colorado

Lydia Olander, PhD, Nicholas Institute for Environmental Policy Solutions, Duke University, Durham, North Carolina

Debra Parkinson, PhD, Monash University and Gender and Disaster Pod, Clayton, Australia

Nick Pidgeon, PhD, MBE, School of Psychology, Cardiff University, Cardiff, United Kingdom

Nikhil A. Ranadive, MD, Emergency Medicine, UCSF Fresno Medical Education, Fresno, California

Justin V. Remais, PhD, School of Public Health, University of California- Berkeley, Berkeley, California

Rosemary Rochford, PhD, University of Colorado, School of Medicine, Aurora, Colorado

Caitlin S. Rublee, MD, MPH, Medical College of Wisconsin, Milwaukee, Wisconsin

Richard Salkowe, DPM, PhD, University of South Florida, School of Public Affairs, Tampa, Florida

Rebekka Schnitter, MCC, Health Canada, Ottawa, Ontario

Jan C. Semenza, PhD, MPH, MS, European Centre for Disease Prevention and Control (ECDC), Solna, Sweden

Ambereen K. Shaffie, JD, LLM, Shaffie Law and Policy, LLC, Overland Park, Kansas

Chris Shaw, DPhil, Climate Outreach, Oxford, United Kingdom

Nicky Sheats, JD, PhD, Trenton, NJ

Cecilia J. Sorensen, MD, University of Colorado School of Medicine, Aurora, Colorado

Carolyn Sotka, MA, College of Charleston, Charleston, South Carolina

N. R. Souza, Brain Chemistry Labs, Jackson, Wyoming

Craig Spencer, MD, MPH, Columbia University Mailman School of Public Health, New York, New York

Sarah Spengeman, PhD, Mill Valley, California

Heather Tallis, PhD, MSc, MS, The Nature Conservancy, Arlington, Virginia

James D. Tamerius, PhD, University of Iowa, Iowa City, Iowa

Cristina Tirado, DVM, MS, PhD, UCLA School of Public Health, Los Angeles, California

Christopher K. Uejio, PhD, Florida State University, Tallahassee, Florida

Carmel Williams, PhD, Harvard FXB Center, Boston, Massachusetts

Xiangmei (May) Wu, PhD, OEHHA/CalEPA, Oakland, California

Lewis H. Ziska, PhD, Mailman School of Public Health, New York, New York

COMMENTARY ON COVID-19, CLIMATE CHANGE, AND HUMAN HEALTH

Jay Lemery, Kim Knowlton, Cecilia Sorensen, and Hanna Linstadt

The COVID-19 pandemic has demonstrably exposed the fault lines in our public health infrastructure and exacerbated the underlying disparities in our communities. For those of us studying climate change and human health, the parallels are all too easy to make: a public health disaster hampered by a lack of preparation and coordination; health effects spilling over to have dire economic consequences; a disproportionate burden falling upon communities of color, those with the fewest resources and the smallest contribution to the causation of the problem.

But in other ways, there has been a remarkable divergence in the public response toward the pandemic and climate change. We have witnessed an historic mobilization of resources and public policy measures, despite the significant effects these global phenomena have had on business as usual and societal norms. Massive economic stimulus packages passed rapidly, with widespread consent from a historically gridlocked, partisan legislature. Prodigious sums of public funds were allocated toward the accelerated development of diagnostics, treatments, and vaccines.

Despite the criticisms that more could be done, there is no doubt our world changed overnight, and that our society mobilized rapidly to address the crisis. We contrast the pandemic response to the slow-motion climate change crisis, for which, despite being evident for decades, effective action remains elusive.

In crisis comes opportunity. Looking to the world we will create after coronavirus disease 2019 (COVID-19), we believe there are historic opportunities to reinvigorate and enhance the resilience of our communities and institutions. We have a once-in-a-generation mandate to reconsider our public health and economic operating systems, and in turn, change the trajectory of our next public health crisis—a rapidly changing climate.

Understanding that the science and impacts of the pandemic are rapidly changing, we have nevertheless endeavored to provide a brief inventory and overview on the many facets of COVID-19 and climate and health issues. We cite the interactions between COVID-19 and climate-related health conditions and how the global recovery from the pandemic has the potential to improve public health and to limit the effects of climate change in the future.

Climate Change Exposure Pathways and COVID-19

Increasing Temperature

Hotter temperatures are known to worsen chronic conditions like cardiovascular disease and respiratory disease, as well as diabetes-related conditions and cerebrovascular disease (Crimmins et al. 2016). Data on environmental temperatures and COVID-19 infections are conflicting. Some studies show that the transmission of the virus may actually decrease with rising temperatures (Le et al. 2020; Liu et al. 2020; Prata, Rodrigues, and Bermejo 2020), so it is possible the increased average temperatures globally could have a positive effect on slowing the spread of COVID-19. On the other hand, there are also studies that refute this notion (Global Heat Health Information Network 2020; Xie and Zhu 2020). Thus, it is currently unclear what the true effect of rising temperatures has on the transmission and/or severity of COVID-19.

Air Quality

Initial data have shown that people with certain underlying respiratory diseases or cardiovascular disease may be at risk for more severe illness from COVID-19 (Centers for Disease Control and Prevention 2020c). Air pollution exposure increases a person's risk of developing an underlying respiratory disease (Crimmins et al. 2016). This history of exposure may lead to more severe disease when infected with COVID-19. Even exposures to a small increase in air pollution—specifically fine particulate matter—have been shown to increase the COVID-19 death rate (Wu, Nethery, Sabath, Braun, and Dominici. 2020).

Concomitant Stressors

The pandemic is already straining the health care and emergency response systems of many regions and countries (Boccia, Ricciardi, and Ioannidis 2020; Uppal et al. 2020). Simultaneously, climate-driven severe weather events such as wildfires, flooding, and hurricanes continue to occur, resulting in injuries and illnesses that also strain the resources of existing health care systems (Crimmins et al. 2016). When faced with "double disaster" scenarios, the health care system is at risk of becoming overburdened to the point at which it is unable to provide the necessary care.

COVID-19 also affects the public health response to disasters like extreme weather events. For example, it is typical for evacuated or displaced persons in an extreme weather event to congregate in large shelters or community centers. However, many of these shelters have needed to reduce their capacity to allow for recommended social distancing (Wendle 2020), creating a challenging problem in the way we respond to disasters. Simultaneously, a large majority of public health and community time and resources are currently being diverted to address the COVID-19 pandemic, leaving less available to address chronic climate change-fueled stressors such as extreme heat, wildfires, and more. There is an imperative to enact an "all hazards" approach to public health risk reduction that encompasses all types of public health emergencies and addresses vulnerabilities within the system as well as within communities.

Climate Change and Future Pandemics

New and Emerging Pathogens

Anthropogenic forces that contribute to climate change also lead to changes in the geographic distribution of certain species (Crimmins et al. 2016), which can place these species in closer contact with humans. Deforestation and clearance of natural habitat for agricultural purposes not only leads to increasing CO_2 levels and loss of biodiversity but also to more frequent interactions between wild animals and humans, subsequently increasing the risk of novel disease transmission to humans (Rohr et al. 2019). Improving forest management practices may help prevent spillover of yet unknown pathogens while simultaneously helping to address climate change.

Migration and Vulnerable Populations

Loss of land and employment from climate-related extreme weather events, such as floods, drought, and hurricanes can lead to forced migration (United Nations High Commissioner for

Refugees n.d.). There were 24.8 million disaster-related displacements in 2019 (Internal Displacement Monitoring Centre 2019). When populations are displaced, they most often end up in very densely populated settlements (Refugees International 2020), and increased density in housing leads to increased risk of spread of communicable disease (Snyder 2018). This is particularly problematic in the era of COVID-19. Living in densely populated communities can make practicing social distancing extremely difficult, and access to health care is often scarce in these communities (Snyder 2018). Poor infrastructure resulting in a lack of clean, reliable water supply for sanitation and hygiene also increases the risk for COVID-19 outbreaks within communities (Poole, Escudero, Gostin, Leblang, and Talbot 2020).

Even in nonmigrant populations the social determinants of health, including socioeconomic factors, ethnicity, age, and health status increase the exposure to climate change-related negative health impacts (Crimmins et al. 2016). For example, communities of color and people living in poverty are at higher risk of exposure to air pollution (United Nations Environment Programme 2019), suffer higher rates of chronic disease, and lack access to health care (Islam and Winkel 2017). According to the Centers for Disease Control and Prevention (CDC), the pandemic has revealed a similar pattern of vulnerability. The CDC states that "long-standing health and social inequities have put some members of ethnic minority groups at increased risk of getting sick and dying from COVID-19" (CDC 2020b). Initial data shows that non-Hispanic American Indian or Alaska Native persons, non-Hispanic black persons, and Hispanic or Latino persons have COVID-19 hospitalization rates about five times that of non-Hispanic white persons (CDC 2020a). In the United States, racial/ethnic minorities have a disproportionate burden of underlying comorbidities and simultaneously suffer from poorer socioeconomic status and are more likely to live in crowded urban conditions, making it incredibly difficult to practice social distancing or work from home (Webb Hooper, Nápoles, and Pérez-Stable 2020).

Water

Climate change threatens water security, as increasingly unpredictable weather conditions and extremes in precipitation will limit reliable access to safe water and sanitation (United Nations Water n.d.b). Access to basic sanitation and water is a fundamental precondition for adequate public health and is vital to prevent the spread of COVID-19 as well as innumerable current and future pathogens (United Nations Environment Programme n.d.; United Nations Water n.d.a).

Crucial Turning Point

COVID-19 has held a mirror up to the inherent injustices of our society. The frightening reality is that in aggregate, our collective society appears to be one that does not invest in public health; one that has not addressed deep racial and socioeconomic inequalities; has an indifference to science; eschews public education; and allows those most vulnerable to bear the greatest burden of a global pandemic disease, all to avoid an imposition upon individual citizen rights. If we as a society wish to thrive in the face of the next great public health crisis, climate change, we owe it to ourselves and to our offspring to demand structural changes in society, and reassess the policies and practices that got us here in the first place.

Therein lies our historic opportunity—to build our post-COVID-19 world to value *all* human life as well as the life of the planet. To do so, we must enact climate-resilient policies that protect the health of generations to come through investing in renewable and efficient energy, decarbonizing the economy (UN News 2020), developing resilient supply chain and agricultural systems, and creating more climate-smart cities. Simultaneously, we must address deeply rooted environmental justice issues in our communities that negatively affect the health of the most vulnerable and rebuild health care and public health systems that allow all citizens to enjoy a healthy life. As custodians of health and wellness, we have a unique voice to share, and one that still holds the public trust (Funk 2020). In this regard, we are well-positioned to advocate for climate solutions that will advance the cause of social justice within our communities—advancing both human capital potential and human dignity in the same effort.

References

Boccia, S., W. Ricciardi, and J. P. A. Ioannidis. 2020. "What Other Countries Can Learn from Italy During the COVID-19 Pandemic." *JAMA Internal Medicine* 180 (7): 927–928.

Centers for Disease Control and Prevention. 2020a. *COVID-19 Hospitalization & Death by Race/ Ethnicity. Coronavirus Disease 2019.* Updated August 18, 2020. https://www.cdc.gov/coronavirus/2019-ncov/covid-data/investigations-discovery/hospitalization-death-by-race-ethnicity.html. Accessed August 21, 2020.

Centers for Disease Control and Prevention. 2020b. *Health Equity Considerations and Racial and Ethnic Minority Groups. Coronavirus Disease 2019.* Updated July 24, 2020. https://www.cdc.gov/coronavirus/2019-ncov/need-extra-precautions/racial-ethnic-minorities.html. Accessed August 10, 2020.

Centers for Disease Control and Prevention. 2020c. *People with Certain Medical Conditions. Coronavirus Disease 2019.* Updated August 14, 2020. https://www.cdc.gov/coronavirus/2019-ncov/need-extra-precautions/people-with-medical-conditions.html. Accessed August 21, 2020.

Crimmins, A., J. Balbus, J. L. Gamble, C. B. Beard, J. E. Bell, D. Dodgen, R. J. Eisen, et al., eds. 2016. *The Impacts of Climate Change on Human Health in the United States: A Scientific Assessment.* Washington, DC: U.S. Global Change Research Program.

Funk, C. 2020. *Polling Shows Signs of Public Trust in Institutions amid the Pandemic. Pew Research Center: Science & Society.* April 7. https://www.pewresearch.org/science/2020/04/07/polling-shows-signs-of-public-trust-in-institutions-amid-pandemic/.

Global Heat Health Information Network. 2020. "Seasonality and Weather." *Updated May 22, 2020.* http://www.ghhin.org/heat-and-covid-19/seasonality-and-weather. Accessed August 19, 2020.

Internal Displacement Monitoring Centre. 2019. *Global Report on Internal Displacement.* https://www.internal-displacement.org/database/displacement-data.

Islam, N. S., and J. Winkel. 2017. *Climate Change and Social Inequality.* DESA Working Paper no. 152. New York: United Nations Department of Economic and Social Affairs.

Le, N. K., A. V. Le, J. Parikh, J. P. Brooks, T. Gardellini, and R. Izurieta. 2020. "Ecological and Health Infrastructure Factors Affecting the Transmission and Mortality of COVID-19." Preprint from Research Square, March 29, 2020. doi: 10.21203/rs.3.rs-19504/v1.

Liu, J., J. Zhou, J. Yao, X. Zhang, L. Li, X. Xu, X. He et al. 2020. "Impact of Meteorological Factors on the COVID-19 Transmission: A Multi-City Study in China." *Science of the Total Environment* 726: 138513.

Poole, D. N., D. J. Escudero, L. O. Gostin, D. Leblang, and E. A. Talbot. 2020. "Responding to the COVID-19 Pandemic in Complex Humanitarian Crises." *International Journal for Equity in Health* 19 (1):41.

Prata, D. N., W. Rodrigues, and P. H. Bermejo. 2020. "Temperature Significantly Changes COVID-19 transmission in (Sub)tropical Cities of Brazil." *Science of the Total Environment* 729:138862.

Refugees International. 2020. *COVID-19 and the Displaced: Addressing the Threat of the Novel Coronavirus in Humanitarian Emergencies.* https://www.refugeesinternational.org/reports/2020/3/29/covid-19-and-the-displaced-addressing-the-threat-of-the-novel-coronavirus-in-humanitarian-emergencies.

Rohr, J. R., C. B. Barrett, D. J. Civitello, M. E. Craft, B. Delius, G. A. DeLeo, P. J. Hudson et al. 2019. "Emerging Human Infectious Diseases and the Links to Global Food Production." *Nature Sustainability* 2 (6):445–456.

Snyder, M. 2018. *Displaced Populations and the Threat of Disease.* January 4. https://www.outbreakobservatory.org/outbreakthursday-1/1/4/2018/displaced-populations-and-the-threat-of-disease.

UN News. 2020. *Parallel Threats of COVID-19, Climate Change, Require "Brave, Visionary and Collaborative Leadership": UN chief.* April 28. https://news.un.org/en/story/2020/04/1062752.

United Nations Environment Programme. 2019. *Air pollution hurts the poorest most.* May 9. https://www.unenvironment.org/news-and-stories/story/air-pollution-hurts-poorest-most.

United Nations Environment Programme. n.d. *Goal 6: Ensure Access to Water and Sanitation for All. Sustainable Development Goals* 2020. https://www.un.org/sustainabledevelopment/water-and-sanitation/. Accessed July 23, 2020.

United Nations Water. n.d.a. *Handwashing/Hand hygiene.* https://www.unwater.org/water-facts/handhygiene/. Accessed July 23, 2020a.

United Nations Water. n.d.b. *Water and Climate Change.* https://www.unwater.org/water-facts/climate-change/. Accessed August 16, 2020b.

United Nations High Commissioner for Refugees. n.d. *Climate change and disaster displacement.* *https://www.unhcr.org/en-us/climate-change-and-disasters.html.Accessed* July 23, 2020.

Uppal, A., D. M. Silvestri, M. Siegler, S. Natsui, L. Boudourakis, R. J. Salway, M. Parikh et al. 2020. "Critical Care and Emergency Department Response at the Epicenter of the COVID-19 Pandemic." *Health Affairs (Millwood)* 39 (8):1443–1449.

Webb Hooper, M., A. M. Nápoles, and E. J. Pérez-Stable. 2020. "COVID-19 and Racial/Ethnic Disparities." *JAMA* 323 (24):2466–2467. doi:10.1001/jama.2020.8598.

Wendle, A. 2020. *U.S. Disaster Response Scrambles To Protect People From Both Hurricanes And COVID-19.* NPR Morning Edition, July 22. https://www.npr.org/2020/07/22/893286668/u-s-disaster-response-scrambles-to-protect-people-from-both-hurricanes-and-covid.

Wu, X., R. C. Nethery, B. M. Sabath, D. Braun, and F. Dominici. 2020. "Exposure to Air Pollution and COVID-19 Mortality in the United States: A Nationwide Cross-Sectional Study." *medRxiv* Preprint. April 7, 2020. doi: 10.1101/2020.04.05.20054502.

Xie, J., and Y. Zhu. 2020. "Association between Ambient Temperature and COVID-19 Infection in 122 Cities from China." *Science of the Total Environment* 724:138201.

CHAPTER 1

PRIMER ON CLIMATE SCIENCE

Christopher K. Uejio, James D. Tamerius, Yoonjung Ahn, and Elaina Gonsoroski

The notion that carbon dioxide (CO_2) and other greenhouse gases (GHG) emissions could accumulate in the Earth's atmosphere and increase global surface temperatures was first proposed in the nineteenth century. In 1856, U.S. scientist Eunice Newton Foote theorized that altering atmospheric CO_2 could change the earth's temperature (Foote 1856). However, the idea was mostly forgotten until rising global temperatures in the middle of the twentieth century sparked renewed interest in the hypothesis.

In the late 1950s, David Keeling began measuring the atmospheric concentration of CO_2 at the Mauna Loa Observatory in Hawaii. The remote location of this observatory is minimally affected by local CO_2 sources and thus best reflects an average global atmospheric CO_2 level. Over decades, repeated measurements at Mauna Loa have shown a consistent upward trend in the concentration of atmospheric CO_2. Indeed, this atmospheric concentration has increased more than 40 percent—from 280 parts per million (ppm) to 405 ppm—since the dawn of the industrial revolution (Siegenthaler and Oeschger 1987). This increase is consistent with the quantity of CO_2 emitted into the atmosphere by humans through the burning of fossil fuels such as oil, coal, and natural gas, and it continues to grow. Worldwide average fossil fuels and industrial CO_2 emissions increased from 3.1 gigatons of carbon (GtC) per year in the 1960s to an average of 9.3 GtC per year over 2006–2015 (Le Quéré et al. 2016).

Scientific Consensus

As a result of increasingly complex mathematical models of climatologic processes and the development of techniques to study past climates, there is now unequivocal evidence among climate scientists that the altered composition of the atmosphere because of emissions of CO_2 and other greenhouse gases (GHG) from human activities is causing an increase in mean global temperatures. An analysis of 11,944 peer-reviewed global warming studies published between 1991 and 2011 found that 97.7 percent of the studies stated that humans are causing global warming (Oreskes 2004; Cook et al. 2013). The science that has shaped this consensus is synthesized by the Intergovernmental Panel on Climate Change (IPCC), a nonpartisan intergovernmental organization that was created in 1988 and was jointly awarded the Nobel Peace Prize in 2007. The IPCC performs periodic assessments on the status of **climate change** science, potential impacts, and mitigation (strategies to limit and or remove GHG) and adaptation (actions to increase the resilience of social and ecologic systems).

The IPCC reports reflect the evolving state of climate science. The IPCC (1990) stated that "the unequivocal detection of the enhanced greenhouse effect from observations is not likely for a decade or more." In the Third Assessment (IPCC 2001), the panel concluded that there was better evidence that human

KEY CONCEPTS

- Climate scientists state that the evidence is unequivocal; increasing global temperatures and climate change in the past century are due to human caused emissions of greenhouse gases.

- Human activities have increased the concentration of greenhouse gases in the atmosphere, which have augmented the greenhouse effect and increased average global temperatures by approximately 0.9°C (1.6°F) since the 1850s.

- Average global temperatures are expected to increase between approximately 0.8°C and 4.9°C (1.4°F and 8.8°F) by the end of this century, and there will likely be an increase in extreme heat events associated with climate change.

- The hydrologic cycle is changing, and extreme rainfall events will likely become more intense and frequent.

- Snow, glaciers, and sea ice cover are decreasing, and the average global sea level will continue to rise.

activities were responsible for the majority of the observed temperature increases. The Fourth Assessment Report (IPCC 2007) collectively determined with "very high confidence" (very low uncertainty) that human activities have increased global temperatures over the past fifty years. Over five hundred scientists and two thousand reviewers voluntarily contributed to the report. The Fifth Assessment (IPCC 2013) issued the strongest statement that observed warming in the past fifty years was "unequivocal." By comparison, the strength of this scientific consensus is similar to the evidence linking smoking to carcinogens and the development of cancer (Shwed and Bearman 2010).

This book examines the climatologic processes that affect human health. This chapter, however, focuses on the physical processes associated with climate change to provide a foundation for subsequent discussions. In particular, we clarify how greenhouse gases alter the Earth's **energy balance** and describe recent climate trends and projections of future climate change. In addition, we present multiple converging lines of evidence that support that the climate is indeed changing and that the changes are primarily caused by human activities.

Weather, Climate Variability, Climate Change, and Scientific Theory

It is important to distinguish the differences between short-term weather changes, natural **climate variability**, and long-term climate change. People are intricately familiar with short-term weather changes in atmospheric conditions from their everyday experiences. However, it can be difficult to sense changes to the climate because of its relatively slow progression amidst the background of natural climatic fluctuations. Confusion about these concepts leads to common misconceptions and incorrect interpretations and conclusions regarding climate change.

We experience weather—the state of the atmosphere at any given moment in time—through changes in temperature, humidity, precipitation, cloudiness, and wind. Although weather may change from moment to moment, weather events such as storms may last from several hours to several days. Specific locations around the world tend to experience relatively unique weather patterns based on features of latitude, proximity to large water bodies, and unique terrain (e.g., mountains). Collectively these features and the general circulation of the Earth's atmosphere and oceans shape a location's climate. Climate can be defined as the long-term average weather patterns for a specific region. More colloquially, Robert Heinlein (1973) stated, "Climate is what on an average we may expect; weather is what we actually get." J. Marshall Shepherd, former president of the American Meteorological Society, analogously stated, "Weather is your mood and climate is your personality." A more precise, operational climate definition is the average weather conditions over a period of thirty to fifty years.

Climate change also has a precise definition: the systematic change in the long-term state of the atmosphere over multiple decades (or longer). In the scientific literature, climate change may refer to a combination of human induced and natural climatic changes or only human-induced changes. Climate change may be ascertained and quantified by probabilistic statistical tests that measure the likelihood that observed changes are outside the range of natural variability. For example, there is at least a 99 percent chance that average global temperatures have significantly increased from 1950 to present (IPCC 2013). There is less than a 1 percent chance that we would randomly observe a similar increase in global temperatures over the same time period. Thus, climate scientists avoid using strict statements such as "I do [do not] believe" in climate change. The most robust examples of climate change exhibit the same unequivocal trend regardless of the choice of reference period (e.g., 1950–1989, 1970–2009), which suggests a long-term phenomenon outside of natural fluctuations in climate variability.

Superimposed on long-term trends in climate is natural climate variability. Natural climate variability is often associated with regular patterns in the Earth system that occur over periods of months to decades. The El Niño Southern Oscillation (ENSO) is the best-known and most important driver of year-to-year climate variability (Trenberth 1997). ENSO is associated with a two- to seven-year oscillation in sea surface temperatures (SST) in the eastern tropical Pacific, with warmer SST during El Niño. Conversely, during a La Niña event, eastern tropical Pacific SST are cooler than normal. Shifts in SST in this region have dramatic effects on the large-scale atmospheric circulation patterns around the world and can influence temperature and precipitation conditions. For example, in the eastern part of South Africa, El Niño events are frequently accompanied by drier-than-normal summers, whereas La Niña is associated with a slightly greater chance of above-average precipitation. However, the distribution, magnitude, and timing of the effects of ENSO vary from event to event (McPhaden, Zebiak, and Glantz 2006; Zebiak et al. 2015). Other analogous ocean atmosphere climate variability features vary over longer periods. For example, the Pacific Decadal Oscillation alters weather throughout the Pacific Ocean and Pacific Rim, whereas the North Atlantic Oscillation influences eastern North America, the Atlantic, and Europe (Vuille and Garreaud 2011). The Northern and Southern annular mode, respectively, alter weather in North America/Eurasia and Antarctica.

The contention that climate change is "just" a theory reflects common confusion about the meaning of the term theory. When used colloquially, a theory is defined as an educated guess. Scientifically, however, a theory is a well-substantiated, evidence-based explanation. By definition, scientific theories begin as hypotheses. Over the course of repeated verifications through experimental testing and observations, some hypotheses are deemed to be so well supported by scientific evidence that they become accepted as theories. This is the case with climate change, an evidence-based theory of science. Other well-known examples that define our understanding of the natural world include the germ theory of disease and the atomic theory of matter (American Association for the Advancement of Science 2006).

CLINICAL CORRELATES 1.1 HEAT WAVES AND OLDER ADULTS

Although no population is completely protected from outdoor and indoor heat, older adults have proven particularly vulnerable (Cheng et al. 2018; Liss, Chui, and Naumova 2017). During the 2003 heat wave in Europe, a majority of the seventy thousand excess deaths were among older persons (age > sixty-five years) who remained alone in their homes, despite warnings to seek cooler environments (Ledrans et al. 2004; Robine et al. 2008). Even excluding these severe heat events, numerous studies have shown older adults remain at high risk of heat-related illness due tobecause of a complex mixture of health and social factors. Geriatric physiologic changes in blood circulation and perspiration, polypharmacy, and lack of adaptive behaviors contribute to increased susceptibility to heat (Lindemann et al. 2018). Limitations in mobility, hearing, vision, and cognition make it difficult for these individuals to adhere to warnings. In addition, co-morbidities common in older adults such as renal, cardiovascular, and respiratory conditions can be exacerbated by high temperatures, while and geographical and social factors, such as isolation, may compound heat risk further (Gronlund 2014; Lindemann et al. 2018).

Knowing which factors make an individual more susceptible to heat and identifying these vulnerabilities in routine health screenings will allow primary care physicians to take an active role in raising awareness among this population and preventing heat-related morbidity and mortality.

Energy Balance

A basic understanding of Earth's energy balance is required to understand the theory of climate change. Our planet's temperature is dependent on how solar energy is transferred within the Earth system. The global temperature remains relatively constant because the total energy entering Earth is balanced by the energy that is released back into space. Specifically, solar energy is transmitted to Earth, and a proportion of the energy is naturally reflected back to space. However, some solar energy that enters the Earth system is absorbed by the atmosphere, oceans, and land surfaces, which causes the planet to warm. Historically however, the Earth system releases (transmits) energy back into space, which precludes the accumulation of energy in the Earth system and sustains homeostasis of global temperatures.

Yet several factors can cause the Earth's energy balance to change over time. We now discuss changes in the concentration of GHG, the **greenhouse effect**, GHG **global warming potential**, and changes in the amount of solar energy reaching Earth. Each of these factors is elaborated in detail.

Greenhouse Gases

We review the main GHGs whose atmospheric levels have increased as a result of human activities, at terrestrial concentrations not seen in hundreds of thousands of years. In order of their contribution to climate change, these GHGs are CO_2, methane (CH_4), nitrous oxide (N_2O), and fluorinated gases: hydrofluorocarbons, perfluorocarbons, and sulfur hexafluoride. The most important greenhouse gas is CO_2 (Figure 1.1). CO_2 is naturally emitted into the atmosphere through animal respiration and volcanic eruptions. Correspondingly, plant photosynthesis and ocean-atmospheric interactions absorb ambient CO_2. Although the cycle of CO_2 from these interactions is a natural process, humans have perturbed this balance by discharging increasing amounts of CO_2 through the burning of fossil fuels (i.e., oil, coal, and natural gas), solid waste, trees, and wood products. We have also disturbed this balance toward increased atmospheric CO_2 through land use changes such as deforestation (Environmental Protection Agency 2017). The result of this is that human activities such as fossil fuel use and land use change have emitted so much CO_2 into the atmosphere that natural CO_2 sinks (sources of CO_2 absorption such as oceans and plants) are no longer able to effectively absorb this excess CO_2 (EPA 2017). Indeed, since the eighteenth century, atmospheric CO_2 concentrations have increased by 40 percent

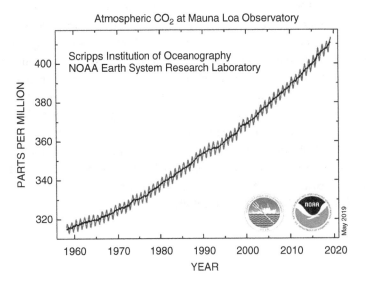

Figure 1.1   Atmospheric CO_2 levels, 1958–2019
Source: "NOAA Earth System" (2019).
Note: Rapid increases in CO_2 concentrations accompanied the industrial revolution.

from approximately 280 parts per million by volume (ppmv) to 407.4 ppmv in 2017. The current CO_2 level has likely not occurred for three million years (National Research Council 2010; Willeit et al. 2019) and is not a result of natural CO_2 variation in the atmosphere.

Methane (CH_4), an another important GHG, is emitted into the atmosphere through several processes. CH_4 is naturally emitted from wetlands and other areas through the decomposition of organic materials and is normally removed from the atmosphere through soil and other chemical reactions. Humans contribute to atmospheric CH_4 through the production and use of fossil fuels and commercial livestock (via decomposition of manure). The processing and decomposition of human solid waste in landfills and treatment facilities also produce CH_4. Atmospheric CH_4 levels have not been as high as they are now for 650,000 years (Environmental Protection Agency 2017).

For the 11,500 years before the industrial revolution, atmospheric nitrous oxide (N_2O) levels remained virtually constant. This gas is naturally released into the atmosphere through the breakdown of nitrogen by bacteria in the soil and ocean waters (denitrification). It is removed from the atmosphere through absorption by bacteria or decomposition by ultraviolet light radiation or other chemical reactions. Human causes of increased N_2O emissions stem from agriculture (e.g., synthetic fertilizers and livestock excrement), industry (e.g., nitric acid fertilizers and other synthetic products), and the combustion of solid waste and fossil fuels (Environmental Protection Agency 2017). After CO_2 and CH_4, increased atmospheric N_2O is the third largest contributor to the greenhouse effect and the largest contributor to depletion of Earth's ozone layer.

The final group of extremely potent GHG are fluorinated gases: hydrofluorocarbons (HFC), perfluorocarbons, and sulfur hexafluoride. Fluorinated gases are used as refrigerants (air conditioning for buildings and vehicles), solvents, propellants, and fire repellants. Perfluorocarbons are produced through industrial by-products of aluminum production and semiconductor manufacturing. Sulfur hexafluoride is produced by way of transmission of electricity through electrical equipment. HFC were designed to replace chlorofluorocarbons which degrade the stratospheric ozone layer. The Montreal Protocol (1987) and Kigali amendment are global agreements to phase out chlorofluorocarbon usage by the middle of the twenty-first century. This amendment spurred new technology development and created plans to steadily reduce consumption and production of chlorofluorocarbon and HFC. The Montreal Protocol has stabilized or decreased ambient concentrations of chlorofluorocarbons (Mäder et al. 2010).

The Greenhouse Effect

The most discussed driver of change in Earth's energy balance is the greenhouse effect, that is, the ability of GHGs to trap heat in the atmosphere. Specifically, when the planet releases or reflects energy into the atmosphere as infrared radiation (i.e., heat), GHGs absorb that radiation and prevent or slow down the loss of energy to space. The result is that GHGs essentially act like a blanket that keeps the planet warm. The greenhouse effect is a naturally occurring phenomenon, and through its capture of the sun's energy, raises the Earth's baseline average temperature by 33°C (60°F). Although the natural greenhouse effect is beneficial, scientists are concerned that higher GHG concentrations in the atmosphere—brought about by recent industrial activity—are intensifying the greenhouse effect to unprecedented levels (Environmental Protection Agency 2017). Ground-based observations observed an enhanced greenhouse effect of 2.6 Watts per meter squared (energy per area) per decade from 1986 to 2000 (Wild 2012; Wacker et al. 2011). Satellites provide a complementary record to ground-based observations of the enhanced greenhouse effect. Since 1970, less heat emitted by the Earth's surface has escaped to space, which strongly suggests more heat is being absorbed by GHGs and transferred back toward the Earth's surface (Harries et al. 2001; Feldman et al. 2015).

Greenhouse Gas Global Warming Potential

Each GHG has a particular potential to absorb energy emitted from the Earth's surface and atmosphere, and is termed its global warming potential (GWP). GWPs are calculated based on the average length of time a GHG remains in the atmosphere and the amount of the heat energy it absorbs. GHGs that have a higher GWP absorb more energy and contribute more toward global warming than GHG with lower GWPs. The GWP of CO_2 is used as a baseline value against which other GHGs are compared. For instance, whereas CO_2 has a GWP of 1, CH_4 has a GWP of 21. This means that 1 pound of CH_4 is equivalent to 21 pounds of CO_2, and CH_4 has the potential to cause 21 times as much warming as the same amount of CO_2 over 100 years. N_2O has a GWP of 300, HFCs 140 to 11,700, perfluorocarbons 6,500 to 9,200, and sulfur hexafluoride to 23,900 (Environmental Protection Agency 2017). Although many molecules have a greater GWP than CO_2, the abundance of CO_2 in the atmosphere and the rate that it is increasing makes it the most important GHG. In concert with CO_2, the emissions of other important GHG have exponentially increased since the industrial revolution. Thus, GHG mitigation policies must also holistically consider non-CO_2 emissions.

The residence time, or amount of time individual GHGs remain in the atmosphere, varies substantially. For instance, CO_2 remains in the atmosphere for 50 to 200 years, methane (CH_4) for approximately 12 years, and nitrous oxide (N_2O) for about 120 years. For the fluorinated gases, HFCs can remain in the atmosphere in the range of 1 to 270 years, perfluorocarbons for 800 to 50,000 years, and sulfur hexafluoride for 3,200 years (Environmental Protection Agency 2017). Cutting edge research attempts to estimate each GHG's contribution to temperature change (Allen et al. 2018). Historic CO_2 emissions account for the vast majority of observed warming. Current, as opposed to historic CH_4, emissions account for a moderate amount and N_2O a modest amount of warming.

Because of long residence times of the GHG, it takes decades for energy in the Earth's system to equilibrate to increased GHG levels. Ocean and land temperatures will continue to increase even if all GHG emissions from human activities abruptly stopped. In other words, society is committed to additional climate changes from GHG that have already been emitted.

CLINICAL CORRELATES 1.2 INNOVATIONS IN EMERGENCY READINESS IN THE ERA OF HEAT WAVES

Epidemiological research shows that mortality in many places increases as the temperature rises (Guo et al. 2017; Heutel, Miller, and Molitor 2017). Models have assessed temperature and humidity variability to implement time-sensitive public health heat warnings. However, there is significant variability in how communities are affected based on factors such as age, architecture, socioeconomic status, prevalence of chronic disease, and relative social isolation (Kravchenko et al. 2013). Thus, different zip code neighborhoods have varying thresholds at which heat-related illness becomes clinically apparent.

Emergency medical systems (Belval et al. 2018; Uejio et al. 2016) and emergency departments (Epstein and Yanovich 2019; Hess, Saha, and Luber 2014) are at the forefront of rapidly recognizing and treating heat-related illnesses. Reliance on these and other public health services increases with rising temperatures, and the public's reliance on these institutions could therefore be an accurate indicator of the appearance of clinically relevant heat-related disease. Researchers continue to develop methods and improved surveillance for rapidly identifying heat-related incidences through use of near real-time data (Mathes et al. 2017; White et al. 2017). The National Oceanic and Atmospheric Administration (NOAA) team also developed an interactive tool that maps extreme heat with vulnerability to assist communities with adapting with cooling centers and urban landscape design, as well as resource allocation (https://maps.esri.com/jg/HeatVulnerability/index.html). Such early warnings can help to ease the toll of health-related illness, and prevention may ease the burden of extreme heat events on the health care system (Vaidyanathan et al. 2019).

Real-time data indicate clinically significant heat events and could be used to generate public warnings and emergency system preparedness.

Solar Radiation Cycles

Solar radiation is the final factor to consider in the Earth's energy balance. Short-term solar cycles such as sunspots marginally alter the solar energy that the Earth receives. Over the past thirty years, short-term solar cycles have increased the energy in the Earth system (0.017 W/m2 per decade), but this is notably less than the greenhouse gas contribution (0.30 W/m2 per decade) (IPCC 2013). Since 1750, there has been a slight increase in the total emitted solar energy 0.05 W/m2 solar energy.

In addition to short-term solar cycles, gradual long-term solar cycles (10,000 to 100,000 years) also modulate the amount of solar energy reaching Earth. These cycles, referred to as Milankovitch cycles, affect the distance, orientation, and axis of the Earth relative to the sun. Indeed, the timing of the ice ages generally corresponds to periods of the Milankovitch cycles when the Earth is receiving less solar energy (Hays, Imbrie, and Shackleton 1976). Based on these predictable solar cycles, the Earth should be in the midst of a gradual cooling trend lasting 23,000 years instead of rapidly warming (Imbrie and Imbrie 1980).

Summary

In summary, there is a strong and consistent physical mechanism linking GHG to observed changes to the Earth's energy balance. GHGs absorb thermal radiation emitted by the Earth's surface and cycle this energy, further warming the Earth's surface. Human activities such as burning fossil fuels, synthesizing fertilizer, and using artificial coolants, and agricultural activities have rapidly increased atmospheric GHG concentrations. These activities have committed the planet to future climate changes due to the intrinsic chemical properties of GHGs interacting with the Earth's energy balance.

Evidence of a Changing Climate

This section focuses on climatic changes that are virtually certain (99 to 100 percent probability), very likely (90 to 100 percent probability), or likely (66 to 100 percent probability) (Mastrandrea et al. 2010). There is no doubt that the climate on Earth is changing. We know this from direct observations of increasing average air and ocean temperatures, melting snow and ice, and rising average sea levels (Figure 1.2). Here we examine the evidence for climate change since the first measurements were recorded in 1959 at Mauna Loa Observatory and from paleoclimate records that provide physical evidence of a changing climate before the nineteenth century.

Temperature

Global surface temperatures have been increasing since the early twentieth century. Indeed, global temperatures increased by 0.85°C (1.8°F) from 1880 to 2012 (IPCC 2013). The rate of warming since 1957 is 0.13°C (0.27°F) per decade, almost twice as fast as it had been during the previous century (Hansen et al. 2010), and nearly all of the warmest years have occurred since 2000 (16 of the 17 warmest years from observations) ("NOAA" 2019). Stated another way, no person under the age of thirty four has experienced a cooler-than-normal month based on global average temperatures ("NOAA" 2019).

Although nearly the entire globe has experienced increasing temperatures over the past century (IPCC 2013), there is significant geographic variation with respect to the magnitude of these increases (Figure 1.3). Observed temperature changes have been greatest in polar regions of the Northern Hemisphere, and air temperatures over land have increased faster than over oceans (Hansen et al. 2010). The ocean's ability to store more heat energy modulates temperature increases compared to the land surface.

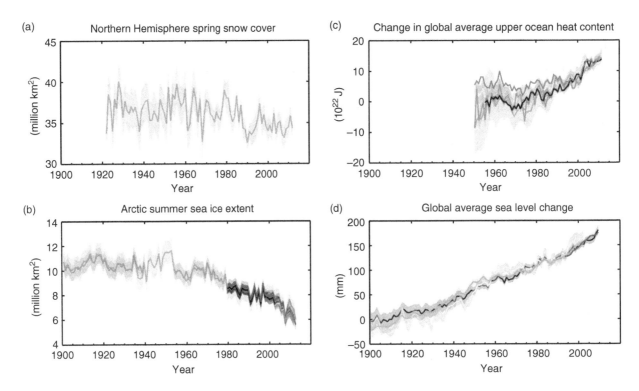

Figure 1.2   Observed changes in the earth system related to climate change
Source: IPCC (2013).
Note: Consistent with warming temperatures, the extent of Northern Hemisphere snow cover (a) from March to April and Arctic summer sea ice extent (b) from July to September are significantly decreasing. The upper ocean (0–700 meters) is also strongly warming (c), as summarized by standardized observational data sets, and (d) global average sea levels are increasing. Each line corresponds to a different data set. The lighter shading captures observational uncertainty.

Precise temperature and systematic observations did not exist before the late nineteenth century. Fortunately, a variety of natural records indirectly measured historic conditions. Tree rings, ocean lake microorganisms, and pollen stored in soil are mechanistically linked and well associated with temperature, moisture, and other physical environmental properties of the past. Although each proxy record has its limitations, all peer-reviewed proxies exhibit the same trend.

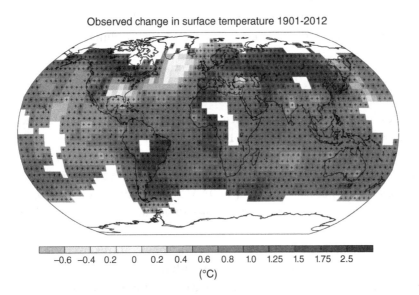

Figure 1.3   Decadal rate of observed temperature changes, 1901–2012
Source: IPCC (2013).
Note: Map of the observed surface temperature change from 1901 to 2012.

Seasonal Temperature Cycles

The onset of many biologically important seasonal events now occurs at a different time of the year from the past. For example, the length of the frost season is declining in many temperate regions, with later onsets and earlier cessations than in the past (McCabe, Betancourt, and Feng 2015; Wang et al. 2017). It is important to note that recent temperature increases have not been evenly distributed across the world or across geographic seasons. For instance, summer-time temperatures in the Southeast and central United States have slightly cooled because of natural climate variability and increased local emissions of aerosols (Mascioli et al. 2017).

Hydrologic Cycle

Precipitation—rainfall and other solid forms of water that fall from the atmosphere to Earth's surface—occurs when the atmosphere absorbs more water vapor than it can hold. The majority of atmospheric water recirculates through surface evaporation or indirectly through plant transpiration. The rest remains in the form of liquid water and runs off the land surface to a body of water such as lakes, rivers, or oceans. Additional waters percolate into groundwater systems. Water may also be temporarily stored on the surface as ice or snow. Glaciers, snowpack, and groundwater are natural reservoirs that can trap water for extended periods of time.

There have been distinct geographical changes in total annual precipitation over the past century (Figure 1.4). Total precipitation has significantly decreased in the Mediterranean and West Africa. Such drier-than-normal conditions may increase the frequency of wildfires, challenge hydropower generation, lower agriculture yields, and impair transportation on waterways. In contrast, precipitation has significantly increased in the midlatitudes of both hemispheres (IPCC 2013). There is also some evidence for precipitation increases in polar areas of the Northern Hemisphere, although the strength of the conclusions is limited by patchy observations. There are inconsistent precipitation trends in the tropics and Southern Hemisphere polar regions due to uncertainties in early records.

Changes to the types and seasonal phase of precipitation may have an adverse impact on societal and ecosystem functioning. The frequency and intensity of heavy precipitation events likely have increased over North America and Europe since 1950. This relationship is well grounded in physical theory because the amount of water the atmosphere can hold increases by approximately 7 percent for each additional degree Celsius of warming (Allan and

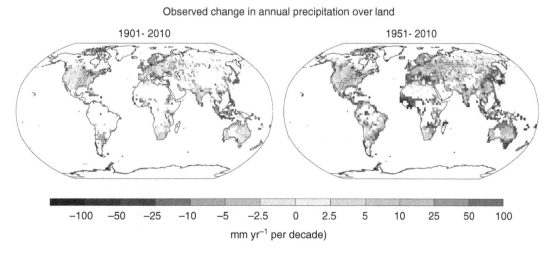

Figure 1.4   Observed precipitation, 1901–2010 and 1951–2010 (rates per decade)
Source: IPCC (2013).

Soden 2008). Furthermore, consistent with observed temperature increases, there is a trend toward less snowfall and more liquid rainfall events. This transition was recorded in North America, Europe, and South and East Asia (Takeuchi, Endo, and Murakami 2008; Kunkel et al. 2016). Satellite and ground-based observations support a significant decrease in snow cover extent (very high confidence) and depth (medium confidence) in spring and early summer (Brown and Mote 2009; Brown and Robinson 2011; Kunkel et al. 2016). In addition, the area, volume, and mass of almost all glaciers are decreasing across the globe (Arendt et al. 2012). Globally, one billion people live in watersheds with rivers fed by glaciers or snowmelt. Ice loss is geographically concentrated in polar regions and high-altitude mountains such as the Andes and Himalayas.

Sea Ice Extent, Sea Level, and Ocean Acidification

Scientists are highly confident that there are significant regional differences in sea ice extent that appear to be controlled by different earth system processes (IPCC 2013). In other words, decreasing Arctic and increasing Antarctic sea ice trends over time are not inconsistent with climate change (Zhang 2007). Since 1978, satellite data have allowed us to observe overall Arctic sea ice shrinkage (Solomon et al. 2007). From 1979 to 2012, annual mean Arctic sea ice area had very likely decreased in the range of 3.5 to 4.1 percent per decade. On the other side of the world, the Antarctic sea ice area slightly increased 1.2 to 1.8 percent per decade from 1979 to 2016. (Zhang 2007; Holland and Kwok 2012). Interestingly, since 2016 Antarctic sea ice has also started to decrease, potentially due to natural climate variability (Meehl et al. 2019).

For approximately the past two thousand years, average sea level changed very little. However, since the start of the twentieth century, the **sea level rise** is accelerating (Environmental Protection Agency 2017). For instance, since 1961, global sea level rose at an average rate of 1.8 millimeters per year. But since the 1990s, that rate has accelerated to 3.1 millimeters per year (Solomon et al. 2007; Dangendorf et al. 2017). Future sea level rise projections have wide variability. For the year 2100, the high GHG emissions pathway (representative concentration pathway 8.5) predicts 0.5m to 2.5m of sea level rise (Jevrejeva et al. 2019).

Thermal water expansion, the melting of mountain glaciers, Greenland and Antarctic ice sheets, and land-water storage all influence global sea levels. Melting of sea ice can marginally increase sea levels because freshwater is less dense than saltwater (Noerdlinger and Brower 2007). Increasing ocean temperatures cause water to thermally expand and historically contributed the most to sea level rise. Since the 1950s, melting glaciers became the most important source of sea level rise (Gregory et al. 2013). The remaining mountain glaciers contain 0.35-0.50m of sea level rise (Marzeion, Jarosch, and Hofer 2012; Grinsted 2013). The Greenland and Antarctic land ice cover over more than 50,000 square kilometers and contains 99 percent of the freshwater stored as ice on earth. Troublingly, Greenland's ice sheet melted six times faster between 2010 and 2018 compared to melting rates in the 1980s (Mouginot et al. 2019).

In addition to increasing sea levels, seawater chemistry has also been altered as the oceans have absorbed increasing amounts of carbon from the atmosphere. Today the oceans are about 26 percent more acidic than they were forty years ago (IPCC 2013). Tiny microscopic creatures on which the marine food chain depends are significantly affected by the calcium chemistry of ocean waters. Increased seawater acidity has also decreased the ability of these creatures to form shells (Rodolfo-Metalpa et al. 2011). This will have cascading impacts on biodiversity, narrowing the range of species, altering predator–prey relationships, changing fish stocks, and disrupting human livelihoods (Gaylord et al. 2015; Nagelkerken et al. 2016).

Urban Heat Island

Warming is becoming a major problem in cities and urban areas through a phenomenon known as the **urban heat island (UHI)** effect: a built environment that is hotter than the surrounding rural areas (Oke 1982). UHI is a result of several distinct processes. The first of these is "waste" heat released from vehicles, power plants, air-conditioning units, and other anthropogenic sources. Second, the urban built environment typically absorbs more radiation than rural areas, as urban streets and tall buildings composed of asphalt, concrete, and metal reflect less solar radiation than vegetated areas. Third, urban areas alter the hydrologic cycle, which also changes the local temperature. Urban surfaces and stormwater infrastructure move water out of the city thus retaining less local water that can moderate surface temperatures through evaporation. UHI effects also cause increases in energy consumption (e.g., using air-conditioning units for extended periods) and elevated levels of ground-level ozone in urban areas.

It is important to note that although UHI effects are changing the climate at the micro-level, they are of little importance to rising temperatures at the global level with less than a 0.006°C impact on land temperatures and no impact on ocean temperatures (Solomon et al. 2007). However, UHI is a massive global health problem as approximately three billion people live in urban areas and are directly affected by it (Rizwan, Dennis, and Liu 2008; Ward et al. 2016). Outdoor extreme heat increases will likely be more pronounced in large, sprawling cities with an enhanced UHI (Stone, Hess, and Frumkin 2010). Furthermore, many of the contributors to UHI also contribute to climate change, including greenhouse gas emissions from vehicles, industrial sources, and air-conditioning units. As the global population continues to urbanize, UHI may become a more serious problem in the future.

The UHI effect on human health is evident from heat events in Phoenix, Arizona (Uejio et al. 2011; Harlan et al. 2013), and Chicago in 1995 (Semenza et al. 1996) when a disproportionate number of deaths occurred among inner-city poor. Poverty is an independent risk factor for illness related to heat. It is associated with a decreased likelihood of access to medical care and associated with decreased access to protective measures, such as air conditioning (Balbus and Malina 2009, Harlan et al. 2013). More resources will be needed to address environmental disparities and provide protective measures against urban heat related illness for this at-risk population.

Summary

Global surface and ocean temperatures and sea levels are significantly increasing, and the rate of change continues to accelerate. Surface temperatures and human heat exposures may be further magnified by the UHI. In turn, increased temperatures alter the timing of the seasons and length of the frost season. Increased temperatures are altering the amount, timing, and phases of precipitation and storage of liquid water. In the latter half of the twentieth century, annual precipitation increased in many midlatitude and polar regions. In North America and Europe, extreme precipitation events are becoming more intense and frequent. In North America, Europe, and South and Southeast Asia, there are fewer snowfall and more liquid precipitation events. Globally almost all glaciers are shrinking. Arctic sea ice area or extent has rapidly decreased. Thus, nonrandom climate changes are already detectable and are starting to challenge biological system stability and societal well-being.

CLIMATE MODELS

How do scientists draw informed conclusions from climatic data and make reasonable predictions about future change? Mathematical computer models and simulations within those models are the current state-of-the-art ways to assess representations of and interactions between the oceans, atmosphere, land surface, and cryosphere.

The backbone of **climate models** consists of physical equations and principles that govern the transfer of energy and mass. Climate models with increasing GHG levels over time have accurately reproduced increasing temperatures, sea ice dynamics, and changing patterns of extreme weather (IPCC 2013). These models also provide additional evidence that observed climate change is caused by human activities. Detection and attribution studies have attempted to determine if climate models can reproduce observed changes without elevated GHG levels (Figure 1.5). Observed climate changes are outside the range of those expected by natural variability, such as by short-term solar radiation changes, volcanic eruptions, and other confounding processes. Only climate models with elevated greenhouse gas levels and reduced stratospheric ozone can reproduce our observed climatic changes, and more than half of the observed changes in average global surface temperature from 1951 to 2010 are due to human activities based on the modeling results.

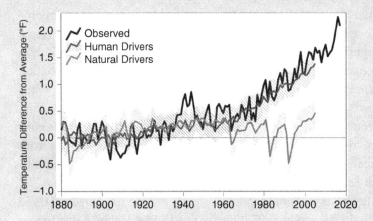

Figure 1.5   Detection and attribution study results

Source: Wuebbles et al. (2017).

Note: Comparison of observed and simulated climate change based. Only climate models that account for human impacts on the atmosphere can reproduce observed temperature and heat content changes.

Climate Projections, Uncertainty, and Climate Feedbacks

Future climate projections are uncertain for multiple reasons. The largest contributors to uncertainty are societal choices and policies, natural climate variability, and scientific uncertainty. The relative contribution of societal versus scientific uncertainty for climate change varies over time and region (Hawkins and Sutton 2009, 2011). Societal choices broadly refers to demographic, economic growth and distribution, technological, and public policy changes. Projecting future societal actions and behaviors is notoriously difficult. For instance, a high population growth rate would increase emitted carbon 12.4 gigatons per year by 2100 over a low growth rate (O'Neill et al. 2010). To put this in perspective, 31.6 gigatons of carbon were emitted in 2012. Climate change and health impact studies work with climate projections over multiple years, and ideally decades, to minimize the influence of natural climate variability.

Scientific uncertainty in climate models is introduced by the modeling techniques and incomplete knowledge of some Earth system processes. Climate modeling techniques use simplified representations of processes smaller than approximately 100 to 300 kilometers. For example, North American summer precipitation changes are more uncertain than temperature changes. Climate models have difficulty resolving clouds, water vapor, and aerosols, which are key components of convective summer precipitation. Similarly, climate projections may be more uncertain in areas with topography, near coastlines, or with large inland water bodies due to their simplified representation in global climate models (GCMs).

Scientific uncertainty also surrounds the ability of climate models to reproduce climate feedback. **Climate feedback** is defined as a forcing in the climate system that is both a cause and effect of itself and either acts to amplify (positive feedback) or dampen the initial forcing (negative feedback). As an example of positive feedback, increasing surface temperatures cause highly reflective snow and ice to melt, thereby exposing dark soil and rock with lower reflectivity. This increases the solar radiation absorbed by Earth's surface, resulting in additional temperature increases and melting. Human-induced global climate change is unprecedented, so many important feedbacks have not been directly observed. Each GCM represents climate change feedback in subtle to moderately different ways.

Major climate feedbacks are related to changes in the distribution of clouds, atmospheric temperature structure (changes to the relationship between temperature and altitude), vegetation type and coverage, the atmospheric concentration and distribution of water vapor, and modification of the carbon and sulfur cycles. There remains considerable uncertainty regarding feedback mechanisms, in particular those associated with clouds and the capacity of terrestrial surfaces and the ocean to absorb CO_2. (The following section provides more information on key feedbacks.)

Robustly projecting the climate change disease burden should account for societal and scientific uncertainty. Climate models provide plausible projections of future conditions based on future GHG emissions trajectories or **representative concentration pathways (RCPs).** Climate projections that use multiple RCPs essentially represent some of the societal uncertainty. Using a suite of projections from ten or more climate models will capture a range of scientific uncertainty. Rather than issue a precise forecast, scientists use scenarios to generate a plausible range of RCPs. The RCPs are bounded on the upper end by rapid GHG emission growth (RCP 8.5 Watts per meter squared, i.e., energy per area) and on the lower end by aggressive limits on GHG emissions (RCP 2.6) (Moss et al. 2010). The middle pathways suggest that GHGs stabilize at different levels (RCP 4.5, 6.0) by the end of the century.

The RCPs were recently updated in the 2013 IPCC assessment. The RCPs replace the Special Report on Emission Scenarios (SRES) used in the third and fourth IPCC assessments (IPCC 2001, 2007). The SRES describes four "scenario families" that reflect distinct and realistic demographic, technological, and economic paths, enabling projections of global GHG emissions (Nakicenovic and Swart 2000). Among the key scenarios are A1F1, A1B, and B1. A1F1 describes a world characterized by intense economic growth, a decrease in global economic disparity, low to decreasing population growth, rapid introduction of efficient technology, and a reliance on fossil energy sources. The A1B scenario is equivalent with the exception that societies use a balance of fossil and nonfossil energy resources. In scenario B1, the demographic changes are identical to those in A1F1 and A1B; however, service and information economies rapidly become predominant, clean and efficient technologies are introduced, and significant decreases in material consumption are observed. There may be some confusion surrounding the transitions in nomenclature. To help interpret the previous literature, RCP 8.5 is analogous to the A1F1, RCP 6.0 to A1B, and RCP 4.5 to B1. The lowest RCP (2.6) is new and did not have a Special Report on Emissions Scenarios analogue.

Cloud Feedbacks

It is worth noting that cloud feedbacks represent a persistent challenge to climate modeling, and it is essential to understand their effects to improve predictions of future climatic conditions. Increasing temperatures will cause changes in the distribution and types of clouds occurring across Earth. Clouds are involved in both positive and negative feedback mechanisms by reflecting short-wave radiation back into space and by absorbing and reradiating outgoing longwave radiation back to the surface, although different types of clouds have different radiative properties (Zelinka et al. 2013). The cumulative effect of feedback related to cloud cover is impeded by our inability to predict how the type, distribution, and characteristics of clouds will change as temperatures increase (Zelinka et al. 2013).

Carbon Sources and Sinks

Carbon sinks such as the ocean, soil, and vegetation remove carbon dioxide from the atmosphere. Slightly less than half of the total CO_2 emissions currently absorbed by land and ocean reservoirs (Le Quéré et al. 2016). Oceans serve as the largest carbon sink as CO_2 dissolves in water and additional amounts are absorbed by marine life. These "blue carbon ecosystems" are some of the most efficient in sequestering carbon (Macreadie et al. 2017). Terrestrial carbon sinks are more variable due to changes in land use and land cover and from natural disasters (Canadell et al. 2007). Through photosynthesis plants absorb CO_2 that can then be passed on to soil through the roots. Soil also stores CO_2 as plants and animals decompose.

Restoration and conservation efforts may increase the amount of carbon absorbed. For example, research into the benefits of tidal marshlands in Australia have shown their capacity for carbon sequestration at about .75 Tg annually (Macreadie et al. 2017). Although estimates of annual sequestration potential and current carbon storage in these ecosystems may vary, research supports their importance. Historically these ecosystems have faced deterioration; however, with the increased urgency of efforts to balance the global carbon budget, there is renewed interest in protecting these valuable ecosystems.

There is evidence that carbon reservoirs are becoming increasingly saturated with CO_2 (Le Quéré et al. 2016) and their rates of uptake are decreasing. Furthermore, physical characteristics of the reservoirs are being altered by increasing temperatures and anthropogenic activity (e.g., land cover change). The mechanisms underlying the uptake of carbon by land and ocean reservoirs are complex, and it remains uncertain how carbon reservoirs will absorb CO_2 in the future.

Permafrost is permanently frozen ground generally located at high latitudes. Within this frozen layer are located the organic remains of plants and animals that in many cases have been frozen for thousands of years (Schuur et al. 2015). However, with increasing temperatures, permafrost is beginning to thaw potentially exposing these organic materials to microbe decomposition. As a result, additional greenhouse gases, mostly carbon and some methane, are released into the atmosphere (Le Quéré et al. 2016; Schuur et al. 2015). Although the impact of this release is likely to be gradual, it may accelerate climate projections over the coming decades. The potential for greenhouse gas release is significant—although an abrupt thaw is unlikely, estimates place the amount of carbon stored in permafrost as double the amount currently in the atmosphere (Schuur et al. 2015). Thus, although permafrost may have been overlooked in the past, researchers have recognized its importance as a source of greenhouse gases as the polar regions continue to warm. As a result, permafrost emissions have more recently been incorporated into climate change projections as studies continue to analyze the impact of thawing permafrost on climate.

Summary

Climate models are multifaceted tools that complement observations and theory. Retrospectively, they show that natural climatic and solar variability cannot explain observed temperature increases. Accounting for increased GHG, however, produces similar changes to what scientists have observed. Prospectively, these models provide a range of plausible future climatic conditions. Future climate projections differ based on the magnitude and timing of climate feedbacks, natural variability, and substantial uncertainty surrounding human behavior. Nonetheless, the models continue to improve and increasingly capture the complexity of Earth's systems.

Projected Future Climate Changes

This section focuses on projected temperature, hydrologic cycle, and cryosphere changes, based on an ensemble of multiple climate model projections, as such composite projections are typically more accurate than any individual climate model projection alone (Pierce et al. 2009).

CLINICAL CORRELATES 1.3 PHYSICIANS SERVING AS CLIMATE CHANGE RESOURCES

According to surveys of hundreds of physicians, up to 97 percent recognize that climate change is happening (Rudolph and Harrison 2016). Furthermore, up to 88 percent state that some of their patients are affected by severe weather-related injuries. Yet, physicians find it difficult to talk about climate change with their patients because of time constraints, uncertainty regarding communication on the issue, and lack of resources. The Physician's Guide to Climate Change, Health and Equity suggests placing climate change educational materials (brochures, fact sheets, and posters) in physicians' offices. These materials can help initiate conversations about the impact of climate change on health. The Medical Consortium on Climate and Health has free material for clinicians to use for patient education. EcoAmerica also provides guidance on communicating climate change with people (ecoAmerica 2013). Climate change can be integrated into disease management plans, discharge materials, and medication sheets. Physicians' offices can help patients interpret extreme weather watch/warning systems and air quality indexes. The Department of Homeland Security offers tips for climate-driven disaster planning at www.ready.gov.

Health professionals can also provide community resources for building climate resilience, especially for low-income populations. The U.S. Department of Health and Human Services provides a Low-Income Home Energy Assistance Program to assist families with energy costs. The U.S. Department of Energy Weatherization Assistance Program increases the energy efficiency of low-income households. Although limited in scope, the programs help low-income people to avoid some harmful effects of extreme weather.

Physicians serve as a clear link to connecting patients with climate-related community resources, educational materials, health messaging, and disaster preparedness.

Increasing Temperatures

Global mean surface air temperatures are expected to increase from 1986–2005 averages by approximately 0.3°C to 0.7°C by the period 2016 to 2030, and 0.8°C to 4.9 °C by the period 2081 to 2100 (Kharin et al. 2013). However, mean temperature increases over land will be double the global mean increase (Figure 1.6). This will be even greater in high latitudes of the Northern Hemisphere. Although mean surface temperatures over the ocean will generally not increase as rapidly as surface temperatures over land, large changes will be observed over the Arctic and the southern oceans, where the reduction of sea ice will be associated with temperature increases of approximately 2°C to 11°C by the period 2081 to 2100 (IPCC 2013). Stated another way, by the middle of this century, average annual temperatures will be higher than the hottest observed annual temperatures from 1860 to 2005 over most of the world (Mora et al. 2013).

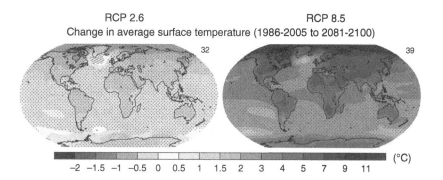

Figure 1.6   Projected changes in average surface temperature difference for 2081–2100 versus 1986–2005 for different RCP
Source: IPCC (2013).
Note: The average change is the mean of thirty-two climate model projections for RCP 2.6 and thirty-nine models for RCP 8.5. The figure also conveys uncertainty. In the dotted areas, the average projected changes is notably larger (two standard deviations) than natural variability. There is less confidence in the areas with hatching.

Seasonal variation of climate will continue to evolve with anthropogenic climate change. In high and middle latitudes, the number of frost days could decrease by up to ninety days in some regions of North America and Western Europe by 2081 to 2100, and the poleward extent of permafrost areas will be reduced (Sillmann et al. 2013). The seasonal modification of temperature and precipitation will modify the seasonal and spatial range of many plants and animals, including disease vectors such as mosquitoes and allergenic plant species. The

diurnal temperature range (DTR) will continue to decrease across much of the world, especially in high and low latitudes, due to increased cloud coverage. Many middle-latitude locations will experience increases or no change in DTR in the coming century (Kharin et al. 2013).

Extreme Heat Events

Extreme heat events (EHE) can be defined as periods with notably greater than-normal surface temperatures and moisture for a specific time of year (Robinson and Dewy 1990). EHE generally occur when very hot and humid air moves into an area where people are not adapted to extreme conditions. The longer air masses linger over a region, the greater the potential for harm to society and the environment. Many heat metrics suggest EHE are already becoming more intense, longer lasting, frequent, and geographically widespread (IPCC 2013), a trend that is likely to continue into the future. By the end of this century, extreme heat events will be even hotter, more likely to last weeks instead of days, and more frequent (Russo et al. 2014; Guo et al. 2017).

Scientists cannot directly link individual weather events to climate change. However, they can determine the extent to which climate change is increasing the odds of an extreme event such as EHE compared to historically normal conditions. For example, climate change has at least doubled the probability (Stott, Stone, and Allen 2003) that an EHE event of the same magnitude as the historic European heat event of 2003 linked to seventy thousand excess deaths (Robine et al. 2008) will occur in the coming years.

Hydrologic Cycle

Climate change is expected to amplify important interactions between energy in Earth's system and the intensity of the hydrologic cycle. With increasing temperatures, average total global precipitation will almost certainly increase by 2050 (IPCC 2013). The rate of annual precipitation increases ranges from 1 to 3 percent per degree average annual temperature increase for all scenarios except RCP 2.5. However, there will be substantial geographical variability in projected changes (Figure 1.7). At high latitudes, precipitation is very likely to increase because warmer air holds more moisture combined with the increased transfer of tropical moisture into the region.

In the midlatitudes, there are distinct total annual precipitation trends for drylands and deserts versus relatively wet and semitropical regions. Under the high RCP 8.5 scenario, dry areas are projected to desiccate further, whereas precipitation is expected to increase in relatively wet midlatitude locations. Summertime monsoon precipitation will likely increase in

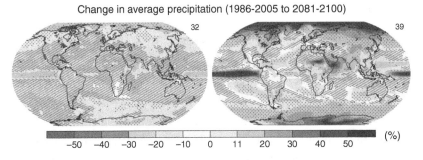

Change in average precipitation (1986-2005 to 2081-2100)

Figure 1.7 Projected changes in average annual precipitation difference for 2081–2100 versus 1986–2005 for different RCP
Source: IPCC (2013).
Note: The average change is the mean of thirty-two climate model projections for RCP 2.6 and thirty-nine models for RCP 8.5. The figure also conveys uncertainty. In the dotted areas, the average projected changes is notably larger (two standard deviations) than natural variability. There is less confidence in the areas with hatching.

Southeast Asia, southern India, southern regions of the West Africa, and northern Australia, whereas summertime precipitation will likely decrease in southern Africa, Mexico, and Central America (IPCC 2013). In dry regions, climate warming will accelerate land surface drying as heat goes into the evaporation of moisture and increase the frequency and severity of droughts.

The frequency and intensity of average daily precipitation events will likely increase across most midlatitude and wet tropical locations. The difference in total annual versus daily precipitation may seem incongruous for drylands and deserts; however, both trends can coexist. These regions may receive fewer precipitation events that are not compensated by the increase in relatively rare extreme precipitation events. More intense precipitation will generally transport more pollutants and pathogens into water bodies (Corsi et al. 2014; Levy et al. 2016). Increasing atmospheric water vapor may also contribute to the greenhouse effect, further increasing the amount of energy in the system.

CLINICAL CORRELATES 1.4 INTEGRATIVE APPROACHES TO HEAT RESILIENCE

Air conditioning has become the mainstay approach to buffer the deleterious health effects of indoor heat in homes, workplaces, and health care facilities (Ito, Lane, and Olson 2018; Williams et al. 2019). Unfortunately, it places major strain on energy supplies and contributes substantially to CO_2 emissions, which in turn increase global surface temperatures. In the United States, air conditioners use 6 percent of the nation's electricity and release 117 million metric tons of carbon dioxide into the air annually (U.S. Department of Energy n.d.). Eighty percent of energy for air conditioning comes from fossil fuels, and according to estimates, total world air conditioning consumes roughly one trillion kilowatt hours annually, more than twice the total energy consumption of the entire continent of Africa (Dahl 2013).

Understanding future trends, we see that the developing world contains thirty-eight of the largest fifty cities on the planet (Sivak 2009). Thus, many opportunities remain to curb the preventable health effects of heat stress in high-exposure areas with limited adaptive capacity. Solutions may include (1) urban planning and building design, (2) alternative cooling, and (3) climate-sensitive attitudes and behaviors (Lundgren-Kownacki et al. 2018). City planners and engineers are challenged with creatively use low-cost energy-saving technologies and integrate traditional technologies that have a small energy footprint. These designs include passive cooling systems—evaporative cooling, night flushing, and passive downdraft evaporative cooling—exterior heat sinks, and modification of existing structures with awnings, reflective paint, and landscaping that maximizes shade (Dahl 2013).

Air conditioning is both a cure for and a cause of heat-related illness. Large commercial buildings like health care facilities should model and promote energy efficiency for community members and employees.

Sea Ice Extent, Sea Level, Ocean Acidification, Glacial Extent, and Snow Cover

The geographical extent of Arctic sea ice will continue to decrease by the end of this century under all RCP scenarios, and in all seasons. During the Arctic sea ice nadir in September, projected decreases range from 43 to 94 percent relative to 1985 to 2006. Similarly, the apex of sea ice extent in February will also be reduced 8 to 34 percent relative to 1985 to 2006 (IPCC 2013).

Since 1870, the global sea level has risen by eight inches due to the thermal expansion of water and melting polar ice and glaciers. In the next century, future sea level rise is expected to occur at a faster rate compared with the past fifty years. Various scenarios estimate different levels of sea level rise (Table 1.1) and will vary by coastal regions. Major factors that affect local and regional sea levels will be subsiding coastal land and the changing gravitational pull of large glaciers (EPA 2017; Slangen et al. 2014). With rising sea levels, coastal populations will

Table 1.1   Projected Changes in Global Mean Sea Level Rise Relative to 1986–2005 for Four Representative Concentration Pathways (in meters)

Scenario	2046-2065		2081-2100	
	Mean	Likely Range	Mean	Likely Range
RCP2.6	0.24	0.17 to 0.32	0.40	0.26 to 0.55
RCP4.5	0.26	0.19 to 0.33	0.47	0.32 to 0.63
RCP6.0	0.25	0.18 to 0.32	0.48	0.33 to 0.63
RCP8.5	0.30	0.22 to 0.38	0.63	0.45 to 0.82

Note: The estimates are based on twenty-one global climate models. Rapid ice sheet changes and altered societal practices such as increasing water storage are not considered in these estimates.

face shore erosion, loss of dry land, flooding, property damage, and displacement. There will also be significant damage to wetlands and coastal ecosystems (EPA 2017).

Ocean acidification is a direct result of the absorption of atmospheric CO_2 as the resulting chemical reactions change the composition of the ocean. When CO_2 interacts with the water, the number of hydrogen ions increase, and the pH levels and the amount of carbonate ions in the water decrease. Ocean acidification has a wide range of consequences for marine life and the ecosystem services these species provide. Carbonite ions are vitally important for the creation and maintaining of seashells and coral (Gattuso et al. 2015; Albright et al. 2016). Without an abundance of carbonite ions, certain species such as oysters, clams, and corals have difficulties maintaining shells and coral skeletons. This in turn adversely affects ecosystems, economies, and communities that rely on these species (Lemasson et al. 2017). As ecosystems are degraded, species populations will decrease. Threats to these species will have harmful impacts on economies and human health. Populations with heavy seafood diets may face food insecurity and lack of nutrition. Additionally economies heavily reliant on aquaculture could face collapse (Weatherdon et al. 2016). While Earth's oceans act as a carbon sink, the negative impacts of resulting ocean acidification will have direct consequences for marine and human communities.

It is virtually certain that the global permafrost area will decrease in response to rising temperatures and less snow cover. Furthermore, the proportion of North America covered by snow in the spring will likely continue to decrease (Brutel-Vuilmet, Ménégoz, and Krinner 2013). Climate models do not explicitly capture local processes like glacier dynamics. Nonetheless, based on projected temperature changes, glacier area, volume, and mass are reasonably expected to continue to recede. Springtime glacier runoff is also expected to decrease.

DISCUSSION QUESTIONS

1. How have the conclusions of scientific assessments (e.g., Intergovernmental Panel on Climate Change) on whether climate change is occurring and what processes are responsible for these changes been updated over time?

2. What is the difference between natural climate variability and long-term climate change?

3. Why is it so difficult for an individual to observe long-term climate change?

4. If society somehow suddenly stopped emitting greenhouse gases, would existing greenhouse gases in the atmosphere continue to alter the climate? If so, for how long?

5. Some proposed public policies to mitigate or limit greenhouse gas emissions focus on methane, nitrous oxide, and fluorinated gases instead of carbon dioxide. What is the scientific rationale for these proposals? Discuss the relative merits and limitations of such a policy?

6. In what regions are temperatures increasing the most rapidly? Most slowly? Why?

7. Why are the most important causes of sea level increases that have already happened?

8. What are the different types of evidence that support that the climate is changing?

9. What are the primary causes of uncertainty in climate model projections?

10. What are representative concentration pathways (RCPs), and why are they used?

KEY TERMS

Climate change: (1) the systematic change in the long-term state of the atmosphere over multiple decades (or longer); (2) a combination of human induced and natural climatic changes or human-induced changes alone.

Climate feedback: Forcing in the climate system that is both a cause and effect of itself and either acts to amplify (positive feedback) or dampen the initial forcing (negative feedback).

Climate models: Multifaceted tools that complement observations and theory.

Climate variability: Regular patterns in the Earth system that occur over periods of months to decades.

Diurnal temperature range (DTR): The difference between daily maximum and minimum temperature

Energy balance: The ability of greenhouse gases to trap heat in the atmosphere.

Extreme heat event: A period with notably greater than-normal surface temperatures and moisture for a specific geographic location and time of year.

Global warming potential (GWP): A particular potential to absorb energy emitted from the Earth's surface and atmosphere.

Greenhouse effect: A naturally occurring phenomenon that, through its capture of the sun's energy, raises the Earth's baseline average temperature by 33°C (60°F).

Ocean acidification: The decrease in the pH values of Earth's oceans primarily due to chemical reactions between seawater and carbon dioxide as it is absorbed from the atmosphere.

Representative concentration pathways (RCPs): Scenarios that take into account different levels of emissions and concentrations of greenhouse gases. Each scenario considers a trajectory over time that would lead to potential future climate conditions.

Sea level rise: Refers to the increase in the average level of all of Earth's oceans. This increase is mainly because of the melting of sea ice and expansion of saltwater as temperatures warm.

Urban heat island (UHI): An urban or metropolitan area that experiences warmer temperatures than surrounding rural areas.

Acknowledgment

We thank the anonymous reviewers for providing critical feedback on earlier drafts of this chapter.

References

Albright, R., L. Caldeira, J. Hosfelt, L. Kwiatkowski, J. K. Maclaren, B. M. Mason, Y. Nebuchina et al. 2016. "Reversal of Ocean Acidification Enhances Net Coral Reef Calcification." *Nature* 531 (7594):362–65. https://doi.org/10.1038/nature17155

Allan, R. P., and B. J. Soden. 2008. "Atmospheric Warming and the Amplification of Precipitation Extremes." *Science* 321(5895):1481–84.

Allen, M. R., K. P. Shine, J. S. Fuglestvedt, R. J. Millar, M. Cain, D. J. Frame et al. 2018. "A solution to the misrepresentations of CO 2-equivalent emissions of short-lived climate pollutants under ambitious mitigation." *NPJ Climate and Atmospheric Science* 1 (1):16.

American Association for the Advancement of Science. 2006. "Evolution on the Front Line: An Abbreviated Guide for Teaching Evolution, from Project 2061 at AAAS." http://www.project2061. org/publications/guides/evolution.pdf.

Arendt, A., T. Bolch, J. Cogley, A. Gardner, J. Hagen, R. Hock, G. Kaser et al. 2012. *Randolph Glacier Inventory [v1. 0]: A Dataset of Global Glacier Outlines. Global Land Ice Measurements from Space.* Boulder, CO: Digital Media.

Balbus, M., and C. Malina. 2009. "Identifying Vulnerable Subpopulations for Climate Change Health Effects in the United States." *Journal of Occupational and Environmental Medicine* 51:33–37.

Belval, L. N., D. J. Casa, W. M. Adams G. T. Chiampas, J. C. Holschen, Y. Hosokawa, J. Jardine et al. 2018. "Consensus Statement–Prehospital Care of Exertional Heat Stroke. *Prehospital Emergency Care* 22(3):392–97. doi:10.1080/10903127.2017.1392666.

Brown, R. D., and P. W. Mote. 2009. "The Response of Northern Hemisphere Snow Cover to a Changing Climate." *Journal of Climate* 22:2124–45.

Brown, R., and D. Robinson. 2011. "Northern Hemisphere Spring Snow Cover Variability and Change over 1922–2010 including an Assessment of Uncertainty." *Cryosphere* 51:219–29.

Brutel-Vuilmet, M. Ménégoz, and G. Krinner. 2013. "An Analysis of Present and Future Seasonal Northern Hemisphere Land Snow Cover Simulated by CMIP5 Coupled Climate Models." *Cryosphere* 7:67–80.

Canadell, J. G., D. E. Pataki, R. Gifford, R. A. Houghton, Y. Luo, M. R. Raupach et al. 2007. "Saturation of the Terrestrial Carbon Sink." In *Terrestrial Ecosystems in a Changing World*, edited by J. G. Canadell, D. E. Pataki, and L. F. Pitelka, 59–78. New York: Springer.

Cheng, J., Z. Xu, H. Bambrick, H. Su, S. Tong, and W. Hu. 2018. "Heatwave and Elderly Mortality: An Evaluation of Death Burden and Health Costs Considering Short-Term Mortality Displacement." *Environment International* 115:334–42. doi:10.1016/j.envint.2018.03.041.

Cook J., D. Nuccitelli, S. A. Green, M. Richardson, B. Winkler, R. Painting, R. Way, P. Jacobs, and A. Skuce. 2013. "Quantifying the Consensus on Anthropogenic Global Warming in the Scientific Literature." *Environmental Research Letters* 8 (2):024024.

Corsi, S. R., M. A. Borchardt, S. K. Spencer, P. E. Hughes, and A. K. Baldwin. 2014. "Human and Bovine Viruses in the Milwaukee River Watershed: Hydrologically Relevant Representation and Relations with Environmental Variables." *Science of the Total Environment* 490:849–60.

Dahl, R. 2013. "Cooling Concepts: Alternatives to Air-Conditioning for a Warm World." *Environmental Health Perspectives* 1 (1):A19–A25

Dangendorf, S., M. Marcos, G. Wöppelmann, C. P. Conrad, T. Frederikse, and R. Riva. 2017. "Reassessment of 20th Century Global Mean Sea Level Rise." *Proceedings of the National Academy of Sciences* 114 (23):5946–51.

ecoAmerica. 2013. "Communicating on Climate: 13 Steps and Guiding Principles." https://ecoamerica. org/wp-content/uploads/2013/11/Communicating-on-Climate-13-steps_ecoAmerica.pdf.

Environmental Protection Agency. 2017. "Climate Change." https://19january2017snapshot.epa.gov/climatechange_.html.

Epstein Y., and R. Yanovich. 2019. "Heatstroke." *New England Journal of Medicine* 380 (25):2449–59.

Feldman D., W. Collins, P. Gero, M. Torn, E. Mlawer, and T. Shippert. 2015. "Observational Determination of Surface Radiative Forcing by CO_2 from 2000 to 2010." *Nature* 519 (7543):339–43.

Foote, E. 1856. "Circumstances Affecting the Heat of the Sun's Rays: Art. XXX." *American Journal of Science and Arts, 2nd series,* 22 (66):382–83. https://ia800802.us.archive.org/4/items/mobot31753002152491/mobot31753002152491.pdf.

Gattuso, J. P., A. Magnan, R. Billé, W. W. L. Cheung, E. L. Howes, F. Joos, D. Allemand et al. 2015. "Contrasting Futures for Ocean and Society from Different Anthropogenic CO2 Emissions Scenarios." *Science* 349 (6243). https://doi.org/10.1126/science.aac4722.

Gaylord, B., K. J. Kroeker, J. M. Sunday, K. M. Anderson, J. P. Barry, N. E. Brown et al. 2015. "Ocean Acidification through the Lens of Ecological Theory." *Ecology* 96 (1):3–15.

Gregory, J. M., N. J. White, J. A. Church, M. Bierkens, J. E. Box, M. R. Van den Broeke, G. Cogley et al. 2013. "Twentieth-Century Global-Mean Sea Level Rise: Is the Whole Greater than the Sum of the Parts?" *Journal of Climate* 26 (13):4476–99.

Grinsted, A. 2013. "An Estimate of Global Glacier Volume." *The Cryosphere* 7 (1):141–51.

Gronlund, C. J. 2014. "Racial and Socioeconomic Disparities in Heat-Related Health Effects and Their Mechanisms: A Review." *Current Epidemiology Reports* 1 (3):165–73. doi: 10.1007/s40471-014-0014-4.

Guo, Y., A. Gasparrini, B. G. Armstrong, B. Tawatsupa, A. Tobias, E. Lavigne, M. Coelho et al. 2017. "Heat Wave and Mortality: A Multicountry, Multicommunity Study." *Environmental Health Perspectives* 125 (8):087006. doi:10.1289/EHP1026.

Guo, X., J. Huang, Y. Luo, Z. Zhao, and Y. Xu. 2017. "Projection of Heat Waves over China for Eight Different Global Warming Targets Using 12 CMIP5 Models." *Theoretical and Applied Climatology* 128 (3–4):507–22.

Hansen, J., R. Ruedy, M. Sato, and K. Lo. 2010. "Global Surface Temperature Change." *Reviews of Geophysics* 48:RG4004.

Harlan, S., J. Declet-Barret, W. Stefanov, and D. Petitti. 2013. "Neighborhood Effects on Heat Deaths: Social and Environmental Predictors of Vulnerability in Maricopa County, Arizona." *Environmental Health Perspectives* 121 (2):197–204.

Harries, J. E., H. E. Brindley, P. J. Sagoo, and R. J. Bantges 2001. "Increases in Greenhouse Forcing Inferred from the Outgoing Longwave Radiation Spectra of the Earth in 1970 and 1997." *Nature* 410:355–57.

Hawkins, E., and R. Sutton. 2009. "The Potential to Narrow Uncertainty in Regional Climate Predictions." *Bulletin of the American Meteorological Society* 90:1095–1107.

Hawkins, E., and R. Sutton. 2011. "The Potential to Narrow Uncertainty in Projections of Regional Precipitation Change." *Climate Dynamics* 37 (1–2):407–18.

Hays J. D., J. Imbrie, and N. J. Shackleton. 1976. *Variations in the Earth's Orbit: Pacemaker of the Ice Ages.* Washington, DC: American Association for the Advancement of Science.

Heinlein, R. A. 1973. *Time Enough for Love.* New York: Putnam.

Hess, J. J., S. Saha, and G. Luber. 2014. "Summertime Acute Heat Illness in U.S. Emergency Departments from 2006 through 2010: Analysis of a Nationally Representative Sample." *Environmental Health Perspectives* 122 (11):1209–15.

Holland, P. R., and R. Kwok. 2012. "Wind-Driven Trends in Antarctic Sea-Ice Drift." *Nature Geoscience* 5 (12):872–75.

Hueutel, G., N. H. Miller, and D. Molitor. 2017. *Adaptation and the Mortality Effects of Temperature across U.S. Climate Regions.* Cambridge, MA: National Bureau of Economic Research.

Imbrie, J., and J. Z. Imbrie. 1980. "Modeling the Climatic Response to Orbital Variations." *Science* 207 (4434):943–53.

Intergovernmental Panel on Climate Change. 1990. *Climate Change: The IPCC Scientific Assessment.* Cambridge: Cambridge University Press.

Intergovernmental Panel on Climate Change. 2001. *Climate Change 2001: Synthesis Report. A Contribution of Working Groups I, II, and III to the Third Assessment Report of the Intergovernmental Panel on Climate Change, edited by R. T. Watson and the Core Writing Team.* Cambridge: Cambridge University Press.

Intergovernmental Panel on Climate Change. 2007. *Climate Change 2007: Synthesis Report. Contribution of Working Groups I, II and III to the Fourth Assessment Report of the Intergovernmental Panel on Climate Change,* edited by R. K. Pachauri and A. Reisinger. Geneva: IPCC.

Intergovernmental Panel on Climate Change. 2013. "Summary for Policymakers." In *Climate Change 2013: The Physical Science Basis,* edited by T. F. Stocker, D. Qin, G.-K. Plattner, M. Tignor, S. K. Allen, J. Boschung, A. Nauels et al., 3–29. Cambridge: Cambridge University Press.

Ito, K., K. Lane, and C. Olson. 2018. "Equitable Access to Air Conditioning: A City Health Department's Perspective on Preventing Heat-related Deaths." *Epidemiology* 29 (6):749–52. doi:10.1097/EDE.0000000000000912.

Jevrejeva, S., T. Frederikse, R. E. Kopp, G. Le Cozannet, L. P. Jackson, and R. van de Wal. 2019. "Probabilistic Sea Level Projections at the Coast by 2100." *Surveys in Geophysics* 40 (6):1673–96.

Kharin, V. V., F. W. Zwiers, X. Zhang, and M. Wehner. 2013. "Changes in Temperature and Precipitation Extremes in the CMIP5 Ensemble." *Climatic Change* 119:345–57.

Kravchenko J., A. P. Abernethy, M. Fawzy, and H. K. Lyerly. 2013. "Minimization of Heatwave Morbidity and Mortality. *American Journal of Preventive Medicine* 44 (3):274–82.

Kunkel, K. E., D. A. Robinson, S. Champion, X. Yin, T. Estilow, and R. M. Frankson. 2016. "Trends and Extremes in Northern Hemisphere Snow Characteristics." *Current Climate Change Reports* 2 (2):65–73.

Ledrans, M., P. Pirard, H. Tillaut, M. Pascal, S. Vandentorren, F. Suzan, G. Salines, et al. 2004. "The Heat Wave of August 2003: What Happened?" *La Revue du Praticien* 54:1289–97.

Lemasson, A. J., S. Fletcher, J. M. Hall-Spencer, and A. M. Knights. (2017). "Linking the Biological Impacts of Ocean Acidification on Oysters to Changes in Ecosystem Services: A Review." *Journal of Experimental Marine Biology and Ecology* 492:49–62. https://doi.org/10.1016/j.jembe.2017.01.019.

Le Quéré, C., R. M. Andrew, J. G. Canadell, S. Sitch, J. I. Korsbakken, G. P. Peters, A. C. Manning et al. 2016. "Global Carbon Budget 2016." *Earth System Science Data* 8 (2). http://www.earth-syst-sci-data.net/8/605/2016/.

Levy, K., A. P., Woster, R. S., Goldstein, and E. J. Carlton. 2016. "Untangling the Impacts of Climate Change on Waterborne Diseases: A Systematic Review of Relationships Between Diarrheal Diseases and Temperature, Rainfall, Flooding, and Drought." *Environmental Science & Technology* 50 (10):4905–22.

Lindemann, U., D. A. Skelton, J. Oksa, N. Beyer, K. Rapp, C. Becker, and J. Klenk. 2018. "Social Participation and Heat-Related Behavior in Older Adults during Heat Waves and on Other Days." *Zeitschrift für Gerontologie und Geriatrie* 51 (5):543–49. doi:10.1007/s00391-017-1338-8.

Liss, A., R. Wu, K. K. Chui, and E. N. Naumova. 2017. "Heat-Related Hospitalizations in Older Adults: An Amplified Effect of the First Seasonal Heatwave." *Scientific Reports* 7: 39581.

Lundgren-Kownacki, K., E. D. Hornyanszky, T. A. Chu, J. A. Olsson, and P. Becker. 2018. "Challenges of Using Air Conditioning in an Increasingly Hot Climate." *International Journal of Biometeorology* 62 (3):401–12. doi:10.1007/s00484-017-1493-z.

Macreadie, P. I., D. A.Nielsen, J. J. Kelleway, T. B. Atwood, J. R. Seymour, K. Petrou, R. M. Connolly et al. 2017. "Can We Manage Coastal Ecosystems to Sequester More Blue Carbon?" *Frontiers in Ecology and the Environment* 15 (4):206–13.

Mäder, J. A., J. Staehelin, T. Peter, D. Brunner, H. E. Rieder, and W. A. Stahel. 2010. "Evidence for the Effectiveness of the Montreal Protocol to Protect the Ozone Layer." *Atmospheric Chemistry and Physics* 10 (24):12161–71.

Marzeion, B.,A. H. Jarosch, and M. Hofer. 2012. "Past and Future Sea-Level Change from the Surface Mass Balance of Glaciers." *The Cryosphere* 6 (6):1295–1322.

Mascioli, N. R., M. Previdi, A. M. Fiore, and M. Ting. 2017. "Timing and Seasonality of the United States 'Warming Hole.'" *Environmental Research Letters* 12 (3):034008.

Mastrandrea, M., C. Field, T. Stocker, O. Edenhofer, K. Ebi, D. Frame, H. Held et al. 2010. *Guidance Note for Lead Authors of the IPCC Fifth Assessment Report on Consistent Treatment of Uncertainties*. Jasper Ridge, CA: Intergovernmental Panel on Climate Change.

Mathes, R. W., K. Ito, K. Lane, and T. D. Matte. 2017. "Real-Time Surveillance of Heat-Related Morbidity: Relation to Excess Mortality Associated with Extreme Heat." *PLoS One* 12 (9):e0184364. doi:10.1371/journal.pone.0184364.

McCabe, G. J., J. L. Betancourt, and S. Feng. 2015. "Variability in the Start, End, and Length of Frost-Free Periods across the Conterminous United States during the Past Century." *International Journal of Climatology* 35 (15):4673–80.

McPhaden, M. J., S. E.Zebiak, and M. H. Glantz. 2006. "ENSO as an Integrating Concept in Earth Science." *Science* 314 (5806):1740–45.

Meehl, G. A., J. M. Arblaster, C. T. Chung, M. M. Holland, A. DuVivier, L. Thompson et al. 2019. "Sustained Ocean Changes Contributed to Sudden Antarctic Sea Ice Retreat in Late 2016." *Nature Communications* 10 (1):14.

Mora, C., A. G. Frazier, R. J. Longman, R. S. Dacks, M. M. Walton, E. J. Tong, J. J. Sanchez et al. 2013. "The Projected Timing of Climate Departure from Recent Variability." *Nature* 502 (7470):183–87.

Moss, R. H., J. A. Edmonds, K. A. Hibbard, M. R. Manning, S. K. Rose, D. P. van Vuuren, T. R. Carter et al. 2010. "The Next Generation of Scenarios for Climate Change Research and Assessment." *Nature* 463:747–56.

Mouginot J., E. Rignot, A. A. Bjørk, M. van den Broeke, R. Millan, M. Morlighem et al. 2019. "Forty-Six Years of Greenland Ice Sheet Mass Balance from 1972 to 2018." *Proceedings of the National Academy of Sciences* 116 (19):9239–44.

Nagelkerken, I., B. D. Russell, B. M. Gillanders, and S. D. Connell. 2016. "Ocean Acidification Alters Fish Populations Indirectly through Habitat Modification." *Nature Climate Change* 6 (1):89–93.

Nakicenovic, N., and R. Swart, eds. 2000. *Special Report on Emissions Scenarios*. Cambridge: Cambridge University Press.

National Research Council. Committee on America's Climate Choices. 2010. *Advancing the Science of Climate Change: America's Climate Choices.* Washington, DC: National Academies Press.

"NOAA Earth System Research Laboratory: Global Greenhouse Gas Reference Network." 2019. *Asheville, NC:* National Oceanic and Atmospheric Administration. https://www.esrl.noaa.gov/gmd/ccgg/ggrn.php.

Noerdlinger, P. D., and K. R. Brower. 2007. "The Melting of Floating Ice Raises the Ocean Level." *Geophysical Journal International* 170 (1):145–50.

Oke, T. R. 1982. "The Energetic Basis of the Urban Heat Island." *Quarterly Journal of the Royal Meteorological Society* 108 (455):1–24.

O'Neill, B. C., M. Dalton, R. Fuchs, L. Jiang, S. Pachauri, and K. Zigova. 2010. "Global Demographic Trends and Future Carbon Emissions." *Proceedings of the National Academy of Sciences* 107 (41):17521–526.

Oreskes, N. 2004. "Beyond the Ivory Tower: The Scientific Consensus on Climate Change." *Science* 306 (5702):686.

Pierce, D. W., T. P. Barnett, B. D. Santer, and P. J. Gleckler. 2009. "Selecting Global Climate Models for Regional Climate Change Studies." *Proceedings of the National Academy of Sciences* 106 (21):8441.

Rhea, S., A. Ising, A. T. Fleischauer, L. Deyneka, H. Vaughan-Batten, and A. Waller. 2012. "Using Near Real-Time Morbidity Data to Identify Heat-Related Illness Prevention Strategies in North Carolina." *Journal of Community Health* 37 (2):495–500.

Rizwan, A. M., Y. C. L. Dennis, and C. Liu. 2008. "A Review on the Generation, Determination and Mitigation of Urban Heat Island." *Journal of Environmental Sciences* 20:120–28.

Robine J. M., S. L. Cheung, S. Le Roy, H. Van Oyen, C. Griffiths, J. P. Michel, and F. R. Herrmann. 2008. "Death Toll Exceeded 70,000 in Europe during the Summer of 2003." *Comptes Rendus Biologies* 331 (2):171–78.

Robinson, D. A., and K. F. Dewy. 1990. "Recent Secular Variations in the Extent of Northern Hemisphere Snow Cover." *Geophysical Research Letters* 17:1557–60.

Rodolfo-Metalpa, R., F. Houlbrèque, E. Tambutté, F. Boisson, C. Baggini, F. P. Patti, R. Jefree et al. 2011. "Coral and Mollusc Resistance to Ocean Acidification Adversely Affected by Warming." *Nature Climate Change* 1:308–12.

Rudolph, L., and C. Harrison. 2016. *A Physician's Guide to Climate Change, Health and Equity.* Oakland, CA: Public Health Institute. http://climatehealthconnect.org/wp-content/uploads/2016/09/FullGuideTEMP.pdf.

Russo, S., A. Dosio, R. G. Graversen, J. Sillmann, H. Carrao, M. B. Dunbar et al. 2014. "Magnitude of Extreme Heat Waves in Present Climate and Their Projection in a Warming World." *Journal of Geophysical Research: Atmospheres* 119 (22):12500–512.

Schuur, E. A., A. D. McGuire, C. Schädel, G. Grosse, J. W. Harden, D. J. Hayes et al. 2015. "Climate Change and the Permafrost Carbon Feedback." *Nature* 520 (7546):171

Semenza, J. C., C. H. Rubin, K. H. Falter, J. D. Selanikio, W. D. Flanders, H. L. Howe, and J. L. Wilhelm. 1996. "Heat-Related Deaths during the July 1995 Heat Wave in Chicago." *New England Journal of Medicine* 335 (2):84–90.

Shwed, U., and P. S. Bearman. 2010. "The Temporal Structure of Scientific Consensus Formation." *American Sociological Review* 75:817–40.

Siegenthaler, U., and H. Oeschger. 1987. "Biospheric CO_2 Emissions during the Past 200 Years Reconstructed by Deconvolution of Ice Core Data." *Tellus B* 39:140–54.

Sillmann, J., V. V. Kharin, F. W. Zwiers, X. Zhang, and D. Bronaugh. 2013. "Climate Extremes Indices in the CMIP5 Multimodel Ensemble: Part 2. Future Climate Projections." *Journal of Geophysical Research: Atmospheres* 118:2473–93.

Sivak, M. 2009. "Potential Energy Demand for Cooling in the 50 Largest Metropolitan Areas of the World: Implications for Developing Countries." *Energy Policy* 37:1382–84.

Slangen, A., M. Carson, C. Katsman, R. van de Wal, A. Köhl, L. Vermeersen, and D. Stammer. 2014. "Projecting Twenty-First Century Regional Sea-Level Changes." *Climate Change* 124:1–16.

Solomon, S., D. Qin, M. Manning, Z. Chen, M. Marquis, K. B. Avery, M. Tignor, and H. L. Miller. 2007. *Contribution of Working Group I to the Fourth Assessment Report of the Intergovernmental Panel on Climate Change, 2007.* Cambridge: Cambridge University Press.

Stone, B., J. J. Hess, and H. Frumkin. 2010. "Urban Form and Extreme Heat Events: Are Sprawling Cities More Vulnerable to Climate Change Than Compact Cities?" *Environmental Health Perspectives* 118 (10):1425.

Stott, P. A., D. A. Stone, and M. R. Allen. 2004. "Human Contribution to the European Heatwave of 2003." *Nature* 432:610–14.

Takeuchi, Y., Y. Endo, and S. Murakami. 2008. "High Correlation between Winter Precipitation and Air Temperature in Heavy-Snowfall Areas in Japan." *Annals of Glaciology* 49 (1):7–10.

Trenberth, K. E. 1997. "The Definition of El Niño." *Bulletin of the American Meteorological Society* 78 (12):2771–77.

Uejio, C. K., J. D. Tamerius, J. Vredenburg, G. Asaeda, D. A. Isaacs, J. A. BraunA. Quinn, and J. P. Freese. 2016. "Summer Indoor Heat Exposure and Respiratory and Cardiovascular Distress Calls in New York City, NY, US." *Indoor Air* 26 (4):594604.

Uejio C. K., O. V. Wilhelmi, J. S. Golden, D. M. Mills, S. P. Gulino, and J. P. Samenow. 2011. "Intra-urban Societal Vulnerability to Extreme Heat: The Role of Heat Exposure and the Built Environment, Socioeconomics, and Neighborhood Stability." *Health Place* 17 (2):498–507.

Uejio, C. K., J. D. Tamerius, J. Vredenburg, G. Asaeda, D. A. Isaacs, J. Braun et al. 2016. "Summer Indoor Heat Exposure and Respiratory and Cardiovascular Distress Calls in New York City, NY, US." *Indoor Air* 26 (4):594–604.

U.S. Department of Energy. n.d. "Air Conditioners." Accessed February 5, 2020. https://www.energy.gov/energysaver/home-cooling-systems/air-conditioning.

Vaidyanathan A., S. Saha, A. M. Vicedo-Cabrera, A. Gasparrini, N. Abdurehman, R. Jordan, M. Hawkins, J. Hess, and A. Elixhauser. 2019. "Assessment of Extreme Heat and Hospitalizations to Inform Early Warning Systems." *Proceedings of the National Academy of Sciences* 116 (12):5420–27. doi:10.1073/pnas.1806393116.

Vuille, M., and R. D. Garreaud. 2011. "Ocean-Atmosphere Interactions on Interannual to Decadal Timescales." In *Handbook of Environmental Change*, edited by J. A. Matthews, P. J. Bartlein, K. R. Briffa, A. G. Dawson, A. De Vernal; T. Denham, S. C. Fritz et al., 469–94. Los Angeles: Sage.

Wacker, S., J. Gröbner, K. Hocke, N. Kämpfer, and L. Vuilleumier. 2011. "Trend Analysis of Surface Cloud-Free Downwelling Long-Wave Radiation from Four Swiss Sites." *Journal of Geophysical Research: Atmospheres* 116 (D10):1–13.

Wang, L., Z. Wu, H. He, F. Wang, H. Du, and S. Zong S. 2017. "Changes in Start, End, and Length of Frost-Free Season Across Northeast China." *International Journal of Climatology* 37:271–83.

Ward, K., S. Lauf, B. Kleinschmit, and W. Endlicher. 2016. "Heat Waves and Urban Heat Islands in Europe: A Review of Relevant Drivers." *Science of the Total Environment* 569: 527–39.

Weatherdon, L. V., A. K. Magnan, A. D. Rogers, U. R. Sumaila, and W. W. L. Cheung. (2016). "Observed and Projected Impacts of Climate Change on Marine Fisheries, Aquaculture, Coastal Tourism, and Human Health: An Update." *Frontiers in Marine Science* 3 (APR). https://doi.org/10.3389/fmars.2016.00048.

White, J. R., V. Berisha, K. Lane, H. Ménager, A. Gettel, and C. R. Braun. 2017. "Evaluation of a Novel Syndromic Surveillance Query for Heat-Related Illness Using Hospital Data from Maricopa County, Arizona, 2015." *Public Health Reports* 132 (1 suppl):39S.

Wild, M. 2012. "Enlightening Global Dimming and Brightening." *Bulletin of the American Meteorological Society* 93 (1):27–37.

Willeit, M., A. Ganopolski, R. Calov, and V. Brovkin. 2019. "Mid-Pleistocene Transition in Glacial Cycles Explained by Declining CO2 and Regolith Removal." *Science Advances* 5 (4):eaav7337.

Williams, A. A., J. D. Spengler, P. Catalano, J. G. Allen, and J. G. Cedeno-Laurent. 2019. "Building Vulnerability in a Changing Climate: Indoor Temperature Exposures and Health Outcomes in Older Adults Living in Public Housing during an Extreme Heat Event in Cambridge, MA." *International Journal of Environmental Research and Public Health* 16 (13):2373. doi:10.3390/ijerph16132373.

Wuebbles, D. J., D. W. Fahey, and K. A. Hibbard. 2017. *Climate science special report: Fourth National Climate Assessment, vol. I*. Washington, DC: U.S. Global Change Research Program.

Zebiak, S. E., B. Orlove, A. G. Muñoz, C. Vaughan, J. Hansen, T. Troy, M. C. Thomson, A. Lustig, and S. Garvin. 2015. "Investigating El Niño-Southern Oscillation and Society Relationships." *Climate Change* 6 (1):17–34.

Zelinka, M. D., S. A. Klein, K. E. Taylor, and T. Andrews. 2013. "Contributions of Different Cloud Types to Feedbacks and Rapid Adjustments in CMIP5." *Journal of Climate* 26:5007–27.

Zhang, J. 2007. "Increasing Antarctic Sea Ice under Warming Atmospheric and Oceanic Conditions." *Journal of Climate* 20 (11):2515–29.

CHAPTER 2

CLIMATE-RELATED DISASTERS: THE ROLE OF PREVENTION FOR MANAGING HEALTH RISK

Mark E. Keim

Introduction

Definition of a Climate-Related Disaster

A **disaster** is "a serious disruption of the functioning of a community or a society causing widespread human, material, economic or environmental losses that exceed the ability of the affected community or society to cope using its own resources" (United NationsOffice for Disaster Risk Reduction n.d.).

Climate-related disasters (**CRDs**) are caused by oceanic and atmospheric hazards that are influenced by the global climate. Warming of the global climate is known to increase the number of extreme weather events (EWE) (i.e., associated with climatologic, hydrologic, and meteorologic hazards) (EM-DAT 2019); and extreme oceanic events (EOE) (i.e., associated with **sea level rise**) (Hoegh-Guldberg et al. 2018; Intergovernmental Panel on Climate Change [IPCC] 2007).

Disasters caused by EWE have been associated with high precipitation, (e.g., **storms, floods,** and **landslides**) or low precipitation (e.g., **heat waves, drought,** and **wildfire**) (Keim 2011). Disasters caused by EOE (e.g., sea level rise) have been associated with soil and groundwater salinification resulting in loss of food and water security (Keim 2010c). CRDs occur as a result of the combination of population **exposure** to a climate-related hazard (e.g., EWE and sea level rise), the conditions of **vulnerability** that are present (e.g., dependence upon local human, shelter, food, and water resources), and insufficient **resilience** to reduce or cope with the negative consequences (e.g., living in a low-resource nation) (Keim 2018a). Without outside assistance, these events often overwhelm the **capacity** of the population to respond effectively, and the resulting mismatch between needs and resources may result in a disaster declaration.

Global Incidence of CRDs

During the past fifty years (1967–2016), 22,173 disasters (i.e., associated with **biological, natural, technological, extraterrestrial and conflict hazards**) caused an estimated 6.2 million deaths and $3.4 trillion in damages worldwide (EM-DAT 2019). Half (50 percent) of these disasters were climate related (i.e., associated with climatologic, hydrologic, or meteorologic hazards) (EM-DAT 2019) (see Figure 2.1).

Fifty percent of these CRDs involved **hydrologic hazards** (**floods** and **landslides**); 40 percent involved **meteorologic hazards** (temperature extremes, fog, and **storms**); and 10 percent were associated with **climatologic hazards** (**drought** and **wildfire**s).[2] Ninety-five percent of all people affected by disasters during this time were affected by CRDs. The world's poor were disproportionately affected by

KEY CONCEPTS

- Climate-related disasters (CRDs) are a major cause contributing to the global burden of disasters.

- There are a predictable number of major public health consequences associated with most CRDs. These consequences vary only in the degree of impact among the various causative hazards.

- Disaster risk management is a comprehensive approach that entails developing and implementing strategies for each phase of the disaster life cycle.

- Disaster risk management as applied to climate change adaptation includes both preimpact disaster risk reduction (prevention and mitigation), postimpact disaster risk transfer (risk pools and insurance policies), and disaster risk retention (preparedness, response, and recovery).

- Health-related disaster risk due to extreme weather events occurs as the result of convergence of three major risk factors:

  ○ The presence of a health *hazard* associated with extreme weather and climate events. (This factor is commonly considered as a function of hazard frequency and impact.)

  ○ The degree of *exposure* to the hazard sustained by the person (or population). (This factor is commonly considered as a function of hazard dose and time.)

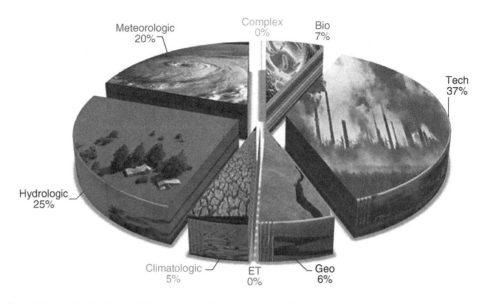

Figure 2.1 Relative incidence of disasters, according to category of hazard, 1969–2018

all disasters. The most vulnerable and marginalized in all societies bear the highest health burden for all CRDs (Brouewer et al. 2007; Clack et al. 2002; International Federation of Red Cross [IFRC] 2005; IFRC and Red Crescent Societies 2009; National Science and Technology 1996; Nelson 1990).

Global Trends

Global Trends in Disasters

The incidence of disasters is increasing worldwide (EM-DAT 2019). Continued global warming is expected to further exacerbate the frequency and/or severity of CRDs (Hoegh-Guldberg et al. 2018; IPCC 2007). The frequency and magnitude of floods and droughts are expected to increase with rising global temperatures. Risks of water scarcity are projected to be greater in some regions. Impacts associated with sea level rise, groundwater salinification, and increased flooding are projected to be critically important in small islands, low-lying coasts, and deltas (Hoegh-Guldberg et al. 2018; IPCC 2007).

Global Trends in Disaster Management

In 1994, the first United Nations World Congress on Disaster Reduction (WCDR) recognized that "disaster prevention, mitigation, and preparedness are better than disaster response in achieving the goals and objectives of the decade. Disaster response alone is not sufficient, as it yields only temporary results at a very high cost" (IPCC 2007). Since then, **disaster risk reduction** has become the mainstay for international development related to disasters (Keim 2018b).

By 2015, at the third WCDR, all members of the United Nations formally accepted the Sendai Framework for Disaster Risk Reduction with a key goal to "substantially reduce global mortality by 2030" (UNISDR 2015). Although disaster risk reduction has now become an internationally accepted standard, it remains largely unimplemented by some nations, including the United States. In 2019, twenty-five years after the first WCDR, the U.S. National Academies of Sciences, Engineering, and Medicine noted that, "while some disaster management and pub- lic health preparedness programming may be viewed as tangentially related, a multi-sectoral and inter-disciplinary national platform for coordination and policy guidance on involving disaster risk reduction in the United States does not exist" (National Academies of Sciences, Engineering, and Medicine 2016). Despite the findings of a 2018 Pew Trust study estimating a 600 percent return on investment for **risk reduction** and **preparedness**, the majority of national-level, disaster-related policies, programming, and investments at the local, state, and national levels are customarily directed more toward responding to and recovering from disasters (National Academies of Sciences, Engineering, and Medicine 2016).

Global Trends in Human Development

Disaster risk reduction has also emerged as a core element of **sustainable development.** The 2002 World Summit on Sustainable Development (WSSD) concluded that "an integrated multi-hazard, inclusive approach to address vulnerability, risk assessment, and disaster management, including prevention, mitigation, preparedness, response and recovery, is an essential part of a safer world in the twenty-first century" (United Nations 2002).

The emerging vision of environmental sustainability as wedded to economic vitality and social equity is becoming an important rationale for reducing natural-hazard risk to human settlements (Beatley 1998). The high property damage levels in recent disasters clearly suggest that current patterns and practices of land use and community building are not sustainable in the long run (Beatley 1998). Economic development achieved in a sustainable manner could itself be regarded as an adaptation measure for climate change (Fankhauser 2009). Addressing CRDs can be viewed as one component of a broad, sustainable development strategy that aims at increasing national and regional **capacity** to deal with long-term climate change (Keim 2011; Schipper and Pelling 2006).

Public Health Impact of Climate-Related Disasters, in General

The Relative Impact of CRDs

Although the hazards that cause disasters may vary, the potential health consequences and subsequent public health and medical needs of the population do not (Federal Emergency Management Agency 1996; Keim 2016a; Keim and Giannone 2006).

Regardless of the hazard, disasters can be conceptualized as causing fifteen public health consequences that are addressed by approximately thirty-five categories of public health and medical capabilities (Keim 2016a; Centers for Disease Control and Prevention 2011).

For example, floods, heat waves, hurricanes, and wildfires all have the potential to displace people from their homes. These hazards require the same sheltering capability with only minor adjustments based on the rapidity of onset, scale, duration, location, and intensity. Table 2.1 identifies the relative impact of these fifteen public health consequences caused by seven major climate-related hazards.

Mortality Associated with CRDs

During the past fifty years, 10,950 CRDs caused an estimated 3.6 million deaths (57 percent of all disaster-related mortality) worldwide and $2.6 trillion (75 percent of all disaster-related losses) worldwide (EM-DAT 2019). The most frequently occurring CRDs (hydrologic hazards consisting mostly of floods) comprised 25 percent of all disasters but were responsible for only 6 percent of global disaster mortality during this time. On the contrary, climatologic disasters (consisting mostly of droughts) comprised only 5 percent of disasters but caused 36 percent of global mortality (EM-DAT 2019) (see Figure 2.2).

The mortality rate is generally lower for CRDs, as compared to other disaster hazard categories. This is largely because of the relatively high incidence of low mortality floods. The

Table 2.1   The Relative Public Health Impacts of CRDs

Public Health Impact	Hydrologic				Meteorologic	Climatologic	
	Sea level rise	High precipitation				Low precipitation	
	Coastal floods	Riverine floods	Landslide	Storms	Heat	Drought	Wildfire
Deaths	Few	Few, but many in poor nations	Few to moderate	Few, but many in poor nations	Moderate to many in rich nations	Few, but many in poor nations	Few
Injuries	Unlikely	Few	Few to moderate	Few	Unlikely	Unlikely	Few
Loss of clean water	Focal to widespread	Focal to widespread	Focal	Focal to widespread	Unlikely	Widespread	Focal
Loss of safe shelter	Unlikely	Focal to widespread	Focal	Focal to widespread	Focal to widespread	Focal to widespread	Focal
Loss of personal/household goods	Unlikely	Focal to widespread	Focal	Focal to widespread	Unlikely	Focal to widespread	Focal
Major population movements	Focal to widespread	Focal to widespread	Focal	Focal to widespread	Unlikely	Focal to widespread	Focal
Loss of routine hygiene	Unlikely	Focal to widespread	Focal	Focal to widespread	Unlikely	Widespread	Focal
Loss of sanitation	Unlikely	Focal to widespread	Focal	Focal to widespread	Unlikely	Focal	Focal
Disruption of solid waste management	Unlikely	Focal to widespread	Focal	Focal to widespread	Unlikely	Focal	Focal
Public concern for safety	Moderate	Moderate to high	Moderate to high	High	Moderate to high	Low to moderate	Moderate to high
Increased pests	Unlikely	Focal to widespread	Unlikely	Focal to widespread	Unlikely	Focal to widespread	Unlikely
Loss or damage of health care system	Unlikely	Focal to widespread	Focal	Focal to widespread	Unlikely	Focal	Focal to widespread
Worsening of chronic illnesses	Focal to widespread	Focal to widespread	Focal	Focal to widespread	Focal to widespread	Widespread	Focal to widespread
Loss of electrical power	Unlikely	Focal to widespread	Focal	Focal to widespread	Focal	Focal to widespread	Unlikely
Toxic exposures	Unlikely	Widespread for carbon monoxide poisoning	Focal	Widespread for carbon monoxide poisoning	Unlikely	Focal	Widespread for air
Food scarcity	Focal to widespread	Focal to widespread	Focal	Common in low-lying coastal areas	Unlikely	Widespread in poor nations	Focal

mean mortality rate for CRDs (60/100,000 affected) is 40 percent lower than that of all disasters in general (101/100,000). Mortality rates also vary according to each climate-related hazard (EM-DAT 2019). The mortality rates of 83/100,000 for climatologic hazards (e.g., drought and wildfire) and 87/100,000 meteorologic hazards (e.g., storms and heat waves) are quite similar, whereas the mortality rate for hydrologic hazards (e.g., floods and landslides) was 8 times less (10/100,000) (EM-DAT 2019).

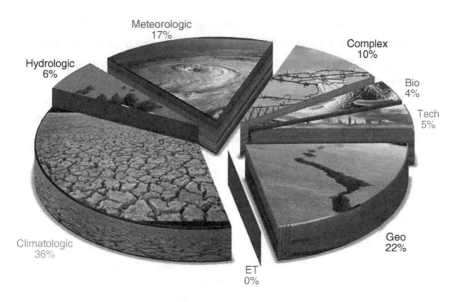

Figure 2.2 Percentage of global disaster-related mortality, according to category of hazard, 1969–2018

Morbidity Associated with CRDs

Most of the morbidity related to CRDs occurs as injuries sustained as a result of exposure to environmental hazards such as water, wind, fire, smoke, debris, and heat or through the absence of a life-sustaining requirement (e.g., air, food, and water).

Communicable disease epidemics are rare following CRDs and risk differs according to the level of economic development of the affected nation (Keim 2016b). Behavioral health effects are commonly reported long-term outcomes of CRDs (Caldera et al. 2001; Goenjian et al. 2001; Keenan et al. 2004; Krug et al. 1998; Sattler et al. 2002).

CRDs can markedly affect the ability of the population to maintain access to adequate shelter, water, sanitation, hygiene, health care, nutrition, security, public services, or utilities in order to maintain their health during a disaster event.

Public Health Impact of Climate-Related Disasters, According to Hazard

During the past fifty years, climatologic hazards caused 1,094 disasters comprising 10 percent of all CRDs, killing 703,416 and affecting an astounding 2.5 billion people (EM-DAT 2019). Droughts comprised 62 percent of these climatologic disasters and were associated with 99.6 percent of their mortality. Wildfires (forest and land fires) caused 36 percent of climatologic disasters and were associated with 0.3 percent of their mortality. Nearly all (99.7 percent) people affected by climatologic disasters during the past 50 years were affected by drought (EM-DAT 2019).

Meteorologic hazards caused 5,865 disasters (comprising 40 percent of all CRDs), were responsible for the deaths of 1.1 million, and affected 2.2 billion people worldwide.

There were 5,368 hydrologic disasters during this time, representing 50 percent of all CRDs, killing 358,177 and affecting 3.7 billion people worldwide (EM-DAT 2019). Floods comprised 88 percent of these hydrologic disasters and were associated with 89 percent of their mortality. Landslides caused 12 percent of hydrologic disasters and were associated with 11 percent of their mortality. Nearly all (99.7 percent) of people affected by hydrologic disasters during the past fifty years were affected by floods (EM-DAT 2019). During the past fifty years, eighty-one coastal flooding events have resulted in the death of 3,269 persons, affected 19.3

million people, and caused $ 10 billion in damage worldwide (EM-DAT 2019). Impacts of acute **sea inundation** events are particularly severe among small island populations. These populations are particularly vulnerable to acute disruptions involving crop productivity and access to freshwater (Keim 2010b).

Most morbidity and mortality associated with CRD-related disease are attributable to injury. Psychological illness is common after CRDs. Communicable disease outbreaks have been reported after floods, **cyclones** (EM-DAT 2019), and droughts. The risk of infectious disease differs by hazard and the resources available to affected populations.

Table 2.2 summarizes causes of morbidity and mortality associated with CRDs.

Table 2.2 Health Consequences of CRDs

Category	Hazard	Causes of morbidity and mortality
Climatologic	Drought	Chronic malnutrition, diarrheal and respiratory infections, toxic gas and algal exposures, vector-borne disease, mental illness, and exacerbations of asthma and chronic obstructive pulmonary disease
	Wildfires	Burns and inhalation injury, exacerbations of asthma and chronic obstructive pulmonary disease, mental illness, lower infant birth weights
Meteorologic	Heat waves	Heat illness, exacerbations of chronic disease, and mental illness
	Storms	Drowning and near drowning; lacerations, blunt trauma, and puncture wounds; animal and insect bites; toxic exposures to carbon monoxide and mold; vector-borne disease; diarrheal illness; infectious disease; exacerbations of chronic cardiovascular and respiratory disease; and mental illness
Hydrologic	Floods	Drowning and near drowning, exacerbations of chronic illness, toxic exposures to carbon monoxide and mold, outbreaks of vector-borne disease and diarrheal illness, mental illness
	Landslides	Traumatic injury, asphyxiation, toxic exposures to hazardous materials, gangrene and necrotizing fasciitis
Oceanic	Sea inundations	Acute malnutrition; diarrheal, parasitic, and respiratory infections; and exacerbations of chronic disease

Sources: Agampodi et al. (2014); Agrawal et al. (2013); Alderman et al. (2012); Alhinai (2011); Amiridis et al. (2012); Anderson et al. (2009); Arlappa et al. (2011); Atuyambe et al. (2011); Azhar et al. (2014); Bai et al. (2014); Bayer et al. (2014); Bei et al. (2013); Berko et al. (2014); Bernstein and Rice (2013); Brunetti et al. (2014); Bustinza et al. (2013); Caamano Isorna et al. (2011); Calzolari and Albieri (2013); Carnie et al. (2011); Cash et al. (2013); Catapano et al. (2001); Chan et al. (2013); Chaturongkasumrit et al. (2013); Chen et al. (2014); Clemens et al. (2013); Collins et al. (2013); Davis (2008); Ding et al. (2013); D'Ippoliti et al. (2010); Doocy et al. (2013); Doocy et al. (2013); Fussell and Lowe (2014); Grimm et al. (2014); Grimsley et al. (2012); Hanigan et al. (2012); Haque et al. (2012); Hartz et al. (2012); Harville et al. (2009); Harville et al. (2011); Horton et al. (2010); Ibrahim et al. (2012); Keim (2010b); Kessler (2012); Kim et al. (2012); Kistin et al. (2010); Kue and Dyer et al. (2013); Lane et al. (2013); Laugharne et al. (2011); Lowe et al. (2014); Mendoza et al. (2013); Morrow et al. (2010); Mosley et al. (2004); Murakami et al. (2012); Nahar et al. (2014); Notes from the field (2012); Ostad Taghizadeh et al. (2013); Papanikolaou et al. (2011); Park et al. (2013); Pascal et al. (2012); Pereira et al. (2013); Perez-Gracia et al. (2013); Price et al. (2013); Rabito et al. (2012); Rando et al. (2012); Rigby et al. (2011); Robinson et al. (2011); Sanchez et al. (2009); Sanguanklin et al. (2014); Schaffer et al. (2012); Seifman et al. (2011); Shaposhnikov et al. (2014); Simpson and Abelsohn (2012); Smith et al. (2014); Stanke et al. (2012); Stanke et al. (2013); Sun et al. (2014); Sunyer (2010); Takaro et al. (2013); Tally et al. (2013); Tees et al. (2010); Tempark et al. (2013); Tian et al. (2013); Vranken et al. (2013); Waite et al. (2014); Wang et al. (2010); Wind et al. (2014); Yelland et al. (2010).

Managing the Health Risk of Climate-Related Disasters

Disaster Risk Management

Risk Management

Risk represents the degree of uncertainty involving the interaction between an event and its outcome. Uncertainty adversely affects our ability to predict the risk of outcome. Management is used to reduce the uncertainty of outcomes through organization of the activities intended to achieve defined objectives. **Risk management** assesses, controls, and monitors risk. Evidence regarding protective and risk factors is analyzed and **risk treatment** measures are implemented using ISO31000, a set of international standards relating to risk management that includes a framework for risk assessment, avoidance, reduction, transfer, and acceptance (International Organization for Standardization [ISO] 2009).

Analytical risk assessments typically guide the most cost-effective options for treatment of the risk. Risk treatment measures include avoiding the risk, reducing the negative effect of the risk, transferring the risk to another party, and accepting some or all of the consequences of a particular risk (ISO 2009).

CLINICAL CORRELATES 2.1 HOUSING SECURITY AND MEDICATIONS AFTER THE STORM

Climate-driven extreme weather events affect the environments that support health and well-being, especially for medically and socially vulnerable populations. Some effects are transient whereas others are major structural or socioeconomic disturbances that may ultimately lead to the uprooting of homes and forced migration (Fussell, Sastry, and Vanlandingham 2010). Equitable housing is one national problems amplified during times of stress (i.e., weak housing infrastructure has a greater risk of damage from floods). Already 11% percent of households spend more than half their income on housing costs, especially in communities of color (University of Wisconsin 2019). The problem is compounded when unemployment and job interruptions create unreliable income streams. Housing insecurity also influences health care utilization. After hurricane Sandy, emergency departments in New York City saw an acute increase use of emergency services for homelessness and inadequate housing, disproportionately affecting older persons (Doran et al. 2016). Disasters can also directly and indirectly disrupt routine tasks such as doctor appointments, medication retrieval, and grocery shopping. Many Americans, especially older adults (Jonkman et al. 2009), are ill prepared for these events. In one survey, 37% percent of Americans could go a week or less without medications before experiencing a "medical crisis." (Health Care Ready 2019). As expected, increases in health care utilization for prescription refills have been demonstrated in the weeks following storms (Malik et al. 2018).

Housing insecurity and medication disruptions have an impact on health care utilization during significant disasters calling for increased preparedness and planning for at-risk populations.

Disaster Risk Management

Disaster risk management applies the general principles of risk management to disasters. It is a comprehensive approach that entails strategies before and after hazard impact (National Science and Technology Council 1996). Disaster risk management includes preimpact measures for **risk avoidance** (e.g., floodplain management); risk reduction (e.g., **land use planning**), and **risk transfer** (insurance) measures, as well as postimpact measures including risk transfer (e.g., external aid) and risk retention (e.g., emergency **response** and **recovery**). Once risks have been identified and assessed, techniques to manage (i.e., prevent and control) the risk fall into one or more of these four major categories (ISO 2009; Keim 2010a).

Figure 2.3 and Table 2.3 describe the components of disaster risk management, in terms of risk assessment and risk treatment.

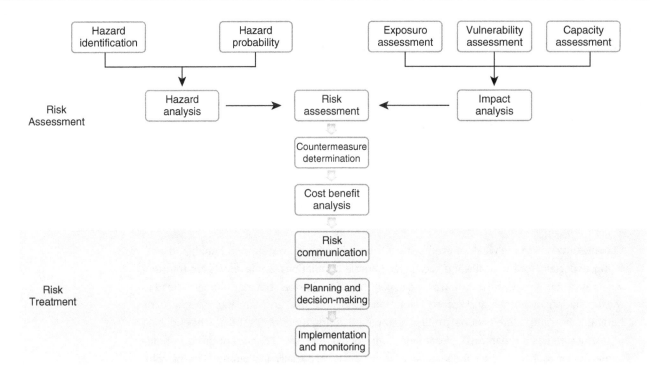

Figure 2.3   Schematic overview of disaster risk management process
Source: Adapted from Keim (2002, 2010a, 2010b).

Table 2.3   Key Components of Disaster Risk Management

Component	Activities
Hazard Analysis • Hazard identification • Hazard probability	Identify health hazards (e.g., drowning) associated with each disaster hazard (e.g., flood) Determine the frequency of past hazard events
Impact Analysis • Assessment • Prioritization	Determine critical assets, (i.e., population, medical facilities, etc.) Identify expected health consequences and impact for each hazard Prioritize subpopulations based on degree of impact
Capacity Assessment	Identify the extent of capabilities (strengths, attributes, and resources) available to counter the adverse health effects (before, during and after the event).
Exposure Assessment	Determine the degree of population exposure to the health hazard
Vulnerability Assessment • Exposure • Susceptibility	Estimate the degree of vulnerability of each subpopulation for each hazard Identify preexisting countermeasures and their level of effectiveness
Countermeasure Determination • avoidance/reduction • transfer/retention	Identify new countermeasures which may be taken to eliminate or lessen hazards and/or exposures and vulnerabilities
Cost - Benefit Analysis	Identify countermeasure costs and benefits Prioritize options
Risk Communication	Prepare a range of recommendations for decision-makers and/or the public.
Risk Management Plan	Develop a disaster risk treatment plan for all four phases of prevention
Implementation and Monitoring	Implement and monitor the risk management program for effectiveness in achieving outcomes (not merely outputs).

Source: Adapted from Keim (2002, 2010a, 2010b, 2011).

CLINICAL CORRELATES 2.2 THE ROAD TO POOR HEALTH: TRANSPORTATION SYSTEM DISRUPTIONS

Transportation systems are vital to health care access, even more so during times of disaster. Ambulances, helicopters, and private vehicles bring patients for use of emergency care, medications, critical supplies, and other health care services. Extreme weather events such as flooding disrupt or destroy infrastructure, making usual roadways or landing areas inaccessible, hindering both primary assessments of patients and critical care transports (to higher levels of care) (Bucher et al. 2018). Transportation systems also interconnect with many other systems—water, electric, information communication technology, and petroleum systems, with direct and indirect influences on patient care and health outcomes (Markolf et al. 2019).

Communities must work to build climate-resilient transportation systems to support patient transport, access to health care facilities, and community resilience during disasters.

Disease Management

Natural History and Causal Factors of Disease   Any disease (including injury), if left untreated, progresses through a natural history that can be broken into a series of stages. But, if an intervention is applied, the natural history is modified to change the outcome. Preventive measures can be applied at any stage along the natural history of a disease, with the goal of preventing further progression of the condition (Association of Faculties of Medicine of Canada 2017).

Disease does not occur randomly. It is caused when hosts are exposed to an environment containing agents that are hazardous to health. It is therefore possible to study the causal factors involving the agent (i.e., hazard), host (i.e., vulnerability), and environment (e.g., exposure), including both risk and protective factors (Keim 2017, 2018a, 2018b).

Natural History and Causal Factors of Disaster-Related Injuries   The time between exposure to the hazard and biological onset of disease (the "**incubation period**") is of critical importance when prioritizing activities intended to reduce disaster-related mortality (Association of Faculties of Medicine of Canada 2017) (see Figure 2.2).

The period for developing a life-threatening injury is commonly measured in minutes to hours, whereas this period for outbreaks of disease is most commonly measured in days to weeks. This rapid onset of disaster-related injuries markedly limits the effectiveness of secondary and tertiary prevention (e.g., emergency medical response and recovery interventions).

However, the character of most large-scale, environmental (e.g., technological, hydro-meteorologic, and geophysical) disasters commonly precludes accessibility of lifesaving surgical care for the overwhelming majority of patients. This is of critical significance considering that 96 percent of the world's disaster deaths during the past fifty years were due to injury (EM-DAT 2019). In the case of food and water insecurity due to sea level rise disasters, geographical isolation, and lack of resources may forestall detection and assistance efforts.

Thus, the natural history of disaster-related injuries often limits the effectiveness of secondary and tertiary prevention following disasters from climate-related hazards. Primary prevention of the exposure (before injury/illness can occur) is therefore of critical importance to reducing mortality risk from these hazards (Huppert and Sparks 2006; Keim 2018b; Schipper and Pelling 2006; World Bank 2007).

CLINICAL CORRELATES 2.3 PROTECTING PREGNANT WOMEN AND INFANTS

Pregnant women and infants are at increased risk of adverse events during times of disaster. The American College of Obstetrics and Gynecology has cited extreme weather events as a risk for care interruption, advising all patients to have awareness of obstetric-centered disaster preparedness plans (ACOG Committee 2017), as such disasters have historically been correlated with an increase in pregnancy complications including threatened or spontaneous abortions, preterm delivery, low birth weight, and abnormal glucose tolerance testing (Abdo et al. 2019; Xiao et al. 2019). Timing of exposure also contributes to specific hazards. For example, wildfire smoke exposure early on in pregnancy had a higher association of decreased birth weight (Abdo et al. 2019) and pregnant women have increased health care utilization for mental health months later in gestation (Xiao et al. 2019). Large interruptions in systems processing influence the peripartum period via power outages, evacuations, and disruptions in services. Neonatal intensive care unit patients, requiring feeding and often oxygen or ventilator support, are arguably one of the most vulnerable groups in the hospital. One facility had to evacuate twenty-one neonates over four and a half hours after a storm surge caused power outages (Espiritu et al. 2014).

Hospitals should have obstetric-centered disaster preparedness plans to support the unpredictability and vulnerability of childbirth for mothers and infants.

Disease Prevention

Disease **prevention** occurs in four main stages: **primordial**, **primary**, **secondary**, and **tertiary** (Association of Faculties of Medicine of Canada 2017). Primordial prevention modifies determinants of health ("the cause of the cause" of disease) in order to prevent health hazards from occurring. Primary prevention focuses on reducing risk factors for exposure to the disease hazard. Secondary prevention reduces disease susceptibility once exposure has occurred. Tertiary prevention seeks to reduce mortality and disease severity once diseases (including injuries) occur (Association of Faculties of Medicine of Canada 2017). (See Table 2.3.)

Primordial Prevention Primordial prevention of disaster-related health effects involves controlling the hazard occurrence and health determinants (i.e., environmental, economic, health, social, behavioral, and cultural factors) known to amplify the risk of disease (Association of Faculties of Medicine of Canada 2017). Primordial prevention seeks first to prevent the disaster hazard from ever occurring. In examples where the hazard cannot be prevented, primordial prevention may be used to guide developmental decisions that avoid placing critical infrastructure and human settlements within hazardous areas.

Primary Prevention The adverse health effect of a hazard is often characterized by a dose-response relationship. Typically, as the degree of exposure to a health hazard increases, the adverse health effect appears in more of the population. Persons receiving a higher dose (magnitude of exposure to the disaster hazard over time) of the hazardous agent have a higher risk for adverse health outcomes as compared with those less exposed. Vulnerability is the degree of observed health impact per dose (concentration/magnitude over time) of the health hazard (e.g., mechanical, chemical, thermal, or restrictive of essential elements like food, air, and water). In other words, vulnerability is the slope of the hazard dose-response curve for disaster-related health effects (Keim 2018a).

Primary prevention involves preventing exposures that lead to disease (Association of Faculties of Medicine of Canada 2017). It involves an interdisciplinary approach for identifying, characterizing, monitoring, and avoiding exposure to human health hazards. This includes those investigational aspects (like monitoring, forecasting, modeling, and dose reconstruction), as well as structural (e.g., engineering controls, construction methods, and architectural design) and nonstructural (e.g., public policy, education, and population protection measures) means for reducing exposures (Keim 2010a). Long-term exposure reduction for all of these hazards most frequently involves disaster-related **mitigation** (United Nations Disaster Relief Office 1991). Mitigation may occur as both **structural mitigation** measures (such as wind and/or flood resistant construction, floodplain management, and planting) and **nonstructural mitigation** measures (such as land use regulation, water conservation, agricultural and forestry practices, and building codes) (Malilay 1997; United Nations Disaster Relief Office 1991).

Secondary Prevention   The goal of secondary prevention is to prevent disease, given that exposure has already occurred (Association of Faculties of Medicine of Canada 2017). These actions typically involve emergency response capabilities (e.g., search and rescue, occupational health, preventive medicine, disease control, and hazardous material response) that enable early detection and appropriate preventive care. Response usually includes those actions immediately necessary to *remove the affected population from ongoing exposure or risk of harm.* Rapid and effective response can prevent adverse health impacts.

This element of risk treatment known as **risk retention** involves accepting disaster loss when it occurs and then attempting to respond and recover (if possible). By default, all residual risks that are not avoided or transferred are retained and will require allocation of resources at some time in the future. Risk acceptance is not considered sustainable because the practice is, in effect, tends to accumulate risk for future generations (Foke et al. 2002; United Nations 2012; United Nations Conference on Environment and Development 1992).

Tertiary Prevention   The goal of tertiary prevention is to prevent permanent impairment, disability, and death given that disease has occurred (Association of Faculties of Medicine of Canada 2017). Tertiary prevention includes capabilities that reduce disease severity, thus minimizing the risk of additional risk in the form of protracted illness, medical complications, disability, and death.

The capabilities involved in the tertiary prevention of disaster-related morbidity and mortality largely involve a network of curative and rehabilitative health, interagency coordination, risk communication, and social services intended to prevent additional or ongoing disability and death after the disease or injury occurs. This rehabilitation and recovery phase is characteristically long in duration (Keim 2010a).

Table 2.4 reveals the means by which disease prevention may be integrated to achieve the mutual goal of reducing health risk associated with CRDs.

Table 2.4   Prevention as an Integrated Approach for Managing the Health Risk of CRDs

Stage of Prevention	Disaster Risk Management Capability	Capabilities that Reduce the Risk of Adverse Health Effects
Primordial Prevention *Preventing Hazards*	Risk assessment	Hazard identification and monitoring Weather forecasting and modeling Health surveillance and risk assessment Hazard analysis and mapping Health impact assessment with new construction

Table 2.4   (Continued)

Stage of Prevention	Disaster Risk Management Capability	Capabilities that Reduce the Risk of Adverse Health Effects
	Hazard avoidance	Land use regulation and building codes Environmental health Urban planning and engineering controls Sustainable development Watershed, coastal, and forestry management Soil and water conservation
Primary Prevention *Preventing Exposures* *after* *Hazards Occur*	Risk assessment	Hazard analysis and mapping Weather forecasting and modeling Health surveillance and risk assessment Hazard analysis and mapping Exposure assessment and dose reconstruction
	Hazard monitoring	Hazard monitoring Environmental monitoring (e.g., air, water, soil) Event surveillance (e.g., commodities, critical infrastructure, economics) Health surveillance (clinical, laboratory, and occupational) Veterinary and vector surveillance
	Exposure reduction	Emergency management Risk communication and public education Public alert and warning systems Structural mitigation and building codes Population protection measures (e.g., evacuation and shelter-in-place) Sheltering and temporary settlement Health surveillance (clinical, laboratory, and occupational) Water, sanitation, and hygiene Clinical and community-based infection control measures Agricultural assistance Food safety, food security and nutritional support Environmental health Social cohesion and neighborhood coalitions
Secondary Prevention *Preventing Disease* *after* *Exposure Occurs*	Risk assessment	Exposure assessment and dose reconstruction Health surveillance and epidemiologic investigation Rapid needs and damage assessments Disease risk assessment (for infections, injuries, and chronic disease)
	Vulnerability reduction (susceptibility)	Emergency management Health surveillance (clinical, laboratory, and occupational) Health promotion Social cohesion and neighborhood coalitions Risk communication and public education Psychosocial and mental health services Prenatal care and maternal-child health Elder health and support services
Tertiary Prevention *Preventing Disability/* *Death after* *Disease Occurs*	Risk assessment	Health surveillance and epidemiologic investigation Rapid needs and damage assessment
	Vulnerability reduction (severity)	Emergency management Emergency, curative, and rehabilitative health services Risk communication and public education Psychosocial and mental health services Social support services

Source: Adapted from Keim (2016b).

Summary

Effective disaster risk management requires not only management of the immediate problem (disaster-related injuries and disease) but also of the patient's risk factors and of the underlying health determinants. This requires the involvement of many sectors and disciplines that contribute to the management of population health risks associated with emergencies and disasters. Disaster-related deaths are effectively reduced by health interventions and other measures that occur within a framework of primary prevention (preventing hazards and exposures), secondary prevention (preventing injury or disease following exposure), and tertiary prevention (preventing disability and death following injury/disease).

The natural history of disaster-related injuries often limits the effectiveness of secondary and tertiary prevention following disasters from technological, geophysical, and hydro-meteorologic hazards, emphasizing the importance of primary prevention before the event occurs. In order to be effective in reducing mortality, health-related actions must be applied during the appropriate window of opportunity. It is important to recognize the value of a comprehensive approach to the prevention of disaster-related mortality.

DISCUSSION QUESTIONS

1. Identify three extreme weather hazards that could potentially occur in your home jurisdiction (city, state/province, or nation). Discuss prior events that may have occurred in the past.

2. Identify three major public health consequences for each of these three disaster hazards.

3. Identify ways that you may be able to reduce your risk of exposure to each of these three hazards.

4. Identify people in your home jurisdiction that may be highly vulnerable to each of these three disaster hazards

5. Identify developmental strategies by which your home jurisdiction could potentially lessen its future risk of morbidity and mortality associated with these three disaster hazards.

KEY TERMS

Adapted from Association of Faculties of Medicine of Canada 2017; Henry 2006; Hoegh-Guldberg et al. 2018; Intergovernmental Panel on Climate Change 2007; Sundnes and Birnbaum 2003; United Nations Office for Disaster Risk Reduction n.d..

Biological hazards: Communicable disease pathogens that when exposed to populations may cause loss of life, injury, or other health impacts.

Capacity: The measure of all the strengths, attributes, and resources available to a community, society, or organization (e.g., people) that can be used to achieve agreed goals.

Climate-related disaster (CRD): Serious disruption influenced by long-term meteorologic conditions caused by changes in long-term weather patterns Disasters caused by oceanic and atmospheric hazards that are influenced by the global climate.

Climatologic hazards: Weather conditions that, when occurring over a period of time, may cause loss of life, injury, or other health impacts.

Conflict hazards: Conditions of human conflict that when exposed to a population may cause loss of life, injury, or other health impacts.

Cyclone: Weather phenomenon featuring a central region of low pressure surrounded by air flowing in an inward spiral and generating maximum sustained winds speeds of 74 mph or greater.

Disaster: A serious disruption involving widespread human morbidity and mortality, which exceeds the ability of the affected community or society to cope using its own resources.

Disaster risk management: The systematic process of lessening the adverse impacts of hazards and the possibility of disaster.

Disaster risk reduction: The concept and practice of reducing disaster risks through systematic efforts to analyze and manage the causal factors of disasters, including through reduced exposure to hazards, lessened vulnerability of people, wise management of land and the environment, and improved preparedness for adverse events.

Drought: A period of deficiency of moisture in the soil such that there is inadequate water required for plants, animals, and human beings.

Exposure: Contact between a person and one or more biological, chemical, or physical stressors, including stressors affected by climate change.

Extraterrestrial hazards: Extraterrestrial objects that, when exposed to populations, may cause loss of life, injury, or other health impacts.

Flood: A significant rise of water level in a stream, lake, reservoir, or coastal region

Hazard: A dangerous phenomenon, substance, human activity, or condition that may cause loss of life, injury, or other health impacts.

Hazard avoidance: The category of risk treatment that seeks to avoid the incidence and prevalence of hazards.

Heat wave: A period of time when daily temperatures rise above a specified threshold high-end temperature (e.g., the 95th or 99th percentile of X-year seasonal or monthly averages) for at least two consecutive days in a given location.

Hydrologic hazards: Movement of water that, when exposed to populations, may cause loss of life, injury, or other health impacts.

Incubation period: Time between exposure to the hazard and biological onset of disease.

Landslides: All types of gravity-induced ground movements, ranging from rock falls through slides/slumps, avalanches, and flows, triggered mainly by precipitation, seismic activity, and volcanic eruptions.

Land use planning: The process undertaken by public authorities to identify, evaluate, and decide on different options for the use of land.

Meteorologic hazards: Acute weather conditions that, when exposed to populations, may cause loss of life, injury, or other health impacts.

Mitigation: The lessening or limitation of the adverse impacts of hazards and related disasters.

Natural hazards: Natural process or phenomenon that may cause loss of life, injury, or other health impacts, property damage, loss of livelihoods and services, social and economic disruption, or environmental damage.

Nonstructural mitigation: Any measure that uses knowledge, practice, or agreement to reduce risks and impacts, in particular through policies and laws, public awareness raising, training, and education.

Preparedness: The knowledge and capacities developed by people to effectively anticipate, respond to, and recover from, the impacts of likely, imminent, or current hazard events or conditions.

Prevention: The outright avoidance of adverse impacts of hazards and related disasters.

Primary prevention: Avoidance of adverse outcomes before they occur at the population level, by reducing risk factors for specific hazards within groups of healthy individuals.

Primordial prevention: Prevention of health hazards from occurring.

Recovery: The restoration, and improvement where appropriate, of facilities, livelihoods, and living conditions (and health status), including efforts to reduce disaster risk factors.

Resilience: The ability of an asset that is exposed to hazards to resist, absorb, accommodate, and recover from the effects of a hazard in a timely and efficient manner, including through the preservation and restoration of its essential basic structures and functions.

Response: The provision of emergency services and public assistance during or immediately after a disaster in order to save lives, reduce health impacts, ensure public safety, and meet the basic subsistence needs of the people affected.

Risk: The probability of harmful consequences, (e.g., morbidity and mortality) resulting from interactions between natural or human-induced hazards and vulnerable conditions.

Risk avoidance: Methods that avoid risk altogether (e.g., hazard avoidance and exposure avoidance).

Risk management: The systematic approach and practice of managing uncertainty to minimize potential harm and loss.

Risk reduction: Methods that reduce the likelihood or impact of a hazard.

Risk retention: Methods that accept the risk (also known as risk acceptance).

Risk transfer: The process of formally or informally shifting the financial consequences of particular risks from one party to another.

Risk treatment: The process of selecting and implementing of measures to modify risk. Risk treatment measures can include avoiding, optimizing, transferring, or retaining risk.

Sea inundation: An acute-onset, coastal flood event, not associated with low pressure weather systems, tides, or top-overs/breaches of barriers.

Sea level rise: The increase in the average level of all of Earth's oceans, mainly because of the melting of sea ice and expansion of saltwater as temperatures warm.

Secondary prevention: Once the exposure/hazard has occurred, secondary prevention aims to avoid adverse outcomes through early detection of disease among high -risk individuals.

Storm: Any disturbed state of an astronomical body's atmosphere, especially affecting its surface, and strongly implying severe weather.

Structural mitigation: Any physical construction to reduce or avoid possible impacts of hazards, or application of engineering techniques to achieve hazard-resistance and resilience in structures or systems.

Sustainable development: Development that meets the needs of the present without compromising the ability of future generations to meet their own needs.

Technological hazards: Human-made technologies that when exposed to populations may cause loss of life, injury, or other health impacts.

Tertiary prevention: Once exposure/hazard has occurred, involves treatment of established conditions in order to avoid further deterioration (which may include permanent disability and/or death).

Vulnerability: Susceptibility to harm and risk.

Wildfire: Fires in forest or brush grasslands that cover extensive areas and usually do extensive damage.

References

Abdo, M., I. Ward, K. O'Dell, B. Ford, J. R. Pierce, E. V. Fischer, and J. L. Crooks. 2019. "Impact of Wildfire Smoke on Adverse Pregnancy Outcomes in Colorado, 2007–2015." *International Journal of Environmental Research and Public Health* 16 (19):3720.

Agampodi, S. B., N. J. Dahanayaka, A. K. Bandaranayaka, M. Perera, S. Priyankara, P. Weerawansa, M. A. Matthias, and J. M. Vinetz. 2014. "Regional Differences of Leptospirosis in Sri Lanka: Observations from a Flood-Associated Outbreak in 2011." *PLoS Neglected Tropical Diseases* 8:e2626.

Agrawal, S., T. Gopalakrishnan, Y. Gorokhovich, and S. Doocy. 2013. "Risk Factors for Injuries in Landslide- and Flood-Affected Populations in Uganda." *Prehospital And Disaster Medicine* 28:314–21.

Alderman, K., L. R. Turner, and S. Tong. 2012. "Floods and Human Health: A Systematic Review." *Environment International* 47:37–47.

Alhinai, M. Y. 2011. "Tropical Cyclone Gonu: Number of Patients and Pattern of Illnesses in the Primary Health Centers in A'seeb Area, Muscat, Sultanate of Oman." *Oman Medical Journal* 26:223–8.

ACOG Committee on Obstetric Practice and the American Academy of Pediatrics' Council on Environmental Health. 2017. "Hospital Disaster Preparedness for Obstetricians and Facilities Providing Maternity Care." *Obstetrics & Gynecology* 130 (6):e291–7.

Amiridis, V., C. Zerefos, S. Kazadzis, E.Gerasopoulos, K.Eleftheratos, M. Vrekoussis, A. Stohlf et al. 2012. "Impact of the 2009 Attica Wild Fires on the Air Quality in Urban Athens." *Atmospheric Environment* 46:536–44.

Anderson, A. H., A. J. Cohen, N. G. Kutner, J. B. Kopp, P. L. Kimmel, and P. Muntner. 2009. "Missed Dialysis Sessions and Hospitalization in Hemodialysis Patients after Hurricane Katrina." *Kidney International* 75:1202–8.

Arlappa, N., K. Venkaiah, and G. N. Brahmam. 2011. "Severe Drought and the Vitamin A Status of Rural Pre-School Children in India." *Disasters* 35:577–86.

Association of Faculties of Medicine of Canada. 2017. "AFMC Primer on Population Health." http://phprimer.afmc.ca/Glossary?l=H.

Atuyambe, L. M., M. Ediau, C. G. Orach, M. Musenero, and W. Bazeyo. 2011. "Land Slide Disaster in Eastern Uganda: Rapid Assessment of Water, Sanitation and Hygiene Situation in Bulucheke Camp, Bududa District." *Environmental Health* 10:38.

Azhar, G., D. Mavalankar, A. Nori-Sarma, A. Rajiva, P. Dutta, A. Jaiswal, P. Sheffield, K. Knowlton, J. J. Hess et al. 2014. "Heat-Related Mortality in India: Excess All-Cause Mortality Associated with the 2010 Ahmedabad Heat Wave." *PloS One* 9:e91831-e.

Bai, L., G. Ding, S. Gu, P. Bi, B. Su, D. Qin, G. Xu, and Q. Liu. 2014. "The Effects of Summer Temperature and Heat Waves on Heat-Related Illness in a Coastal City of China, 2011–2013." *Environmental Research* 132:212–9.

Bayer, A. M., H. E. Danysh, M. Garvich, G. Gonzálvez, W. Checkley, M. Alvarez, and R. H Gilman. 2014. "An Unforgettable Event: A Qualitative Study of the 1997–98 El Nino in Northern Peru." *Disasters* 38:351–74.

Beatley, T. 1998. "The Vision of Sustainable Communities." In *Cooperating with Nature: Confronting Natural Hazards with Land-Use Planning for Sustainable Communities*, edited by R. Burby, 233–62. Washington, DC: Joseph Henry Press.

Bei, B., C. Bryant, K. M. Gilson, J. Koh, P. Gibson, A. Komiti, H. Jackson, and F. Judd. 2013. "A Prospective Study of the Impact Of Floods on the Mental and Physical Health of Older Adults." *Aging & Mental Health* 17:992–1002.

Berko, J., D. D. Ingram, S. Saha, and J. D. Parker. 2014. "Deaths Attributed to Heat, Cold, and Other Weather Events in the United States, 2006–2010." *National Health Statistics Reports* 2014:1–16.

Bernstein, A. S., and M. B. Rice. 2013. "Lungs in a Warming World: Climate Change and Respiratory Health." *Chest* 143:1455–9.

Brouewer, R., S. Akter, L. Brander, and E. Haque. 2007. "Socioeconomic Vulnerability and Adaptation to Environmental Risk: A Case Study of Climate Change and Flooding in Bangladesh." *Risk Analysis* 27:313–26.

Brunetti, N., D. Amoruso, L. De Gennaro, G. Dellegrottaglie, G. Di Giuseppe, G. Antonelli, and M. Di Biase. 2014. "Hot Spot: Impact of July 2011 Heat Wave in Southern Italy (Apulia) on Cardiovascular Disease Assessed by Emergency Medical Service and Telemedicine Support." *Telemedicine and e-Health* 20:272–81.

Bucher, J., J. McCoy, C. Donovan, S. Patel, P. Ohman-Strickland, and A. Dewan. 2018. "EMS Dispatches during Hurricanes Irene and Sandy in New Jersey." *Prehospital Emergency Care* 22 (1):15–21.

Bustinza, R., G. Lebel, P. Gosselin, D. Bélanger, and F. Chebana. 2013. "Health Impacts of the July 2010 Heat Wave in Québec, Canada." *BMC Public Health* 13:56.

Caamano Isorna, F., A. Figueiras, I. Sastre, A. Montes Martínez, M. Taracido, and M. Piñeiro-Lamas. 2011. "Respiratory and Mental Health Effects of Wildfires: An Ecological Study in Galician Municipalities (North-West Spain)." *Environmental Health* 10:48.

Caldera, T., L. Palma, U. Penayo, and G. Kullgren. 2001. "Psychological Impact of the Hurricane Mitch in Nicaragua in a One-Year Perspective." *Social Psychiatry and Psychiatric Epidemiology* 36:108–14.

Calzolari, M., and A. Albieri. 2013. "Could Drought Conditions Trigger Schmallenberg Virus and Other Arboviruses Circulation?" *International Journal of Health Geographics* 12:7.

Carnie, T. L., H. L. Berry, S. A. Blinkhorn, and C. R. Hart. "In Their Own Words: Young People's Mental Health in Drought-Affected Rural and Remote NSW." *Australian Journal of Rural Health* 19:244–8.

Cash, R. A., S. R. Halder, M. Husain, S. Islam, F. H. Mallick, M. A. May, M. Rahman, and M. A. Rahman. 2013. "Reducing the Health Effect of Natural Hazards in Bangladesh." *Lancet* 382:2094–103.

Catapano, F., R. Malafronte, F. Lepre, P. Cozzolino, R. Arnone, E. Lorenzo, G. Tartaglia, F. Starace, L. Magliano, and M. Maj. 2001. "Psychological Consequences of the 1998 Landslide in Sarno, Italy: A Community Study." *Acta Psychiatrica Scandinavica* 104:438–42.

Centers for Disease Control and Prevention. 2011. *Public Health Preparedness Capabilities: National Standards for State and Local Planning.* Atlanta, GA: CDC.

Chan, E. Y. Y., W. Goggins, J. S. K. Yue, and P. Lee. 2013. "Hospital Admissions as a Function of Temperature, Other Weather Phenomena and Pollution Levels in An Urban Setting in China." *Bulletin of the World Health Organization* 91:576–84.

Chaturongkasumrit, Y., P. Techaruvichit, H. Takahashi, B. Kimura, and S. Keeratipibul. 2013. "Microbiological Evaluation of Water during the 2011 Flood Crisis in Thailand." *Science of the Total Environment* 463-464:959–67.

Chen, H., Y. Chen, M. Au, L. Feng, Q. Chen, H. Guo, Y. Li, and X. Yang. 2014. "The Presence of Post-Traumatic Stress Disorder Symptoms in Earthquake Survivors One Month after a Mudslide in Southwest China." *Nursing & Health Sciences* 16:39–45.

Clack, Z., M. Keim, A. MacIntyre, and K. Yeskey. 2002. "Emergency Health and Risk Management in Sub-Saharan Africa: A Lesson from the Embassy Bombings in Tanzania and Kenya." *Prehospital and Disaster Medicine* 17:59–66.

Clemens, S. L., H. L. Berry, B. M. McDermott, and C. M. Harper. 2013. "Summer of Sorrow: Measuring Exposure to and Impacts of Trauma after Queensland's Natural Disasters of 2010–2011." *Medical Journal of Australia* ;199:552–5.

Collins, T. W., A. M. Jimenez, and S. E. Grineski. 2013. "Hispanic Health Disparities after a Flood Disaster: Results of a Population-Based Survey of Individuals Experiencing Home Site Damage in El Paso (Texas, USA)." *Journal of Immigrant and Minority Health* 15:415–26.

Cusack, L., C. de Crespigny, and P. Athanasos. 2011. "Heatwaves and Their Impact on People with Alcohol, Drug and Mental Health Conditions: A Discussion Paper on Clinical Practice Considerations." *Journal of Advanced Nursing* 67:915–22.

Davis, L. 2008. *Famines and Droughts. Natural Disasters.* New York: Checkmark Books.

Ding, G., Y. Zhang, L. Gao, W. Ma, X. Li, J. Liu, Q. Liu, and B. Jiang. 2013. "Quantitative Analysis of Burden of Infectious Diarrhea Associated with Floods in Northwest of Anhui Province, China: A Mixed Method Evaluation." *PloS One* 8:e65112.

D'Ippoliti, D., P. Michelozzi, C. Marino, F. de'Donato, B. Menne, K. Katsouyanni, U. Kirchmayer et al. 2010. "The Impact of Heat Waves on Mortality in 9 European Cities: Results from the Euroheat Project." *Environmental Health* 9:37.

Doocy, S., A. Daniels, S. Murray, and T. D. Kirsch. 2013a. "The Human Impact of Floods: A Historical Review of Events 1980–2009 and Systematic Literature Review." *PLoS Currents* 5.

Doocy, S., A. Dick, A. Daniels, and T. D. Kirsch. 2013b. "The Human Impact of Tropical Cyclones: A Historical Review of Events 1980–2009 and Systematic Literature Review. *PLoS Currents* 5.

Doran, K. M., R. P. McCormack, E. L. Johns, B. G. Carr, S. W. Smith, L. R. Goldfrank, and D. C. Lee. 2016. "Emergency Department Visits for Homelessness or Inadequate Housing in New York City before and after Hurricane Sandy." *Journal of Urban Health* 93 (2):331–344.

EM-DAT: The International Disaster Database. 2019. Ecole se Sante Publique, Universite Catholique de Louvain. Accessed April 10, 2019. http://www.emdat.be/.

Espiritu, M., U. Patil, H. Cruz, A. Gupta, H. Matterson, Y. Kim, M. Caprio, and P. Mally. 2014. "Evacuation of a Neonatal Intensive Care Unit in a Disaster: Lessons from Hurricane Sandy." *Pediatrics* 134 (6):e1662–1669.

Fankhauser, S. 2009. *The Costs of Adaptation*. London, UK: London School of Economics.

Federal Emergency Management Agency. 1996. *Guide for All-Hazard Emergency Operations Planning, State & Local Guide 101*. Washington, DC: FEMA.

Foke, C., S. Carpenter, T. Elmqvist, L. Gunderson, C. S. Holling, and B. Walker. 2002. "Resilience and Sustainable Development: Building Adaptive Capacity in a World of Transformation." *Ambio* 31 (5):437–40.

Fussell, E., and S. R. Lowe. 2014. "The Impact of Housing Displacement on the Mental Health of Low-Income Parents after Hurricane Katrina." *Social Science & Medicine* 113:137–44.

Goenjian, A. K., L. Molina, A. M. Steinberg, L. A. Fairbanks, M. L. Alvarez, H. A. Goenjian, and R. S. Pynoos. 2001. "Posttraumatic Stress and Depressive Reactions among Nicaraguan Adolescents after Hurricane Mitch." *American Journal of Psychiatry* 158:788–94.

Fussell, E., N. Sastry, and M. Vanlandingham. 2010. "Race, Socioeconomic Status, and Return Migration to New Orleans after Hurricane Katrina." *Population and Environment* 31 (1–3):20–42. doi:10.1007/s11111-009-0092-2.

Grimm, A., L. Hulse, M. Preiss, and S. Schmidt. 2014. "Behavioural, Emotional, and Cognitive Responses in European Disasters: Results of Survivor Interviews." *Disasters* 38:62–83.

Grimsley, L. F., P. C. Chulada, S. Kennedy, L. White, J. Wildfire, R. D. Cohn, H. Mitchell et al. 2012. "Indoor Environmental Exposures for Children with Asthma Enrolled in the HEAL Study, Post-Katrina New Orleans." *Environmental Health Perspectives* 120:1600–6.

Hanigan, I. C., C. D. Butler, P. N. Kokic, and M. F. Hutchinson. 2012. "Suicide and Drought in New South Wales, Australia, 1970–2007." *Proceedings of the National Academy of Sciences of the United States of America* 109:13950-5.

Hartz, D., J. Golden, C. Sister, W,-C. Chuang, and A. Brazel. 2012. "Climate and Heat-Related Emergencies in Chicago, Illinois (2003–2006)." *International Journal of Biometeorology* 56:71–83.

Harville, E. W., X. Xiong, and P. Buekens. 2009. "Hurricane Katrina and Perinatal Health." *Birth (Berkeley, Calif)* 36:325–31.

Harville, E. W., X. Xiong, B. W. Smith, G. Pridjian, K. Elkind-Hirsch, and P. Buekens. 2011. "Combined Effects of Hurricane Katrina and Hurricane Gustav on the Mental Health of Mothers of Small Children." *Journal of Psychiatric And Mental Health Nursing* 18:288–96.

Haque, U., M. Hashizume, K. N. Kolivras, H. J. Overgaard, B. Das, and T. Yamamoto. 2012. "Reduced Death Rates from Cyclones in Bangladesh: What More Needs to Be Done?" *Bulletin of the World Health Organization* 90:150–6.

Health Care Ready. 2019. *Fourth Annual Preparedness Poll*. May 29, 2019. Accessed November 19, 2019. https://www.healthcareready.org/press-release/poll-reveals-lack-of-preparedness-in-the-face-of-increasingly-frequent-disasters.

Henry, R. 2006. *Defense Transformation and the 2005 Quadrennial Defense Review*. Washington, DC: Department of Defense.

Hoegh-Guldberg, O., D. Jacob, M. Taylor, M. Bindi, S. Brown, I. Camilloni, A. Diedhiou et al. 2018. "Impacts of 1.5°C Global Warming on Natural and Human Systems." In *Global Warming of 1.5°C. An IPCC Special Report*, edited by V. Masson-Delmotte et al., 175–311. Geneva, Switzerland: Intergovernmental Panel on Climate Change.

Horton, G., L. Hanna, and B. Kelly. 2010. "Drought, Drying and Climate Change: Emerging Health Issues for Ageing Australians in Rural Areas." *Australasian Journal on Ageing* 29:2–7.

Huppert, H. E., and R. S. J. Sparks. 2006. "Extreme Natural Hazards: Population Growth, Globalization And Environmental Change." *Philosophical Transactions of the Royal Society. A, Mathematical, Physical, and Engineering Sciences* 364:1875–88.

Ibrahim, J., J. McInnes, N. Andrianopoulos, and S. Evans. 2012. "Minimising Harm from Heatwaves: A Survey of Awareness, Knowledge, and Practices of Health Professionals and Care Providers in Victoria, Australia." *International Journal of Public Health* 57:297–304.

Intergovernmental Panel on Climate Change. 2007. *Climate Change 2007: Impacts, Adaptation, and Vulnerability*. Cambridge, UK: Cambridge University Press.

International Federation of Red Cross. 2005. "Disaster Data: Building a Foundation for Disaster Risk Reduction." *In* World Disasters *Report 2005*, 172–81. Geneva: IFRC.

International Federation of Red Cross and Red Crescent Societies. 2009. *World Disasters Report 2009*. Geneva: IFRC.

International Organization for Standardization. 2009. *ISO 31000—Risk Management: A Practical Guide for Subject Matter Experts*. Geneva: ISO. https://www.iso.org/standard/43170.html

Jonkman, S. N., B. Maaskant, E. Boyd, and M. L. Levitan. 2009. "Loss of Life Caused by the Flooding of New Orleans after Hurricane Katrina: Analysis of the Relationship Between Flood Characteristics and Mortality." *Risk Analysis* 29 (5):676–98.

Keenan, H. T., S. W. Marshall, M. A. Nocera, and D. K. Runyan. 2004. "Increased Incidence of Inflicted Traumatic Brain Injury in Children after a Natural Disaster." *American Journal of Preventive Medicine* 26:189–93.

Keim, M. 2002. "Intentional Chemical Disasters." In *Disaster Medicine*, edited by D. Hogan and J. Burstein, 340–9. Philadelphia, PA: Lippincott, Williams & Wilkins.

Keim, M. 2010a. "Disaster Risk Management for Health." In *Textbook of Emergency Medicine*, edited by S. David, 1309–18. Chicago, IL: Wolters Kluwer Health (Lippincott).

Keim, M. E. 2010b. "Sea-Level-Rise Disaster in Micronesia: Sentinel Event for Climate Change? *Disaster Medicine and Public Health Preparedness* 4:81–7.

Keim, M. E. 2011. "Preventing Disasters: Public Health Vulnerability Reduction as a Sustainable Adaptation to Climate Change." *Disaster Medicine and Public Health Preparedness* 5 (2):140–8.

Keim, M. 2016a."Disaster Preparedness." In *Disaster Medicine*, 2d ed., edited by G. Ciottone, 200–14. Philadelphia, PA: Mosby-Elsevier.

Keim, M. 2016b. "Environmental Disasters." In *Environmental Health from Global to Local*, 3rd ed., edited by H. Frumkin, 667–92. San Francisco, CA: John Wiley and Sons.

Keim, M. 2017. "Assessing Disaster-Related Health Risk: Appraisal for Prevention." *Prehospital and Disaster Medicine* 33:317–25.

Keim, M. E. 2018a. "Defining Disaster-Related Health Risk: A Primer for Prevention." *Prehospital and Disaster Medicine* 33:308–16.

Keim, M. E. 2018b. "Managing Disaster-Related Health Risk: A Process for Prevention." *Prehospital and Disaster Medicine* 33:326–34.

Keim, M., and P. Giannone. 2006. "Disaster Preparedness." In *Disaster Medicine*, edited by G. Ciottone, P. Anderson, E. Auf Der Heide, R. Darling, I. Jacoby, E. Noji, and S. Suneret, 164–73. Philadelphia, PA: Mosby-Elsevier.

Kessler, R. 2012. "Followup in Southern California: Decreased Birth Weight Following Prenatal Wildfire Smoke Exposure." *Environmental Health Perspectives* 120:A362-A.

Kim, J. J., and D. Guha-Sapir. 2012. "Famines in Africa: Is Early Warning Early Enough?" *Global Health Action* 5. doi: 10.3402/gha.v5i0.18481.

Kistin, E. J., J. Fogarty, R. S. Pokrasso, M. McCally, and P. G. McCornick. 2010. "Climate Change, Water Resources and Child Health." *Archives of Disease in Childhood* 95:545–9.

Krug, E. G., M. Kresnow, J. P. Peddicord, L. L. Dahlberg, K. E. Powell, A. E. Crosby, and J. L. Annest. 1998. "Suicide after Natural Disasters." *New England Journal of Medicine* 338:373–8.

Kue, R., and K. S. Dyer. 2013. "The Impact of Heat Waves on Transport Volumes in an Urban Emergency Medical Services System: A Retrospective Review." *Prehospital and Disaster Medicine* 28:610–5.

Lane, K., K. Charles-Guzman, K. Wheeler, Z. Abid, N. Graber, and T. Matte. 2013. "Health Effects oOf Coastal Storms and Flooding in Urban Areas: A Review and Vulnerability Assessment." *Journal of Environmental and Public Health* 2013:913064.

Laugharne, J., G. van der Watt, and A. Janca. 2011. "After the Fire: The Mental Health Consequences of Fire Disasters." *Current Opinion in Psychiatry* 24:72–7.

Lowe, S. R., M. Willis, and J. E. Rhodes. 2014. "Health Problems among Low-Income Parents in the Aftermath of Hurricane Katrina." *Health Psychology* 33:774–82.

Malik, S., D. C. Lee, K. M. Doran, C. R. Grudzen, J. Worthing, I. Portelli, L. R. Goldfrank et al. 2018. "Vulnerability of Older Adults in Disasters: Emergency Department Utilization by Geriatric Patients After Hurricane Sandy." *Disaster Medicine and Public Health Preparedness.* 12 (2):184–193.

Malilay, J. 1997. "Tropical Cyclones." In *The Public Health Consequences of Disasters*, edited by E. Noji, 207–27. New York: Oxford University Press.

Markolf, S. A., C. Hoehne, A. Fraser, M. V. Chester, and B. S. Underwood. 2019. "Transportation Resilience to Climate Change and Extreme Weather Events—Beyond Risk and Robustness." *Transport Policy* 74:174–186.

Mendoza, M. T., E. A. Roxas, J. K. Ginete, M. M. Alejandria, A. Dessi, E. Roman, K. T. Leyritana, M. A. D. Penamora, and C. C. Pineda. 2013. "Clinical Profile of Patients Diagnosed with Leptospirosis after a Typhoon: A Multicenter Study." *Southeast Asian Journal of Tropical Medicine and Public Health* 44:1021–35.

Morrow, M. G., R. N. Johnson, J. Polanco, and D. M. Claborn. 2010. "Mosquito Vector Abundance Immediately Before and After Tropical Storms Alma and Arthur, Northern Belize, 2008." *Pan American Journal of Public Health* 28:19–24.

Mosley, L. M., D. S. Sharp, and S. Singh. 2004. "Effects of a Tropical Cyclone on the Drinking-Water Quality of a Remote Pacific Island." *Disasters* 28:405–17.

Murakami, S., N. Miyatake, and N. Sakano. 2012. "Changes in Air Temperature and Its Relation to Ambulance Transports due to Heat Stroke in All 47 Prefectures of Japan." *Journal of Preventive Medicine and Public Health* 45:309–15.

Nahar, N., Y. Blomstedt, B. Wu, I. Kandarina, L. Trisnantoro, and J. Kinsman. 2014. "Increasing the Provision of Mental Health Care for Vulnerable, Disaster-Affected People in Bangladesh." *BMC Public Health* 14:708.

National Academies of Sciences, Engineering, and Medicine. 2016. *Exploring Disaster Risk Reduction Through Community-Level Approaches to Promote Healthy Outcomes: Proceedings of a Workshop—in Brief.* Washington, DC: NAS. https://www.nap.edu/read/23600/chapter/1.

National Science and Technology Council. 1996. *Natural Disaster Reduction: A Plan for the Nation.* Washington, DC: Committee on the Environment and Natural Resources, Subcommittee on Natural Disaster Reduction.

Nelson, D. 1990. "Mitigating Disasters: Power to the Community." *International Nursing Review* 37 (6):371.

"Notes from the Field: Carbon Monoxide Exposures Reported to Poison Centers and Related to Hurricane Sandy–Northeastern United States, 2012." 2012. *MMWR Morbidity and Mortality Weekly Report* 61:905.

Ostad Taghizadeh, A., S. V. Soleimani, and A. Ardalan. 2013. "Lessons from a Flash Flood in Tehran Subway, Iran." *PLoS Currents* 2013;5.

Papanikolaou, V., G. Leon, J. Kyriopoulos, J. Levett, and E. Pallis. 2011. "Surveying the Ashes: Experience from the 2007 Peloponnese Wildfires Six Months after the Disaster." *Prehospital and Disaster Medicine* 26:79–89.

Park, K. J., J. Y. Moon, J. S. Ha, S. D. Kim, B. Y. Pyun, T. K. Min, and Y. H. Park. 2013. "Impacts of Heavy Rain and Typhoon on Allergic Disease." *Osong Public Health and Research Perspectives* 4:140–5.

Pascal, M., A. Le Tertre, and A. Saoudi. 2012. "Quantification of the Heat Wave Effect on Mortality in Nine French Cities during Summer 2006." *PLoS Currents* 4:RRN1307-RRN.

Pereira, B. M. T., W. Morales, R. Cardoso, R. Fiorelli, G. Fraga, and S. Briggs. 2013. "Lessons Learned from a Landslide Catastrophe in Rio De Janeiro, Brazil." *American Journal of Disaster Medicine* 8:253–8.

Perez-Gracia, M. T., M. L. Mateos Lindemann, and M. C. Montalvo Villalba. 2013. "Hepatitis E: Current Status." *Reviews in Medical Virology* 23:384–98.

Price, K., S. Perron, and N. King. 2013. "Implementation of the Montreal Heat Response Plan during the 2010 Heat Wave." *Canadian Journal of Public Health* 104:e96–100.

Rabito, F. A., S. Iqbal, S. Perry, W. Arroyave, and J. C. Rice. 2012. "Environmental Lead after Hurricane Katrina: Implications for Future Populations." *Environmental Health Perspectives* 120:180–4.

Rando, R. J., J. J. Lefante, L. M. Freyder, and R. N. Jones. 2012. "Respiratory Health Effects Associated with Restoration Work in Post-Hurricane Katrina New Orleans." *Journal of Environmental and Public Health* 2012:462478.

Rigby, C. W., A. Rosen, H. L. Berry, and C. R. Hart. 2011. "If the Land's Sick, We're Sick: The Impact of Prolonged Drought on the Social and Emotional Well-Being of Aboriginal Communities in Rural New South Wales." *Australian Journal of Rural Health* 19:249–54.

Robinson, B., M. Alatas, A. Robertson, and H. Steer. 2011. "Natural Disasters and the Lung." *Respirology* 16:386–95.

Sanchez, C., T. S. Lee, S. Young, D. Batts, J. Benjamin, and J. Malilay. 2009. "Risk Factors for Mortality during the 2002 Landslides in Chuuk, Federated States of Micronesia." *Disasters* 33:705–20.

Sanguanklin. N., B. L. McFarlin, C. G. Park, C. Giurgescu, L. Finnegan, R. White-Traut, and J. L Engstrom. 2014. "Effects of the 2011 Flood in Thailand on Birth Outcomes and Perceived Social Support." *Journal of Obstetric, Gynecologic, and Neonatal Nursing* 43:435–44.

Sattler, D. N., A. J. Preston, C. F. Kaiser, V. E. Olivera, J. Valdez, and S. Schlueter. 2002. "Hurricane Georges: A Cross-National Study Examining Preparedness, Resource Loss, and Psychological Distress in the US Virgin Islands, Puerto Rico, Dominican Republic, and the United States." *Journal of Traumatic Stress* 15:339–50.

Schaffer, A., D. Muscatello, R. Broome, S. Corbett, and W. Smith. 2012. "Emergency Department Visits, Ambulance Calls, and Mortality Associated with an Exceptional Heat Wave in Sydney, Australia, 2011: A Time-Series Analysis." *Environmental Health* 11 (1):3.

Schipper, L., and M. Pelling. 2006. "Disaster Risk, Climate Change and International Development: Scope for, and Challenges to, Integration." *Disasters* 30:19–38.

Seifman, M., E. W. Ek, H. Menezes, W. M. Rozen, I. S. Whitaker, and H. J. Cleland. 2011. "Bushfire Disaster Burn Casualty Management: The Australian "Black Saturday" Bushfire Experience." *Annals of Plastic Surgery* 67:460–3.

Shaposhnikov, D., B. Revich, T. Bellander, G. B. Bedada, M. Bottai, T. Kharkova, E. Kvasha et al. 2014. "Mortality Related to Air Pollution with the Moscow Heat Wave and Wildfire of 2010." *Epidemiology* 25:359–64.

Simpson, C., and A. Abelsohn. 2012. "Heat-Induced Illness." *Canadian Medical Association Journal* 184 (10):1170.

Smith, L. T., L. E. Aragao, C. E. Sabel, and T. Nakaya. 2014. "Drought Impacts on Children's Respiratory Health in the Brazilian Amazon." *Scientific Reports* 4:3726.

Stanke, C., M. Kerac, C. Prudhomme, J. Medlock, and V. Murray. 2013. "Health Effects of Drought: A Systematic Review of the Evidence. *PLoS Currents* 5. doi: 10.1371/currents.dis.7a2cee9e980f91ad769 7b570bcc4b004.

Stanke, C., V. Murray, R. Amlot, J. Nurse, and R. Williams. 2012. "The Effects of Flooding on Mental Health: Outcomes and Recommendations from a Review of the Literature." *PLoS Currents* 4:e4f9f1fa9c3cae.

Sun, X., Q. Sun, X. Zhou, X. Li, M. Yang, A. Yu, and F. Geng. 2014. "Heat Wave Impact on Mortality in Pudong New Area, China in 2013." *Science of the Total Environment* 493:789–94.

Sundnes, K. O., and P. L. Birnbaum. 2003. "Health Disaster Management Guidelines for Evaluation and Research in the Utstein Style." *Prehospital and Disaster Medicine* 17 (suppl 3):1–177.

Sunyer, J. 2010. "Geographical Differences on the Mortality Impact of Heat Waves in Europe." *Environmental Health* 9:38.

Takaro, T., K. Knowlton, and J. Balmes. 2013. "Climate Change and Respiratory Health: Current Evidence and Knowledge Gaps." *Expert Review of Respiratory Medicine* 7:349–61.

Tally, S., A. Levack, A. Sarkin, T. Gilmer, and E. Groessl. 2013. "The Impact of the San Diego Wildfires on a General Mental Health Population Residing in Evacuation Areas." *Administration and Policy in Mental Health* 40:348–54.

Tees, M. T., E. W. Harville, X. Xiong, P. Buekens, G. Pridjian, and K. Elkind-Hirsch. 2010. "Hurricane Katrina-Related Maternal Stress, Maternal Mental Health, and Early Infant Temperament." *Maternal and Child Health Journal* 14:511–8.

Tempark, T., S. Lueangarun, S. Chatproedprai, and S. Wananukul. 2013. "Flood-Related Skin Diseases: A Literature Review." *International Journal of Dermatology* 52:1168–76.

Tian, Z., S. Li, J. Zhang, and Y. Guo. 2013. "The Characteristics of Heat Wave Effects on Coronary Heart Disease Mortality in Beijing, China: A Time Series Study." *PLoS One* 8:e77321-e.

United Nations. 2002. *Plan of Implementation of the World Summit on Sustainable Development.* New York: UN.

United Nations. 2012. *Resolution 66/28 The Future We Want.* New York: United Nations General Assembly.

United Nations. 1992. *United Nations Conference on Environment and Development—Agenda 21.* New York: United Nations. https://sustainabledevelopment.un.org/content/documents/Agenda21.pdf

United Nations Disaster Relief Office. 1991. *Mitigating Natural Disasters: Phenomena, Effects and Options.* New York: United Nations.

United Nations International Strategy for Disaster Risk Reduction. 2015. *Sendai Framework for Disaster Reduction: 2015–2030.* New York New York: United Nations.

United Nations Office for Disaster Risk Reduction. n.d. "Terminology." https://www.undrr.org/terminology.

University of Wisconsin Population Health Institute. 2019. "County Health Rankings Key Findings 2019." Accessed November 28, 2019. https://www.countyhealthrankings.org/reports/2019-county-health-rankings-key-findings-report.

Vranken, L., P. Van Turnhout, M. Van Den Eeckhaut, L. Vandekerckhove, and J. Poesen. 2013. "Economic Valuation of Landslide Damage in Hilly Regions: A Case Study from Flanders, Belgium." *Science of the Total Environment* 447:323–36.

Waite, T., V. Murray, and D. Baker. 2014. "Carbon Monoxide Poisoning and Flooding: Changes in Risk Before, During and After Flooding Require Appropriate Public Health Interventions." *PLoS Currents* 6. doi: 10.1371/currents.dis.2b2eb9e15f9b982784938803584487f1.

Wang, G., R. B. Minnis, J. L. Belant, and C. L. Wax. 2010. "Dry Weather Induces Outbreaks of Human West Nile Virus Infections." *BMC Infectious Diseases* 10:38.

Wind, T. R., P. C. Joshi, R. J. Kleber, I. H. Komproe. 2014. "The Effect of the Postdisaster Context on the Assessment of Individual Mental Health Scores." *American Journal of Orthopsychiatry* 84:134–41.

World Bank. 2007. *Climate Change and Adaptation.* Washington, DC: International Bank for Reconstruction and Development/World Bank.

Xiao, J., M. Huang, W. Zhang, A. Rosenblum, W. Ma, X. Meng, and S. Lin. 2019. "The Immediate and Lasting Impact of Hurricane Sandy on Pregnancy Complications in Eight Affected Counties of New York State." *Science of the Total Environment* 678:755–60.

Yelland, C., P. Robinson, C. Lock, A. M. La Greca, B. Kokegei, V. Ridgway, and B. Lai. 2010. "Bushfire Impact on Youth." *Journal of Traumatic Stress* 23:274–7.

CHAPTER 3

HEALTH IMPACTS OF EXTREME HEAT

Xiangmei (May) Wu and Rupa Basu

Introduction

- "Extreme heat kills more people on average (approximately 600 deaths per year in the United States) than hurricanes, floods, tornadoes, earthquakes, and lightning combined." —Centers for Disease Control and Prevention (CDC)[1]

- "In 2003, the European Union suffered its strongest heat wave ever. Over 70,000 excess deaths were reported from 12 European countries. The elderly are most at risk of death." —World Health Organization (WHO)[2]

- "Between 2000 and 2016, the number of vulnerable people (around the world) exposed to heat wave events increased by about 125 million, with a record 175 million more people exposed to heatwaves in 2015." —The *Lancet* Countdown on Health and Climate Change 2018 Report (Watts et al. 2018)

The U.S. National Oceanic and Atmospheric Administration (NOAA) has confirmed a warming of 0.9°C (1.6°F) of the global average surface temperature by 2017 relative to 1951–1980 average temperatures (Figure 3.1). At the current rate of progression, the Earth's long-term average temperature will increase 1.5°C (2.7°F) above the 1850–1900 average by 2040, 2°C (3.6°F) by 2065, and 3°C by 2100 (http://berkeleyearth.org/global-temperatures-2017/).

Heat waves, which are continuous extreme hot days, form when high pressure in the upper atmosphere remains over a region for several days or weeks. Although there is no standardized definition, the U.S. NOAA defines a heat wave as a period when daily mean temperatures go above a specified high threshold temperature (e.g., 95th or 99th of the distribution) for at least two consecutive days in a given location. Therefore, a heat wave is usually reported relative to the historical weather patterns and temperatures for the season in a specific area. In the summer of 2018, severe heat waves were observed across the northern hemisphere, setting new all-time high temperature records in several locations (Freedman 2018) (Figure 3.2).

Elevated temperature and heat waves have already increased mortality and morbidity, creating a global health burden and enormous economic loss. Epidemiologic studies have reported associations between heat with increases in mortality and hospitalizations or emergency department (ED) visits from various causes, not only limited to "classic" heat-related diseases but also including

KEY CONCEPTS

- Heat may trigger many kinds of health outcomes beyond classified heat-related illnesses, including cardiovascular and cerebrovascular diseases as well as adverse birth outcomes.

- Health effects from heat exposure generally occur immediately within three to five days and often the same day, requiring a rapid public health response.

- Age, physical condition, and socioeconomic status could affect susceptibility to health complications from heat.

- Temperature thresholds that trigger health Impacts vary by region, by population characteristics, and by timing within the season.

---

[1]https://www.cdc.gov/disasters/extremeheat/index.html. Note that this number is only for deaths from heat illness, not including cases triggered by heat that may have another disease designated as the primary cause of death. Thus, this number is likely to be severely underestimated.

[2]World Health Organization, Regional Office for Europe, http://www.euro.who.int/en/health-topics/environment-and-health/Climate-change/data-and-statistics.

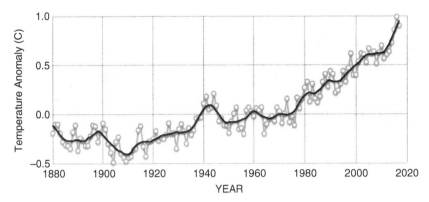

Source: climate.nasa.gov

Figure 3.1   Global land-ocean temperature index
Source: NASA's Goddard Institute for Space Studies, https://climate.nasa.gov/vital-signs/global-temperature/.

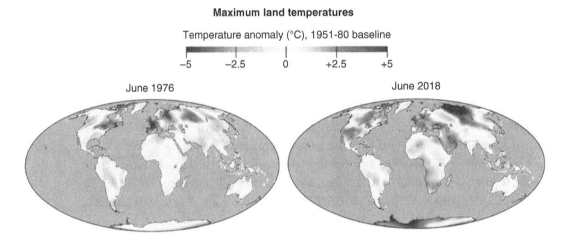

Figure 3.2   Comparison between maximum June land temperatures in 1976, when Europe had a major heat wave, and 2018.
Source: Adapted from Zeke Hausfather/Berkeley Earth, berkeleyearth.org; Graphic: Axios Visuals, https://www.axios.com/global-heat-wave-stuns-scientists-as-records-fall-4cad71d2-8567-411e-a3f6-0febaa19a847.html.

cardiovascular and respiratory diseases as well as mental health and adverse birth outcomes. Because there is no systematic definition of heat-related deaths or illnesses in the United States, the statistics of "heat illness" we usually see are likely to be highly underreported. Heat illnesses are often not listed as the primary cause of death unless there is a heat wave and no other cause of death can be determined. In this chapter, we explain health impacts from excessive ambient heat exposure by the type of outcomes, discuss factors influencing heat exposure, and briefly review adaptation and mitigation plans.

Heat-Triggered Health Effects

Humans typically thermoregulate their core body temperatures to maintain an internal temperature of around (37°C), mostly through **vasodilation** and sweating. In this physiologic process heat is initially sensed by the skin, brain, and spinal cord. As body temperature increases, the brain, specifically the hypothalamus, sends signals to dilate the blood vessels and increase blood circulation flow to trigger sweating (Parsons 2014). Through vasodilation, venous blood returns closer to the skin, carrying fluid to the sweat glands and increasing the heat loss from the skin to the environment. Evaporation of sweat from the skin occurs in an extremely efficient manner to cool the body to maintain a stable body temperature.

Under extreme heat, the ability to lose heat by sweating may be compromised, especially with concomitant high humidity. Illness and death caused by heat stress may occur in many scenarios from both indoor and outdoor exposures, such as extreme outdoor temperatures via military training and action, industrial activity (e.g., miners, workers in the oil and construction industries), and normal civilian activity, including tourism, outdoor physical exercise, or playing sports in hot weather.

In the next section, we discuss the health effects from heat stress, starting with classic heat illnesses, followed by changes in other health outcomes associated with temperature increase based primarily on epidemiologic evidence. Many morbidity and mortality cases triggered by heat exposure may be classified into other categories for the primary diagnoses, and thus, an accurate measure of heat-related morbidity and mortality is difficult to obtain (Kilbourne 1999; Semenza et al. 1999).

Heat Illness

Heat stress occurs in humans when the body is unable to cool itself down effectively in a process known as **thermoregulation**. When multiple organs experience heat stress, the body will still attempt to thermoregulate as efficiently as possible. However, excessive sweating may lead to **dehydration**, and vasodilation is usually maintained regardless of low blood pressure (**hypotension**), which could result in **heat syncope**.

As body temperature increases and/or under high humidity, sweat will not evaporate as quickly and hidromeiosis (a reduction in sweating) may occur when the skin is completely wet. The decrease in sweating further inhibits cooling and at a body temperature of 100–102°F (38–39°C), heat collapse may occur. Once heat exposure increases beyond these limits, the risks of morbidity and mortality increase substantially (Hall 2015). Although temperature thresholds vary by region, it is generally accepted that when body temperatures go beyond 105°F (41°C), **heatstroke** and even death may occur. The pathophysiology of thermoregulation is summarized in Figure 3.3.

The traditionally considered heat illnesses include heatstroke, heat syncope, heat cramp, heat exhaustion, heat fatigue, heat edema, and heat rash (Lipman et al. 2014). Some illnesses triggered by heat exposure may be classified under metabolic disorders and genitourinary diseases based on the primary diagnosis. This was supported by increased hospital admissions and ED visits for heat-related illnesses, including dehydration, fluid and electrolyte disorders, renal failure, urinary tract infection, septicemia, and heatstroke (Bobb et al. 2014a; Gronlund et al. 2014; Hansen et al. 2008; Knowlton et al. 2009; Levy et al. 2015). Vulnerable subgroups, including African-Americans, + elderly, and those residing in cities with lower air conditioning prevalence—all markers of lower socioeconomic status, face greater health risks from heat waves (Gronlund et al. 2016). Studies in California have found that with a 10°F increase in mean daily apparent temperature (a combination of temperature and relative humidity), the number of ED visits increased 393.3 percent (95 percent CI, 331.2 percent, 464.5 percent) for heat illness, 25.6 percent (21.9 percent, 29.4 percent) for dehydration, and 15.9 percent (12.7 percent, 19.3 percent) for acute renal failure (Basu et al. 2012). Hospital admissions for these diseases also increased correspondingly, as well as cardiovascular and respiratory diseases mentioned in the following sections (Green et al. 2010; Ostro et al. 2010). In previous studies, risk varied by age or racial/ethnic group and remained relatively stable after adjustment for criteria air pollutants.

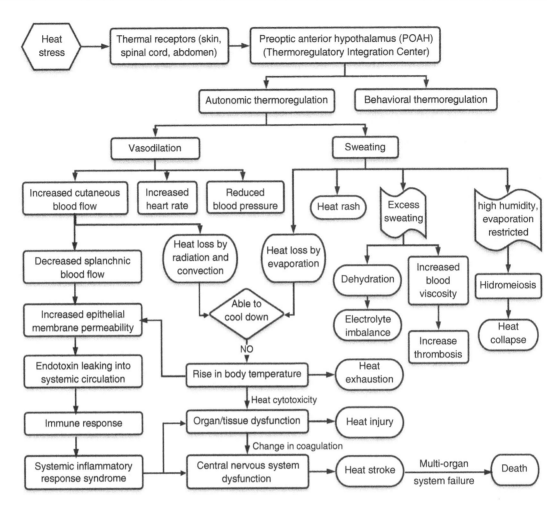

Figure 3.3 Major mechanisms of heat stress on the body
Source: Developed from Leon and Kenefick (2017) and Parsons (2014).

Cardiovascular and Cerebrovascular Diseases

As mentioned previously, the primary response to thermoregulation stress is vasodilation, which reduces blood pressure and increases the risk of hypotension. Subcutaneous blood flow escalates to dissipate heat. Rising blood flow volume to the extremities increases the heart rate leading to stress on the cardiovascular system. Further, increased blood viscosity due to body water loss or changes in coagulation may lead to increased thrombosis. All of these changes could contribute to ischemic stroke and heart disease. Thus, high associations between temperature increases and ischemic stroke and heart disease were observed in numerous epidemiologic studies (Bayentin et al. 2010; Dawson et al. 2008; Nitschke, Tucker, and Bi 2007; Ye et al. 2012). A study conducted in California found that the number of ED visits increased 12.7 percent (8.3 percent, 17.4 percent) for hypotension, 2.8 percent (0.9 percent, 4.9 percent) for cardiac dysrhythmia, 2.8 percent (0.9 percent, 4.7 percent) for ischemic stroke, and 1.7 percent (0.2 percent, 3.3 percent) for ischemic heart disease with a 10°F increase in mean daily apparent temperature, a combination of temperature and relative humidity (Basu et al. 2012). A meta-analysis of sixty-four independent studies reported that the overall risk for cardiovascular hospitalizations increased 2.2 percent (relative risk [RR] = 1.022, 1.006–1.039) from exposure to heat waves (Phung et al. 2016). Similar increments (RR = 1.016, 1.004–1.028 per 1°C increase) in the risk of myocardial infarction, which is a heart attack triggered by blockage of blood flow to the heart, was obtained in a recent systematic review and meta-analysis (Sun et al. 2018).

Subtypes of cardiovascular and cerebrovascular diseases may react to temperature via different pathways (Dawson et al. 2008; Lian et al. 2015; Lin et al. 2009; Ye et al. 2001). As the subcutaneous vessels dilate, central nervous blood volume decreases, i.e. high temperatures increase the risk of ischemic stroke, while the risk of hemorrhagic stroke decreases (Lavados, Olavarria, and Hoffmeister 2018; X. Wang et al. 2016), supported by the reduction of hospital admissions and ED visits from hemorrhagic stroke and hypertension with higher same-day apparent temperature, regardless of heat wave (Basu et al. 2012; Green et al. 2010). Koken et al. (2003) also reported that hospitalization rates of coronary atherosclerosis and pulmonary heart disease decreased with same-day apparent temperature among the elderly, while acute myocardial infarction rates increased. The opposite associations of specific diseases with temperature, for example, increase of ischemic stroke versus decrease of hemorrhagic stroke and increase of hypotension versus decrease of hypertension, could be numerically canceled. As a result, when pooling all cardiovascular morbidity together, the associations with temperature were usually not statistically significant (Bunker et al. 2016; Michelozzi et al. 2009; Song et al. 2017; Turner et al. 2012). Therefore, it is important to consider subtypes of cardiovascular or cerebrovascular diseases in epidemiologic studies of heat exposure, rather than relying only on all diseases combined.

Respiratory Diseases

Evidence on respiratory morbidity has been inconsistent across studies (Anderson et al. 2013; Bunker et al. 2016; Kovats, Hajat, and Wilkinson 2004; Lin et al. 2009; Turner et al. 2012), and the mechanisms behind them remain uncertain. Some researchers hypothesize that increased temperatures may trigger the release of inflammatory factors as well as enhance the growth of allergens and/or the transmission of viruses (Pica and Bouvier 2014). Air pollutants, such as ozone, which are positively correlated with ambient temperature especially during the summer, may also cause or exacerbate respiratory symptoms and may have synergistic effects in combination with temperature (Amegah, Rezza, and Jaakkola 2016; Basu 2009).

Compared to the general population, the elderly were found to be more vulnerable to respiratory morbidity associated with heat due to their high prevalence of chronic obstructive pulmonary disease (COPD) (Leon and Helwig 2010; Mannino 2011; Song et al. 2017). Inhaling hot air for a few minutes may trigger adverse airway responses in the elderly, exacerbating existing COPD (Anderson et al. 2013). Based on a meta-analysis of sixteen studies, each 1°C temperature rise increased respiratory mortality for the elderly (age sixty-five and over) by 3.6 percent (3.2 percent, 4.0 percent) (Bunker et al. 2016). Using U.S. Medicare billing records in 213 counties between 1999 and 2008, Anderson et al. (2013) reported a 4.3 percent (3.8 percent, 4.8 percent) increase in emergency hospitalizations for respiratory diseases among the elderly per 10°F increase in same-day temperature. Another meta-analysis of twelve studies found a similar magnitude of association between temperature and respiratory morbidity, including asthma, but the finding was not statistically significant (Turner et al. 2012).

Birth Outcomes (Reproductive and Developmental Effects)

Heat impacts on adverse birth outcomes, such as preterm delivery, low birth weight, and stillbirth have been consolidated in several review articles. Higher temperatures exacerbate the risk of preterm delivery (20 to less than 37 gestational weeks), low birth weight (less than 2,500 grams), and stillbirth (fetal death 20 or more gestational weeks) (Beltran, Wu, and Laurent 2013; Carolan-Olah and Frankowska 2014; Poursafa, Keikha, and Kelishadi 2015; Strand, Barnett, and Tong 2011; Zhang, Yu, and Wang 2017). In California, each 10°F increase in average apparent temperature the week before delivery was found to be associated with 8.6 percent (6.0

percent, 11.3 percent) and 10.4 percent (4.4 percent, 16.8 percent) increased risks of preterm delivery and stillbirth, respectively (Basu, Malig, and Ostro 2010; Basu, Sarovar, and Malig 2016). Mothers who were younger, belonged to a race/ethnic minority group, were less educated at the time of giving birth, or had preexisting conditions such as diabetes, hypertension, or preeclampsia, had greater risks of preterm delivery associated with heat (Basu, Chen, and Avalos 2017). Similar associations were observed in nationwide studies (Ha et al. 2017a, 2017b, 2018).

The specific mechanisms behind these associations have not yet been fully established. Some researchers postulate that pregnant women and their fetuses are more vulnerable to heat exposure because pregnant women are not able to thermoregulate their body temperatures efficiently. Blood flow from the developing fetus may be averted to underneath the skin in an effort to cool down. Dehydration from heat exposure also likely contributes to increased oxytocin in the mother's body, which induces labor, often prematurely.

Given these adverse birth outcomes that have been reported with increasing temperatures, pregnant women and their health care providers (e.g., obstetricians/gynecologists, midwives, nurses, physicians' assistants, etc.) are advised to be aware of reduced heat tolerance in pregnant women, recognize that symptoms such as dehydration may be triggered by heat, and take special precautions to avoid heat stress.

Mental Health and Neurological Outcomes

Heat stress may lead to behavioral changes and decrement in cognitive function, including mental performance, information processing, and memory, although the findings vary by specific task (Hancock and Vasmatzidis 2003). Extreme heat exposure may lead to heat collapse or heatstroke with neurological sequelae, such as acute mental confusion and behavioral changes. Available evidence has been inconsistent, and mechanisms behind them are unclear.

Individuals with existing mental health issues (e.g., depression, dementia, Parkinson's disease) are more at risk when faced with high temperatures, as cognitive performance has been shown to be differentially affected by heat, especially among people who take medications such as anti-depressants or beta-blockers and/or have impaired mobility (Hancock and Vasmatzidis 2003). A recent systematic review found an increased suicide risk associated with heat, with RR ranging from 1.014 to 1.370 per 1°C increase, and increases of mental-health related admissions and ED visits at higher temperatures (Thompson et al. 2018). A study conducted in California by Basu et al. (2018) also found positive associations between temperature and daily counts of ED visits for all mental health disorders, psychoses, neurotic outcomes, self-injury/suicide, and intentional injury/homicide. In this study, greatest risks were observed for Hispanics, Whites, six- to eighteen-year-olds, and females for most outcomes.

In addition, increased temperatures reduced emotional well-being (Gao et al. 2019; Noelke et al. 2016). Compared to average daily temperatures in the 50–60°F (10–16°C) range, temperatures above 70°F (21°C) reduced positive emotions (e.g., joy, happiness), increased negative emotions (e.g., stress, anger), and increased fatigue (e.g., feeling tired, low energy) (Noelke et al. 2016). Greater associations were observed among less educated and older populations. Heat effects on mental well-being exist across regions regardless of mild or hot weather, suggesting limited variation in heat adaptation.

Infectious Diseases

Increases in some vector-borne diseases have been associated with increased temperature, such as Lyme disease, dengue fever, and malaria, as vector habitats are highly influenced by temperature. Two reviews illustrated the associations between temperature and dengue fever, with an odds ratio (OR) of 1.35 (95 percent CI, 1.18-1.52) per 1°C increase, with a steep increase from 72°F (22°C) to 84°F (29°C) (Fan et al. 2014; Viana and Ignotti 2013).

Some waterborne and foodborne diseases also thrive in warmer temperatures. For example, Carlton et al. (2016) had demonstrated the association between temperature and all-cause diarrhea and bacterial diarrhea in a review article. In Vietnam, pooled estimates showed that heat waves were significantly associated with a 2.5 percent (0.8 percent, 4.3 percent) and 3.8 percent (1.5 percent, 6.2 percent) increase in all causes and infectious diseases admissions on the same day, respectively (Phung et al. 2017). A study conducted in California found that the number of ED visits increased 6.1 percent (3.3 percent, 9.0 percent) for intestinal infections for every 10°F increase in mean daily apparent temperature (Basu et al. 2012), particularly among children five to eighteen years of age because they spend more time outdoors doing recreational activities such as swimming, boating and picnicking in hotter temperatures.

Other morbidity studies

With higher temperatures, hospital admissions and ED visits for many diseases have been observed to be significantly increased. Continued hot weather has a cumulative effect on morbidity, as such conditions could result in not only heat-related events but also an exacerbation of underlying conditions. Extreme heat, for example, 99th percentile of apparent temperature, could increase all-cause hospital admissions 2–4 percent over the subsequent eight days (Gronlund et al. 2014). Similarly, ED visits could increase by approximately 2 percent when the mean heat index approached 100°F for three days (Levy et al. 2015). During the 2006 heat wave in California, there were 16,166 (3 percent) excess ED visits and 1,182 (1 percent) excess hospitalizations (Knowlton et al. 2009). In a study in Adelaide, Australia, Nitschke et al. (2007) reported a 4 percent and 7 percent increase in total ambulance transport and hospital admissions during heat waves, respectively, compared with non-heat wave periods. During the 1995 heat wave in Chicago, Illinois, a total of 838 (35 percent) more hospital admissions of the elderly (age sixty-five and over) occurred compared with the average number of admissions during comparable weeks (Semenza et al. 1999). Health effects from heat exposure generally occur more immediately, often on the same day or up to three days following heat exposure, than those due to cold exposures, requiring a rapid public health response (Green et al. 2010; Koken et al. 2003; Lin et al. 2009).

Increases of metabolic diseases, such as diabetes mellitus, associated with heat exposure have also been reported. For example, Basu et al. (2012) reported a 4.3 percent (2.8 percent, 5.9 percent) increase in the number of ED visits for diabetes in California for every 10°F increase in mean daily apparent temperature. However, given the limited evidence to date, metabolic outcomes are not presented in a separate section.

Mortality

Increase in mortality during heat waves have been observed throughout the world (Åström, Forsberg, and Rocklov 2011; Bobb et al. 2014b; Gasparrini and Armstrong 2011; Xu et al. 2016; Yu et al. 2012). The 2003 European heat wave resulted in over 70,000 excess deaths, mostly among the elderly (World Health Organization 2017). A study of 50 U.S. cities found that extreme heat was associated with a 5.7 percent (3.4 percent, 8.2 percent) increase in mortality, and these effects were heterogeneous across cities (Medina-Ramon and Schwartz 2007). Another study covering 43 U.S. communities also found that mortality increased 3.7 percent (2.3 percent, 5.2 percent) during heat waves compared with non-heat wave days (Anderson and Bell 2011). A meta-analysis following the 2006 heat wave in California revealed a 9.0 percent (1.6 percent, 16.3 percent) increase in daily mortality during the heat wave per 10°F change in apparent temperature in seven major California counties combined (Ostro et al. 2009). This estimate was almost three times greater than the association estimated during the entire warm season from May through September including both non-heat wave and heat wave periods.

Evidence suggests that heat waves especially increased risks of cardiovascular and respiratory mortality, including myocardial infarction, ischemic stroke (rather than hemorrhagic stroke), and chronic obstructive pulmonary disease (Amegah et al. 2016; Åström et al. 2011; Xu et al. 2016). Based on a meta-analysis of twenty-three studies, Sun et al. (2018) estimated that the mortality due to myocardial infarction increased by 63.9 percent (RR=1.639, 1.087, 2.470) during a heat wave. Again, the risks generally occurred immediately and lasted for up to three to five days.

Part of the mortality observed during a heat wave may be attributed to a **harvesting effect** (also known as mortality displacement), which refers to a short-term increase in mortality followed by reduced mortality, especially among susceptible people who may have died within the next few days anyway regardless of heat exposure. However, studies that have considered the harvesting effect have found no compensatory decrease in overall mortality during the subsequent weeks, so the associations that were found between temperature and mortality represent true risks to the populations studied (Basu and Malig 2011), although may vary by region and age group (Baccini, Kosatsky, and Biggeri 2013).

In addition to heat waves, elevated average surface temperature was also associated with increases in mortality (Figure 3.4) (Arbuthnott and Hajat 2017; Baccini et al. 2008; Bunker et al. 2016; Song et al. 2017; Ye et al. 2012). Bunker et al. (2016) conducted a thorough review on studies worldwide and their meta-analysis suggested that 1°C increase in temperature was associated with increases of 3.4 percent (3.1 percent, 3.8 percent), 3.6 percent (3.2 percent, 4.0 percent), and 1.4 percent (0.1 percent, 2.8 percent) in cardiovascular, respiratory, and cerebrovascular mortality, respectively. A recent U.S. study reported an increase of 1.5 percent (1.3 percent, 1.7 percent) in daily nonaccidental mortality per 10°F (5.6°C) increase in **diurnal temperature range** (the difference between the daily maximum and minimum temperature) across 95 large U.S. communities between 1987 and 2000 (Lim et al. 2015). This increase was mainly a result of cardiovascular and respiratory mortality in the elderly above sixty-five years of age. The impacts of diurnal temperature range varied by region, with the strongest association

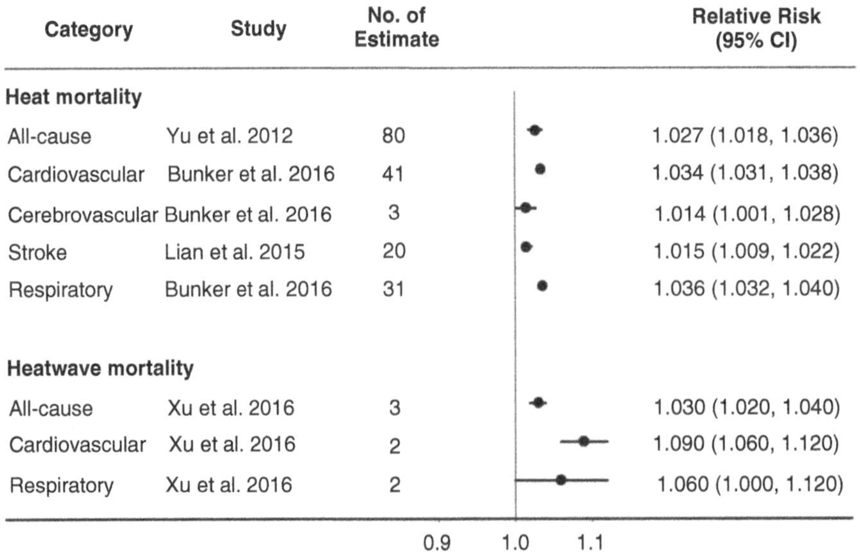

Category	Study	No. of Estimate		Relative Risk (95% CI)
Heat mortality				
All-cause	Yu et al. 2012	80		1.027 (1.018, 1.036)
Cardiovascular	Bunker et al. 2016	41		1.034 (1.031, 1.038)
Cerebrovascular	Bunker et al. 2016	3		1.014 (1.001, 1.028)
Stroke	Lian et al. 2015	20		1.015 (1.009, 1.022)
Respiratory	Bunker et al. 2016	31		1.036 (1.032, 1.040)
Heatwave mortality				
All-cause	Xu et al. 2016	3		1.030 (1.020, 1.040)
Cardiovascular	Xu et al. 2016	2		1.090 (1.060, 1.120)
Respiratory	Xu et al. 2016	2		1.060 (1.000, 1.120)

0.9   1.0   1.1

Figure 3.4   Forest plot for the association between temperature (heat) or heat wave exposure on mortality
Source: Song et al. (2017).

observed in southern California (1.7 percent; 1.2 percent, 2.4 percent). Studies focusing on California reported that each 10°F increase in daily mean apparent temperature was associated with a 2.3 percent increase in nonaccidental mortality (1.0 percent, 3.6 percent) (Basu, Feng, and Ostro 2008), with the most significant risk found for ischemic heart disease (Basu and Ostro 2008). These associations were independent of air pollution and were observed even without extremes in apparent temperature or heat waves.

When both general increase of temperature and heat waves were considered, mortality risks increased as heat waves were longer or more intense. Gasparrini and Armstrong (2011) decomposed the risk of temperature into the main effect due to daily high temperature and the added effect due to sustained duration of heat waves and concluded that **most excess risk was explained by the main effect, and a smaller added effect was found if heat waves lasted more than four days.**

Indirect Health Impacts of Extreme Heat

Increasing global surface temperature may trigger other extreme weather or natural disasters, such as hurricanes, rainstorms, floods, droughts, and wildfires. These events have become more frequent and intense and have resulted in direct and indirect health impacts. As a result of heat waves in 2018, thousands of lakes in Europe have dried up; Australia experienced its record-breaking drought, western Canada and the United States observed their biggest wildfires in history, and thus, the worst air quality from wildfire smoke. Heat is also related to air pollution, increasing levels of carbon monoxide, nitrogen oxides, particulate matter, and volatile organic compounds. These pollutants combined with high temperature could increase the production of ozone, a greenhouse gas that also has been linked with various adverse health effects (USEPA 2019).

Health effects of extreme climate events are still under scientific investigation. Precipitation and flooding affect diseases transmitted through water and via vectors such as mosquitoes. Climate-sensitive diseases, for example, diarrhea and malaria, are among the largest global killers. Drought could compromise the supply of freshwater and increase the chance of water contamination, which in turn, compromises hygiene and health. Wildfires have destroyed numerous properties and natural environments as well as threatened human and animals' lives. Fire smoke could cause severe air pollution, triggering several cardiorespiratory diseases. Furthermore, forced evacuation, loss of homes, and/or loss of lives due to extreme weather or natural disasters could overwhelm the survivors, causing mental stress and trauma.

Factors Influencing Health Effects of Heat Exposure

Vulnerable Populations

As many studies have pointed out, some groups are more susceptible to health complications from heat because of physical and physiological characteristics, including the elderly over sixty-five years of age, young children, infants, pregnant women, and people with pre-existing illnesses (Åström et al. 2011; Balbus and Malina 2009; Basu and Malig 2011; Knowlton et al. 2009; Kovats et al. 2004; Lin et al. 2009; Semenza et al. 1999). These vulnerable populations may have higher sweating thresholds, making them slow to react and adjust to external temperature change, which may result in adverse health outcomes. Children, especially infants, were more susceptible to renal and genitourinary disease, fever, and electrolyte imbalances during heat waves (Xu et al. 2012; Xu et al. 2014). Infant mortality increased by 4.4 percent (0.3 percent, 9.2 percent) per 10°F increase for an average of the three previous days of apparent temperature, and African-American infants faced the highest risk for deaths from all causes

(13.3 percent; 0.6 percent, 27.6 percent) and gestation duration (23.7 percent; 3.3 percent, 58.2 percent) (Basu et al. 2016).

People belonging to racial/ethnicity minority groups, which is often a proxy for lower socioeconomic status, were observed to be more sensitive to morbidity from temperature. Although there are many possible explanations, some may be due to the exposure itself. For example, more African-Americans and Hispanics live in areas with greater environmental exposures, including heat, traffic, and air pollutants (Basu 2009; Green et al. 2010). Another reason for higher morbidity and mortality may be poorer housing conditions, such as lacking air conditioners. Even if air conditioners are available, many people may not be able to afford using them because of the cost of electricity.

Urban Heat Island

An **urban heat island** (**UHI**) is defined as a city or metropolitan area that is significantly warmer than its surrounding rural areas, for example, typically 1–3°C warmer for a city with 1 million people or more, between the center of the city and surrounding fields, and the difference could be up to 12°C in the evening (EPA 2020). A UHI exists because of human activities, absorbance of heat by blacktops and buildings, as well as generally less greenspace in urban areas. UHIs can potentially increase the magnitude and duration of heat waves within its domain and thus, exacerbate excess mortality and morbidity associated with high temperatures. The nighttime effect of a UHI can be particularly harmful during a heat wave, as it deprives urban residents the chance to cool down during the night, as was observed during the July 2006 heat wave in California (Guirguis et al. 2014; Ostro et al. 2009). Because of the demographics of urban areas, UHIs disproportionately affect vulnerable subgroups, especially those with lower socioeconomic including the elderly and racial/ethnic minorities.

CLINICAL CORRELATES 3.1 URBAN HEAT ISLANDS

The urban heat island phenomenon is a term used to describe elevated temperatures in high exposure areas with large populations and developed infrastructure, that is, paved roads and buildings. Heat islands are associated with communities of lower socioeconomic means and greater physiologic vulnerability (medical comorbidities, age) (Voelkel et al. 2018). Local public health interventions are increasingly using maps to identify people at the greatest risk of heat-related illness due to environmental factors and social determinants of health. When mapping temperature data with sociodemographic factors in Oregon, the hottest locations were in neighborhoods identified as having populations with less ability to adapt to heat stress (Voelkel et al. 2018). The city of Richmond, Virginia also mapped out neighborhoods of increased heat vulnerability related to income to target interventions that would advance equity in their community (Hoffman and USGCRP 2019). Other adaptive changes to reduce and maintain temperatures in urban areas, especially for communities of color and low socioeconomic status, include decreasing paved surfaces and increasing open green space, canopy and vegetation (Makido, Hellman, and Shandas 2019).

With warming temperatures and rapid urbanization, mapping sociodemographic factors with heat data represents an opportunity to identify, intervene, and protect those at heightened risk of heat-related illness.

Local Climate

Numerous studies have centered around an effective definition for "heat wave" regarding temperature threshold, duration, and metric used (Kent et al. 2014; Xu et al. 2016). There is considerable variability and uncertainty about definitions for a given location and population. **The temperature threshold at which an impact is observed varies by region, by population characteristics, and by timing within the season.** This is complicated by the fact that background climates for a particular region or community greatly differ by latitude, terrain, proximity to the coast, and other local factors.

Although there has been evidence of increased resilience to temperature-related mortality (Bobb et al. 2014b), populations in areas with cooler summer temperatures were less acclimated to heat (Nordio et al. 2015). They may lack consciousness of heat-related health impacts or lack the ability to take possible mitigation strategies. Also, they may have lower tolerance to heat exposure, both physiologically and psychologically, making it harder for them to adapt to sudden heat waves. Air conditioning use has been found to significantly reduce morbidity effects of heat (Ostro et al. 2010). However, areas with milder climates generally have low prevalence of air conditioners as well as less acclimatization to heat, and thus, less resistance to high temperatures.

There are several examples of differential heat exposure and acclimatization throughout the world. Northern European countries are cooler and appear to be more vulnerable to heat waves than southern European countries (Ward et al. 2016). A study observed increased hospital admissions for respiratory diseases at temperatures greater than 28.9°C in New York City (Lin et al. 2009), whereas the threshold of respiratory hospital admissions was only 23°C in London, United Kingdom (Kovats et al. 2004), as the cooler climate corresponded to lower acclimatization rates to high temperatures (Ye et al. 2012). Residents of the west coast of the United States demonstrated stronger health impacts associated with high temperatures compared to the U.S. national average (Lim et al. 2015; Nordio et al. 2015), with higher heat-related hospitalization rates among counties with cooler average summer temperatures, like those on the California coast (Anderson et al. 2013). Furthermore, the north coast of California contributes disproportionately to the statewide health impact during heat waves, with a 10.5 percent increase in daily morbidity during heat wave peaks compared with 8.1 percent for the Central Valley and 5.6 percent for the southern coast of California, demonstrating the influence of local climate on heat resistance (Guirguis et al. 2014).

Greater heat associations with mortality are generally observed during the spring and early summer compared to later in the year (Anderson and Bell 2011; Lee et al. 2014). According to previous studies, the first heat wave of the season could cause two times more increase in mortality rate (Anderson and Bell 2010) and three to four times more heat-related hospitalization among the elderly (Liss et al. 2017), than subsequent heat waves. People are less adaptive to sudden increases of temperature in the spring and early summer, and there is a greater number of the susceptible population still alive compared to later in the summer or fall, a phenomenon known as the "loss of susceptibles" (Basu and Samet 2002). It is essential to consider short-term monthly associations in local areas instead of longer-term seasonal relationships, as was done in a previous study (Sherbakov et al. 2018).

Occupational Exposures

Occupations that involve long hours of outdoor operations, for example, agricultural workers, construction workers, and delivery drivers, are subject to higher risks of heat exposure. Though people in such occupations are predominantly male and healthy, the long working hours may bring on health burdens that they cannot afford physically and for financial reasons, they may not be able to take day(s) off from work. There are recognized heat prevention strategies and international thermal ergonomic standards to protect workers, such as the U.S. Occupational Safety and Health Act (OSHA) and European Union Safety and Health Legislation. Figure 3.5 presents the heat index system developed by NOAA, by which OSHA defines heat hazards and requires employers to protect their employees. However, such standards have been developed largely in temperate western settings, and often not regulated well enough to protect workers'

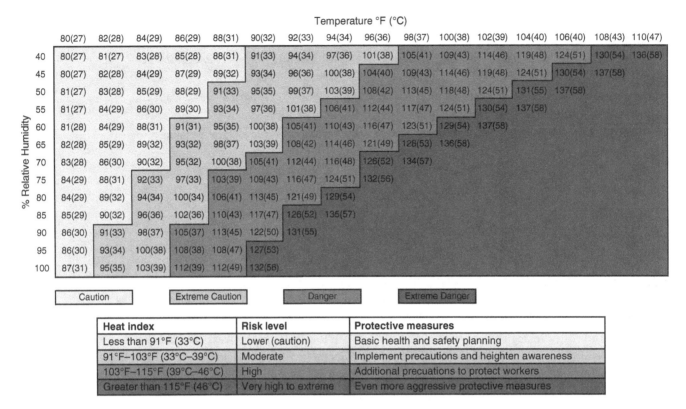

Temperature °F (°C)

% Relative Humidity	80(27)	82(28)	84(29)	86(29)	88(31)	90(32)	92(33)	94(34)	96(36)	98(37)	100(38)	102(39)	104(40)	106(40)	108(43)	110(47)
40	80(27)	81(27)	83(28)	85(28)	88(31)	91(33)	94(34)	97(36)	101(38)	105(41)	109(43)	114(46)	119(48)	124(51)	130(54)	136(58)
45	80(27)	82(28)	84(29)	87(29)	89(32)	93(34)	96(36)	100(38)	104(40)	109(43)	114(46)	119(48)	124(51)	130(54)	137(58)	
50	81(27)	83(28)	85(29)	88(29)	91(33)	95(35)	99(37)	103(39)	108(42)	113(45)	118(48)	124(51)	131(55)	137(58)		
55	81(27)	84(29)	86(30)	89(30)	93(34)	97(36)	101(38)	106(41)	112(44)	117(47)	124(51)	130(54)	137(58)			
60	81(28)	84(29)	88(31)	91(31)	95(35)	100(38)	105(41)	110(43)	116(47)	123(51)	129(54)	137(58)				
65	82(28)	85(29)	89(32)	93(32)	98(37)	103(39)	108(42)	114(46)	121(49)	128(53)	136(58)					
70	83(28)	86(30)	90(32)	95(32)	100(38)	105(41)	112(44)	116(48)	126(52)	134(57)						
75	84(29)	88(31)	92(33)	97(33)	103(39)	109(43)	116(47)	124(51)	132(56)							
80	84(29)	89(32)	94(34)	100(34)	106(41)	113(45)	121(49)	129(54)								
85	85(29)	90(32)	96(36)	102(36)	110(43)	117(47)	126(52)	135(57)								
90	86(30)	91(33)	98(37)	105(37)	113(45)	122(50)	131(55)									
95	86(30)	93(34)	100(38)	108(38)	108(47)	127(53)										
100	87(31)	95(35)	103(39)	112(39)	112(49)	132(56)										

Caution   Extreme Caution   Danger   Extreme Danger

Heat index	Risk level	Protective measures
Less than 91°F (33°C)	Lower (caution)	Basic health and safety planning
91°F–103°F (33°C–39°C)	Moderate	Implement precautions and heighten awareness
103°F–115°F (39°C–46°C)	High	Additional precautions to protect workers
Greater than 115°F (46°C)	Very high to extreme	Even more aggressive protective measures

Figure 3.5   Heat Index System Developed by National Oceanic Atmospheric Administration (NOAA)

Note: The heat index serves as the basis for NOAA to issue heat advisories. It combines both air temperature and relative humidity into apparent temperature to better estimate true exposure (i.e., how hot it actually feels).

health. Low- and middle-income countries and counties in tropical and subtropical zones still face great challenges in protecting workers from excessive heat exposure, given the dense populations, under-regulated work environments, and projected temperature increases due to climate change (Lucas, Epstein, and Kjellstrom 2014).

Adaptation, Mitigation, and Resilience

As heat waves become more frequent and severe, people have been developing adaptations to heat. In a multicountry study including 305 locations in ten countries, consistent reductions in heat-related mortality were observed in the majority of the world (Vicedo-Cabrera et al. 2018). Wang et al. (2016) found that heat-wave-associated heatstroke risks decreased substantially over the time span from 1999 to 2010, suggesting a potential for heat acclimatization in the population. Such improvement is also attributed to heat-health prevention policies and improvement of health care and emergency response resources (Arbuthnott et al. 2016). However, there is evidence that there are more temperature and heat wave increases predicted for the future and thus more expected health impacts. Differential acclimatization with full understanding of heat exposure scenarios and adaptive strategies that prioritize the protection of vulnerable populations is critical to minimize health threats.

The increased frequency of heat wave events has prompted governments worldwide to take action by developing heat-health action plans focused on susceptible populations. The WHO Regional Office for Europe published guidance to prevent morbidity and mortality following heat events in "Heat-Health Action Plans," including "meteorologic early warning systems, timely public and medical advice, improvements to housing and urban planning and ensuring that health care and social systems are ready to act" (Matthies et al. 2008). Many developed countries (Canada, France, Italy, and Spain) have implemented preventive measures and provided guidelines on extreme heat, which have effectively reduced heat-related mortality and morbidity (Benmarhnia et al. 2016; Boeckmann and Rohn 2014; de'Donato et al. 2015; Schifano et al. 2012). For example, the Heat Health Prevention Plan in Spain greatly reduced extreme heat-related mortality over the past twenty years, especially among vulnerable subgroups (Martinez-Solanas and Basagaña 2019). Developing countries and regions, like many countries in Africa, Asia, and Central and South America, have not yet or been in the process of adapting policies due to limited economy, governance, social commitment, and readiness for climate change (Sarkodie and Strezov 2019). Vulnerabilities inherent in the ethnic, cultural, and economic diversity of populations need to be considered in any action plan.

As mentioned previously, one potential strategy to mitigate heat impacts is to implement heat warning systems on extremely hot days so that targeted, vulnerable populations can take preventive actions. However, a recent study in California revealed that **the majority of impactful heat wave events were not accompanied by a heat advisory or warning from the National Weather Service** (Guirguis et al. 2014). Current official warning/guidance systems do not address local variability of heat tolerance, and thus, has limited effectiveness on the reduction of adverse health effects (Weinberger et al. 2018; Wellenius et al. 2017).

Furthermore, there are many health impacts of mortality or morbidity attributable to heat observed when temperatures are below extreme levels. In fact, most of the burden related to exposure to hot temperatures comes from non-extreme temperatures because of a higher frequency of occurrence. Therefore, focusing only on very extreme days would be insufficient for mitigating heat-related health impacts, and long-term actions to reduce exposure to more typical hot temperatures are fundamental (Markevych et al. 2017; Schinasi, Benmarhnia, and De Roos 2018).

Apart from heat preparedness plans and heat warning systems, other mitigation and resilience strategies include opening cooling centers during extreme heat, identifying vulnerable populations and their distributions, and increasing health care system resilience. City/community design and building design should incorporate the considerations of heat resilience, such as increased tree and shrub coverage, improving building materials, using green roofs and shaded building construction. These strategies could reduce the heat effects while achieving energy efficiency. Public education and science communication may help promote public awareness of heat-related health effects and prepare individuals for potential heat events.

Summary

Increased mortality and morbidity associated with heat exposure have been observed throughout the world. The health effects were not limited to "classic" heat illness but also include cardiovascular, cerebrovascular, respiratory, neurological, and infectious diseases as well as adverse birth outcomes, and thus, are often underestimated when considering only heat-related deaths and/or illnesses. Ongoing temperature increases are expected to exacerbate this burden. Governments at the local, national, and international levels have the responsibility to implement heat preventive actions and emergency-response policies to help their populations acclimate to more frequent heat waves and other related climate events and reduce heat-related health effects.

KEY TERMS

Dehydration: A significant loss of body fluid that impairs normal body functions.

Diurnal temperature range: The difference between the daily maximum and minimum temperature.

Harvesting effect: Also referred to as mortality displacement, a short-term increase in mortality followed by reduced mortality, especially among susceptible people who may have died regardless of heat exposure within the next few days.

Heat syncope: Fainting or dizziness as a result of overheating (*syncope* is the medical term for fainting). It is a type of *heat* illness. The basic symptom of *heat syncope* is fainting, with or without mental confusion.

Heat wave: A period when daily mean temperatures go above a specified threshold high-end temperature (e.g., 95th or 99th) for at least two consecutive days in a given location.

Heatstroke: Also known as sun stroke, is a severe heat illness, defined as hyperthermia with a body temperature greater than 40.6 °C (105.1 °F) because of environmental heat exposure with lack of thermoregulation. This is distinct from a fever, where there is a physiological increase in the temperature set point of the body. The term "stroke" is a misnomer in that it does not involve a blockage or hemorrhage of blood flow to the brain.

Hypotension: Low blood pressure, which can cause fainting or dizziness because the brain does not receive enough blood.

Thermoregulation: A process to maintain a relatively constant core body temperature, which is critical to the survival of the creature, even when the surrounding temperature is different.

Urban heat island: An urban or metropolitan area that is significantly warmer than its surrounding rural areas.

Vasodilation: The dilatation of blood vessels, which decreases blood pressure.

DISCUSSION QUESTIONS

1. Describe the known mechanisms of heat-related health effects.

2. How can we develop a systematic definition for heat-related deaths so that they are not so grossly underestimated? Can we include deaths and illnesses from other causes that may not be the underlying cause of death (i.e., secondary causes of death)? How about for heat-related illnesses?

3. How can heat warnings be more effective? Can a standardized definition for heat waves be implemented for specific regions and populations?

4. Given what is known from the research to date, how can morbidity and mortality be prevented for a certain location? What heat-action plans would be most effective for each population, particularly to protect vulnerable subgroups?

References

Amegah, A. K., G. Rezza, and J. J. Jaakkola. 2016. "Temperature-Related Morbidity and Mortality in Sub-Saharan Africa: A Systematic Review of the Empirical Evidence." *Environment International* 91:133–49.

Anderson, G. B., and M. L. Bell. 2011. "Heat Waves in the United States: Mortality Risk During Heat Waves and Effect Modification by Heat Wave Characteristics in 43 U.S. Communities." *Environmental Health Perspectives* 119:210–18.

Anderson, G. B., F. Dominici, Y. Wang, M. C. McCormack, M. L. Bell, and R. D. Peng. 2013. "Heat-Related Emergency Hospitalizations for Respiratory Diseases in the Medicare Population." *American Journal of Respiratory and Critical Care Medicine* 187:1098–1103.

Arbuthnott, K., S. Hajat, C. Heaviside, and S. Vardoulakis. 2016. "Changes in Population Susceptibility to Heat and Cold over Time: Assessing Adaptation to Climate Change." *Environmental Health* 15 (suppl 1):1:33.

Arbuthnott, K. G., and S. Hajat. 2017. "The Health Effects of Hotter Summers and Heat Waves in the Population of the United Kingdom: A Review of the Evidence." *Environmental Health* 16 (suppl 1):119.

Åström, D. O., B. Forsberg, and J. Rocklov. 2011. "Heat Wave Impact on Morbidity and Mortality in the Elderly Population: A Review of Recent Studies." *Maturitas* 69:99–105.

Auerbach, P. S., T. A. Cushing, and N. S. Harris. 2017. *Auerbach's Wilderness Medicine*, 7th ed. Philadelphia, PA: Elsevier/Mosby.

Baccini, M., A. Biggeri, G. Accetta, T. Kosatsky, K. Katsouyanni, A. Analitis, H. R. Anderson et al. 2008. "Heat Effects on Mortality in 15 European Cities." *Epidemiology* 19:711–19.

Baccini, M., T. Kosatsky, and A. Biggeri. 2013. "Impact of Summer Heat on Urban Population Mortality in Europe During the 1990s: An Evaluation of Years of Life Lost Adjusted for Harvesting." *PLoS One* 8:e69638.

Balbus, J. M., and C. Malina. 2009. "Identifying Vulnerable Subpopulations for Climate Change Health Effects in the United States." *Journal of Occupational and Environmental Medicine* 51:33–7.

Basu, R. 2009. "High Ambient Temperature and Mortality: A Review of Epidemiologic Studies from 2001 to 2008." *Environmental Health* 8:40. doi: 10.1186/1476-1069X-1188-1140.

Basu, R., H. Chen, D. K. Li, and L. A. Avalos. 2017. "The Impact of Maternal Factors on the association Between Temperature and Preterm Delivery." *Environmental Research* 154:109–14.

Basu, R., W. Y. Feng, and B. D. Ostro. 2008. "Characterizing Temperature and Mortality in Nine California Counties." *Epidemiology* 19:138–45.

Basu, R., L. Gavin, D. Pearson, K. Ebisu, and B. Malig. 2018. "Examining the Association Between Apparent Temperature and Mental Health-Related Emergency Room Visits in California." *American Journal of Epidemiology* 187:726–35.

Basu, R., and B. Malig. 2011. "High Ambient Temperature and Mortality in California: Exploring the Roles of age, Disease, and Mortality Displacement." *Environmental Research* 111:1286–92.

Basu, R., B. Malig, and B. Ostro. 2010. "High Ambient Temperature and the Risk of Preterm Delivery." *American Journal of Epidemiology* 172:1108–17.

Basu, R., and B. D. Ostro. 2008. "A Multicounty Analysis Identifying the Populations Vulnerable to Mortality Associated with High Ambient Temperature in California." *American Journal of Epidemiology* 168:632–37.

Basu, R., D. Pearson, B. Malig, R. Broadwin, R. Green. 2012. "The Effect of High Ambient Temperature on Emergency Room Visits." *Epidemiology* 23:813–20.

Basu, R., and J. M. Samet. 2002. "Relation Between Elevated Ambient Temperature and Mortality: A Review of the Epidemiologic Evidence." *Epidemiologic Reviews* 24:190–202.

Basu, R., V. Sarovar, and B. J. Malig. 2016. "Association between High Ambient Temperature and Risk of Stillbirth in California." *American Journal of Epidemiology* 183 (10): 894–901.

Bayentin, L., S. El Adlouni, T. B. Ouarda, P. Gosselin, B. Doyon, and F. Chebana. 2010. "Spatial Variability of Climate Effects on Ischemic Heart Disease Hospitalization Rates for the Period 1989–2006 in Quebec, Canada." *International Journal of Health Geographics* 9:5.

Beltran, A. J., J. Wu, and O. Laurent. 2013. "Associations of Meteorology with Adverse Pregnancy Outcomes: A Systematic Review of Preeclampsia, Preterm Birth and Birth Weight." *International Journal of Environmental Research and Public Health* 11:91–172.

Benmarhnia, T., Z. Bailey, D. Kaiser, N. Auger, N. King, and J. S. Kaufman. 2016. "A Difference-in-Differences Approach yo Assess the Effect of a Heat Action Plan on Heat-Related Mortality, and Differences in Effectiveness According to Sex, Age, and Socioeconomic Status (Montreal, Quebec)." *Environmental Health Perspectives* 124:1694–99.

Bobb, J. F., Z. Obermeyer, Y. Wang, and F. Dominici. 2014a. "Cause-Specific Risk of Hospital Admission Related to Extreme Heat in Older Adults." *JAMA* 312:2659–67.

Bobb, J. F., R. D. Peng, M. L. Bell, and F. Dominici. 2014b. "Heat-Related Mortality and Adaptation to Heat in the United States." *Environmental Health Perspectives* 122:811–16.

Boeckmann, M., and I. Rohn. 2014. "Is Planned Adaptation to Heat Reducing Heat-Related Mortality and Illness? A Systematic Review." *BMC Public Health* 14:1112.

Bunker, A., J. Wildenhain, A, Vandenbergh, N. Henschke, J. Rocklov, S. Hajat, and R. Sauerborn. 2016. "Effects of Air Temperature on Climate-Sensitive Mortality and Morbidity Outcomes in the Elderly; A Systematic Review and Meta-analysis of Epidemiological Evidence." *EBioMedicine* 6:258–68.

Carlton, E. J., A. P. Woster, P. DeWitt, R. S. Goldstein, and K. Levy. 2016. "A Systematic Review and Meta-analysis of Ambient Temperature and Diarrhoeal Diseases." *International Journal of Epidemiology* 45:117–30.

Carolan-Olah, M., and D. Frankowska. 2014. "High Environmental Temperature and Preterm Birth: A Review of the Evidence." *Midwifery* 30:50–59.

Dawson, J., C. Weir, F. Wright, C. Bryden, S. Aslanyan, K. Lees, W. Bird, and M. Walters. 2008. "Associations between Meteorological Variables and Acute Stroke Hospital Admissions in the West of Scotland." *Acta Neurologica Scandinavica* 117:85–89.

De'Donato, F. K., M. Leone, M. Scortichini, M. De Sario, K. Katsouyanni, T. Lanki, X. Basagaña et al. 2015. "Changes in the Effect of Heat on Mortality in the Last 20 Years in Nine European Cities. Results from the Phase Project." *International Journal of Environmental Research and Public Health* 12:15567–83.

Environmental Protection Agency. 2019. "Health Effects of Ozone Pollution." Updated July 30, 2019. https://www.epa.gov/ground-level-ozone-pollution/health-effects-ozone-pollution.

Environmental Protection Agency. 2020. Heat Island Effect. Updated May 18, 2020. https://www.epa.gov/heat-islands

Fan, J., W. Wei, Z. Bai, C. Fan, S. Li, Q. Liu, and K. Yang. 2014. "A Systematic Review and Meta-analysis of Dengue Risk with Temperature Change." *International Journal of Environmental Research and Public Health* 12:1–15.

Freedman, A. 2018. "2018's Global Heat Wave Is So Pervasive It's Surprising Scientists." *aXIOS* July 27, 2018.

Gao, J., Q. Cheng, J. Duan, Z. Xu, L. Bai, Y. Zhang, H. Zhang et al. 2019. "Ambient Temperature, Sunlight Duration, and Suicide: A Systematic Review and Meta-analysis." *Science of the Total Environment* 646:1021–29.

Gasparrini, A., and B. Armstrong. 2011. "The Impact of Heat Waves on Mortality." *Epidemiology* 22:68–73.

Green, R. S., R. Basu, B. Malig, R. Broadwin, J. J. Kim, and B. Ostro. 2010. "The Effect of Temperature on Hospital admissions in Nine California Counties." *International Journal of Public Health* 55:113–21.

Gronlund, C. J., A. Zanobetti, J. D. Schwartz, G. A. Wellenius, and M. S. O'Neill. 2014. "Heat, Heat Waves, and Hospital Admissions among the Elderly in the United States, 1992–2006." *Environmental Health Perspectives* 122 (11): 1187–92.

Gronlund, C. J., A. Zanobetti, G. A. Wellenius, J. D. Schwartz, and M. S. O'Neill. 2016. "Vulnerability to Renal, Heat and Respiratory Hospitalizations During Extreme Heat among U.S. Elderly." *Climate Change* 136:631–45.

Guirguis, K., A. Gershunov, A. Tardy, and R. Basu. 2014. "The Impact of Recent Heat Waves on Human Health in California." *Journal of Applied Meteorology and Climatology* 53:3–19.

Ha, S., D. Liu, Y. Zhu, S. Soo Kim, S. Sherman, K. L. Grantz, and P. Mendola. 2017a. "Ambient Temperature and Stillbirth: A Multi-Center Retrospective Cohort Study." *Environmental Health Perspectives* 125:067011.

Ha, S., Y. Zhu, D. Liu, S. Sherman, and P. Mendola. 2017b. "Ambient Temperature and Air Quality in Relation Too Small for Gestational Age and Term Low Birthweight." *Environmental Research* 155:394–400.

Ha, S., D. Liu, Y. Zhu, S. Sherman, and P. Mendola. 2018. "Acute Associations between Outdoor Temperature and Premature Rupture of Membranes." *Epidemiology* 29:175–82.

Hall, J. E. 2015. *Guyton and Hall Textbook of Medical Physiology*, 13th ed. Philadelphia: Saunders.

Hancock, P. A., and I. Vasmatzidis. 2003. "Effects of Heat Stress on Cognitive Performance: The Current State of Knowledge." *International Journal of Hyperthermia* 19:355–72.

Hansen, A. L., P. Bi, P. Ryan, M. Nitschke, D. Pisaniello, and G. Tucker. 2008. "The Effect of Heat Waves on Hospital Admissions for Renal Disease in a Temperate City of Australia." *International Journal of Epidemiology* 37:1359–65.

Hoffman, J. S. and the USGCRP. 2019. *U.S. Climate Resilience Toolkit Case Study: Where Do We Need Shade? Mapping Urban Heat Islands in Richmond, Virginia*. Updated October 28, 2019. https://toolkit.climate.gov/case-studies/where-do-we-need-shade-mapping-urban-heat-islands-richmond-virginia.

Kent, S. T., L. A. McClure, B. F. Zaitchik, T. T. Smith, and J. M. Gohlke JM. 2014. "Heat Waves and Health Outcomes in Alabama (USA): The Importance of Heat Wave Definition." *Environmental Health Perspectives* 122:151–58.

Kilbourne, E. M. 1999. "The Spectrum of Illness During Heat Waves." *American Journal of Preventive Medicine* 16:359–60.

Knowlton, K., M. Rotkin-Ellman, G. King, H. G. Margolis, D. Smith, G. Solomon, R. Trent, and P. English. 2009. "The 2006 California Heat Wave: Impacts on Hospitalizations and Emergency Department Visits. *Environmental Health Perspectives* 117:61–67.

Koken, P. J., W. T. Piver, F. Ye, A. Elixhauser, L. M. Olsen, and C. J. Portier. 2003. "Temperature, air Pollution, and Hospitalization for Cardiovascular Diseases among Elderly People in Denver." *Environmental Health Perspectives* 111:1312–17.

Kovats, R. S., S. Hajat, and P. Wilkinson. 2004. "Contrasting Patterns of Mortality and Hospital Admissions During Hot Weather and Heat Waves in Greater London, UK." *Occupational and Environmental Medicine* 61:893–98.

Lavados, P. M., V. V. Olavarria, and L. Hoffmeister. 2018. "Ambient Temperature and Stroke Risk: Evidence Supporting a Short-Term Effect at a Population Level from Acute Environmental Exposures." *Stroke* 49:255–61.

Lee, M., F. Nordio, A. Zanobetti, P. Kinney, R. Vautard, and J. Schwartz. 2014. "Acclimatization across Space and Time in the Effects of Temperature on Mortality: A Time-Series Analysis." *Environmental Health* 13:89.

Leon, L. R., and B. G. Helwig. 2010. "Heat Stroke: Role of the Systemic Inflammatory Response." *Journal of Applied Physiology* 109:1980–88.

Leon, L. R., and R. W. Kenefick. 2017. "Chapter 12: Pathophysiology of Heat-Related Illnesses." In *Auerbach's Wilderness Medicine*, 7th ed., edited by P. S. Auerbach, T. A. Cushing, and N. S. Harris, 249–67. Philadelphia, PA: Elsevier/Mosby.

Levy, M., M. Broccoli, G. Cole, J. L. Jenkins, and E. Y. Klein. 2015. "An Analysis of the Relationship between the Heat Index and Arrivals in the Emergency Department." *PLoS Currents* 7.

Lian, H., Y. Ruan, R. Liang, X. Liu, and Z. Fan. 2015. "Short-Term Effect of Ambient Temperature and the Risk of Stroke: A Systematic Review and Meta-analysis." *International Journal of Environmental Research and Public Health* 12:9068–88.

Lim, Y. H., C. E. Reid, J. K. Mann, M. Jerrett, and H. Kim. 2015. "Diurnal Temperature Range and Short-Term Mortality in Large US Communities." *International Journal of Biometeorology* 59:1311–19.

Lin, S., M. Luo, R. J. Walker, X. Liu, S. Hwang, and R. Chinery. 2009. "Extreme High Temperatures and Hospital Admissions for Respiratory and Cardiovascular Diseases." *Epidemiology* 20:738–46.

Lipman, G. S., K. P. Eifling, M. A. Ellis, F. G. Gaudio, E. M. Otten, and C. K. Grissom. 2014. "Wilderness Medical Society Practice Guidelines for the Prevention and Treatment of Heat-Related Illness: 2014 Update." *Wilderness and Environmental Medicine* 25:S55–S65.

Liss, A., R. Wu, K. Chui, and E. N. Naumova. 2017. "Heat-Related Hospitalizations in Older Adults: An Amplified Effect of the First Seasonal Heatwave." *Scientific Reports* 7:39581. https://doi.org/10.1038/srep39581

Lucas, R. A. I., Y. Epstein, and T. Kjellstrom. 2014. "Excessive Occupational Heat Exposure: A Significant Ergonomic Challenge and Health Risk for Current and Future Workers." *Extreme Physiology & Medicine* 3:14.

Makido, Y., D. Hellman, and V. Shandas. 2019. "Nature-Based Designs to Mitigate Urban Heat: The Efficacy of Green Infrastructure Treatments in Portland, Oregon." *Atmosphere* 10:282.

Mannino, D. M. 2011. "The Natural History of Chronic Obstructive Pulmonary Disease." *Pneumonologia i alergologia polska* 79:139–43.

Markevych, I., J. Schoierer, T. Hartig, A. Chudnovsky, P. Hystad, A. M. Dzhambov, S. de Vries et al. 2017. "Exploring Pathways Linking Greenspace to Health: Theoretical and Methodological Guidance." *Environmental Research* 158:301–17.

Martinez-Solanas, E., Basagaña. 2019. "Temporal Changes in Temperature-Related Mortality in Spain and Effect of the Implementation of a Heat Health Prevention Plan." *Environmental Research* 169:102–13.

Matthies, F., G. Bickler, N. Cardeñosa Marín, and S. Hales. 2008. *Heat–Health Action Plans*. Geneva: World Health Organization. https://www.euro.who.int/en/publications/abstracts/heathealth-action-plans

Medina-Ramon, M., and J. Schwartz. 2007. "Temperature, Temperature Extremes, and Mortality: A Study of Acclimatisation and Effect Modification in 50 US Cities." *Occupational and Environmental Medicine* 64:827–33.

Michelozzi, P., G. Accetta, M. De Sario, D. D'Ippoliti, C. Marino, M. Baccini, A. Biggeri et al. 2009. "High Temperature and Hospitalizations for Cardiovascular and Respiratory Causes in 12 European Cities." *American Journal of Respiratory and Critical Care Medicine* 179:383–9.

Nitschke, M., G. R. Tucker, and P. Bi. 2007. "Morbidity and Mortality during Heatwaves in Metropolitan Adelaide." *Medical Journal of Australia* 187:662–5.

Noelke, C., M. McGovern, D. J. Corsi, M. P. Jimenez, A. Stern, I. S. Wing, and L. Berkman. 2016. "Increasing Ambient Temperature Reduces Emotional Well-Being." *Environmental Research* 151:124–9.

Nordio, F., A. Zanobetti, E. Colicino, I. Kloog, and J. Schwartz. 2015. "Changing Patterns of the Temperature-Mortality Association by Time and Location in the US, and Implications for Climate Change." *Environment International* 81:80–86.

Ostro, B., S. Rauch, R. Green, B. Malig, and R. Basu. 2010. "The Effects of Temperature and Use of Air Conditioning on Hospitalizations." *American Journal of Epidemiology* 172:1053–61.

Ostro, B. D., L. A. Roth, R. S. Green, and R. Basu. 2009. "Estimating the Mortality Effect of the July 2006 California Heat Wave." *Environmental Research* 109:614–9.

Parsons, K. 2014. *Human Thermal Environments: The Effects of Hot, Moderate, and Cold Environments on Human Health, Comfort, and Performance*, 3rd ed. Boca Raton, FL: CRC Press.

Phung, D., C. Chu, S. Rutherford, H. L. T. Nguyen, C. M. Do, and C. Huang. 2017. "Heatwave and Risk of Hospitalization: A Multi-Province Study in Vietnam." *Environmental Pollution* 220:597–607.

Phung, D., P. K. Thai, Y. Guo, L. Morawska, S. Rutherford, and C. Chu. 2016. "Ambient Temperature and Risk of Cardiovascular Hospitalization: An Updated Systematic Review and Meta-analysis." *Science of the Total Environment* 550:1084–1102.

Pica, N., and N. M. Bouvier. 2014. "Ambient Temperature and Respiratory Virus Infection." *Pediatric Infectious Disease* 33:311–13.

Poursafa, P., M. Keikha, and R. Kelishadi. 2015. "Systematic Review on Adverse Birth Outcomes of Climate Change." *Journal of Research in Medical Sciences* 20:397–402.

Sarkodie, S. A., and V. Strezov. 2019. "Economic, Social and Governance Adaptation Readiness for Mitigation of Climate Change Vulnerability: Evidence from 192 Countries." *Science of the Total Environment* 656:150–64.

Schifano, P., M. Leone, M. De Sario, F. de'Donato, A. M. Bargagli, D. D'Ippoliti, C. Marino, and P. Michelozzi. 2012. "Changes in the Effects of Heat on Mortality among the Elderly from 1998-2010: Results from a Multicenter Time Series Study in Italy." *Environmental Health* 11:58.

Schinasi, L. H., T. Benmarhnia, and A. J. De Roos. 2018. "Modification of the Association Between High Ambient Temperature and Health by Urban Microclimate Indicators: A Systematic Review and Meta-analysis." *Environmental Research* 161:168–80.

Semenza, J. C., J. E. McCullough, W. D. Flanders, M. A. McGeehin, and J. R. Lumpkin. 1999. "Excess Hospital Admissions During the July 1995 Heat Wave in Chicago." *American Journal of Preventive Medicine* 16:269–77.

Sherbakov, T., B. Malig, K. Guirguis, A. Gershunov, and R. Basu. 2018. "Ambient Temperature and Added Heat Wave Effects on Hospitalizations in California from 1999 to 2009." *Environmental Research* 160:83–90. doi: 10.1016/j.envres.2017.08.052.

Song, X., S. Wang, Y. Hu, M. Yue, T. Zhang, Y. Liu, J. Tian, and K. Shang. 2017. "Impact of Ambient Temperature on Morbidity and Mortality: An Overview of Reviews." *Science of the Total Environment* 586:241–54.

Strand, L. B., A. G. Barnett, and S. Tong. 2011. "The Influence of Season and Ambient Temperature on Birth Outcomes: A Review of the Epidemiological Literature." *Environment Research* 111:451–62.

Sun, Z., C. Chen, D. Xu, and T. Li. 2018. "Effects of Ambient Temperature on Myocardial infarction: A Systematic Review and Meta-analysis." *Environmental Pollution* 241:1106–14.

Thompson, R., R. Hornigold, L. Page, and T. Waite. 2018. "Associations between High Ambient Temperatures and Heat Waves with Mental Health Outcomes: A Systematic Review." *Public Health* 161:171–91.

Turner, L. R., A. G. Barnett, D. Connell, and S. Tong. 2012. "Ambient Temperature and Cardiorespiratory Morbidity: A Systematic Review and Meta-analysis." *Epidemiology* 23:594–606.

Viana, D. V., and E. Ignotti. 2013. "The Occurrence of Dengue and Weather Changes in Brazil: A Systematic Review." *Brazilian Journal of Epidemiology* 16:240–56.

Vicedo-Cabrera, A. M., F. Sera, Y. Guo, Y. Chung, K. Arbuthnott, S. Tong, A. Tobias et al. 2018. "A Multi-Country Analysis on Potential Adaptive Mechanisms to Cold and Heat in a Changing Climate." *Environment International* 111:239–46.

Voelkel, J., D. Hellman, R. Sakuma, and V. Shandas. 2018. "Assessing Vulnerability to Urban Heat: A Study of Disproportionate Heat Exposure and Access to Refuge by Socio-Demographic Status in Portland, Oregon." *International Journal of Environmental Research and Public Health* 15(4).

Wang, X., Y. Cao, D. Hong, D. Zheng, S. Richtering, E. C. Sandset, T. H. Leong et al. 2016. "Ambient Temperature and Stroke Occurrence: A Systematic Review and Meta-analysis." *International Journal of Environmental Research and Public Health* 13.

Wang, Y., J. F. Bobb, B. Papi, Y. Wang, A. Kosheleva, Q. Di, J. D. Schwartz, and F. Dominici. 2016. "Heat Stroke Admissions During Heat Waves in 1,916 US Counties for the Period from 1999 to 2010 and Their Effect Modifiers." *Environmental Health* 15:83.

Ward, K., S. Lauf, B. Kleinschmit, and W. Endlicher. 2016. "Heat Waves and Urban Heat Islands in Europe: A Review of Relevant Drivers." *Science of the Total Environment* 569–570:527–39.

Watts, N., M. Amann, S. Ayeb-Karlsson, K. Belesova, T. Bouley, M. Boykoff, P. Byass et al. 2018. "The Lancet Countdown on Health and Climate Change: From 25 Years of Inaction to a Global Transformation for Public Health." *Lancet* 391:581–630.

Weinberger, K. R., A. Zanobetti, J. Schwartz, and G. A. Wellenius. 2018. "Effectiveness of National Weather Service Heat Alerts in Preventing Mortality in 20 US Cities." *Environment International* 116:30–38.

Wellenius, G. A., M. N. Eliot, K. F. Bush, D. Holt, R. A. Lincoln, A. E. Smith, and J. Gold 2017. "Heat-Related Morbidity and Mortality in New England: Evidence for Local Policy." *Environmental Research* 156:845–53.

World Health Organization. 2017. *Fact Sheet on SDGs—Climate Change.* Geneva: World Health Organization, Regional Office for Europe.

Xu, Z., R. A. Etzel, H. Su, C. Huang, Y. Guo, and S. Tong. 2012. "Impact of Ambient Temperature on Children's Health: A Systematic Review." *Environmental Research* 117:120–31.

Xu, Z., G. FitzGerald, Y. Guo, B. Jalaludin, and S. Tong. 2016. "Impact of Heatwave on Mortality under Different Heatwave Definitions: A Systematic Review and Meta-analysis." *Environment International* 89–90:193–203.

Xu, Z., P. E. Sheffield, H. Su, X. Wang, Y. Bi, and S. Tong. 2014. "The Impact of Heat Waves on Children's Health: A Systematic Review." *International Journal of Biometeorology* 58:239–47.

Ye, F., W. T. Piver, M. Ando, and C. J. Portier. 2001. "Effects of Temperature and Air Pollutants on Cardiovascular and Respiratory Diseases for Males and Females Older than 65 Years of Age in Tokyo, July and August 1980–1995." *Environmental Health Perspectives* 109:355–59.

Ye, X., R. Wolff, W. Yu, P. Vaneckova, X. Pan, and S. Tong. 2012. "Ambient Temperature and Morbidity: A Review of Epidemiological Evidence. *Environmental Health Perspectives* 120:19–28.

Yu, W., K. Mengersen, X. Wang, X. Ye, Y. Guo, X. Pan, and S. Tong. 2012. "Daily Average Temperature and Mortality among the Elderly: A Meta-analysis and Systematic Review of Epidemiological Evidence." *International Journal of Biometeorology* 56:569–81.

Zhang, Y., C. Yu, and L. Wang. 2017. "Temperature Exposure during Pregnancy and Birth Outcomes: An Updated Systematic Review of Epidemiological Evidence." *Environmental Pollution* 225:700–12.

CHAPTER 4

CLIMATE CHANGE IMPACTS ON THE HYDROLOGIC CYCLE AND WATERBORNE DISEASES

Jan C. Semenza

Changes in Hydrology Caused by Climate Change

The climate system is composed of several interconnected subsystems including the **atmosphere**, the **hydrosphere** (rivers, lakes, and oceans), the **cryosphere** (ice and snow), the **lithosphere** (soils), and the **biosphere** (ecosystems). Historically, many factors have influenced the climate such as volcanic activity, atmospheric composition, the earth's orbit around the sun, and solar activity. However, human activities are responsible for approximately 1.0°C of global warming since preindustrial times, according to the Intergovernmental Panel on Climate Change (IPCC) Special Report on warming of 1.5°C and if it continues to increase at the current rate, warming is likely to reach 1.5°C between 2030 and 2052 (IPCC 2018). Yet, increasing temperatures due to anthropogenic activity are only one manifestation; another is the changes to the **hydrologic cycle**, which describes the continuous movement of water on earth (Figure 4.1). The IPCC report concluded that climate change will continue to increase the frequency and intensity of heavy precipitation events globally as well as the risk of droughts (IPCC 2018). The water-holding capacity of the atmosphere is a function of temperature and has been calculated to increase by about 8 percent per degree Celsius (Trenberth 1999). The most important **greenhouse gas** (GHG) in the atmosphere is water vapor, which, although it allows visible light to pass through, will absorb part of the infrared radiation from the earth and thus retain heat in the earth's systems. A warming hydrologic cycle will not only cause increases in temperature but also in evaporation, which enhances the atmospheric moisture content; changes in both the frequency and the intensity of extreme (high and low) precipitation are expected to occur (Semenza 2012). Another manifestation of global climate change is the increasing heat content of the oceans. The capacity of water to absorb heat is approximately twenty times greater than that of the atmosphere (Levitus et al. 2012). The frequency and duration of marine heat waves, characterized by prolonged periods of anomalously high sea surface temperatures, have increased significantly in the last century (Oliver et al. 2018). The hydrology of freshwater quantity and quality is also affected by global climate change. High river flows are projected to increase significantly, specifically in South and Southeast Asia and Central Africa at 1.5°C (2.7°F), with this effect intensifying and including parts of South America at 2°C (3.6°F) (Döll et al. 2018), which has implications for flood hazard. These changes to the hydrologic cycle can affect waterborne diseases because their **environmental exposure**

KEY CONCEPTS

- Early warning systems that rely on environmental or climatic precursors of disease can guide climate change adaptation strategies.

- Vulnerability, impact, and adaptation assessment can improve risk management of water resources and prepare society for changes in the hydrologic cycle such as failures of the water supply.

- Monitoring and reporting of contaminated beaches and enforcing beach closures can reduce illnesses from swimming in contaminated recreational waters.

- Upgrading aging water treatment and distribution systems including improved water filter operations is warranted to cope with extremes of the hydrologic cycle and prevent breakthrough of filters.

- Risk assessments by municipal water providers to help manage heavy precipitation discharge by augmenting sewer system storage capacity or droughts through increasing supplies of drinking water.

- Adjustments of existing surveillance practices for infectious diseases is necessary for monitoring climate change related threats to public health.

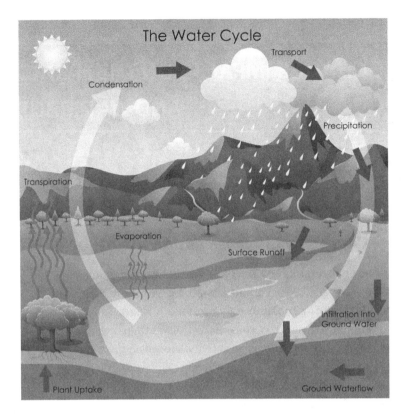

Figure 4.1   As part of the "water cycle" or "hydrologic cycle," water evaporates from the sea and lakes and transpires from vegetation. While the water vapor rises in the atmosphere it cools, condenses, and returns to earth as rain where it enters waterways and starts the cycle again

pathways are intricately linked to local climate and weather conditions (Figure 4.1) (Boxall et al. 2009). Certain waterborne pathogens cannot multiply outside of the human/animal host (e.g., norovirus, *Cryptosporidium*, *Campylobacter*) whereas others can multiply in the environment (e.g., *Vibrio*, *Salmonella*)(Semenza, Herbst et al. 2012). This chapter discusses the **climate change impacts** on the hydrologic cycle and waterborne diseases; it touches on elevated water temperature, precipitation extremes, and flooding and discusses specific waterborne disease in more detail.

Water Temperature

The link between water temperature and *Vibrio* and *Campylobacter* has been extensively investigated in the peer-reviewed literature but much less so for other waterborne pathogens such as *Cryptosporidium*, *Salmonella*, or norovirus (Semenza, Herbst et al. 2012). Elevated river water temperature and lower flow rates during the warmer summer months result in inactivation of certain waterborne pathogens such as norovirus and *Campylobacter* (Table 4.1) (Schijven and de Roda Husman 2005). Conversely, these pathogens can survive longer during the colder winter months, which explains in part the higher concentrations in river water. However, *Listeria*, *Vibrio*, and *Salmonella* concentrations can increase at elevated temperatures, which is of particular concern in marine environments where indigenous *Vibrio* can readily replicate above temperatures of 16°C (Table 4.1) (Semenza et al. 2017).

For example, environmental monitoring of *Campylobacter* from rivers, showed that inactivation was fastest in spring and summer, when temperature and solar radiation were at their highest (Rodriguez and Araujo 2012). Although *Campylobacter* does not readily die off at 4°C

Table 4.1   Climate Change and Waterborne Diseases; Environmental Effects, Pathogen Fate, and Microbial Risk

Climate Change	Effects	Consequences	Microbial Risk
Water temperature increase	Replication of marine bacteria (*Vibrio*)	Bacterial blooms in marine environments	Increased risk
	Dieoff of enteric pathogens (Norovirus, *Campylobacter*, etc.)	Lower concentrations of pathogens in surface water	Decreased risk
	Water purification at the treatment plant more efficient	Elimination of pathogens from drinking water	Decreased risk
	Organic matter/nutrients dissolve better	Challenges for water treatment: less efficient	Increased risk
Extended seasons for agriculture and leisure activities	Altered demand on water treatment plant	Opportunities for exposures (e.g., contamination of irrigation water)	Increased/decreased risk
	Shortened winter season with lower snow cover and reduced flooding due to snow melt	Reduced stress on water treatment plants	Decreased risk
Precipitation increase	Runoff, sediments, organic matter, nutrients	Challenges for water treatment: less efficient	Increased risk
	Peak concentrations of pathogens in surface water	Challenges for water treatment: less efficient	Increased risk
	Flooding of wells or water treatment plants	Water treatment at risk	Increased risk
	Stormwater runoff and combined sewage overflow	Water treatment at risk Recreational water contamination	Increased risk
	Groundwater contamination with fecal pathogens	Water treatment insufficient	Increased risk
Drought	Changes in water sources	Insufficient treatment options	Increased risk
	Concentration of pathogens	Challenges for water treatment: less efficient	Increased risk

Adapted from Schijven and de Roda Husman. (2005).

in water, it is nonetheless very vulnerable to environmental stresses such as freezing, desiccation, elevated temperatures, or exposure to ultraviolet (UV) light (Blaser 2000; Jones 2001). In contrast, concentration of *Vibrio* bacteria increase during times of elevated surface water temperatures and zooplankton blooms (Lipp, Huq, and Colwell 2002). In fact, *Vibrio* bacteria are most abundant in the warmest periods of the year (Urquhart et al. 2016). Peak concentrations are found primarily in the later parts of the summer and early autumn and reveal a direct association with salinity and water temperatures (Semenza et al. 2017). *Vibrio* propagates with mounting surface water temperatures during continued periods of advantageous environmental conditions. The seasonal window was related to water temperatures from 12 to 15°C, up to an optimum of 26°C (Randa, Polz, and Lim 2004). In Israel, infections were significantly associated with elevated temperatures during the preceding month; indeed, in hot climates the minimum temperature is the determining factor contributing to the growth of *Vibrio* (Paz et al. 2007a). Not surprisingly, 78 percent of all infections occur between May and October (Daniels et al. 2000). In diabetics or immunocompromised individuals swimming in contaminated waters with open wounds, infection can lead to severe necrotic ulcers, septicemia, and death (Lindgren et al. 2012).

CLINICAL CORRELATES 4.1 OYSTERS AND MARINE WATER "FLESH-EATING BACTERIA"

Vibrio bacteria can infect open wounds in humans, especially those with diabetes or immunocompromised individuals, recreating in contaminated salt or brackish waters. Although rare, infection may lead to severe necrotic ulcers, septic shock, and death (Lindgren et al. 2012). Most cases occur during the warmer summer months. The number of cases is trending upward and data supports climate-influenced warming water temperatures, increasing water salinity, sea level rise, and changing environmental factors as key influences (Deeb et al. 2018). Traditionally nonendemic areas are reporting an increase in the number of cases of *Vibrio vulnificus* infections in the United States (King et al. 2019). An increase in cases have also been reported following hydrological events like hurricane Katrina with five deaths (Centers for Disease Control and Prevention [CDC] 2005; Liang and Messenger 2018). There are also thousands of cases of vibriosis per year related to consuming undercooked seafood, usually oysters (Froelich and Noble 2016). Symptoms often are a self-limited diarrheal illness, abdominal cramping, nausea, and vomiting making it difficult to capture true impact. The National Shellfish Sanitation Program (NSSP) is a collaboration with the Food and Drug Administration and Interstate Shellfish Sanitation Conference to regulate shellfish for human consumption and reduce risks to health.

Warm water loving *Vibrio* bacteria are on the rise in marine environments causing a diarrheal illness with raw seafood consumption or life-threatening wound infections.

Precipitation

In the scientific literature the effect of precipitation has been studied extensively for *Campylobacter* and *Cryptosporidium* but less so for other waterborne pathogens such as *Vibrio*, norovirus, *Salmonella*, or *Listeria* (Semenza, Herbst et al. 2012). Rain events can flush pathogens from surrounding areas into streams or lakes and contaminate the water source of water treatment plants (Table 4.1). The intensity of such rain events can exceed or simply overwhelm the capacity of the treatment plant and result in water treatment failure. Infiltration of pathogenic *Cryptosporidium* oocysts into drinking water reservoirs poses a technical challenge because the oocysts are resistant to chlorination. Heavy rain events have been associated with a number of waterborne outbreaks in many countries (Guzman Herrador et al. 2015; Guzman Herrador et al. 2016; Semenza and Nichols 2007).

In developing countries, the pathogens involved and the exposure pathways might differ. For example, a number of cholera outbreaks have been associated with heavy rain in developing countries (Camacho et al. 2018; Eisenberg et al. 2013; Finger et al. 2016; Lemaitre et al. 2019). It is important to note that rain can trigger widespread cholera transmission only after the region has already been seeded with the pathogen.

Heavy rain has also been associated with a hepatitis A outbreak in Korea due to contamination of the water source (Lee, Lee, and Kwon, 2008) and with outbreaks of enterovirus infections in Taiwan (Jean et al. 2006). If the sewage collection system simultaneously collects surface runoff in a shared infrastructure, then the surface runoff flow can exceed the capacity of the sewage treatment plant during extreme precipitation events. Thus, large rainstorms can result in **combined sewer overflows** of a toxic sewage-runoff mixture contaminating beaches, shellfish production, and drinking water sources (Figure 4.2). The presence of fecal coliform in drinking water is an indication of water treatment failure and has been linearly associated with rainfall during the preceding day (Richardson et al. 2009). Elevated concentrations of enteric pathogens due to runoff is particularly a problem during the first heavy rain event of the season. Open water reservoirs are at risk for post-treatment contamination during rain events with fecal matter from domestic or wild animals that can shed *Giardia* and *Cryptosporidium*.

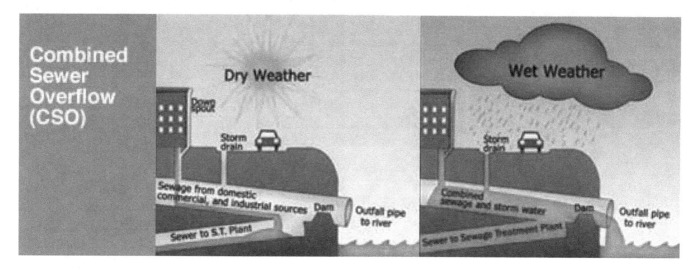

Figure 4.2 Combined sewer overflow
Source: Environmental Protection Agency; http://www.beachapedia.org/File:Cso-ss0-524.jpg

Precipitation events have also been associated with coastal water contamination from surface runoff (Aguilera, Gershunov, and Benmarhnia 2019; Ahmed et al. 2018). Seawater contamination is of particular concern during heavy precipitation events when outfalls from urban stormwater contaminate the beaches (He et al. 2019; Semenza, Herbst et al. 2012).

These storm events can result in runoff and loading of coastal waters with pathogens, nutrients, and toxic chemicals that may adversely affect aquatic life and public health. This is particularly concerning in coastal watersheds where human development and population increases have led to urbanization of coastal areas (Gaffield et al. 2003; Mallin et al., 2000). In southern California, urban runoff affects coastal water quality most significantly during the storm season (Dwight et al. 2002; He and He 2008; Noble et al. 2003). The intensity of storms, a manifestation of global climate change, has been related to greater bacterial concentrations in ocean water at beaches in Santa Monica, California (Ackerman and Weisberg 2003; Schiff, Morton, and Weisberg 2003). **Storm runoff** also carries other pathogens including viruses and parasites, into the coastal waters (Griffin et al. 2003; Schiff et al. 2003). For example, a positive link has been established between measured precipitation and observed coastal water contamination with *Enterococcus* bacteria in southern California (Semenza, Herbst et al. 2012). Exposure to elevated concentrations of bacteria in waters at southern California beaches has been associated with an increased health risk (Dwight et al. 2004; Haile et al. 1999). An estimated 1.4 million enteric and respiratory illnesses occur at these beaches each year as a result of exposure to contaminated water, but surveillance data for this region do not exist (Brinks et al. 2008).

Mathematical climate change models of future precipitation project a decrease in *Enterococcus* levels through most of the twenty-first century (Semenza, Herbst et al. 2012). These findings hold potentially beneficial implications for public health although the variability of storminess might actually increase in southern California in the twenty-first century (California Climate Adaptation Strategy 2009), which calls for innovative adaptation and surveillance strategies (Lindgren et al. 2012).

Droughts

Precipitation extremes include both high and low extremes (Figure 4.3; Semenza, Höser et al. 2012). Interestingly, one study found that in the last century, 10 percent of waterborne disease outbreaks from Wales and England were indeed associated with heavy precipitation, but 20 percent of waterborne outbreaks were actually associated with prolonged periods of low

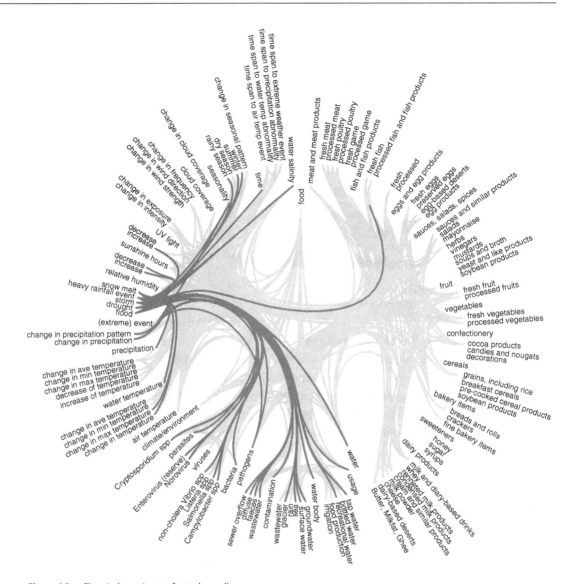

Figure 4.3 Climatic determinants of waterborne diseases
Source: Adapted from Semenza, Höser et al. (2012).

rainfall (Senhorst and Zwolsman 2005). Drought-related health risks were also observed in the Australian Capital Territory (Southeast Australia): cryptosporidiosis was associated with prolonged drought conditions between 2001 and 2009 (Lal and Konings 2018). Increasing droughts in Africa related to climate change are projected to increase the incidence and transmission of *Cryptosporidium, Giardia,* and other protozoa (Ahmed, Guerrero Florez, and Karanis, 2018). Low extremes, that is, prolonged dry periods or droughts, can significantly diminish river discharge and thus augment the concentration of effluent pathogens. River discharge was significantly reduced during the dry summer of 2003, which affected water quality (Senhorst and Zwolsman 2005). Reductions in the rate of water flow can pose problems for the clearance capacity of water treatment plants (Table 4.1) (Senhorst and Zwolsman). Water quality can also be affected by the fact that residues and minerals are more concentrated in dwindling water supplies. Less mobile, disabled, or the elderly might be particularly at risk due to lack of access to safe water. The use of poor-quality water sources due to increased demand can create microbiological threats, such as the use of contaminated irrigation water on crops in the field.

However, water availability may or may not be associated with the microbiological water quality. For example, extended periods of low precipitation levels in more southern latitude countries might also result in reductions in the pathogen load of river water due to longer residence time and higher inactivation of these pathogens. For example, norovirus is inactivated through UV light, drought, or reductions in relative humidity.

Flooding

Heavy precipitation can generate excessive runoff and cause natural disasters such as flooding (Figure 4.3; Semenza 2020). However, flooding can also occur because of river overflow, rapid snow melt, tidal or storm surge, flash flood, tsunami, etc. As society is increasingly interconnected, these interdependencies and vulnerabilities contribute to a cascade effect succeeding a natural disaster where a sequence of events in human subsystems can result in physical, social, or economic disruption (Suk et al. 2019; Semenza 2020). An initial impact from an extreme weather event can trigger a cascading effect with other consequences of significant magnitude, even larger than the initial event. These cascading effects are a function of the magnitude of the existing vulnerabilities rather than of the initial hazard. Thus, even a low-level hazard can generate unexpected secondary events of significant impact if there are widespread vulnerabilities in human subsystems. Climate change adaptation aims to anticipate and address unresolved vulnerabilities in order to avoid the amplification of subsequent and unanticipated public health crises. For example, floods can cause waterborne outbreaks, because of the cascade effects on the diverse risk drivers of infectious diseases that in turn can have disruptive effects on society, including on trade, tourism, and health care provision. Flooding of agricultural land contaminated with waterborne pathogens, poor drainage, and backed-up sewage systems can quickly become a public health emergency (Semenza 2020). The contaminated floodwaters can transport the pathogens to drinking water wells and infiltrate the water distribution system (Table 4.1). Standing water can also become a breeding ground for vector-borne diseases. Floods and increased water flows can lead to contamination of drinking, recreational, irrigation, or drinking water supplies and thus increase the risk of waterborne epidemics (Sinisi and Aertgeerts 2011). Occupational risk cascaded down to the cleanup crew of a flooding event in Denmark where 22 percent of workers suffered from infectious disease, 16 percent visited a doctor, and 7 percent missed a day or more of work as a result (Wojcik et al. 2013).

A number of microbial agents have been associated with floods; these include cholera (Jutla, Khan, and Colwell 2017), cryptosporidiosis (Lal, Fearnley, and Wilford 2019), leptospirosis (Naing et al. 2019); unspecified diarrhea (Heller, Colosimo, and Antunes 2003; Kunii et al. 2002; Mondal, Biswas, and Manna 2001; Zhang et al. 2019), rotavirus (Jones et al. 2016; Masciopinto et al. 2019); and typhoid and paratyphoid (Liu et al. 2018; Vollaard et al. 2004). The majority of these outbreaks due to flooding have occurred in developing countries but have also been observed in developed countries where epidemics followed such natural disasters (Semenza and Menne 2009; Suk et al. 2019).

Waterborne Pathogens Sensitive to Climate Change

Selected waterborne pathogens are discussed here in light of their relationship with climatic conditions. Bacteria (*Campylobacter, Salmonella,* and *Vibrio*), parasites *(Cryptosporidium),* and viruses (norovirus) are discussed next in more detail.

Campylobacter

Campylobacteriosis is caused by thermophilic *Campylobacter,* with *C. jejuni* being the most common species in humans (Blaser 2000). Symptoms include watery, sometimes bloody diarrhea;

abdominal pain; fever; headache; and nausea (Young, Davis, and Dirita 2007). *Campylobacter* are incapable of reproducing outside animal hosts, such as poultry or pigs, and cannot grow in the presence of air. These bacteria are extremely susceptible to a number of environmental stressors, including heat and cold stress, UV light, acidic conditions, etc. *C. jejuni* tends to survive in various biological environments better at 4°C (39°F) than at 25°C (77°F). Lakes, rivers, streams, or other surface water sources can become polluted with *Campylobacter* by defecating wild birds or domestic animals that harbor the bacteria. Humans can be exposed through contaminated food or water but also through exposure to sewage effluent during combined sewer overflows (Murphy, Carroll, and Jordan 2006). Risk factors for campylobacteriosis are a function of age, season, and degree of urbanization (Doorduyn et al. 2010).

Ambient temperature has been associated with the incidence of campylobacteriosis although not consistently (Bi et al. 2008; Djennad et al. 2019; Fleury et al. 2006; Kovats et al. 2005; Lake et al. 2019; Patrick et al. 2004; Sheppard et al. 2009). As noted previously, *Campylobacter* is not capable of reproducing outside of its animal host and the seasonal incidence peak does not occur during the hottest time of the year, which might explain in part the inconsistent findings in the literature. Rain in early spring can also trigger campylobacteriosis outbreaks (Bi et al. 2008; Djennad et al. 2019; Kovats et al. 2005; Lake et al. 2019; Louis et al. 2005). Households with private water sources tend to be more susceptible to contamination during extreme weather events; indeed, outbreaks tend to occur more often in rural areas than in metropolitan areas with a municipal water source (Hearnden et al. 2003; Pebody, Ryan, and Wall 1997). Extreme rainfall events as a result of climate change might therefore augment the risk of surface and ground water contamination. Conversely, in more temperate and southern latitude countries, climate change might increase the reliance on rainwater during dry spells or droughts. If the harvesting of rainwater increases, *Campylobacter* in untreated roof runoff water might contribute to an increased risk of both animal and human disease (Palmer et al. 1983; Savill et al. 2001).

However, in spite of public health interventions to control foodborne illness, the timing and magnitude of campylobacteriosis peaks have remained essentially the same over the past ten years, which indicates that still unidentified drivers are in part responsible for these infections (Djennad et al. 2019; Lake et al. 2019).

CLINICAL CORRELATES 4.2   SUMMER RAIN, FLOODING, WELLS, AND CAMPYLOBACTER

Campylobacter bacteria is one of the most common causes of food and waterborne infections. It usually causes a self-limited diarrheal illness but can have long-term complications including hemolytic uremic syndrome and Guillain-Barré—conditions that affect the blood and neurologic systems, respectively. Infections are seasonally mediated, worse during warmer summer months and with heavy rainfall, and are more severe in young children (Kuhn et al. 2018; Rosenberg et al. 2018). Prevention is through proper hand hygiene, avoiding untreated water consumption, monitoring drinking wells for contamination from septic tanks and livestock, and adequately cooking poultry (CDC 2019a). Drinking water becomes contaminated by waste via several potential routes. During heavy or prolonged rain, wells—especially shallow or old wells—can leak and get contaminated by feces in storm or agricultural runoff or via disrupted sewage systems nearby (CDC 2015).

Campylobacteriosis is a common bacterial cause of diarrheal illness during warmer months that can have long-term health sequelae in young children.

Salmonella

Among all the *Salmonella* species, S. *enterica* is the species that mostly affects humans and causes gastroenteritis, with nausea, vomiting, and diarrhea, six to forty-eight hours after ingestion. Although the disease tends to be self-limited, the elderly and immunocompromised can suffer from bacteremia or endovascular complications (Crum Cianflone 2008). Food is a major source of exposure for humans because *Salmonella* has the ability to persist and reproduce outside of the host (European Food Safety Authority [EFSA] and European Centre for Disease Prevention and Control [ECDC] 2014). The water can become contaminated through fecal pollution by infected individuals but also by other vertebrates, such as birds and reptiles, poultry, cattle, and sheep. Environmental sampling has documented that the bacteria can persist in a dry environment over extended periods of time; it has been recovered from two and a half year old dried excrement (Stine et al. 2005). In wet environments, in soil, and in sediment, *Salmonella* can also survive relatively long and even multiply for up to a year (Winfield and Groisman 2003).

Salmonella usually grows within a temperature range of between 10–47°C (50–116°F), where temperature accelerates the growth rate, but growth at 6–8°C (43–46°F) is still possible. Temperature is a biological determinant, which manifests itself in the highly seasonal incidence of *Salmonella*. An increase in weekly temperatures has been linked with elevated incidence in different countries (Akil, Ahmad, and Reddy 2014; D'Souza et al. 2004; Fleury et al. 2006; Jiang et al. 2015; Kovats et al. 2004; Naumova et al. 2007; Nichols 2010; Uejio 2017; Wang, Goggins, and Chan 2018a; Zhang, Bi, and Hiller 2008). Under climate change scenarios, a warmer world should experience a mounting disease burden. However, *Salmonella* incidence has decreased in many countries over the last few years (EFSA and ECDC 2014). This decrease is in part due to effective public health interventions such as vaccination of animal hosts of culling of infected poultry flocks. It is also possible that the influence of temperature on *Salmonella* incidence has been attenuated by other measures, such as health education and health promotion, which has resulted in a decline of salmonellosis over the years (Lake et al. 2009). Seasonal *Salmonella* concentrations in water environments are related to monthly maximum precipitation in summer and fall following fecal contamination events (Craig, Fallowfield, and Cromar 2003; Martinez-Urtaza et al. 2004). Floods caused by heavy rainfall events may disrupt water treatment and sewage systems and contribute to increased exposure to *Salmonella* and other pathogens (Table 4.1). Thus, effective public health interventions should be able to mitigate adverse impacts of climate change.

Vibrio (noncholera)

Bacteria of the genus *Vibrio* includes several species, the most important being *V. cholerae*, which causes cholera. *V. vulnificus* and *V. parahaemolyticus* are other clinically important species that, unlike *V. cholerae*, are endemic in Europe and the United States and can infect open wounds that can necrotizee and cause septicemia in individuals bathing in marine waters (Semenza et al. 2017). Vibrios are halophytic organisms known to have their natural habitat in the warm waters of coastal areas (Lipp, Huq, and Colwell 2002); their growth is mainly dependent on temperature and salinity (Morris and Kris 2008). Because of higher temperatures the bacteria reach their highest concentrations in summer and early autumn (Lipp et al. 2002); if the environmental conditions are unfavourable for growth and multiplication, *Vibrio* enter a dormant phase. The occurrence of *V. vulnificus* and *V. parahaemolyticus* in the marine environment is clearly associated with the growth of zooplankton, shellfish, and fish. Relatively higher *Vibrio* concentrations are observed in zooplankton than in the surrounding water column (Lipp et al. 2002). In Spain, Vibrios are frequently isolated during red tides (Lipp et al. 2002). An increase in water temperature promotes the growth of *Vibrio*, which become particularly concentrated in shellfish. The largest known outbreak of illness caused by *V. parahaemolyticus* occurred in Alaska in 2004 (McLaughlin et al. 2005). Passengers on a cruise ship ate raw local Alaskan oysters and developed diarrhea. This outbreak demonstrated a change in the spatial distribution of Vibrios and the correlation between *Vibrio* growth and high temperatures. Rising ocean water temperatures allowed the spread of subtropical *Vibrio* to the north. The northernmost documented oyster source contaminated with *V. parahaemolyticus* was immediately extended by 1,000 km (McLaughlin et al. 2005).

In Israel a high number of *V. vulnificus* wound infections and bacteremia were noted during the summer months of 1996, which was the hottest ever recorded in Israel in the previous 40 years (Paz et al. 2007). Infections were significantly correlated with high temperatures during the preceding weeks. It was noted by Paz et al. that in hot climates the minimum temperature is the most important factor contributing to the growth of Vibrios (Paz et al. 2007). During daytime temperature is always higher than 15°C (59°F), so the growth of Vibrios is unlimited. Minimum temperatures occur during the night and if they drop below 15°C the growth of Vibrios will be interrupted.

In the Baltic Sea, notified *V. vulnificus* infections occur during hot summer months and augment with water temperatures above 20°C (68°F) (Baker-Austin et al. 2012; Baker-Austin et al. 2016; Semenza et al. 2017). The Baltic Sea has experienced an unprecedented rate of warming over the last three decades with recent peak temperatures never documented since the inception of instrumental measurements in this region. Simultaneously, Northern Europe witnessed an unexpected emergence of *Vibrio* infections with a clear link between elevated sea surface temperatures during extended summer seasons (Andersson and Ekdahl 2006; Dalsgaard et al. 1996; Frank et al. 2006; Lukinmaa et al. 2006; Ruppert et al. 2004). These open wound infections from recreational water use can necrotize and cause septicemia; in immunocompromised individuals these infections can be fatal (Andersson and Ekdahl 2006; Frank et al. 2006; Lukinmaa et al. 2006). There is strong empirical evidence that anthropogenic climate change drives the emergence of *Vibrio* infections in this region of the world (Baker-Austin et al. 2012; Semenza et al. 2017).

Cryptosporidium

Cryptosporidium is an intestinal parasite that causes watery diarrhea that spontaneously resolves over a couple of weeks in otherwise healthy patients but can be severe and even life threatening in immunocompromised individuals. In humans, the disease is predominantly caused by the two species *C. parvum* and *C. hominis*, although a number of other species are pathogenic for humans (Khan, Shaik, and Grigg 2018). *Cryptosporidium* generates sturdy oocysts that can sustain significant environmental impacts such as chlorine. Once released, the oocysts can survive in moist soil or water for months and remain infectious even under varying temperatures (Jaskiewicz et al. 2018). *Cryptosporidium* oocysts appear to be very widespread in drinking water resources, including rivers, streams, lakes, and reservoirs, being found in most wastewater discharge (Nasser 2016). The small size of *Cryptosporidium* makes their removal by filtration during water and wastewater treatment a difficult task (Nasser 2016). Die-off can be achieved using UV light and dry heat. Chlorine is not an appropriate disinfectant but ozone is more effective in inactivating *Cryptosporidium* oocysts, than chlorine (Nasser 2016).

Over 60 percent of water-related disease outbreaks worldwide from 2011 to 2016 were caused by the parasite *Cryptosporidium* spp. (Efstratiou, Ongerth, and Karanis 2017). Contamination of water supplies and subsequent outbreaks of cryptosporidiosis have been linked to heavy rainfall events (Aksoy et al. 2007; Hoek et al. 2008; Mohammed and Seidu 2019;

Semenza and Nichols 2007; Smith et al. 2006), as the concentration of *Cryptosporidium* oocysts in river water increases significantly during rainfall events. Thus, heavy precipitation can result in persistence of oocysts in the water distribution system and the contamination of drinking water reservoirs from springs and lakes. A rise in precipitation is predicted to lead to an increase in cryptosporidiosis, although the strength of the relationship varies with the kind of climate category (Jagai et al. 2009; Sterk, et al. 2016). As noted previously, dry weather conditions preceding a heavy rain event has also been associated with drinking water outbreaks (Nichols et al. 2009).

CLINICAL CORRELATES 4.3 PARASITIC WATERBORNE WOES

Cryptosporidium is an underdiagnosed intestinal waterborne parasite that causes diarrhea, which can be particularly severe and even life threatening in immunocompromised individuals and children. Common transmission is through drinking water contaminated by feces such as in swimming pools or from person to person, and infection has broad-ranging effects on the health of people around the world (Checkley et al. 2015). Exposed individuals may be asymptomatic whereas others suffer a persistent course of abdominal cramping, fever, nausea, and profuse watery diarrhea. Diarrhea contributes to dehydration, reduced oral intake, and altered absorption of nutrients. Patients with significantly compromised immune system function, classically those with human immunodeficiency virus (HIV) not on antiretroviral therapy, suffer more severe symptoms, wasting, and a prolonged duration of illness (O'Connor et al. 2011). Patients with transplanted organs or receiving treatments for cancer are also often at risk. The environment and public health processes contribute to parasite transmission and human exposure. Basic sanitation, socioeconomic factors (poverty, population densities), seasonality with extreme rainfall events, and climate-related factors have all been implicated in disease transmission and risk (Ahmed, Florez, and Karanis 2018; Lal, Fearnley, and Wilford 2019; Semenza et al. 2012; Young, Smith, and Fazil 2015).

Waterborne parasitic infections can cause severe, life-threatening diarrheal illnesses in children and immunocompromised patients.

Norovirus

Noroviruses cause acute gastroenteritis in humans. Symptoms include projectile vomiting, watery non-bloody diarrhea with abdominal cramps, nausea, myalgia, malaise, and headaches, occasionally also with low-grade fever. Noroviruses are ubiquitous and highly resistant in the environment. They can survive for long periods on different surfaces, at temperatures below 0°C (32°F) and up to 60°C (140°F) and in fluids with up to 10 ppm chlorine. In many surface waters, norovirus can be detected during all seasons (Miura, Gima, and Akiba 2019). Transmission during outbreaks is complex. Often, an initial food or waterborne transmission is followed by secondary person-to-person transmission. Waterborne Norovirus outbreaks are less common but well investigated and are often caused by sewage contamination of wells and groundwater or recreational water (Carrique-Mas et al. 2003; Kauppinen, Pitkanen, and Miettinen 2018; Nygard et al. 2003). Foodborne norovirus outbreaks have been linked to climate and weather events; for example, heavy rainfall has been associated with more norovirus hospitalizations among young children in Hong Kong (Wang, Goggins, and Chan 2018b). In a hotel in Austria, flooding with water contaminated with sewage caused by heavy rainfall, resulted in twenty-six out of thirty-six hotel guests and six out of ten firefighters who assisted in the cleanup falling ill with symptoms of norovirus (Schmid et al. 2005). The magnitude of rainfall has also been related to viral contamination of the marine environment with peaks in diarrhea incidence (Miossec et al. 2000). The predicted increase of heavy rainfall events under climate change scenarios could lead to an increase in norovirus infections, because floods are known to be linked to norovirus outbreaks.

Other infectious diseases

Listeriosis is a serious infection caused by food or drinking water contaminated with the bacterium *Listeria* (Semenza, Herbst et al. 2012). About three to seventy days (average three weeks) after ingestion the infected person suffers from fever, muscle aches, and sometimes gastrointestinal symptoms such as nausea or diarrhea. The only relevant human pathogenic species is *L. monocytogenes*, which is found in soil, surface water, plants, animals, and food. Under optimal conditions the bacteria multiply at temperatures ranging from –0.4°C to +45°C and they are considered as a psychrophilic bacteria capable to multiply in a refrigerator at +4°C (Greifenhagen and Noland 2003). However, growth rates increase at elevated temperatures. During heat waves a breakdown of the cold chain for (processed) food could not only propagate the (re-) growth of *Listeria* but also of other pathogens such as *Clostridium perfringens* and *Staphylococcus aureus.*

Another health concern is the free-living amoeba *Naegleria fowleri* that can cause primary amoebic meningoencephalitis and death (Hara, Yagita, and Sugita 2019). It is often found in warm freshwater environments such as pools, hot springs, lakes, natural mineral water, and resort spas (Heggie 2010). During an unusually hot summer month in 2010 a Minnesota resident, aged seven years, was infected by this amoeba and subsequently died of rapidly progressive meningoencephalitis after local freshwater exposures, with no history of travel outside the state. This local freshwater exposure occurred at much higher latitude than previously described (Kemble et al. 2012). It is possible that hot weather conditions due to climate variability and long-term climate change could affect the distribution and frequency of primary amoebic meningoencephalitis. Algal blooms are likely to become more prevalent in recreational waters under climate change scenarios.

CLINICAL CORRELATES 4.4 BRAIN-EATING AMOEBAS

The free-living amoeba *Naegleria fowleri* can cause primary amoebic meningoencephalitis—a serious brain infection—and is almost universally fatal. It is a rare disease with 143 cases (0–8 per year) documented from 1962 to 2017 (CDC 2019b; Cooper et al. 2019). The parasite lives in warm, untreated freshwater nutrient-rich lakes, ponds, and reservoirs (Yoder et al. 2010). Water enters the noses of recreational water enthusiasts and subsequently migrates to the brain. Death occurs days after symptom onset, which leaves clinicians with a narrow window of opportunity to intervene. Most cases are in warm weather states where sunlight influences parasite prevalence and food sources; however, cases have been reported in northern latitudes such as Minnesota, and there are growing concerns that a warming climate may influence the incidence rates of this deadly disease (Cooper et al.; Yoder et al.). ,

Parasitic amoebas living in warm, nutrient-rich freshwater sources can transmit a rare but serious brain infection sending caution to recreational swimmers in a warming climate.

Community-acquired pneumonia caused by *Legionella pneumophila* has been associated with air conditioners and water systems in buildings, such as water taps, shower heads, and other sources of aerosol (Cunha, Burillo, and Bouza 2016). Wet periods with elevated humidity and temperature have been linked to Legionnaires' disease in several locations (Fisman et al. 2005; Ricketts et al. 2009). Climate change projects a higher frequency, intensity, and duration of heat waves. During periods of excessive heat, the temperature of water in buildings might increase as well as might air conditioner use. Whether this will lead to growth of *L. pneumophila,* and pose a threat to the health of the public has not yet been ruled out.

Vector-borne diseases that are transmitted by insect vectors are also water-related diseases because many insects complete part of their life cycle in water. These insect species include mosquitoes, black flies, and a number of biting midge species that transmit diseases such as dengue, chikungunya, West Nile Fever, malaria, Rift valley fever, or river blindness. The arthropod vectors are subjected to abiotic conditions such as increased temperature, which influences vector capacity, boosts mosquito reproduction rates, prolongs their breeding season but also accelerates virus replication within vectors. Europe has experienced a number of dengue and chikungunya outbreaks in recent years, related to favorable climatic conditions (Lillepold et al. 2019). Moreover, precipitation patterns, floods, and droughts are also important determinants of these diseases. The association of these diseases with climate change is covered in Chapter 8 and has been discussed extensively elsewhere (Semenza and Menne 2009).

Adaptation Strategies

Even in the absence of conclusive evidence, public health practitioners are obliged to address credible risks from climate change through adaptation strategies, particularly for vulnerable populations such as migrants (Semenza 2013; Semenza and Ebi 2019). **Vulnerability**, impact, and adaptation assessment can help prepare society for changes in the hydrologic cycle (ECDC 2010; Semenza, Suk et al. 2012).

A particular problem arises for *Vibrio* (noncholera) infections (discussed previously) because they are not reportable in many parts of the world. In and around the Baltic Sea and the Eastern North Sea area, which is characterized by low salinity, the number of *Vibrio* cases has increased because of a climate change-related upsurge in temperature (Baker-Austin et al. 2012; Semenza et al. 2017). Climate change projections up to 2060 indicate that this upsurge is projected to continue (Semenza et al. 2017). The monthly projection of sea surface temperature (SST) suitability for *Vibrio* in the Baltic Sea is provided in Figure 4.4. A marked upward trend is observed for SST during July, August, and September but even more so during the months immediately before and after the summer (June and October). Periods of reported infections are closely associated with areas of maximum warming of the Baltic Sea and a highly significant statistical association was found between the annual number of human cases and mean summer SST increase (Semenza et al. 2017). Can forecasts of SST be used as climatic precursors of these *Vibrio* infections as part of an **early warning system** for climate change

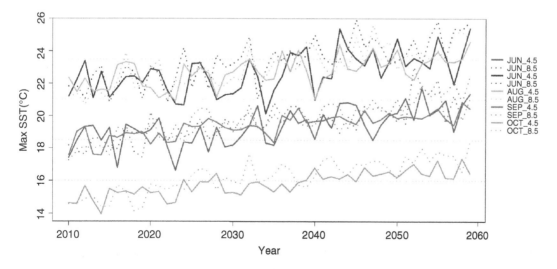

Figure 4.4   Suitability for *Vibrio* based on SST in the Baltic Sea for RCP 4.5 and RCP 8.5, from 2010 until 2058, by month
Source: Semenza et al. (2017).

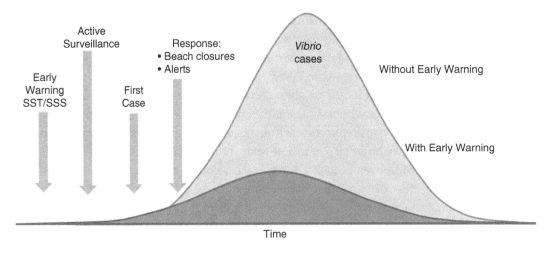

Figure 4.5   Early warning system for *Vibrio*: Environmental monitoring of sea surface temperature (SST) and salinity (SSS)
Source: Adapted from Semenza (2020).

adaptation? Early detection and response to climate change-sensitive pathogens can reduce the burden of disease as opposed to passive surveillance systems (Morin et al. 2018). However, it relies on the monitoring of SST and other environmental conditions (e.g., salinity) at scales useful for implementation of interventions, timely sharing of the information with public health professionals, and performing of continuous evaluation of this interconnected system to maximize its efficiency and improve its efficacy (Figure 4.5).

A suitability model was developed, using SST and salinity to estimate the environmental suitability for *Vibrio* spp. in coastal waters (Baker-Austin et al. 2012; Semenza et al. 2017). The output of the model defines coastal areas with climatic and environmental conditions suitable for the occurrence of human pathogenic *Vibrio* species that can propagate the emergence of infections. ECDC developed the ECDC Vibrio Map Viewer as an early warning system for public health (ECDC 2019). It is intended to help reduce human exposure to *Vibrio* bacteria in coastal waters and consequently reduce the disease burden from *Vibrio* infections (Semenza et al. 2017). By using SST records from earth observations, the influence of recent warming trends on the emergence and dynamics of vibriosis in the Baltic could be assessed (Ebi et al. 2017; Semenza et al. 2017). The assessment analyzed epidemiological data together with long-term SST records and shorter-term data from the National Oceanic and Atmospheric Administration (NOAA) that integrates satellite SST retrieval (Semenza et al. 2017). The ECDC Vibrio Map Viewer from the European Environment and Epidemiology (E3) network has provided environmental suitability maps of *Vibrio* spp. through the E3 Geoportal since 2013 (ECDC 2019). The ECDC Vibrio Map Viewer provides global environmental suitability maps for *Vibrio* spp. that are based on a real-time model that has been calibrated to the Baltic Region in Northern Europe (Semenza et al. 2017). It uses daily updated remote sensing data to provide information about environmentally suitable conditions such as salinity and SST for *Vibrio* spp. However, the model can also be used and calibrated for any other region of the world.

At ECDC, the epidemic intelligence team monitors the Vibrio Map Viewer on a daily basis during the summer months in order to identify coastal areas with increased environmental suitability. The monitoring findings are reported biweekly in the ECDC Communicable Disease Threats Report (CDTR), which is distributed to national state epidemiologists in Europe. The CDTR also presents options for public health prevention and control actions. For example, these might include beach closures, issuing alerts when the environmental suitability of *Vibrio* infections is predicted to increase, notifying health care providers, and encouraging

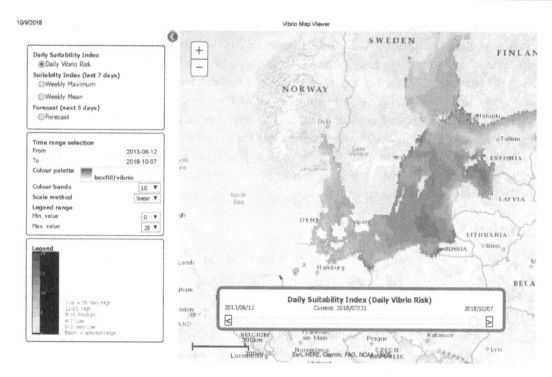

Figure 4.6   Sample display of the daily *Vibrio* risk map viewer provided by the ECDC Vibrio Map Viewer from the European Environment and Epidemiology (E3) Network for the Baltic Sea on July 31, 2018

Source: European Centre for Disease Prevention and Control, https://e3geoportal.ecdc.europa.eu/SitePages/Home.aspx.

Note: Areas depicted in dark grey indicate high to very high risk and areas in light grey indicate low to very low risk.

at-risk individuals (e.g., children, the elderly, cancer patients, and immune-compromised individuals) to avoid exposure to *Vibrio* bacteria through recreational water use. Delineating areas of environmental suitability for *Vibrio* bacteria in the near future can inform public health decision-making. For example, in 2018, the model detected a significant increase in the geographic extent of environmental suitability for *Vibrio* bacteria in coastal areas of the Baltic Sea and the Gulf of Bothnia, both daily and forecasted values (Figure 4.6). This was linked to abnormally high temperatures and drought conditions in several countries around the Baltic Sea. At the beginning of August 2018, ECDC sent a notice to state epidemiologists around the Baltic Sea through the Epidemic Intelligence Information System for Food-and Waterborne Diseases and Zoonoses (EPIS FWD), alerting them to the possibility of an increase in *Vibrio* cases.

Other adaptation strategies include augmenting sewer system storage capacity to minimize wet weather discharges (David and Matos 2005). Storage and advanced physical-chemical treatment of stormwater could significantly reduce overflow volumes. Even though settling in sedimentation tanks would reduce the overflow, microorganism concentrations could nevertheless remain high, which could potentially be treated with UV disinfection (Soyeux, Blanchet, and Tisserand 2007). Holding tanks for stormwater, water diversion, levees, reservoirs, dikes, or mechanical barriers are all measures that need to be reconsidered under the changing circumstances of climate change. They need to be judiciously applied because many of these measures are mutually exclusive. For example, a drinking water reservoir cannot simultaneously act as a stormwater holding tank; they are supposed to be either full or empty, respectively, in order to be functional.

The challenges outlined in this chapter call for a number of adaptation interventions such as higher water quality standards, prudent use of desalination, grey water reclamation, but also greater public outreach and education campaigns. Moreover, monitoring meteorologic conditions and epidemiologic intelligence will increasingly be part of public health practice aiming to protect the health of the public (Semenza 2013). **Climate change impacts** on the hydrologic cycle and waterborne diseases calls for adjustments to existing surveillance practices (Lindgren et al. 2012). For example, enhanced collaboration between surveillance for human cases of *Vibrio* and laboratory monitoring of bivalve shellfish could prevent *Vibrio* outbreaks caused by seafood consumption. Climate change adaptation strategies should be designed to enhance public health preparedness and facilitate the response to emerging threats from waterborne diseases and thereby help contain human and economic costs. Society will have to accept these adaptive strategies to mitigate the negative consequences of the anticipated extremes of the hydrologic cycle.

Summary

Rising mean temperatures, heat waves, drought, sea level rise or flooding from extremes of the hydrologic cycle—the continuous movement of water on earth—are some of the manifestations of global climate change. Moreover, an increase in ambient temperature augments the water-holding capacity of the atmosphere, which affects the hydrologic cycle. The most significant greenhouse gas in the atmosphere is in fact water vapor, which lets visible light pass through but absorbs part of the infrared radiation from the earth and thus retains heat. This perpetual cycle not only increases temperature but also accelerates evaporation and thus enhances the atmospheric moisture content. The consequences of climate change therefore also include changes in the frequency, intensity, duration, and variability of extreme (high and low) precipitation events.

Precipitation events have been associated with an increase in the incidence of waterborne diseases, in the majority of epidemiological studies, throughout the world. During such precipitation events, waterborne parasites such as *Cryptosporidium* can infiltrate the water treatment plant and persist in the water distribution system because of the resistance of *Cryptosporidium* oocysts to chlorine disinfection. Buildup and accumulation of pathogens in the environment during drought conditions can exacerbate the impact of subsequent rain events.

An increase in ambient temperature has also been associated epidemiologically with a rise in the incidence of *Salmonella*. In contrast, the association with *Campylobacter* is not as well understood because in some countries campylobacteriosis incidence peaks before the ambient temperature reaches a high and in some countries after. In warm marine waters with low salinity, such as in the Baltic Sea or Chesapeake Bay, pathogenic *Vibrio* bacteria thrive and *Vibrio* infections in humans spike during hot summer months if the water temperature surpasses 18°C (64°F).

The meteorologic ability of forecasting weather conditions has improved significantly and can now be harnessed for public health practice. Early warning systems can monitor meteorologic conditions and predict heavy rain events or a rise in sea surface temperature in coastal waters. Essential to such an early warning system is an exposure-response relationship in order to compute the epidemic risk based on meteorologil conditions. Once a threshold for meteorologic conditions is predicted to be exceeded, active surveillance can be established and infected individuals can be identified. These alerts can also trigger interventions, such as temporary beach closures for public safety purposes or information for health care providers and at-risk populations about how to avoid exposure. Climate change adaptation entails intercepting the cascading risks from climate change and early warning systems can help to minimize the impact on public health.

Discussion Questions

1. Describe climate change impacts on the hydrologic cycle and the associated health risks.

2. Name vulnerable groups who are most at risk for experiencing negative health outcomes from climate change impacts on the hydrologic cycle and explain why.

3. Describe how early warning systems can protect population health from climate change impacts on the hydrologic cycle.

4. Discuss the cascading effects of extreme weather events and how climate change adaptation can prevent them.

Key Terms

Atmosphere: The gaseous envelope of a planet such as Earth.

Biosphere: The regions of a planet in which life can exist.

Climate change impact: Any of a number of effects of the long-term variation in average weather conditions occurring across the globe.

Combined sewer overflow: The untreated and partially treated human and industrial waste, toxic materials, stormwater, and debris that exceed the holding capacity of the sewer system. Resulting runoff pollutes nearby and downstream rivers, streams, and other bodies of water.

Cryosphere: The frozen water parts of a planet such as Earth.

Early warning system: Predictive modeling tool used by epidemiologists, meteorologists, and others to anticipate environmental hazards such as heat waves and hurricanes. Early warning systems are also being developed to predict occurrences and health impacts of vector-borne and foodborne infections.

Environmental exposure pathways: The physical course taken by hazardous substances from point of origin through human contact.

Global climate change: The long-term variation in average weather conditions that occur across the globe.

Hydrologic cycle: The sequence of conditions through which water passes, from vapor to precipitation in the form of liquids and solids then back to vapor through the process of evaporation and transpiration.

Hydrosphere: The solid, liquid, and gaseous water parts of a planet such as Earth.

Lithosphere: The rocky, outer part of the Earth.

Storm runoff: Rainfall and snowmelt that flows across impervious surfaces.

Vulnerability: The Intergovernmental Panel on Climate Change defines vulnerability as the degree to which a system is susceptible to, or unable to cope with, adverse effects of climate change, including climate variability and extremes. Vulnerability is a function of the character, magnitude, and rate of climate variation to which a system is exposed, its sensitivity, and its adaptive capacity.

Acknowledgment

I would like to acknowledge my collaborators, without whom none of this work would have been possible; in particular, Jonathan Suk, Bertrand Sudre, Tolu Oni, and Massimiliano Rossi at ECDC. The work on the knowledge base was performed with Christoph Höser, Andrea Rechenburg, Susanne Herbst, and Thomas Kistemann at the University of Bonn. ECDC Vibrio Map Viewer was developed with Joacim Rocklöv, Joaquin Trinanes, Bertrand Sudre, and Jaime Martinez Urtaza. The adaptation handbook was developed with Elisabet Lindgren and Kris Ebi at Karolinska Institutet and University of Washington, respectively.

Online Resources

European Centre for Disease Prevention and Control: Climate Change, https://www.ecdc.europa.eu/en/climate-change

Intergovernmental Panel on Climate Change, http://www.ipcc.ch/

UK Government: Flooding: Health Guidance and Advice, http://www.hpa.org.uk/Topics/EmergencyResponse/ExtremeWeatherEventsAndNaturalDisasters/EffectsOfFlooding/

UK Government: Climate Change: Health Effects in the UK, http://www.hpa.org.uk/hecc2012

Centers for Disease Control and Prevention Climate and Health Program, http://www.cdc.gov/climateandhealth/default.htm

European Environment Agency: Climate Change Migration, http://www.eea.europa.eu/themes/climate

NRDC: Global Warming 101, http://www.nrdc.org/globalwarming/

References

Ackerman, D., and S. Weisberg. 2003. "Relationship between Rainfall and Beach Bacterial Concentrations on Santa Monica Bay Beaches." *Journal of Water and Health* 1 (2):85–89.

Aguilera, R., A. Gershunov, and T. Benmarhnia. 2019. "Atmospheric Rivers Impact California's Coastal Water Quality via Extreme Precipitation." *Science of the Total Environment* 671:488–94. doi:10.1016/j.scitotenv.2019.03.318

Ahmed, S. A., M. Guerrero Florez, and P. Karanis. 2018a. "The Impact of Water Crises and Climate Changes on the Transmission of Protozoan Parasites in Africa." *Pathogens and Global Health* 112 (6):281–93. doi:10.1080/20477724.2018.1523778.

Ahmed, W., Q. Zhang, A. Lobos, J. Senkbeil, M. J. Sadowsky, V. J. Harwood, N. Saeidi, O. Marinoni, and S. Ishii. 2018b. "Precipitation Influences Pathogenic Bacteria and Antibiotic Resistance Gene Abundance in Storm Drain Outfalls in Coastal Sub-Tropical Waters." *Environment International* 116:308–18. doi:10.1016/j.envint.2018.04.005

Akil, L., H. A. Ahmad, and R. S. Reddy. 2014. "Effects of Climate Change on Salmonella Infections." *Foodborne Pathogens and Disease* 11 (12):974–80. doi:10.1089/fpd.2014.1802.

Aksoy, U., C. Akisu, S. Sahin, S. Usluca, G. Yalcin, F. Kuralay, and A. M. Oral. 2007. "First Reported Waterborne Outbreak of Cryptosporidiosis with Cyclospora Co-Infection in Turkey." *Eurosurveillance* 12 (7). https://doi.org/10.2807/esw.12.07.03142-en.

Andersson, Y., and K. Ekdahl. 2006. "Wound Infections due to Vibrio Cholerae in Sweden after Swimming in the Baltic Sea, Summer 2006." *Eurosurveillance* 11 (8):E060803.2.

Baker-Austin, C., J. A. Trinanes, S. Salmenlinna, M. Lofdahl, A. Siitonen, N. G. Taylor, and J. Martinez-Urtaza. 2016. "Heat Wave-Associated Vibriosis, Sweden and Finland, 2014." *Emerging Infectious Diseases* 22 (7):1216–20. doi:10.3201/eid2207.151996.

Baker-Austin, C., J. Trinanes, N. Taylor, R. Hartnell, A. Siitonen, and J. Martinez-Urtaza. 2012. "Emerging Vibrio Risk at High Latitudes in Response to Ocean Warming." *Nature Climate Change* 13:73–77. doi:doi:10.1038/nclimate1628

Bi, P., A. Cameron, Y. Zhang, and K. Parton. 2008. "Weather and Notified Campylobacter Infections in Temperate and Sub-Tropical Regions of Australia: An Ecological Study." *Journal of Infection* 57 (4):317–23.

Blaser, M. J. 2000. *Campylobacter jejuni and Related Species*, 5th ed. Philadelphia, PA: Churchill Livingstone.

Boxall, A. B., A. Hardy, S. Beulke, T. Boucard, L. Burgin, P. D. Falloon, P. M. Haygarth et al. 2009. "Impacts of Climate Change on Indirect Human Exposure to Pathogens and Chemicals from Agriculture." *Environmental Health Perspectives* 117 (4):508–14. doi:10.1289/ehp.0800084 [doi].

Brinks, M., R. Dwight, N. Osgood, G. Sharavanakumar, D. Turbow, M. El-Gohary, J. S. Caplan et al. 2008. "Health Risk of Bathing in Southern California Coastal Waters." *Archives of Environmental and Occupational Health* 63 (3):123–35.

California Climate Adaptation Strategy. 2009. *A Report to the Governor of the State of California in Response to Executive Order S-13-2008*. Sacramento: California Natural Resources Agency.

Camacho, A., M. Bouhenia, R. Alyusfi, A. Alkohlani, M. A. M. Naji, X. de Radigues, A. M. Abubakar et al. 2018. "Cholera Epidemic in Yemen, 2016–18: An Analysis of Surveillance Data." *Lancet Global Health* 6 (6):e680–e690. doi:10.1016/s2214-109x(18)30230-4.

Carrique-Mas, J., Y. Andersson, B. Petersen, K. O. Hedlund, N. Sjogren, and J. Giesecke. 2003. "A Norwalk-Like Virus Waterborne Community Outbreak in a Swedish Village During Peak Holiday Season." *Epidemiology and Infection* 131 (1):737–44.

Centers for Disease Control and Prevention. 2005. "Vibrio Illnesses after Hurricane Katrina—Multiple States, August–September 2005." *MMWR. Morbidity and Mortality Weekly Report* 54:928–31.

Centers for Disease Control and Prevention. 2015. "Drinking Water: Campylobacter." https://www.cdc.gov/healthywater/drinking/private/wells/disease/campylobacter.html.

Centers for Disease Control and Prevention. 2019a. "*Campylobacter* (Campylobacteriosis) Prevention." https://www.cdc.gov/campylobacter/prevention.html.

Centers for Disease Control and Prevention. 2019b. "*Naegleria fowleri*: Case report data & graphs." https://www.cdc.gov/parasites/naegleria/graphs.html.

Checkley, W., A. C. White, D. Jaganath, M. J. Arrowood, R. M. Chalmers, X.-M. Chen, R. Fayer, et al. 2015. "A Review of the Global Burden, Novel Diagnostics, Therapeutics, and Vaccine Targets for Cryptosporidium." *Lancet Infectious Diseases* 15 (1):85–94.

Cooper, A. M., S, Aouthmany, K, Shah, and P. P. Rega. 2019. "Killer Amoebas: Primary Amoebic Meningoencephalitis in a Changing Climate." *JAAPA* 32 (6):30–35.

Craig, D., H. Fallowfield, and N. Cromar. 2003. "Effectiveness of Guideline Faecal Indicator Organism Values in Estimation of Exposure Risk at Recreational Coastal Sites." *Water Science and Technology* 47 (3):191–98.

Crum Cianflone, N. F. 2008. "Salmonellosis and the GI Tract: More than Just Peanut Butter." *Current Gastroenterology Reports* 10:424–31.

Cunha, B. A., A. Burillo, and E. Bouza. 2016. "Legionnaires' Disease." *Lancet* 387 (10016):376–85. doi:10.1016/s0140-6736(15)60078-2.

D'Souza, R., N. Becker, G. Hall, and K. Moodie. 2004. "Does Ambient Temperature Affect Foodborne Disease? *Epidemiology* 15 (1):86–92.

Dalsgaard, A., N. Frimodt-Møller, B. Bruun, L. Høi, and J. L. Larsen. 1996. "Clinical Manifestations and Molecular Epidemiology of Vibrio Vulnificus Infections in Denmark." *European Journal of Clinical Microbiology & Infectious Diseases* 15 (3):227–32.

Daniels, N. A., B. Ray, A. Easton, N. Marano, E. Kahn, A. L. I. McShan, L. Del Rosario et al. 2000. "Emergence of a New Vibrio Parahaemolyticus Serotype in Raw Oysters: A Prevention Quandary." *JAMA* 284:1541–45.

David, L. M., and J. S. Matos. 2005. "Combined Sewer Overflow Emissions to Bathing Waters in Portugal. How to Reduce in Densely Urbanised Areas?" *Water Science and Technology* 52 (9):183–90.

Deeb, R., D. Tufford, G. I. Scott, J. G. Moore, and K. Dow. 2018. "Impact of Climate Change on Vibrio Vulnificus Abundance and Exposure Risk." *Estuaries and Coasts* 41 (8):2289–2303.

Djennad, A., G. Lo Iacono, C. Sarran, C. Lane, R. Elson, C. Höser, I. R. Lake et al. 2019. "Seasonality and the Effects of Weather on Campylobacter Infections." *BMC Infectious Diseases* 19 (1):255. doi:10.1186/s12879-019-3840-7.

Döll, P., T. Trautmann, D. Gerten, H. Muller Schmied, S. Ostberg, F. Saaed, and C. F. Schleussner. 2018. "Risks for the Global Freshwater System at 1.5°C and 2°C Global Warming." *Environmental Research Letters* 13(044038).

Doorduyn, Y., W. E. Van Den Brandhof, Y. T. Van Duynhoven, B. J. Breukink, J. A. Wagenaar, and W. Van Pelt. 2010. "Risk Factors for Indigenous Campylobacter Jejuni and Campylobacter Coli Infections in the Netherlands: A Case-Control Study." *Epidemiology and Infection* 138 (10):1391–1404.

Dwight, R., J. Semenza, D. Baker, and B. Olson. 2002. "Association of Urban Runoff with Coastal Water Quality in Orange County, California." *Water Environment Research* 74:82–89.

Dwight, R. H., D. B. Baker, J. C. Semenza, and B. H. Olson. 2004. "Health Effects Associated with Recreational Coastal Water Use in Urban Vs. Rural California." *American Journal of Public Health* 94 (4):565–7.

Ebi, K. L., N. H. Ogden, J. C. Semenza, and A. Woodward. 2017. "Detecting and Attributing Health Burdens to Climate Change." *Environmental Health Perspectives.* 125 (8):085004. doi:10.1289/EHP1509.

Efstratiou, A., J. E. Ongerth, and P. Karanis. 2017. "Waterborne Transmission of Protozoan Parasites: Review of Worldwide Outbreaks—An Update 2011–2016." *Water Research* 114:14–22. doi:10.1016/j.watres.2017.01.036.

Eisenberg, M. C., G. Kujbida, A. R. Tuite, D. N. Fisman, and J. H. Tien. 2013. "Examining Rainfall and Cholera Dynamics in Haiti Using Statistical and Dynamic Modeling Approaches." *Epidemics* 5 (4):197–207. doi:10.1016/j.epidem.2013.09.004.

European Centre for Disease Prevention and Control. 2010. *Climate Change and Communicable Diseases in the EU Member Countries. Handbook for National Vulnerability, Impact and Adaptation Assessments.* Stockholm: ECDC. https://www.ecdc.europa.eu/en/publications-data/climate-change-and-communicable-diseases-eu-member-states.

European Centre for Disease Prevention and Control. 2019. *ECDC Vibrio Map Viewer from the European Environment and Epidemiology (E3) Network.* https://e3geoportal.ecdc.europa.eu/SitePages/Home.aspx.

European Food Safety Authority and European Centre for Disease Prevention and Control. 2014. "The European Union Summary Report on Trends and Sources of Zoonoses, Zoonotic Agents and Food-borne Outbreaks in 2012." *EFSA Journal* 12 (2)(3547): 312. doi:10.2903/j.efsa.2014.3547.

Finger, F., T. Genolet, L. Mari, G. C. de Magny, N. M. Manga, A. Rinaldo, and E. Bertuzzo. 2016. "Mobile Phone Data Highlights the Role of Mass Gatherings in the Spreading of Cholera Outbreaks." *Proceedings of the National Academy of Sciences of the USA* 113 (23):6421–26. doi:10.1073/pnas.1522305113.

Fisman, D. N., S. Lim, G. A. Wellenius, C. Johnson, P. Britz, M. Gaskins, J. Maher et al. 2005. "It's Not the Heat, It's the Humidity: Wet Weather Increases Legionellosis Risk in the Greater Philadelphia Metropolitan Area." *Journal of Infectious Diseases* 192 (12):2066–73.

Fleury, M., D. F. Charron, J. D. Holt, O. B. Allen, and A. R. Maarouf. 2006. "A Time Series Analysis of the Relationship of Ambient Temperature and Common Bacterial Enteric Infections in Two Canadian Provinces." *International Journal of Biometeorology* 50 (6):385–91.

Frank, C., M. Littman, K. Alpers, and J. Hallauer. 2006. "Vibrio Vulnificus Wound Infections after Contact with the Baltic Sea, Germany." *Eurosurveillance* 11(8:E060817.1.).

Froelich, B. A., and R. T. Noble. 2016. "Vibrio Bacteria in Raw Oysters: Managing Risks to Human Health." *Philosophical Transactions of the Royal Society of London. Series B, Biological Sciences* 371 (1689):20150209. doi:10.1098/rstb.2015.0209.

Gaffield, S., R. Goo, L. Richards, and R. Jackson. 2003. "Public Health Effects of Inadequately Managed Stormwater Runoff." *American Journal of Public Health* 93 (9):1527–33.

Greifenhagen, S., and T. L. Noland. 2003. *A Synopsis of Known and Potential Diseases and Parasites Associated with Climate Change.* Forest Research Information Paper 154. Sault Ste. Marie, ON: Ontario Forest Research Institute. https://collections.ola.org/mon/31011/232549.pdf.

Griffin, D., K. Donaldson, J. Paul, and J. Rose. 2003. "Pathogenic Human Viruses in Coastal Waters." *Clinical Microbiology Reviews* 16:129–43.

Guzman Herrador, B., B. F. de Blasio, A. Carlander, S. Ethelberg, H. O. Hygen, M. Kuusi, V. Lund et al. 2016. "Association between Heavy Precipitation Events and Waterborne Outbreaks in Four Nordic Countries, 1992–2012." *Journal of Water and Health* 14 (6):1019–27. doi:10.2166/wh.2016.071.

Guzman Herrador, B. R., B. F. de Blasio, E. MacDonald, G. Nichols, B. Sudre, L. Vold, J. C. Semenza, and K. Nygard. 2015. "Analytical Studies Assessing the Association between Extreme Precipitation or Temperature and Drinking Water-Related Waterborne Infections: A Review." *Environmental Health* 14:29. doi:10.1186/s12940-015-0014-y.

Haile, R., J. Witte, M. Gold, R. Cressey, C. McGee, R. Millikan, A. Glasser et al. 1999. "The Health Effects of Swimming in Ocean Water Contaminated by Storm Drain Runoff." *Epidemiology* 10 (4):355–63.

Hara, T., K. Yagita, and Y. Sugita. 2019. "Pathogenic Free-Living Amoebic Encephalitis in Japan." *Neuropathology* 39 (4):251–58. doi:10.1111/neup.12582.

He, L., and Z. He. 2008. "Water Quality Prediction of Marine Recreational Beaches Receiving Watershed Baseflow and Stormwater Runoff in Southern California, USA." *Water Research* 42 (10–11):2563–73.

He, Y., Y. He, B Sen, H. Li, J. Li, Y. Zhang, J. Zhang, S. C. Jiang, and G. Wang. 2019. "Storm Runoff Differentially Influences the Nutrient Concentrations and Microbial Contamination at Two Distinct Beaches in Northern China." *Science of the Total Environment* 663:400–7. doi:10.1016/j. scitotenv.2019.01.369.

Hearnden, M., C. Skelly, R. Eyles, and P. Weinstein. 2003. "The Regionality of Campylobacteriosis Seasonality in New Zealand." *International Journal of Environmental Research and Public Health* 13 (4):337–48.

Heggie, T. 2010. "Swimming with Death: *Naegleria fowleri* Infections in Recreational Waters." *Travel Medicine and Infectious Disease* 8 (4):201–6.

Heller, L., E. Colosimo, and C. Antunes. 2003. "Environmental Sanitation Conditions and Health Impact: A Case-Control Study." *Revista da Sociedade Brasileira de Medicina Tropical* 36 (1):41–50.

Hoek, M. R., I. Oliver, M. Barlow, L. Heard, R. Chalmers, and S. Paynter. 2008. "Outbreak of Cryptosporidium Parvum among Children after a School Excursion to an Adventure Farm, South West England." *Journal of Water and Health* 6 (3):333–38.

Intergovernmental Panel on Climate Change. 2018. "Summary for Policymakers." In *Global Warming of 1.5°C. An IPCC Special Report on the Impacts of Global Warming of 1.5°C above Pre-Industrial Levels and Related Global Greenhouse Gas Emission Pathways, in the Context of Strengthening the Global Response to the Threat of Climate Change, Sustainable Development, and Efforts to Eradicate Poverty,* 3–24. Geneva: IPCC. https://www.ipcc.ch/sr15/.

Jagai, J. S., D. A. Castronovo, J. Monchak, and E. N. Naumova. 2009. "Seasonality of Cryptosporidiosis: A Meta-Analysis Approach." *Environmental Research* 109 (4):465–78.

Jaskiewicz, J. J., Sandlin, R. D., Swei, A. A., Widmer, G., Toner, M., and Tzipori, S. (2018). "Cryopreservation of Infectious *Cryptosporidium parvum* Oocysts." *Nature Communications* 9 (1):2883. doi:10.1038/s41467-018-05240-2.

Jean, J., Guo, H., Chen, S., Liu, C., Chang, W., Yang, Y., and Huang, M. (2006). "The association between Rainfall Rate and Occurrence of an Enterovirus Epidemic due to a Contaminated Well." *Journal of Applied Microbiology* 101(6):1224–31.

Jiang, C., K. S. Shaw, C. R. Upperman, D. Blythe, C. Mitchell, R. Murtugudde, A. R. Sapkota, and A. Sapkota. 2015. "Climate Change, Extreme Events and Increased Risk of Salmonellosis in Maryland, USA: Evidence for Coastal Vulnerability." *Environment International* 83:58–62. doi:10.1016/j. envint.2015.06.006.

Jones, F. K., A. I. Ko, C. Becha, C. Joshua, J. Musto, S. Thomas, A. Ronsse et al. 2016. "Increased Rotavirus Prevalence in Diarrheal Outbreak Precipitated by Localized Flooding, Solomon Islands, 2014." *Emerging Infectious Diseases* 22 (5):875–79. doi:10.3201/eid2205.151743.

Jones, K. 2001. "Campylobacters in Water, Sewage and the Environment." *Symposium Series (Society for Applied Microbiology* 30:68S–79S.

Jutla, A., R. Khan, and R. Colwell. 2017. "Natural Disasters and Cholera Outbreaks: Current Understanding and Future Outlook." *Current Environmental Health Reports* 4 (1):99–107. doi:10.1007/s40572-017-0132-5.

Kauppinen, A., T. Pitkanen, I. T. and Miettinen. 2018. "Persistent Norovirus Contamination of Groundwater Supplies in Two Waterborne Outbreaks." *Food and Environmental Virology* 10 (1):39–50. doi:10.1007/s12560-017-9320-6.

Kemble, S., R. Lynfield, A. DeVries, D. Drehner, W. Pomputius, M. Beach, G. S. Visvesvara et al. 2012. "Fatal *Naegleria fowleri* Infection Acquired in Minnesota: Possible Expanded Range of a Deadly Thermophilic Organism." *Clinical Infectious Diseases* 54 (6):805–09.

Khan, A., J. S. Shaik, and M. E. Grigg. 2018. "Genomics and Molecular Epidemiology of Cryptosporidium Species." *Acta Tropica* 184:1–14. doi:10.1016/j.actatropica.2017.10.023.

King, M., L. Rose, H. Fraimow, M. Nagori, M. Danish, and K. Doktor. 2019. "*Vibrio vulnificus* Infections from a Previously Nonendemic Area." *Annals of Internal Medicine* 171 (7):520–21.

Kovats, R., S. Edwards, D. Charron, J. Cowden, R. D'Souza, K. L. Ebi, C. Gauci et al. 2005. "Climate Variability and Campylobacter Infection: An International Study." *International Journal of Biometeorology* 49 (4):207–14.

Kovats, R., S. Edwards, S. Hajat, B. Armstrong, K. Ebi, and B. Menne. 2004. "The Effect of Temperature on Food Poisoning: A Time-Series Analysis of Salmonellosis in Ten European Countries." *Epidemiology and Infection* 132 (3):443–53.

Kuhn, K., E. Nielsen, K. Molbak, and S. Ethelberg. 2018. "Epidemiology of Campylobacteriosis in Denmark 2000–2015." *Zoonoses and Public Health* 65:59–66.

Kunii, O., S. Nakamura, R. Abdur, and S. Waka. 2002. "The Impact on Health and Risk Factors of the Diarrhoea Epidemics in the 1998 Bangladesh Floods." *Public Health* 116 (2):68–74.

Lake, I. R., F. J. Colon-Gonzalez, J. Takkinen, M. Rossi, B. Sudre, J. G. Dias, L. Tavoshi et al. 2019. Exploring "Campylobacter Seasonality across Europe Using the European Surveillance System (TESSy), 2008 to 2016." *Eurosurveillance* 24 (13). doi:10.2807/1560-7917.es.2019.24.13.180028.

Lake, I. R., I. A. Gillespie, G. Bentham, G. L. Nichols, C. Lane, G. K. Adak, and E. J. Threlfall. 2009. "A Reevaluation of the Impact of Temperature and Climate Change on Foodborne Illness." *Epidemiology and Infection* 137 (11):1538–47.

Lal, A., E. Fearnley, and E. Wilford. 2019. "Local Weather, Flooding History and Childhood Diarrhoea Caused by the Parasite *Cryptosporidium* spp.: A Systematic Review and Meta-Analysis." *Science of the Total Environment* 674:300–6. doi:10.1016/j.scitotenv.2019.02.365.

Lal, A., and P. Konings. 2018. "Beyond Reasonable Drought: Hotspots Reveal a Link between the 'Big Dry' and Cryptosporidiosis in Australia's Murray Darling Basin." *Journal of Water & Health* 16 (6):1033–37. doi:10.2166/wh.2018.199.

Lee, C. S., J. H. Lee, and K. S. Kwon. 2008. "Outbreak of Hepatitis A in Korean Military Personnel." *Japanese Journal of Infectious Diseases* 61 (3):239–41.

Lemaitre, J., D. Pasetto, J. Perez-Saez, C. Sciarra, J. F. Wamala, and A. Rinaldo. 2019. "Rainfall as a Driver of Epidemic Cholera: Comparative Model Assessments of the Effect of Intra-Seasonal Precipitation Events." *Acta Tropica* 190:235–43. doi:10.1016/j.actatropica.2018.11.013.

Levitus, S., J. I. Antonov, T. P. Boyer, O. K. Baranova, H. E. Garcia, R. A. Locarnini, A. V. Mishonov et al. 2012 "World Ocean Heat Content and Thermosteric Sea Level Change (0–2000 m), 1955–2010." *Geophysical Research Letters* 39 (10). doi:10.1029/2012GL051106.

Liang, S. Y., and N. Messenger. 2018. "Infectious Diseases after Hydrologic Disasters." *Emergency Medicine Clinics of North America* 36 (4):835–51.

Lillepold, K., J. Rocklov, J. Liu-Helmersson, M. Sewe, and J. C. Semenza. 2019. "More Arboviral Disease Outbreaks in Continental Europe Due to the Warming Climate?" *Journal of Travel Medicine* 26 (5). doi:10.1093/jtm/taz017.

Lindgren, E., Y. Andersson, J. E. Suk, B. Sudre, and J. C. Semenza. 2012. "Monitoring EU Emerging Infectious Disease Risk Due to Climate Change." *Science* 336:418–19.

Lipp, E. K., A. Huq, and R. R. Colwell. 2002. "Effects of Global Climate on Infectious Disease: The Cholera Model." *Clinical Microbiology Reviews* 15:757–70.

Liu, Z., J. Lao, Y. Zhang, Y. Liu, J. Zhang, H. Wang, and B. Jiang. 2018. "Association between Floods and Typhoid Fever in Yongzhou, China: Effects and Vulnerable Groups." *Environmental Research* 167:718–24. doi:10.1016/j.envres.2018.08.030.

Louis, V., I. Gillespie, S. O'Brien, E. Russek-Cohen, A. Pearson, and R. Colwell. 2005. "Temperature-Driven Campylobacter Seasonality in England and Wales." *Applied and Environmental Microbiology* 71 (1):85–92.

Lukinmaa, S., K. Mattila, V. Lehtinen, M. Hakkinen, M. Koskela, and A. Siitonen. 2006. "Territorial Waters of the Baltic Sea as a Source of Infections Caused by Vibrio Cholerae Non-O1, Non-O139: Report of 3 Hospitalized Cases." *Diagnostic Microbiology and Infectious Disease* 54 (1):1–6.

Mallin, M., K. Williams, E. Esham, and R. Lowe. 2000. "Effect of Human Development on Bacteriological Water Quality in Coastal Watersheds." *Ecological Applications* 10:1047.

Martinez-Urtaza, J., M. Saco, J. de Novoa, P. Perez-Pineiro, J. Peiteado, A. Lozano-Leon, and O. Garcia-Martin. 2004. "Influence of Environmental Factors and Human Activity on the Presence of Salmonella Serovars in a Marine Environment." *Applied and Environmental Microbiology* 70 (4):2089–97.

Masciopinto, C., O. De Giglio, M. Scrascia, F. Fortunato, G. La Rosa, E. Suffredini, C. Pazzani, R. Prato, and M. T. Montagna. 2019. "Human Health Risk Assessment for the Occurrence of Enteric Viruses in Drinking Water from Wells: Role of Flood Runoff Injections." *Science of the Total Environment* 666:559–71. doi:10.1016/j.scitotenv.2019.02.107.

McLaughlin, J., A. DePaola, C. Bopp, K. Martinek, N. Napolilli, C. Allison, S. L. Murray et al. 2005. "Outbreak of Vibrio Parahaemolyticus Gastroenteritis Associated with Alaskan Oysters." *New England Journal of Medicine* 353 (14):1463–70.

Miossec, L., F. Le Guyader, L. Haugarreau, and M. Pommepuy. 2000. "Magnitude of Rainfall on Viral Contamination of the Marine Environment during Gastroenteritis Epidemics in Human Coastal Population." *Revue d'épidémiologie et de santé publique* 48 (2):S62–S71.

Miura, T., A. Gima, and M. Akiba. 2019. "Detection of Norovirus and Rotavirus Present in Suspended and Dissolved Forms in Drinking Water Sources." *Food and Environmental Virology* 11 (1):9–19. doi:10.1007/s12560-018-9361-5.

Mohammed, H., and R. Seidu. 2019. "Climate-Driven QMRA Model for Selected Water Supply Systems in Norway Accounting for Raw Water Sources and Treatment Processes." *Science of the Total Environment* 660:306–20. doi:10.1016/j.scitotenv.2018.12.460.

Mondal, N., R. Biswas, and A. Manna. 2001. "Risk Factors of Diarrhoea among Flood Victims: A Controlled Epidemiological Study." *Indian Journal of Public Health* 45 (4):122–27.

Morin, C. W., J. C. Semenza, J. M. Trtanj, G. E. Glass, C. Boyer, and K. L. Ebi. 2018. "Unexplored Opportunities: Use of Climate- and Weather-Driven Early Warning Systems to Reduce the Burden of Infectious Diseases." *Current Environmental Health Reports* 5 (4):430–38. doi:10.1007/s40572-018-0221-0.

Morris, J., and H. Kris. 2008. *Cholera and Other Vibrios.* Oxford, UK: Academic Press.

Murphy, C., C. Carroll, and K. Jordan. 2006. "Environmental Survival Mechanisms of the Foodborne Pathogen *Campylobacter jejuni.*" *Journal of Applied Microbiology* 100 (4):623–32.

Naing, C., S. A. Reid, S. N. Aye, N. H. Htet, and S. Ambu. 2019. "Risk Factors for Human Leptospirosis Following Flooding: A Meta-Analysis of Observational Studies." *PLoS One* 14 (5):e0217643. doi:10.1371/journal.pone.0217643.

Nasser, A. M. 2016. "Removal of Cryptosporidium by Wastewater Treatment Processes: A Review." *Journal of Water and Health* 14 (1):1–13. doi:10.2166/wh.2015.131.

Naumova, E. N., J. S. Jagai, B. Matyas, A. DeMaria, Jr., I. B. MacNeill, and J. K. Griffiths. 2007. "Seasonality in Six Enterically Transmitted Diseases and Ambient Temperature." *Epidemiology and Infection* 135 (2):281–92.

Nichols, G. 2010. *Mapping Out the Causes of Infectious Diseases: A Case Study on the Multiple Factors Involved in Salmonella Enteritidis Infections.* London: Hodder.

Nichols, G., C. Lane, N. Asgari, N. Q. Verlander, and A. Charlett. 2009. "Rainfall and Outbreaks of Drinking Water Related Disease and in England and Wales." *Journal of Water and Health* 7 (1):1–8.

Noble, R., S. Weisberg, M. Leecaster, C. McGee, J. Dorsey, P. Vainik, and V. Orozco-Borbón. 2003. "Storm Effects on Regional Beach Water Quality along the Southern California Shoreline." *Journal of Water and Health* 1 (1):23–31.

Nygard, K., M. Torven, C. Ancker, S. B. Knauth, K. O. Hedlund, J. Giesecke, Y. Andersson, and L. Svensson. 2003. "Emerging Genotype (GGIIb) of Norovirus in Drinking Water, Sweden." *Emerging Infectious Diseases* 9 (12):1548–52.

O'Connor, R. M., R. Shaffie, G. Kang, and H. D. Ward. 2011. "Cryptosporidiosis in Patients with HIV/AIDS." *AIDS* 25 (5):549–60.

Oliver, E. C. J., M. G. Donat, M. T. Burrows, P. J. Moore, D. A. Smale, L. V. Alexander, J. A. Benthuysen et al. 2018. "Longer and More Frequent Marine Heatwaves over the Past Century." *Nature Communications* 9 (1):1324. doi:10.1038/s41467-018-03732-9.

Palmer, S., P. Gully, J. White, A. Pearson, W. Suckling, D. Jones, J. C. Rawes, and J. L. Penner. 1983. "Waterborne Outbreak of Campylobacter Gastroenteritis. *Lancet* 1 (8319):287–90.

Patrick, M., L. Christiansen, M. Waino, S. Ethelberg, H. Madsen, and H. Wegener. 2004. "Effects of Climate on Incidence of *Campylobacter* spp. on Humans and Prevalence in Broiler Flocks in Denmark." *Applied and Environmental Microbiology* 70 (12):7474–80.

Paz, S., N. Bisharat, E. Paz, O. Kidar, and D. Cohen. 2007. "Climate Change and the Emergence of Vibrio Vulnificus Disease in Israel." *Environmental Research* 103:390–96.

Pebody, R., M. Ryan, and P. Wall. 1997. "Outbreaks of Campylobacter Infection: Rare Events for a Common Pathogen." *Communicable Disease Report. CDR Review* 7 (3):R33–37.

Randa, M. A., M. F. Polz, and E. Lim. 2004. "Effects of Temperature and Salinity on Vibrio Vulnificus Population Dynamics as Assessed by Quantitative PCR." *Applied and Environmental Microbiology* 70:5469–76.

Richardson, H., G. Nichols, C. Lane, I. Lake, and P. Hunter. 2009. "Microbiological Surveillance of Private Water Supplies in England: The Impact of Environmental and Climate Factors on Water Quality." *Water Research* 43 (8):2159–68.

Ricketts, K. D., A. Charlett, D. Gelb, C. Lane, J. V. Lee, and C. A. Joseph. 2009. "Weather Patterns and Legionnaires' Disease: A Meteorological Study." *Epidemiology and Infection* 137 (7):1003–12.

Rodriguez, S., and R. Araujo. 2012. "Effect of Environmental Parameters on the Inactivation of the Waterborne Pathogen Campylobacter in a Mediterranean River." *Journal of Water and Health* 10 (1):100–7. doi:10.2166/wh.2011.044.

Rosenberg, A., M. Weinberger, S. Paz, L. Valinsky, V. Agmon, and C. Peretz. 2018. "Ambient Temperature and Age-Related Notified Campylobacter Infection in Israel: A 12-Year Time Series Study." *Environmental Research* 164:539–45.

Ruppert, J., B. Panzig, L. Guertler, P. Hinz, G. Schwesinger, S. Felix, and S. Friesecke. 2004. "Two Cases of Severe Sepsis due to Vibrio Vulnificus Wound Infection Acquired in the Baltic Sea." *European Journal of Clinical Microbiology & Infectious Diseases* 23 (12):912–15.

Savill, M., J. Hudson, A. Ball, J. Klena, P. Scholes, R. Whyte, R. E. McCormick, and D. Jankovic. 2001. "Enumeration of Campylobacter in New Zealand Recreational and Drinking Waters." *Journal of Applied Microbiology* 91 (1):38-46.

Schiff, K., J. Morton, and S. Weisberg. 2003. "Retrospective Evaluation of Shoreline Water Quality along Santa Monica Bay Beaches." *Marine Environmental Research* 56 (1–2):245–53.

Schijven, J., and A. de Roda Husman. 2005. "Effect of Climate Changes on Waterborne Diseases in the Netherlands." *Water Science and Technology* 51 (5):79–87.

Schmid, D., I. Lederer, P. Much, A.-M. Pichler, and F. Allerberger. 2005. "Outbreak of Norovirus Infection Associated with Contaminated Flood Water, Salzburg." *Eurosurveillance* 10 (24).

Semenza, J. C. 2012. *Human Health Effects of Extreme Weather Events. Vol. 3: Water, Air, and Solid Waste*. Santa Barbara, CA: Praeger; ABC-CLIO, LLC.

Semenza, J. C. 2013. *Climate Change Adaptation to Infectious Diseases in Europe*. Wallingford, UK: CABI.

Semenza, J. C. 2020. "Cascading Risks of Waterborne Diseases from Climate Change." *Nature Immunology* 21 (5):484–87.

Semenza, J. C., J. S. Caplan, G. Buescher, T. Das, M. V. Brinks, and A. Gershunov. 2012a. "Climate Change and Microbiological Water Quality at California Beaches." *Ecohealth* 9 (3):293–97.

Semenza, J. C., and K. L. Ebi. 2019. "Climate Change Impact on Migration, Travel, Travel Destinations and the Tourism Industry." *Journal of Travel Medicine* 26 (5). doi:10.1093/jtm/taz026.

Semenza, J. C., S. Herbst, A. Rechenburg, J. E. Suk, C. Höser, C. Schreiber, and T. Kistemann. 2012b. "Climate Change Impact Assessment of Food- and Waterborne Diseases." *Critical Reviews in Environmental Science and Technology* 42 (8):857–90. doi:10.1080/10643389.2010.534706.

Semenza, J. C., C. Höser, S. Herbst, A. Rechenburg, J. E. Suk, T. Frechen, and T. Kistemann. 2012c. "Knowledge Mapping for Climate Change and Food and Waterborne Diseases." *Critical Reviews in Environmental Science and Technology* 42:378–411. doi: 10.1080/10643389.2010.518520.

Semenza, J. C., and B. Menne. 2009. "Climate Change and Infectious Diseases in Europe." *Lancet. Infectious Diseases* 9 (6):365–75. doi:10.1016/s1473-3099(09)70104-5.

Semenza, J. C., and G. Nichols. 2007. "Cryptosporidiosis Surveillance and Water-Borne Outbreaks in Europe." *Eurosurveillance* 12 (5):E13–14.

Semenza, J. C., J. E. Suk, V. Estevez, K. L. Ebi, and E. Lindgren. 2012d. "Mapping Climate Change Vulnerabilities to Infectious Diseases in Europe." *Environmental Health Perspectives* 120 (3):385–92. doi:10.1289/ehp.1103805.

Semenza, J. C., J. Trinanes, W. Lohr, B. Sudre, M. Lofdahl, J. Martinez-Urtaza, G. L. Nichols, and J. Rocklov. 2017. "Environmental Suitability of Vibrio Infections in a Warming Climate: An Early Warning System." *Environmental Health Perspectives* 125 (10):107004. doi:10.1289/ehp2198.

Senhorst, H., and J. Zwolsman. 2005. "Climate Change and Effects on Water Quality: A First Impression." *Water Science and Technology* 51 (5):53–9.

Sheppard, S. K., J. F. Dallas, N. J. Strachan, M. MacRae, N. D. McCarthy, D. J. Wilson, F. J. Gormley et al. 2009. "Campylobacter Genotyping to Determine the Source of Human Infection." *Clinical Infectious Diseases* 48 (8):1072–78. doi:10.1086/597402.

Sinisi, L., and R. Aertgeerts. 2011. *Guidance on Water Supply and Sanitation in Extreme Weather Events*. Copenhagen, Denmark: World Health Organization, Regional Office for Europe. http://www.euro.who.int/__data/assets/pdf_file/0016/160018/WHOGuidanceFVLR.pdf.

Smith, A., M. Reacher, W. Smerdon, G. K. Adak, G. Nichols, and R. M. Chalmers. 2006. "Outbreaks of Waterborne Infectious Intestinal Disease in England and Wales, 1992–2003." *Epidemiology and Infection* 134 (6):1141–49.

Soyeux, E., F. Blanchet, and B. Tisserand. 2007. "Stormwater Overflow Impacts on the Sanitary Quality of Bathing Waters." *Water Science and Technology* 56 (11):43–50.

Sterk, A., J. Schijven, A. M. de Roda Husman, and T. de Nijs. 2016. "Effect of Climate Change on Runoff of Campylobacter and Cryptosporidium from Land to Surface Water." *Water Research* 95:90–102. doi:10.1016/j.watres.2016.03.005.

Stine, S. W., I. Song, C. Y. Choi, and C. P. Gerba. 2005. "Effect of Relative Humidity on Preharvest Survival of Bacterial and Viral Pathogens on the Surface of Cantaloupe, Lettuce, and Bell Peppers." *Journal of Food Protection* 68 (7):1352–58.

Suk, J. E., E. C. Vaughan, R. G. Cook, and J. C. Semenza. 2019. "Natural Disasters and Infectious Disease in Europe: A Literature Review to Identify Cascading Risk Pathways." *European Journal of Public Health* doi:10.1093/eurpub/ckz111.

Trenberth, K. 1999. "Conceptual Framework for Changes of Extremes of the Hydrological Cycle with Climate Change." *Climatic Change* 42:327–39.

Uejio, C. 2017. "Temperature Influences on Salmonella Infections across the Continental United States." *Annals of the American Association of Geographers* 107 (3):751–64.

Urquhart, E. A., S. H. Jones, J. W. Yu, B. M. Schuster, A. L. Marcinkiewicz, C. A. Whistler, and V. S. Cooper. 2016. "Environmental Conditions Associated with Elevated *Vibrio parahaemolyticus* Concentrations in Great Bay Estuary, New Hampshire." *PLoS One* 11 (5):e0155018. doi:10.1371/journal.pone.0155018.

Vollaard, A., S. Ali, H. van Asten, S. Widjaja, L. Visser, C. Surjadi, and J. van Dissel. 2004. "Risk Factors for Typhoid and Paratyphoid Fever in Jakarta, Indonesia." *JAMA* 291 (21):2607–15.

Wang, P., W. B. Goggins, and E. Y. Y. Chan. 2018a. "Associations of Salmonella Hospitalizations with Ambient Temperature, Humidity and Rainfall in Hong Kong." *Environment International* 120:223–30. doi:10.1016/j.envint.2018.08.014.

Wang, P., W. B. Goggins, and E. Y. Y. Chan. 2018b. "A Time-Series Study of the Association of Rainfall, Relative Humidity and Ambient Temperature with Hospitalizations for Rotavirus and Norovirus Infection among Children in Hong Kong." *Science of the Total Environment* 643:414–22. doi:10.1016/j.scitotenv.2018.06.189.

Winfield, M. D., and E. A. Groisman. 2003. "Role of Nonhost Environments in the Lifestyles of Salmonella and *Escherichia coli*." *Applied and Environmental Microbiology* 69 (7):3687–94.

Wojcik, O. P., J. Holt, A. Kjerulf, L. Muller, S. Ethelberg, and K. Molbak. 2013. "Personal Protective Equipment, Hygiene Behaviours and Occupational Risk of Illness after July 2011 Flood in Copenhagen, Denmark." *Epidemiology and Infection* 141 (8):1756–63. doi:10.1017/s0950268812002038.

Yoder, J. S., B. A. Eddy, G. S. Visvesvara, L. Capewell, and M. J. Beach. 2010. "The Epidemiology of Primary Amoebic Meningoencephalitis in the USA, 1962–2008." *Epidemiology and Infection* 138 (7):968–75.

Young, I., B. Smith, and A. Fazil. 2015. "A Systematic Review and Meta-Analysis of the Effects of Extreme Weather Events and Other Weather-Related Variables on Cryptosporidium and Giardia In Fresh Surface Waters." *Journal of Water and Health* 13:1–17.

Young, K. T., L. M. Davis, and V. J. Dirita. 2007. "*Campylobacter jejuni*: Molecular Biology and Pathogenesis." *Nature Reviews. Microbiology* 5 (9):665–79.

Zhang, N., D. Song, J. Zhang, W. Liao, K. Miao, S. Zhong, S. Lin et al. 2019. "The Impact of the 2016 Flood Event in Anhui Province, China on Infectious Diarrhea Disease: An Interrupted Time-Series Study." *Environment International* 127:801–9. doi:10.1016/j.envint.2019.03.063.

Zhang, Y., P. Bi, and J. Hiller. 2008. "Climate Variations and Salmonellosis Transmission in Adelaide South Australia: A Comparison between Regression Models." *International Journal of Biometeorology* 52 (3):179–87.

CHAPTER 5

DEGRADED AIR QUALITY

Kim Knowlton and Vijay S. Limaye

Climate Change and Air Quality

Climate change is caused by human-made (**anthropogenic**) heat-trapping pollution emitted by burning **fossil fuels** in the two hundred years since the dawn of the industrial revolution. In the last fifty years, atmospheric temperatures have risen at an accelerating pace, particularly across the Northern Hemisphere. Rising atmospheric (and ocean) temperatures in turn influence global and regional precipitation, humidity, wind patterns and pollution **dispersion**, and pressure systems in ways that affect local meteorology and air quality (Bernard et al. 2001; Kinney 2008; Jacob and Winner 2009). Accelerating climate change is anticipated to affect **ambient air** pollution levels by altering atmospheric chemical reaction rates, boundary layer conditions affecting the vertical mixing of pollutants, and changes in air flow affecting the transport of pollution (Ebi and McGregor 2008). Climate change will likely offset some of the expected improvements in air quality that would be otherwise enjoyed from reductions in **primary pollution** sources and precursor emissions (Avise et al. 2009; Hogrefe 2012, Kinney 2018).

Air Pollutants Affected by Climate Change

Several major air pollutants, notably ground-level **ozone**, **particulate matter**, and **aeroallergens**, are sensitive to climatic conditions and are affected by climate change. These pollutants increase the number of air pollution days that can be hazardous to health and exacerbate underlying respiratory and cardiovascular disease, causing increases in emergency room visits, hospitalizations, and premature mortality (Pope et al. 2002; Archer et al. 2019).

Ground-Level Ozone

Ozone (O_3) is the most frequently cited climate-sensitive air pollutant. It is not emitted directly from tailpipes or smokestacks but instead is a **secondary pollutant** formed in the atmosphere from **photochemical** reactions between **ozone precursor** compounds that include **nitrogen oxides** (NO_x) and **volatile organic compounds (VOCs)**, themselves health-harming pollutants.

In urban settings, power plants, industrial and vehicle-based fossil fuel emissions, and chemical solvents provide ample sources for the NO_x and VOCs that are the precursors of O_3. In the presence of sunlight, these precursor compounds undergo temperature-dependent photochemical reactions that form O_3, the major component of the ground-level air pollution commonly known as smog. Higher temperatures drive both ozone formation and destruction (Jacob and Winner 2009); anticipated climate-fueled increases in ozone, caused by warmer conditions

KEY CONCEPTS

- Climate change, often in combination with local topography and population growth, may affect weather patterns to reduce atmospheric mixing and make oppressive, health-harming air pollution episodes occur more frequently.

- Ground-level ozone smog is a widespread threat to respiratory health because of rising temperatures that enhance the formation of ground-level ozone in the atmosphere.

- Heat-trapping carbon pollution from burning fossil fuels is the key driver of climate change; that combustion is also the direct source for numerous other health-harming air pollutants, notably ozone precursors and a variety of air toxins and microscopic particles. These particles are also formed in the atmosphere from a variety of other climate-sensitive sources, including wildfires, drought, and dust storms.

- Climate change fuels extreme rainfall events and increases global sea levels, which worsen coastal storm surge damage. Mold and moisture from weather-related flooding can compromise indoor air quality and harm respiratory health and have been linked to longer-term psychosocial impacts.

- Strategies to control stagnant air masses and improve degraded air quality focus on limiting carbon and associated air pollutants and preparing for those health-harming effects that cannot be avoided. These include identifying local vulnerabilities to air pollution, tracking air pollution–related health threats, designing communities and transportation systems (encompassing **mobile sources** of air pollution) to be more resilient to climate change, and mobilizing public health practitioners' and clinicians' involvement in proactive outreach on these issues.

and heightened **biogenic emissions** of ozone precursors, are collectively known as the "**climate penalty**" effect.

The most abundant atmospheric VOC, methane (CH_4), a potent greenhouse gas, is typically outpaced by anthropogenic nonmethane VOCs (NMVOCs) in urban and suburban ozone formation chemistry (Shea et al. 2008). Globally, methane has a key role in determining atmospheric concentrations of ozone because it reacts slowly and affects global background concentrations of O_3. Thus, reducing CH_4 reduces O_3 concentrations in both polluted urban regions and rural areas (West et al. 2006). Strategies to reduce methane could provide cost-effective ways to reduce O_3 internationally and yield air quality, public health, and climate **co-benefits** (Fann et al. 2018). One study suggests that by reducing about 20 percent of global anthropogenic methane, an estimated 30,000 premature deaths could be prevented globally in 2030 or an estimated 370,000 deaths between 2010 and 2030 (West et al. 2006).

CLINICAL CORRELATES 5.1 HUMAN HEALTH EFFECTS OF OZONE

Acute and chronic ozone exposure has been associated with significant adverse health effects in humans, including cardiopulmonary and respiratory morbidity and premature mortality (Berman et al. 2012; Wang et al. 2019). Increases in ozone concentrations have been shown to decrease pulmonary function (Mudway and Kelly 2000), increase asthma exacerbations (Strickland et al. 2010; Zheng et al. 2015), and emergency department visits (Choi et al. 2011; Pratt et al. 2019). Ozone is also associated with an increased relative risk of death from all cardiopulmonary causes (Jerrett et al. 2009). A health impact assessment found that, annually, 2,650 ozone-related premature deaths could have been avoided nationally by full **attainment** of the current 70 parts per billion (ppb) **National Ambient Air Quality Standard** for ground-level ozone (Cromar et al. 2016). Similar studies in other countries support significant increases in premature deaths and overall years of life lost with ozone exposure (Nuvolone, Petri, and Voller 2018). Even greater health benefits could be achieved with a more stringent primary standard based on professional society and scientific recommendations (Balmes 2017).

Ozone not only contributes to global warming but also causes measurable negative health effects during periods of acute and chronic exposure (Limaye and Knowlton 2019).

Particulate Matter

Whereas **coarse, fine,** and **ultrafine particles** come from natural and anthropogenic sources, diesel and fossil-fuel burning vehicles and industries are the major sources in cities and suburban areas (Shea et al. 2008). Particulate matter is also generated by several climate-sensitive environmental changes, including forest fires, drought, and desertification (Achakulwisut et al. 2019). Airborne particles come from many sources: secondary pollutants formed by chemical reactions of pollutant gases, dust particles suspended from road surfaces by traffic, and particles emitted by industrial and agricultural activities. Another important source of particulate matter worldwide is the combustion of charcoal, animal dung, and plant matter in indoor cooking and heating. An estimated four billion people are exposed to these sources, which are dramatically increasing mortality from children's respiratory infections and chronic obstructive pulmonary disease worldwide (Pinkerton et al. 2012; Balakrishnan, Cohen, and Smith 2014). It is estimated that 3.5 million people annually die from exposures to cookstove and cooking fire smoke, mostly children and women, because of indoor use patterns and cultural traditions that place these family members in close contact with smoke, often in relatively unvented conditions (Lim et al. 2012). Exposures to extremely high levels of particle pollution contribute to respiratory illnesses such as pneumonia, emphysema, lung cancer, and heart disease and reduce lifespan significantly in some developing countries (Smith 2000; Haines 2007; Smith et al. 2013; Limaye, Schöpp, and Amann 2018; Balakrishnan et al. 2019). The warming effect of **soot**, whether from cookstoves, industrial boilers, power plants, or ship boilers, is twice as great as previously estimated by the 2007 Intergovernmental Panel on Climate Change (IPCC) report, according to a 2013 study by Bond et al. 2013. Roughly eight million tons of **soot** are produced annually worldwide, and soot particles can have various warming effects. They can absorb solar energy, pass it on to the atmosphere, and exacerbate global warming caused by anthropogenic greenhouse gases; they can shrink cloud droplet size and brighten clouds; they can land on ice and snow and darken it sufficiently to absorb more sunlight and melt; but now it is understood that soot's net warming effect is second only to carbon dioxide (CO_2) (Bond et al. 2013). Understanding the amount of soot being produced by developing regions and these particles' interactions with clouds will help fill important research gaps.

CLINICAL CORRELATES 5.2 HEALTH EFFECTS OF FINE PARTICULATE MATTER

Fine particulate matter, generated through diesel and fossil-fuel burning vehicles, industrial processes, and climate-sensitive environmental changes, causes negative acute and chronic health problems. Studies show that elevations in ambient particulate matter are associated with increases in heart attacks and accelerated atherosclerosis, stroke, lung cancer mortality, and health care utilization from acute on chronic disease exacerbations (Zhang et al. 2009; Shah et al. 2013; Shah et al. 2016; Cakmak et al. 2018). Disproportionate health impacts have been demonstrated in low- and middle-income settings further illustrating global health inequities from air pollution (Newell et al. 2018). Other studies indicate that a 10 micrograms per cubic meter elevation in fine particulate air pollution is associated with approximately a 4 percent, 6 percent, and 8 percent increased risk of all-cause, cardiopulmonary, and lung cancer mortality, respectively (Pope et al. 2002). Overall in the United States, air quality problems caused by particulate matter remain a serious public health challenge (American Lung Association n.d.). Average fine particulate matter increased 5.5 percent between 2016 and 2018 (compared with a decrease of 24 percent from 2009 to 2016) resulting in an estimated 9,700 additional premature deaths in 2018 (Clay and Muller 2019).

In addition to accelerating global climate change, ambient fine particulate matter has a significant negative impact on human health.

Wildfires

Wildfire smoke is a complex and toxic brew of hundreds of different of chemical compounds, from fine particles to ozone precursors to mercury, many of them potentially health-harming (Johnston et al. 2002; Shea et al. 2008; Delfino et al. 2009; Dennekamp and Abramson 2011; Johnston et al. 2012; Marlier et al. 2013). Premature death from injuries, burns, smoke inhalation, and cardiovascular and respiratory illness; increased hospital and emergency room visits; exacerbation of asthma, allergies, and chronic obstructive pulmonary disease; and displacement and loss of homes with associated mental stress are among the adverse health impacts of wildfires (Kinney 2008; Shea et al. 2008; Dennekamp and Abramson 2011).

The observed increase in western U.S. wildfire activity since the 1980s has caused atmospheric organic carbon concentrations to increase 30 percent relative to 1970 to 1984, and in future decades, climate change is likely to exacerbate wildfires further (Spracklen et al. 2007; Abatzoglou and Williams 2016; Ford et al. 2018). Research suggests that some western forests will become more susceptible to wildfire as high concentrations of O_3 air pollution increase plant transpiration and exacerbate tree drought stress (Grulke and Schilling 2008). This could increase their vulnerability to both insect pest attacks and wildfire. The particulate and carbonaceous **aerosol** components of wildfire smoke could increase as air pollutants of concern in the future, due to climate change (Spracklen et al. 2009; Marlier et al. 2013). By the 2050s, climate change could increase concentrations of summer organic carbon aerosols over the western United States by an estimated 40 percent and elemental carbon by 20 percent, with important consequences for air quality (Spracklen et al. 2009).

The range of **air toxins** included in wildfire smoke surprises most people, even clinicians: wildfire smoke produces large amounts of carbon monoxide, carbon dioxide, NO_x, ozone precursors and O_3, particulate matter or PM (both coarse PM_{10} and finer $PM_{2.5}$), VOCs, metals including mercury, organic acids, and other air toxics (Shea et al. 2008; Dennekamp and Abramson 2011). Associations between bushfire smoke, PM_{10}, and respiratory hospitalizations and emergency room visits in Australian studies are consistent with those found in urban air pollution exposure studies (Dennekamp and Abramson 2011). Worldwide, an estimated 339,000 people annually perish from the combined effects of wildfire and landscape fire smoke (Johnston et al. 2012).

People exposed to smoke from wildfires or landscape fires may not realize the health risks to which they are being exposed. The Children's Health Study found that after the 2003 California wildfires, even the smell of fire smoke, having penetrated indoors, could persist for more than six days and has been associated with continued respiratory symptoms: sore throat, cough, bronchitis, wheezing, and asthma attacks (Kunzli et al. 2006). Clinicians should take care to both diagnose and counsel carefully, even at locations far distant and downwind of fire source areas, because fire smoke can travel hundreds of miles downwind and still affect air quality measurably (Natural Resources Defense Council 2013; Larsen et al. 2018). One study found that $PM_{2.5}$ from 2002 wildfires in northern Quebec, Canada, traveled over one thousand kilometers southward to affect air quality in Baltimore, Maryland (Kinney 2008).

Aeroallergens

Climate change affects levels of allergenic pollen, as higher temperatures, increased humidity, and elevated levels of carbon dioxide in the Earth's atmosphere have been shown to stimulate the growth of certain plant species. Climate change is also expected to extend the pollen production season (Reid and Gamble 2009; Ziska et al. 2011; Neumann et al. 2018; Sapkota et al. 2019; Ziska et al. 2019). Higher pollen levels from specific trees, grasses, and weeds are associated with asthma exacerbations (Sun et al. 2016). Because millions of people suffer from allergies to pollen, a longer allergy season in which plants have more time to grow, flower, and produce pollen could worsen symptoms. It is estimated that allergies cost the United States about $18 billion each year, including the cost of emergency room care for asthma exacerbations (Frenkel and Hermoni 2002). According to another study by U.S. Department of Agriculture researchers, higher levels of carbon dioxide in the Earth's atmosphere levels increase the potency of ragweed pollen for allergic people (Singer et al. 2005).

Drought

A devastating drought struck much of the United States in 2011 and 2012, the most widespread in fifty years. Over thirteen hundred counties across twenty-nine states were declared by the U.S. Department of Agriculture as drought disaster areas in 2012. Billion-dollar disasters in 2011 and 2012 affected 67 percent of U.S. counties in forty-three states, and the combined heat and drought damage estimates were among the highest (Weiss, Weidman, and Bronson 2012). Drought affects not only the farm households that are directly involved in production and agriculturally based communities in the Midwest and Great Plains states. Rising food prices affect families across the country and globally (Redman 2012). Drought has a wide range of respiratory effects on health that, until now, have not often been seen as a whole spectrum (Stanke et al. 2013). Climate change may exacerbate these health impacts in the future across many regions (Achakulwisut et al. 2019).

Drought Effects on Respiratory Health

Periods of drought have long affected North America, and the memory of the 1930s Dust Bowl is vivid still for many. Since then, periods of drought hit the Great Plains in the 1950s and 1980s, with "significant negative economic and societal consequences" (Centers for Disease Control and Prevention [CDC] 2010). However, the ongoing effects of climate change are likely to increase the severity of future droughts into this century (Dai 2011; Schwalm et al. 2012). Increasing air temperatures (even in nondrought periods) can lead to excessive soil and vegetation drying and loss of ground cover (National Weather Service 2013), poor soil quality, diminishing soil and surface water, and reduced crop yields. The interspersed extreme rainfall events that can punctuate drought periods increase runoff and erosion, compounding the effects of enhancing drought. This cycle can lead to soils, dusts, and soil-borne pathogens that can become airborne and have far-reaching health impacts (CDC 2010).

The potentially health-harming respiratory effects of droughts include increased mobilization of dust from dry soils that can irritate bronchial passages and lungs, exacerbating asthma symptoms and increasing risks of acute respiratory infection, bronchitis, and bacterial pneumonia. Because associated dry soils and hot temperatures also increase wildfire risks, risk of smoke inhalation means potentially increased exposures to $PM_{2.5}$, ozone, and a host of air toxins that can harm respiratory health. During drought periods, harmful algal blooms in freshwater bodies can increase, and some species generate aerosolized toxins. Transmission patterns of vector-borne illnesses like West Nile virus, hantavirus, coccidiomycosis, and dengue fever can be affected by drought, because these periods can put animal and insect vectors into closer contact with human hosts as both species vie for shrinking water resources (Gage et al. 2008).

CLINICAL CORRELATES 5.3 WILDFIRES AND HUMAN HEALTH

Although direct impacts of wildfires tend to occur in restricted geographical regions, they have potential to affect the health of populations hundreds of miles away (Le et al. 2014; Dreesen, Sullivan, and Delgado 2016; Larsen et al. 2018). Smoke from the combustion of biomass contains a myriad of chemicals known to be detrimental to human health (Naeher et al. 2007). Examples include carbon monoxide, organic acids, mercury, and fine particulate matter. Some experts compare the impact of particulate matter produced by wildfires to that of industrial urban environments where fine particulate matter is associated with a wide range of adverse health effects, including neonatal and cardiorespiratory mortality, exacerbations of respiratory and cardiovascular conditions, and pathophysiological changes such as inflammation, oxidative stress, and coagulation (Pope and Dockery 2006). Carbon monoxide poisoning can manifest as headache, confusion, coma, and death in severe cases. Mercury can cause neurological toxicity, and a study from the National Center for Atmospheric Research found that 48 tons of mercury are redistributed by wildfires annually in the United States (Lipsher 2007). It is unclear exactly how the metal is affecting human health, although experts suspect it is entering waterways and drinking water.

Wildfire smoke has direct and indirect impacts on health through carbon monoxide production, toxic chemicals, and fine particulate matter.

Clinicians should take care to both diagnose and counsel carefully, even at locations far distant and downwind of fire source areas, because fire smoke can travel hundreds of miles downwind and still affect air quality measurably.

Coccidiomycosis and Respiratory Health

A recently reemergent fungal infectious illness, coccidiodomycosis or "valley fever," is on the rise, with rapidly increasing numbers in the US southwestern border region (CDC 2019). Coccidiomycosis was first recognized and reported over one hundred years ago, but since the early 1990s, its incidence has increased dramatically. Valley fever is caused by inhalation of fungal spores that reside in desert soils, which can become airborne during periods of drought, when soils are more easily crumbled or pulverized, and can subsequently become airborne and be dispersed by high winds. Between these dry periods that contribute to airborne pathogen transport, the spores reside and thrive in relatively moist soils, leading to the phrase "grow and blow" to describe the life cycle of coccidiomycosis. It is estimated that in endemic regions, 30 to 60 percent of residents are exposed to the fungus at some time in their lives (CDC 2019).

For most people, the infection clears on its own, but medical treatment is needed for those few who develop severe infections with its flulike symptoms that can last for weeks or turn into chronic pneumonia. The infection can spread from the lungs throughout the body, causing meningitis or even death. Fever, chest pain, coughing, rash, and muscle aches are among its range of symptoms. Groups most at risk for the more severe disseminated infection form of valley fever are women in their third trimester of pregnancy, people with weakened immune systems, or who are of African-American, Asian, Hispanic, or Filipino descent (CDC 2010). California state prisons have seen high incidence rates as the construction of new prison facilities in endemic areas disturbed spores and then put large numbers of inmates in potential contact with dusty, fungus-laden soil (Pappagianis 2007). Approximately 20,000 new cases are reported nationally each year in the United States, but an estimated 150,000 may be infected. Far fewer cases are diagnosed across the Arizona-Mexico border, although the pathogen's progress obviously does not stop at the border (CDC 2019).

This evidence highlights the need for more health care providers and laboratories to be trained to recognize and diagnose valley fever and prevent its spread beyond the areas in which it is now endemic in the United States. Expanding awareness of valley fever among clinicians and the public can help minimize delays in diagnosis and treatment (CDC 2019).

Summers in and around Phoenix, Arizona, have taken a new twist in recent years. Besides the searing temperatures that summer brings to the region, residents turn to the horizon with an eye to the towering dust storms, or haboobs, which have appeared out of the desert landscape in summer to darken the air with massive columns of particulates and dusts (American Meteorology Society 2016). Named for the Arabic term for "blasting," these large-scale haboobs, intense dust storms with sometimes blasting winds, have become a more regular feature of summers in the desert Southwest. Although dust storms have long been part of desert life, more of them seem to be occurring recently. Some of the meteorologic conditions that can contribute to the formation of major dust storms and haboobs include drought, which can diminish the amount of ground-covering vegetation, leaving more open fields that can serve as sources of dust. The widespread drought and heat of recent summers, notably 2011 and 2012, contributed to some ideal local conditions in parts of the desert Southwest. Eye and respiratory protection and taking shelter is advisable in the face of these approaching clouds.

Mold and Fungi

Extreme rainfall events, along with sea level rise that can worsen storm surge and coastal flooding, are being fueled by climate change (IPCC 2012;, Horton et al. 2015). Together, they can cause moisture damage in residences, businesses, schools, and other institutions. The associated growth of indoor molds can have health-harming respiratory effects (Institute of Medicine 2004, 2011; Fisk, Lei-Gomez, and Mendell 2007; Mudarri and Fisk 2007; Reid and Gamble 2009; Sheffield et al. 2011), and exposure to dampness and mold in homes has also been linked to depression (Shenassa et al. 2007). Exposure to *Alternaria alternata* in U.S. homes is associated with higher prevalence of current asthma symptoms. In a survey of 831 U.S. housing units, higher levels of *A. alternata* antigens measured in indoor dust increased the odds of having asthma symptoms in the past year, relative to the lowest tertile (adjusted odds ratio was 1.84, 95 percent confidence interval, 1.18 to 2.85 for the third tertile) (Salo et al. 2006). Besides prevalence, asthma's persistence and severity of symptoms have been strongly associated with sensitization and exposure to the widespread fungus *A. alternata*, though few studies have assessed indoor exposure.

Increasing carbon dioxide levels in the atmosphere can also exacerbate spore production and total antigen production in molds like *Alternaria*, an allergenic fungus so ubiquitous that this response may contribute to the increasing prevalence of allergies and asthma (Wolf et al. 2010). Furthermore, mold and moisture are exacerbated by flooding associated with tropical storms and intense rainfall events that are fueled by climate change.

Challenges exist in characterizing mold exposures in indoor environments. These allergens have not been characterized as well as other indoor allergens such as dust mites, cockroaches, and pets (Salo et al. 2006). Measuring moisture conditions indoors, evaluating damage to home building materials, and surveying for mold growth visually are the current means of establishing potential mold health issues when respiratory symptoms are reported. Human exposures to fungal allergens have been estimated by indirect methods using spore or fungal colony counts in air or dust samples as a proxy of exposure. Thus, the absence of standardized measurement techniques for evaluation of fungal allergen exposures has been a major constraint in risk assessment. Because interpretation of fungal exposure data is both complex and contentious, no universally recognized exposure thresholds exist, but these would be tremendously helpful in guiding remediation efforts to reestablish healthy indoor environments after flooding (Salo et al. 2006).

Air Pollution—Vulnerable Populations

Some of the groups most susceptible to air pollution are children, people with preexisting heart or lung disease, people with diabetes, athletes, and outdoor workers (Bateson and Schwartz 2007; Makri and Stilianakis 2008; Balbus and Malina 2009; Siddique et al. 2010; Sheffield and Landrigan 2011; Pinkerton et al. 2012). Socioeconomic factors and economic disadvantage increase people's susceptibility to air pollution health effects in terms of both increased, disproportionate exposures and reduced coping capacities and access to health care (Makri and Stilianakis 2008; Mikati et al. 2018; Limaye et al. 2019; Limaye et al. 2020).

Homeless people are especially vulnerable to the harmful health effects of air pollution, with high rates of respiratory infections and self-reported lung diseases including asthma, chronic bronchitis, and emphysema that are double the rates in the general population; asthma rates in homeless children have been reported as six times the national rate (Ramin and Svoboda 2009). However, homeless people may be a challenging population to locate, protect, and serve, and comorbidities including mental illness are also common in this population. Developing strategies to communicate climate health risks widely and in ways that speak to local community needs will be essential in the years ahead. The active engagement of leaders from highly vulnerable communities in developing effective outreach will be critical.

Double-Whammy for People with Asthma

Climate change is projected to worsen many of the existing health issues that face Americans and the clinicians who serve them. One season that is already challenging is the dog days of summer, which include the hottest, most sultry months—typically July and August in the Northern Hemisphere. Heat can compound respiratory and cardiovascular illnesses, increasing rates of emergency room visits and hospitalizations. Late summer sees rampant seasonal allergy symptoms from ragweed pollen beginning in August and lasting into October. An estimated thirty-six million people in the United States have seasonal allergies (Natural Resources Defense Council 2007), and ragweed causes more allergies than any other plant pollen. Among people with asthma, approximately 70 percent also have allergies (American Academy of Allergy, Asthma and Immunology/National Allergy Bureau 2013), making the possibility of both allergy and asthma symptoms far more than an inconvenience for some patients.

Ground-level ozone concentrations tend to be higher in the hotter temperatures of late summer, because the underlying formation chemistry for ozone is temperature-dependent. So the health "double-whammy" of higher exposures to ozone smog plus ragweed pollen can be a challenge to children and adults trying to enjoy sports, back-to-school activities, or just a day in the late-summer sun. Clinicians should take note that in future decades, climate change could make those hot, cloudless days even tougher. Rising CO_2 concentrations make ragweed grow larger and produce more pollen per plant (D'Amato et al. 2014). In the years ahead, especially in and around cities where vehicle and industrial sources are concentrated, with ragweed pollen seasons increasing in length (Ziska et al. 2011; Ziska et al. 2019), there could be more people sensitized to ragweed, more severe symptoms if peak pollen concentrations increases, or the need to counsel patients to sustain allergy medication over a longer time period, beginning earlier and lasting later into the season (D'Amato et al. 2014).

CLINICAL CORRELATES 5.4 DROUGHT AND REEMERGENCE OF DISEASE: COCCIDIOIDOMYCOSIS

Coccidioidomycosis, often called valley fever, is a fungal infection common in the southwestern United States, South America, the Middle East, and Africa that is capable of causing severe respiratory failure and disseminated disease (Shriber et al. 2017; CDC 2019). Exposure occurs from inhalation of the fungal spores that reside in desert soils and dust. Periods of drought cause the spores to become airborne and dispersed by winds. Although a majority of residents living in endemic regions are exposed, certain populations including pregnant women and immunocompromised individuals are susceptible to more severe disease (Zhang et al. 2016). Symptoms include a flulike illness initially and pneumonia followed by the possibility of spread throughout the body and central nervous system. Clinicians in endemic and even nearby drought-affected areas should be aware of the potential for this disease. Its distribution is subject to change with warming temperatures, droughts, and wind including worsening of extreme weather events like dust storms (Weaver and Kolivras 2018).

Drought, dust storms, and changing climate in the desert regions mean that local clinicians must be attuned to symptoms of reemergent disease such as coccidioidomycosis to avoid missed and delayed diagnosis.

Future Projections of Climate Change Effects on Air Pollution

Studies have modeled temperature-dependent ozone air pollution into future decades taking into account the influence of climate change. These forward-looking ozone modeling efforts suggest that climate change alone will increase summertime surface ozone in polluted regions of the United States by 1 to 10 ppb this century, with the largest effects in urban areas during pollution episodes (Wu et al. 2008; Jacob and Winner 2009; Fiore et al. 2012). Changes in extreme climate conditions may intensify the extreme meteorologic conditions that encourage high-ozone episodes in many parts of the world. Changes in regional high-ozone episodes by the 2050s appear to depend mainly on assumptions about precursor inventories: three major pollutant regions—North America, Europe, and East Asia—would see increases in the number of days with hazardous eight-hour ozone concentrations (thirty-nine to seventy-nine days per summer by the 2050s) under a fossil fuel-intensive, high greenhouse gas-emissions A1F1 scenario (Lei, Wuebbles, and Liang 2012). The A1 storyline and scenario family describe a future world of very rapid economic growth, global population that peaks in midcentury and declines thereafter, and the rapid introduction of new and more efficient technologies. Major underlying themes are convergence among regions, capacity building, and increased cultural and social interactions, with a substantial reduction in regional differences in per capita income. A1F1 is fossil fuel intensive (https://www.ipcc.ch/site/assets/uploads/2018/03/sres-en.pdf).

Several studies have used a combination of the output from current-day epidemiological studies' air pollution exposure-response coefficients and future climate-health risk assessments to estimate health impacts from future climate-sensitive air pollution model projections. Bell et al. (2007) modeled temperature-dependent ozone by the 2050s in fifty large eastern cities, assuming constant precursor emissions, and found a 68 percent increase in unhealthy summertime ozone days by the 2050s relative to the 1990s and a 2.1 percent increase in asthma hospitalizations across all the cities, ranging as high as 4.7 percent from O_3 exposures. Sheffield et al. (2011) considered potential effects of climate change on ozone-related emergency room visits for asthma in the 2020s, driven by climate-sensitive temperature changes, and found a median 7.3 percent increase occurring in fourteen metropolitan New York City counties by the 2020s (Sheffield et al. 2011).

A study that looked at the metropolitan New York City region and the effects of climate change on human health found that by the 2050s, projected ozone-related premature mortality could increase by 4.5 percent across the region, compared to the 1990s (Knowlton et al. 2004). Other studies have estimated that globally by 2050, there could be four thousand additional premature deaths each year attributable to climate change-connected PM increases, and three hundred due to O_3 increases (Russell et al. 2010; Tagaris et al. 2010).

Mitigation: Health Benefits of Reducing Carbon Pollution and Associated Co-Pollutant Air Pollution

It is important to remember that many of the fossil fuel combustion sources of heat-trapping carbon pollution are also sources of local-scale co-pollutants like PM, ozone precursors, air toxins, and metals that can have health-harming effects on local air quality. By reducing carbon pollution and moving away from fossil fuel use, those co-pollutants can simultaneously be reduced in ways that can provide substantial health co-benefits in terms of immediate air quality improvements and through initiatives that provide more access to walkable, bikeable local transportation networks, enhanced exercise and fitness opportunities, and increased social contacts in the community (Patz et al. 2020).

Achieving Cleaner Air

Nationally, the 1970 **Clean Air Act** (CAA) is the foundational statute that protects human health and welfare from air pollution, via the National Ambient Air Quality Standards. The CAA limits major climate-sensitive air pollutants or precursors in the United States. Since being enacted in 1970, the CAA plus its 1990 amendments prevented more than 160,000 premature deaths in 2010 and will prevent a projected 450,000 deaths in 2030 (EPA 2011; Mui and Levin 2020).

Local initiatives to reduce health-harming air pollution exposures include strategies to improve local air quality and reduce emissions of heat-trapping carbon pollution. For example, the New York City West Harlem Environmental Action, along with the Natural Resources Defense Council and Environmental Defense Fund, were instrumental in developing initiatives to take diesel buses off the streets and reduce the high concentrations of bus depots in residential neighborhoods among communities of color.

New York City is also among the communities that prohibit trucks and buses from idling their engines when they stop for more than a few minutes. Passage of these local laws and making enforcement a neighborhood priority can lead to appreciable differences to health. New York City, for example, not only allows agents of the Department of Parks and Recreation and the Department of Sanitation to issue idling summonses, appearance tickets, and violation notices but gives citizens the ability to report truck violations (New York City 2019).

Triple Wins: Cutting Carbon Pollution and Air Pollution, and Improving Community Health

The transportation systems that communities plan and operate, as well as overall community form and proximities of living, working, recreational and community spaces, have enormous impacts on transportation energy demand, associated air pollution emissions, overall air quality, and community health. For example, one study of ninety-eight U.S. communities suggests that for every 10 percent of the population that takes public transportation to work, long-term ozone levels decrease by 9 percent (Bell and Dominici 2008).

Eliminating short automobile trips (eight or fewer kilometers or about five miles round trip) and substituting bicycle trips instead can help limit average urban $PM_{2.5}$ and O_3 concentrations. In a study that considered this switch for eleven Upper Midwest cities, $PM_{2.5}$ would decline and summer O_3 would increase slightly in cities but decline regionally, resulting in net annual health co-benefits of $4.9 billion (in 2010 dollars). Making 50 percent of short trips by bicycle would save approximately $3.8 billion annually from avoided mortality and reduced health care costs. The combined co-benefits of improved air quality and physical fitness were estimated at over $8 billion annually (in 2010 dollars; Grabow et al. 2012).

Cutting Pollution with Walkable, Bikeable, Active Transit in New York City

Even in New York City, where residents have long prided themselves on getting a bit more exercise than their fellow Americans might expect—sprints to catch the bus, walking blocks from apartment to subway station—obesity and type 2 diabetes are epidemic, with 40 percent of elementary and middle school children overweight or obese. This exceeds the 30 percent rate nationwide (Lee 2012). Moreover, obesity is the second leading cause of deaths in the United States behind tobacco. Physical inactivity not only contributes to the second through fourth leading causes—obesity, high blood pressure, and high blood glucose—it is the fifth leading cause itself. The built environment—the streets, buildings, and neighborhoods where we work and live—can play a vital role in encouraging healthy physical activities (Patz et al. 2007). When cities are redesigned to promote fitness and discourage fossil fuel–based transit, the triple win of personal fitness, better air quality today, and reductions in heat-trapping carbon pollution combines to limit the worst of climate change's effects (Patz et al.).

Nationwide, 40 percent of car trips are less than two miles (Patz et al. 2007), and 62 percent of all trips are less than six miles (U.S. Department of Energy 2013); these could easily be translated into a bike trip. In 2009, 5 percent of walk trips and 11 percent of bike trips were to or from work (U.S. Department of Energy 2013). Active transport has the potential to move past recreation and become a way of life for many Americans.

In May 2013, New York City began its first public subscription bikeshare program, CitiBike, with sponsorship from Citibank to place six thousand bikes at 330 stations in Manhattan and parts of Brooklyn. Within less than a month, over one million rider-miles had been logged by CitiBike participants (Donohue 2013). Bike share kiosk programs in other locations have found that well-planned, ongoing community engagement is needed to reach a wide variety of residents and make these programs a long-term success accessible to a wide cross-section of city residents (Stewart et al. 2013). Although CitiBike represents an innovative effort to reduce emissions and promote physical activity in New York City, it is not yet accessible in many poorer neighborhoods to members of the subpopulations who are most vulnerable to asthma. The fate of active transport in the Big Apple may depend on the support of people whose lives and health it is changing for the better.

Adaptation: Climate Health Preparedness and Reducing Air Pollution Vulnerability

Despite increasing exposures to climate-sensitive air pollution and a rise in underlying population vulnerability, several strategies are available to mitigate against climate change (Natural Resources Defense Council 2017):

- Identifying local vulnerabilities to air pollution at an individual, neighborhood, and community level by conducting vulnerability assessments

- Tracking air pollution-related health threats and establishing publicly available resources that allow easily access to daily monitoring data and forecasts

- Designing buildings, communities, and transportation systems to be more resilient to climate change

- Promoting outreach, communication, and active engagement of health care providers, communities, and policymakers in discussing strategies to limit carbon pollution and its associated air pollutants as well as adaption strategies to effects that cannot be avoided

There is no legislation or federal mandate that requires states to have a climate and health **adaptation** plan. In fact, just over half of states have identified evidence-based interventions to protect public health from climate change (McKillop et al. 2020)—illustrating a need for more policymaker awareness in this area. In recent years, online interactive mapping tools of climate health vulnerabilities (including air pollution) have been developed, which can be used as a screening tool for local vulnerability assessment needs (Natural Resources Defense Council 2017).

Creating healthier, more vibrant communities reflects the triple co-benefit "wins" of reducing air pollution; living healthier, more active lifestyles; and reducing community carbon footprints with cleaner, more sustainable transportation and energy systems. Furthermore, reductions in fossil fuel combustion have the additional benefit of simultaneously reducing other health-harming air pollutants, such as $PM_{2.5}$ and air toxins. Such changes will manifest long-term benefits of healthier, more climate-secure communities for generations to come.

Conclusion

Research is needed to better assess the links between climate change, meteorology, air pollution, and health outcomes and to improve upon modeling simulations of the respiratory health effects of a changing climate. (Grulke and Schilling 2008; Gamble 2009; Pinkerton et al. 2012; Reid and Abel et al. 2018). To accomplish this, some knowledge gaps and research merit further investigation:

- Gaps in environmental data, such as future projections of global **ozone precursor** emissions, especially regarding lower- and middle-income countries

- Studying how climate change and its effects on meteorology will affect fine particle concentrations locally, in co-pollutant hot spots near **stationary sources** of fossil fuel emissions and **peaker plants**

- Experimental and field studies to examine how allergen content, distribution, growth, and genetic variation of pollens and of molds (indoor and outdoor) may be altered in response to changing CO_2 concentration, bioavailability, and temperature

- Evaluating how the impacts of urban warming or land use changes may exacerbate climate change's effects on desertification and loss of vegetation, which increase the likelihood and extent of dust storms

Other knowledge gaps include the current understanding of human health impacts from air pollution exposures and local variations in both exposures and underlying vulnerabilities. For example:

- Health impact assessments for air pollution exposures that account for cumulative, long-term exposures to multiple air pollutants species

- Studies of how changes in humidity, precipitation, and extreme weather events affect respiratory exposures to mold, especially those brought on by flooding

- How underlying population vulnerability factors may change in the future, especially given a combination of vulnerability factors in some locations or among certain communities

- Local evaluations into how climate change could affect the frequency, intensity, and extent of forest fires and smoke production; associated smoke impact on human respiratory exposures; and possible interventions to limit harmful effects

- How climate change affects the frequency and intensity of forest fires regionally and, in turn, their impacts on local and downwind exposures to respiratory irritants

- Analyses of how drought conditions enhance wildfire risks and affect transport and subsequent case incidence of coccidiomycosis or other infectious illnesses

- Evaluation of the extent to which climate change could alter time spent indoors versus outside, and time-behavior patterns for air pollution exposure assessments

Finally, a third type of knowledge gap comes from the need for monitoring data and ensuring better compatibility and consistency of meteorologic, air quality/environmental, and health impact data sets across timescales. These might include:

- Creating a network of monitoring sites capable of detecting wildfire smoke downwind of source areas and estimating the smoke origins' effects on public health as a way to inform development of an early warning systems to affected communities

- Linking existing long-term data sets on the occurrence of molds, fungi, and valley fever to those on respiratory illness and diseases that are available through the Environmental Public Health Tracking Network (CDC 2018)

- Quantifying wildfire smoke exposures with more centralized, real-time environmental monitoring linked with health tracking data at similar spatial and timescales nationwide

- Establishing a larger network of continuous or daily monitoring sites in air pollution-vulnerable communities across the United States

Despite advances in improving air quality overall in recent decades, climate change is challenging healthy air for communities everywhere. The effects of heat-trapping and carbon pollution not only increase atmospheric temperatures but also alter key meteorologic characteristics and flow patterns, and affect how pollutants are dispersed and how widely they affect human health. These changes involve frequent extreme rainfalls, flood damage, drought, heat waves, and windstorms affect respiratory health. Adaptation and health preparedness strategies must be developed, because while these climate-sensitive effects on air quality and related exposures are increasing, many of the population's underlying health vulnerabilities are also on the rise: asthma prevalence increasing in all age categories, a rapidly aging American demographic, poverty, and communities facing long-term cumulative exposures to multiple air pollutants. Better preparedness to face tomorrow's climate changes can be achieved by making climate health preparedness a national priority and also by becoming part of everyday conversation.

Online Resources

Centers for Disease Control and Prevention. "National Environmental Public Health Tracking." https://www.cdc.gov/nceh/tracking/default.htm.

U.S. Environmental Protection Agency. "AirNow." https://airnow.gov/.

U.S. Environmental Protection Agency. "Climate Adaptation and Outdoor Air Quality." Overviews and Factsheets. https://www.epa.gov/arc-x/climate-adaptation-and-outdoor-air-quality.

World Health Organization. "Air Pollution Portal." http://www.who.int/airpollution/en/.

United Nations Environment. "Climate & Clean Air Coalition." http://ccacoalition.org/en.

American Lung Association. "State of the Air Reports." http://www.stateoftheair.org/ .

Health Effects Institute, and Institute for Health Metrics and Evaluation. "State of Global Air." https://www.stateofglobalair.org/.

University of Chicago Energy Policy Institute. "Air Quality Life Index." https://aqli.epic. uchicago.edu/.

National Geographic. "Air Pollution 101." https://www.youtube.com/watch?v=e6rglsLy1Ys.

DISCUSSION QUESTIONS

1. America is in the midst of a national obesity health crisis. An estimated 17 percent of children aged two to nineteen years are obese, or 12.5 million kids. Since 1980, prevalence has almost tripled (Ogden and Carroll 2010). No matter what a person's age, getting daily physical exercise is important, and for many people making exercise a priority remains challenging. With climate change, are the messages becoming mixed? For example, encouraging children to go outdoors and get more exercise and play to stay physically fit flies in the face of concerns that in warmer summer months, ground-level ozone can threaten respiratory health, even for healthy athletes, especially in late afternoon hours after school in many parts of the country. And early-morning hours can be high-pollen hours during certain seasons of the year. How might clinicians, public health professionals, teachers, and parents work with available knowledge sources to best counsel their patients or their children to make the most health-enhancing choices about outdoor activities?

2. In trying to make decisions about how to project the future effects of climate change on air quality and the associated human health effects, how would you decide what combination of assumptions to use about, for example, precursor emissions inventories, population projections, changing prevalence over time of the health outcome being studied, and land use and land cover changes that can affect air quality? If incorporating each of these future projections introduces some level of uncertainty into modeling, should you include any at all?

3. India is in the midst of an air pollution crisis and in recent years, stories in the international press have shown compelling images of the visibly high concentrations of particulate and other air pollution in India's booming cities. Yet some have argued that the visible need for improved regulation to improve air quality and reduce "traditional" air pollutants also affords a golden opportunity to make advances in limiting heat-trapping carbon pollution (see the *New York Times* article "Silver Lining in China's Smog As It Puts Focus on Emissions" [Buckley 2013]). Do you think that an air quality or health crisis is what it takes to act as a policy lever to enact more long-lasting, health-protective policies? Why or why not? Can you name any parallels in domestic pollution regulation policies? What do you think it would take to go beyond crises and move toward more health protective air pollution policies before public health is endangered?

4. One argument forwarded to avoid deeper regulation of air pollution is that society cannot afford to cut air pollution more significantly, not more than the gains already accomplished in the forty-plus years since the Clean Air Act was first passed, because stricter regulation of air pollution from industry or vehicles will cost jobs. This argument has been made by business and industrial interests regarding regulation of toxic air pollutants; today, it is also applied in continuing efforts to limit carbon pollution from power plants. Others (often those in the public health and environmental justice community) counter that society cannot afford not to limit air pollutants and/or carbon pollution, because the associated health effect costs run into the billions in health effects and lives lost. Play devil's advocate and write a paragraph defending each side of the issue of figuring costs into air pollution regulation issues.

5. Go to the U.S. Environmental Protection Agency website or other sources to gather some supporting information on costs related to air pollution regulation. Develop one to three points with supporting evidence on each side of the argument about why we should or should not limit either air toxics or carbon pollution. On the basis of your own evidence, select which you think is the more convincing argument; and state why you were convinced of its merits.

KEY TERMS

Adaptation: The process of adjusting to new conditions; in the climate literature, used in reference to actions taken to help communities and ecosystems cope with changing climate conditions.

Aeroallergen: Any airborne substance, such as pollen or spores, which triggers an allergic reaction.

Aerosol: A suspension of fine solid particles or liquid droplets, in air or another gas.

Air toxins: Airborne pollutants that cause or may cause cancer or other serious health effects, such as reproductive effects or birth defects, or adverse environmental and ecological effects.

Ambient air: Regulatory term within EPA's National Ambient Air Quality Standards that refers to "the atmosphere, external to buildings, to which the general public has access."

Anthropogenic: Originating from human activity.

Attainment area: A location with concentrations of criteria pollutants that are below the levels established by the EPA's National Ambient Air Quality Standards.

Biogenic: Originating from natural sources. Often used in the climate literature to describe emissions including volatile organic compounds released from trees and vegetation, such as monoterpenes and isoprenes, as well as emissions of nitrogen compounds from soil.

Clean Air Act (CAA): A U.S. federal law that regulates air emissions from stationary and mobile sources. Among other things, this law authorizes EPA to establish National Ambient Air Quality Standards to protect public health and public welfare and to regulate emissions of hazardous air pollutants.

Climate penalty: Increase in surface ozone resulting from regional climate warming in the absence of precursor emission changes.

Coarse particles: A type of particulate matter found near roadways and dusty industries, with an aerodynamic diameter larger than 2.5 micrometers and smaller than 10 micrometers in diameter (PM_{10}).

Co-benefits: Positive benefits (air quality, health, economic, aesthetic, ecosystem) related to the reduction of greenhouse gases.

Dispersion: Distribution of air pollution into the atmosphere.

Fossil fuels: A natural fuel such as coal or gas, formed in the geological past from the remains of living organisms.

Mitigation: The process of reducing the severity or seriousness of something; used in the climate literature in reference to the reduction of climate-altering pollutant concentrations either through reductions in emissions or increases in gas capture processes.

Mobile source: Sources of air pollution including on-road vehicles and nonroad vehicles and engines.

National Ambient Air Quality Standards: Clean Air Act-mandated ambient air limits for air pollutants considered harmful to public health and the environment.

Nitrogen oxides (NO_x): A class of precursor compounds that, when combined in the atmosphere in the presence of sunlight along with VOCs, can form ground-level ozone, a major component of smog.

Ozone (O_3): A major air pollutant and colorless, unstable gas with a pungent odor. Ozone is a powerful lung irritant that harmful in the lower atmosphere (troposphere) but a beneficial component of the upper atmosphere (stratosphere).

Particulate matter (PM): A major air pollutant comprised of a complex mixture of extremely small particles and liquid droplets. Particle pollution is made up of a number of components, including acids (such as nitrates and sulfates), organic chemicals, metals, and soil or dust particles. Fine particles such as those found in smoke and haze, are 2.5 micrometers in diameter and smaller ($PM_{2.5}$).

Peaker plants: Power plants that generally run only when there is a high demand, known as peak demand, for electricity.

Photochemical: A chemical reaction initiated by the absorption of energy in the form of light.

Precursor: An air pollutant emitted directly from a source, this term is often used in describing the pollutant building blocks that drive formation of secondary pollutants.

Primary pollutant: An air pollutant emitted directly from a source.

Secondary pollutant: An air pollutant that forms when other (primary) pollutants react in the atmosphere

Soot: A black, carbonaceous substance produced during incomplete combustion of fossil fuels.

Stationary source: Place-bound emitters of air pollution including factories, refineries, boilers, and power plants.

Stratosphere: The layer of the earth's atmosphere above the troposphere, extending to about 50 km above the earth's surface.

Troposphere: The lowest region of the atmosphere, extending from the earth's surface to a height of about 6–10 km, which is the lower boundary of the stratosphere.

Ultrafine particles: Particulate matter of nanoscale size (less than 0.1 μm or 100 nm in diameter), which are not distinctly regulated by the National Ambient Air Quality Standards.

Volatile organic compounds (VOCs): Along with nitrogen oxides, precursor compounds of ozone, a major component of smog.

References

Abatzoglou, J. T., and A. P. Williams. 2016. "Impact of Anthropogenic Climate Change on Wildfire across Western US Forests." *Proceedings of the National Academy of Sciences* 113 (42):11770–75. https://doi.org/10.1073/pnas.1607171113.

Abel, D. W., T. Holloway, M. Harkey, P. Meier, D. Ahl, V. S. Limaye, and J. A. Patz. 2018. "Air-Quality-Related Health Impacts from Climate Change and from Adaptation of Cooling Demand for Buildings in the Eastern United States: An Interdisciplinary Modeling Study." *PLOS Medicine* 15 (7):e1002599. https://doi.org/10.1371/journal.pmed.1002599.

Achakulwisut, P., S. C. Anenberg, J. E. Neumann, S. L. Penn, N. Weiss, A. Crimmins, N. Fann, J. Martinich, H. Roman, and L. J. Mickley. 2019. "Effects of Increasing Aridity on Ambient Dust and Public Health in the U.S. Southwest under Climate Change." *GeoHealth*, April, 2019GH000187. https://doi.org/10.1029/2019GH000187.

American Academy of Allergy, Asthma and Immunology/National Allergy Bureau. 2013. "Allergy Statistics." https://www.aaaai.org/about-aaaai/newsroom/allergy-statistics.

American Lung Association. n.d. "State of the Air." Accessed March 1, 2020. https://www.lung.org/our-initiatives/healthy-air/sota/.

Archer, Cristina L., Joseph F. Brodie, and Sara A. Rauscher. 2009. "Global Warming Will Aggravate Ozone Pollution in the U.S. Mid-Atlantic." *Journal of Applied Meteorology and Climatology* 58 (6): 1267–78. https://doi.org/10.1175/JAMC-D-18-0263.1.

Avise, J., J. Chen, B. Lamb, C. Wiedinmyer, A. Guenther, E. Salathé, and C. Mass. 2009. "Attribution of Projected Changes in Summertime US Ozone and $PM_{2.5}$ Concentrations to Global Changes." *Atmospheric Chemistry and Physics* 9 (4):1111–24. https://doi.org/10.5194/acp-9-1111-2009.

Balakrishnan, K., A. Cohen, and K. R. Smith. 2014. "Addressing the Burden of Disease Attributable to Air Pollution in India: The Need to Integrate across Household and Ambient Air Pollution Exposures." *Environmental Health Perspectives* 122 (1). https://doi.org/10.1289/ehp.1307822.

Balakrishnan, K., S. Dey, T. Gupta, R. S. Dhaliwal, M. Brauer, A. J. Cohen, J. D. Stanaway et al. 2019. "The Impact of Air Pollution on Deaths, Disease Burden, and Life Expectancy across the States of India: The Global Burden of Disease Study 2017." *Lancet Planetary Health* 3 (1):e26–39. https://doi.org/10.1016/S2542-5196(18)30261-4.

Balbus, J. M., and C. Malina. 2009. "Identifying Vulnerable Subpopulations for Climate Change Health Effects in the United States." *Journal of Occupational and Environmental Medicine* 51:33–37.

Balmes, J. R. 2017. "EPA's New Ozone Air Quality Standard: Why Should We Care?" *Annals of the American Thoracic Society* 14 (11):1627–29.

Bateson, T. F., and J. Schwartz. 2007. "Children's Response to Air Pollutants." *Journal of Toxicology and Environmental Health, Part A* 71 (3):238–43. https://doi.org/10.1080/15287390701598234.

Bell, M. L., and F. Dominici. 2008. "Effect Modification by Community Characteristics on the Short-Term Effects of Ozone Exposure and Mortality in 98 US Communities." *American Journal of Epidemiology* 167:986–97.

Bell, M. L., R. G. Goldberg, C. Hogrefe, P. L. Kinney, K. Knowlton, B. Lynn, J. Rosenthal, C. Rosenzweig, and J. A. Patz. 2007. "Climate Change, Ambient Ozone, and Health in 50 US Cities." *Climatic Change* 82:61–76. doi:10.1007/ s10584–006–9166–7.

Berman, J. D., N. Fann, J. W. Hollingsworth, K. E. Pinkerton, W. N. Rom, A. M. Szema, P. N. Breysse, R. H. White, and F. C. Curriero. 2012. "Health Benefits from Large-Scale Ozone Reduction in the United States." *Environmental Health Perspectives* 120:1404–10. http://dx.doi.org/10.1289/ehp.1104851.

Bernard, S. M., J. M. Samet, A. Grambsch, K. L. Ebi, and I. Romieu. 2001. "The Potential Impacts of Climate Variability and Change on Air Pollution-Related Health Effects in the United States." *Environmental Health Perspectives* 109 (May):199. https://doi.org/10.2307/3435010.

Bond, T. C., S. J. Doherty, D. W. Fahey, P. M. Forster, T. Berntsen, B. J. DeAngelo, M. G. Flanner, et al. 2013. "Bounding the Role of Black Carbon in the Climate System: A Scientific Assessment." *Journal of Geophysical Research: Atmospheres* 118:5380–5552. doi:10.1002/jgrd.50171.

Cakmak, S., C. Hebbern, L. Pinault, E. Lavigne, J. Vanos, D. Lawson Crouse, and M. Tjepkema. 2018. "Associations between Long-Term PM2.5 and Ozone Exposure and Mortality in the Canadian Census Health and Environment Cohort (CANCHEC), by Spatial Synoptic Classification Zone." *Environment International* 111:200–11. doi:10.1016/j.envint.2017.11.030.

Centers for Disease Control and Prevention. Environmental Protection Agency, National Oceanic and Atmospheric Agency, and American Water Works Association. 2010. *When Every Drop Counts: Protecting Public Health during Drought Conditions—A Guide for Public Health Professionals.* Atlanta: U.S. Department of Health and Human Services. http://www.cdc.gov/nceh/ehs/Publications/Drought.htm.

Centers for Disease Control and Prevention. 2018. "National Environmental Public Health Tracking." https://www.cdc.gov/nceh/tracking/default.htm.

Centers for Disease Control and Prevention. 2019. "Valley Fever (Coccidiomycosis)." https://www.cdc.gov/fungal/diseases/coccidioidomycosis/index.html.

Choi, M., F. C. Curriero, M. Johantgen, M.E.C. Mills, B. Sattler, and J. Lipscomb. 2011. "Association between Ozone and Emergency Department Visits: An Ecological Study." *International Journal of Environmental Health Research* 21:201–21. doi:10.1080/096–3123.2010.533366.

Clay, K., and N. Muller. 2019. *Recent Increases in Air Pollution: Evidence and Implications for Mortality.* Cambridge, MA: National Bureau of Economic Research.

Cromar, K. R., L. A. Gladson, L. D. Perlmutt, M. Ghazipura, and G. W. Ewart. 2016. "American Thoracic Society and Marron Institute Report. Estimated Excess Morbidity and Mortality Caused by Air Pollution above American Thoracic Society–Recommended Standards, 2011–2013." *Annals of the American Thoracic Society* 13 (8):1195–1201. https://doi.org/10.1513/AnnalsATS.201602-103AR.

Dai, A. 2011. "Drought under Global Warming: A Review." *WIREs Climate Change* 2:45–65. doi:10.1002/wcc81.

D'Amato, G., L. Cecchi, M. D'Amato, and I. Annesi-Maesano. 2014. "Climate Change and Respiratory Diseases." *European Respiratory Review* 23 (132):161–69. https://doi.org/10.1183/09059180.00001714.

Delfino R. J., S. Brummel, J. Wu, H. Stern, B. Ostro, M. Lispett, A. Winer, et al. 2009. "The Relationship of Respiratory and Cardiovascular Hospital Admissions to the Southern California Wildfires of 2003." *Occupational and Environmental Medicine* 66(3):189–97.

Dennekamp, M., and M. J. Abramson. 2011. "The Effects of Bushfire Smoke on Respiratory Health." *Respirology* 16:198–209.

Donohue, P. 2013. "Citi Bike Program Will Soon Top Mark of 1 Million Miles Traveled." *New York Daily News*, June 20. http://www.nydailynews.com/new-york/citi-bike-program-speeding-1st-milestone-article-1.1378709.

Dreessen, J., J. Sullivan, and R. Delgado. 2016. "Observations and Impacts of Transported Canadian Wildfire Smoke on Ozone and Aerosol Air Quality in the Maryland Region on June 9–12, 2015." *Journal of the Air & Waste Management Association* 66(9):842–62.

Ebi, K. L., and G. McGregor. 2008. "Climate Change, Tropospheric Ozone and Particulate Matter, and Health Impacts." *Environmental Health Perspectives* 116 (11):1449–55. https://doi.org/10.1289/ehp.11463.

Environmental Protection Agency. 2011. "The Benefits and Costs of the Clean Air Act 1990–2020, the Second Prospective Study." https://www.epa.gov/clean-air-act-overview/benefits-and-costs-clean-air-act-1990-2020-second-prospective-study.

Fann, N., K. R. Baker, E. A. W. Chan, A. Eyth, A. Macpherson, E. Miller, and J. Snyder. 2018. "Assessing Human Health PM2.5 and Ozone Impacts from U.S. Oil and Natural Gas Sector Emissions in 2025." *Environmental Science & Technology* 52 (15):8095–8103. https://doi.org/10.1021/acs.est.8b02050.

Fiore, A. M., V. Naik, D. V. Spracklen, A. Steiner, N. Unger, M. Prather, D. Bergmann, et al. 2012. "Global Air Quality and Climate." *Chemical Society Reviews* 41:6663–83.

Fisk, W. J., Q. Lei-Gomez, and M. J. Mendell. 2007. "Meta-Analyses of the Associations of Respiratory Health Effects with Dampness and Mold in Homes." *Indoor Air* 17:284–96.

Ford, B., M. V. Martin, S. E. Zelasky, E. V. Fischer, S. C. Anenberg, C. L. Heald, and J. R. Pierce. 2018. "Future Fire Impacts on Smoke Concentrations, Visibility, and Health in the Contiguous United States." *GeoHealth* 2 (8):229–47. https://doi.org/10.1029/2018GH000144.

Frenkel, M., and Hermoni, D. (2002). Effects of homeopathic intervention on medication consumption in atopic and allergic disorders. *Alternative therapies in health and medicine* 8(1), 76.

Gage, K. L., T. R. Burkot, R. J. Eisen, and E. B. Hayes. 2008. "Climate and Vectorborne Diseases." *American Journal of Preventive Medicine* 35 (5):436–50. https://doi.org/10.1016/j.amepre.2008.08.030.

Grabow, M. L., S. N. Spak, T. Holloway, B. Stone Jr., A. C. Mednick, and J. A. Patz. 2012. "Air Quality and Exercise-Related Health Benefits from Reduced Car Travel in the Midwestern United States." *Environmental Health Perspectives* 120(1):68–76.

Grulke, N., and S. Schilling. 2008. Air Pollution and Climate Change. Washington, DC: U.S. Department of Agriculture, Forest Service, Climate Change Resource Center. http://www.fs.fed.us/ccrc/topics/air-pollution.shtml.

Haines, A. 2007. "Energy and Health Series." *Lancet* 370 (9591):922. https://doi.org/10.1016/S0140-6736(07)61259-8.

Hogrefe, C. 2012. "Emissions versus Climate Change." *Nature Geoscience* 5(10):685–86.

Horton, R., C. Little, V. Gornitz, D. Bader, and M. Oppenheimer. 2015. "New York City Panel on Climate Change 2015 Report Chapter 2: Sea Level Rise and Coastal Storms: NPCC 2015 Report Chapter 2." *Annals of the New York Academy of Sciences* 1336 (1):36–44. https://doi.org/10.1111/nyas.12593.

Institute of Medicine. 2004. *Damp Indoor Spaces and Health*. Washington, DC: Committee on Damp Indoor Spaces and Health, Institute of Medicine, National Academies of Sciences.

Institute of Medicine. 2011. *Climate Change, the Indoor Environment, and Health*. Washington, DC: Committee on the Effect of Climate Change on Indoor Air Quality and Public Health. Institute of Medicine, National Academies of Sciences.

Intergovernmental Panel on Climate Change. 2012. *Managing the Risks of Extreme Weather Events and Disasters to Advance Climate Change Adaptation (SREX): A Special Report of Working Groups I and II of the IPCC*, edited by C. Field and coauthors. Cambridge: Cambridge University Press.

Jerrett, M., R. T. Burnett, C. A. Pope III, K. Ito, G. Thurston, D. Krewski, Y. Shi, et al. 2009. "Long-Term Ozone Exposure and Mortality." *New England Journal of Medicine* 360:1085–95. doi:10.1056/NEJMoa0803894.

Johnston, F. H., S. B. Henderson, Y. Chen, J. T. Randerson, M. Marlier, R. DeFries, P. Kinney, et al. 2012. "Estimated Global Mortality Attributable to Smoke from Landscape Fires." *Environmental Health Perspectives* 120:695–701. http://dx.doi.org/10.1289/ehp.1104422.

Johnston, F. H., A. M. Kavanagh, D. M. Bowman, and R. K. Scott. 2002. "Exposure to Bushfire Smoke and Asthma: An Ecological Study." *Medical Journal of Australia* 176:535–38.

Kinney, P. L. 2008. "Climate Change, Air Quality, and Human Health." *American Journal of Preventive Medicine* 35:450–67.

Kinney, P. L. 2018. "Interactions of Climate Change, Air Pollution, and Human Health." *Current Environmental Health Reports* 5 (1):179–86. https://doi.org/10.1007/s40572-018-0188-x.

Knowlton, K., J. E. Rosenthal, C. Hogrefe, B. Lynn, S. Gaffin, R. Goldberg, C. Rosenzweig, et al. 2004. "Assessing Ozone-Related Health Impacts under a Changing Climate." *Environmental Health Perspectives* 112:1557–63.

Kunzli, N., E. Avol, J. Wu, W. J. Gauderman, E. Rappaport, J. Millstein, J. Bennion, et al. 2006. "Health Effects of the 2003 Southern California Wildfires on Children." *American Journal of Respiratory and Critical Care Medicine* 174:1221–28.

Larsen, A. E., B. J. Reich, M. Ruminski, and A. G. Rappold. 2018. "Impacts of Fire Smoke Plumes on Regional Air Quality, 2006–2013." *Journal of Exposure Science & Environmental Epidemiology* 28 (4):319–27. https://doi.org/10.1038/s41370-017-0013-x.

Le, G., P. Breysse, A. McDermott, S. E. Eftim, A. Geyh, J. D. Berman, and F. C. Curriero. 2014. "Canadian Forest Fires and the Effects of Long-Range Transboundary Air Pollution on Hospitalizations among the Elderly." *ISPRS International Journal of Geo-Information* 3(2):713–31.

Lee, K. K. 2012. "Developing and Implementing the Active Design Guidelines in New York City." *Health and Place* 18:5–7.

Lei, H., D. J. Wuebbles, and X.-Z. Liang. 2012. "Projected Risk of High-Ozone Episodes in 2050." *Atmospheric Environment* 59:567–77.

Lim, S. S, T. Vos, A. D Flaxman, G. Danaei, K. Shibuya, H. Adair-Rohani, M. A. Al-Mazroa et al. 2012. "A Comparative Risk Assessment of Burden of Disease and Injury Attributable to 67 Risk Factors and Risk Factor Clusters in 21 Regions, 1990–2010: A Systematic Analysis for the Global Burden of Disease Study 2010." *Lancet* 380 (9859):2224–60. https://doi.org/10.1016/S0140-6736(12)61766-8.

Limaye, Vijay S., "Bitter Pill: The High Health Costs of Climate Change." Natural Resources Defense Council, September 18, 2019. https://www.nrdc.org/resources/bitter-pill-high-health-costs-climate-change.

Limaye, Vijay S, and Kim Knowlton. "Shining New Light on Long-Term Ozone Harms." *JAMA Internal Medicine*, 2019, 2. https://doi.org/10.1001/jamainternmed.2019.5967.

Limaye, V. S., W. Max, J. Constible, and K. Knowlton. 2019. "Estimating the Health-Related Costs of 10 Climate-Sensitive U.S. Events During 2012." *GeoHealth* 3 (9):245–65. https://doi.org/10.1029/2019GH000202.

Limaye, Vijay S, Wendy Max, Juanita Constible, and Kim Knowlton. 2020. "Estimating the Costs of Inaction and the Economic Benefits of Addressing the Health Harms of Climate Change." *Health Affairs* 39(12): 2098–2104. https://doi.org/10.1377/hlthaff.2020.01109.

Limaye, V. S., W. Schöpp, and M. Amann. 2018. "Applying Integrated Exposure-Response Functions to PM2.5 Pollution in India." *International Journal of Environmental Research and Public Health* 16 (1): 60. https://doi.org/10.3390/ijerph16010060.

Lipsher, S. "Wildfire Smoke a Culprit in Mercury's Spread." Denver Post, October 19, 2007.

Makri, A., and N. I. Stilianakis. 2008. "Vulnerability to Air Pollution Health Effects." *International Journal of Hygiene and Environmental Health* 211:326–36.

Marlier, M. E., R. S. DeFries, A. Voulgarakis, P. L. Kinney, J. T. Randerson, D. T. Shindell, Y. Chen, et al. 2013. "El Niño and Health Risks from Landscape Fire Emissions in Southeast Asia." *Nature Climate Change* 3:131–36.

McKillop, Matt, Jonathan M. Links, Crystal R. Watson, Rachel Pittluck, Megan Weil Latshaw, and Tara Kirk Sell. "Climate Change & Health: Assessing State Preparedness." *Trust for America's Health and the Johns Hopkins Bloomberg School of Public Health*, December 9, 2020. https://climateandhealthreport.org/assets/pdfs/JHU-004_Climate_Change_and_Health_Report_FINAL_112520.pdf.

Mikati, I., A. F. Benson, T. J. Luben, J. D. Sacks, and J. Richmond-Bryant. 2018. "Disparities in Distribution of Particulate Matter Emission Sources by Race and Poverty Status." *American Journal of Public Health* 108 (4):480–85. https://doi.org/10.2105/AJPH.2017.304297.

Mudarri, D., and W. J. Fisk. 2007. "Public Health and Economic Impact of Dampness and Mold." *Indoor Air* 17:226–35.

Mui, Simon, and Levin, Amanda. "Clearing The Air: The Benefits Of The Clean Air Act." *Natural Resources Defense Council*, May 2020. https://www.nrdc.org/sites/default/files/benefitsclean-air-act-ib.pdf.

Naeher, L. P., M. Brauer, M. Lipsett, J. T. Zelikoff, C. D. Simpson, J. Q. Koenig, and K. R. Smith. 2007. "Woodsmoke Health Effects: A Review." *Inhalation Toxicology* 19 (1):67–106.

National Weather Service, Lubbock, Texas. 2013. "Intense Cold Front Produces Severe Winds and Blowing Dust—17 October 2011." http://www.srh.noaa.gov/lub/?n=events-2011–20111017-haboob.

Natural Resources Defense Council. 2007. *Sneezing and Wheezing: How Global Warming Could Increase Ragweed Allergies, Air Pollution, and Asthma*, by K. Knowlton, M. Rotkin-Ellman, and G. Solomon. https://www.nrdc.org/sites/default/files/sneezing-report-2015.pdf.

Natural Resources Defense Council. 2013. "Where There's Fire, There's Smoke: Wildfire Smoke Affects Communities Distant from Deadly Flames." New York: NRDC. https://www.nrdc.org/sites/default/files/wildfire-smoke-IB.pdf.

Natural Resources Defense Council. 2017. "Climate Change Threatens Health." https://www.nrdc.org/climate-change-and-health

Neumann, J. E., S. C. Anenberg, K. R. Weinberger, M. Amend, S. Gulati, A. Crimmins, Henry Roman, N. Fann, and P. L. Kinney. 2018. "Estimates of Present and Future Asthma Emergency Department Visits Associated with Exposure to Oak, Birch, and Grass Pollen in the United States." *GeoHealth*. https://doi.org/10.1029/2018GH000153.

New York City. 2019. "Vehicle Idling Complaint. NYC 311." https://www1.nyc.gov/site/dep/environment/idling-citizens-air-complaint-program.page.

New York City Department of Environmental Protection. 2019. "Emissions from Transportation." https://www1.nyc.gov/site/dep/environment/transportation-emissions.page.

Newell, K., C. Kartsonaki, K. B. H. Lam, and O. Kurmi. 2018. "Cardiorespiratory Health Effects of Gaseous Ambient Air Pollution Exposure in Low and Middle Income Countries: A Systematic Review and Meta-Analysis." *Environmental Health* 17 (1):41. doi:10.1186/s12940-018-0380-3.

Nuvolone, D., D. Petri, and F. Voller. 2018. "The Effects of Ozone on Human Health." *Environmental Science and Pollution Research International* 25 (9):8074–88. doi:10.1007/s11356-017-9239-3.

Ogden, C., and M. Carroll. 2010. "Prevalence of Obesity among Children and Adolescents: United States, Trends 1963–1965 through 2007–2008." Division of Health and Nutrition Examination Surveys. http://www.cdc.gov/nchs/data/hestat/obesity_child_07_08/obesity_child_07_08.pdf.

Pappagianis, D. 2007. "Coccidiomycosis in California State Correctional Institutions." *Annals of the New York Academy of Sciences* 1111:103–11.

Patz, J. A., H. K. Gibbs, J. A. Foley, J. A. Rogers, and K. R. Smith. 2007. "Climate Change and Global Health: Quantifying a Growing Ethical Crisis." *EcoHealth* 4:397–405. doi:10.1007/s10393-007-0141-1.

Patz, Jonathan A., Valerie J. Stull, and Vijay S. Limaye. 2020. "A Low-Carbon Future Could Improve Global Health and Achieve Economic Benefits." *JAMA*, 2. https://doi.org/10.1001/jama.2020.1313.

Pinkerton, K. E., W. N. Rom, M. Akpinar-Elci, J. R. Balmes, H. Bayram, O. Brandli, J. W. Hollingsworth, et al. 2012. "An Official American Thoracic Society Workshop Report: Climate Change and Human Health." *Proceedings of the American Thoracic Society* 9 (1):3–8.

Pope, C. A. III, and D. W. Dockery. 2006. "Health Effects of Fine Particulate Air Pollution: Lines That Connect." *Journal of the Air and Waste Management Association* 56:709–42.

Pope, C. A. III, R. T. Burnett, M. J. Thun, E. E. Calle, and G. D. Thurston. 2002. "Lung Cancer, Cardiopulmonary Mortality and Long Term Exposure to Fine Particulate Air Pollution." *Journal of the American Medical Association* 287:1132–41.

Pratt, J. R., R. W. Gan, B. Ford, S. Brey, J. R. Pierce, E. V. Fischer, and S. Magzamen. 2019. "A National Burden Assessment of Estimated Pediatric Asthma Emergency Department Visits that May Be Attributed to Elevated Ozone Levels Associated with the Presence of Smoke." *Environmental Monitoring and Assessment* 191 (suppl 2):269. doi:10.1007/s10661-019-7420-5.

Redman, J. 2012. "Connecting the Dots of Extreme Weather." *Albert Lea Tribune*, July 20. http://www.albertleatribune.com/2011/07/20/connecting-the-dots-of-extreme-weather/ .

Reid, C. E., and J. L. Gamble. 2009. "Aeroallergens, Allergic Disease, and Climate Change: Impacts and Adaptation." *EcoHealth* 6 (3):458–70. https://doi.org/10.1007/s10393-009-0261-x.

Russell, A. G., E. Tagaris, K. Liao, and P. Amar. 2010. "Climate Impacts on Air Pollution and the Related Health Impacts and Increased Control Costs." Paper presented at the American Meteorological Association's 12th Conference on Atmospheric Chemistry and the 2nd Symposium on Aerosol-Cloud-Climate Interactions as part of the 90th American Meteorological Society Annual Meeting, January 16–21, Atlanta, GA.

Salo, P. M., S. J. Arbes Jr., M. Sever, R. Jaramillo, R. D. Cohn, S. J. London, and D. C. Zeldin. 2006. "Exposure to Alternaria alternata in US Homes Is Associated with Asthma Symptoms." *Journal of Allergy and Clinical Immunology* 118:892–98.

Sapkota, A., R. Murtugudde, F. C. Curriero, C. R. Upperman, L. Ziska, and C. Jiang. 2019. "Associations between Alteration in Plant Phenology and Hay Fever Prevalence among US Adults: Implication for Changing Climate." *PLOS One* 14 (3):e0212010. https://doi.org/10.1371/journal.pone.0212010.

Schwalm, C. R., C. A. Williams, K. Schaefer, D. Baldocchi, T. A. Black, A. H. Goldstein, B. E. Law et al. 2012. "Reduction in Carbon Uptake during Turn of the Century Drought in Western North America." *Nature Climate Change* 5:551–56.

Shah, A. S., J. P. Langrish, H. Nair, D. A. McAllister, A. L. Hunter, K. Donaldson, D. E. Newby, and N. L. Mills. 2013. "Global Association of Air Pollution and Heart Failure: A Systematic Review and Meta-Analysis." *Lancet* 382 (9897):1039–48. doi:10.1016/S0140-6736(13)60898-3.

Shah, A. S., K. K. Lee, D. A. McAllister, A. Hunter, H. Nair, W. Whiteley, J. P. Langrish, D. E. Newby, and N. L. Mills. 2015. "Short Term Exposure to Air Pollution And Stroke: Systematic Review and Meta-Analysis [published correction appears in 2016 Sep 06;354:i4851]." *BMJ* 350:h1295. doi:10.1136/bmj.h1295.

Shea, K. M., R. T. Truckner, R. W. Weber, and D. B. Peden. 2008. "Climate Change and Allergic Disease." *Journal of Allergy and Clinical Immunology* 122:443–53.

Sheffield, P. E., K. Knowlton, J. L. Carr, and P. L. Kinney 2011. "Modeling of Regional Climate Change Effects on Ground-Level Ozone and Childhood Asthma." *American Journal of Preventive Medicine* 41:251–57.

Sheffield, P. E., and P. J. Landrigan. 2011. "Global Climate Change and Children's Health: Threats and Strategies for Prevention." *Environmental Health Perspectives* 119:291–98. doi:10.1289/ehp.1002233.

Shenassa, E. D., C. Daskalakis, A. Liebhaber, M. Braubach, and M. J. Brown. 2007. "Dampness and Mold in the Home and Depression: An Examination of Mold-Related Illness and Perceived Control of One's Home as Possible Depression Pathways." *American Journal of Public Health* 97:1893–99.

Shriber, J., K. C. Conlon, K. Benedict, O. Z. McCotter, and J. E. Bell. 2017. "Assessment of Vulnerability to Coccidioidomycosis in Arizona and California." *International Journal of Environmental Research and Public Health* 147):680. doi:10.3390/ijerph14070680.

Siddique, Shabana, Madhuchanda Banerjee, Manas Ranjan Ray, and Twisha Lahiri. 2010. "Air Pollution and Its Impact on Lung Function of Children in Delhi, the Capital City of India." *Water, Air, & Soil Pollution* 212 (1–4):89–100.

Singer, B. D., L. H. Ziska, D. A. Frenz, D. E. Gebhard, and J. G. Straka. 2005. "Increasing Amb a 1 Content in Common Ragweed (Ambrosia artemisiifolia) Pollen as a Function of Rising Atmospheric CO2 Concentration." *Functional Plant Biology* 32 (7):667–70.

Smith, K. R. 2000. "National Burden of Disease in India from Indoor Air Pollution." *Proceedings of the National Academy of Sciences* 97 (24):13286–93. https://doi.org/10.1073/pnas.97.24.13286.

Smith, Kirk R., Howard Frumkin, Kalpana Balakrishnan, Colin D. Butler, Zoë A. Chafe, Ian Fairlie, Patrick Kinney, Tord Kjellstrom, Denise L. Mauzerall, and Thomas E. McKone. 2013. "Energy and Human Health." *Annual Review of Public Health* 34:159–88.

Spracklen, D. V., J. A. Logan, L. J. Mickley, R. J. Park, R. Yevich, A. L. Westerling, and D. A. Jaffe. 2007. "Wildfires Drive Interannual Variability of Organic Carbon Aerosol in the Western US in Summer." *Geophysical Research Letters* 34 (16). L16816. doi:1029/2007GL030037.

Spracklen, D. V., L. J. Mickely, J. A. Logan, R. C. Judman, R. Yevich, M. D. Flannigan, and A. J. Westerling. 2009. "Impacts of Climate Change from 2000 to 2050 on Wildfire Activity and Carbonaceous Aerosol

Concentrations in the Western United States." *Journal of Geophysical Research* 114:D20301. doi:10.1029/2008JD010966.

Stanke, C., M. Kerac, C. Prudhomme, J. Medlock, and V. Murray. 2013. "Health Effects of Drought: A Systematic Review of the Evidence." *PLoS Currents* https://doi.org/10.1371/currents.dis.7a2cee9e980 f91ad7697b570bcc4b004.

Stewart, S. K., D. C. Johnson, and W. P. Smith. 2013. "Bringing Bike Share to a Low-Income Community: Lessons Learned through Community Engagement, Minneapolis, Minnesota, 2011." *Preventing Chronic Disease* 10:E138.

Strickland, M. J., L. A. Darrow, M. Klein, W. D. Flanders, J. A. Sarnat, L. A. Waller, S. E. Sarnat, J. A. Mulholland, and P. E. Tolbert. 2010. "Short-Term Associations between Ambient Air Pollutants and Pediatric Asthma Emergency Department Visits." *American Journal of Respiratory and Critical Care Medicine* 182:307–16.

Sun, X., A. Waller, K. B. Yeatts, and L.n Thie. 2016. "Pollen Concentration and Asthma Exacerbations in Wake County, North Carolina, 2006–2012." *Science of the Total Environment* 544 (February):185–91. https://doi.org/10.1016/j.scitotenv.2015.11.100.

Tagaris, E., K.-J. Liao, A. J. DeLucia, L. Deck, P. Amar, and A. G. Russell. 2010. "Sensitivity of Air Pollution–Induced Premature Mortality to Precursor Emissions under the Influence of Climate Change." *International Journal of Environmental Research and Public Health* 7:2222–37.

U.S. Department of Energy. 2013. *Transportation Energy Data Book: Edition 32*, edited by S. C. Davis and S. W. Diegel. Oak Ridge, TN: Oak Ridge National Laboratory.

Wang, M., C. P. Aaron, J. Madrigano, E. A Hoffman, E. Angelini, J. Yang, A. Laine et al. 2019. "Association Between Long-term Exposure to Ambient Air Pollution and Change in Quantitatively Assessed Emphysema and Lung Function." *JAMA* 322 (6):546–56.

Weaver, E. A., and K. N. Kolivras. 2018. "Investigating the Relationship between Climate and Valley Fever (Coccidioidomycosis)." *EcoHealth* 15:840–52. https://doi.org/10.1007/s10393-018-1375-9.

Weiss, D. J., J. Weidman, and M. Bronson. 2012. *Heavy Weather: How Climate Destruction Harms Middle and Low-Income Americans*. Washington, DC: Center for American Progress. http://www.american-progress.org/wp-content/uploads/2012/11/ExtremeWeather.pdf.

West, J. J., A. M. Fiore, L. W. Horowitz, and D. L. Mauzerall. 2006. "Global Health Benefits of Mitigating Ozone Pollution with Methane Emission Controls." *Proceedings of the National Academies of Sciences of the United States of America* 103:3988–93.

Wolf, J., N. R. O'Neill, C. A. Rogers, M. L. Muilenberg, and L. H. Ziska. 2010. "Elevated Atmospheric Carbon Dioxide Concentrations Amplify Alternaria alternata Sporulation and Total Antigen Production." *Environmental Health Perspectives* 118:1223.

Wu, S., L. J. Mickley, E. M. Leibensperger, D. J. Jacob, D. Rind, and D. G. Streets. 2008. "Effects of 2000–2050 Global Change on Ozone Air Quality in the United States." *Journal of Geophysical Research* 113 (D6). https://doi.org/10.1029/2007JD008917.

Zhang, X., L. Zhao, D. Tong, G. Wu, M. Dan, and B. Teng. 2016. "A Systematic Review of Global Desert Dust and Associated Human Health Effects." *Atmosphere* 7 (12).

Zhang, Z., E. Whitsel, P. M. Quibrera, R. Smith, D. Liao, G. L. Anderson, and R. Z. J. Prineas. 2009. "Ambient Fine Particulate Matter Exposure and Myocardial Ischemia in the Environmental Epidemiology of Arrhythmogenesis in the Women's Health Initiative (EEAWHI) Study." *Environmental Health Perspectives* 117:751–56.

Zheng, M. Qiu, Y. Zhou, Q. Chen, and W. Guan. 2015. "Association between Air Pollutants and Asthma Emergency Room Visits and Hospital Admissions in Time Series Studies: A Systematic Review and Meta-Analysis." *PLoS One* 10 (9):e0138146. doi:10.1371/journal.pone.0138146.

Ziska, L. H., K. Knowlton, C. A. Rogers, D. Dalan, N. Tierney, M. A. Elder, W. Filley et al. 2011. "Recent Warming by Latitude Associated with Increased Length of Ragweed Pollen Season in Central North America." *Proceedings of the National Academies of Sciences of the United States of America* 108:4248–51.

Ziska, L. H., L. Makra, S. K. Harry, N. Bruffaerts, M. Hendrickx, F. Coates, A. Saarto et al. 2019. "Temperature-Related Changes in Airborne Allergenic Pollen Abundance and Seasonality across the Northern Hemisphere: A Retrospective Data Analysis." *Lancet Planetary Health* 3 (3):e124–31. https://doi.org/10.1016/S2542-5196(19)30015-4.

CHAPTER 6

POTENTIAL RISKS FROM CYANOBACTERIAL AND ALGAL BLOOMS

J. S. Metcalf and N. R. Souza

Introduction

Cyanobacteria and algae are photosynthetic organisms that occur in a wide variety of environments, including marine and freshwaters. These essential primary producers are the basis for freshwater and marine food chains and webs. Within the microalgae, diatoms, dinoflagellates, euglenoids, haptophytes and cyanobacteria all have the potential to adversely affect water quality (Hallegraeff 2003). This is largely through the production of toxins, comprising both high and low molecular weight compounds. Some algal groups have the ability to cause fish kills through the blockage of gills, as spines on the physical structure of the algae become lodged in the gills, rendering fish unable to breathe (Bell 1961; Kent, White, and LaTrace 1995). Other adverse aspects of algae and cyanobacteria are a result of heterotrophic bacterial oxygenic respiration to decay dead or **senescing** mass populations of algae, microalgae, or cyanobacteria (i.e., scum) resulting in decreased oxygen concentrations in water, causing fish deaths due to suffocation (Barica 1978). Large concentrations of microalgae also have the ability to cause shading in waters (Barros et al. 2003), potentially affecting other aquatic organisms. Depending on the light climate of the water, marine and freshwater microalgae have a variety of photosynthetic pigments that allow them to adapt to their environment.

Nutrients are the principal drivers of algal growth, and the availability of carbon, nitrogen and phosphorous—according to the **Redfield ratio**—are the necessary components to allow microalgae to bloom (Geider and La Roche 2002). Although microalgae and cyanobacteria are natural constituents of freshwater and marine ecosystems, problems arise when mass populations develop. This is largely as a result of their capacity to produce toxins that have been associated with acute and chronic health problems (Metcalf and Codd 2012).

This chapter focuses on the possible effects of climate change on eukaryotic microalgae and cyanobacteria. The potential effects of climate change are extensive and may be direct or indirect when other **biotic** and **abiotic** factors are considered. Some of the potential effects are summarized here, with a greater emphasis on cyanobacteria because of their adverse effects in freshwater ecosystems.

Toxin Producing Groups of Algae

Diatoms

Although there are few data on the production of toxins by freshwater diatoms, marine diatom toxin production is very well documented. The major problematic genus is most likely *Pseudo-nitzschia* with a number of species being able to produce the marine toxin domoic acid (Lelong et al. 2012). An analog of

KEY CONCEPTS

- Cyanobacteria and microalgae are essential ecosystem components providing the basis of food chains and food webs.

- They are capable of producing a range of toxic compounds of risk to human and animal health.

- Intoxications may increase with blooms that are geographically larger and more extensive and that can persist for longer periods of time.

- Climate change is considered to increase the likelihood of blooms forming.

kainic acid (Armstrong et al. 1998; Nanao et al. 2005), and originally isolated from red algae (Sato et al. 1996), domoic acid can cause **amnesic shellfish poisoning** (ASP), mostly through the consumption of contaminated shellfish (Lelong et al. 2012). This occurs through destruction of cells within the brain, in particular in the regions of the amygdala and hippocampus, through activation of **AMPA** receptors, kainate receptors, and uncontrolled calcium influx (Strain and Tasker 1991; Costa, Giordano, and Faustman 2010). As the name indicates, permanent loss of short-term memory can occur and in high enough doses, death can result (Perl et al. 1990).

Dinoflagellates

A phylum within the Protista, the dinoflagellates are a diverse group of photosynthetic microalgae (Hackett et al. 2004). Of relevance to human health is their capacity to produce a wide range of toxic compounds with associated intoxications, mostly observed as a result of consuming contaminated seafood. The various toxins produced by dinoflagellates were traditionally split along symptoms observed after exposure but now are classified via the causative agent/compound of the illness or intoxication. Azaspiracids, produced by, for example, *Protoperidinium* spp. (James et al. 2003) and *Azadinium spinosum* (Tillman et al. 2009), can cause azaspiracid poisoning (AZP), largely observed as gastrointestinal upset (James et al. 2004). Similarly, **diarrhetic shellfish poisoning** (DSP) is caused by ingestion of okadaic acid and dinophysis toxins (Vale and Botana 2008), the former an inhibitor of protein phosphatases. DSP toxins are largely produced by *Procentrum* spp. (Hu et al. 1995; Heredia-Tapia et al. 2002) and *Dinophysis* spp. (Cembella 1989).

Saxitoxins can be produced by *Alexandrium* and *Pyrodinium* spp., and result in **paralytic shellfish poisoning** (PSP) through blockage of **voltage-gated sodium channels** (Lefebvre et al. 2008; Wiese et al. 2010). Palytoxins have been shown to be produced by *Ostreopsis* spp. (Usami et al. 1995) and can cause palytoxin poisoning (PTX) with gastrointestinal and systemic effects, including muscle breakdown (Okano et al. 1998). Yessotoxin poisoning (YTX) can be caused by exposure to yessotoxins, **polyether** compounds produced by dinoflagellates, including *Proroceratium* spp., *Gonyaulax* spp. and *Lingulodinium* spp. (Satake, MacKenzie, and Yasumoto 1997; Paz et al. 2004, 2008; Rhodes et al. 2006). Although more toxic when administered intraperitoneally versus orally (Tubaro et al. 2003), these compounds are known to accumulate in shellfish and bivalves. Similarly, spirolides produced by *Alexandrium* spp. (e.g. Cembella, Lewis, and Quilliam 2000) also show high toxicity when administered intraperitoneally to mice during routine toxicity testing (Richard et al. 2000).

Species of the genus *Gambierdiscus* (e.g., *G. toxicus*, *G. polynesiensis*; Holmes et al. 1991; Chinain et al. 2010) and *Fukuyoa* (e.g., *F. ruetzleri*; Litaker et al. 2017) are known to produce ciguatoxins (CTXs), a neurotoxic compound causing CFP (ciguatera fish poisoning) and CSP (ciguatera shellfish poisoning) through the ingestion of contaminated tropical and subtropical reef fish and mollusks, respectively (Larsson et al. 2019, Gatti et al. 2018). Other toxins such as maitotoxins (MTX) and CTX-like toxins have also been reported (Murray et al. 2018).

Of increasing concern and one of the most common dinoflagellate phenomena are **red tides**. These are generally orange to red-coloured blooms of microalgae, often comprised of *Karenia brevis*, that can overwinter or germinate from cysts to form mass populations in marine environments (Kubanek et al. 2005). Of particular concern is their ability to produce brevetoxins, potent sodium channel blocking compounds that are responsible for mass deaths of shellfish, fish and mammals (Landsberg, Flewelling, and Naar 2009).

Some nonphotosynthetic dinoflagellates are known to exist including *Oodinium* and *Pfiesteria*. These are largely problematic because of their ability to parasitize fish for nutrition resulting in damage, disease, and death to these vertebrates (Burkholder et al. 2001; Levy et al. 2007; Gómez and Skovgaard 2015).

Haptophytes

Haptophytes are a clade of algae that form mass blooms in marine environments; coccolithophores are a common type (Moore, Dowell, and Franz 2012). Of the haptophytes, perhaps the most problematic are species of the genus *Prymnesium* (Manning and La Claire 2010). Species of *Prymensium* such as *P. parvum* are capable of producing prymnesin toxins, which often result in fish deaths due to their high cellular toxicity and their capacity to cause hemolysis (Igarashi, Sataka, and Yasumoto 1996).

Euglenoids

Euglenoids are flagellated freshwater algae with *Euglena* spp. being one of the most common. Although little research has been conducted on the toxic potential of these photosynthetic organisms, *Euglena sangiunea* has been shown to be capable of producing euglenophycins, a toxin with necrotic activity to mammalian cells (Zimba et al. 2017).

Cyanobacteria

Cyanobacteria, Gram-negative bacteria, are found in many terrestrial and aquatic environments. Genera such as *Synechococcus* and *Prochlorococcus* are common cyanobacterial components of marine environments (Flombaum et al. 2013) along with e.g. occasional blooms of *Trichodesmium*. This latter genus has been shown to have toxicity when collected from the marine environment (Hawser et al. 1992; Ramos et al. 2005). Cyanobacteria are mostly known for their occurrence in freshwater (Figure 6.1), largely because of the input of nutrients such as nitrogen and phosphorous, which can allow mass populations to form. With the ability of some to regulate buoyancy, they are able to float to the surface where the action of wind can create scums, resembling thick paint. Often, these accumulations occur on shorelines where humans and animals enter and leave the water (Fogg et al. 1973; Metcalf and Codd 2012). In the case of dogs, such animals can also be attracted to the scums by taste and odor compounds that cyanobacteria can produce, such as geosmin and methylisoborneol (Codd et al. 1992, 2005). Because of the high biomass that can result when scums occur, only small amounts of toxin-producing material need to be ingested to result in toxic effects. Furthermore, a collapse of the bloom and subsequent breakdown of the organic material can cause a decrease in the oxygen concentration of the water leading to fish mortalities (Barica 1978).

Cyanobacteria are capable of producing a wide range of compounds with differing toxicological modes of action (Metcalf and Codd 2012). Termed cyanotoxins, the most commonly reported are the microcystins and nodularins, cyclic peptides, which are hepatotoxic and able to inhibit protein phosphatase enzymes. Although the 5-amino acid containing nodularins have been reported only in *Nodularia* and *Hapalosiphon* in marine and brackish environments, the 7-amino acid microcystins have been shown to be more widely distributed among freshwater cyanobacterial genera including *Microcystis*, *Dolichospermum*, and *Planktothrix* (Catherine et al. 2017). Other toxins with hepatotoxic and cytotoxic effects are cylindrospermopsins, again produced by a range of cyanobacteria such as *Cylindrospermopsis*, *Anabaena*, and

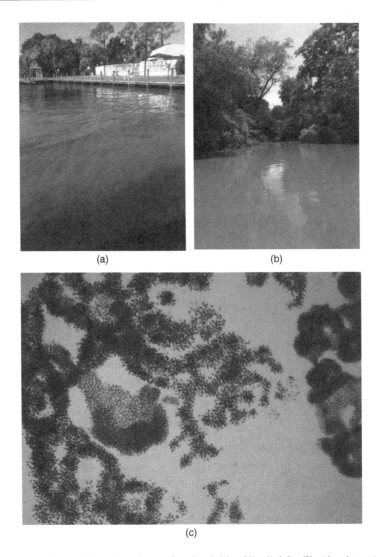

Figure 6.1   Examples of cyanobacterial blooms in freshwaters from Florida (A) and New York City (B) with a photo micrograph of *Microcystis* spp. (C)

Aphanizomenon (Metcalf and Codd 2012). Cyanobacteria are also capable of producing a variety of highly neurotoxic compounds such as anatoxin-a, anatoxin-a(S), and saxitoxins, the latter also produced by marine dinoflagellates (Metcalf and Codd 2012). More recent discoveries include β-N-methylamino-L-alanine (BMAA) and isomers N-(2-aminoethyl)glycine (AEG) and 2,4-diaminobutyric acid (DAB), with administration of BMAA shown to result in the production of neuropathologies consistent with human neurodegenerative disease (Cox et al. 2016; Davis et al. 2020). Research indicates that BMAA may also be produced by diatoms and dinoflagellates (Jiang et al. 2014; Lage et al. 2014; Violi et al. 2019). As cyanobacteria are Gram-negative photo-synthetic bacteria, they also possess lipopolysaccharide (LPS) in their outer cell wall which can result in gastrointestinal upset if ingested (Metcalf and Codd 2012). Dermatotoxins are also known to be produced by marine (e.g., *Moorea*) and freshwater cyanobacteria (e.g., *Lyngbya*) with adverse effects reported, largely presenting as rashes or skin irritation such as itching (Osborne and Shaw 2008; Puschner, Bautista, and Wong 2017). Further research continues to develop an understanding of other bioactive compounds that are produced by cyanobacteria, such as anabaenopeptins, microginins, and nostocylin, as examples (Elersek et al. 2017).

CLINICAL CORRELATES 6.1 MICROCYSTINS AND PRIMARY LIVER CANCER

The ability of microcystins to inhibit protein phosphatases (MacKintosh et al. 1990), essential mammalian cellular enzymes, raised the possibility that such compounds may have carcinogenic potential. Although the risks associated with short-term acute exposure to microcystins were known, the issue of long-term exposure to low concentrations was not understood. Ultimately, a World Health Organization Guideline value of 1μg/l for microcystin-LR in drinking water was proposed to protect human health over a lifetime (Falconer 2005). As people may be exposed long-term to low concentrations of microcystins, the possibility exists that inhibition of protein phosphatases may result in the loss of key cellular safeguards. As microcystins can covalently bind to these enzymes and inhibit them (MacKintosh et al. 1995), it raises the possibility that they may be tumor promoters (Falconer and Humpage 1996). Consequently, if people are exposed to a tumor initiator, then subsequent exposure to microcystin may cause a more-rapid development of the tumor.

With climate change, the incidence of blooms containing microcystins may well increase with increased human exposures. Work by Ueno et al. (1996) using an immunoassay for microcystins showed the presence of this toxin in 17 percent of pond/ditch water, 32 percent of river water, and 4 percent of deep well water. Conclusions were that microcystin exposure was considered to be a risk factor for primary liver cancer after initiation of the tumor from exposure to compounds such as aflatoxin. Other studies examining blooms in Serbia also indicated a connection between the incidence of this disease and the preparation and consumption of water from reservoirs containing cyanobacterial blooms (Svircev et al. 2013). Further studies in China have indicated that chronic exposure to microcystins may cause liver damage (Li et al. 2011) and serum microcystin concentrations correlate with cases of hepatocellular carcinoma (Zheng et al. 2017).

If climate change affects cyanobacterial blooms to result in increased exposure to microcystins, then long-term damage to human liver function, including primary liver cancer, may be expected.

Effects of Cyanobacterial and Algal Toxins

The majority of cyanobacterial and algal toxins are known for their ability to adversely affect health, largely acting in minutes to hours or occasionally days in their adverse effects. This toxicity is largely due to the ability of such toxins to inhibit enzymes and ion channels, leading to organ failure in a short time (e.g., Metcalf and Codd 2012). Acute effects attributed to cyanobacterial and algal toxins have been observed with mortality of a variety of animals such as fish, dogs, cattle, and sheep (Codd et al. 2005). In addition to direct human health effects, the death of large numbers of animals can have a negative impact on local economies and industries such as tourism and fisheries (Hoagland and Scatasta 2006). As acute exposures to cyanobacterial and algal toxins have increasingly been reported, public understanding of the risks has increased, as has the introduction of legislation and guidelines to help protect people from future toxin exposures (Codd et al. 2005; Metcalf and Codd 2012).

In addition to the acute health effects of algal and cyanobacterial toxins, research is now focused on the long-term effects of these toxic exposures. Many algal and cyanobacterial toxins are increasingly thought to be carcinogens and tumor promoters (Nishiwaki-Matsushima et al. 1992; Ohta et al. 1994; Zegura, Straser, and Filipic 2011). Higher incidences of primary liver cancer have been attributed to exposure to microcystin in China (Ueno et al. 1996) and Eastern Europe (Svircev et al. 2013) and may occur through the inhibition of protein phosphatases, which is also a mode of action of okadaic acid (Metcalf, Bell, and Codd 2001), a primary cause of marine DSP toxicity events. Other tumor promoters include palytoxin, teliocidin, and aplysiatoxin (Fujiki and Sugimura 1987). Long-term exposure to BMAA is now considered to be a possible causative agent of human neurodegenerative diseases (Cox et al. 2016). With

ASP, exposure to domoic acid can result in permanent loss of short-term memory, which can have drastic chronic effects for people who have been exposed to sufficient doses of this marine toxin (Perl et al. 1990). Furthermore, chronic or long-term exposure to domoic acid is also suspected of causing cognitive decline (Lefebvre et al. 2017).

CLINICAL CORRELATES 6.2 BMAA AND HUMAN NEURODEGENERATIVE DISEASE

Progressive neurodegenerative diseases, including amyotrophic lateral sclerosis/motor neuron disease (ALS/MND), Alzheimer's, and Parkinson's disease, are devastating illnesses, which in many cases result in death. Analysis of the genetics of those who suffer from such diseases indicate that, in the case of ALS for example, only 8–10 percent of these have a familial history of the disease, with half of those patients having a known mutation and the remaining 90–92 percent represent sporadic cases (e.g., Forsberg et al. 2010). In both familial and sporadic cases, exposure to environmental toxins may play a role in disease etiology. One risk factor that has been identified is the cyanobacterial toxin β-N-methylamino-L-alanine (BMAA), which is produced by cyanobacteria in laboratory cultures and environmental blooms (Metcalf et al. 2008; Bishop et al. 2018). Furthermore, freshwater diatoms, along with marine diatoms and dinoflagellates may also produce this neurotoxic amino acid (Lage et al. 2014; Jiang et al. 2014; Violi et al. 2019). BMAA appears to accumulate in contaminated marine shellfish. On the Pacific island of Guam, the Chamorro Indigenous people suffered from a high incidence of a neurodegenerative disease now known as ALS/PDC that has clinical and neuropathological characteristics of ALS, Alzheimer's and Parkinson's Disease (Reed et al. 1966). People who died of this disease in Guam and other neurological diseases in Canada and the USA had BMAA present within brain samples, whereas people who died of diseases unrelated to neurodegeneration or suffered from Huntington's Disease, which is purely a genetic disease did not (Murch et al. 2004; Pablo et al. 2009). Low-dose chronic administration of BMAA to non-human primates triggered neuropathologies such as β-amyloid plaques and neurofibrillary tangles consistent with the degenerative disease on Guam and also of Alzheimer's (Cox et al. 2016). Recent research examining the spinal cords of these animals revealed microglial activation, and proteinopathies of TDP-43, FUS, and Ubiquitin consistent with early stages of ALS in human beings (Davis et al. 2020). Therefore, chronic exposure to BMAA over many years at low doses through food or water may increase the risk of people developing a debilitating neurodegenerative disease.

Climate change may increase the frequency of blooms and may affect the production of BMAA in such blooms that could result in an increase in environmentally-induced human neurodegenerative disease.

How Will Climate Change Affect Algal and Cyanobacterial Blooms and Toxins?

Global climate change is likely to have a wide variety of impacts on ecosystems and environments. Primarily, this is considered to be a result of increased water and air temperatures around the world (Hansen et al. 2006). Other predictions include the potential for short-term localized chaotic weather events such as cyclones and thunderstorms (Easterling et al. 2000). Such changes to global climate are likely to affect the development of cyanobacterial and algal blooms.

Temperature and Nutrients

With climate change, an increase in the global temperature is expected (Intergovernmental Panel on Climate Change 2018). Most algae and cyanobacteria have an optimum growth temperature and will grow slower at temperatures lower and higher than this optimum, due to adverse effects on the metabolism of the cell. Cyanobacteria such as *Aphanizomenon flos-aquae* can grow at temperatures of 30°C (86°F) (Butterwick, Heaney, and Talling 2004). As a group, cyanobacteria can exhibit optimal growth at higher temperatures and are most likely to outcompete eukaryotic algae (Paerl and Huisman 2008; Paerl, Hall, and Calandrino 2011).

Changes in temperature will also affect weather patterns and associated conditions that may influence periods during which cyanobacteria and algae bloom. As a general rule, cold and dark conditions (such as in winter) are less favorable for bloom development than calm, warm sunny weather. In temperate freshwater environments, cyanobacteria generally bloom during the summer and autumn and then disappear when autumnal conditions turn over the water, disrupting the thermocline (Xu et al. 2009). With climate change, the likely effects might be an extension in the duration of the bloom season and a geographic expansion of blooms and species (Peeters et al. 2007; Wiedner et al. 2007). This may increase the risk of toxic exposures as toxin-containing blooms may exist for longer time periods. Certain species such as *Cylindrospermopsis raciborskii*, a tropical and subtropical species known to produce toxins (Hawkins et al. 1985), have been shown to be present in temperate regions (Antunes et al. 2015). The appearance of this invasive species in cooler regions may be attributable to climate change (Antunes et al. 2015).

The increased frequency of extreme weather events from climate change, specifically precipitation downpours, may have the increased effect of flushing cyanobacterial blooms from waterways (Elliott 2010). Although such discharges can prevent blooms by flushing algae and mixing waters, in the long term this phenomenon may promote blooms due to surface runoff, ground water discharges, and erosion of soil, all leading to a potential increase of nutrients in the water. With an ever-increasing human population that needs to abstract water, many lakes and rivers may suffer from a loss of or reduced flows of water. As cyanobacteria proliferate slowly, they prefer low flows and calm conditions in waters with long **residence times** (Romo et al. 2012) and may benefit from reduced flows in waters as a result of climate change.

Another manner in which climate change is driving cyanobacterial and algal blooms is through carbon sequestration into the oceans from the atmosphere, considered to be a factor in an observed increase in ocean acidification (Orr et al. 2005). Algae that contain calcium carbonate as a structural component of their skeletons require carbonate from waters for their synthesis. Ocean acidification will affect the chemical equilibrium of the formation of these nutrients possibly affecting the growth of certain types of algae, potentially disrupting the algae ecosystem (Raven 2011). It has been hypothesized that ocean acidification may preferentially adversely affect non-toxin-producing algae, therefore creating conditions that may shift the balance towards more toxin-producing algae and algae that can adapt to increasing temperatures and a tolerance of acidification (Doney et al. 2009).

In addition to carbon for photosynthesis, algae and cyanobacteria also require nutrients such as nitrogen and phosphorous for optimal growth. In the case of cyanobacteria, some genera are capable of fixing atmospheric **diazotrophic** nitrogen, negating the requirement to obtain organic forms of this nutrient from water (Fogg et al. 1973). As nutrients are often the drivers of bloom formation in marine and freshwater ecosystems, influxes of essential elements will permit the production of or may enhance the development of blooms. Pressures caused by human populations due to the release of nutrients such as through sewage and agriculture, which often end up in water sources, are likely to promote the formation of blooms (Paerl and Paul 2012).

Increased nutrient inputs into marine environments are occurring, partly as a result of agricultural fertilizers. Nitrogen and phosphorous are primary drivers of eutrophication and can result in the formation of **"dead zones"** within marine and freshwater environments (Dodds 2006; Diaz and Rosenberg 2008). Dead zones have been reported in coastal regions, where the majority of marine life is often found, near highly urbanized areas such as in North America, Europe, and Japan (Diaz and Rosenberg 2008; Altieri and Gedan 2015). A further aspect of these zones is that the oxygen concentration in the water is often extremely low (Dodds 2006; Diaz and Rosenberg 2008). Consequently, marine life struggles to survive under these conditions, removing potential consumers of algae such as fish. With little biological competition and high nutrient concentrations, these are ideal conditions for the development of toxic harmful algal and cyanobacterial blooms (Conley et al. 2009). Coupled with rising temperatures through global climate change, these conditions may allow the mass algal and cyanobacterial populations to exist for longer periods of time and cover a greater area than previously occupied. Such conditions have been observed in the Gulf of Mexico, where large blooms of *Karenia brevis* occur with associated brevetoxin production, affecting fish and marine mammals with the potential for mass animal and fish mortalities (Hu et al. 2006).

Sea levels are expected to rise with increasing temperatures through global climate change (Nicholls and Cazanave 2010). This is mostly because of two synergistic factors, namely the melting of ice and glaciers, such as in Antarctica and Greenland (Alley et al. 2005), and the thermal expansion of water (Wigley and Raper 1987). Both of these processes are predicted to cause rises in sea level around the world with the risk that low-lying coastlines and islands may ultimately be submerged (Nicholls and Cazanave 2010). Although very little work has been carried out on the effects of flooding on algal blooms, flooding of urban areas may result in the washing of nutrients into marine and freshwater ecosystems, in addition to increasing the likelihood of harmful algal and cyanobacterial exposures *via* floodwaters (Cook, Holland, and Longmore 2010). Adverse health effects under these flooding scenarios are most likely to present as skin irritations from cyanobacterial compounds such as aplysia-toxins and gastrointestinal symptoms. The latter scenario would most likely occur from Gram-negative bacteria, including cyanobacteria (Monteiro et al. 2017) and heterotrophic Gram-negative bacteria such as *Vibrio cholerae*. Reports from Bangladesh have shown a correlation between freshwater blooms of cyanobacteria and outbreaks of cholera (Islam, Drasar, and Sack 1994).

Polar Marine Environments and Algal Blooms

With increasing water temperatures in marine environments as a consequence of global climate change, effects on the occurrence of sea ice in polar latitudes are being observed. One effect of diminishing sea ice is that the transparency of the water will increase as ice can absorb sunlight, which may have the ultimate effect of increasing the potential for photosynthesis (Arrigo, van Dijken, and Pabi 2008; Popova et al. 2012) and the development of harmful algal and cyanobacterial blooms.

Although changes to water temperatures are likely to significantly affect ice in polar environments, the different poles may ultimately behave differently. In Antarctica, the most likely effect of increased temperatures will be the melting of glaciers (Pritchard et al. 2012), which will result in pulses of freshwater entering these marine systems (Dierrsen, Smith, and Vernet 2002). Such freshwater inputs may significantly affect the salinity of the water, which may affect the production of harmful cyanobacterial and algal blooms, in addition to potential sea level rises. In the Arctic, ice is mostly present as floating sea ice, which when it melts will result in increasingly open waters. Even though this will mostly have little effect on sea level height, the increase of open water will ultimately permit the establishment of new navigation routes between the Atlantic and Pacific Oceans (Smith and Stephenson 2013). Consequently, with marine currents and ballast transfer by ships, macro and microalgae have the potential to move between the two oceans (Hoegh-Guldberg and Bruno 2010). The influx of potentially invasive species into new oceans may result in novel blooms that can significantly adversely affect marine life and people.

Dust Storms, Deserts and Winds

With climate change, there will likely be dramatic effects concerning heating and cooling of land and water. These may bring changes to airborne weather patterns, which may have significant effects on marine and freshwater systems. For example, the windborne transportation of Saharan dust to Europe has been known for some time. The transfer of such iron-laden dust could therefore have significant effects on harmful cyanobacterial and algal blooms. In marine environments, iron is often a limiting nutrient and when deposited can result in the development of blooms. This was shown by the presence of a large bloom of microcystin-containing *Trichodesmium erythraeum* around the Canary Islands, caused by a combination of iron deposition with a nutrient upwelling off the West African coast (Ramos et al. 2005). With global climate change, such depositions could possibly increase and result in further development, extension, and longevity of harmful algal and cyanobacterial blooms.

In addition to aquatic environments, terrestrial environments may also be affected by dust storms. In desert environments cyanobacteria are often pioneering organisms that produce **cryptobiotic crusts** that cover the surface (Richer et al. 2012). Once these crusts stabilize the substrate then plant species can grow and develop into an ecosystem (Richer et al. 2012). Although useful ecologically, cyanobacterial crusts have been shown to contain cyanotoxins including BMAA, microcystins, and anatoxin-a(S) (Cox et al. 2009; Metcalf et al. 2012) and have been implicated in animal intoxications (Chatziefthimiou et al. 2014). Furthermore, in countries such as Qatar, they have been shown to cover up to 87 percent of the land surface showing how significant and important they are to the biology of these environments (Richer et al. 2012). With global climate change, droughts and desertification are considered likely to occur, with the potential to destroy cyanobacterial crusts and make cyanotoxin-containing particles airborne with possible adverse human health effects (Metcalf et al. 2012). Once crusts have been degraded through climate change, the substrate beneath may then be exposed, increasing the likelihood of erosion. As cyanobacterial crusts in desert environments have potentially been created over long periods of time, the possibility also exists that toxins may be present within the soil profile. Analysis of such horizons in Qatar showed that cyanotoxins were present at up to 25 cm below the surface of the crusts, indicating long-term persistence and production, potentially posing a risk to human and animal health (Richer et al. 2015).

Although microalgae are best known for their occurrence in aquatic environments, research is understanding their presence in air (Sharma et al. 2007). This may allow the seeding or transfer of microalgae to new environments and, depending on the algal/cyanobacterial concentration and composition in the air sample, could also potentially lead to adverse human health effects (Caller et al. 2009). This theory is supported through a possible link between BMAA exposure and the development of neurodegenerative diseases such as amyotrophic lateral sclerosis (ALS). The risk of developing this disease is higher when living in close proximity to water with cyanobacterial blooms (Caller et al. 2009).

Likewise, storms and their associated sprays and wave action have the potential to generate aerosols with microcystins and brevetoxins (Pierce et al. 2003; Cheng et al. 2005, 2007; Backer et al. 2008, 2010). Assessment of certain cyanobacterial toxins via intranasal administration has shown equal, if not greater toxicity via this exposure route (Fitzgeorge, Clark, and Keevil 1994). The increased likelihood of storms as a consequence of climate change may also result in more harmful algae and cyanobacteria becoming aerosolized due to increased sprays and wave action (e.g., Cheng et al. 2007).

Long-Term Solutions and Remediation

Microalgae and cyanobacteria are common components of freshwater, marine, and terrestrial environments. They perform essential ecological processes such as primary production and nitrogen fixation, they are food sources for a variety of organisms and food webs, and their presence is integral to a healthy and functioning ecosystem. Although certain algal and cyanobacterial species produce toxins, ultimately the toxicological risk is a function of dose and exposure route. Therefore, managing the concentration of algal and cyanobacterial cells through catchment practices, smart agriculture and water practices, and water treatment technologies will ultimately result in minimizing health threats from algal and cyanobacterial blooms (e.g., Westrick et al. 2010).

Emerging Questions and Conclusions

In order to understand the potential effects of climate change on harmful algal and cyanobacterial blooms, many questions require further investigation. These are largely related to the effects of climate change on temperature and the supply of nutrients to blooms, as well as the impacts of different species' interactions within food webs on microalgae and cyanobacterial homeostasis. Likewise, ocean carbon dioxide sequestration and acidification and its effects on marine and freshwater organisms and photosynthesis remains an area of active research. Climate change is likely to increase the effects of harmful algal and cyanobacterial blooms. Further scientific investigation, monitoring, remediation, and legislation is required to protect human and animal health from these adverse effects.

DISCUSSION QUESTIONS

1. Is climate change likely to increase the frequency and intensity of algal blooms?

2. Are humans and animals more likely to suffer adverse effects from exposure to algae and toxins as a result of climate change?

3. Could climate change result in the movement of algae and toxins to new geographical areas?

4. How do we manage the effects of climate change on algal blooms?

KEY TERMS

Abiotic factor: Non-living chemical or physical factor that can affect an ecosystem.

Amnesic shellfish poisoning: Poisoning syndrome occurring from the consumption of shellfish contaminated with domoic acid.

AMPA: α-amino-3-hydroxy-5-methyl-4-isoxazolepropionic acid, a neurotransmitter that has an action similar to that of glutamate.

Biotic factor: A living factor that can affect an ecosystem.

Cryptobiotic crusts: Communities of living organisms, often containing fungi and cyanobacteria that form crusts on soils in arid regions such as deserts.

Dead zones: Areas of oceans and lakes that contain little or no oxygen because of nutrient inputs.

Diarrhetic shellfish poisoning: Poisoning syndrome that occurs from the consumption of shellfish contaminated with okadaic acid.

Diazotrophic: With reference to atmospheric N_2, and the organisms able to use (fix) this atmospheric gas to make more complex forms of nitrogen such as ammonia.

Paralytic shellfish poisoning: Poisoning syndrome occurring from the consumption of shellfish contaminated with saxitoxin and related compounds.

Polyether: Polymeric, often chain-like, organic compounds containing ether linkages.

Red tides: Common term for blooms of microalgae and cyanobacteria that contain red pigments, causing an appearance of "red paint" on the surface of the water.

Redfield ratio: Molar ratio of carbon:nitrogen:phosphorous of 106:16:1 as found in seawater and phytoplankton.

Residence time: Relative measure of the average amount of time that a water molecule would be expected to be present within a waterbody before being lost or removed.

Senescing: In the case of algae, refers to the aging and breakdown of a bloom, and the release of pigments (and toxins) into water.

Voltage-gated sodium channels: Transmembrane proteins that allow sodium ions to travel across membranes and cause depolarization of neurons, resulting in an action potential.

References

Alley, R. B., P. U. Clark, P. Huybrechts, and I. Joughin. 2005. "Ice-Sheets and Sea-Level Changes." *Science* 310:456–60.

Altieri, A. H., and K. B. Gedan. 2015. "Climate Change and Dead Zones." *Global Change Biology* 21:1395–1406.

Antunes, J. T., P. N. Leão, and V. M. Vasconcelos. 2015. "*Cylindrospermopsis raciborskii*: Review of the Distribution, Phylogeography, and Ecophysiology of A Global Invasive Species." *Frontiers in Microbiology* 6:article 473.

Armstrong, N., Y. Sun, G.-Q. Chen, and E. Gouaux. 1998. "Structure of a Glutamate-Receptor Ligand-Binding Core in Complex with Kainate." *Nature* 395:913–17.

Arrigo, K. R., G. van Dijken, and S. Pabi. 2008. Impact of a shrinking ice cover on marine primary production. *Geophysical Research Letters* 35:L19603. doi:10.1029/2008GL35028.

Backer, L. C., W. Carmichael, B. Kirkpatrick, C. Williams, M. Irvin, Y. Zhou, T. B. Johnson et al. 2008. "Recreational Exposure to Low Concentrations of Microcystins During an Algal Bloom in a Small Lake." *Marine Drugs* 6:389–406.

Backer, L. C., S. V. McNeel, T. Barber, B. Kirkpatrick, C. Williams, M. Irvin, Y. Zhou, et al. 2010. "Recreational Exposure to Microcystins during Algal Blooms in Two California Lakes." *Toxicon* 55:909–21.

Barica, J. 1978. "Collapses of *Aphanizomenon flos-aquae* Blooms Resulting in Massive Fish Kills in Eutrophic Lakes: Effect of Weather." *Internationale Vereinigung für Theoretische und Angewandte Limnologie: Verhandlungen.* 20:208–13.

Barros, M. P., M. Pedersén, R. Colepicolo, and P. Snoeijs. 2003. "Self-Shading Protects Phytoplankton Communities against H_2O_2-Induced Oxidative Damage." *Aquatic Microbial Ecology* 30:275–82.

Bell, G. R. 1961. "Penetration of Spines from a Marine Diatom into the Gill Tissues of Lingcod (*Ophiodon elongatus*)." *Nature* 192:279–80.

Bishop, S.L., J. K. Kerkovius, F. Menard, S. J. Murch. 2018. "N-β-methylamino-L-alanine and its naturally occurring isomers in cyanobacterial blooms in Lake Winnipeg. *Neurotox. Res.* 33:133–142.

Burkholder, J. M., H. B. Glasgow, N. J. Deamer-Melia, J. Springer, M. W. Parrow, C. Zhang, and P. J. Cancellieri. 2001. "Species of the Toxic *Pfiesteria* Complex, and the Importance of Functional Type in Data Interpretation." *Environmental Health Perspectives* 109:667–79.

Butterwick, C., S. I. Heaney, and J. F. Talling. 2004. "Diversity in the Influence of Temperature on the Growth of Freshwater Algae, and Its Ecological Relevance." *Freshwater Biology* 50:291–300.

Caller, T. A., J. W. Doolin, J. F. Haney, A. J. Murby, K. G. West, H. E. Farrar, A. Ball, B. T. Harris, and E. W. Stommel. 2009. "A Cluster of Amyotrophic Lateral Sclerosis in New Hampshire: A Possible Role for Toxic Cyanobacteria Blooms." *Amyotrophic Lateral Sclerosis* 10:101–08. doi: https://doi.org/10.3109/174829609.

Catherine, A., C. Bernard, L. Spoof, and M. Bruno. 2017. "Microcystins and Nodularins." In *Handbook of Cyanobacterial Monitoring And Cyanotoxin Analysis*, edited by J. Meriluoto, L. Spoof, G. A. Codd, 109–26. London: John Wiley and Sons.

Cembella, A. D. 1989. "Occurrence of Okadaic Acid, a Major Diarrheic Shellfish Toxin, in Natural Populations of *Dinophysis* spp. from the Eastern Coast of North America." *Journal of Applied Phycology* 1:307–11.

Cembella, A. D., N. I. Lewis, and M. A. Quilliam. 2000. "The Marine Dinoflagellate *Alexandrium Ostenfeldii* (Dinophyceae) as the Causative Organism of Spirolide Shellfish Toxins." *Phycologia* 39:67–74.

Chatziefthimiou, A. D., R. Richer, H. Rowles, J. T. Powell, and J. S. Metcalf. 2014. "Cyanotoxins as a Potential Cause of Dog Poisonings in Desert Environments." *Veterinary Record* 174 (19):484–85.

Cheng, Y. S., Y. Zhou, C. M. Irvin, B. Kirkpatrick, and L. C. Backer. 2007. "Characterization of Aerosols Containing Microcystin." *Marine Drugs* 5:136–50.

Cheng, Y. S., Y. Zhou, C. M. Irvin, R. H. Pierce, J. Naar, L. C. Backer, and L. E. Fleming. 2005. "Characterization of Marine Aerosol for Assessment of Human Exposure to Brevetoxins." *Environmental Health Perspectives* 113:638–43.

Chinain, M., H. T, Darius, A. Ung, P. Cruchet, Z. Wang, D. Ponton, D. Laurent, and S. Pauillac. 2010. "Growth and Toxin Production in the Ciguatera-Causing Dinoflagellate *Gambierdiscus polynesiensis* (Dinophyceae) in Culture." *Toxicon* 56:739–50.

Codd, G. A., C. Edwards, K. A. Beattie, W. M. Barr, and G. J. Gunn. 1992. "Fatal Attraction to Cyanobacteria?" *Nature* 359:110–1.

Codd, G. A., J. Lindsay, F. M. Young, L. F. Morrison, and J. S. Metcalf. 2005. "Harmful Cyanobacteria: From Mass Mortalities to Management Measures." In *Harmful Cyanobacteria*, edited by J. Huisman, H. C. P. Matthijs, and P. M. Visser, 1–23. Dordrecht, the Netherlands: Springer.

Conley, D. J., H. W. Paerl, R. W. Howart, D. F. Boesch, S.P. Seitzinger, K. E. Havens, C. Lancelot, and G. E. Likens. 2009. "Controlling Eutrophication: Nitrogen and Phosphorus." *Science* 323:1014–15.

Cook, P. L. M., D. P. Holland, and A. R. Longmore. (2010). "Effect of a Flood Event on the Dynamics of Phytoplankton and Biogeochemistry in a Large Temperate Australian Lagoon." *Limnology and Oceanography* 55: 1123–33.

Costa, L. G., G. Giordano, and E. M. Faustman. 2010. "Domoic Acid as a Developmental Neurotoxin." *Neurotoxicology* 31:409–23.

Cox, P. A., D. A. Davis, D. C. Mash, J. S. Metcalf, and S. A. Banack. 2016. "Dietary Exposure to an Environmental Toxin Triggers Neurofibrillary Tangles and Amyloid Deposits in the Brain." *Proceedings of the Royal Society of London. Series B* 283:2015–97.

Cox, P. A., R. Richer, J. S. Metcalf, S. A. Banack, G. A. Codd, and W. G. Bradley. 2009. "Cyanobacteria and BMAA Exposure from Desert Dust: A Possible Link to Sporadic ALS among Gulf War Veterans." *Amyotrophic Lateral Sclerosis* 10 (suppl 2): 09–17.

Davis, D. A., P. A. Cox, S. A. Banack, P. D. Lecusay, S. P. Garamszegi, M. J. Hagan, J. T. Powell, J. S. Metcalf, R. M. Palmour, A. Beierschmitt, W. G. Bradley and D. C. Mash. (2020). L-serine reduces spinal cord pathology in a vervet model of preclinical ALS/MND. *J. Neuropath. Exp. Neurol.* 79: 393–406.

Diaz, R. J., and R. Rosenberg. 2008. "Spreading Dead Zones and Consequences for Marine Ecosystems." *Science* 321:926–29.

Dierssen, H. M., R. C. Smith, and M. Vernet. 2002. "Glacial Meltwater Dynamics in Coastal Waters West of the Antarctic Peninsula." *Proceedings of the National Academy of Sciences of the USA* 99:1790–95.

Dodds, W. K. 2006. "Nutrients and the 'Dead Zone': The Link between Nutrient Ratios and Dissolved Oxygen in the Northern Gulf of Mexico." *Frontiers in Ecology and the Environment* 4:211–17.

Doney, S. C., V. J. Fabry, R. A. Feely, and J. A. Kleypas. 2009. "Ocean Acidification: The Other CO_2 Problem." *Annual Review of Marine Science* 1:169–92.

Easterling, D. R., J. L. Evans, P. Y. Groisman, T. R. Karl, K. E. Kunkel, and P. Ambenje. 2000. "Observed Variability and Trends in Extreme Climate Events: A Brief Review." *Bulletin of the American Meteorological Society* 81:417–25.

Elersek, T., L. Blaha, H. Mazur-Marsec, W. Schmidt, and S. Carmeli. 2017. "Other Cyanobacterial Bioactive Substances." In *Handbook of Cyanobacterial Monitoring And Cyanotoxin Analysis*, edited by J. Meriluoto, L. Spoof, and G. A. Codd, 179–95. London: John Wiley and Sons.

Elliott, J. A. 2010. The Seasonal Sensitivity of Cyanobacteria and Other Phytoplankton to Changes in Flushing Rate and Water Temperature." *Global Change Biology* 16:864–76.

Falconer, I.R. (2005). Is there a human health hazard from microcystins in the drinking water supply? *Acta Hydrochim. Hydrobiolog.* 33: 64–71.

Falconer, I.R. & A. R. Humpage. (1996). Tumour promotion by cyanobacterial toxins. Phycologia 35: 74–79.

Fitzgeorge, R. B., I. A. Clark, and C. W. Keevil. 1994. "Routes of Intoxication." In *Detection Methods for Cyanobacterial Toxins*, edited by G. A. Codd, T. M. Jeffries, C. W. Keevil, and E. Potter, 69–74. Cambridge, UK: Royal Society of Chemistry.

Flombaum, P., J. L. Gallegos, R. A. Gordillo, J. Rincón, L. L. Zabala, N. Jiao, D. M. Karl et al. 2013. "Present and Future Global Distributions of the Marine Cyanobacteria *Prochlorococcus* and *Synechococcus*." *Proceedings of the National Academy of Sciences of the USA* 110:9824–29.

Fogg, G., W. D. P. Stewart, P. Fay, and A. E. Walsby. 1973. *The Blue-Green Algae*. London: Academic Press.

Forsberg, K., P.A. Jonsson, P. M. Andersen, D. Bergemalm & T. Brannstrom. (2010). Novel antibodies reveal inclusions containing non-native SOD1 in sporadic ALS patients. *PLoS ONE* 5(7):e11552.

Fujiki, H., and T. Sugimura. 1987. "New Classes of Tumor Promoters: Teleocidin, Aplysiatoxin and Palytoxin." *Advances in Cancer Research* 49:223–64.

Gatti, C. M., D. Lonati, H. T. Darius, A. Zancan, M. Roué, A. Schicchi, C. A. Locatelli, and M. Chinain. 2018. "*Tectus niloticus* (Tegulidae, Gastropod) as a Novel Vector of Ciguatera Poisoning: Clinical Characterization and Follow-Up of a Mass Poisoning Event in Nuku Hica Island (French Polynesia)." *Toxins* 10 (2): 102. https://doi.org/10.3390/toxins10030102.

Geider, R. J., and J. La Roche. 2002. "Redfield Revisited: Variability of C:N:P in Marine Microalgae and Its Biochemical Basis." *European Journal of Phycology* 37:1–17.

Gómez, F., and A. Skovgaard. 2015. "The Molecular Phylogeny of the Type-Species of *Oodinium* Chatton, 1912 (Dinoflagellata: Oodiniaceae), a Highly Divergent Parasitic Dinoflagellate with Non-Dinokaryotic Characters." *Systematic Parasitology* 90:125–35.

Hackett, J. D., D. M. Anderson, D. L. Erdner, and D. Bhattacharya. 2004. "Dinoflagellates: A Remarkable Evolutionary Experiment." *American Journal of Botany* 91:1523–34.

Hallegraeff, G. M. 2003. "Harmful Algal Blooms: A Global Overview." In *Manual on Harmful Marine Microalgae*, edited by G. M. Hallegraeff, D. M. Anderson, and A. D. Cembella. Monographs on Oceanographic Methodology 11:25–50.

Hansen, J., M. Sato, R. Ruedy, K. Lo, D. W. Lea, and M. Medina-Elizade. 2006. "Global Temperature Change." *Proceedings of the National Academy of Sciences of the USA* 103:14288–293.

Hawkins, P. R., M. T. Runnegar, A. R. Jackson, and I. R. Falconer. 1985. "Severe Hepatotoxicity Caused by the Tropical Cyanobacterium (Blue-Green Alga) Cylindrospermopsis Raciborskii (Woloszynska) Seenaya and Subba Raju Isolated from a Domestic Water Supply Reservoir." *Applied and Environmental Microbiology* 50:1292–95.

Hawser, S. P., J. M. O'Neil, M. R. Roman, and G. A. Codd. 1992. "Toxicity of Blooms of the Cyanobacterium *Trichodesmium* to Zooplankton." *Journal of Applied Phycology* 4:79–86.

Heredia-Tapia, A., B. O. Arredondo-Vega, E. J, Nuñez-Vázquez, T. Yasumoto, M. Yasuda, and J. L. Ochoa. 2002. "Isolation of *Prorocentrum lima* (Syn. *Exuviaella lima*) and Diarrhetic Shellfish Poisoning (DSP) Risk Assessment in the Gulf of California, Mexico." *Toxicon* 40:1121–27.

Hoagland, P., and S. Scatasta. 2006. "The Economic Effects of Harmful Algal Blooms." In *Ecology of Harmful Algae. Ecological Studies vol. 189*, edited by E. Graneli and J. T. Turner, 391–402. Heidelberg, Germany: Springer-Verlag.

Hoegh-Guldberg, O., and J. F. Bruno. 2010. "The Impact of Climate Change on the World's Marine Ecosystems." *Science* 328:1523–28.

Holmes, M. J., R. J. Lewis, M. A. Poli, and N. C. Gillespie. 1991. "Strain Dependent Production Of Ciguatoxin Precursors (Gambiertoxins) by *Gambierdiscus toxicus* (Dinophyceae) in Culture." *Toxicon* 29:761–75.

Hu, T., J. M. Curtis, J. A. Walter, J. L. McLachlan, and J. L. C. Wright. 1995. "Two New Water Soluble DSP Toxin Derivatives from the Dinoflagellate *Prorocentrum maculosum*: Possible Storage and Excretion Products." *Tetrahedron Letters* 36 9273–76.

Hu, C., F. E. Muller-Karger, and P. W. Swarzenski. 2006. "Hurricanes, Submarine Groundwater Discharge, and Florida's Red Tides." *Geophysical Research Letters* 33:L11601, doi:10.1029/2005GL025449.

Igarashi, T., M. Sataka, and T. Yasumoto. 1996. "Prymnesin-2: A Potent Ichtyotoxic and Hemolytic Glycoside from the Red Tide Alga *Prymnesium parvum*." *Journal of the American Chemical Society* 118:479–80.

Intergovernmental Panel on Climate Change. 2018. "Summary for Policymakers." In *Global Warming of 1.5°C. An IPCC Special Report on the Impacts of Global Warming of 1.5°C above Pre-Industrial Levels and Related Global Greenhouse Gas Emission Pathways, in the Context of Strengthening the Global Response to the Threat of Climate Change, Sustainable Development, and Efforts to Eradicate Poverty*, edited by V. Masson-Delmotte, P. Zhai, H. O. Pörtner, D. Roberts, J. Skea, P. R. Shukla, A. Pirani et al., 3–24. Geneva, Switzerland: IPCC.

Islam, M. S., B. S. Drasar, and B. Sack. 1994. "Probable Role of Blue-Green Algae in Maintaining Endemicity and Seasonality of Cholera in Bangladesh: A Hypothesis." *Journal of Diarrhoeal Diseases Research* 12 (4):245–56.

James, K. J., M. J. Fidalgo Sáez, A. Furey, and M. Lehane. (2004). "Azaspiracid Poisoning, The Food-Borne Illness Associated with Shellfish Consumption. *Food Additives and Contaminants* 21:879–92.

James, K. J., C. Moroney, C. Roden, M. Satake, T. Yasumoto, M. Lehane, and A. Furey. 2003. "Ubiquitous 'Benign' Alga Emerges as the Cause of Shellfish Contamination Responsible for the Human Toxic Syndrome, Azaspiracid Poisoning." *Toxicon* 41:145–51.

Jiang, L., J. Eriksson, S. Lage, S. Jonasson, S. Shams, M. Mehine, L. L. Ilag, and U. Rasmussen. 2014. "Diatoms: A Novel Source for the Neurotoxin BMAA in aquatic Environments." *PLoS ONE* 9 (8):e 106696. https://doi.org/10.1371/journal.pone.0084578 .

Kent, M. L., J. N. C. Whyte, and C. LaTrace. 1995. "Gill Lesions and Mortality in Seawater Pen-Reared Atlantic Salmon *Salmo salar* Associated with a Dense Blooms of *Skeletonema costatum* and *Thalassiosira* Species." *Diseases of Aquatic Organisms* 22:77–81.

Kubanek, J., M. K. Hicks, J. Naar, and T. A. Villareal. 2005. "Does the Red Tide Dinoflagellate *Karenia brevis* Use Allelopathy to Outcompete Other Phytoplankton?" *Limnology and Oceanography* 50:883–95.

Lage, S., P. R. Costa, T. Moita, J. Eriksson, U. Rasmussen, and S. J. Rydberg. 2014. "BMAA in Shellfish from Two Portuguese Transitional Water Bodies Suggest the Marine Dinoflagellate *Gymnodinium catenatum* as a Potential BMAA Source." *Aquatic Toxicology* 152:131–38.

Landsberg, J. H., L. J. Flewelling, and J. Naar. 2009. "*Karenia brevis* Red Tides, Brevetoxins in the Food Web, and Impacts on Natural Resources: Decadal Advancements." *Harmful Algae* 8:598–607.

Larsson, M. E., T. D. Harwood, R .J. Lewis, S. W. A. Himaya, and M. A. Doblin. 2019. "Toxicological Characterization of *Fukuyoa paulensis* (Dinophyceae) from Temperate Australia." *Phycology Research* 67:65–71.

Lefebvre, K. A., B. D. Bill, A. Erickson, K. A. Baugh, L. O'Rourke, P. R. Costa, S. Nance, and V. L. Trainer. 2008. "Characterization of Intracellular and Extracellular Saxitoxin Levels in Both Field and Cultured *Alexandrium* spp. Samples from Sequim Bay, Washington." *Marine Drugs* 6:103–16.

Lefebvre, K. A., P. S. Kendrick, W. Ladiges, E. M. Hiolski, B. E. Ferriss, D. R. Smith, and D. J. Marcinek. 2017. "Chronic Low-Level Exposure to the Common Seafood Toxin Domoic Acid Causes Cognitive Deficits in Mice." *Harmful Algae* 64:20–29.

Lelong, A., H. Hégaret, P. Soudant, and S. S. Bates. 2012. "*Pseudo-nitzschia* (Bacillariophyceae) Species, Domoic Acid and Amnesic Shellfish Poisoning: Revisiting Previous Paradigms." *Phycologia* 51:168–216.

Levy, M. G., R. W. Littaker, R. J. Goldstein, M. J. Dykstra, M. W. Vandersea, and E. J. Noga. 2007. "*Piscinoodinium*, a Fish-Ectoparasitic Dinoflagellate, Is a Member of the Class Dinophyceae, Subclass Gymnodiniphycidae: Convergent Evolution with *Amyloodinium*." *Journal of Parasitology* 93:1006–15.

Li, Y., J-A. Chen, Q. Zhao, C. Pu. Z. Qiu, R. Zhang, W. Shu. (2011). A cross-sectional investigation of chronic exposure to microcystin in relationship to childhood liver damage in the Three Gorges Reservoir region, China. *Env. Hlth. Perspec.* 119: 1483–1488.

Litaker, R. W., W. C. Holland, D. R. Hardison, F. Pisapia, P. Hess, S. R. Kibler, and P. A. Tester. 2017. "Ciguatoxicity and *Gambierdiscus* and *Fukuyoa* species from the Caribbean and Gulf of Mexico." *PLoS ONE* 12(10):e0185776. http://doi.org/10.371/journal.pone.0185776.

MacKintosh, C., Beattie, K. A., Klumpp, S., Cohen, P., Codd, G. A. 1990. "Cyanobacterial microcystin-LR is a potent and specific inhibitor of protein phosphatases 1 and 2A from both mammals and higher plants." *FEBS Letts* 264:187–192.

MacKintosh, R.W., K. N. Dalby, D. G. Campbell, P. T. W. Cohen, P. Cohen & C. MacKintosh. (1995). The cyanobacterial toxin microcystin binds covalently to cysteine-273 on protein phosphatase 1. *FEBS Letts.* 371: 236–240.

Manning, S. R., and J. W. La Claire. 2010. "Prymnesins: Toxic Metabolites of the Golden Alga, *Prymnesium parvum* Carter (Haptophyta)." *Marine Drugs* 8:678–704.

Metcalf, J. S., S. G. Bell, and G. A. Codd. 2001. "Colorimetric Immuno-Protein Phosphatase Inhibition Assay for Specific Detection of Microcystins and Nodularins of Cyanobacteria." *Applied and Environmental Microbiology* 67:904–09.

Metcalf, J. S., and G. A. Codd. 2012. "Cyanotoxins." In *Ecology of Cyanobacteria II*, edited by B. A. Whitton, 651–75. Dordrecht: Springer.

Metcalf, J. S., R. Richer, P. A. Cox, and G. A. Codd. 2012. "Cyanotoxins in Desert Environments May Present a Risk to Human Health." *Science of the Total Environment* 421–22:118–23.

Metcalf, J.S., S. A. Banack, J. Lindsay, L. F. Morrison, P. A. Cox & G. A. Codd (2008). Co-occurrence of beta-N-methylamino-L-alanine, a neurotoxic amino acid with other cyanobacterial toxins in British waterbodies, 1990-2004. *Env. Microbiol.* 10: 702–708.

Monteiro, S., R. Santos, L. Blaha, and G. A. Codd. 2017. "Lipopolysaccharide Endotoxins." In *Handbook of Cyanobacterial Monitoring and Cyanotoxin Analysis*, edited by J. Meriluoto, L. Spoof, and G. A. Codd, 109–26. Chichester, UK: John Wiley & Sons.

Moore, T. S., M. D. Dowell, and B. A. Franz. 2012. "Detection of Coccolithophore Blooms in Ocean Color Satellite Imagery: A Generalized Approach for Use with Multiple Sensors." *Remote Sensing of Environment* 117:249–63.

Murch, S. J., P. A. Cox, S. A. Banack, J. C. Steele & O. W. Sacks. 2004. "Occurrence of β-methylamino-l-alanine (BMAA) in ALS/PDC patients from Guam." *Acta Neurologica Scand.* 110: 267–269.

Murray, J. S., M. J. Boundy, A. I. Selwood, and D. T. Harwood. 2018. "Development of an LC-MS/MS Method to Simultaneously Monitor Maitotoxins and Selected Ciguatoxins in Algal Cultures and P-CTX-1B in Fish." *Harmful Algae* 80:80–87.

Nanao, M. H., T. Green, Y. Stern-Bach, S. F. Heinemann, and S. Choe. 2005. "Structure of the Kainate Receptor Subunit GluR6 Agonist-Binding Domain Complexed with Domoic Acid. *Proceedings of the National Academy of Sciences of the USA* 102:1708–13.

Nicholls, R. J., and A. Cazenave. 2010. "Sea-Level Rise and Its Impact on Coastal Zones." *Science* 328:1517–20.

Nishiwaki-Matsushima, R., T. Ohta, S. Nishiwaki, M. Suganuma, K. Kohyama, T. Ishikawa, W. W. Carmichael, and H. Fujiki. 1992. "Liver Tumor Promotion by the Cyanobacterial Peptide Toxin Microcystin-LR." *Journal of Cancer Research and Clinical Oncology* 118:420–24.

Ohta, T., E. Sueoka, N. Lida, A. Komori, M. Suganuma, R. Nishiwaki, M. Tatematsu et al. 1994. "Nodularin, a Potent Inhibitor of Protein Phosphatases 1 and 2A, Is a New Environmental Carcinogen in Male F344 Rat Liver." *Cancer Research* 54:6402–06.

Okano, H., H, Masuoka, S. Kamei, T. Seko, S. Koyabu, K. Tsuneoka, T. Tamai et al. 1998. "Rhabdomyolysis and Myocardial Damage Induced by Palytoxin, a Toxin of Blue Humphead Parrotfish." *Internal Medicine* 37:330–33.

Orr, J. C., V. J. Fabry, O. Aumont, L. Bopp, S. C. Doney, R. A., Feely, A. Gnanadesikan et al. (2005). "Anthropogenic Ocean Acidification over the Twenty-First Century and Its Impact on Calcifying Organisms." *Nature* 437:681–86.

Osborne, N. J., and G. R. Shaw. 2008. "Dermatitis Associated with Exposure to a Marine Cyanobacterium during Recreational Water Exposure." *BMC Dermatology* 8:5.

Pablo, J., S. A. Banack, P. A. Cox, T. E. Johnson, S. Papapetropoulos, W. G. Bradley, A. Buck & D. C. Mash (2009). Cyanobacterial neurotoxin BMAA in ALS and Alzheimer's disease. *Acta Neurologica Scand.* 120: 216–225.

Paerl, H. W., and J. Huisman. 2008. "Blooms Like It Hot." *Science* 320:57–58.

Paerl, H. W., and V. J. Paul. 2012. "Climate Change: Links to Global Expansion of Harmful Cyanobacteria." *Water Research* 46:1349–63.

Paerl, H. W., N.S. Hall, and E. S. Calandrino. 2011. "Controlling Harmful Cyanobacterial Blooms in a World Experiencing Anthropogenic and Climatic-Induced Change." *Science of the Total Environment* 409:1739–45.

Paz, B., A. H. Daranas, M. Norte, P. Riobó, J. M. Franco, and J. J. Fernández. 2008. "Yessotoxins, a Group of Marine Polyether Toxins: An Overview." *Marine Drugs* 6:73–102.

Paz, B., P. Riobó, M. L. Fernández, S. Fraga, and J. M. Franco. 2004. "Production and Release of Yessotoxins by the dinoflagellates *Prorocentrum reticulatum* and *Lingulodinium polyedrum* in Culture." *Toxicon* 44:251–58.

Peeters, F., D. Straile, A. Lorke, and D. M. Livingstone. 2007. "Earlier Onset of the Spring Phytoplankton Bloom in Lakes of the Temperate Zone in a Warmer Climate." *Global Change Biology* 13:1898–1909.

Perl, T. M., L. Bedard, T. Kosatsky, J. C. Hockin, E. C. Todd, and R. S. Remis. 1990. "An Outbreak of Encephalopathy Caused by Eating Mussels Contaminated with Domoic Acid." *New England Journal of Medicine* 322:1775–80.

Pierce, R. H., M. S. Henry, P. C. Blum, J. Lyons, Y. S. Cheng, D. Yazzie, and Y. Zhou. 2003. "Brevetoxin Concentrations in Marine Aerosol: Human Exposure Levels during a *Karenia brevis* Harmful Algal Bloom." *Bulletin of Environmental Contamination and Toxicology* 70: 61–65.

Popova, E. E., A. Yool, C. Coward, F. Dupont, C. Deal, S. Elliott, E. Hunke et al. 2012. "What Controls Primary Production in the Arctic Ocean? Results from an Intercomparison of Five General Circulation Models with Biogeochemistry." *Journal of Geophysical Research* 117:C00D12. doi:10.1029/2011JC007112.

Pritchard, H. D., S. R. M. Ligtenberg, H. A, Fricker, D. G. Vaughan, M. R. van den Broeke, and L. Padman. 2012. "Antarctic Ice-Sheet Loss Driven by Basal Melting of Ice Shelves." *Nature* 484:502–05.

Puschner, B., A. C. Bautista, and C. Wong. 2017. "Debromoaplysiatoxin as the Causative Agent of Dermatitis in a Dog after Exposure to Freshwater in California." *Frontiers in Veterinary Science* 4:50. doi: 10.3389/fvets.2017.00050.

Ramos, A. G., A. Martel, G. A. Codd, E. Soler, J. Coca, A. Redondo, L. F. Morrison et al. 2005. "Bloom of the Marine Diazotrophic Cyanobacterium *Trichodesmium erythraeum* in the Northwest African Upwelling." *Marine Ecology Progress Series* 301:303–05.

Raven, J. A. 2011. "Effects on Marine Algae of Changed Seawater Chemistry with Increasing Atmospheric CO_2." *Biology and Environment: Proceedings of the Royal Irish Academy* 111B:1–17.

Reed, D., C. Plato, T. Elizan & L. T. Kurland. (1966). The amyotrophic lateral sclerosis/parkinsonism dementia complex: A ten-year follow-up on Guam: Part I. Epidemiological studies. *Am J. Epidemiol.* 83: 54–73.

Richard, D., E. Arsenault, A. Cembella, and M. Quilliam. 2000. "Investigations into the Toxicology and Pharmacology of Spirolides, a Novel Group of Shellfish Toxins." In *Harmful Algal Blooms 2000*, edited by G .M. Hallegraeff, S. I. Blackbum, C. J. Bolch, and R. J. Lewis, 383–86. Paris: Intergovernmental Oceanographic Commission of UNESCO.

Rhodes, L., P. McNabb, M. de Salas, L. Briggs, V. Beuzenberg, and M. Gladstone. 2006. "Yessotoxin Production by *Gonyaulax spinifera*." *Harmful Algae* 5:148–55.

Richer, R., D. Anchassi, I. El-Assaad, M. El-Matbouly, F. Ali, I. Makki, and J. S. Metcalf. 2012. "Variation in the Coverage of Biological Soil Crusts in the State of Qatar." *Journal of Arid Environments* 78:187–90.

Richer, R., S. A. Banack, J. S. Metcalf, and P. A. Cox. 2015. "The Persistence of Cyanobacterial Toxins in Desert Soils." *Journal of Arid Environments* 112B:134–39.

Romo, S., J. Soria, F. Fernández, Y. Ouahid, and A. Barón-Solá. 2012. "Water Residence Time and the Dynamics of Toxic Cyanobacteria." *Freshwater Biology* 58:513–22.

Satake, M., L. MacKenzie, and T. Yasumoto. 1997. "Identification of *Prororceratium reticulatum* as the Biogenetic Origin of Yessotoxin." *Natural Toxins* 5:164–67.

Sato, M., T. Nakano, M. Takeuchi, N. Kanno, E. Nagahisa, and Y. Sato. 1996. "Distribution of Neuroexcitatory Amino Acids in Marine Algae." *Phytochemistry* 42:1595–97.

Sharma, N. K., A. K. Rai, S. Singh, and R. M. Brown, Jr. 2007. "Airborne Algae: Their Present Status and Relevance." *Journal of Phycology* 43:615–27.

Smith, L. C., and S. R. Stephenson. 2013. "New Trans-Arctic Shipping Routes Navigable by Midcentury." *Proceedings of the National Academy of Sciences of the USA* 110:E1191–E1195.

Strain, S. M., and R. A. R. Tasker. 1991. "Hippocampal Damage Produced by Systemic Injection of Domoic Acid." *Neuroscience* 44:343–52.

Svircev, Z., D. Drobac, N. Tokodi, M. Vidovic, J. Simeunovic, M. Miladinov-Mikov, and V. Baltic. 2013. "Epidemiology of Primary Liver Cancer in Serbia and Possible Connection with Cyanobacterial Blooms." *Journal of Environmental Science and Health. Part C, Environmental Carcinogenesis & Ecotoxicology Reviews* 31:181–200.

Tillman, U., M. Elbrächter, B. Krock, U. John, and A. Cembella. 2009. "*Azadinium spinosum* gen. et sp. nov. (Dinophyceae) Identified as a Primary Producer of Azaspiracid Toxins." *European Journal of Phycology* 44:63–79.

Tubaro, A., S. Sosa, M. Carbonatto, G. Altinier, F. Vita, M. Melato, M. Satake, and T. Yasumoto. 2003. "Oral and Intraperitoneal Acute Toxicity Studies of Yessotoxin and Homoyessotoxins in Mice." *Toxicon* 41:783–92.

Ueno, Y., S. Nagata, T. Tsutsumi, A. Hasegawa, M. F. Watanabe, H. D., Park, G. C. Chen, G. Chen, and S. Z. Yu. 1996. "Detection of Microcystins, a Blue-Green Algal Hepatotoxin, in Drinking Water Sampled in Haimen and Fusui, Endemic Areas of Primary Liver Cancer in China, by Highly Sensitive Immunoassay." *Carcinogenesis,* 17:1317–21.

Usami, M., M. Satake, S. Ishida, A. Inoue, Y. Kan, and T. Yasumoto. 1995. "Palytoxin Analogs from the Dinoflagellate *Ostreopsis siamensis*." *Journal of the American Chemical Society* 117:5389–90.

Vale, C., and L. M. Botana. 2008. "Marine Toxins and the Cytoskeleton: Okadaic Acid and Dinophysistoxins." *The FEBS Journal* 275:6060–66.

Violi, J. P., J. A. Facey, S. M, Mitrovic, A. Colville, and K. J. Rodgers. 2019. "Production of β-methylamino-L-alanine (BMAA) and Its Isomers by Freshwater Diatoms." *Toxins* 11 (9):pii:E512. doi:10.3390/toxins11090512.

Westrick, J. A., D. C. Szlag, B. J. Southwell, and J. Sinclair. 2010. "A Review of Cyanobacteria and Cyanotoxins Removal/Inactivation in Drinking Water Treatment." *Analytical and Bioanalytical Chemistry* 397:1705–14. doi:10.1007/s00216-010-3709-5.

Wiedner, C., J. Rücker, R. Brüggemann, and B. Nixdorf. 2007. "Climate Change Affects Timing and Size of Populations of an Invasive Cyanobacterium in Temperate Regions." *Oecologia* 152:473–84.

Wiese, M., P. M. D'Agostino, T. K. Mihali, M. C. Moffitt, and B. A. Neilan. 2010. "Neurotoxic Alkaloids: Saxitoxin and Its Analogs." *Marine Drugs* 8:2185–2211.

Wigley, T. M. L., and S. C. B. Raper. 1987. "Thermal Expansion of Sea Water Associated with Global Warming." *Nature* 330:127–31.

Xu, Y., Q. Cai, L. Ye, S. Zhou, and X. Han. 2009. "Spring Diatom Blooming Phases in a Representative Eutrophic Bay of the Three-Gorges Reservoir, China." *Journal of Freshwater Ecology* 24:191–98.

Zegura, B., A. Straser, and M. Filipic. 2011. "Genotoxicity and Potential Carcinogenicity of Cyanobacterial Toxins—A Review." *Mutation Research* 727:16–41.

Zheng, C., H. Zeng, H. Lin, J. Wang, X. Feng, Z. Qiu, J-A. Chen, J. Luo, Y. Luo, Y. Huang, L. Wang, W. Liu, Y. Tan, A. Xu, Y. Yao & W. Shu. (2017). Serum microcystin levels positively linked with risk of hepatocellular carcinoma: A case-control study in southwest China. *Hepatology* 66: 1519–1528.

Zimba, P. V., I.S. Huang, D. Gutierrez, W. Shin, M. S. Bennett, and R. E. Triemer. 2017. "Euglenophycin Is Produced in at Least Six Species of Euglenoid Algae and Six of Seven Strains of *Euglena sanguinea*." *Harmful Algae* 63:79–84.

CHAPTER 7

CLIMATE CHANGE, CARBON DIOXIDE, AND PUBLIC HEALTH: THE PLANT BIOLOGY PERSPECTIVE

Lewis H. Ziska and Kristie L. Ebi

Introduction

Because carbon dioxide absorbs and reradiates heat back to the earth's atmosphere, there is widespread scientific agreement that the ongoing rise in CO_2 levels will result in increasing surface temperatures (Intergovernmental Panel on Climate Change [IPCC] 2007, 2014). The magnitude and extent of current and projected increases in temperature and the potential consequences for public health, from undernutrition to the spread of malaria, are the principal theme of this book, as well as the subject of ongoing medical and epidemiological research (Haines and Ebi 2019; IPCC 2014).

However, the role of increasing CO_2 and concomitant temperature increases is also likely to alter plant biology with subsequent consequences, direct and indirect, for human health. Human well-being and even existence are fundamentally dependent on the ability of plants to generate complex carbohydrates and chemical energy from just four basic resources: sunlight, nutrients (e.g., nitrogen, phosphorous), water, and carbon dioxide. At present, approximately 95 percent of all plant species are deficient in the amount of CO_2 needed to operate at maximum efficiency; therefore, the rapid rise in an essential resource (atmospheric CO_2 has increased 27 percent since 1970 and is now at approximately 412 ppmv) is likely to alter many aspects of plant biology—in addition to any concurrent temperature changes resulting from the role of CO_2 as a greenhouse gas (Ziska and Bunce 2006).

Any acknowledgment of these changes should examine their impacts beyond a simple "CO_2 is plant food" meme. The recognition that CO_2 is a promoter of plant growth has been used by critics of anthropogenic climate change to argue that rising atmospheric CO_2 will lead to an Eden-like plant environment, ignoring, among other likely environmental interactions, that any increase in CO_2 is indiscriminate with respect to which plant species may respond and to whether the nutrient content of plants will remain constant (Loladze 2014, Zhu et al. 2018).In this review, we provide an up-to-date assessment of both CO_2 and temperature as likely drivers of quantitative and qualitative changes in plant chemistry and physiology and delineate, wherever possible, the role that such changes play in the context of public health. Such effects range in scope from plant-based pollen to contact dermatitis to nutrition to plant-based medicines. Assuming efforts to mitigate the ongoing increase in CO_2 will be limited, we indicate limitations of current studies and emphasize several crucial needs that will reduce vulnerability to the ongoing challenges associated with climate, CO_2, plant function, and public health.

KEY CONCEPTS

- Interactions between climate change, rising carbon dioxide (CO_2) levels and plant biology can directly influence human health, through changes in plant-based production of aeroallergens, contact dermatitis, or toxicology.

- Similar, but indirect effects may occur with food security, including changes in production, nutritional quality, or pesticide contamination.

- Increasing CO_2 can alter plant-based pharmacological and narcotic compounds.

- CO_2 and/or climate may also alter food supply and demography of known human disease vectors, such as mosquitoes and rodents.

- CO_2 and climate can affect fire frequency, with consequences for air quality.

- CO_2 and/or climate can reduce the efficacy of pesticides, especially herbicidal control of weeds, with potential changes in environmental and economic consequences.

Direct Consequences

The role of plant biology in human health may seem obscure to many public health professionals. Yet there are many processes by which plants directly affect human physiology, including **aerobiology**, contact dermatitis, pharmacology and toxicology, and physical contact (e.g., thorns, spines), among others. Many of these processes are, or will be, affected by the ongoing rise in atmospheric carbon dioxide and subsequent changes in climate.

Aeroallergens

One of the most recognized plant-induced health effects is associated with aeroallergens. Contact with plant-based pollen can induce sneezing, inflammation of nasal and eye membranes, and wheezing. Complications, including nasal polyps, asthma, or permanent bronchial obstructions, can occur in severe cases. Results from a four-year study by Quest Diagnostics (2011) in the United States indicated that sensitivity to ragweed and mold may have increased by 15 and 12 percent, respectively. The same study also indicated that allergies may be affecting 53 percent of children between the ages of two and seventeen. This is consistent with other work by the International Study of Asthma and Allergies in Childhood indicating that the global prevalence of asthma is continuing to increase (Weinmayr et al. 2007).

The role of rising CO_2 and temperature, or both, in eliciting quantitative or qualitative changes in aeroallergens is still being elucidated but recent work suggests that it may be a global phenomenon (Ziska et al. 2019) and that temporal shifts may be associated with increased symptoms of hay fever (Sapkota et al. 2019). For example, Neumann et al. (2019) project that climate change will increase season length of oak, birch, and grass pollen in the United States, resulting in associated increases in asthma-related emergency department (ED) visits of 14 percent by 2090 under a high emissions scenario and 8 percent under a moderate emissions scenario. Overall, sufficient information is now available to recognize that anthropogenic-driven climate change (i.e., CO_2 and temperature) is altering season length and pollen load for three distinct plant-based contributions to allergenic pollen: trees in the spring, grasses and weeds in the summer, and ragweed (*Ambrosia* spp.) in the fall (autumn).

Trees

A number of empirical studies indicate a clear association between anthropogenic climate change and temporal advances in **phenology** as evidenced by early anthesis and pollen shedding in the spring (Fitter and Fitter 2002; Elwood et al. 2013). For trees, multiyear records have shown earlier floral initiation for oak (*Quercus* species) and birch (*Betula* species) (Emberlin et al. 2002; Garcia-Mozo et al. 2006). Additional studies have projected an advance of pollen initiation of one to three weeks for olive (*Olea europea*) and up to four weeks for Quercus with further warming (Garcia-Mozo et al.).

Research conducted on loblolly pine (*Pinus taeda*) at the Duke University forest using free-air CO_2 enrichment (FACE) demonstrated that elevated CO_2 concentrations (200 ppm above ambient CO_2 levels) resulted in earlier pollen production from younger trees and greater seasonal pollen production (LaDeau and Clark 2006). Consistent with warmer spring temperatures, European pollen data have shown increases in hazel (*Corylus* species) and birch pollen counts in Switzerland and Denmark (Rasmussen 2002; Clot 2003; Frei and Gassner 2008). Severe climate change could increase oak pollen season length and associated asthma ED visits with associated increases in public health costs (Anenberg et al. 2017). Currently, no data are available regarding warming or CO_2 effects on potential qualitative changes in the allergenicity of tree pollen.

Weeds and Grasses

Plant species are also recognized as significant sources of allergenic pollen during the summer months. Overall, warmer temperatures and earlier springs are altering pollen production of mugwort (*Artemisia* species) (Stach et al. 2007), nettle (Frenguelli 2002), and some grasses (Burr 1999; Emberlin et al. 1999). There is an association between pollen production and increasing temperature for other summer flowering plant species (e.g., *Parietaria*; Ariano, Canonica, and Passalacqua 2010). Work by Albertine et al. (2014) also demonstrates a clear link to rising CO_2 levels and increasing pollen and allergen exposure in timothy grass (*Phleum pratense*).

Ragweed

One of the most studied plant species regarding pollen production is ragweed (*Ambrosia* species). This may in part reflect the large numbers of individuals in the United States and elsewhere who exhibit seasonal ragweed allergies (Burbach et al. 2009; Centers for Disease Control and Prevention [CDC] 2011). Indoor studies examining temperature and increased CO_2 as treatment variables indicate consistent stimulation in plant growth and pollen production of common ragweed (*Ambrosia artemisiifolia*) (Ziska and Caulfield 2000; Wan et al. 2002; Wayne et al. 2002) and a potential increase in allergenic content (Singer et al. 2005; El Kelish et al. 2014). Manipulation of both temperature and CO_2 concentration in a glasshouse study to simulate future climate change resulted in earlier flowering, greater floral numbers, and greater pollen production in common ragweed (Rogers et al. 2006).

Because these initial results indicated that common ragweed may respond significantly to anthropogenic climate change and increased CO_2, attempts were made to quantify changes in ragweed biology at greater spatial and temporal scales. To this end, differences in regional microclimate (CO_2/temperature gradient between urban and rural locales) were used as a surrogate of near-term climate change projections to quantify the growth and pollen production of common ragweed for Baltimore, Maryland, and the surrounding environs (Ziska et al. 2003). Data from this study indicated that urban ragweed plants grew faster, flowered earlier, and produced significantly greater above-ground biomass and pollen relative to the same plants growing in a rural location. Similar microclimatic effects of urbanization were linked to longer pollen seasons and earlier floral initiation in European cities (Rodríguez-Rajo et al. 2010). To scale up from regional to continental effects, pollen data collected from the National Allergy Bureau in the United States and the Aerobiology Research Laboratories in Canada were collected to determine whether recent surface warming had resulted in a lengthening of the duration of the ragweed pollen season in North America. An analysis of these data demonstrated that the duration of the season has been increasing since the mid-1990s but only as a function of increasing latitude, consistent with differential anthropogenic warming as postulated by the IPCC (Ziska et al. 2011) (Figure 7.1). Although this study did not examine quantitative and qualitative measures, it does suggest that length of exposure is likely to increase with continued anthropogenic warming, particularly in northern latitudes. However, a recent analysis has indicated that ongoing increases in temperature extremes (Tmin and Tmax) may already be contributing to extended seasonal duration and increased pollen load for multiple aero-allergenic pollen taxa in diverse locations across the northern hemisphere (Ziska et al. 2019)

Plants and Fungi

It is generally recognized that climate, particularly humidity and precipitation, plays a fundamental role in the induction and spread of allergenic molds (Burch and Levetin 2002). However,

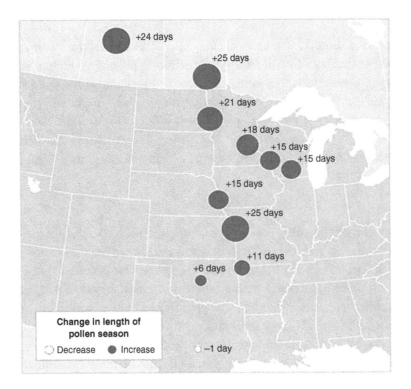

Figure 7.1   Change in the length of ragweed pollen season at 11 locations in the central United States and Canada between 1995 and 2015
Source: Ziska et al. (2011).
Note: Black circles represent a longer pollen season; the white circle represents a shorter season. Larger circles indicate larger changes.

it is important to also recognize the role of plants in fungal biology. For example, *Alternaria alternata* is a well-known source of aeroallergens (as spores) with over 350 known plant hosts, including hay. Given that CO_2 and temperature will alter plant (host) biology, a question is how this will alter sporulation of *A. alternata.*

Indirectly, climate change, particularly warming temperatures, could alter the timing of agricultural harvests with subsequent effects on *Alternaria* exposure times (Corden and Millington 2001). For example, differences between two UK towns, Derby and Cardiff, in *Alternaria* spore counts were associated with increased cereal production and changes in climate since the 1970s (Corden and Millington, 2001; Corden, Millington, and Mullins 2003). For quaking aspen (*Populus tremuloides*) grown at projected increases of atmospheric CO_2, a significant increase in fungal propagules (including a doubling of *A. alternata*) was observed in the leaf litter (Klironomos et al. 1997). A similar experiment was conducted with timothy grass (*Phleum pratense*) to quantify the effects of recent and projected increases in atmospheric CO_2 (300, 400, 500, and 600 ppm) on the quantity and quality of *Alternaria* spores (Wolf et al. 2010). Results from this study indicated that at 500 and 600 ppm CO_2, *A. alternata* produced nearly three times the number of spores and more than twice the total antigenic protein per plant than at lower CO_2 concentrations. Wolf et al. suggested that recent and projected increases in CO_2 could increase the carbon to nitrogen ratio in leaves of timothy grass (*Phleum pratense*), with subsequent quantitative and qualitative changes in *A. alternata* sporulation.

Contact Dermatitis

Plants have evolved numerous defensive chemicals, including those associated with contact dermatitis, an immune-mediated (immunoglobulin E) allergenic response. Plants may also induce **photodermatitis,** a form of allergic contact dermatitis where light is needed to activate the allergen. Contact dermatitis is associated with over one hundred different plant species (e.g., poison ivy, *Toxicodendron radicans*), whereas photodermatitis is associated principally with plant members of the Apiaceal or Umbelliferae family (e.g., giant hogweed, *Heracleum mantegazzianum*). It is estimated that sensitivity to urushiol, the principal allergen in poison ivy, occurs in about two out of every three individuals, and amounts as small as one nanogram (ng) are sufficient to induce a reaction (Tanner 2000). Each year, approximately 300,000 people in the United States suffer from contact with member of the poison ivy family (e.g., poison ivy, oak, and sumac) (Mohan et al. 2006).

Can anthropogenic climate change, rising CO_2 levels, or both alter the ability of such plants to induce contact dermatitis? Laboratory trials for poison ivy examined the range of growth responses and simulated herbivory (leaf consumption by herbivores) at recent and projected CO_2 changes—300, 400, 500, and 600 parts per million (ppm)—that is, the approximate CO_2 concentrations that existed during the middle of the twentieth century, the current concentration, and near- and long-term projections for this century (2050 and 2090, respectively) (Ziska et al. 2007). These data indicated that poison ivy can respond to even small (approximately 100 ppm) increases in CO_2 concentration above the mid-twentieth-century carbon dioxide level, suggesting that its rate of spread, its ability to recover from herbivory, and its production of urushiol may be enhanced in a future, higher CO_2 environment. Outdoor trials of poison ivy using Free-Air CO_2 Enrichment (FACE at Duke University) showed that poison ivy responded significantly to projected increases in atmospheric CO_2 (approximately 700 ppm) (Mohan et al. 2006). Interestingly, in addition to growth changes, the ratio of unsaturated to saturated urushiol increased as a function of CO_2 concentration, indicating a more virulent form of urushiol (Mohan et al.). Although information on temperature or temperature-CO_2 interactions is lacking, other known allergenic species such as stinging nettle (*Urtica dioica*) and leafy spurge (*Euphorbia esula*) also showed significant increases in growth in response to recent and projected CO_2 changes (Hunt et al. 1991; Ziska 2003).

Physical Contact

Many plants can be associated with physical injury. Spines or other sharp appendages can puncture the skin. Removing or encountering plants such as Canada thistle (*Cirsium arvense*) or puncture vine (*Tribulus terrestris*) can be particularly painful. As with toxicology, few studies have quantified changes in physical appendages as a function of CO_2 or temperature. One exception is for Canada thistle: data demonstrate that an increase in the number and length of leaf spines as CO_2 increased from preindustrial levels (285 ppm) to projected twenty-first-century levels (721 ppm) (Ziska 2004).

Toxicology

In addition to plant-based allergens, plants can produce numerous toxic substances; more than seven hundred plant species are known to be poisonous for human or animal consumption. The amount and location of the poison, as with dermatitis, varies by species; however, some plants, such as poison hemlock (*Conium maculatum*), oleander (*Nerium aleander*), and castor bean (*Ricinus communis*), are sufficiently toxic so that even small quantities can result in death. Accidental ingestion of plant material is recognized as a source of toxic exposure and accounts for nearly 100,000 calls to national poison centers annually (Watson et al. 2004), with approximately 80 percent of plant-related exposures associated with pediatric patients.

At present, little information is available regarding anthropogenic climate-CO_2 impacts on toxicology. One seminal study by Ros Gleadow (Gleadow et al., 2009) indicated that for cassava (*Manihot esculentum*), a primary caloric source for approximately eight hundred million people globally, rising levels of CO_2 above ambient (550 and 710 ppm CO_2) resulted in nearly doubling the concentration of cyanogenic glycosides in the edible leaves at the highest CO_2 concentration. This suggested that cyanide poisoning could increase as a function of rising atmospheric CO_2 levels. The impact of CO_2 or temperature, or both, on toxicological effects of other plant species has not been examined. Ziska. Emche et al. (2005) showed that increasing CO_2 above early twentieth-century levels increased tobacco growth but decreased the concentration of nicotine, a toxic alkaloid, in tobacco leaves.

Indirect Consequences

At present, there are several clear examples whereby rising CO_2 per se or in conjunction with rising temperatures will directly affect human health. However, the role of CO_2 and/or climate can be indirect, altering different environmental aspects with secondary consequences with respect to human health. Such consequences can include changes in food security (e.g., food safety, nutrition) or medicine (pharmacology).

Food Security

Although various definitions of food security exist, there are three categories of special concern in the context of rising CO_2 and/or climate: production, quality (nutrition) and safety. All three aspects are likely to be affected by CO_2 or climatic changes. (Additional details as to the range and extent of these impacts, as well as potential adaptation measures, can be found in Lobell et al. 2008; Lobell and Burke 2010; and Beddington et al. 2012.)

Production

Water and temperature are among the climatic factors that can significantly affect crop production; both are in turn, likely to be affected by climatic change (IPCC 2007, 2014). Water availability, particularly drought, has been a factor in noteworthy reductions in corn, soybean, and wheat production for the United States in 2012 (Boyer et al. 2013) and Russia in 2010 and 2011 (Wegren 2011). Irrigation, which is essential to maintaining production of cereal crops with drought, particularly in populous areas (e.g., India, East Asia), may also be at risk as precipitation decreases in many regions and water supply declines as ice and snow reserves diminish in mountainous regions with warming (e.g., Kerr 2007) or ground water reserves diminish (Panda and Wahr 2016). Record-high spring and summer temperatures observed in the United States during 2012 may also be of concern in agronomic production, as flowering is one of the most thermal-sensitive stages of crop growth (Lobell et al. 2013); there is additional concern that rising CO_2 may also reduce transpirational canopy cooling, increasing pollen sterility with warmer air temperatures (Matsui et al. 1997). Chronic or short-term exposure to higher temperatures during flowering can result in reduced pollen viability, inadequate fertilization, and aborted fruit development (Hatfield et al. 2011). Given the current level of one billion individuals who are food insecure and the additional two billion who will be added to the global population by 2040, understanding, quantifying, and adapting global agriculture to maintain crop production is a crucial, if underappreciated, aspect of plant biology and public health.

Nutrition

The role of nutrition in all aspects of public health and human wellness is universally acknowledged. The latest Food and Agriculture Organization food security report estimated that as of 2019, over 820 million people are suffering from hunger (http://www.fao.org/state-of-food-security-nutrition/en/).

Malnutrition increases the risk of disease and early death. Protein-energy malnutrition plays a major role in half of all under-five deaths each year in developing countries (Bernstein 2017). Undernutrition generally results from a lack of protein that is needed for muscle development and maintenance, or micronutrients such as iodine, vitamin A, or iron that boost immunity and healthy development. Therefore, it is necessary to also consider the quality, or nutritional aspects, of the food supply in the framework of climate change, CO_2, and plant biology.

As CO_2 increases, photosynthesis requires less nitrogen (i.e., nitrogen use efficiency, the ratio of carbon to nitrogen, or C:N, typically increases) (Loladze 2014). Numerous studies, including meta-analyses have examined the role of rising CO_2 on protein concentration of major crops, including barley, potato, rice, soybean, and wheat (Taub, Miller, and Allen 2008). Overall, among crops examined, a significant decline (about 10 to 15 percent) in protein content was observed if atmospheric CO_2 increases rose to between 540 and 960 ppm (Taub et al. 2008), a range anticipated before the end of this century (IPCC 2007). In addition to this dilution of protein levels, rising CO_2 may also reduce water flow through the crop plant due to its physiological effect of closing stomata. As a result, uptake of key micro- and macronutrients from the soil (e.g., iron, zinc, and manganese) may also be negatively affected; micronutrient deficiency is a much larger problem globally than undernutrition (Loladze 2002, 2014; Myers et al. 2014). Recent work for multiple, genetically diverse cultivars indicated significant declines in protein and B vitamin concentration (Zhu et al. 2018) (Figure 7.2). Conversely, some studies indicate an improvement in some aspects of nutritional quality, such as an increase in antioxidants in strawberries with rising CO_2 (Wang, Bunce, and Maas 2003).

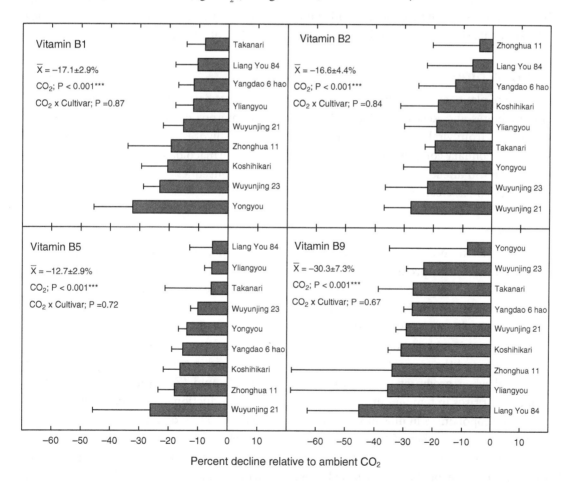

Figure 7.2 CO_2-induced reductions in vitamins B1 (thiamine), B2 (riboflavin), B5 (pantothenic acid), and B9 (folate) by cultivar. No significant effect was observed for vitamin B6 (pyridoxine), and results are not shown. Analysis was conducted only for the China FACE location. Bars are ±SE. *$P < 0.05$ and **$P < 0.01$ for a given cultivar. CO_2; **$P < 0.01$ is based on all cultivars.

For many populations in the developing world, meat is scarce, and plants provide the primary source of both protein and micronutrients. If, as we expect, rising CO_2 levels decrease the protein concentration and affects the nutritional quality of crops, then it is possible that impoverished areas of the world already threatened by deficiency in food supply may face an additional burden of nutritional shortfall (Lloyd, Kovats, and Chalabi 2011; Myers et al. 2014). Overall, changes in food quality and nutritional value have been well described in the context of CO_2 or climate; however, application of that information to the global population is only beginning (Beach et al. 2019).

Food Safety

Post-harvest food safety could be negatively affected by climatic disruption (e.g., temperature, rainfall extremes) when, for example, pathogens are washed into food sources, or higher temperatures facilitate the reproduction of pathogens on produce or seafood (Ziska et al. 2016). Climate change could increase human exposure to chemical contaminants in food through rising sea surface temperatures or greater accumulation of mercury in seafood or via extreme weather events (e.g., flooding).

Agriculture and pesticide use are dependent on climate, which means that rising carbon dioxide concentrations and warming may alter the incidence and distribution of pests, parasites, and microbes, leading to changes in the use and timing of pesticides applications and veterinary drugs that could affect food safety (Noyes et al. 2009). In addition, there is increasing evidence that CO_2 and/or climate may reduce the chemical efficacy of pesticides for crop-based pests, especially for weeds, with potential increases in pesticide usage and chemical contaminants (Refatti et al. 2019; Ziska 2016, Waryszak et al. 2018)

Pharmacology

The use of plants as medicinal sources for human ailments dates to the beginning of civilization (Schultes and Reis 1995). Plants have evolved numerous chemical pathways to protect themselves from viral diseases, fungal pathogens, and herbivores. Diversity in the production of these secondary compounds has been an important pharmacological resource. As CO_2 and/or climate will affect plant biology, there are potential consequences as well regarding plant chemistry and associated pharmacology.

Medicine

Only a small number of studies have examined how pharmacological compounds could respond to recent or projected increases in atmospheric CO_2 or temperature. Among these, growth of wooly foxglove (*Digitalis lanata*) and production of digoxin were increased at 1000 ppmv CO_2 relative to ambient conditions (Stuhlfauth and Fock 1990). Production of morphine in wild poppy (*Papaver setigerum*) (Ziska et al. 2008) showed significant increases with both recent and projected carbon dioxide concentrations. Growth of St. John's wort (*Hypericum perforatum)* and the concentration of hypericin, a drug used in treatment of depression, were increased when grown at CO_2 concentrations of 1,000 ppm (Zobayed and Saxena 2004). Concurrent rises in temperature or CO_2 increased the production and concentration of atropine and scopolamine in jimson weed (*Datura stromonium*) (Ziska, Emche et al. 2005); however, a synergistic effect of CO_2 and temperature on either concentration or production of these compounds was not observed. Overall, CO_2 and/or climate can alter the concentration of known pharmacological plant-based substance, with consequences regarding their efficacy in human physiology.

Narcotics

Although pharmaceuticals contribute significantly to public health, plants are a known source of narcotic compounds whose abuse constitutes a significant global health problem including nicotine in tobacco, tetrahydrocannabinol (THC) in *Cannabis* spp., and cocaine chlorohydrate in *Erythoxylum coca*.

Although the growth of narcotic plants can be stimulated by rising CO_2 and temperature (e.g., *Cannabis sativa*; Chandra et al., 2008); few peer-reviewed studies have quantified the impact on the narcotic compound per se. One exception is nicotine in tobacco (*Nicotiana* spp.), which was quantified in response to rising CO_2 and temperature (Ziska, Emche et al. 2005). In this study increasing CO_2 above the early twentieth-century baseline (approximately 295 ppm) reduced the concentration of nicotine; however, CO_2 stimulated overall plant growth so that while concentration was reduced, production per plant increased (Ziska et al. 2005).

Many of the most used plant compounds are bicyclic alkaloids (e.g., cocaine, nicotine, caffeine, and atropine). It has been suggested (Bryant, Chapin, and Klein et al. 1983) that as CO_2 increases, the resulting increase in the C:N ratio of plant leaves will reduce the concentration of nitrogen-based secondary compounds (e.g., caffeine in coffee) while increasing compounds that have little or no nitrogen (e.g., scopolamine in jimson weed). If true, this implies that concentrations of these compounds could decrease in a warming climate. However, insufficient data exist at present to confirm this hypothesis.

CLINICAL CORRELATES 7.1 MEDICINES FROM NATURE

More than half of prescribed medications and most medicines approved by the Food and Drug Administration can be traced to natural origins (Tables 7.1 and 7.2) (Grifo 1997). In developing areas of the world, people rely primarily on natural medicines, in some places deriving as much as 90 percent of their healing substances directly from the local environment (Patwardhan 2005). Habitat destruction and climate change threaten biodiversity and the use of medicines from nature as well as availability of natural medicines for local use and future development (Intergovernmental Science-Policy Platform on Biodiversity and Ecosystem Services 2019). Rising carbon dioxide levels also alter plants (Zhu et al. 2015) and the environments required for optimal plant growth (Boretti and Florentine 2019). Loss of biodiversity affects Indigenous communities and low-income countries specifically where plants are relied upon more so for treatments. The loss of these treatments is anticipated to be faster than the development of new drug products, which notoriously is a lengthy and costly process. Further concern is raised for securing land in these communities as large drug companies become challenged and research pressures amplify globally (Neergheen-Bhujun et al. 2017).

Plant biodiversity is vital to the myriad of plant-based medicines relied upon globally and especially in Indigenous communities and low- and middle-income countries.

Table 7.1 Examples of Drugs Derived from Natural Sources

Plant	Location	Drug	Use
Willow	Worldwide	Aspirin	Fever and pain
Digitalis purpurea	Eurasia, Africa	Digoxin	Cardiac arrhythmia
Catharanthus roseus	Madagascar	Vinblastine	Hodgkin's lymphoma
Taxus brevifolia	Pacific Northwest	Taxol	Ovarian cancer
Cinchona sp.	Tropical Andes, South America	Quinine	Malaria
Atropa Belladonna	Europe, Western Asia, North America	Atropine	Cholinergic
Papaver somniferum	Cultivated worldwide	Morphine, codeine	Pain reliever
Curare	Central and South America	Tubocurarine	Nondepolarizing muscle relaxant

Table 7.2   Examples of Noncommercialized, Medically Important Plants

Plant	Location	Uses
Ucaria tormentosa	Tropical forests of South and Central America	Arthritis, rheumatism, gastric ulcers, and wounds
Arnica montana	North America	Anti-inflammatory
Actaea racemosa	Eastern North America	Premenstrual tension, menopause, anti-inflammatory
Cassia occidentalis	West Africa	Antibacterial/antiparasitic
Pilocarpus	Neotropics of South America	Breast milk inducer, glaucoma, diuretic

Air Quality

It is well recognized that when insects land on and chew leaves, plants can release volatile organic compounds (VOCs) into the air—compounds that are "detected" by other plants who ramp up their production of chemical "weapons" in response. Kudzu, an invasive vine present over millions of acres, produces two key VOCs (Wiberley et al. 2005). The first is isoprene, released from kudzu leaves. The second is from kudzu roots, which convert atmospheric nitrogen into ammonia, converted in turn by soil bacteria into nitric oxide. If sunlight is present, isoprene and nitric oxide mix together to make ground level ozone. (Nitric oxide is also a powerful greenhouse gas.)

There are several studies indicating more CO_2 induces a strong growth response in kudzu (Weltzin, Belote, and Sanders 2003) and that warmer temperatures may be associated with the northward migration of this species (Coiner et al. 2018). Such changes could significantly alter VOC concentration and trophic ozone levels but additional work is necessary to quantify likely impacts.

Fires and particulate matter are recognized as altering air quality. For the western United States, the introduction of an invasive grass species, *Bromus tectorum* (cheatgrass), is associated with increased fire frequency (Bradley et al. 2018). There are additional studies (Ziska, Reeves, and Blank 2005; Blank, White, and Ziska 2006) indicating that recent and projected CO_2 levels can stimulate biomass, seed production, and flammability of this species, with subsequent effects on fire frequency and air quality.

Pesticide Use

Climate-induced changes in pest distribution and populations may exacerbate pest pressures and lead to increases in pesticide use and human exposure to those pesticides. Although the link between pesticide application, exposure, and human health will depend on the type of chemical used, amount of exposure, genetic predisposition, and other factors, it is reasonable to question whether changes in climate or CO_2 may reduce the efficacy or increase the need for chemical applications.

Temperature and precipitation are known abiotic factors that can affect chemical application rates and overall efficacy (Ziska 2016 for herbicides; Whiten and Peterson 2016 for insecticides). There is also increasing evidence that rising CO_2 levels can decrease chemical efficacy for the control of some annual and perennial weeds (Ziska, Teasdale, and Bunce 2000; Archambault 2007; Manea, Leishman, and Downey 2011; Jugulam et al. 2018). The basis for a reduction in efficacy with climate is likely related to changes in physical parameters such as increased wind speed and greater frequency of heavy precipitation (Ziska 2016). A basis for the reduction in efficacy with increasing CO_2 is less clear. At the biological level, increased CO_2 may alter carbon distribution with consequences for translocation (within plant mobility) of the herbicide and potential effects on its chemical efficacy. For example, in Canada thistle, increasing CO_2 resulted in greater carbon allocation to the roots. The increase in the root-to-shoot biomass may have diluted the recommended dosage of glyphosate so that roots were not killed by the pesticide. Because roots of Canada thistle can regenerate the plant asexually, glyphosate efficacy was reduced to zero in an elevated CO_2 environment (Ziska, Faulkner, and Lydon 2004). In addition to the effect of CO_2 on efficacy, there is also evidence that seasonal changes may increase pesticide use. For example, soybeans grown over a north-south transect in the Midwest (Minnesota to Louisiana) showed that pesticide applications increased for soybeans as winters warmed and pest survival over winter increased (Ziska 2014).

Overall, on a global basis, pests, pathogens, and weeds currently consume some 42 percent of growing and stored crops annually (Pimentel 1997), and this figure could escalate as a function of CO_2 or climate disruption. Increased use of petrochemicals for control, combined with reduced efficacy of application, carries additional risks for human and animal health because it could increase the presence of these chemicals in the environment and the risk of toxic exposures.

Uncertainties and Research Priorities

We have reviewed published interactions illustrating the range and scope of plant-based links between climate change and public health. Further inquiry is warranted because the initial observations are often based on a handful of studies, many of which did not capture the complexity of interactions, address the ambiguity underlying the empirical observation, or explore local interactions that could exacerbate or ameliorate possible negative impacts. The priorities given here are not inclusive, but indicative as to future research needs.

Aerobiology and Public Health

Studies evaluating climate and/or rising CO_2 on aeroallergen production and seasonality are ongoing. Initial trials relating these changes to health impacts (rhinitis, asthma) are beginning and should be encouraged. However, there are a number of key research issues that remain minimally or unexplored. These include the role of warmer winters on **vernalization** and floral production for tree species; the role of rising CO_2 per se on pollen allergen content; the role of climate on aeroallergenic plant species distribution (e.g., ragweed in Europe). Integration of these studies with other meteorological factors likely to change, such as ozone or flooding, is needed to provide regional estimates of the production and dissemination of plant- and fungal-based allergens (Albertine et al. 2014; Beggs 2016). Such information would also be invaluable in providing clinical and epidemiological knowledge as to the seasonality and occurrence of allergic disease in the context of climate or CO_2 concentration; as such, this information could facilitate better recognition of vulnerability and disease management.

Research priorities include:

- The development of long-term (multidecadal) pollen and spore data sets that use consistent methods for quantification, qualification, and monitoring of pollen counts and aeroallergen concentrations at regional and national levels

- Sharing of this data with health officials (e.g., CDC)

- Surveillance information from emergency department visits to help clarify the epidemiology of extreme weather events and climate in the context of aeroallergen exposure and asthma
- Increased recognition of the role of plant-based pollen production in international assessments of climate change impacts
- Initiation of urban ecological studies (which can mimic projected climate change) to help identify and manage allergenic plants to minimize aeroallergen exposure
- Additional research to determine potential synergies between aeroallergens and human pollution
- Using environmental information to develop early warning systems of aeroallergen exposure
- Cooperation and quantitative comparisons between health care professionals and plant biologists to establish a common set of pollen and climate indexes for additional research and modeling efforts

Contact Dermatitis

For plant-based contact dermatitis, additional experimental data are necessary to determine the ubiquity of potential changes in urushiol and similar chemical compounds from related plant species (e.g., poison sumac, poison ivy) with climate and CO_2. Such information should also be collected to determine climate-induced changes in the current and future distribution of known toxicological plant species. Warmer temperatures, higher CO_2 concentrations, and longer growing seasons could also facilitate increasing contact with urushiol or similar compounds in urban areas. Climatic shifts in temporal contact and dermatitis should also be quantified or projected.

Toxicology

From pharmacology to toxicology, it is well established that secondary plant compounds significantly affect human health (Schultes and Reis 1995). It is also clear that rising CO_2 and temperature are altering or will alter the concentration or temporal production of these compounds. However, several fundamental research priorities remain to be addressed regarding the influence of climate and CO_2. Can we expect toxicological changes in poisonous plants? Will plants that are known sources of either medicine or narcotics change their global distribution or in response to climate? Will the concentration or efficacy of the pharmacological compound change? There are also questions regarding management. For example, do current government efforts to reduce acreage for illegal poppy production consider the role of climate and/or CO_2 on those efforts?

Food Security

Because of the enormity of and potential vulnerability to food security (access to sufficient, safe, and nutritious food that provides the full range of necessary calories and micronutrients), there are clear and compelling issues related to climate change that have drawn the attention of scientists, the general public, and policymakers. These issues have been extensively examined in a variety of public and academic forums, from the medical community (Watts et al. 2017, Swinburn et al. 2019) to the U.S. Government (Howden et al. 2007) to the international community (IPCC 2014) to business leaders (Myers 2015).

Surprisingly, however, the role of rising CO_2 in the context of food security is still unclear. Will rising CO_2 alter interactions with drought or flooding? How? Does CO_2 increase vulnerability to rising temperatures by limiting transpirational cooling and exacerbating pollen sterility? Does CO_2 favor weeds over crops, with concomitant reductions in crop yields? Does CO_2 alter susceptibility of crops to pathogens? To insects? Can varieties of wheat or rice be selected that will be able to use additional CO_2 more effectively as a resource to increase seed yields? What is the role of rising CO_2 on food allergens? Is the reduction in protein and/or micronutrients with additional CO_2 a linear response? These are simply a small subset of research priorities that have been recognized but largely, to date, unaddressed at the scientific, modeling, or policy level. A related issue is the fate of cash crops in a changed climate. For subsistence farmers relying on cash crops to purchase agricultural inputs, any change in productivity could affect their ability to continue to feed their families (Ebi et al. 2011).

CLINICAL CORRELATES 7.2 PLANT BIOLOGY AND DISEASE VECTORS

Although plants generally do not transmit human disease, they are food and habitats for animal vectors that do spread disease, such as rodents and mosquitoes, and an integral part of the greater ecosystem including livestock and humans. Many animal vectors rely on plants as a principal food source (although female mosquitoes require blood proteins to lay eggs). The rich biodiversity offered creates environments that directly and indirectly support human health (Aerts, Honnay, and Van Nieuwenhuyse 2018). In a changing climate, rising carbon dioxide will stimulate plant growth, including pollen and seed production, and influence plant demography and biodiversity. The question remains on how these changes will influence disease ecology including to what extent diseases will expand (Caminade, McIntyre, and Jones 2019). As one example, a change in climate may influence seed sources for rodents, thus potentially altering the occurrence and spread of hantavirus (Plowright et al. 2008). Hantavirus is transmitted via rodent droppings or saliva and can cause acute respiratory failure. Another example is pollen on open ponds that serve as food for mosquito larvae (Ye-Ebiyo, Pollack, and Spielman 2000). There are variable effects on mosquito growth based on several variables (Asmare et al. 2017) and unknown influence on fecundity or disease prevalence.

Understanding the links regarding climate and carbon dioxide, plant biology, and the resulting changes in vector range and disease transmission, remain a little recognized, if highly desirable, research goal.

Conclusion

Potential serious consequences of a warmer planet include concurrent increases in extreme events, increases in disease outbreaks, reductions in air and water quality, decreases in food availability, and increases in respiratory illness (IPCC 2014; McMichael and Lindgren 2011; McMichael, Montgomery, and Costello 2012). However, in our estimation, the nexus of climate-CO_2, plant biology, and human health are not always considered or evaluated in that context. Yet, plant biology affects every aspect of civilization, from air, to water, to clothing, to food, to shelter, to medicine. As this review illustrates, the consequences for public health of climate change and rising CO_2 on plant biology, from aeroallergens, to pharmacology to food safety are, and will continue to be, extensive. The hope is that this chapter has illustrated the critical nature of these relationships among plants, climate, and health; highlighted critical research areas; and acted as a clear and timely appeal for additional resources to address these challenges.

DISCUSSION QUESTIONS

1. How will CO_2-induced changes in plant nutrition alter global nutritional availability and health?

2. How will climate change alter the spatial and temporal occurrence of plant-based aeroallergens? Does rising CO_2 alter the allergenic content of pollen?

3. If agricultural pest threats increase, how will that alter pesticide exposure rates?

4. How will climate and/or CO_2 alter plant based medicinal use for developed regions?

KEY TERMS

Aerobiology: A subset of biology that studies the dynamics of organic particles and small organisms that can be passively transported by air. Aerobiologists are associated with the measuring and reporting of airborne pollen and fungal spores as a public health service.

Demography: The statistical study of living populations in regard to dynamic changes in their size, structure, and distribution in time and space.

Phenology: The study of periodic plant and animal lifecycle events and how these are influenced by seasonal and interannual variations in climate.

Photodermatitis: A form of allergic contact dermatitis whereby the allergen is activated by light to order to induce the allergic response.

Vernalization: The biological requirement of cold temperature exposure required by some plants prior to spring flowering.

References

Aerts, R., O. Honnay, and A. Van Nieuwenhuyse. 2018. "Biodiversity and Human Health: Mechanisms and Evidence of the Positive Health Effects of Diversity in Nature and Green Spaces." *British Medical Bulletin* 127 (1):5–22. doi:10.1093/bmb/ldy021.

Albertine, J. M., W. J. Manning, M. DaCosta, K. A. Stinson, M. L. Muilenberg, and C. A. Rogers. 2014. "Projected Carbon Dioxide to Increase Grass Pollen and Allergen Exposure Despite Higher Ozone Levels." *PloS One* 9:e111712.

Anenberg, S. C., K. R. Weinberger, H. Roman, J. E. Neumann, A. Crimmins, N. Fann, J., Martinich, J. and P. L. Kinney. 2017. "Impacts of Oak Pollen on Allergic Asthma in the United States and Potential Influence of Future Climate Change. *GeoHealth* 1:80K.R., 92.

Archambault, D. J. 2007. "Efficacy of Herbicides under Elevated Temperature and CO_2." In *Agroecosystems in a Changing Climate*, edited by P. C. D. Newton et al. Boca Raton, FL: CRC Press.

Ariano, R., G. W. Canonica, and G. Passalacqua. 2010. "Possible Role of Climate Changes in Variations in Pollen Seasons and Allergic Sensitizations during 27 Years." *Annals of Allergy Asthma and Immunology* 104:215–22.

Asmare, Y., R. J. Hopkins, H. Tekie, S. R. Hill, and R. Ignell. 2017. "Grass Pollen Affects Survival and Development of Larval *Anopheles arabiensis* (Diptera: Culicidae)." *Journal of Insect Science* 17(5):93. doi:10.1093/jisesa/iex067.

Beach, R. H., T. B. Sulser, A. Crimmins, N. Cenacchi, J., Cole, N. K. Fukagawa, D. Mason-D'Croz et al. 2019. "A Modeling Approach Combining Elevated Atmospheric CO_2 Effects on Protein, Iron and Zinc Availability with Projected Climate Change Impacts on Global Diets." *Lancet Planetary Health* 3:e307–17.

Beddington, J. R., M. Asaduzzaman, M. E. Clark, A. Fernandez Bremauntz, M. D. Guillou, D. J. B. Howlett et al. 2012. "What Next for Agriculture after Durban?" *Science* 335:289–90.

Beggs, P. J., 2016. *Impacts of Climate Change on Allergens and Allergic Diseases*. Cambridge: Cambridge University Press.

Bernstein, L. H. 2017. "The Global Problem of Malnutrition." *Food Nutrition Journal* 10:2575-7091.

Blank, R. R., R. H. White, and L. H. Ziska. 2006. "Combustion Properties of *Bromus tectorum* L.: Influence of Ecotype and Growth under Four CO_2 Concentrations." *International Journal of Wildland Fire* 15:227–36.

Boretti, A., and S. Florentine. 2019. "Atmospheric CO_2 Concentration and Other Limiting Factors in the Growth of C_3 and C_4 Plants." *Plants (Basel)* 8(4):92. doi:10.3390/plants8040092.

Boyer, J. S., P. Byrne, K. G. Cassman, M. Cooper, D. Delmer, T. Greene, F. Gruis et al. 2013. "The US Drought of 2012 in Perspective: A Call to Action." *Global Food Security* 2:139–43.

Bradley, B. A., C. A. Curtis, E. J. Fusco, J. T. Abatzoglou, J. K. Balch, S. Dadashi, and M. N. Tuanmu. 2018. "Cheatgrass (*Bromus tectorum*) Distribution in the Intermountain Western United States and Its Relationship to Fire Frequency, Seasonality, and Ignitions." *Biological Invasions* 20:1493–1506.

Bryant, J. P., F. S. Chapin, and D. R. Klein. 1983. "Carbon/Nutrient Balance of Boreal Plants in Relation to Vertebrate Herbivory." *Oikos* 40:357–68.

Burbach, G. J., L. M. Heinzerling, C. Röhnelt, K.-C. Bergmann, H. Behrendt, and T. Zuberbier. 2009. "Ragweed Sensitization in Europe: GALEN Study Suggests Increasing Prevalence." *Allergy* 64:664–65.

Burch, M., and E. Levetin. 2002. "Effects of Meteorological Conditions on Spore Plumes." *International Journal of Biometeorology* 46:107–17.

Burr, M. L. 1999. "Grass Pollen: Trends and Predictions." *Clinical and Experimental Allergy* 29:735–38.

Caminade, C., K. M. McIntyre, and A. E. Jones. 2019. "Impact of Recent and Future Climate Change on Vector-Borne Diseases." *Annals of the New York Academy of Sciences* 1436(1):157–73. doi:10.1111/nyas.13950.

Centers for Disease Control and Prevention. 2011. "Allergies and Hay Fever." http://www.cdc.gov/nchs/fastats/allergies.htm.

Chandra, S., H. Lata, I. A. Khan, and M. A. Elsohly. 2008. "Photosynthetic Response of *Cannabis sativa l.* to Variations in Photosynthetic Photon Flux Densities, Temperature and CO_2 Conditions." *Physiological and Molecular Biology of Plants* 14:299–306.

Coiner, H. A., K. Hayhoe, L. H. Ziska, J. Van Dorn, and R. F. Sage. 2018. "Tolerance of Subzero Winter Cold in Kudzu (Pueraria montana var. lobata)." *Oecologia* 187: 839–49.

Corden, J. M., and W. M. Millington. 2001. "The Long-Term Trends and Seasonal Variation of the Aeroallergen *Alternaria* in Derby, UK." *Aerobiologia* 17:127–36.

Corden, J. M., W. M. Millington, and J. Mullins. 2003. "Long-Term Trends and Regional Variation in the Aeroallergen *Alternaria* in Cardiff and Derby UK: Are Differences in Climate and Cereal Production Having an Effect?" *Aerobiologia* 19:191–99.

Clot, B. 2003. "Trends in Airborne Pollen: An Overview of 21 Years of Data in Neuchâtel (Switzerland)." *Aerobiologia* 19:227–34.

Ebi, K. L., J. Padgham, M. Doumbia, A. Kergna, J. Smith, T. Butt, and B. McCarl. 2011. "Smallholders Adaptation to Climate Change in Mali." *Climatic Change* 108:423–36.

El Kelish A., F. Zhao, W. Heller, J. Durner, J. B. Winkler, H. Behrendt, C. Traidl-Hoffmann et al. 2014. "Ragweed (*Ambrosia artemisiifolia*) Pollen Allergenicity: SuperSAGE Transcriptomic Analysis upon Elevated CO_2 and Drought Stress." *BMC Plant Biology* 14:176–90.

Ellwood, E. R., S. A. Temple, R. B. Primack, N. L. Bradley, and C. C. Davis. 2013. "Record-Breaking Early Flowering in the Eastern United States. *PLoS ONE* 8:e53788.

Emberlin, J., M. Detandt, R. Gehrig, S. Jaeger, N. Nolard, and A. Rantio-Lehtimäki. 2002. "Responses in the Start of the Betula (Birch) Pollen Seasons to Recent Changes in Spring Temperatures across Europe." *International Journal of Biometeorology* 46:159–70.

Emberlin, J., J. Mullins, J. Corden, S. Jones, W. Millington, M. Brooke, and M. Savage. 1999. "Regional Variations in Grass Pollen Seasons in the UK, Long-Term Trends and Forecast Models." *Clinical and Experimental Allergy* 29:347–56.

Fitter, A. H., and R. S. R. Fitter. 2002. "Rapid Changes in Flowering Time in British Plants." *Science* 296:1689–91.

Frei, T., and E. Gassner. 2008. "Climate Change and Its Impact on Birch Pollen Quantities and the Start of the Pollen Season: An Example from Switzerland for the Period 1969–2006." *International Journal of Biometeorology* 52:667–74.

Frenguelli, G. 2002. "Interactions between Climatic Changes and Allergenic Plants." *Monaldi Archives for Chest Disease* 57:141–43.

García-Mozo, H., C. Galán, V. Jato, J. Belmonte, C. D. De La Guardia, D. Fernández, M. Gutiérrez et al. 2006. "*Quercus* Pollen Season Dynamics in the Iberian Peninsula: Response to Meteorological

Parameters and Possible Consequences of Climate Change." *Annals of Agricultural and Environmental Medicine* 13:209–224.

Gleadow, R. M., J. R. Evans, S. Mccaffery, and T. R. Cavagnaro. 2009. "Growth and Nutritive Value of Cassava (*Manihot esculenta* Cranz.) Are Reduced When Grown in Elevated CO_2." *Plant Biology* 11:76–82.

Haines, A., and K. Ebi. 2019. "The Imperative for Climate Action to Protect Health." *New England Journal of Medicine* 380 (3): 263–73.

Hatfield, J. L., K. J. Boote, B. A. Kimball, L. H. Ziska, R. C. Izaurralde, D. Ort, A. M. Thomson, and D. Wolfe, 2011. "Climate Impacts on Agriculture: Implications for Crop Production." *Agronomy Journal* 103:351–70.

Howden, S. M., J. F. Soussana, F. N. Tubiello, N. Chetri, M. Dunlop, and H. Meinke. 2007. "Adapting Agriculture to Climate Change." *Proceedings of the National Academy of Sciences of the USA* 104:9691–96.

Hunt, R., D. W. Hand, M. A. Hannah, and A. M. Neal. 1991. "Response to CO_2 Enrichment in 27 Herbaceous Species." *Functional Ecology* 5:410–21.

Intergovernmental Panel on Climate Change. 2007. *Climate Change 20007: Impacts, Adaptation and Vulnerability*. Geneva: IPCC Secretariat.

Intergovernmental Panel on Climate Change. 2014. *Climate Change 2014: Synthesis Report. Contribution of Working Groups I, II and III to the Fifth Assessment Report of the Intergovernmental Panel on Climate Change*. Geneva: IPCC.

Intergovernmental Science-Policy Platform on Biodiversity and Ecosystem Services. 2019. *Summary for Policymakers of the Global Assessment Report on Biodiversity and Ecosystem Services of the Intergovernmental Science-Policy Platform on Biodiversity and Ecosystem Services*. Bonn, Germany: IPBES Secretariat.

Jugulam, M., A. K. Varanasi, V. K. Varanasi, and P. V. V. Prasad. 2018. "Climate Change Influence on Herbicide Efficacy and Weed Management." In *Food Security and Climate Change*, edited by S. S. Yadav, R. J. Redden, J. L. Hatfield, A. W. Ebert, and D. Hunter, 433–48. Hoboken, NJ: Wiley.

Kerr, R. A. 2007. "Global Warming Coming Home to Roost in the American West." *Science* 318:1859.

Klironomos, J. N., M. C. Rillig, M. F. Allen, D. R. Zak, K. S. Pregitzer, and M. E. Kubiske. 1997. "Increased Levels of Airborne Fungal Spores in Response to *Populus tremuloides* Grown under Elevated Atmospheric CO_2." *Canadian Journal of Botany* 75:1670–73.

LaDeau, S. L., and J. S. Clark, 2006. "Pollen Production by *Pinus taeda* Growing in Elevated Atmospheric CO_2." *Functional Ecology* 20:541–47.

Lloyd, S. J., R. S. Kovats, and Z. Chalabi. 2011. "Climate Change, Crop Yields and Undernutrition: Development of a Model to Quantify the Impact of Climate Scenarios on Child Undernutrition." *Environmental Health Perspectives* 119:1817–23.

Lobell, D. B., and M. B. Burke. 2010. "On the Use of Statistical Models to Predict Crop Yield Responses to Climate Change." *Agricultural and Forest Meteorology* 150:1443–52.

Lobell, D. B., M. B. Burke, C. Rebaldi, M. D. Mastrandrea, W. P. Falcon, and R. L. Naylor. 2008. "Prioritizing Climate Change Adaptation Needs for Food Security in 2030." *Science* 319:607–10.

Lobell, D. B., G. L. Hammer, McLean, C. Messina, M. J. Roberts, and, W. Schlenker. 2013. "The Critical Role of Extreme Heat for Maize Production in the United States." *Nature Climate Change* 3:497–501.

Loladze, I. 2002 "Rising Atmospheric CO_2 and Human Nutrition: Toward Globally Imbalanced Plant Stoichiometry?" *Trends in Ecology and Evolution* 17:457–61.

Loladze, I. 2014. "Hidden Shift of the Ionome of Plants Exposed to Elevated CO_2 Depletes Minerals at the Base of Human Nutrition." *eLife* 1–30. doi:10.7554/eLife.02245.

Manea, A., M. R. Leishman, and P. O. Downey. 2011. "Exotic C_4 Grasses Have Increased Tolerance to Glyphosate under Elevated Carbon Dioxide." *Weed Science* 59:28–36.

Matsui, T., Namuco, O.S., Ziska, L.H. and Horie, T., 1997. Effects of High Temperature and CO_2 Concentration on Spikelet Sterility in Indica Rice." *Field Crops Research* 51:213–19.

McMichael, A. J., and E. Lindgren. 2011. "Climate Change: Present and Future Risks to Health, and Necessary Responses." *Journal of Internal Medicine* 270:401–13.

McMichael, A. J., H. Montgomery, and A. Costello. 2012. "Health Risks, Present and Future, from Global Climate Change." *British Medical Journal* 344. doi:10.1136/bmj.e1359.

Mohan, J. E., L. H. Ziska, W. H. Schlesinger, R. B. Thomas, R. C. Sicher, K. George, and J. S. Clark. 2006. "Biomass and Toxicity Responses of Poison Ivy (*Toxicodendron radicans*) to Elevated Atmospheric CO_2." *Proceedings of the National Academy of Science USA* 103:9086–89.

Myers, J. 2015. "How Will Climate Change Affect Food Security?" Geneva, Switzerland: World Economic Forum. https://www.weforum.org/agenda/2015/12/how-will-climate-change-affect-food-security.

Myers, S. S., A. Zanobetti, I. Kloog, P. Huybers, A. D. B. Leakey, A. J. Bloom, E. Carlisle et al. 2014. "Increasing CO$_2$ Threatens Human Nutrition." *Nature* 510:139–44.

Neergheen-Bhujun, V., A. T. Awan, Y. Baran, N. Bunnefeld, K. Chan, T. E. de la Cruz, D. Egamberdieva et al. "Biodiversity, Drug Discovery, and the Future of Global Health: Introducing the Biodiversity to Biomedicine Consortium, a Call to Action." *Journal of Global Health* 7(2):020304. doi:10.7189/jogh.07.020304.

Neumann, J. E., S. C. Anenberg, K. R. Weinberger, M. Amend, S. Gulati, A. Crimmins, H. Roman, N. Fann, and P. L. Kinney. 2019. "Estimates of Present and Future Asthma Emergency Department Visits Associated with Exposure to Oak, Birch, and Grass Pollen in the United States." *GeoHealth* 3 (1): 11–27.

Noyes, P. D., M. K. McElwee, H. D. Miller, B.W. Clark, L. A. Van Tiem, K. C. Walcott, K. N. Erwin, and E. D. Levin. 2009. "The Toxicology of Climate Change: Environmental Contaminants in a Warming World." *Environment International* 35 (6):971–86.

Panda, D. K., and J. Wahr. 2016. "Spatiotemporal Evolution of Water Storage Changes in India from the Updated GRACE-Derived Gravity Records." *Water Resources Research* 52:135–49.

Pimentel, D. 1997. *Techniques for Reducing Pesticides: Environmental and Economic Benefits.* Chichester, UK: Wiley.

Quest Diagnostics Health Trends. 2011. *Allergy Report 2011.* Allergies Across America. http://www.questdiagnostics.com/dms/Documents/Other/allergy-report-executive-summary.pdf.

Rasmussen, A. 2002. "The Effects of Climate Change on the Birch Pollen Season in Denmark." *Aerobiologia* 18:253–65.

Refatti, J. P., L. A. Avila, E. R. Camargo, L. H. Ziska, C. Oliveira, R. Salas-Perez, and N. R. Burgos. 2019. "High [CO$_2$] and Temperature Increase Resistance to Cyhalofop-Butyl in Multiple-Resistant *Echinochloa colona.*" *Frontiers in Plant Science* 10:529–36.

Rodríguez-Rajo, F. J., D. Fdez-Savilla, A. Stach, and V. Jato. 2010. "Assessment between Pollen Seasons in Areas with Different Urbanization Level Related to Local Vegetation Sources and Differences in Allergen Exposure." *Aerobiologia* 26:1–14

Rogers, C. A., P. M. Wayne, E. A. Macklin, M. L. Mullenberg, C. J. Wagner, P. R. Epstein, and F. A. Bazzaz. 2006. "Interaction of the Onset of Spring and Elevated Atmospheric CO$_2$ on Ragweed (*Ambrosia artemisiifolia* L.) Pollen Production." *Environmental Health Perspectives* 114:865–69.

Sapkota, A., Murtugudde, R., Curriero, F.C., Upperman, C.R., Ziska, L. and Jiang, C., 2019. "Associations between Alteration in Plant Phenology and Hay Fever Prevalence among US Adults: Implication for Changing Climate." *PloS One* 14 (3):p.e0212010.

Schultes, R. E., and S. V. Reis. 1995. *Ethnobotany: The Evolution of a Discipline.* Portland, OR: Dioscorides Press.

Singer, B. D., L. H. Ziska, D. A. Frenz, D. E. Gebhard, and J. G. Straka 2005. "Increasing Amb a 1 Content in Common Ragweed (*Ambrosia artemisiifolia*) Pollen as a Function of Rising Atmospheric CO$_2$ Concentration." *Functional Plant Biology* 32:67–70.

Stach, A., García-Mozo, H., Prieto-Baena, J.C., Czarnecka-Operacz, M., Jenerowicz, D., Silny, W. and Galán, C. 2007. "Prevalence of *Artemisia* Species Pollinosis in Western Poland: Impact of Climate Change on Aerobiological Trends, 1995–2004." *Journal of Allergologia Clinical Immunology* 17:39–45.

Stuhlfauth, T., and H. P. Fock. 1990. "Effect of Whole Season CO$_2$ Enrichment on the Cultivation of a Medicinal Plant, *Digitalis lanata.*" *Journal of Agronomy and Crop Science* 164:168–73.

Swinburn, B. A., V. I. Kraak, S. Allender, V. J. Atkins, P. I. Baker, J. R. Bogard, H. Brinsden et al. 2019. "The Global Syndemic of Obesity, Undernutrition, and Climate Change: The Lancet Commission Report. *The Lancet.*" 393:791–846.

Tanner, T. 2000. "Rhus (Toxicodendron) Dermatitis." *Primary Care* 27:493–501.

Taub, D., B. Miller, and H. Allen. 2008. "Effects of Elevated CO$_2$ on the Protein Concentration of Food Crops: A Meta-Analysis." *Global Change Biology* 14:565–75.

Wan, S., T. S. Yuan, Bowdish, L. Wallace, S. D. Russell, and Y. Luo. 2002. "Response of an Allergenic Species, *Ambrosia psilostachya* (*Asteraceae*), to Experimental Warming and Clipping: Implications for Public Health." *American Journal of Botany* 89:1843–46.

Wang, S. Y., J. A. Bunce, and J. L. Maas. 2003. "Elevated Carbon Dioxide Increases Contents of Antioxidant Compounds in Field-Grown Strawberries." *Journal of Agriculture and Food Chemistry* 51:4315–20.

Waryszak, P., T. I. Lenz, M. R. Leishman, and P. O. Downey. 2018. "Herbicide Effectiveness in Controlling Invasive Plants under Elevated CO$_2$: Sufficient Evidence to Rethink Weeds Management." *Journal of Environmental Management* 226:400–7.

Watson, W. A., T. L. Litovitz, W. Klein-Schwartz, G. C. Rodgers, J. Youniss, N. Reid, W. G. Rouse, R. S. Rembert, and D. Borys. 2004. "2003 Annual Report of the American Association of Poison Control Centers Toxic Exposure Surveillance System." *American Journal of Emergency Medicine* 22:335–404.

Watts, N., W. N. Adger, S. Ayeb-Karlsson, Y. Bai, P. Byass, D. Campbell-Lendrum, T. Colbourn et al. 2017. "The Lancet Countdown: Tracking Progress on Health and Climate Change." *Lancet* 389:1151–64.

Wayne, P., S. Foster, J. Connolly, F. A. Bazzaz, and P. R. Epstein, 2002. "Production of Allergenic Pollen by Ragweed (*Ambrosia artemisiifolia* L.) Is Increased in CO_2-Enriched Atmospheres." *Annals of Allergy Asthma and Immunology* 80:669–79.

Wegren, S. K. 2011. "Food Security and Russia's 2010 Drought." *Eurasian Geography and Economics* 52:140–56.

Weinmayr, G., S. K. Weiland, B. Bjorksten, B. Brunekreef, G. Büchele, W. O. Cookson, L. Garcia Marcos, et al. 2007. "Atopic Sensitization and the International Variation of Asthma Symptom Prevalence in Children." *American Journal of Respiratory and Critical Care Medicine* 176:565–74.

Weltzin, J. F., R. T. Belote, and N. J. Sanders. 2003. "Biological Invaders in a Greenhouse World: Will Elevated CO_2 Fuel Plant Invasions?" *Frontiers in Ecology and the Environment* 1:146–53.

Whiten, S. R., and R. K. Peterson. 2015. "The Influence of Ambient Temperature on the Susceptibility of Aedes aegypti (Diptera: Culicidae) to the Pyrethroid Insecticide Permethrin." *Journal of Medical Entomology* 53:139–43.

Wiberley, A. E., A. R. Linskey, T. G. Falbel, and T. D. Sharkey. 2005. "Development of the Capacity for Isoprene Emission in Kudzu." *Plant, Cell & Environment* 28:898–905.

Wolf, J., N. R. O'Neill, C. A. Rogers, M. L. Muilenberg, and L. H. Ziska. 2010. "Elevated Atmospheric Carbon Dioxide Concentrations Amplify *Alternaria alternata* Sporulation and Total Antigen Production." *Environmental Health Perspectives* 118:1223–28.

Zhu, C., K. Kobayashi, I. Loladze, J. Zhu, Q. Jiang, X. Xu, and G. Liu et al. 2018. "Carbon Dioxide (CO_2) Levels This Century Will Alter the Protein, Micronutrients, and Vitamin Content of Rice Grains with Potential Health Consequences for the Poorest Rice-Dependent Countries." *Science Advances* 4 (5):eaaq1012. doi: 10.1126/sciadv.aaq1012.

Ziska, L. H. 2003. "Evaluation of the Growth Response of Six Invasive Species to Past, Present and Future Atmospheric Carbon Dioxide." *Journal of Experimental Botany* 54:395–404.

Ziska, L. H. 2004. "Influence of Rising Atmospheric CO_2 since 1900 on Early Growth and Photosynthetic Response of a Noxious Invasive Weed, Canada Thistle (*Cirsium arvense*)." *Functional Plant Biology* 29:1387–92.

Ziska, L. H. 2014. "Increasing Minimum Daily Temperatures are Associated with Enhanced Pesticide Use in Cultivated Soybean along a Latitudinal Gradient in the Mid-Western United States." *PloS One* 9:e98516.

Ziska, L.H. 2016. "The Role of Climate Change and Increasing Atmospheric Carbon Dioxide on Weed Management: Herbicide Efficacy." *Agriculture, Ecosystems & Environment* 231:304–9.

Ziska, L. H., and J. A. Bunce, 2006. "Plant Responses to Rising Carbon Dioxide." In *Plant Growth and Climate Change*, edited by J. Morison Morecroft, 17–47. Oxford: Blackwell.

Ziska, L. H., and F. A. Caulfield. 2000. "Rising CO_2 and Pollen Production of Common Ragweed (*Ambrosia artemisiifolia*), a Known Allergy-Inducing Species: Implications for Public Health." *Australian Journal of Plant Physiology* 27:893–98.

Ziska, L. H., A. Crimmins, A. Auclair, S. Degrasse, J. F. Garofalo, A. S. Khan, I. Loladze et al. 2016. "Food Safety, Nutrition and Distribution." In *The Impacts of Climate Change on Human Health in the United States: A Scientific Assessment*, edited by A. Crimmins, J. Balbus, J. L. Gamble, C. B. Beard, J. E. Bell, D. Dodgen, R. J. Eisen et al., 189–216. Washington, DC: U.S. Global Change Research Program. http://dx.doi.org/10.7930/J0ZP4417

Ziska, L. H., S. D. Emche, E. L. Johnson, K. George, D. R. Reed, and R. C. Sicher. 2005. "Alterations in the Production and Concentration of Selected Alkaloids as a Function of Rising Atmospheric Carbon Dioxide and Air Temperature: Implications for Ethno-Pharmacology." *Global Change Biology* 11:1798–1807.

Ziska, L. H., S. S. Faulkner, and J. Lydon. 2004 "Changes in Biomass and Root: Shoot Ratio of Field-Grown Canada Thistle (*Cirsium arvense*), a Noxious, Invasive Weed, with Elevated CO_2: Implications for Control with Glyphosate." *Weed Science* 52:584–88.

Ziska, L. H., Gebhard, D.E., Frenz, D.A., Faulkner, S., Singer, B.D. and Straka, J.G., 2003. Cities as harbingers of climate change: common ragweed, urbanization, and public health. *Journal of Allergy and Clinical Immunology* 111: 290–95.

Ziska, L., K. Knowlton, C. Rogers, D. Dalan, N. Tierney, M. A. Elder, W. Filley et al. 2011. "Recent Warming by Latitude Associated with Increased Length of Ragweed Pollen Season in Central North America." *Proceedings of the National Academy of Sciences* 108:4248–51.

Ziska, L. H., L. Makra, S. K. Harry, N. Bruffaerts, M. Hendrickx, F. Coates, A. Saarto et al. 2019. "Temperature-Related Changes in Airborne Allergenic Pollen Abundance and Seasonality across the Northern Hemisphere: A Retrospective Data Analysis." *Lancet Planetary Health* 3:e124–e131.

Ziska, L. H., S. Panicker, and H. L. Wojno. 2008. "Recent and Projected Increases in Atmospheric Carbon Dioxide and the Potential Impacts on Growth and Alkaloid Production in Wild Poppy (*Papaver setigerum* DC.)." *Climatic Change* 91:395.

Ziska, L.H., J. B. Reeves III, and B. Blank. 2005. "The Impact of Recent Increases in Atmospheric CO_2 on Biomass Production and Vegetative Retention of Cheatgrass (*Bromus tectorum*): Implications for Fire Disturbance." *Global Change Biology*, 11:1325–32.

Ziska, L. H., R. C. Sicher, K. George, and J. E. Mohan, J.E., 2007. "Rising Atmospheric Carbon Dioxide and Potential Impacts on the Growth and Toxicity of Poison Ivy (*Toxicodendron radicans*)." *Weed Science* 55 (4):288–92.

Ziska, L. H., J. R. Teasdale, and J. A. Bunce. 1999. "Future Atmospheric Carbon Dioxide May Increase Tolerance to Glyphosate." *Weed Science* 47 (5): 608–15.

Zobayed, S. S. P. K., and P. K. Saxena. 2004. "Production of St. John's Wort Plants under Controlled Environment for Maximizing Biomass and Secondary Metabolites." *In Vitro Cellular & Developmental Biology-Plant* 40:108–14.

CHAPTER 8

CLIMATE AND ITS IMPACTS ON VECTOR-BORNE DISEASES

Andrea G. Buchwald, Jada F. Garofalo, Kenneth L. Gage, Charles B. Beard, and Rosemary Rochford

Vector-borne diseases (VBD) are infectious diseases transmitted by arthropod vectors (e.g., insects and ticks). The arthropods that can transmit pathogens to humans include mosquitoes, ticks, flies, and fleas. VBDs account for close to 20 percent of all infectious diseases affecting the human population. Because vector-borne pathogens that cause disease in humans utilize an arthropod vector, environmental factors that affect the vector can affect the transmission of the pathogens to humans. To understand the impact of climate change on VBDs then, it is useful to first understand how vectors are sensitive to their environment.

Arthropods are coldblooded (i.e., ectothermic), which means they do not regulate their own temperature and are highly susceptible to variations in climate. In more temperate regions, warming trends increase the duration of favorable conditions for ectotherm development and reproduction. Temperature influences insect development, mortality, reproduction, and behavior. Likewise, precipitation, humidity, and vapor pressure are all important for reproductive success. Variability or alterations in any of these factors can lead to changes in availability of habitats and, in most regions of the world, variations in weather patterns associated with climate change are contributing to changes in insect habitat suitability. For example, temperature affects how long mosquitoes live, how quickly they mature to adulthood, how often they bite, and population density. Precipitation is essential to mosquito breeding as mosquito eggs are laid in or near water and mosquito larva mature in water. Humidity, which is related to precipitation, increases the lifespan of mosquitoes, giving them more opportunities to carry pathogens from one person or host to another. Ticks are similarly dependent on temperature and precipitation, requiring humid environments to prevent desiccation, and thriving within a narrow temperature range.

Although environmental factors can affect the insect host, it should be noted that pathogen survival and success are a product of both vector and human host ecology. Several variables including host and vector biology, density, and behavior, as well as the development of the pathogens within the vector, can affect the rate or probability of transmission of the pathogen. For example, immunity in existing human populations can decrease infection transmission rates as compared to the introduction of a new pathogen into a population of naive hosts that have never experienced the infection. Thus, the immune status of human populations is one of many factors that can affect how rapidly a pathogen can cause epidemics. Another important variable affecting transmission is the **extrinsic incubation period (EIP)**. The **EIP** is the time required for the pathogen to (1) establish an infection in a blood-feeding vector and (2) multiply or develop to the point where it can be further transmitted during subsequent vector feedings.

KEY CONCEPTS

- The transmission and distribution of vector-borne diseases (VBDs) are strongly influenced by environmental conditions including climate.

- VBDs are climate sensitive diseases.

- The arthropods that transmit disease, the pathogens that cause disease, and the human hosts that are susceptible to disease are linked in complex ecological systems.

- Our ability to anticipate and react effectively to the impacts of climate change on VBDs is dependent upon the availability of appropriate surveillance, demographic, land use, and environmental data

- Climate change is characterized by changing temperature trends, modified precipitation patterns, increasing weather variability, and increased frequency of extreme weather events.

- Even small changes in important climatic factors can affect the incidence, transmission, and distribution of VBD, as insect vectors depend on optimal conditions of temperature, humidity, and precipitation.

- The nature of this climatic influence suggests the potential for long-term shifts in VBD patterns due to changes in temperature, extreme weather events, and seasonal shifts associated with climate change.

Finally, another factor to consider when assessing the impact of climate change on VBD is the role of the public health infrastructure in mitigation of impacts. Vector control is a key part of public health infrastructure. For example, because of rapid implementation of insecticide spraying, Zika virus transmission in Florida was halted within months of detecting signs of local transmission (Likos et al. 2016). Climate change may allow for movement of disease vectors to new areas, but the level of public health capacity or preexisting vector control measures in those areas will dictate the potential for and severity of outbreaks when they occur.

This chapter discusses how climate change might affect the spread and distribution of VBDs. It explores how climate change is likely to act in conjunction with other drivers of global change to influence the transmission and complex ecological cycles of the agents responsible for VBDs. Although a wide variety of VBDs exist, this chapter focuses on select representative examples (**malaria**, **arboviruses**, and **Lyme disease**). Finally, this chapter discusses the importance of formulating effective response plans for responding to changing distributions of VBDs. This process necessitates the timely collection of reliable surveillance data on human and animal cases of disease. Consistent and accurate data help identify potential climate-related changes in disease incidence, support the implementation of targeted research to identify areas at greatest risk for VBD emergence or outbreaks, and create accessible environmental data sets at appropriate spatial and temporal scales for both researchers and policymakers to identify high-risk areas and populations.

CLINICAL CORRELATES 8.1 CHALLENGES OF VECTOR-BORNE DISEASES FOR CLINICIANS

Diseases from infected ticks, mosquitoes, and fleas tripled between 2004 to 2016 (Salas, Knappenberger, and Hess 2019). Climate-driven changes are only expected to increase worldwide mosquito-borne arboviruses such as Zika, dengue virus, yellow fever, and chikungunya with North America projected to be affected the worst (Monaghan et al. 2016; Sukhralia et al. 2019). Shifts in infections will require clinicians to be aware of dynamic geographic distributions and seasonality. Obtaining appropriate travel histories and timing of potential exposures will also be important in assessing risk to patients. Clinicians and public health officials will be integral to identifying new cases and communicating these risks to their communities.

Vector-borne diseases are changing geographic distributions challenging clinicians to identify new cases via travel histories, symptoms, and appropriate testing for accurate reporting to public health officials.

CLINICAL CORRELATES 8.2 WEST NILE VIRUS

West Nile virus (WNV) is a common arbovirus disease in the United States with broad geographic distribution. Transmission occurs through the bite of an infected mosquito, via infected birds serving as a reservoir. Usually symptoms are mild and similar to a flu-like illness, but the most serious cases of WNV invade the central nervous system. Neuroinvasive WNV incidence increased almost 25 percent in 2018 from the previous years 2008–2017 (McDonald et al. 2018). Scientists and certain states have incorporated vector surveillance through monitoring different mosquito species and bird necropsies (California Vectorborne Disease Surveillance System 2020). Mosquito control remains crucial to reducing WNV, most commonly through reduction of standing water pools and use of larvicides.

Health care and public health professionals should recognize seasonality, climate variability, and geography on the incidence of West Nile virus and other arboviruses.

Arboviruses

Arthropod-borne viruses (arboviruses) are so-called as they are transmitted to humans primarily through the bites of infected mosquitoes, ticks, sand flies, or midges. The focus of this chapter is on arboviruses transmitted by the *Aedes* species mosquito. *Aedes* species mosquitoes are notable for the breadth of infectious pathogens they can carry and transmit, both between humans and from a variety of other vertebrate hosts. *Ae. (Stegomyia) aegypti* and *Ae. (Stegomyia) albopictus* are two species with the greatest global impact on human health, as they act as the predominant mosquito vectors of important arboviruses including yellow fever virus (YFV), **dengue** virus (DENV), chikungunya virus (CHIKV), and Zika virus (ZIKV), among many other pathogens. DENV is the most prevalent *Aedes*-borne virus and is believed to have afflicted human populations for centuries. It has expanded from endemicity in only nine countries before 1970 (World Health Organization 2020) to over one hundred countries in 2013 with an estimated 390 million people infected annually (Bhatt et al. 2013). ZIKV, first isolated in 1947 from a Rhesus monkey in Uganda, has circulated relatively unnoticed for decades, causing only sporadically detected infections in Africa and Asia (Gubler, Vasilakis, and Musso 2017). The first large ZIKV outbreak occurred in Yap State in 2007, followed by another large epidemic in French Polynesia (Cao-Lormeau et al. 2014). The virus caused global public health concern starting in 2014 when a large ZIKV outbreak in the Americas coincided with a noticeable rise in severe neurological outcomes among newborns and led to the first description of congenital Zika syndrome (Mlakar et al. 2016). All *Aedes*-borne viruses cause acute febrile illness, which may be easily misdiagnosed as malaria in malaria-endemic regions (Stoler et al. 2014).

Aedes Mosquito Vector

Although there are many species of Aedes mosquito, most do not transmit pathogens to humans. However, as noted, two species are the main contributors to human disease, *Ae. aegypti* and *Ae. albopictus* and they are the focus of this chapter. Historically, *Ae. aegypti* were the primary vector of global arboviral outbreaks. This species primarily feeds on humans, efficiently transmits DENV and YFV, and is widely found in anthropogenic environments. Until recently, *Ae. albopictus* were considered a secondary vector, as they historically transmitted DENV less efficiently and were less host specific. While *Ae. albopictus* can feed on a variety of animals including birds, reptiles, and amphibians, more recent research has found, given the option they preferentially choose to feed on humans (Delatte et al. 2010; Kamgang et al. 2012; Nibyelski et al. 2004; Ponlawat and Harrington 2005; Richards et al. 2006). Independent of climatic factors, the range of *Ae. aegypti* and *albopictus* and their associated viruses all have the potential to increase over time with changes in climate, land use patterns, and other factors. Development affects the distribution of both primary vectors because they are adapted to human development and are uniquely suited to urban environments, with a preference for urbanized breeding grounds and domestic containers for egg laying (Chang et al. 2016; Fikrig et al. 2017; Kamgang et al. 2012; Li et al. 2014).

Ae. aegypti and albopictus are active primarily during daylight hours and rest in shaded sites (Schultz 1993). Both vectors lay eggs just above the water line in artificial containers including bottles, flowerpots, or other containers partially filled with water. *Ae. albopictus* eggs are commonly found in discarded tires, the transport of which is believed to be one of the primary sources of *Ae. albopictus* expansion globally (Cornel and Hunt 1991; Reiter and Sprenger 1987). For both species, the eggs are resistant to desiccation after water evaporates from the container, with eggs surviving up to one year (Estrada-Franco and Craig 1995; Juliano et al. 2002). They are dependent on precipitation to progress to their next life stage: when next it rains, the water floods the container and, if eggs are submerged, this leads to hatching and releasing of larval mosquitoes. The requirements of the *Aedes* life cycle makes these viral vectors particularly sensitive to climatic conditions including temperature, humidity, and precipitation.

Aedes-borne infections can lead to severe sequelae including joint pain and arthritis (Paul et al. 2011), severe birth defects (Hall et al. 2017), and fatal hemorrhagic fever (Simmons et al. 2012). There is currently no curative treatment available for any of the *Aedes*-borne arboviruses; thus, medical care for affected individuals is focused on treatments that alleviate symptoms as well as prevent severe complications of the diseases. There is a highly effective vaccine available for YFV, but no effective vaccines are currently available to protect against ZIKV, DENV, or CHIKV.

Ae. aegypti and *albopictus* Vector Distribution Globally

Aedes species mosquitoes are currently found worldwide throughout the tropics and extending into North America and Europe. *Ae. aegypti* is believed to have originated in Africa but is now distributed widely around the world, primarily found in the tropics between degrees 40N and 40S (Kraemer et al. 2015). Similarly, *Ae. albopictus* is believed to have originated in Asia, and rapid range expansion has occurred in recent years, with *Ae. albopictus* now found throughout North and South America, Africa, Europe, and Australia (Paupy et al. 2009). Movement and range expansion of both mosquitoes has been linked to a variety of factors including human behavior (Kraemer et al. 2019) (e.g., deforestation, shipping, travel, urban expansion, and migration), population growth, and changing climatic suitability linked with both long-term climate and short-term weather patterns (Figure 8.1).

Climate Impact on Arbovirus Transmission

On a global scale, temperature and precipitation are the two variables most strongly correlated with *Aedes*-borne disease risk (Banu et al. 2011; Bhatt et al. 2013; Estallo et al. 2015). Temperature has been found to have complex nonlinear effects on both *Aedes* mosquito spp.

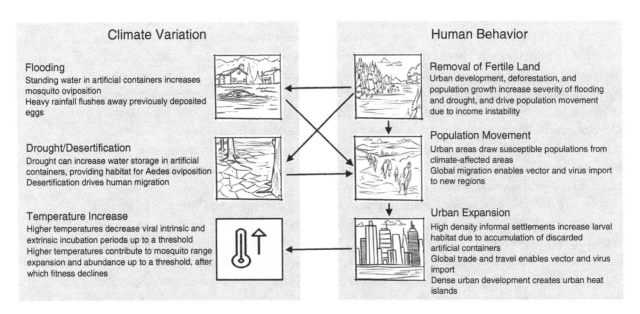

Figure 8.1 Conceptual model of the interaction between climate variation and human factors affecting *Aedes* mosquitoes distribution
Source: Buchwald et al. (2020).

life cycles and fitness (Mordecai et al. 2017; Shragai et al. 2017; Tun-Lin, Burkot, and Kay 2000). Ideal temperatures are between 20° and 30°C, with temperatures both lower and higher associated with decreased egg laying and decreased adult survival (Alto and Juliano 2001a, 2001b; Costa et al. 2010; Rueda et al. 1990; Tun-Lin, Burkot, and Kay 2000). Conversely, higher temperatures decrease the development time from egg hatching to adult, with the shortest development times seen between 35° and 39°C. (Tun-Lin, Burkot, and Kay 2000).

As a result of temperature constraints, *Ae. aegypti* cannot tolerate prolonged freezing temperatures, preventing them from establishing year-round breeding outside their current range, though outbreaks do occur seasonally. *Ae. albopictus*, on the other hand, has a greater ability to survive low temperatures and lengthy winters with mean winter temperature as low as 0°C (Nawrocki and Hawley 1987) and can become established in temperate regions with winters too cold for *Ae. aegypti*.

The effects of temperature on mosquito survival and reproduction are further complicated by an interaction with humidity (Alto and Juliano 2001a). Humidity has impacts on adult mosquito survival, egg viability, number of eggs laid, and the number of days over which females will lay eggs, all decreasing with lower humidity (Costa et al. 2010). Precipitation affects *Aedes* mosquito populations by altering the availability of preferred breeding environments. Rain may fill breeding sites with water, providing new breeding habitat for mosquitoes, or can wash away previously deposited eggs, decreasing *Aedes* populations as a result. Periods of drought may limit availability of natural mosquito breeding sites.

In addition to the effects on the mosquito life cycle, climatic variables also have independent effects on the development and transmission of *Aedes*-borne viruses, as the EIP is directly related to temperature. The shorter the EIP, the more likely a mosquito is to be able to transmit the virus from one human host to another. Increasing temperatures have been demonstrated to shorten the EIP for DENV, ZIKV, and CHIKV (Mbaika et al. 2016; Tesla et al. 2018; Watts et al. 1987), increasing the probability of a given mosquito transmitting the virus from one host to another, as well as increasing the probability of a human encountering an infectious mosquito in the population. Additionally, increased EIP at higher temperatures may counter the effect of decreased survival of the mosquito at higher temperatures, allowing for transmission to occur even when the adult mosquito is suffering a shortened lifespan.

Increasing periods of drought associated with climate change may limit availability of natural mosquito breeding sites; however, this may be offset by *Aedes* mosquitoes' distinct preference for anthropogenic habitats. Water storage during dry periods may lead to increases in available *Ae. aegypti* breeding sites (Beebe et al. 2009). Thus, environments with substantial human development and a wide availability of man-made containers may see limited decreases of *Aedes* populations during drought. This makes the lower limits of precipitation for *Aedes* habitat suitability difficult to define in urban areas and other anthropogenic environments.

Climate Change and Arbovirus Risk

Distribution of *Ae. aegypti and albopictus* is expected to increase their geographic range by up to 8.5 percent by 2050. This places more than one billion new people at risk of *Aedes*-borne disease, under climate change projections (Kamal et al. 2018; Ryan et al. 2019). Climate change is expected to alter the distribution of arboviruses—by either increasing climatic suitability for the vectors and pathogens in previously unsuitable regions or decreasing climatic suitability in previously habitable regions—and affect the movement of infected people. Climate change and variability is thought to have been a key driver of the expansion and emergence of recent ZIKV and CHIKV outbreaks in Southeast Asia and the Americas (Ebi and Nealon 2016; Paz and Semenza 2016) and has been credited for newly established DENV endemicity in the

Middle East (Altassan et al. 2019). Despite these impacts, there is uncertainty about the relative importance of climate change on changing arbovirus infection risk as compared to other global drivers of disease spread, including human population movement, urbanization, and human behavioral changes.

Extreme or unusual weather events have been linked to increases in arboviral disease through various potential pathways (Beard et al. 2016). CHIKV outbreaks have been linked to unusually dry, hot weather (Chretien et al. 2007; Subra 1983), possibly as a result of increased water storage, as well as periods of heavy precipitation (Ditsuwan et al. 2011). Flooding, due to extreme precipitation events can increase arbovirus risk by increasing water accumulation in artificial containers and increasing the number of preferred *Aedes* breeding sites (Chinery 1969). Increasing temperatures globally may simultaneously lead to range expansion of *Aedes* mosquitoes into more temperate climes, as well as range contraction in some tropical, previously hospitable regions (Khormi and Kumar 2014). Increases in average winter temperatures could allow for year-round survival of *Aedes* populations where vectors have previously been introduced but were unable to become established, as seen with expansion of *Aedes albopictus'* range into the Alps and North America (Roiz et al. 2011). Increasing temperatures can additionally accelerate larval growth rate, decrease mosquito generation times, and lead to a greater density of vectors in regions where the mosquitoes are already established. Increasing temperatures may also lead to decreases and contractions in *Ae. aegypti* range, particularly in hot, dry areas that currently host *Ae. aegypti* (Khormi and Kumar 2014). However, extreme weather events can also decrease severity of a disease outbreak. For example, high winds associated with hurricanes can kill infected adult mosquitoes. Urban/suburban flooding can wash away container-breeding mosquito larvae around homes, which can be beneficially disruptive during an actual outbreak. This has also been seen with West Nile virus that is transmitted by the mosquito *Culex quinquefasciatus* (Beard et al. 2016). In the United States, because hurricanes typically occur in the late summer/fall, which is toward the end of mosquito season, the risk for outbreaks is somewhat less.

Mathematical models have been developed to project global changes in arbovirus presence under various climate change scenarios. Most projections for *Aedes*-borne viruses point to expansion of endemic areas and increased incidence globally due to climate change (Bogoch et al. 2016; Hales et al. 2002; Kraemer et al. 2019; Mweya et al. 2016; Tjaden et al. 2017). Although climate and *Aedes* population dynamics are inextricably linked, projections of *Aedes*-borne disease outbreaks based on weather and climate alone may not tell a complete story. A variety of nonclimatic variables, including increased urbanization, economic and population growth, land and water use changes, population movement, and public health responses (or a lack thereof), are thought to strongly influence *Aedes* mosquito distribution and consequent arboviral infection exposure.

Urbanization is a dominant force altering the ecological landscape of the planet. Urban cities are now the primary ecosystem around the globe, and the characteristics of urban growth work in concert with climatic forces to alter risk of *Aedes*-borne diseases (Santos-Vega, Martinez, and Pascua 2016). *Aedes* mosquitoes thrive in urban environments and the global growth of urban centers is considered a primary driver of *Aedes*-borne disease outbreaks (Ebi and Nealon 2016; Gubler 2011; Mayer, Tesh, and Vasilakis 2017). Increasing urban density and expanding urban footprints lead to the replacement of natural foliage with manmade structures. These changes create heterogeneous climatic environments, such as urban heat zones (Santos-Vega et al. 2016) and allow for *Aedes* mosquitoes to thrive in previously inhospitable environments.

Socioeconomic factors are another major driver of *Aedes*-borne disease risk. Human behaviors may place humans in contact with mosquitoes, and failure to implement mosquito-reduction measures may increase risk of *Aedes*-borne disease exposure. For instance, many underdeveloped areas have insufficient or difficult to access water supplies, which results in water storage in containers such as clay jars and cisterns and creates more potential mosquito breeding opportunities. Individuals living in low-income settings have increased frequency of exposure to *Aedes*-borne viruses; the absence of air-conditioning or screens, the absence of street drainage, proximity to low-income urban centers, and low family income are all associated with increased risk of DENV, and ZIKV burden has been found to disproportionately affect individuals of low socioeconomic status (Bhatt et al. 2013; Brunkard et al. 2007; United Nations Development Programme 2017). In contrast, higher socioeconomic development is protective against *Aedes*-borne disease risk in areas that are otherwise hospitable to *Aedes* mosquitoes. For instance, the range of *Ae. aegypti* in North America extends well north of the U.S.-Mexico border. However, there is a distinct lack of DENV transmission north of the U.S.-Mexico border because of vector barriers such as air conditioners and window screens (Hayden et al. 2010; Ramos et al. 2008; Reiter et al. 2003). Due to the strong link between poverty and arboviral disease, one study found that rising income levels with increasing global development would offset the effect of climate change, such that arboviral disease could actually decrease by 2050 (Åström et al. 2012).

Malaria

Etiology/Disease in Humans

The World Health Organization (WHO) estimates that in 2017 more than 200 million illnesses and approximately 435,000 deaths from malaria occurred, with nearly one half of the world's population at risk for malaria (WHO 2018b). Although a majority of malaria deaths occur in Africa, populations in Asia and Latin America are at risk as well. Malaria is a disease that ranges from asymptomatic to severe. Symptoms include repeated fever and chills, mild to severe anemia, acute respiratory distress syndrome, and cerebral malaria. In individuals that have never experienced an infection with a malaria parasite, infection can result in a high degree of morbidity and mortality. Repeated infections ultimately reduce the severity of disease but do not affect resistance to infection.

There are five species of *Plasmodium* parasites that cause malaria in humans: *P. falciparum*, *P. vivax*, *P. malariae*, *P. knowesi*, and *P. ovale*. Of these, infections with *P. falciparum* and *P. vivax* cause the greatest burden of disease. *Plasmodium* parasites have a complex life cycle in the human host. The *Plasmodium* parasite is transmitted when an infected female *Anopheles* mosquito bites a human. The *Plasmodium* sporozoite travels to the liver where it establishes an infection. This early-stage infection is silent and not associated with disease. After seven to ten days (depending on the species), parasites erupt from infected liver cells into the bloodstream. Red blood cells become infected with the emerging asexual-stage *Plasmodium* parasite (the merozoite) and a cyclic infection of red blood cells ensues, resulting in the classic symptoms of malaria. Transmission to a new human host occurs when the parasites enter the sexual-stage of its life cycle (called gametocytes), which are taken up when another female mosquito bites an infected human, thus completing the life cycle in the human host.

Anopheles Vector Distribution

With over 400 described species, *Anopheles* mosquitoes are found throughout the world. Seventy species are known transmitters of the *Plasmodium* parasites to humans, and forty of those species are considered to be the dominant vectors for *Plasmodium* parasites. *Anopheles* species that are capable of transmitting malaria are found on every continent (Sinka et al. 2012). However, as a result of malaria control programs, malaria is currently not found in all countries where the *Anopheles* mosquito is present. Anopheles are "night biters" and live both outside and within homes. In the last twenty years, significant reduction in malaria transmission has occurred through introduction of insecticide treated bed-nets and indoor residual spraying of insecticide for anopheles mosquito control (O'Meara et al. 2010).

Climate Change and Malaria Risk

As with arboviruses, the three key features of climate—temperature, precipitation, and humidity—can affect the transmission of malaria. Temperature changes affect malaria transmission by affecting both the *Anopheles* mosquito life cycle and the parasite's replication in the mosquito vector. Precipitation and humidity are both important factors in *Anopheles* distribution and abundance and thus may alter malaria disease risk by causing variations in mosquito abundance.

Development and survival of both *Anopheles* mosquitoes and *Plasmodium* parasites within the mosquito are temperature dependent. Similar to *Aedes* mosquitoes, increasing temperature is associated with increasing survival and development rates of *Anopheles* mosquitoes to varying thresholds, after which increasing temperature is associated with decreases in both survival and development (Bayoh and Lindsay 2004). Once a female mosquito ingests the blood of an infected human host, the parasite undergoes a new phase of its life cycle, and this phase is dependent on temperature (Paaijmans and Thomas 2011). Like arboviruses, transmission of the *Plasmodium* parasite from a female mosquito is dependent on the EIP. If the temperature is too cold, the parasite will be unable to complete its life cycle within the mosquito and the mosquito will not be able to transmit the infection to a susceptible human host. As temperature increases, transmission is enhanced. At higher threshold temperatures, mortality increases. It is important to note that humidity is also crucial to mosquito survival (Lindsay and Birley 1996).

Precipitation provides necessary water sources for the larval stage of the mosquito to develop. Increased precipitation is generally associated with an increase in abundance of mosquitos and incidence of malaria. As a result of this relationship, the rainy season is often referred to as the malaria season in places where the burden of malaria is high. Humidity, which is related to precipitation, is associated with mosquito lifespan. Although the relationship between mosquito lifespan and humidity is not linear, *Anopheles* survival and lifespan decrease precipitously below certain thresholds of humidity (Yamana and Eltahir 2013). In arid regions, increases in humidity may give *Anopheles* mosquitoes more opportunities to carry malaria infections from one person to another. Thus, changes in climate can affect the intensity of malaria transmission within a given region.

Because there is a clear linkage between the environment and mosquito development, there were early studies arguing that increases in temperature at the lower range of vector survival would increase malaria transmission to vulnerable populations (Lindsay and Birley 1996). In support of this, models using predicted changes in temperature and past malaria mortality estimates suggest that under certain predicted climate change conditions, there is an expected increase in childhood malaria mortality of up to 20 percent in some areas of the world (Dasgupta 2018). Modeling data suggest that climate change will increase the range of areas suitable for malaria transmission into the Americas (Caminade 2014). However, the areas with predicted future suitability for malaria transmission are areas that previously struggled with malaria transmission. Notably, it was through malaria control programs that malaria transmission in these regions was eliminated (Mendis et al. 2009). This point highlights the challenge involved when attempting to link changes in malaria distribution to climate change alone. Ultimately, to understand how climate change may have an impact on malaria risk, it is important to account for other factors that affect susceptibility of a given population to malaria transmission (Figure 8.2). These

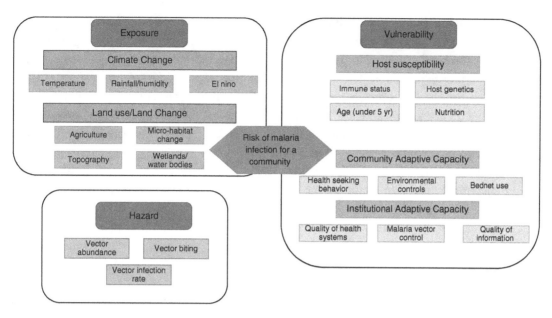

Figure 8.2   Integrated model to evaluate malaria risk within a community
Source: Onyango et al. (2016), p. 551.

factors include those that influence human exposure to the *Plasmodium* parasite and increase human vulnerability to infection. Human exposure to mosquitos carrying the *Plasmodium* parasite is linked to climate change, as described previously but is also dependent on the distance to suitable mosquito habitat and the availability and efficacy of control measures. Land use change has been linked to changes in malaria prevalence; urban development may decrease the availability of suitable mosquito habitat (Trape and Zoulani 1987). Conversely, construction of dams and irrigation canals may increase the presence of mosquito breeding grounds (Keiser et al. 2005). As with other mosquito-borne diseases, socioeconomic status predicts exposure to malaria because household factors linked to socioeconomic status, such as living in houses with screens and closed eaves, can prevent entry of mosquitoes into the household. Finally, the availability and efficacy of control measures, such as insecticide treated bed nets and indoor residual spraying of insecticides, can reduce human–mosquito interaction and decrease malaria risk.

Susceptibility of the human host to infection can be related to age (in regions with high transmission levels, younger individuals are more vulnerable than older), but it is always dependent on whether a person was previously infected with malaria because previous infections result in acquired immunity. For instance, repeated infections throughout childhood result in resistance to malaria disease in areas where *Plasmodium* transmission is endemic and highly prevalent. However, in areas where *Plasmodium* transmission is either epidemic or present at a low rate, outbreaks of malaria can occur in a larger portion of the population, irrespective of host age (Carneiro et al. 2010). A good way to think of the paradoxes surrounding the incidence of malaria is that whereas climate (e.g., temperature, precipitation, and humidity) can shape the potential for malaria transmission, humans (through susceptibility and interventions) can affect whether malaria transmission occurs. In areas where transmission is currently endemic, small changes in temperature are unlikely to affect the burden of disease within a community; rather, interventions to mitigate malaria exposure will likely have a greater impact.

It is also important to consider that in many malaria endemic and epidemic areas of the world the public health infrastructure is not sophisticated, which makes it difficult to accurately detect how many cases occurred in the past. This makes predictions of the potential impacts of climate change—determined in decades-long time-scales—difficult to correlate with changes in the malaria burden within communities. A good example of the challenges presented when predicting the impact of climate change on malaria risk is demonstrated by studies of climate change impact on malaria in the Kenyan highlands.

The Kenyan highlands have a cooler climate than other parts of the country due to the elevation and do not sustain endemic malaria transmission. One group of studies reported that climate variability in the early 1980s resulted in malaria epidemics in this highland region (Zhou et al. 2005). Other scientists argued that the methodology used was not appropriate for making this claim (Hay et al. 2005). These challengers argued that there was an absence of strong epidemiologic data to support the conclusion that slight temperature increases were correlated with malaria epidemics. The issues raised by these opposing studies demonstrate how a lack of long-term, well-validated malaria data within communities presents challenges for future climate studies. Nonetheless, most agree that it is the regions that currently experience only periodic epidemic malaria that are most likely to be affected by the changing climate (Caminade 2014).

Malaria is undoubtedly a climate-sensitive disease. However, the malaria risk within a community is dependent on many factors in addition to climate change—human exposure to the vector, the vulnerability of the human population, the capacity of the public health infrastructure to mitigate malaria transmission, and the burden of disease (Gething et al. 2010; Onyango et al. 2016).

Lyme Disease in the United States

Etiology

Lyme disease is a tick-borne spirochetal infection caused by *Borreliella* species *B. burgdorferi* and *Borrelia mayonii* in the United States and by *B. burgdoferi*, *B. afzelii* and *B. garinii*, in Europe and Asia. Lyme borreliosis is maintained in nature in a zoonotic cycle that involves small rodents and birds as reservoirs for the spirochete, ticks in the genus *Ixodes* (*I. scapularis* and *pacificus* in the United States and *I. ricinus* and *I. persulcatus* in Europe and Asia, respectively) as vectors, and a variety of mammals and birds, which serve as host for the tick vectors. Humans are accidental hosts, incidentally infected when bitten by infected *Ixodes* ticks, and do not contribute to the spirochete life cycle. Symptoms typically include fever, headache, fatigue, and erythema migrans, a characteristic skin rash that appears at the site of the initial tick bite and often resembles a target bull's-eye. If treated promptly with appropriate antibiotics, patients usually recover quickly and without complications. If unrecognized or treated improperly, however, the spirochetes can spread to the joints, where they can cause arthritis, and to the heart and nervous system, which can result in more serious complications.

Lyme disease, also referred to as Lyme borreliosis, was first recognized as a clinical entity in the late 1970s in coastal Connecticut, appearing in a cluster of juvenile rheumatoid arthritis cases (Steere et al. 1977). Tick-bite associated rash illness cases were also reported in Wisconsin during the same time period (Scrimenti 1970). It was not until the early 1980s, however, that the etiological agent *B. burgdorferi* was discovered in ticks from Shelter Island, New York (Burgdorfer et al. 1982). Since that time, Lyme disease cases have been increasing steadily in the United States, both in number and in geographic distribution (https://www.cdc.gov/lyme/datasurveillance/maps-recent.html).

Currently, over 30,000 cases of Lyme disease are reported each year in the United States, making it the nation's seventh most commonly reported infectious disease and the most frequently reported VBD (Figure 8.3; Centers for Disease Control and Prevention 2019). Over 95 percent of these cases occur in 15 states located primarily in the northeastern and upper

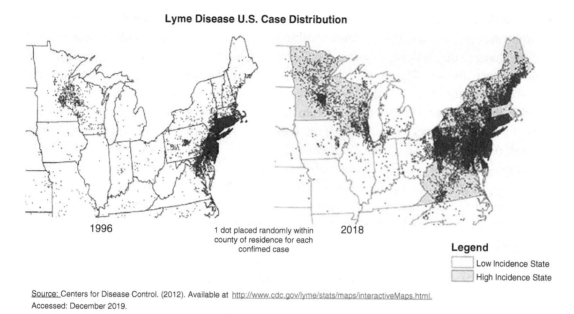

Lyme Disease U.S. Case Distribution

1996   1 dot placed randomly within   2018
                        county of residence for each
                        confimed case

Legend
☐ Low Incidence State
▨ High Incidence State

Source: Centers for Disease Control. (2012). Available at http://www.cdc.gov/lyme/stats/maps/interactiveMaps.html. Accessed: December 2019.

Figure 8.3   U.S. case distribution of Lyme disease 1996 and 2018

midwestern regions of the United States where *I. scapularis* ticks are common and bite humans. Fewer (about 100–150 cases per year) cases occur annually in the Pacific coast region, where the tick vector is *I. pacificus*. Lyme disease is relatively uncommon in the southern United States despite the presence of *I. scapularis* in many areas of the southeast and south-central states. This is primarily due to two factors associated with host preferences of southern *I. scapularis* populations:that larval ticks often feed on lizards, which are incompetent hosts for *Borrelia* and that nymphal ticks, which are small and difficult to detect, rarely bite humans in this region of the country.

This increase in Lyme disease cases, a trend also seen for the other major nationally notifiable tick-borne diseases, has resulted in efforts over the last few decades aimed at determining the drivers of tick-borne disease emergence in the United States (Hoen et al. 2009). Clearly, these drivers are multifactorial, involving changes in land use patterns, demographics, and human behavior. It is likely that Lyme disease was broadly enzootic throughout portions of the northern United States during precolonial days, but with widespread clearing of land for agricultural purposes the causative agent of the disease was apparently pushed back into local pockets or refuges where sufficient populations of deer or other large mammals remained to support survival of tick vector (*I. scapularis*) populations (Margos et al. 2012). Continuation of the industrial revolution in the United States during the 1900s resulted in the movement of rural populations to more urbanized areas and increased reforestation of previously cultivated regions of the northern United States, a trend that was followed in the second half of the century by the suburbanization of much of the secondary growth forest found on lands that previously were farmed.

Linkages to the Climate

Reforestation, overabundant deer, increased tick populations, and suburban encroachment on wooded areas in the northeastern and upper Midwest states, have led collectively to increased tick exposures and a subsequent increase in Lyme disease in residents of these regions. Although this series of events provides a plausible explanation for the emergence of this disease in the northeastern United States, some concern has been raised about how climate change will influence its rate of spread and geographic range. It is not unreasonable to suspect that climate change could affect both the distribution of *B. burgdorferi* and the human risk of acquiring this disease. Similar to the mosquito vectors described previously, the survival, reproduction and behavior of the *Ixodes* ticks that transmit *B. burgorferi* are strongly influenced by the abiotic environment, with precipitation and temperature significantly influencing mortality in off-host tick populations (Figure 8.4) (Bertrand and Wilson 1996; Brownstein, Holford, and Fish 2005; Needham and Teel 1991). However, tick dependency on acute variability in temperature and precipitation is substantially less than with mosquito vectors (Ogden and Lindsay 2016). Only a small portion of a typical tick's life cycle (about 2 percent) is actually spent on the host (Brownstein, Holford, and Fish 2003). Because ticks spend only limited time on hosts, they are likely to be exposed at all life stages (e.g., as eggs, larvae, nymphs, and adults) to varying and potentially harmful environmental conditions (Bertrand and Wilson 1996). For example, hot, dry conditions can increase mortality, especially among larvae, nymphs, or adults as they leave the more stable and high humidity microclimates found in leaf litter or moist soil in order to quest for hosts. The group of *Ixodes* ticks responsible for transmitting *B. burgdorferi* and other closely related spirochetes are especially vulnerable, requiring at least 80 percent relative humidity to prevent death by desiccation (Gray et al. 2009). Egg hatching success for ticks also decreases markedly at low temperatures ($\leq 10°$ C) (Dorr and Gothe 2001). Because ticks are poikilothermic ("coldblooded"), their metabolic activity, development, hatching success, and oviposition behavior are influenced by changes in ambient temperatures (Bertrand and Wilson 1996; Dorr and Gothe 2001).

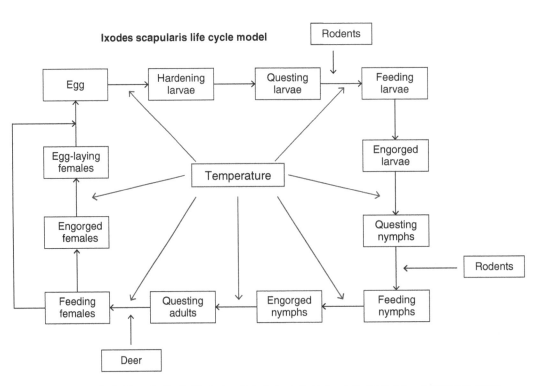

Adapted from: Ogden, N. H., Bigras-Poulin, M., O'callaghan, C. J., Barker, I. K., Lindsay, L. R., Maarouf, A.,... & Charron, D. (2005). A dynamic population model to investigate effects of climate on geographic range and seasonality of the tick *Ixodes scapularis*. *International journal for parositology*, 35(4), 375-389.

Figure 8.4   The varied impacts of temperature on *Ixodes scapularis* life cycle
Source: adapted from Ogden et al. (2005).

Models of future climate change and environmental factors affecting tick distributions have been used to predict the impact of a changing climate on the distribution of Lyme borreliosis in the United States (Brownstein et al. 2005; Monaghan et al. 2015) and in southern Canada (McPherson et al. 2017; Ogden and Lindsay 2016; Ogden et al. 2008). Outputs of these models show the geographic range of the tick vectors and subsequent areas at risk for Lyme disease significantly expanding, primarily as a result of a northward expansion into areas such as southern Canada, which were previously too cold for maintenance of *I. scapularis* populations (Figure 8.4). These models have also suggested a possible increase in the duration of Lyme disease risk because of early onset of springtime leading to increasing vector activity in current Lyme-endemic regions. Simultaneously, the southern limit of this tick's geographic range is predicted to retract, resulting in its disappearance of *I. scapularis* from some areas within the southeastern and south-central states of the United States. Although this prediction could eventually prove true, it should be noted that the distribution and frequency of Lyme disease has increased recently not only northward into Canada but also southward along the mid-Atlantic coast (Diuk-Wasser et al. 2012), possibly as a result of earlier springs leading to increasing duration of vector activity (Levi et al. 2015).

Lyme disease is maintained in a complex cycle involving ticks, multiple mammal and bird species, and humans. Although reforestation, increasing biodiversity, and expanding deer populations have been proposed as significant drivers in the emergence of Lyme and other tick-borne diseases over the last fifty years at larger spatial scales, it is likely that at local scales, habitat fragmentation, encroaching suburban development, and reduced biodiversity have contributed to increased disease risk (Allan, Keesing, and Ostfeld 2003; Margos et al. 2012; Wood and Lafferty 2013). The challenge that must be addressed is in determining how climate variability and disruption interact with the numerous and diverse factors, both ecological and epidemiologic and at local and regional scales, that contribute to Lyme disease transmission and subsequent disease emergence.

CLINICAL CORRELATES 8.3 RIFT VALLEY FEVER

Rift Valley Fever (RVF) is a zoonotic disease transmitted from mosquitoes to animals and subsequently through blood or body fluids of infected animals (sheep, cattle, camels, goats) to humans. Transmission is usually during slaughtering activities, veterinary services or animal births. It has been documented throughout sub-Saharan Africa, Saudi Arabia, and Yemen with concerns for future spread to Europe. Most cases are mild flulike illnesses, but severe forms occur manifesting as hemorrhagic fever, meningoencephalitis, or ocular disease (WHO 2018a). Mosquito vectors vary in abundance based on biotopes, rainfall, and humidity, which contribute to animal transmission (Biteye et al. 2018). Increased precipitation events such as El Niño are associated with RVF outbreaks. Enhanced syndromic surveillance has successfully been implemented in Kenya using animal data from farmers to warn humans of disease risk and to initiate preventative measures (Oyas et al. 2018). Efforts continue using mobile technology to expand reporting as part of a global health initiative in Kenya.

Emerging technologies and improved communication with veterinary and medical teams allow for improved surveillance of suspected animal Rift Valley Fever outbreaks as a way to warn humans and reduce spread.

Summary and Conclusions

Climate change is likely to act in concert with other environmental and anthropogenic factors to increase the transmission and risk of infectious disease. Because of the interactive nature of the determinants of disease, without years of longitudinally collected data, it is much more difficult to link annual disease trends to climate change than it is to link individual outbreak events to weather patterns, such as extreme precipitation, mild winters, or early springs. It is essential to understand the interactions of the climate (humidity, temperature, and precipitation) with other nonclimate factors and across different geographic locations in order to effectively prepare for the effects on infectious disease occurrence.

It is still uncertain how much climate variability contributes to human-pathogen exposure; however, certain trends have become apparent. Sustained increases in average temperatures due to climate change are causing infectious disease transmission to spread to higher elevations and latitudes and may support long-term establishment and spread of VBD. Recent advances in mathematical modeling have provided numerous predictions of potential for disease expansion and retraction under varying climate change scenarios and have allowed researchers to identify regions most at risk of VBD emergence.

These models should help shape public health investments for the future and help guide at-risk areas in implementing early prevention measures, such as local vector control. In conjunction, large-scale public health infrastructure should support these local efforts by establishing state control measures for their establishment or funding mechanisms for their maintenance. Surveillance is needed for disease cases, vectors, reservoir hosts, as well as the determinants of disease. Reporting systems also require further development to promote a more streamlined and consistent approach to quantifying disease risk and disseminating warning messages. In addition, scientists should strive for consensus regarding their methodology of data collection and its application to research; this will encourage consistency and progress.

CLINICAL CORRELATES 8.4 LEPTOSPIROSIS

Leptospirosis is a zoonotic bacterial infection spread from infected animals urinating in the water or soil that humans subsequently come in contact. During extreme precipitation events such as floods and hurricanes, disruption of drinking water integrity increases risk of human exposure (Centers for Disease Control and Prevention 2018; Ehelepola, Ariyaratne, and Dissanayake 2019). There are more than one million cases per year and an estimated 58,900 deaths from severe complications of the disease including pulmonary hemorrhage and Weil's syndrome—a rare form of kidney failure (Costa et al. 2015). Rural farmers and those living in urban slums are especially at- risk of exposure. Treatments are available but prevention of the disease is critical: after flooding events people should avoid exposure to runoff, swimming or bathing, especially with open wounds, and above all ensure consumption of safe drinking water. Rodent control is also important as a preventive step for disease transmission.

Zoonotic diseases including leptospirosis are a growing concern with increased flooding events with transmission from animals to people coming in contact with infected water or soil.

DISCUSSION QUESTIONS

1. What mosquito species typically carries dengue, and where does the mosquito prefer to lay its eggs?

2. Which climate factors affect the transmission cycle of the dengue virus?

3. What is the vector agent that transmits malaria to humans and what characteristics allow it to be effective?

4. Describe EIP and why it is temperature dependent.

5. List some of the factors that contributed to the emergence of tick-borne disease in the United States in the last century and few decades. In which regions of the United States do most cases of Lyme disease occur?

KEY TERMS

Arboviruses: Viruses transmitted by mosquitoes, ticks, and midges. They include the important human pathogens, yellow fever virus (YFV), dengue virus (DENV), chikungunya virus (CHIKV), and Zika virus (ZIKV).

Dengue: A term used to refer both to a virus and to the disease caused when this virus infects humans. Dengue is an arbovirus primarily transmitted to humans by *Aedes* species. Dengue infection typically manifests as a self-limited acute febrile illness; however, a range of symptoms are possible, including life-threatening hemorrhagic shock. No specific treatment exists beyond supportive care.

Extrinsic incubation period (EIP): The EIP is the time required for the pathogen to (1) establish an infection in a blood-feeding vector and (2) multiply or develop to the point where it can be further transmitted during subsequent vector feedings.

Lyme disease: A tick-borne illness primarily caused by three species of the *Borreliella* bacteria. Infection is typically divided into three clinical phases—early localized, early disseminated, and late—based on time from the primary tick bite. Rash is the most typical finding of early localized disease, whereas early disseminated disease can manifest with cardiac and/or neurologic symptoms anywhere from weeks to months after the initial bite. If left untreated, late disease can develop months to years after initial exposure and most typically manifests as a relapsing polyarticular arthritis, though chronic fatigue and neurologic symptoms can also occur. Early localized infections are easily treated with antibiotics, whereas treatment for later stages is more nuanced.

Malaria: A febrile illness caused by the *Plasmodium* parasites *P. falciparum, P. vivax, P. malariae, P. ovalae,* and *P. knowelsi.* The uncomplicated illness typically manifests as fever in addition to a range of nonspecific symptoms. Complicated infections may affect any or a number of organ system(s), Antiparasitic treatment varies according to the causative species. Inadequately or untreated infections can recur after apparent cure.

Vector-borne diseases (VBD): Infectious diseases transmitted by arthropod vectors (e.g., insects and ticks).

References

Allan, B. F., F. Keesing, and R. S. Ostfeld. 2003. "Effect of Forest Fragmentation on Lyme Disease Risk." *Conservation Biology* 17 (1):267–72.

Altassan, K. K., C. Morin, M. S. Shocket, K. Ebi, and J. Hess. 2019. "Dengue Fever in Saudi Arabia: A Review of Environmental and Population Factors Impacting Emergence and Spread." *Travel Medicine and Infectious Disease* 30:46–53.

Alto, B. W., and S. A. Juliano. 2001a. "Precipitation and Temperature Effects on Populations of *Aedes albopictus* (Diptera: Culicidae): Implications for Range Expansion." *Journal of Medical Entomology* 38 (5):646–56.

Alto, B. W., and S. A. Juliano. 2001b. "Temperature Effects on the Dynamics of *Aedes albopictus* (Diptera: Culicidae) Populations in the Laboratory". *Journal of Medical Entomology* 38 (4):548–56.

Åström, C., J. Rocklöv, S. Hales, A. Béguin, V. Louis, and R. Sauerborn. 2012. "Potential Distribution of Dengue Fever under Scenarios of Climate Change and Economic Development." *Ecohealth 2012.* 9 (4): p. 448–54.

Banu, S., W. Hu, C. Hurst, and S. Tong. 2011. "Dengue Transmission in the Asia-Pacific Region: Impact of Climate Change and Socio-Environmental Factors." *Tropical Medicine & International Health* 16 (5):598–607.

Bayoh, M. N., and S. W. Lindsay. 2004. "Temperature-Related Duration of Aquatic Stages of the Afrotropical Malaria Vector Mosquito Anopheles Gambiae in the Laboratory." *Medical and Veterinary Entomology* 18 (2):174–9.

Beard, C. B., R. J. Eisen et al. 2016. "Vector-Borne Diseases." In *Impacts of Climate Change on Human Health in the United States: A Scientific Assessment*, 129–57. Washington, DC: U.S. Global Change Research Program.

Beebe, N. W., R, D. Cooper, P. Mottram, and A. W. Sweeney. 2009. "Australia's Dengue Risk Driven by Human Adaptation to Climate Change." *PLoS Neglected Tropical Diseases* 3 (5):e429.

Bertrand, M. R., and M. L. Wilson. 1996. "Microclimate-Dependent Survival of Unfed Adult *Ixodes scapularis* (Acari:Ixodidae) in Nature: Life Cycle and Study Design Implications." *Journal of Medical Entomology* 33 (4):619–27.

Bhatt, S., P. W. Gething, O. J. Brady, J. P. Messina, A. W. Farlow, C. L. Moyes, J. M. Drake et al. 2013. "The Global Distribution and Burden of Dengue." *Nature* 496 (7446):504–7.

Biteye, B., A. G. Fall, M. Ciss, M. T Seck, A. Apolloni, M. Fall, A. Tran, and G. Gimonneau. 2018. "Ecological Distribution and Population Dynamics of Rift Valley Fever Virus Mosquito Vectors (Diptera, Culicidae) in Senegal." *Parasite Vectors* 11 (1):27. doi:10.1186/s13071-017-2591-9.

Bogoch, I. I., O. J. Brady, M. U. G. Kraemer, M. German, M. I. Creatore, S. Brent, A. G. Watts et al. 2016. "Potential for Zika Virus Introduction and Transmission in Resource-Limited Countries in Africa and the Asia-Pacific Region: A Modelling Study." *Lancet Infectious Diseases* 16 (11):1237–45.

Brownstein, J. S., T. R. Holford, and D. Fish. 2003. "A Climate-Based Model Predicts the Spatial Distribution of the Lyme Disease Vector *Ixodes scapularis* in the United States." *Environmental Health Perspectives* 111 (9):1152–7.

Brownstein, J. S., T. R. Holford, and D. Fish. 2005. "Effect of Climate Change on Lyme Disease Risk in North America." *Ecohealth 2005* 2 (1):38–46.

Brunkard, J. M., J. L. Robles López, J. Ramirez, E. Cifuentes, S. J. Rothenberg, E. A. Hunsperger, C. G. Moore et al. 2007. "Dengue Fever Seroprevalence and Risk Factors, Texas–Mexico Border." *Emerging Infectious Diseases* 13 (10):1477.

Buchwald, A. G., Hayden, M. H., Dadzie, S. K., Paull, S. H. & Carlton, E. J. 2020. "Aedes-borne disease outbreaks in West Africa: A call for enhanced surveillance." *Acta Trop* 209:1054–68.

Burgdorfer, W., A. G. Barbour, S. F. Hayes, J. L. Benach, E. Grunwaldt, and J .P. Davis 1982. "Lyme Disease—a Tick-Borne Spirochetosis?" *Science* 216 (4552):1317–9.

California Vectorborne Disease Surveillance System. Updated 2020. Accessed February 1, 2020. https://vectorsurv.org.

Caminade, C., S. Kovats, J. Rocklov, A. M. Tompkins, A. P. Morse, F. J. Colón-González, H. Stenlund, P. Martens, and S. J. Lloyd "Impact of Climate Change on Global Malaria Distribution." 2014. *Proceedings of the National Academy of Sciences of the USA* 111 (9):3286–91.

Cao-Lormeau, V.-M., C. Roche, A. Teissier, E. Robin, A.-L. Berry, H.-P. Mallet, A. A. Sall, and D. Musso 2014. "Zika Virus, French Polynesia, South Pacific, 2013." *Emerging Infectious Diseases* 20 (6):1085.

Carneiro, I., A. Roca-Feltrer, J. T. Griffin, L. Smith, M. Tanner, J. A. Schellenberg, B. Greenwood, and D. Schellenberg. 2010. "Age-Patterns of Malaria Vary with Severity, Transmission Intensity and Seasonality in Sub-Saharan Africa: A Systematic Review and Pooled Analysis." *PLoS One* 5 (2):e8988.

Centers for Disease Control and Prevention. 2018. "Hurricanes, Floods, and Leptospirosis." *Updated September* 12, 2018. https://www.cdc.gov/leptospirosis/pdf/hurricanes-lepto-fact-sheet-H.pdf.

Centers for Disease Control and Prevention, National Center for Emerging and Zoonotic Infectious Diseases, Division of Vector-Borne Diseases. 2019. *Lyme Disease Data Tables: Most Recent Year.* https://www.cdc.gov/lyme/datasurveillance/tables-recent.html.

Chang, C., K. Ortiz, A. Ansari, and M. E. Gershwin. 2016. "The Zika Outbreak of the 21st Century." *Journal of Autoimmunity* 68:1–13.

Chinery, W. 1969. "A survey of Mosquito Breeding in Accra, Ghana, during a Two-Year Period of Larval Mosquito Control. I. The Mosquitoes Collected and Their Breeding Places." *Ghana Medical Journal* 8 (4):266–74.

Chretien, J.-P., A. Anyamba, S. A. Bedno, R. F. Breiman, R. Sang, K. Sergon, A. M. Powers et al. 2007. "Drought-Associated Chikungunya Emergence along Coastal East Africa." *American Journal of Tropical Medicine and Hygiene* 76 (3):405–7.

Cornel, A., and R. Hunt. 1991. "*Aedes albopictus* in Africa? First Records of Live Specimens in Imported Tires in Cape Town." *Journal of the American Mosquito Control Association* 7 (1):107–8.

Costa, E. A. P. de A., E. M. de M. Santos; J. C. Correia; and C. M. R. de Albuquerque. 2010. "Impact of Small Variations in Temperature and Humidity on the Reproductive Activity and Survival of *Aedes aegypti* (Diptera, Culicidae)." *Revista Brasileira de Entomologia* 54 (3):488–93.

Costa, F., J. E. Hagan, J. Calcagno, M. Kane, P. Torgerson, M. S. Martinez-Silveira, C. Stein, B. Abela-Ridder, and A. I. Ko. 2015. "Global Morbidity and Mortality of Leptospirosis: A Systematic Review." *PLoS Neglected Tropical Diseases* 9 (9):e0003898.

Dasgupta, S. 2018. "Burden of Climate Change on Malaria Mortality." *International Journal of Hygiene and Environmental Health* 221 (5):782–91.

Delatte, H., A. Desvars, A. Bouétard, S. Bord, G. Gimonneau, G. Vourc'h, and D. Fontenille. 2010. "Blood-Feeding Behavior of *Aedes albopictus*, a Vector of Chikungunya on La Réunion." *Vector-Borne and Zoonotic Diseases* 10 (3):249–58.

Ditsuwan, T., T. Liabsuetrakul, V. Chongsuvivatwong, S. Thammapalo, and E. McNeil. 2011. "Assessing the Spreading Patterns of Dengue Infection and Chikungunya Fever Outbreaks in Lower Southern Thailand Using a Geographic Information System." *Annals of Epidemiology* 21 (4):253–61.

Dorr, B., and R. Gothe. 2001. "Cold-Hardiness of *Dermacentor marginatus* (Acari: Ixodidae)." *Experimental & Applied Acarology* 25 (2):151–69.

Diuk-Wasser, M. A., A. G. Hoen, P. Cislo, R. Brinkerhoff, S. A. Hamer, M. Rowland, and R. Cortinas. 2012. "Human Risk of Infection with *Borrelia burgdorferi*, the Lyme Disease Agent, in Eastern United States." *American Journal of Tropical Medicine and Hygiene* 86 (2):320–7.

Ebi, K. L., and J. Nealon. 2016. "Dengue in a Changing Climate." *Environmental Research* 151:115–23.

Ehelepola, N. D. B., K. Ariyaratne, and W. P. Dissanayake. 2019. "The Correlation between Local Weather and Leptospirosis Incidence in Kandy District, Sri Lanka from 2006 to 2015." *Global Health Action* 12 (1):1553283.

Estallo, E. L., F. F. Ludueña-Almeida, M. V. Introini, M. Zaidenberg, and W. R. Almirón. 2015. "Weather Variability Associated with *Aedes* (Stegomyia) *aegypti* (Dengue vector) Oviposition Dynamics in Northwestern Argentina." *PLoS One* 10 (5):e0127820.

Estrada-Franco, J. G., and G. B. Craig. 1995. "Biology, Disease Relationships, and Control of *Aedes albopictus*." In *OPS Cuaderno Técnico*. Washington, DC: Pan American Health Organization.

Fikrig, K., B. J. Johnson, D. Fish, and S. A. Ritchie. 2017. "Assessment of Synthetic Floral-Based Attractants and Sugar Baits to Capture Male And Female *Aedes aegypti* (Diptera: Culicidae)." *Parasites & Vectors* 10 (1):32.

Gething, P. W., D. L. Smith, A. P. Patil, A. J. Tatem, R. W. Snow, and S. I. Hay. 2010. "Climate Change and the Global Malaria Recession." *Nature* 465 (7296):342–5.

Gray, J. S., H. Dautel, A. Estrada-Peña, O. Kahl, and E. Lindgren. 2009. "Effects of Climate Change on Ticks and Tick-Borne Diseases in Europe." *Interdisciplinary Perspectives on Infectious Diseases* 2009:593232. doi: 10.1155/2009/593232.

Gubler, D. J. 2011. "Dengue, Urbanization and Globalization: The Unholy Trinity of the 21st century." *Tropical Medicine and Health* 39(4 suppl):S3–S11.

Gubler, D. J., N. Vasilakis, and D. Musso. 2017. "History and Emergence of Zika Virus." *Journal of Infectious Diseases* 216 (suppl 10):S860–S867.

Hales, S., N. de Wet, J. Maindonald, and A. Woodward. 2002. "Potential Effect of Population and Climate Changes on Global Distribution of Dengue Fever: An Empirical Model." *Lancet* 360 (9336):830–34.

Hall, N. B., K. Broussard, N. Evert, and M. Canfield. 2017. "Notes from the Field: Zika Virus-Associated Neonatal Birth Defects Surveillance—Texas, January 2016–July 2017." *MMWR. Morbidity and Mortality Weekly Report* 66 (31):835.

Hay, S. I., G. D. Shanks, D. I. Stern, R. W. Snow, S. E. Randolph, and D. J. Rogers.2005. "Climate Variability and Malaria Epidemics in the Highlands of East Africa." *Trends in Parasitology* 21 (2):52–3.

Hayden, M. H., C. K. Uejio, K. Walker, F. Ramberg, R. Moreno, C. Rosales, M. Gameros et al. 2010. "Microclimate and Human Factors in the Divergent Ecology of *Aedes aegypti* along the Arizona, US/ Sonora, MX Border." *EcoHealth* 7 (1):64–77.

Hoen, A. G., G. Margos, S. J. Bent, M. A. Diuk-Wasser, A. Barbour, K. Kurtenbach, D. Fish. 2009. "Phylogeography of Borrelia burgdorferi in the Eastern United States Reflects Multiple Independent Lyme Disease Emergence Events." *Proceedings of the National Academy of Sciences of the USA* 106 (35):15013–18.

Juliano, S. A., G. F. O'Meara, J. R. Morrill, and M. M. Cutwa. 2002. "Desiccation and Thermal Tolerance of Eggs and the Coexistence of Competing Mosquitoes." *Oecologia* 130 (3):458–69.

Kamal, M., M. A. Kenawy, M. H. Rady, A. S. Khaled, and A. M. Samy. 2018. "Mapping the Global Potential Distributions of Two Arboviral Vectors *Aedes aegypti* and *Ae. albopictus* under Changing Climate." *PloS One* 13 (12):e0210122.

Kamgang, B., E. Nchoutpouen, F. Simard, and C. Paupy. 2012. "Notes on the Blood-Feeding Behavior of *Aedes albopictus* (Diptera: Culicidae) in Cameroon." *Parasites & Vectors* 5:57.

Keiser, J., M. C. De Castro, M. F. Maltese, R. Bos, M. Tanner, B. H. Singer, and J. Utzinger. 2005. "Effect of Irrigation and Large Dams on the Burden of Malaria on a Global and Regional Scale." *American Journal of Tropical Medicine and Hygiene* 72 (4):392–406.

Khormi, H. M., and L. Kumar. 2014. "Climate Change and the Potential Global Distribution of *Aedes aegypti*: Spatial Modelling using Geographical Information System and CLIMEX." *Geospatial Health* 8 (2):405–15.

Kraemer, M. U., M. E. Sinka, K. A. Duda, A. Q. N. Mylne, F. M. Shearer, C. M. Barker, C. G. Moore et al. 2015. "The Global Distribution of the Arbovirus Vectors *Aedes aegypti* and *Ae. albopictus*." *Elife* 4:e08347.

Kraemer, M. U., R. C. Reiner Jr., O. J. Brady, J. P. Messina, M. Gilbert, D. M. Pigott, D. Yi, et al. 2019. "Past and Future Spread of the Arbovirus Vectors *Aedes aegypti* and *Aedes albopictus*." *Nature Microbiology* 2019:1.

Levi, T., F. Keesing, K. Oggenfuss, and R. S. Ostfeld. 2015. "Accelerated Phenology of Blacklegged Ticks under Climate Warming." *Philosophical Transactions of the Royal Society of London. Series B, Biological Sciences* 370(1665):20130556.

Li, Y., F. Kamara, G. Zhou, S. Puthiyakunnon, C. Li, Y. Liu, Y. Zhou et al. 2014. "Urbanization Increases *Aedes albopictus* Larval Habitats and Accelerates Mosquito Development and Survivorship." *PLoS Neglected Tropical Diseases* 8 (11):e3301.

Likos, A., I. Griffin, A. M. Bingham, D. Stanek, M. Fischer, S. White, J. Hamilton et al. 2016. "Local Mosquito-Borne Transmission of Zika Virus—Miami-Dade and Broward Counties, Florida, June-August 2016." *MMWR. Morbidity and Mortality Weekly Report* 65 (38):1032–8.

Lindsay, S. W., and M. H. Birley. 1996. "Climate Change and Malaria Transmission." *Annals of Tropical Medicine & Parasitology* 90 (5):573–88.

Margos, G., J. I. Tsao, S. Castillo-Ramírez, Y. A. Girard, S. A. Hamer, A. G. Hoen, R. S. Lane, S. L. Raper, and N. H. Ogden 2012. "Two Boundaries Separate *Borrelia burgdorferi* Populations in North America." *Applied and Environmental Microbiology* 78 (17):6059–67.

Mayer, S. V., R. B. Tesh, and N. Vasilakis. 2017. "The Emergence of Arthropod-Borne Viral Diseases: A Global Prospective on Dengue, Chikungunya and Zika Fevers." *Acta Tropica* 166:155–63.

Mbaika, S., J. Lutomiah, E. Chepkorir, F. Mulwa, C. Khayeka-Wandabwa, C. Tigoi, E. Oyoo-Okoth et al. 2016. "Vector Competence of *Aedes aegypti* in Transmitting Chikungunya Virus: Effects and Implications of Extrinsic Incubation Temperature on Dissemination and Infection Rates." *Virology Journal* 13 (1):114.

McDonald, E., S. W. Martin, K. Landry, C. V. Gould, J. Lehman, M. Fischer, and N. P. Lindsey. 2018. "West Nile Virus and Other Domestic Nationally Notifiable Arboviral Diseases—United States, 2018." *MMWR. Morbidity and Mortality Weekly Report* 68 (31):673–8.

McPherson, M., A. García-García, F. J. Cuesta-Valero, H. Beltrami, P. Hansen-Ketchum, D. MacDougall, and N. H. Ogden. 2017. "Expansion of the Lyme Disease Vector *Ixodes scapularis* in Canada Inferred from CMIP5 Climate Projections." *Environmental Health Perspectives* 125 (5):057008.

Mendis, K., A. Rietveld, M. Warsame, A. Bosman, B. Greenwood, and W. H. Wernsdorfer. 2009. "From Malaria Control to Eradication: The WHO Perspective." *Tropical Medicine & International Health* 14 (7):802–9.

Mlakar, J., M. Korva, N. Tul, M. Popović, M. Poljšak-Prijatelj, J. Mraz, M. Kolencet al. 2016. "Zika Virus Associated with Microcephaly." *New England Journal of Medicine* 374 (10):951–58.

Monaghan, A. J., S. M. Moore, K. M Sampson, C. B. Beard, and R. J. Eisen. 2015. "Climate Change Influences on the Annual Onset of Lyme Disease in the United States." *Ticks and Tick-Borne Diseases* 6 (5):615–22.

Monaghan. A. J., K. M. Sampson, D. F. Steinhoff, K. C. Ernst, K. L. Ebi, B. Jones, and M. H. Hayden. 2016. "The Potential Impacts of 21st Century Climatic and Population Changes on Human Exposure to the Virus Vector Mosquito *Aedes aegypti*." *Climatic Change* 146 (3–4):487–500.

Mordecai, E. A., J. M. Cohen, M. V. Evans, P. Gudapati, L. R. Johnson, C. A. Lippi, K. Miazgowicz et al. 2017. "Detecting the Impact of Temperature on Transmission of Zika, Dengue, and Chikungunya Using Mechanistic Models." *PLoS Neglected Tropical Diseases* 11 (4):e0005568.

Mweya, C. N., S. I. Kimera, G. Stanley, G. Misinzo, and L. E. G. Mboera. 2016. "Climate Change Influences Potential Distribution of Infected *Aedes aegypti* Co-Occurrence with Dengue Epidemics Risk Areas in Tanzania." *PloS One* 11 (9):e0162649.

Nawrocki, S., and W. Hawley. 1987. "Estimation of the Northern Limits of Distribution of *Aedes albopictus* in North America." *Journal of the American Mosquito Control Association* 3 (2):314–17.

Needham, G. R., and P. D. Teel. 1991. "Off-Host Physiological Ecology of Ixodid Ticks." *Annual Review of Entomology* 36:659–81.

Niebylski, M. L., H. M. Savage, R. S. Nasci, and G. B. Craig Jr. 1994. "Blood Hosts of *Aedes albopictus* in the United States." *Journal of the American Mosquito Control Association* 10 (3):447–50.

Ogden, N. H., M. Bigras-Poulin, C. J. O'Callaghan, I. K. Barker, L. R. Lindsay, A. Maarouf, K. E. Smoyer-Tomic, D. Waltner-Toews, and D. Charron. 2005. "A Dynamic Population Model to Investigate Effects of Climate on Geographic Range and Seasonality of the Tick *Ixodes scapularis*." *International Journal of Parasitology* 35 (4):375–89.

Ogden, N. H., and L.R. Lindsay. 2016. "Effects of Climate and Climate Change on Vectors and Vector-Borne Diseases: Ticks Are Different." *Trends in Parasitology* 32 (8):646–56.

Ogden, N.H., L. R. Lindsay, K. Hanincová, I. K. Barker, M. Bigras-Poulin, D. F. Charron, A. Heagy et al. 2008. "Role of Migratory Birds in Introduction and Range Expansion of *Ixodes scapularis* Ticks and of *Borrelia burgdorferi* and *Anaplasma phagocytophilum* in Canada." *Applied and Environmental Microbiology* 74 (6):1780–90.

O'Meara, W. P., J. N. Mangeni, R. Steketee, and B. Greenwood. 2010. "Changes in the Burden of Malaria in Sub-Saharan Africa." *Lancet. Infectious Diseases* 10 (8):545–55.

Onyango, E. A., O. Sahin, A. Awiti, C. Chu, and B. Mackey. 2016. "An Integrated Risk and Vulnerability Assessment Framework for Climate Change and Malaria Transmission in East Africa." *Malaria Journal* 15 (1):551.

Oyas, H., L. Holmstrom, N. P. Kemunto, M. Muturi, A. Mwatondo, E. Osoro, A. Bitek et al. 2018. "Enhanced Surveillance for Rift Valley Fever in Livestock during El Niño Rains and Threat of RVF Outbreak, Kenya, 2015–2016." *PLoS Neglected Tropical Diseases* 12 (4):e0006353. https://doi.org/10.1371/journal.pntd.0006353.

Paaijmans, K. P., and M. B. Thomas. 2011. "The Influence of Mosquito Resting Behaviour and Associated Microclimate for Malaria Risk." *Malaria Journal* 10:183.

Paul, B. J., G. Pannarkady, S. P. Moni, and E. J. Thachil. 2011. "Clinical Profile and Long-Term Sequelae of Chikungunya Fever." *Indian Journal of Rheumatology* 6 (1):12–19.

Paupy, C., H. Delatte, L. Bagny, V. Corbel, and D. Fontenille. 2009. "*Aedes albopictus*, an Arbovirus Vector: From the Darkness to the Light." *Microbes and Infection* 11 (14–15):1177–85.

Paz, S., and J. C. Semenza. 2016. "El Niño and Climate Change—Contributing Factors in the Dispersal of Zika Virus in the Americas?" *Lancet* 387 (10020):745.

Ponlawat, A., and L. C. Harrington. 2005. "Blood Feeding Patterns of *Aedes aegypti* and *Aedes albopictus* in Thailand." *Journal of Medical Entomology* 42 (5):844–49.

Ramos, M. M., H. Mohammed, E. Zielinski-Gutierrez, M. H. Hayden, J. L. Robles Lopez, M. Fournier, A. Rodríguez Trujillo, et al. 2008. "Epidemic Dengue and Dengue Hemorrhagic Fever at the Texas–Mexico Border: Results of a Household-Based Seroepidemiologic Survey, December 2005." *American Journal of Tropical Medicine and Hygiene* 78 (3):364–69.

Reiter, P., and D. Sprenger, The Used Tire Trade: A Mechanism for the Worldwide Dispersal of Container Breeding Mosquitoes." *Journal of the American Mosquito Control Association* 3 (3):494–501.

Reiter, P., S. Lathrop, M. Bunning, B. Biggerstaff, D. Singer, T. Tiwari, L. Baber, et al. 2003. "Texas Lifestyle Limits Transmission of Dengue Virus." *Emerging Infectious Diseases* 9 (1):86.

Richards, S. L., L. Ponnusamy, T. R. Unnasch, H. K. Hassan, and C. S. Apperson. 2006. "Host-Feeding Patterns of *Aedes albopictus* (Diptera: Culicidae) in Relation to Availability of Human and Domestic Animals in Suburban Landscapes of Central North Carolina." *Journal of Medical Entomology* 43 (3):543–51.

Roiz, D., M. Neteler, C. Castellani, D. Arnoldi, and A. Rizzoli. 2011. "Climatic Factors Driving Invasion of the Tiger Mosquito (*Aedes albopictus*) into New Areas of Trentino, Northern Italy." *PLoS One* 6 (4):e14800.

Rueda, L., K. J. Patel, R. C. Axtell, and R. E. Stinner. 1990. "Temperature-Dependent Development and Survival Rates of *Culex quinquefasciatus* and *Aedes aegypti* (Diptera: Culicidae)." *Journal of Medical Entomology* 27 (5):892–98.

Ryan, S. J., C. J. Carlson, E. A. Mordecai, and L. R. Johnson. 2019. "Global Expansion and Redistribution of Aedes-Borne Virus Transmission Risk with Climate Change." *PLoS Neglected Tropical Diseases* 13 (3):e0007213.

Salas, R. N., P. Knappenberger, and J. Hess. 2018. *2018 Lancet Countdown on Health and Climate Change Brief for the United States of America*. London: Lancet Countdown.

Santos-Vega, M., P. P. Martinez, and M. Pascual. 2016. "Climate Forcing and Infectious Disease Transmission in Urban Landscapes: Integrating Demographic and Socioeconomic Heterogeneity." *Annals of the New York Academy of Sciences* 1382 (1):44–55.

Schultz, G. 1993. "Seasonal Abundance of Dengue Vectors in Manila, Republic of the Philippines." *Southeast Asian Journal of Tropical Medicine and Public Health* 24 (2):369–75.

Scrimenti, R. J. 1970. "Erythema Chronicum Migrans." *Archives of Dermatology* 102 (1):104-5.

Shragai, T., B. Tesla, C. Murdock, and L. C. Harrington. 2017. "Zika and Chikungunya: Mosquito-Borne Viruses in a Changing World." *Annals of the New York Academy of Sciences* 1399 (1):61–77.

Simmons, C. P., J. J. Farrar, N. V. Chau, and B. Wills. 2012. "Dengue." *New England Journal of Medicine* 366 (15):1423–32.

Sinka, M. E., M. J. Bangs, S. Manguin, Y. Rubio-Palis, T. Chareonviriyaphap, M. Coetzee, C. M Mbogo et al. 2012. "A Global Map of Dominant Malaria Vectors." *Parasites & Vectors* 5:69.

Steere, A. C., S. E. Malawista, J. A. Hardin, S. Ruddy, W. Askenase, and W. A. Andiman. 1977. "Erythema Chronicum Migrans and Lyme Arthritis. The Enlarging Clinical Spectrum." *Annals of Internal Medicine* 86 (6):685–98.

Stoler, J., R. Al Dashti, F. Anto, J. N. Fobil, and G. A. Awandare. 2014. "Deconstructing 'Malaria': West Africa as the Next Front for Dengue Fever Surveillance and Control." *Acta Tropica* 134:58–65.

Subra, R. 1983. "The Regulation Of Preimaginal Populations of *Aedes aegypti* L.(Diptera: Culicidae) on the Kenya Coast: I. Preimaginal Population Dynamics and the Role of Human Behaviour." *Annals of Tropical Medicine & Parasitology* 77 (2):195–201.

Sukhralia, S., M. Verma, S. Gopirajan, V. Mansi, S. Gopirajan, P. S. Dhanaraj, R. Lal, N. Mehla, and C. R. Kant. 2019. "From Dengue to Zika: The Wide Spread of Mosquito-Borne Arboviruses." *European Journal of Clinical Microbiology & Infectious Diseases* 38 (1):3–14.

Tesla, B., L. R. Demakovsky, E. A. Mordecai, S. J. Ryan, M. H. Bonds, C. N. Ngonghala, M. A. Brindley, and C. C. Murdock. 2018. "Temperature Drives Zika Virus Transmission: Evidence from Empirical and Mathematical Models." *Proceedings of the Royal Society B: Biological Sciences* 285 (1884):20180795.

Tjaden, N. B., J. E. Suk, D. Fischer, S. M. Thomas, C. Beierkuhnlein, and J. C. Semenza. 2017. "Modelling the Effects of Global Climate Change on Chikungunya Transmission in the 21st Century." *Scientific Reports* 7 (1):3813.

Trape, J. F., and A. Zoulani. 1987. "Malaria and Urbanization in Central Africa: The Example of Brazzaville. Part III: Relationships between Urbanization and the Intensity of Malaria Transmission." *Transactions of the Royal Society of Tropical Medicine and Hygiene* 81 (suppl 2):19–25.

Tun-Lin, W., T. Burkot, and B. Kay. 2000. "Effects of Temperature and Larval Diet on Development Rates and Survival of the Dengue Vector *Aedes aegypti* in North Queensland, Australia." *Medical and Veterinary Entomology* 14 (1):31–37.

United Nations Development Programme. 2017. *A Socio-economic Impact Assessment of the Zika Virus in Latin America and the Caribbean: with a focus on Brazil, Colombia and Suriname.* New York: UNDP.

Watts, D. M., D. S. Burke, B. A. Harrison, R. E. Whitmire, and A. Nisalak. 1987. "Effect of temperature on the Vector Efficiency of *Aedes aegypti* for Dengue 2 Virus." *American Journal of Tropical Medicine and Hygiene* 36 (1):143–52.

World Health Organization. 2018a. "Rift Valley Fever." https://www.who.int/news-room/fact-sheets/detail/rift-valley-fever.

World Health Organization. 2018b. *World Malaria Report 2018.* Geneva: WHO. https://apps.who.int/iris/bitstream/handle/10665/275867/9789241565653-eng.pdf?ua=1

World Health Organization. 2020. "Dengue and Severe Dengue Fact Sheet." https://www.who.int/news-room/fact-sheets/detail/dengue-and-severe-dengue.

Wood, C. L., and K. D. Lafferty. 2013. "Biodiversity and Disease: A Synthesis of Ecological Perspectives On Lyme Disease Transmission." *Trends in Ecology and Evolution* 28 (4):239–47.

Yamana, T. K., and E. A. Eltahir. 2013. "Incorporating the Effects of Humidity in a Mechanistic Model of *Anopheles gambiae* Mosquito Population Dynamics in the Sahel Region of Africa." *Parasites & Vectors* 6:235.

Zhou, G., N. Minakawa, A. K. Githeko, and G. Yan. 2005. "Climate Variability and Malaria Epidemics in the Highlands of East Africa." *Trends in Parasitology* 21 (2):54–6.

CHAPTER 9

FOOD SYSTEMS TRANSFORMATION: TOWARD SUSTAINABLE AND HEALTHY DIETS FOR ALL

Cristina Tirado

Overview

Climate change, variability, and the consequent environmental degradation have had and will continue to have significant impacts on food systems, food security and **malnutrition**, particularly in low-income populations in developing countries in Africa and Asia. At the same time our global food system and dietary trends toward greater consumption of animal foods are linked to environmental degradation and climate change and contribute to the increase of noncommunicable diseases (NCDs). Globally, more than 820 million people remain undernourished, 151 million children are stunted and more than two billion people are micronutrient deficient. Nearly half of all deaths in children under five are attributable to **undernutrition** (Global Nutrition Report [GNR] 2018; United Nations Children's Fund [UNICEF]/World Health Organization [WHO]/World Bank Group 2019). At the same time, prevalence of diseases associated with high-calorie, unhealthy diets are increasing globally, with 2.1 billion adults and 38.5 million children are overweight or obese and the global prevalence of diabetes almost doubling in the past thirty years (Swinburn et al. 2019).

Climate change and variability affect all four dimensions of food security: food availability, stability of food supplies, access to food, and food utilization. Declining food availability leads to increasing food cost with low-income consumers particularly at risk of food insecurity and hunger. Climate change and variability also affect the key underlying causes of children's undernutrition including household food security, access to maternal and childcare, environmental health, water quality, and food safety, leading to disease and stunting. Climate variability and extremes have been leading causes of recent severe food crises requiring humanitarian assistance of millions of people in developing countries during the last years. Poor access to healthy food contributes not only to undernutrition but also to overweight, obesity and NCDs, thus slowing progress toward the eradication of malnutrition in all its forms in many low-income countries.

The food system is responsible for approximately 30 percent of the global greenhouse gas (GHG) emissions, and changing dietary patterns toward greater consumption of animal foods, particularly meat, are linked to environmental degradation, climate change, and NCDs. To meet climate targets below 2°C by 2050, it is necessary to reduce the GHG emissions related to the food system, and these changes have significant co-benefits for health.

Adaptation is key to address the impact of climate change on the food system and nutrition. A combination of nutrition-sensitive climate adaptation, mitigation, and disaster risk reduction could lessen the threats to nutrition from the impacts of

KEY CONCEPTS

- Climate change and variability can affect all the dimensions of food security including food availability, stability of food supplies, access to food, and food utilization.

- Climate change has an impact on the key underlying causes of undernutrition: household food access, access to maternal and childcare and feeding practices and environmental health, water, and food safety.

- The protection of nutrition under climate change requires a multisectoral integrated adaptation involving the food system, social protection, and the health system among others.

- A combination of transformative food systems and healthy diets, nutrition-sensitive agriculture, health and social protection schemes and safety nets, nutrition-sensitive risk reduction, policy coherence and cross-sectoral collaboration are proposed to address climate impacts to malnutrition.

- Current food systems and dietary patterns contribute to 30 percent of the Global greenhouse gas emissions. A transformation into sustainable and healthy and diets (more plant-based), in line with World Health Organization recommendations, can substantially reduce food-related greenhouse gas emissions and prevent mortality related to noncommunicable diseases.

climate change. Mitigation strategies to reduce food-related GHG emissions from the food system—such as sustainable food production, sustainable and healthy diets, and reduction of food waste—have co-benefits for climate mitigation, nutrition, human health, and the environment and need to be a critical component in climate policies. Transformative approaches toward healthier, sustainable, plant-based dietary patterns require integrated strategies, policies. and measures including economic incentives for the production and consumption of more fruits, vegetables, and pulses; inclusion of sustainability criteria in dietary guidelines; product labeling; public education programs; and promotion of collaboration, good governance, and policy coherence.

Impacts of Climate Change and Variability on Food Security and Malnutrition

Impacts on Food Security

Climate change has an impact on food security as it can adversely affect food production, availability, quality, food access, stability, and food utilization (Mbow et al. 2019). Global temperature increases have a negative impact on the yields of major production crops such as wheat, rice, maize, and soybeans—which provide two thirds of human caloric intake—on a global scale. It is estimated that each degree-Celsius increase in global mean temperature would, on average, reduce global yields of wheat by 6.0 percent, rice by 3.2 percent, maize by 7.4 percent, and soybeans by 3.1 percent (without considering carbon dioxide [CO_2] fertilization and effective adaptation) (Zhao et al., 2017). Climate variability and extremes have the strongest direct impact on food security through the impacts on the production and availability, given the sensitivity of agriculture and fisheries to climate impacts and the primary role of these sectors as a source of food and livelihoods.

Declining food availability caused by climate change is likely to lead to increasing food cost affecting consumers globally through higher prices and reduced purchasing power, with low-income consumers particularly at risk from hunger (Springmann, Godfray et al. 2016; Nelson et al. 2018). Higher prices depress consumer demand, which in turn will not only reduce energy intake (calories) globally but will also likely lead to less healthy diets with lower availability of key micronutrients and increase diet-related mortality in lower and middle-income countries (Springmann, Godfray et al. 2016).

Impacts on Malnutrition

Nutritional status is determined by the interaction between dietary intake and health status. Climate change and variability can affect the main underlying causes of **malnutrition** including (1) household food access, dietary diversity, and nutrient quality; (2) impacts on environmental health, water, and foodborne diseases; and (3) changes in maternal and childcare access and breastfeeding (Tirado 2017; Food and Agriculture Organization [FAO]/International Fund for Agricultural Development [IFAD]/UNICEF/World Food Programme [WFP]/WHO 2018). Climate change can also affect the socioeconomic factors that determine food security and nutrition, such as livelihoods, assets, income, health access, education, food aid, institutions, inequities, human rights, infrastructure, resources, and political structures (Tirado 2017; FAO/IFAD/UNICEF/WFP/WHO 2018). (See Figure 9.1.) Poor access to healthy food contributes not only to undernutrition but also to overweight and obesity and NCDs, and high rates of these multiple forms of malnutrition coexist in many countries and within households. The higher cost of healthy foods, the stress of living with food insecurity, and physiological adaptations to food restrictions contribute to explain why food-insecure families may have a higher

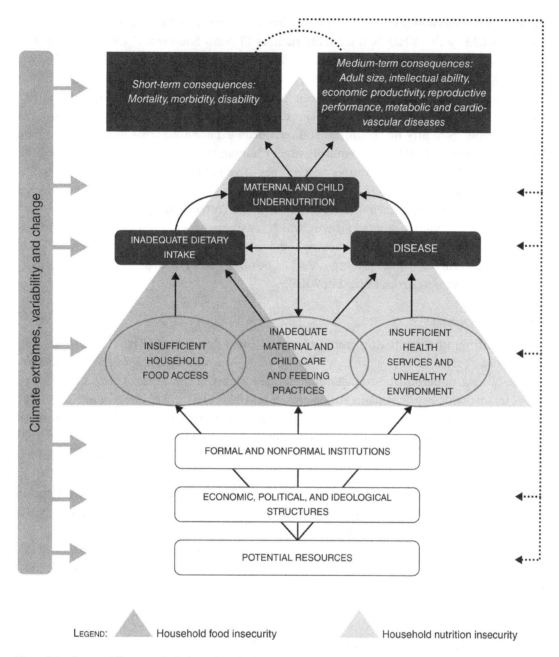

Figure 9.1   Framework Illustrating the Pathways Through Which Climate Change Affects Nutrition
Source: Tirado et al. (2013).

risk of overweight and obesity (FAO/IFAD/UNICEF/WFP/WHO 2018; Swinburn et al. 2019). Additionally, maternal and child food deprivation and low breastfeeding rates can increase the risk of obesity and diet-related non-communicable diseases later in life (Swinburn et al.).

Observed Impacts

Climate variability and extremes can exacerbate seasonal food shortages, thus affecting diet quality and diversity. They are key drivers behind the recent rise in global hunger and one of the leading causes of severe food crises, affecting millions of people and requiring humanitarian assistance (FAO/IFAD/UNICEF/WFP/WHO 2018; Food Security Information Network [FSIN] 2018). In the last twenty years, climate shocks caused by droughts, floods, storms, and heat spells have increased in frequency and intensity in low- and middle-income countries, where **undernourishmen**t and food production are vulnerable to climate extremes (FAO/IFAD/UNICEF/WFP/WHO 2018). Events such as El Niño Southern Oscillation (ENSO)—which is the most significant driver of climate variability across the tropics—affected the food and nutrition security of millions of people in 2015–2016 contributing to the recent increase in undernourishment at the global level, particularly in Eastern and Southern Africa (FAO 2016). Climate extremes were a major driver of global food crises in 2017; almost 124 million people from fifty-one countries and territories experienced crisis levels of acute food insecurity or worse (FSIN 2018) requiring urgent humanitarian assistance to safeguard their lives. In thirty-four of these countries nearly ninety-five million people were also affected by climate shocks and extremes (FSIN 2018). These impacts can be lifelong for children affected by undernutrition during their first 1,000 days of life (International Food Policy Research Institute 2016), leading to stunted growth, which is associated with impaired cognitive ability and reduced school and work performance in the future (UNICEF 2019). The associated costs of stunting in terms of lost economic growth can be on the order of 10 percent of gross domestic product per year in Africa (Wagstaff 2016).

Projected Impacts

Child stunting, undernutrition, and undernutrition-related mortality   Global-level predictive studies conclude climate change will have adverse impacts on childhood undernutrition, severe stunting, undernutrition-related childhood mortality, and increase of disability-adjusted life years lost with largest risks in Africa and Asia (Hales et al. 2014; Lloyd et al. 2018). The WHO assessment of the burden of disease due to climate projected global additional deaths of 95,000 children because of childhood undernutrition in 2030 with highest impact in sub-Saharan countries (Hales et al. 2014). In countries with lower incomes and relatively high food prices, it is projected that rising food prices would tend to increase stunting (Lloyd et al. 2018). Moderate and severe stunting in children under five has been projected at the national level in 2030 under low and high climate change scenarios, combined with poverty and prosperity scenarios in forty-four countries (Lloyd et al. 2018). The mean climate-change attributable stunting projected in 2030 will be between 570,000 children (under a global prosperity and low climate scenario) and one million children (under a global poverty and high climate scenario) (Lloyd et al. 2018).

CLINICAL CORRELATES 9.1 CHILD STUNTING, UNDERNUTRITION, AND UNDERNUTRITION-RELATED MORTALITY

Climate change is predicted to increase childhood undernutrition, and severe stunting, contribute to undernutrition-related childhood mortality, and increase disability-adjusted life years lost, with greatest risks in Africa and Asia (Lloyd et al. 2018; Hales et al. 2014). WHO (Hales et al. 2014) assessment of the burden of disease due to climate change projected additional deaths of 95,000 children worldwide by 2030 as a result of undernutrition, with the greatest impact in sub-Saharan countries.

The impacts are multifaceted: rising carbon dioxide levels reduce nutritional benefits of food (Ebi and Ziska 2018); locust and other insect outbreaks exacerbated by climate change damage crops and land (Zhang et al. 2019); extreme weather events such as droughts, floods, or wildfires disrupt agricultural yields and lead to food shortages. In low- to middle-income countries, it is projected that rising food prices will increase stunting (Lloyd et al. 2018), and the mean climate change attributable to stunting projected that by 2030, there will be between 570,000 children (under a global prosperity and low climate scenario) and one million children (under a global poverty and high climate scenario) affected.

Young children are particularly vulnerable to death and nutritional deficiencies causing acute and chronic adverse health impacts, notably stunted growth.

Diets and mortality related to dietary and weight-related risk factors The greatest nutrition security challenge in 2050 will be providing nutritious diets rather than adequate calories (Springmann, Godfray et al. 2016; Nelson et al. 2018). Agricultural production and regional food availability affect the composition of diets, which can have major consequences for NCDs and health. Springmann projected the excess mortality attributable to agriculturally mediated changes in dietary and weight-related risk factors by cause of death for 155 world regions in the year 2050. The model projected that by 2050, climate change will lead to per person reductions of 3.2 percent in global food availability, 4.0 percent in fruit and vegetable consumption, and 0.7 percent in red meat consumption. These changes will be associated with 529,000 climate-related deaths worldwide; twice as many were associated with reductions in fruit and vegetable consumption than with climate-related increases in the prevalence of underweight (Springmann, Godfray et al. 2016). Most climate-related deaths were projected to occur in South and East Asia.

CLINICAL CORRELATES 9.2 DIETS AND MORTALITY RELATED TO DIETARY AND WEIGHT-RELATED RISK FACTORS

The greater nutrition security challenge in 2050 will be providing nutritious diets rather than adequate calories (Springmann, Godfray et al. 2016). Agricultural production and regional food availability affect the composition of diets, which can have major consequences for non-communicable diseases and health. Springmann et al. projected excess mortality attributable to agriculturally mediated changes in dietary and weight-related risk factors by cause of death for 155 world regions in the year 2050. The model projected that by 2050, climate change will lead to 3.2 percent per person reductions in global food availability, 4.0 percent in fruit and vegetable consumption, and 0.7 percent in red meat consumption. These changes will be associated with 529,000 climate-related deaths worldwide. Twice as many deaths were associated with reductions in fruit and vegetable consumption than with climate-related increases in the prevalence of underweight (Springmann, Godfray et al. 2016). Most climate-related deaths were projected to occur in South and East Asia.

Ensuring sustainable and healthy foods production and consumption represents an opportunity to improve global food security in the face of climate change.

CO$_2$ and Nutritional Quality

The nutritional content, such as the protein content and micronutrients of important food crops, is affected negatively by higher CO$_2$ concentrations, thus affecting food utilization. Micronutrients like iron and zinc will be less accumulated and less available in food (Mbow et al. 2019). Under elevated CO$_2$, the protein content of rice, wheat, barley and potatoes is expected to decrease by 7.6 percent, 7.8 percent, 14.1 percent, and 6.4 percent, respectively by 2050, creating a risk of protein deficiency for an additional 148.4 million people (assuming today's diets and levels of income inequality; Medek 2017). Increased CO$_2$ levels in the 2080s are projected to reduce the protein, micronutrient, and B vitamin content of the eighteen rice cultivars more widely grown in Southeast Asia, creating nutrition-related health risks for 600 million people (Zhu et al. 2018). Assuming population and CO$_2$ emission projections for 2050, the estimated CO$_2$ increase is projected to cause an additional 175 million people to be zinc deficient and an additional 122 million people to be protein deficient globally (Smith and Myers 2018). Around 1.4 billion women of reproductive age and children under five are in countries with greater than 20 percent anemia prevalence, and they would lose more than 4 percent of their dietary iron. Regions at highest risk include South and Southeast Asia, Africa, and the Middle East (Smith and Myers).

Vulnerability to Climate Impacts on Food Insecurity and Malnutrition

Vulnerability to the impacts of climate shocks or extremes on food security and nutrition refers to the inability to cope with external changes, including inability to avoid harm when exposed to shocks, anticipate them, cope with them, and recover from them (Hardoy and Panidella 2009). Various vulnerability assessments have concluded that climate change and extreme weather events are among the largest contributors to food and nutrition insecurity, with the highest vulnerabilities in sub-Saharan Africa, Asia, and Latin America (Betts et al. 2018).

Climate impacts on food security and nutrition have strong gender and equity dimensions (Mbow et al. 2019). Some population groups are more vulnerable, and at greater risk, of increased impacts of climate shocks on livelihoods and assets, depending on age, ethnicity, gender, wealth, and class, thus contributing to food insecurity and malnutrition. These groups include low-income smallholder farmers, pastoralists, agriculture laborers, poorer population groups, groups that suffer greater inequality and marginalization, refugees, Indigenous groups, poor women and children, the elderly, and the socially isolated (FAO/IFAD/UNICEF/WFP/ WHO 2018). Men, women, children, the elderly, and the sick have different nutritional needs (e.g., during pregnancy or breastfeeding, HIV infected, etc.).

Gendered norms and differential gendered access, determines that men and women are affected differently by climate shocks, have differentiated vulnerability, risk perception, behaviors and have different capacities to cope and adapt to long-term changes (Bryan et al. 2016; Mbow et al. 2019). Extreme climate events have immediate and long-term impacts on livelihoods and food and nutrition insecurity of poor and vulnerable communities, and women and girls in low-income countries often experience additional duties as laborers and caregivers because of, for instance, male outmigration (FAO/IFAD/UNICEF/WFP/WHO 2018). Droughts and water scarcity can particularly affect women and girls because they need to spend more time and energy to fetch and collect water, where they may be more exposed to physical and sexual violence (FAO/IFAD/UNICEF/WFP/WHO 2018).

Foodborne and Waterborne Diseases and Emerging Risks

Climate change has the potential to cause and modify the occurrence and intensity of several foodborne and waterborne diarrheal diseases that affect nutrient absorption and aggravate malnutrition. Most of the projected climate-related disease burden in poor children in low-income countries will result from increases in diarrheal diseases and malnutrition.

Climate-sensitive emerging food, human health, and animal health risks have been identified globally (FAO 2020; Mbow et al. 2019). Priority emerging risks include marine biotoxins, mycotoxins, salmonellosis, vibriosis, transfer of contaminants due to floods, increased use of chemicals (plant protection products, fertilizers, veterinary drugs) in the food chain and potential residues in food (FAO 2020).

Gastrointestinal infections from bacterial pathogens such as *Salmonella* are positively correlated with ambient temperature, and high temperatures enable more rapid replication (Lake 2017). The risk of other enteric pathogens could rise in those regions where precipitation or extreme flooding is projected to increment (European Environmental Agency 2016). Compared with a future without climate change, the WHO assessment of the burden of disease due to climate change projected global additional deaths of 48,000 children under five caused by diarrhea in 2030 with highest impact in sub-Saharan countries (Hales et al. 2014).

Elevated risks of water and food contamination and corresponding diseases are directly related to climate change through increase prevalence of pathogens and harmful algal blooms, marine toxins, and increased contaminant bioaccumulation under warming and high CO_2 conditions (Mbow et al. 2019). Coastal areas that are projected to experience warming, changes in precipitation, and increases in nutrient inputs would have an increase in prevalence and expansion of *Vibrio* pathogens and an increased risk of *Vibrio* infections as a result of human exposure to the pathogen (Mbow et al.). Warming, excessive nutrient and seawater inundation due to sea level rise are projected to exacerbate the expansion and threat of *Vibrio* cholera (Bindoff et al. 2019).

Increases in the incidence of harmful algal blooms (HABs) are related to climate change and are projected to increase in the twenty-first century, thus increasing the risk of associated diseases (Mbow et al. 2019). These include the following types of poisoning: amnesic shellfish, diarrheic shellfish, neurotoxic shellfish, azaspiracid shellfish, paralytic shellfish, ciguatera fish, and cyanobacteria. This affects local traditional fisheries and livelihoods.

Climate change–contaminant interactions may alter the bioaccumulation and biomagnification of some contaminant classes: the toxic and fat-soluble persistent organic pollutants (POPs) such as polychlorinated biphenyls (PCBs), as well as the neurotoxic and protein-binding organic form of mercury, methylmercury (MeHg). Of particular concern is the pollution risks influenced by climate change in the Arctic ecosystems and Indigenous communities because of the protracted bioamplification of POPs and MeHg with associated long-term contamination of their traditional foods leading to public health issues (Tirado 2010; Alava et al. 2018).

Integrated Multisectoral Adaptation for Malnutrition

The protection and promotion of nutrition under climate change require a multisectoral integrated adaptation involving the food system, social protection, and health systems among others (Tirado et al. 2013; Mbow et al. 2019; Swinburn et al. 2019). Within broad efforts of climate-resilient development, a combination of healthy food systems and diets, nutrition-sensitive agriculture, health and social protection schemes and safety nets, nutrition-sensitive risk reduction, community-based development, nutrition-smart investments in direct nutrition interventions, increased policy coherence, and institutional and cross-sectoral collaboration have been proposed as a means to address the impacts of climate change to food and nutrition security (Tirado et al. 2013; FAO/IFAD/UNICEF/WFP/WHO 2018; Mbow et al. 2019).

Transformation of the Food System

Transforming the food system, considering nutrition outcomes, is an important lever to address the complex interactions between climate change, food security, nutrition and acting on food demand and supply adaptation can improve human and planetary health (Mbow et al.2019). (See the section Sustainable and Healthy Food Systems and Dietary Patterns.) Nutrition-sensitive agriculture practices including supply-side options and diversification of the food system are part of supply adaptation solutions. Demand-side adaptation such as adoption of healthy and sustainable diets, along with food waste reduction *can contribute to adaptation* through reduction in additional land area needed for food production and associated food system vulnerabilities (Mbow et al. 2019).

Access to Health, Nutrition Services, and Healthy Environments

Access to health care, maternal and child health care, water, and sanitation systems direct nutrition interventions, and adequate, safe food can contribute to reducing vulnerability and building resilience to climate change consequences (Tirado et al. 2013; FAO/IFAD/UNICEF/WFP/WHO 2018). The World Bank has identified highly cost-effective interventions, focusing on the window of opportunity for children under two years of age and including maternal undernutrition, such as promotion of good nutrition, care, and hygiene practices, such as breastfeeding, complementary feeding for infants over six months of age, improved hygiene practices, including handwashing, and deworming programs; micronutrient supplementation for young children and their mothers (e.g., periodic vitamin A supplements and therapeutic zinc supplements for diarrhea management); provision of micronutrients through food fortification for all (e.g., salt iodization, iron fortification, etc.); and therapeutic feeding of malnourished children with special foods, including the prevention or treatment of moderate undernutrition and the treatment of severe undernutrition, with ready-to-use therapeutic foods (RUTF) (Alderman 2016). Food assistance targeted to meet immediate food and nutritional requirements of vulnerable people, increase their productive potential and adaptive capacity, and protect them from climate-related disasters.

Nutrition-Sensitive Social Protection

Social protection mechanisms typically entail cash or asset transfers to households or individuals that meet a particular vulnerability threshold such as malnutrition (Carter and Janzen 2018). Commonly used instruments include cash transfers or public work programs, land reforms and extension of credit and insurance services. The use of these tools, especially conditional cash and asset transfers, has been shown to reduce impacts of climate-related vulnerability to food insecurity and malnutrition during acute environmental stress (Johnson et al. 2013); cash transfers tend to increase household expenditure on good-quality food—often more than other income sources (Alderman 2016). School feeding programs have been shown to improve nutritional outcomes, especially among girls, by promoting education and reducing child pregnancy and fertility rates (Drake et al. 2017). Social protection can be used to build livelihoods and resilience in the face of long-term climate change—especially if the social protection program engages the beneficiaries in activities that increase community resilience (such as water catchment technologies to address drought risk) or if they engage in behavior that increases adaptive capacity (such as reducing production of water-intensive crops to reduce water stress) (Béné et al. 2018). Such *adaptive social protection* programs that combine *social protection, disaster risk reduction, and climate adaptation* objectives in an integrated program are more likely to foster preventive and longer-term adaptive and/or transformational interventions to address climate risks than schemes focusing on social protection and disaster risk reduction alone (Steinbach et al. 2016).

Early Warning Systems to Prevent Adverse Effects on Malnutrition

Early warning systems for food security and nutrition (such as the U.S. Agency for International Development Famine Early Warning System, FAO's Global Information and Early Warning System, and the World Food Programme's Corporate Alert System) are fundamental for anticipating when a crisis might occur and provide essential inputs for prioritizing interventions to avert nutrition and food security crises (Funk et al. 2019). Investment in early warning is cost-effective and can help reduce human suffering induced by climate-related (and other) shocks. For instance, during the 2017 drought-induced food crisis in Kenya, 500,000 fewer people required humanitarian assistance than would be expected by similar droughts—largely due to effective interventions triggered by early warning (Funk et al. 2018). As the magnitude of climate-related events increases under climate change, and their potential impact on food and nutrition security intensifies, so does the need to better anticipate when an extreme weather event might trigger a crisis. Investments will be needed to forecast crises and prioritize limited resources (Choularton and Krishnamurthy 2019). Although early warning systems have been primarily developed to address shorter-term climate risks, usually on seasonal scales, they offer adaptation benefits (Cools, Innocenti, and O'Brien 2016). The information produced through the early warning system has also provided communities with solutions for climate adaptation, enhancing food security, building drought management capacities, nature conservation and protecting human health.

Nutrition-Sensitive Disaster Risk Reduction and Management

With increasing evidence that climate change-related disasters affect **malnutrition**, and that impacts will exacerbate given climate change that is already underway (e.g., Richardson et al. 2018), there is a need to support communities that are vulnerable to nutrition insecurity *and* disaster risk. Current efforts have focused on risk assessments (Challinor, Adger, and Benton 2017), improving emergency and contingency planning efforts (Michalska et al. 2015), and promoting livelihood resilience (Tanner et al., 2015). Such approaches are based on the assumption that solutions required to manage risks associated with future climate change are politically and financially feasible.

Resilience to increasing extreme events can be accomplished through risk sharing and transfer mechanisms such as insurance markets and index-based weather insurance (Mbow et al. 2019). Financial transfer mechanisms and microinsurance schemes targeting nutrition-insecure households hold great potential (Wilkinson et al. 2018), especially when combined with other risk reduction approaches. The World Food Programme-Oxfam R4 Rural Resilience Initiative incorporates improved resource management (risk reduction), insurance (risk transfer), microcredit (prudent risk-taking), and savings (risk reserves) (Peterson and Osgood 2016). Communities participating in this initiative engage in activities that reduce vulnerability to climate change while enhancing their livelihoods and may choose to be paid in kind (through food, insurance, or microcredits). In doing so, communities attempt to reduce key climate risks while also insuring their livelihoods against unavoidable impacts (Osgood et al. 2018).

Cross-Cutting Factors of Successful Climate Resilient Pathways to Address Malnutrition

Multisectoral Approach, Policy Coherence, and Good Governance

Different tools and interventions make it possible to implement climate resilient policies, programs, and practices to address malnutrition such as risk monitoring and early warning systems; emergency preparedness and response; vulnerability reduction measures, shock-responsive social protection, risk transfers, and forecast-based financing; and strengthened governance structures in the environment–food–health nexus (FAO/IFAD/UNICEF/WFP/WHO 2018). Public health policies to improve nutrition such as school procurement, health insurance incentives, and awareness-raising campaigns can potentially change demand, reduce health-care costs, and contribute to lower GHG emissions.

Targeting the Most Vulnerable Groups and Ensuring Social Inclusion and Resilience

Major climate impacts on food security and nutrition disproportionately affect the poor such as Indigenous populations, women and girls, female-headed households, and those with limited access to land, modern agricultural inputs, infrastructure, and education. To meet the nutrition needs of most vulnerable groups, cross-institutional partnerships, responsibility sharing, and information flow need to be at the center of an inclusive climate resilience strategy within and across sectors (FAO/IFAD/UNICEF/WFP/WHO 2018).

Women's Empowerment

Strengthening women's roles in promoting sustainable and diverse diets, resilient livelihoods, local food systems is key to empowering women to address climate change impacts on nutrition. When women are empowered and valued in their societies their capacity to improve food security under climate change and make substantial contributions to their own well-being and that of their families and of their communities is increased (Langer et al. 2015). Women's empowerment includes economic, social, and institutional arrangements and may include targeting men in integrated agriculture programs to change gender norms and improve nutrition (Bezner Kerr et al. 2016).

Sustainable and Healthy Food Systems and Dietary Patterns

The current food system accounts for up to 30 percent of total GHG emissions (Mbow et al. 2019). Current dietary patterns in most high-income countries with increasing consumption of meat and animal products are not sustainable and will be environmentally detrimental if continued and expanded globally (Springmann et al. 2018b). To meet climate targets below 2C by 2050, it is necessary to reduce the GHG emissions related to food production (supply) food consumption and food waste (demand side); these changes have significant co-benefits to health and needs to be a critical component in climate mitigation policies (Hedenus, Wirsenius, and Johansson 2014: Ripple et al. 2014; Tirado et al. 2017; Springmann et al. 2018a; IPCC 2018).

Co-Benefits of Healthy and Sustainable Diets

Healthy diets, high in vegetables, fruits, whole grains, pulses, nuts, and seeds, with modest amounts of meat and dairy, promote health and well-being while also helping to reduce GHG emissions (Tilman and Clark 2014; Springmann et al. 2018b; Willett et al. 2019). Reduction of red meat helps reduce the risk of cardiovascular disease and colorectal cancer; and the consumption of more fruits and vegetables can reduce the risk of cardiovascular disease, type 2 diabetes, cancer, and all causes of mortality (Tilman and Clark 2014; Sabate and Soret 2014; Willett et al. 2019). Globally, it is estimated that transitioning to more plant-based diets, in line with WHO recommendations on healthy eating, could reduce global mortality by 6–10 percent and food-related greenhouse gas emissions by 29–70 percent compared with a reference scenario for 2050 (Springmann et al. 2016b). A transformation to healthy diets by 2050 will require substantial dietary shifts (which differ regionally), including a greater than 50 percent reduction in global consumption of foods, such as red meat and sugar, and a greater than 100 percent increase in consumption of healthy foods, such as nuts, fruits, vegetables, and legumes (Willett et al. 2019). This could prevent up to 11.1 million deaths per year in 2030, a 19.9 percent reduction of all premature mortality due to prevention of cardiovascular disease, diabetes, and cancer, among other diseases (Willett et al.).

Food System Transformation

The EAT-Lancet Commission outlines five implementable strategies supported by a strong evidence for achieving a food system transformation toward healthy diets: (1) international and national commitment to shift towards healthy diets by investment in public health information and sustainability education and improved coordination between departments of health and environment; (2) reorient agricultural priorities from producing high quantities of food to producing healthy food; (3) sustainably intensify food production to increase high-quality output; (4) strong and coordinated governance of land and oceans; and (5) halve food losses and waste, in line with global sustainable development goals, across the food supply chain from production to consumption (Willet et al. 2019).

Transformative approaches toward healthier, sustainable, plant-based dietary patterns require strategies, policies, and measures including economic incentives for the production and consumption of more fruits, vegetables, and pulses; eliminating subsidies of unhealthy foods; taxing unhealthy foods; including sustainability criteria in dietary guidelines; conducting public education campaigns and educational programs in schools; promoting traditional food cultural heritage and gastronomy; labeling; establishing healthy and sustainable institutional food procurement and urban services; and promoting collaboration and shared agreements among others (Garnett 2015; Fischer and Garnett 2016; Springmann et al. 2017, 2018b; Tirado 2017; Nordic Council Food Policy Lab 2018; Willett et al. 2019; Swinburn et al. 2019).

Ensuring access to and affordability of healthy diets from sustainable food systems for all requires reducing volatility of food prices at the regional or local level and particularly in rural areas. Key policies to reduce this volatility include removing market barriers across local regions or markets, ensuring access to price information and early warning systems, implementing strict regulations against speculation, instituting international management of food stocks, revising biofuel subsidies and tariffs to avoid diversion of food to energy use, and establishing social protection schemes, insurance programs, and other safety nets (Torero et al. 2015).

Conclusions

Climate change and the consequent global environmental change can have significant impacts on food and water security and eventually on undernutrition, particularly in developing countries in the sub-Sahara and in Southeast Asia. Climate change and variability affect all four dimensions of food security: food availability, stability of food supplies, access to food, and food utilization. Climate change and variability influence the key determinants of malnutrition, including food access, maternal and childcare, access to health services, and environmental health. The determinants of malnutrition are shaped, in turn, by other socioeconomic factors that are also affected by climate including income, education, social safety nets, food aid, inequities, trade, economic, infrastructure, resources, political structures, and the full realization of human rights.

Current food systems and dietary patterns high in animal products and processed foods are key determinants of ill health and play a significant role in environmental degradation and climate change. The global food system, spanning food production, consumption, and waste, accounts for a substantial portion of the GHG emissions that are leading to climate and environmental change. Climate change mitigation is critical to limit the impact on food security and nutrition. The steadily increasing global demand for meat and animal products, particularly in developed countries and the urban developing world, presents complex challenges for mitigation, agriculture, and nutrition. Reducing food overconsumption, changing dietary preferences toward less meat and more plant-based protein, and avoiding food waste at consumption can contribute significantly to provide healthy diets for all, reduce the food system environmental footprint, and mitigate climate impacts.

A combination of nutrition-sensitive adaptation and mitigation measures, supported by research and technological development, nutrition-smart investments, increased policy coherence, and institutional and cross-sectoral collaboration, can contribute to addressing the threats to food and nutrition security and safety from climate change.

Sustainable food production, sustainable food consumption, and food waste reduction have co-benefits for nutrition, health, and the environment. These measures should be further analyzed and integrated within development strategies and programs.

CLINICAL CORRELATES 9.3 LOCUST SWARMS DESTROY CROPS

Locusts are species of grasshoppers that periodically come together as large swarms, with devastating consequences to agricultural production. Historical examples of plagues demonstrate the widespread destruction they cause on crops, contributing to famines and food insecurity. Swarms can be miles wide and long, travel far distances, and destroy crops sufficient to feed thousands of people every day. Climate change may promote these outbreaks through disruptions to normal breeding cycles through warmer and wetter conditions (Zhang et al. 2019). Outbreaks are controlled through prevention to reduce swarms, monitoring, weather forecasting, biopesticides, and insecticides (FAO 2005).

Locusts are one of the most dangerous threats to crops and food security in low- and middle-income countries, and climate change may provide more favorable conditions for breeding and swarms.

KEY TERMS

Malnutrition: A broad term that refers to all forms of poor nutrition, and it includes **undernutrition** as well as overweight and obesity. Malnutrition is caused by a complex array of factors, including dietary inadequacy (deficiencies, excesses, or imbalances in energy, protein, and micronutrients), infections, and sociocultural factors (GNR 2018).

Undernutrition: Exists when a combination of insufficient food intake, health, and care conditions results in one or more of the following: underweight for age, short for age (stunted), thin for height (wasted), or functionally deficient in vitamins and/or minerals (micronutrient malnutrition).

Undernourishment: The condition in which an individual's habitual food consumption is insufficient to provide the amount of dietary energy required to maintain a normal, active, healthy life (GNR 2018). Prevalence of undernourishment (PoU) is a complex, aggregated measure of undernourishment at national level.

References

Alava, J. J., A. M. Cisneros-Montemayor, U. R. Sumaila, and W. Cheung. 2018. "Projected Amplification of Food Web Bioaccumulation of MeHg and PCBs under Climate Change in the Northeastern Pacific." *Scientific Reports* 8 (1):13460.

Alderman, H. 2016. *Leveraging Social Protection Programs for Improved Nutrition: Summary of Evidence Prepared for the Global Forum on Nutrition-Sensitive Social Protection Programs, 2015.* Washington, DC: World Bank.

Béné, C., S. D. Prager, H. A. E. Achicanoy, P. Alvarez Toro, L. Lamotte, C. Bonilla Cedrez, et al. 2019. "Understanding Food Systems Drivers: A Critical Review of the Literature." *Global Food Security* 23:149–59.

Betts, R. A., L. Alfieri, C. Bradshaw, J. Caesar, L. Feyen, P. Friedlingstein, L. Gohar et al. 2018. "Changes in Climate Extremes, Fresh Water Availability and Vulnerability to Food Insecurity Projected at 1.5 C and 2 C Global Warming with a Higher-Resolution Global Climate Model." *Philosophical Transactions of the Royal Society A: Mathematical, Physical and Engineering Sciences* 376 (2119):20160452.

Bezner Kerr, R. E., L. Lupafya, L. Shumba, R. Dakishoni, A. Msachi, P. Chitaya, M. Nkhonjera et al. 2016. "'Doing Jenda Deliberately' in a Participatory Agriculture and Nutrition Project in Malawi." In *Transforming Gender and Food Security in the Global South*, edited by J. Njuku, A. Kaler, and J. Parkins, 241–59. London: Routledge.

Bindoff, N. L., W. W. L. Cheung, J. G. Kairo, J. Arístegui, V. A. Guinder, R. Hallberg, N. Hilmi et al. 2019. "Changing Ocean, Marine Ecosystems, and Dependent Communities." In *IPCC Special Report on the Ocean and Cryosphere in a Changing Climate*, edited by H.-O. Pörtner, D. C. Roberts, V. Masson-Delmotte, P. Zhai, M. Tignor, E. Poloczanska et al., 447–587. Geneva: Intergovernmental Panel on Climate Change.

Bryan, E., Q. Bernier, M. Espinal, and C. Ringler. 2016. *Integrating Gender in Climate Change Adaptation Programmes. A Research and Capacity Needs Assessment for Sub-Saharan Africa.* Working Paper No. 163. Copenhagen: CGIAR Research Program on Climate Change, Agriculture and Food Security. https://cgspace.cgiar.org/handle/10568/72482).

Carter, M. R., and S. A. Janzen. 2018. "Social Protection in the Face of Climate Change: Targeting Principles and Financing Mechanisms." *Environment and Development Economics* 23 (3):369–89.

Challinor, A. J., W. N. Adger, and T. G. Benton. 2017. "Climate Risks across Borders and Scales." *Nature Climate Change* 7 (9):621.

Choularton, R. J., and P. K. Krishnamurthy. 2019. "How Accurate Is Food Security Early Warning? Evaluation of FEWS NET Accuracy in Ethiopia." *Food Security* 1–12. doi:10.1007/s12571-019-00909-y.

Cools, J., D. Innocenti, and S. O'Brien. 2016. "Lessons from Flood Early Warning Systems." *Environmental Science & Policy* 58:117–22.

Drake, L., M. Fernandes, E. Aurino, J. Kiamba, B. Giyose, C. Burbano, H. Alderman et al. 2017. "School Feeding Programs in Middle Childhood and Adolescence." In *Disease Control Priorities, 3rd. ed. Vol. 8: Child and Adolescent Health and Development*, edited by D. A. P. Bundy, N. de Silva, S. Horton, D. T. Jamison, and G. C. Patton147–64. Washington, DC: World Bank.

Ebi, K. L., and L. H. Ziska. 2018. "Increases in Atmospheric Carbon Dioxide: Anticipated Negative Effects on Food Quality." *PLoS Medicine* 15 (7):e1002600. doi:10.1371/journal.pmed.1002600.

European Environmental Agency. 2016. *Climate Change, Impacts and Vulnerability in Europe 2016.* Copenhagen: EEA.

Fischer, C. G., and T. Garnett. 2016. *Plates, Pyramids and Planets. Developments in National Healthy and Sustainable Dietary Guidelines: A State of Play Assessment.* Rome: Food and Agriculture Organization; Oxford, UK: Food Climate Research Network, University of Oxford.

Food and Agriculture Organization. 2005. *Pesticides in Desert Locust Control.* Rome: FAO. http://www.fao.org/ag/locusts/common/ecg/812_en_FightingDLsafelyE.pdf.

Food and Agriculture Organization. 2016. *The State of Food and Agriculture. Climate Change, Agriculture and Food Security.* Rome: FAO.

Food and Agriculture Organization. 2020. *Climate Change: Unpacking the Burden on Food Safety. Food Safety and Quality Series No. 8.* Rome. FAO. https://doi.org/10.4060/ca8185en.

Food and Agriculture Organization/International Fund for Agricultural Development/UNICEF/World Food Programme/World Health Organization. 2018. *The State of Food Security and Nutrition in the World 2018. Building Climate Resilience for Food Security and Nutrition.* Rome: FAO.

Food Security Information Network. 2018. *Global Report on Food Crises.* Rome: World Food Programme.

Funk, C., F. Davenport, G. Eilerts, N. Nourey, and G. Galu. 2018. *Contrasting Kenyan Resilience to Drought: 2011 and 2017. USAID Special Report.* Washington, DC: U.S. Agency for International Development.

Funk, C., S. Shukla, W. M. Thiaw, J. Rowland, A. Hoell, A. McNally, G. Husak, N. Novella et al. 2019. "Recognizing the Famine Early Warning Systems Network (FEWS NET): Over 30 Years of Drought Early Warning Science Advances and Partnerships Promoting Global Food Security." *Bulletin of the American Meteorological Society* 100 (6):1011–27.

Global Nutrition Report. 2018. *Global Nutrition Report: Shining a Light to Spur Action on Nutrition.* Bristol, UK: Development Initiatives.

Hales, S. S. Kovats, S. Lloyd, and D. Campbell-Lendrum. 2014. *Quantitative Risk Assessment of the Effects of Climate Change on Selected Causes of Death, 2030s and 2050s.* Geneva: World Health Organization.

Hardoy, J., and G. Pandiella. 2009. "Urban Poverty and Vulnerability to Climate Change in Latin America." *Environment and Urbanization* 21 (1):203–24. https://doi.org/10.1177/0956247809103019.

Hedenus, F., S. Wirsenius, and D. J. A. Johansson. 2014. "The Importance of Reduced Meat and Dairy Consumption for Meeting Stringent Climate Change Targets." *Climatic Change* 124 (1):79–91. doi:10.1007/s10584-014-1104-5.

Intergovernmental Panel on Climate Change. 2018. *Summary for Policymakers. In: Global Warming of 1.5°C. An IPCC Special Report on the Impacts of Global Warming of 1.5°C above Pre-Industrial Levels and Related Global Greenhouse Gas Emission Pathways, in the Context of Strengthening the Global Response to the Threat of Climate Change, Sustainable Development, and Efforts to Eradicate Poverty*, edited by V. Masson-Delmotte, P. Zhai, H.-O. Pörtner, D. Roberts, J. Skea, P. R. Shukla, A. Pirani et al., 3–24. Geneva: IPCC.

International Food Policy Research Institute. 2016. *Global Nutrition Report 2016: From Promise to Impact: Ending Malnutrition by 2030*. Washington, DC: IFPRI.

Johnson, C., H. Bansha Dulal, M. Prowse, K. Krishnamurthy, and T. Mitchell. 2013. "Social Protection and Climate Change: Emerging Issues for Research, Policy and Practice." *Development Policy Review* 31:o2–o18.

Lake, I. R. 2017. "Food-Borne Disease and Climate Change in the United Kingdom." *Environmental Health* 16 (suppl 1):117. doi:10.1186/s12940-017-0327-0.

Langer, A., A. Meleis, F. M. Knaul, R. Atun, M. Aran, H. Arreola-Ornelas, Z. A. Bhutta et al. 2015. "Women and Health: The Key for Sustainable Development." *Lancet* 386 (9999):1165–1210. doi:10.1016/S0140-6736(15)60497-4.

Lloyd, S. J., M. Bangalore, Z. Chalabi, R. S. Kovats, S. Hallegatte, J. Rozenberg, H. Valin, and P. Havlík. 2018. "A Global-Level Model of the Potential Impacts of Climate Change on Child Stunting via Income and Food Price in 2030." *Environmental Health Perspectives* 126 (9):097007. doi:10.1289/EHP2916.

Mbow, C., C. Rosenzweig, L. G. Barioni, T. G. Benton, M. Herrero, M. Krishnapillai, E. Liwenga et al. 2019. "Food Security." In *Climate Change and Land: An IPCC Special Report on Climate Change, Desertification, Land Degradation, Sustainable Land Management, Food Security, and Greenhouse Gas Fluxes in Terrestrial Ecosystems*, edited by P. R. Shukla, J. Skea, E. Calvo Buendia, V. Masson-Delmotte, H.-O. Pörtner, D. C. Roberts, P. Zhai et al., 437–550. Geneva: Intergovernmental Panel on Climate Change.

Medek, D. E., J. Schwartz, and S. S. Myers. 2017. "Estimated Effects of Future Atmospheric CO_2 Concentrations on Protein Intake and the Risk of Protein Deficiency by Country and Region." *Environmental Health Perspectives* 125 (8):087002. doi:10.1289/EHP41.

Michalska, A., E. Leidman, S. Fuhrman, L. Mwirigi, O. Bilukha, and C. Basquin. 2015. "Nutrition Surveillance in Emergency Contexts: South Sudan Case Study." *Field Exchange* 50:73.

Nelson, G. C., J. S. Bogard, K. Lividini, J. Arsenault, M. Riley, T. B. Sulser, D. Mason-D'Croz et al. 2018. "Income Growth and Climate Change Effects on Global Nutrition Security to Mid-Century." *Nature Sustainability* 1:773–81.

Nordic Food Policy Lab. 2018. *Guidelines for Sustainable Food Policies*. Copenhagen: Nordic Council.

Osgood, D., B. Powell, R. Diro, C. Farah, M. Enenkel, M. E. Brown, G. Husak et al. 2018. *Farmer Perception, Recollection, and Remote Sensing in Weather Index Insurance for Agriculture in the Developing World: An Ethiopia Case Study*. Available at SSRN: https://doi.org/10.3390/rs10121887 or http://dx.doi.org/10.2139/ssrn.3242142.

Peterson, N. D., and D. Osgood. 2016. "Insuring the Rain as Climate Adaptation in an Ethiopian Agricultural Community." In *Anthropology and Climate Change: From Actions to Transformations*, edited by S. A. Crate and M. Nuttall, 373–87. New York: Routledge.

Richardson, K. J., K. H. Lewis, P. K. Krishnamurthy, C. Kent, A. J. Wiltshire, and H. M. Hanlon. 2018. "Food Security Outcomes under a Changing Climate: Impacts of Mitigation and Adaptation on Vulnerability to Food Insecurity." *Climatic Change* 147 (1–2):327–41.

Ripple, W. J., P. Smith, H. Haberl, S. A. Montzka, C. McAlpine, and D. H. Boucher. 2013. "Ruminants, Climate Change and Climate Policy." *Nature Climate Change* 4:2. doi:10.1038/nclimate2081.

Sabate, J., and S. Soret. 2014. *Sustainability of Plant-Based Diets: Back to the Future*. Rockville, MD: American Society for Nutrition.

Smith, M. R., and S. S. Myers. 2018. "Impact of Anthropogenic CO2 Emissions on Global Human Nutrition." *Nature Climate Change* 8 (9):834–39. doi:10.1038/s41558-018-0253-3.

Springmann, M., M. Clark, D. Mason-D'Croz, K. Wiebe, B. L. Bodirsky, L. Lassaletta, W. de Vries et al. 2018b. "Options for Keeping the Food System within Environmental Limits." *Nature* 562 (7728):519–25. doi:10.1038/s41586-018-0594-0.

Springmann, M., H. C. J. Godfray, M. Rayner, and P. Scarborough. 2016a. "Analysis and Valuation of the Health and Climate Change Cobenefits of Dietary Change." *Proceedings of the National Academy of Sciences of the USA* 113 (15):4146–51. https://doi.org/10.1073/pnas.1523119113.

Springmann, M., D. Mason-D'Croz, S. Robinson, T. Garnett, H. C. J. Godfray, D. Gollin, M. Rayner et al. 2016b. "Global and Regional Health Effects of Future Food Production under Climate Change: A Modelling Study." *Lancet* 387 (10031):1937–46. doi:10.1016/S0140-6736(15)01156-3.

Springmann, M., D. Mason-D'Croz, S. Robinson, K. Wiebe, H. C. J. Godfray, M. Rayner, and P. Scarborough. 2017. "Mitigation Potential and Global Health Impacts from Emissions Pricing of Food Commodities." *Nature Climate Change* 7:69. doi:10.1038/nclimate3155. https://www.nature.com/articles/nclimate3155#supplementary-information.

Springmann, M., K. Wiebe, D. Mason-D'Croz, T. B. Sulser, M. Rayner, and P. Scarborough. 2018a. "Health and Nutritional Aspects of Sustainable Diet Strategies and Their Association with Environmental Impacts: A Global Modelling Analysis with Country-Level Detail." *Lancet Planetary Health* 2 (10):e451–e461. doi:10.1016/S2542-5196(18)30206-7.

Springmann, M., M. Clark, D. Mason-D'Croz, K. Wiebe, B. L. Bodirsky, L. Lassaletta, W. De Vries et al. 2018c. "Options for Keeping the Food System within Environmental Limits." *Nature* 562 (7728):519–25.

Steinbach, D., R. G. Wood, N. Kaur, S. D'Errico, J. Choudhary, S. Sharma, V. Rahar, and V. Jhajharia. 2016. *Aligning Social Protection and Climate Resilience*. London, UK: International Institute for Environment and Development.

Swinburn, B. A., V. I. Kraak, S. Allender, V. J. Atkins, P. I. Baker, J. R. H. Bogard, H. Brindsen et al. 2019. "The Global Syndemic of Obesity, Undernutrition, and Climate Change: *The Lancet* Commission report." *Lancet* 393 (10173):791–846. doi:10.1016/S0140-6736(18)32822-8.

Tanner, T., D. Lewis, D. Wrathall, R. Bronen, N. Cradock-Henry, S. Huq, C. Lawless et al. 2015. "Livelihood Resilience in the Face of Climate Change." *Nature Climate Change* 5 (1):23.

Tilman, D., and M. Clark. 2014. "Global Diets Link Environmental Sustainability and Human Health." *Nature* 515 (7528):518–22. doi:10.1038/nature13959. http://www.nature.com/nature/journal/v515/n7528/abs/nature13959.html#supplementaryinformation.

Tirado, C. 2017. "Sustainable Diets for Healthy People and a Healthy Planet." *Discussion Paper*. Rome: United Nations System Standing Committee on Nutrition.

Tirado, M. C., R. Clarke, L. A. Jaykus, A. McQuatters-Gollop, and J. M. Frank. 2010. "Climate Change and Food Safety: A Review." *Food Research Journal* 43:1745–65.

Tirado, M. C., P. Crahay, L. Mahy, C. Zanev, M. Neira, S. Msangi, R. Brown et al. (2013). "Climate Change and Nutrition: Creating a Climate for Nutrition Security." *Food and Nutrition Bulletin* 34 (4):533–47. doi:10.1177/156482651303400415.

Torero, M., and A. Viceisza. 2015. "To Remit, or Not to Remit: That Is the Question. A Remittance Field Experiment." *Journal of Economic Behavior & Organization* 112:221–36. https://doi.org/10.1016/j.jebo.2015.01.012.

United Nations Children's Fund, World Health Organization, International Bank for Reconstruction and Development/World Bank Group. 2019. *Levels and Trends in Child Malnutrition: Key Findings of the 2019 Edition Joint Child Malnutrition Estimates*. Geneva: World Health Organization.

Wagstaff, G. A. 2016. *The Economic Costs of Stunting and How to Reduce Them. Policy Research Note No. 5*. Washington, DC: World Bank Group.

Wilkinson, E., L. Weingärtner, R. Choularton, M. Bailey, M. Todd, D. Kniveton, and C. Cabot Venton. 2018. *Forecasting Hazards, Averting Disasters: Implementing Forecast-Based Early Action at Scale*. London: Overseas Development Institute.

Willett, W., J. Rockström, B. Loken, M. Springmann, T. Lang, S. Vermeulen, T. Garnett et al. 2019. "Food in the Anthropocene: The EAT–*Lancet* Commission on Healthy Diets from Sustainable Food Systems." *Lancet* 393 (10170):447–92. doi:10.1016/S0140-6736(18)31788-4.

Zhang, L., M. Lecoq, A. Latchininsky, and D. Hunter. 2019. "Locust and Grasshopper Management." *Annual Review of Entomology* 64:15–34. doi:10.1146/annurev-ento-011118-112500.

Zhao, C., B. Liu, S. Piao, X. Wang, D. B. Lobell, Y. Huang, M. Huang et al. 2017. "Temperature Increase Reduces Global Yields of Major Crops in Four Independent Estimates." *Proceedings of the National Academy of Sciences of the USA* 114 (35):9326–31. doi:10.1073/pnas.1701762114.

Zhu, C., K. Kobayashi, I. Loladze, J. Zhu, Q. Jiang, X. Xu, G. Liu et al. 2018. "Carbon Dioxide (CO_2) Levels This Century Will Alter the Protein, Micronutrients, and Vitamin Content of Rice Grains with Potential Health Consequences for the Poorest Rice-Dependent Countries." *Science Advances* 4 (5):eaaq1012.

CHAPTER 10

CLIMATE CHANGE AND POPULATION MENTAL HEALTH

Salma M. Abdalla, Abdulrahman M. El-Sayed, and Sandro Galea

Overview

Global surface temperatures have increased by approximately 1 degree Celsius since the late nineteenth century (pre-industrial age). Other features of global climate change include rising global sea levels, extreme heat waves and precipitation, acidification of oceans, and reduction in glacier mass, among others (Intergovernmental Panel on Climate Change [IPCC] 2018). These changes have demonstrably serious consequences for human well-being. For example, about thirty countries are currently experiencing a downward trend in crop yield, which has great implications on global food security (Watts et al. 2018). Climate change is therefore among the most important challenges facing the global community today. As what were once thought to be long-term effects of climate change begin to occur in real time, understanding the causes and consequences of this challenge takes on particular urgency.

Among the most serious and direct consequences of climate change will be its toll on human health, including the rising burden of mental disorders. Already, mental disorders result in substantial morbidity and financial cost worldwide. In a recent global burden of disease analysis, mental and substance use disorder was the largest contributor to disability among young adults (Naghavi et al. 2017). The World Health Organization (WHO) estimates that 322 million people (4.4 percent of the global population) suffer from depression—making depression a leading cause of disability worldwide (Friedrich 2017). In middle- and high-income countries, more than half of the general population will experience a mental disorder at some point in their lives (Trautmann, Rehm, and Wittchen 2016). Mental disorder is also profoundly expensive, imposing substantial costs—direct and indirect—on individuals, families, industries, health systems, and national economies alike (Luppa et al. 2007; Trautmann et al. 2016).

In this chapter, we explore the mechanisms by which climate change may affect global **mental health**. We then discuss how climate change can contribute to deepening inequities in global mental health. We conclude with a discussion regarding the possible reciprocal mechanisms by which mental disorders may potentiate climate change.

Climate Change Effect on Mental Health: Mechanisms

There are several mechanisms, both direct and indirect, by which climate change may influence global mental health, as indicated in Figure 10.1. First, climate change will lead to higher average ambient temperatures and increase the frequency and severity of heat waves. Among their many effects on health, heat waves are associated with higher burden of mental disorder and suicide rates. Second, climate

KEY CONCEPTS

- There are several mechanisms by which climate change affects population mental health, including natural disasters, heatwaves, forced migration, conflict over scarce resources, and physical comorbidity.

- The burden of psychopathology resulting from climate change is borne disproportionately by the poor and marginalized who lack the resources to protect themselves.

- Climate change and population psychopathology have shared causes and consequences that should be considered in policy conversations about either.

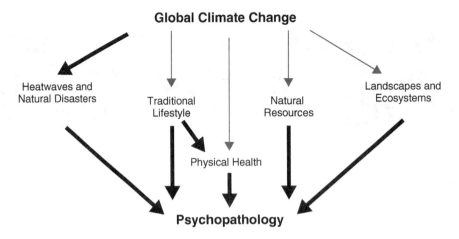

Figure 10.1 A mechanistic map relating global climate change and psychopathology
Note: Thick, black arrows indicate increases, and thin, grey arrows indicate decreases in variables to which arrows point.

change will increase the frequency and severity of natural disasters such as windstorms, flooding, and droughts (Aumann et al. 2008). More frequent disasters will increase exposure to trauma, which may threaten mental health, as well as harm the material well-being of victims. Third, climate change will degrade landscapes, ecosystems, and habitats, thereby undermining agricultural productivity and ethnic, cultural, and religious traditions. Fourth, climate change will intensify global competition for resources, which could increase the rate and consequences of global conflict, especially in areas of poor governance. Fifth, climate change will have important influences on physical health, such as increasing the prevalence of noncommunicable diseases (NCDs) such as obesity, which will in turn increase the burden of mental comorbidity. We discuss each of these mechanisms in turn.

High Ambient Temperature and Heatwaves

The rise in the global average temperature and number and intensity of heat waves is one of the most direct and overwhelming consequence of climate change (European Consortium of Innovative Universities 2017). Heat waves constitute nearly half (46 percent) of the climate change-related extreme weather events. In 2017, 157 million more people were exposed to heatwaves compared to the year 2000 (Watts et al. 2018). By way of example, in 2015, India and Pakistan experienced a heat wave for several days. One study looking at two events reported that in Karachi (one of the areas where the heat waves occurred), the unusual increase in humidity level contributed to a heat index of 7–12°C (12.7°F) above the usual temperature for that time of year (Wehner et al. 2016).

Heat waves are associated with a number of adverse mental health outcomes. High ambient temperature and heat waves are associated with higher rates of hospital admissions for bipolar disorder and dementia, exacerbations of schizophrenic symptoms, mortality due to alcohol and substance abuse, and suicide (Thompson et al. 2018). By way of example, researchers in Australia found that above a threshold of 26.7° C (80°F), hospital admissions due to mental disorders increased by 7.3 percent during heat waves compared to non-heat wave periods (Hansen et al. 2008). Another study in India found that high temperature was responsible for 59,300 suicides between 1980 and 2013. The same study found that for temperatures above 20°C (68°F), a 1°C (1.8°F) increase in a temperature was associated with about seventy suicides in the country per day (Carleton 2017).

The rise in the frequency and severity of heat waves is the most common consequence of climate change. Heat waves are also an important mechanism by which climate change will increase the burden of mental disorders. Increasing ambient temperature and heat waves are associated with several mental health disorders, particularly higher rates of suicide. As such, the effects of heat waves on mental health are of particular concern.

Natural Disasters

One of the most important implications of climate change for human health is the increase in the frequency and severity of natural disasters (e.g., storms, flooding, and droughts) (Carbon Brief 2017). There were three times as many natural disasters between 2000 and 2009 compared to 1980 to 1989. As the frequency and severity of natural disasters increase, their mental health sequelae will as well. Victims of natural disasters are at high risk for several mental health problems. The medical literature has many studies supporting the high burden of **post-traumatic stress disorder** (**PTSD**) after disasters (Galea, Nandi, and Vlahov 2005; Neria, Nandi, and Galea 2008). For example, the prevalence of PTSD in the community following the 2010 Haiti earthquake was 25 percent (National Oceanic and Atmospheric Administration [NOAA] 2013). Similarly, following Hurricane Katrina, the prevalence of PTSD among residents of the twenty-three southernmost counties in Mississippi was 23 percent (Galea et al. 2008). Beyond PTSD, exposure to natural disasters can carry other deleterious mental health risks as well. For example, along with the substantial burden of PTSD, the burden of **major depressive disorder** (**MDD**) in Haiti was nearly 30 percent (Cerdá et al. 2018).

Natural disasters take the lives of loved ones, destroy homes and workplaces, and obliterate livelihoods. Although the bulk of psychopathologic sequelae of disasters may occur in their immediate to short-term aftermath, their long-term implications should not to be overlooked. In the aftermath of Hurricane Katrina, for example, one study demonstrated that the prevalence of both suicidal ideation and severe mental illness among survivors nearly tripled among respondents between five months and one year following the disaster (NOAA 2013). The investigators found that unresolved hurricane-related stresses accounted for over 60 percent of the increase in suicidality and nearly 90 percent of the increase in severe mental illness. In this regard, chronic stressors, or life circumstances that are difficult to cope with—the residual of natural disasters—may have important long-term implications for the burden of psychopathology as survivors struggle to cope with difficult new realities. As the frequency and severity of disasters increase and greater relative and absolute numbers of people are exposed to them, it is clear that the mental health sequelae of natural disasters caused by climate change will be an important mechanism through which the changing environment will influence mental health.

Forced Migration

Climate change will cause substantial changes in the ways in which populations interact with their surroundings—from both sudden events (i.e., disasters) as well as slow, creeping alterations to microenvironments around the globe. These changes will include the loss of coastal environments as the polar ice caps continue to melt and the sea level continues to rise and changes in the crop potential of agricultural lands important to human survival. In this regard, a substantial proportion of the mental health consequences of climate change will result from the **forced migration** of communities—as their habitats and livelihoods degrade—and the associated vulnerabilities to which these communities will be exposed.

Glaciers and the polar ice caps are melting (Li and Lin 2017). It is clear that this will have serious implications for coastal communities as rising sea levels threaten coastal human habitats. The vulnerability of inhabitants of particular environmental regions to climate change is already well established (Wright, Syvitski, and Nichols 2019). For example, small island states are particularly vulnerable to natural disasters (Briguglio 1995; Pelling and Uitto 2001). Moreover, residents of these islands and other coastal residents, particularly in low-income countries, are disproportionately poor, and not as resilient to change (McGranahan, Balk, and Anderson 2007). Mountain communities may also be vulnerable to water insecurity given that glaciers provide freshwater resources to such communities (Fell, Carrivick, and Brown 2017). Social scientists have warned of the potential for forced migration and deep exploitation of poor coastal communities in vulnerable countries (Piguet 2008; Poncelet et al. 2010). Although displacement is likely to occur over time, climate change, in this regard, is a serious potential cause of forced migration in the future. For example, an American Community Survey conducted following Hurricane Katrina—which led to severe damage to the city of New Orleans due to extensive flooding— found that the city's population about four months after the hurricane was about one third of the prehurricane population. Another paper reported that, one year after the hurricane, only 53 percent of adults had returned to or remained in the area (Sastry 2007; Sastry and Gregory 2014).

Loss of habitat is not the only migratory force that climate change will create. Desertification in areas that had been arable and supported generations of agricultural families is also occurring through droughts and as dry-season rainfall continues to drop (Lawrence and Vandeca 2015; Reed, Stringer, and Stringer 2016). This will force communities away from their ancestral homelands in an effort to find new means of self-support. This type of forced migration has already begun to occur in several countries in sub-Saharan Africa where, by 2014, 40 percent of grassland and 26 percent of forestland had already experienced degradation compared to the 1980s (Nkonya et al. 2016).

Moreover, there is clear evidence that climate variability over the past several decades has had tangible effects on crop yields in various contexts. Between the years 1980 and 2008, climate trends led to a 3.5 and 5.5 percent decline in the global production of maize and wheat, respectively. The effects of climate change in some countries were large enough to offset a significant portion of the increase in crop yields due to carbon dioxide fertilization and technology advances (Lobell, Schlenker, and Costa-Roberts 2011). One case study followed the migration of nomadic peoples in remote drylands of Ethiopia resulting from climate-related droughts (Thompson et al. 2018). Similarly, during the last half of the twentieth century, social scientists tracked the movement of heads of household in southern Sudan in relation to climatic events, suggesting that poor agricultural yields have forced male heads of household to leave the countryside for the city in search of labor opportunities (Afolayan and Adelekan 1999; McLeman and Smit 2006). Similar findings were noted among communities in Burkina Faso (Henry, Schoumaker, and Beauchemin 2003).

The effects of climate change on crop yields do not uniquely affect low-income settings. For example, crop yields in Mexico may be an important contributor to cross-border emigration to the United States (Feng, Krueger, and Oppenheimer 2010). Moreover, studies have suggested that U.S. crop yields stand to suffer substantial losses due to climate change as well, potentiating the trend toward coastal migration within the country as agricultural life becomes even less tenable (Schlenker and Roberts 2009).

Forced migration has several important consequences for mental health. First, migration itself—and the implicit requirement to adapt socially, financially, and structurally to a new context—is a powerful stressor. Second, the vast majority of those forced to migrate have few social or economic resources to leverage in their new contexts, and therefore they are vulnerable to exploitation, which itself carries tremendous mental health consequences. Compounding this potential is that much of the forced migration resulting from climate change will move agricultural communities whose skills may be ill matched for employment opportunities available in the contexts to which they are migrating.

Several studies have considered the mental health consequences of migration. One study, for example, found that the rate of PTSD among Somali and Rwandan refugees in African refugee settlements to be nearly 50 percent (Onyut et al. 2009). A systematic review of the literature found that refugees resettled in western countries could be about ten times more likely to have PTSD than the—age-matched—general population of these countries (Fazel, Wheeler, and Danesh 2005). In addition to PTSD, migrants experience a number of other mental health consequences. For example, the prevalence of depression, anxiety, and suicidality among Mexican migrant workers is high (Hiott et al. 2008; Hovey 2000; Hovey and Magaña 2003; Sullivan and Rehm 2005). A systematic review measuring the prevalence of depression and anxiety among labor migrants and refugees found that 20 percent of labor migrants around the world were depressed and 21 percent suffered anxiety disorders. Rates of depression and anxiety among refugees were nearly twice as high (Lindert et al. 2009).

The same review found that the income of the country in which migrant laborers migrated was an important modifier of the risk for depression and anxiety—the higher income the country, the lower the likelihood of adverse outcomes (Lindert et al. 2009). In this regard, the literature is also clear that resources available for coping are an important predictor of the mental health risks of forced migration. One systematic review concluded that although migration is associated with a substantial amount of stress, the translation of this stress to adverse mental health was a consequence of the coping resources available (Bhugra 2004). Coping is highly influenced by the structural and legal resources/obstacles into which communities migrate (Lindert et al. 2008). Unfortunately, in many circumstances, forced migrants are "otherized" by the communities into which they migrate (Grove and Zwi 2006).

Forced migrants are often victims of exploitation, including economic and sexual exploitation and human trafficking, with devastating mental health consequences (Andrees and Belser 2009; Belser 2005; Decker et al. 2009; Ottisova et al. 2016). For example, one study showed that exploitation-related trauma was associated with high risk for adverse mental health outcomes among trafficked women in seven European countries (Hossain et al. 2010).

Among the most important mental health consequences of climate change, therefore, will be the migration it forces. In uprooting coastal communities that lose their homes and agricultural communities whose lands erode, climate change will expose large communities to migration-associated stressors, such as acculturation and exploitation, which will have deleterious consequences for population mental health.

Economics, Geopolitics, and Violent Conflict

As climate change intensifies, the relative availability of commodities will shift, heightening competition for natural resources that are already scarce. This competition is likely to be a geopolitically destabilizing force, increasing the probability of violent conflict as geopolitical actors vie for access to increasingly important commodities (Barnett and Adger 2007; Rademaker et al. 2016; Scheffran 2012).

Changing demand for freshwater is among the most important potential climate-related causes of conflict. As the rate of drought increases, access to freshwater for drinking and irrigation will be at a premium. At the same time, climate change is likely to alter the courses of rivers and the accessibility of other freshwater sources (Mearns and Norton 2009; Tir and Stinnett 2012). Water scarcity increases the likelihood of armed conflict. One study, for example, demonstrated that deviations in rainfall in either direction—expected to increase as climate change follows its current course—were associated with increasing incidence of violent events on the African continent (Hendrix and Salehyan 2012). Other important commodities over which conflict is likely to occur include food, arable land, and fisheries (Adano et al. 2012; Allison et al. 2009; Klare 2002; Mearns and Norton 2009).

Armed conflict is among the most important causes of severe mental trauma and resulting psychopathology among both combatants and civilians. For example, in a longitudinal study of active and reserve soldiers returning from the Iraq war, 20 percent of active-duty soldiers and 40 percent of reservists met screening requirements for care from a mental health professional (Milliken, Auchterlonie, and Hoge 2007). A similar study among over 100,000 veterans of the U.S. wars in Iraq and Afghanistan found that nearly one in four was diagnosed with a mental disorder (Seal et al. 2007).

More problematic are the mental health consequences among civilian victims of conflict. For example, a study among Kosovar Albanians following the 1998–1999 war in Kosovo showed that over 17 percent reported symptoms that met the criteria for PTSD. Particularly affected were those who had firsthand exposure to traumatic events and those who had been internally displaced during the war (Lopes Cardozo et al. 2000). Another study assessed the prevalence of PTSD among over 13,000 adult survivors of the civil war in Liberia nearly two decades following the end of the conflict and found that 50 percent of the study sample had PTSD (Galea et al. 2010). Armed conflict is also linked to other mental health sequalae. A study of more than 6,000 civilians in Colombia between 2010–2011, found a clear effect from the conflict on mental health. Exposure to conflict-related violence was highly related to anxiety-related psychopathology (Bell et al. 2012).

The mental health consequences of war are particularly pronounced in children. Alarmingly high prevalence of psychopathology also has been documented among children in war-torn contexts (Dyregrov et al. 2000). For example, one study found the prevalence of PTSD was 73 percent among children in Gaza who had experienced siege by Israeli forces (Thabet and Vostanis 1999). Another study in the same population found that 21.9 and 50.6 percent of children had anxiety and depression, respectively (Thabet, Thabet, and Vostanis 2016). These consequences last into adulthood. Several studies have demonstrated that exposure to childhood trauma increases the risk for adulthood psychopathology (Spatz Widom, DuMont, and Czaja 2007; Widom 1999). For example, one study found that separation from parents during wartime increased risk of depressive symptoms in adulthood (Pesonen et al. 2007).

Conflict is an important mechanism by which climate change will increase the burden of mental disorders. Climate change stands to increase the scarcity of important natural resources, such as food, and freshwater, and, as a consequence, increase violent conflict and subject millions to the horrors of war, as well as its mental health sequelae.

CLINICAL CORRELATES 10.1 PHYSICAL PAIN AND PSYCHOLOGICAL TRAUMA

Natural disasters can result in significant physical and emotional trauma. Symptoms of trauma can be expressed in many forms, which may complicate accurate clinical diagnosis and compound existing medical comorbidities, including chronic pain and posttraumatic stress disorder (PTSD). Experts in the field of trauma have begun to unravel the ways in which different cultures express of psychological distress. Behavioral health specialists have designed unique screening tools in different countries to detect PTSD across various cultures. In many cases neurological, somatic, and visceral pains become physical manifestations of psychological trauma.

Data show a barriers to effective treatment is the fact that health care professionals often shy away from asking patients about their history of trauma because they "believe they won't have the tools or the time to help survivors once they've elicited their history" (Mollica 2004). However, such a history is imperative and will become more so in the future. Effective treatment of PTSD has been shown to lower a patient's perception of pain (Plagge et al. 2013), improve quality of life, and decrease dependence on narcotic pain medications.

Climate change has the potential to result in widespread physical and psychological trauma. Thus, clinicians must be well versed in properly diagnosing and treating stress syndromes.

CLINICAL CORRELATES 10.2 STRESS AND PHYSICAL HEALTH: IMPLICATIONS FOR CURRENT AND FUTURE GENERATIONS

Extreme stress may be defined as the passing of a mental, emotional, or physiological threshold after which a person can no longer cope and adapt (Haushofer and Fehr 2014). On a physiological level, higher levels of cortisol correlate with poor physical health, manifested through decreased immune function, high blood pressure, and reproductive disturbances, among other physiological responses (Damti et al. 2008). In an era of global climate change, stress levels are expected to rise because of the real and perceived threats of drought, famine, severe weather, overpopulation, and forced migration, to name a few.

For example, in a study of Kenyan farmers subject to drought conditions, cortisol levels were found to be significantly elevated (Chemin, de Laat, and Haushofer 2013). Droughts can also lead to loss of unemployment and job insecurity, which have an effect on the neuroendocrine and immune systems (Arnetz et al. 1991). Even perceived stress may have negative health implications. In one study, participants who reported that stress was affecting their health were found to be twice as likely to suffer from a heart attack as those who believed that stress had no effect on their physical well-being (Nabi et al. 2013).

Higher stress levels have implications for current as well as future generations. Children are recognized as one group suffering mental health consequences from concerns of climate change with resultant disruptions in learning, behaviors, and development (Burke, Sanson, and Van Hoorn 2018). Another study found that women living in war-torn regions of the Democratic Republic of the Congo experience high levels of stress during pregnancy that may directly influence birth weight and lead to epigenetic modification of the glucocorticoid receptor NR3C1 of the infant (Rodney and Mulligan 2014). These epigenetic changes could affect how the child responds to stress and thus his or her long-term health profile.

Climate change causes real and perceived threats of food scarcity, job insecurity, natural disasters, and more. Stress has wide-reaching effects on health that clinicians must be able to diagnose and treat promptly and accurately .

Physical Health

Poor physical health is among the most important determinants of psychopathology. For example, one study found that seventeen physical health conditions were associated with an increased suicide risk (Ahmedani et al. 2017). Those with chronic physical maladies have substantially higher risk for mood and anxiety disorders and, in some circumstances, suicidality. For example, a study of a nationally representative U.S. sample showed that the risk of psychopathology was up to four times higher among those with chronic pain than those without (McWilliams, Cox, and Enns 2003). In another study, 35 percent of those with chronic back or neck pain had comorbid psychopathology (Von Korff et al. 2005). One study assessed the relation between chronic disease diagnoses and suicidality in the elderly and found that several diseases, including chronic obstructive lung disorder, congestive heart failure, seizure disorder, moderate pain, and severe pain, were predictive of suicide risk (Juurlink et al. 2004).

Each of the mechanisms by which climate change may directly contribute to population psychopathology that we have previously discussed—heatwaves, natural disasters, forced migration, and violent conflict—will also increase physical morbidity. The physical morbidity associated with these mechanisms will act as a multiplier of the mental health burden of climate change. Not only will these mechanisms provide acute and chronic stressors that directly lead to mental disorder, but their physical sequelae will act as chronic stressors that indirectly contribute to mental disorder as well.

One condition that may be particularly important for the transmission of mental health is obesity. First, it is clear that obesity and mental disorder are syndemic, meaning that they potentiate one another, disproportionately among certain vulnerable populations. The literature about the directionality of the relationship suggests that obesity is more likely to cause depression than depression is to cause obesity (Faith et al. 2011). Climate change could increase the population burden of obesity through several mechanisms (Blaine 2008). First, climate change has the potential to reduce physical activity (Townsend et al. 2003). As ambient temperatures increase, the viability of outdoor recreational activity will diminish. Moreover, concomitant with the trend toward urbanization, access to, and availability of, green space is likely to decrease with climate change as well. Climate change may also influence population dietary patterns (Parry, Rosenzweig, and Livermore 2005). As larger swathes of arable land deteriorate, the production and quality of nutrients, such as vegetables, are projected to decrease (Scheelbeek et al. 2018). Simultaneously, research predicts that the prices of food are likely to increase (Wiebe et al. 2015). Evidence suggests that when the prices for healthy food are high, people often consume unhealthy alternatives (Kern et al. 2017). As such, climate change may drive the consumption of high-caloric-density foods, particularly among the poor. In this regard, the consumption of refined carbohydrates and fats—important drivers of obesity—is likely to increase. With obesity comes a host of other high-burden diseases, including hypertension, diabetes, cardiovascular disease, and several types of cancers (Must and McKeow 2000). Therefore, climate change may contribute to increased population mental disorders through an increase in the obesity rate and its chronic disease sequelae.

A Disproportionate Burden

Climate change will have broad effects on population mental health through several important mechanisms. These mechanisms have in common the limitations they impose on the availability of important resources, limitations that create emotional and psychological stressors in the population as communities attempt to cope with their scarcity. In that respect, lack of resources is a unifying theme in the translation of climate change to mental disorder. It should be no surprise, then, that the mental health influence of climate change will disproportionately affect the poor and marginalized.

The health consequences of harmful exposures—such as climate change—are never borne equally because higher socioeconomic status affords people the means to insulate themselves from these exposures through access to knowledge, money, capital, power, social connectedness, and prestige (Link and Phelan 1996; Phelan and, Link 2005; Subramanian and Kawachi 2004). It follows that these resources can be used to insulate against potentially harmful exposures, regardless of what they are. An understanding of the mechanisms through which climate change may affect population mental health makes it clear that in each circumstance, socioeconomic resources could mitigate potentially harmful effects.

To illustrate, let's examine the effects of heat waves on society. The poor, minorities, and other vulnerable groups (particularly the elderly [Kovats and Hajat 2008]) are more likely to be exposed to the consequences of heatwaves. Researchers have found an association between level of exposure to heat and lower socioeconomic, and minority status (Mitchell and Chakraborty 2015). For example, African Americans/blacks in Los Angeles are more vulnerable to the effects of heat waves as they often live in the inner city where temperature is magnified by concrete and asphalt. Moreover, this population is less likely to have access to air conditioning or cars. It follows that African Americans/blacks were almost twice as likely to die during a heat wave in Los Angeles than their white counterparts (Fischer 2009). The elderly are another group that is far more likely to be influenced by the effects of heat waves than the general population due to both their increased biological susceptibility (i.e., less physiologic reserve and ability to thermoregulate) and social factors such as lower quality of housing conditions and lack of mobility. During a heat wave that hit Italy during the summer of 2003, the greatest increase in mortality was among the elderly, especially those seventy-five or older (Conti et al. 2005). Given their disproportionate exposure to heat waves, it follows that disadvantaged groups are at a particular risk for the mental health consequences related to heat waves. For example, during a heat wave in 2008 in a city in Australia, the area witnessed an increased rate of mortality attributed to mental disorders among the elderly (Hansen et al. 2008).

Similarly, the population health effects of natural disasters are not borne equally in society. In most coastal cities and towns, for instance, the wealthy occupy high grounds, whereas the poor and minorities generally live in low-lying areas, which are more vulnerable to storm damage (Cutter 1996). To illustrate, the devastation of Hurricane Katrina is known to have disproportionately affected low-income African-Americans/blacks in New Orleans because they were most likely to live in the low-lying center of the city, whereas higher-income whites generally occupied suburbs on higher ground (Snyder 2005). Following the storm, 53 percent of African-American/black residents reported "losing everything," compared to 19 percent of white residents (Jones 2006). Moreover, because government officials provided no means of public transportation out of New Orleans before Katrina's landfall, evacuation was dependent on car ownership: 33 percent of African Americans/blacks (and 52 percent of poor African-Americans/blacks) in the city had no car, compared to 10 percent of whites (Berube and Raphael 2005). It follows that on exposure to Katrina's ravages, African-American/black race and lower income predicted higher risk for PTSD (Galea et al. 2007).

Likewise, forced migration is one means by which climate change may influence population mental health. Climate change is likely to force migration because it may degrade the agricultural viability of lands and associated livelihoods for communities that rely on these for sustenance. Forced migration is, in this way, a function of the lack of wealth, influence, or transferrable skill sets that enable self-support—a function of poverty and marginalization. What is more, the potentially negative consequences of forced migration, such as exploitation and abuse, are tied implicitly to the absence of resources that force individuals into potentially exploitative situations to begin with. The costs of war are also disproportionately borne by the poor. Conflict is more common in resource-limited contexts because of poverty and direct dependence on natural resources for survival (Elbadawi and Sambanis 2000). Moreover, the consequences of war are more devastating among the poor, who often lack the ability to escape conflict and for whom relative losses are more pronounced. There is also clear evidence that physical health is a function of socioeconomic position(Dalstra et al. 2005), suggesting that the influence of climate change on physical health, as well as the mental health burden it mediates, is likely to bear more strongly on the poor as well.

Given that low socioeconomic position is itself a stressor (Zimmerman and Katon 2005), the disproportionate influence of climate change on the mental health of the poor is concerning. As much of the mental health consequence of climate change will be borne by the poor and marginalized, a particular focus on the mental health of this population is warranted as the consequences of climate change ensue.

Common Causes of Climate Change and Mental Health

Although we have focused in this chapter on the unidirectional influence of climate change on mental health, it is important to recognize that the relationship between the two may also share common causes. **Consumerism** is a determinant of adverse mental health, as higher consumerism in highly inequitable societies is thought to mediate the relation between income inequality and mental disorder (Pickett and Wilkinson 2010; Pickett, James, and Wilkinson 2006). The overconsumption associated with consumerism is also a clear driver of climate change. For example, the excess combustion of fossil fuels for transport and the overconsumption of greenhouse-gas emitting foods (both are estimated to be responsible for up to 24 and 14 percent of global emissions, respectively) (IPCC 2014) are cornerstones of a consumerist lifestyles. In that respect, materialism and overconsumption may concomitantly drive both climate change and population psychopathology.

Solutions should account for all the mechanisms by which the two pathologies are related. In that respect, understanding the reciprocal mechanisms by which mental pathology may drive climate change, as well as the common causes of both, may yield insight into avenues to mitigate the concomitant pathologies.

Conclusion

Throughout this chapter, we discussed several mechanisms by which climate change may influence mental health and how the consequences of these mechanisms would fall inequitably across the socioeconomic continuum. We discussed how heat waves and natural disasters resulting from climate change will create traumatic stressors that will harm population mental health. Similarly, climate change will degrade arable lands and inundate coastal regions, challenging communities and pressuring them to migrate in search of new livelihoods; exposing them, in the process, to stressors that will have negative consequences for their mental well-being. Global competition over resources depleted by climate change, such as arable land and foodstuffs, and freshwater, will inspire violent conflict with hazardous consequences for mental health. Finally, climate change will increase physical morbidity and the subsequent mental disorder that accompanies it as more people struggle with the realities of chronic disease.

Importantly, the consequences of climate change will not be equitable. Because each of these mechanisms functions through the changing availability of resources, those who have the least will suffer most. The question of human well-being is intimately tied to the Earth that we share, and its well-being is a consequence of our own. Without a full appreciation of that reciprocity, attempts to intervene on either are likely to be ineffectual.

DISCUSSION QUESTIONS

1. What can be done, if anything, to mitigate the population mental health consequences of climate change?

2. Are some of the mechanisms relating climate change to mental health more amenable to intervention than others? If so, which of the mechanisms? And why?

3. Which mechanisms relating climate change to mental health can have an acute effect on an individual's mental health? And which are more likely to have a gradual effect on mental health?

4. Why will the burden of population mental health resulting from climate change be unequal, and what can be done to address this?

5. How would understanding of the common causes of climate change and mental health effect our approach to mitigate both?

KEY TERMS

Consumerism: A preoccupation with and an inclination toward the buying of consumer goods.

Forced migration: The involuntary movements of refugees and internally displaced people (those displaced by conflict within their country of origin) and people displaced by natural or environmental disasters, famine, chemical or nuclear disasters, or development projects.

Major depressive disorder (MDD): A mood disorder characterized by a pervasive and persistent sense of hopelessness and despair.

Mental health: A state of well-being in which every individual realizes their own potential, can cope with the normal stresses of life, can work productively and fruitfully, and is able to contribute to the community.

Posttraumatic stress disorder (PTSD): A mental health condition triggered by a terrifying event—war, disaster, or physical or emotional trauma.

References

Adano, W. R., T. Dietz, K. Witsenburg, and F. Zaal. 2012. "Climate Change, Violent Conflict and Local Institutions in Kenya's Drylands." *Journal of Peace Research* 49(1):65–80. doi:10.1177/0022343311427344.

Afolayan, A. A., and I. O. Adelekan. 1999. "The Role of Climatic Variations on Migration and Human Health in Africa." *Environmentalist* 18 (4):213–18. doi:10.1023/A:1006581002775.

Ahmedani, B. K., E. L. Peterson, Y. Hu, R. C. Rossom, F. Lynch, C. Y. Lu, B. E Waitzfelder et al. 2017. "Major Physical Health Conditions and Risk of Suicide." *American Journal of Preventive Medicine* 53 (3):308–15. doi:10.1016/j.amepre.2017.04.001.

Allison, E. H., A. L. Perry, M.-C. Badjeck, W. N. Adger, K. Brown, D. Conway, A. S. Halls et al. 2009. "Vulnerability of National Economies to the Impacts of Climate Change on Fisheries." *Fish and Fisheries* 10 (2):173–96. doi:10.1111/j.1467-2979.2008.00310.x.

Andrees, B., and P. Belser. 2009. *Forced Labor : Coercion and Exploitation in the Private Economy.* Boulder, CO: Lynne Rienner Publishers.

Arnetz, B. B., S.-O. Brenner, L. Levi, R. Hjelm, I. L. Petterson, J. Wasserman, B. Petrini, P. Eneroth et al. 1991. "Neuroendocrine and Immunologic Effects of Unemployment and Job Insecurity." *Psychotherapy and Psychosomatics* 55 (2–4):76–80. doi:10.1159/000288412.

Aumann, H. H., A. Ruzmaikin, and J. Teixeira. 2008. "Frequency of Severe Storms and Global Warming." *Geophysical Research Letters* 35 (19):L19805. doi:10.1029/2008GL034562.

Barnett, J., and W. N. Adger. 2007. "Climate Change, Human Security and Violent Conflict." *Political Geography* 26 (6):639–55. doi:10.1016/J.POLGEO.2007.03.003.

Bell, V., F. Méndez, C. Martínez, P. P. Palma, and M. Bosch. 2012. "Characteristics of the Colombian Armed Conflict and the Mental Health of Civilians Living in Active Conflict Zones." *Conflict and Health* 6 (1):10. doi:10.1186/1752-1505-6-10.

Belser, P. 2005. "Forced Labour and Human Trafficking: Estimating the Profits." *SSRN Electronic Journal* March 2005. doi:10.2139/ssrn.1838403.

Berube, A., and S. Raphael. 2005. *Access to Cars in New Orleans.* Washington, DC: Brookings Institution. https://trid.trb.org/view/771719.

Bhugra D. 2004. "Migration and Mental Health." *Acta Neurologica Scandinavica* 109 (4):243–58. http://www.ncbi.nlm.nih.gov/pubmed/15008797.

Blaine B. 2008. "Does Depression Cause Obesity?" *Journal of Health Psycholology* 13 (8):1190–97. doi:10.1177/1359105308095977.

Briguglio, L. 1995. "Small Island Developing States and Their Economic Vulnerabilities." *World Development* 23 (9):1615–32. doi:10.1016/0305-750X(95)00065-K.

Carbon Brief. 2017. "Mapped: How Climate Change Affects Extreme Weather around the World." *Published* July 2017. https://www.carbonbrief.org/mapped-how-climate-change-affects-extreme-weather-around-the-world.

Carleton, T. A. 2017. "Crop-Damaging Temperatures Increase Suicide Rates in India." *Proceedings of the National Academy of Sciences of the USA* 114 (33):8746–51. doi:10.1073/pnas.1701354114.

Cerdá, M., M. Paczkowski, S. Galea, K. Nemethy, C. Péan, and M. Desvarieux. 2013. "Psychopathology in the Aftermath of the Haiti Earthquake: A Population-Based Study of Posttraumatic Stress Disorder and Major Depression." *Depression and Anxiety* 30 (5):413–24. doi:10.1002/da.22007.

Chemin, M., J. de Laat, and J. Haushofer. 2013. "Negative Rainfall Shocks Increase Levels of the Stress Hormone Cortisol among Poor Farmers in Kenya." *SSRN Electronic Journal* July 2013. doi:10.2139/ssrn.2294171.

Conti, S., P. Meli, G. Minelli, R. Solimini, V. Toccaceli, M. Vichi, C. Beltrano, and L. Perini. 2005. "Epidemiologic Study of Mortality during the Summer 2003 Heat Wave in Italy." *Environmental Research* 98 (3):390–9. doi:10.1016/J.ENVRES.2004.10.009.

Cutter, S. L. 1996. "Vulnerability to Environmental Hazards." *Progress in Human Geography* 20 (4):529–39. doi:10.1177/030913259602000407.

Dalstra, J., A. Kunst, C. Borrell, E. Breeze, E. Cambois, G. Costa, J. J. M. Geurts et al. 2005. "Socioeconomic Differences in the Prevalence of Common Chronic Diseases: An Overview of Eight European Countries." *International Journal of Epidemiology* 34 (2):316–26. doi:10.1093/ije/dyh386.

Damti, O. B., O. Sarid, E. Sheiner, T. Zilberstein, and J. Cwikel. 2008. [Stress and Distress in Infertility among Women]. *Harefuah* 147 (3):256–60, 276. http://www.ncbi.nlm.nih.gov/pubmed/18488870.

Decker, M. R., S. Oram, J. Gupta, and J. G. Silverman. 2009. "Forced Prostitution and Trafficking for Sexual Exploitation among Women and Girls in Situations of Migration and Conflict: Review and Recommendations for Reproductive Health Care Personnel." In *Women, Migration, and Conflict*, edited by S. Forbes Martin and J. Tirman, 63–86. Dordrecht: Springer Netherlands. doi:10.1007/978-90-481-2825-9_4.

Dyregrov, A., L. Gupta, R. Gjestad, and E. Mukanoheli. 2000. "Trauma Exposure and Psychological Reactions to Genocide among Rwandan Children." *Journal of Traumatic Stress* 13 (1):3–21. doi:10.1023/A:1007759112499.

Elbadawi, E., and N. Sambanis. 2000. "Why Are There So Many Civil Wars in Africa? Understanding and Preventing Violent Conflict." *Journal of African Economies* 9 (3):244–69. doi:10.1093/jae/9.3.244.

Energy & Climate Intelligence Unit. 2017. *Heavy Weather: Tracking the Fingerprints of Climate Change, Two Years after the Paris Summit.* London: ECIU. https://eciu.net/analysis/reports/2017/heavy-weather.

Faith, M. S., M. Butryn, T. A. Wadden, A. Fabricatore, A. M. Nguyen, and S. B. Heymsfield. 2011. "Evidence for Prospective Associations among Depression and Obesity in Population-Based Studies." *Obesity Reviews* 12 (5):e438–e453. doi:10.1111/j.1467-789X.2010.00843.x.

Fazel, M., J. Wheeler, and J. Danesh. 2005. "Prevalence of Serious Mental Disorder in 7000 Refugees Resettled in Western Countries: A Systematic Review." *Lancet* 365 (9467):1309–14. doi:10.1016/S0140-6736(05)61027-6.

Fell, S. C., J. L. Carrivick, and L. E. Brown. 2017. "The Multitrophic Effects of Climate Change and Glacier Retreat in Mountain Rivers." *Bioscience.* 67 (10):897–911. doi:10.1093/biosci/bix107.

Feng, S., A. B. Krueger, and M. Oppenheimer. 2010 "Linkages among Climate Change, Crop Yields and Mexico-US Cross-Border Migration." *Proceedings of the National Academy of Sciences of the USA* 107 (32):14257–62. doi:10.1073/pnas.1002632107.

Fischer, D. 2009. "Climate Change Hits Poor Hardest in U.S." *Scientific American.* Published May 29, 2009. https://www.scientificamerican.com/article/climate-change-hits-poor-hardest/.

Friedrich, M. J. 2017. "Depression Is the Leading Cause of Disability around the World." *JAMA* 317 (15):1517. doi:10.1001/jama.2017.3826.

Galea, S., C. R. Brewin, M. Gruber, R. T. Jones, D. W. King, L. A. King, R. J. McNally, et al. 2007. "Exposure to Hurricane-Related Stressors and Mental Illness after Hurricane Katrina." *Archives of General Psychiatry* 64 (12):1427. doi:10.1001/archpsyc.64.12.1427.

Galea, S., A. Nandi, and D. Vlahov. 2005. "The Epidemiology of Post-Traumatic Stress Disorder after Disasters." *Epidemiologic Reviews* 27 (1):78–91. doi:10.1093/epirev/mxi003.

Galea, S., P. C. Rockers, G. Saydee, R. Macauley, S. T. Varpilah, and M. E. Kruk. 2010. "Persistent Psychopathology in the Wake of Civil War: Long-Term Posttraumatic Stress Disorder in Nimba County, Liberia." *American Journal of Public Health* 100 (9):1745–51. doi:10.2105/AJPH.2009.179697.

Galea, S, M. Tracy, F. Norris, and S. F. Coffey. 2008. "Financial and Social Circumstances and the Incidence and Course of PTSD in Mississippi during the First Two Years after Hurricane Katrina." *Journal of Traumatic Stress* 21 (4):357–68. doi:10.1002/jts.20355.

Grove, N. J., and A. B. Zwi. 2006. "Our Health and Theirs: Forced Migration, Othering, and Public Health." *Social Science & Medicine* 62 (8):1931–42. doi:10.1016/j.socscimed.2005.08.061.

Hansen, A., P. Bi, M. Nitschke, P. Ryan, D. Pisaniello, and G. Tucker. 2008. "The Effect of Heat Waves on Mental Health in a Temperate Australian City." *Environmental Health Perspectives* 116 (10):1369–75. doi:10.1289/ehp.11339.

Haushofer, J., and E. Fehr. 2014. "On the Psychology of Poverty." *Science* 344 (6186):862–7. doi:10.1126/science.1232491.

Hendrix, C. S., and I. Salehyan. 2012. "Climate Change, Rainfall, and Social Conflict in Africa." *Journal of Peace Research* 49 (1):35–50. doi:10.1177/0022343311426165.

Henry, S., B. Schoumaker, and C. Beauchemin. 2003. "The Impact of Rainfall on the First Out-Migration: A Multi-level Event-History Analysis in Burkina Faso." *Population and Environment* 25 (5):423–60. doi:10.1023/B:POEN.0000036928.17696.e8.

Hiott, A. E., J. G. Grzywacz, S. W. Davis, S. A. Quandt, and T. A. Arcury. 2008. "Migrant Farmworker Stress: Mental Health Implications." *Journal of Rural Health* 24 (1):32-39. doi:10.1111/j.1748-0361.2008.00134.x.

Hossain, M., C. Zimmerman, M. Abas, M. Light, and C. Watts. 2010. "The Relationship of Trauma to Mental Disorders among Trafficked and Sexually Exploited Girls and Women." *American Journal of Public Health* 100 (12):2442–49. doi:10.2105/AJPH.2009.173229.

Hovey, J. D. 2000. "Acculturative Stress, Depression, and Suicidal Ideation in Mexican Immigrants." *Cultural Diversity & Ethnic Minority Psychology* 6 (2):134–51. http://www.ncbi.nlm.nih.gov/pubmed/10910528.

Hovey, J. D., and C. G. Magaña. 2003. "Suicide Risk Factors among Mexican Migrant Farmworker Women in the Midwest United States." *Archives of Suicide Research* 7 (2):107–21. doi:10.1080/13811110301579.

Intergovernmental Panel on Climate Change. 2014. *AR5 Synthesis Report: Climate Change 2014*. Geneva, Switzerland: IPCC. https://www.ipcc.ch/report/ar5/syr/.

Intergovernmental Panel on Climate Change. 2018. *Global Warming of 1.5 oC. Special Report*. Geneva, Switzerland: IPCC. https://www.ipcc.ch/sr15/chapter/summary-for-policy-makers/.

Jones, J. F. 2006. *One in Three New Orleans Residents Lost Everything Following Hurricane*. Gallup. https://news.gallup.com/poll/21703/one-three-new-orleans-residents-lost-everything-following-hurricane.aspx.

Juurlink, D. N., N. Herrmann, J. P. Szalai, A. Kopp, and D. A. Redelmeier. 2004. "Medical Illness and the Risk of Suicide in the Elderly." *Archives of Internal Medicine* 164 (11):1179. doi:10.1001/archinte.164.11.1179.

Kern. D., A. Auchincloss, M. Stehr, A. V. Diez Roux, L. V. Moore, G. P. Kanter, and L. F. Robinson. 2017. "Neighborhood Prices of Healthier and Unhealthier Foods and Associations with Diet Quality: Evidence from the Multi-Ethnic Study of Atherosclerosis." *International Journal of Environmental Research and Public Health* 14 (11):1394. doi:10.3390/ijerph14111394.

Kip, K. E., L. Rosenzweig, D. F. Hernandez, A. Shuman, D. M. Diamond, S. A. Girling, K. L. Sullivan, et al. 2014. "Accelerated Resolution Therapy for Treatment of Pain Secondary to Symptoms of Combat-Related Posttraumatic Stress Disorder." *European Journal of Psychotraumatology* 7:5. doi:10.3402/ejpt.v5.24066.

Klare, M. T. 2002. "The Deadly Nexus: Oil, Terrorism, and America's National Security." *Current History* 101 (414):20. http://www.currenthistory.com/pdf_org_files/101_659_414.pdf.

Kovats, R. S., and S. Hajat. 2008. "Heat Stress and Public Health: A Critical Review." *Annual Review of Public Health* 29 (1):41–55. doi:10.1146/annurev.publhealth.29.020907.090843.

Lawrence, D., and K. Vandecar. 2015. "Effects of Tropical Deforestation on Climate and Agriculture." *Nature Climate Change* 5 (1):27–36. doi:10.1038/nclimate2430.

Li, G., and H. Lin. 2017. "Recent Decadal Glacier Mass Balances over the Western Nyainqentanglha Mountains and the Increase in Their Melting Contribution to Nam Co Lake Measured by Differential Bistatic SAR Interferometry." *Global and Planetary Change* 149:177–90. doi:10.1016/J.GLOPLACHA.2016.12.018.

Lindert, J., O. S. von Ehrenstein, S. Priebe, A. Mielck, and E. Brähler. 2009. "Depression and Anxiety in Labor Migrants and Refugees—A Systematic Review and Meta-Analysis." *Social Science & Medicine* 69 (2):246–57. doi:10.1016/j.socscimed.2009.04.032.

Lindert, J., M. Schouler-Ocak, A. Heinz, and S. Priebe. 2008. "Mental Health, Health Care Utilisation of Migrants in Europe." *European Psychiatry* 23:14–20. doi:10.1016/S0924-9338(08)70057-9.

Link, B. G., and J. C. Phelan. 1996. "Understanding Sociodemographic Differences in Health—The Role of Fundamental Social Causes." *American Journal of Public Health* 86 (4):471–73. http://www.ncbi.nlm.nih.gov/pubmed/8604773.

Lobell, D. B., W. Schlenker, and J. Costa-Roberts. 2011. "Climate Trends and Global Crop Production since 1980." *Science* 333 (6042):616–20. doi:10.1126/science.1204531.

Lopes Cardozo, B., A. Vergara, F. Agani, and C. A. Gotway. 2000. "Mental Health, Social Functioning, and Attitudes of Kosovar Albanians Following the War in Kosovo." *JAMA* 284 (5):569–77. http://www.ncbi.nlm.nih.gov/pubmed/10918702.

Luppa, M., S. Heinrich, M. C. Angermeyer, H.-H. König, and S. G. Riedel-Heller. 2007. "Cost-of-Illness Studies of Depression." *Journal of Affective Disorders* 98 (1–2):29–43. doi:10.1016/j.jad.2006.07.017.

Mcgranahan, G., D. Balk, and B. Anderson. 2007. "The Rising Tide: Assessing the Risks of Climate Change and Human Settlements in Low Elevation Coastal Zones." *Environment and Urbanization* 19 (1):17–37. doi:10.1177/0956247807076960.

McLeman, R., and B. Smit. 2006. "Migration as an Adaptation to Climate Change." *Climate Change* 76 (1–2):31–53. doi:10.1007/s10584-005-9000-7.

McWilliams, L. A., B. J. Cox, and M. W. Enns. 2003. "Mood and Anxiety Disorders Associated with Chronic Pain: An Examination in a Nationally Representative Sample." *Pain* 106(1–2):127–33. http://www.ncbi.nlm.nih.gov/pubmed/14581119.

Mearns, R., and A. Norton, eds. 2009. *The Social Dimensions of Climate Change*. Washington, DC: World Bank. doi:10.1596/978-0-8213-7887-8.

Milliken, C. S., J. L. Auchterlonie, and C. W. Hoge. 2007. "Longitudinal Assessment of Mental Health Problems among Active and Reserve Component Soldiers Returning from the Iraq War." *JAMA* 298 (18):2141. doi:10.1001/jama.298.18.2141.

Mitchell, B. C., and J. Chakraborty. 2015. "Landscapes of Thermal Inequity: Disproportionate Exposure to Urban Heat in the Three Largest US Cities." *Environmental Research Letters* 10 (11):115005. doi:10.1088/1748-9326/10/11/115005.

Mollica, R. F. 2004. "Surviving Torture." *New England Journal of Medicine* 351 (1):5–7. doi:10.1056/NEJMp048141.

Must, A., and N. M. McKeown. 2000. *The Disease Burden Associated with Overweight and Obesity*. South Dartmouth, MA: MDText.com, Inc. http://www.ncbi.nlm.nih.gov/pubmed/25905320.

Nabi, H., M. Kivimäki, G. D. Batty, et al. 2013. "Increased Risk of Coronary Heart Disease among Individuals Reporting Adverse Impact of Stress on Their Health: The Whitehall II Prospective Cohort Study." *European Heart Journal* 34 (34):2697–2705. doi:10.1093/eurheartj/eht216.

Naghavi, M., A. A. Abajobir, C. Abbafati, et al. 2017. "Global, Regional, and National Age-Sex Specific Mortality for 264 Causes Of Death, 1980–2016: A Systematic Analysis for the Global Burden of Disease Study 2016." *Lancet* 390 (10100):1151–1210. doi:10.1016/S0140-6736(17)32152-9.

National Oceanic and Atmospheric Administration. 2013. *National Coastal Population Report: Population Trends from 1970 to 2020*. https://coast.noaa.gov/digitalcoast/training/population-report.html.

Neria, Y., A. Nandi, and S. Galea. 2008. "Post-Traumatic Stress Disorder Following Disasters: A Systematic Review." *Psychological Medicine* 38 (4):467–80. doi:10.1017/S0033291707001353.

Nkonya, E., T. Johnson, H. Y. Kwon, and E. Kato. 2016. "Economics of Land Degradation in Sub-Saharan Africa." In *Economics of Land Degradation and Improvement—A Global Assessment for Sustainable Development*, 215–59. Cham: Springer International Publishing. doi:10.1007/978-3-319-19168-3_9.

Onyut, L. P., F. Neuner, V. Ertl, E. Schauer, M. Odenwald, and T. Elbert. 2009. "Trauma, Poverty and Mental Health among Somali and Rwandese Refugees Living in an African Refugee Settlement—An Epidemiological Study." *Conflict and Health* 3 (1):6. doi:10.1186/1752-1505-3-6.

Ottisova, L., S. Hemmings, L. M. Howard, C. Zimmerman, and S. Oram. 2016. "Prevalence and Risk of Violence and the Mental, Physical and Sexual Health Problems Associated with Human Trafficking: An Updated Systematic Review." *Epidemiology and Psychiatric Sciences* 25 (04):317–41. doi:10.1017/S2045796016000135.

Parry, M., C. Rosenzweig, and M. Livermore. 2005. "Climate Change, Global Food Supply and Risk of Hunger." *Philosophical Transactions of the Royal Society of London. Series B, Biological Sciences* 360 (1463):2125–38. doi:10.1098/rstb.2005.1751.

Pelling, M., and J. I. Uitto. 2001. "Small Island Developing States: Natural Disaster Vulnerability and Global Change." *Global Environmental Change Part B: Environmental Hazards* 3 (2):49-62. doi:10.1016/S1464-2867(01)00018-3.

Pesonen, A.-K., K. Raikkonen, K. Heinonen, E. Kajantie, T. Forsen, and J. G. Eriksson. 2007. "Depressive Symptoms in Adults Separated from Their Parents as Children: A Natural Experiment during World War II." *American Journal of Epidemiology* 166 (10):1126–33. doi:10.1093/aje/kwm254.

Phelan, J. C., and B. G. Link. 2005. "Controlling Disease and Creating Disparities: A Fundamental Cause Perspective." *Journals of Gerontology: Series B* 60(special issue 2):S27–S33. doi:10.1093/geronb/60.Special_Issue_2.S27.

Pickett, K. E., O. W. James, and R. G. Wilkinson. 2006. "Income Inequality and the Prevalence of Mental Illness: A Preliminary International Analysis." *Journal of Epidemiology and Community Health* 60 (7):646–7. doi:10.1136/jech.2006.046631.

Pickett, K.E., and R. G. Wilkinson. 2010. "Inequality: An Underacknowledged Source of Mental Illness and Distress." *British Journal of Psychiatry* 197 (06):426–8. doi:10.1192/bjp.bp.109.072066.

Piguet, E. 2008. *Climate Change and Forced Migration.* Geneva, Switzerland: United Nations High Commissioner for Refugees. http://citeseerx.ist.psu.edu/viewdoc/summary?doi=10.1.1.430.9162.

Plagge, J. M., M. W. Lu, T. I. Lovejoy, A. I. Karl, and S. K. Dobscha. 2013. "Treatment of Comorbid Pain and PTSD in Returning Veterans: A Collaborative Approach Utilizing Behavioral Activation." *Pain Medicine* 14 (8):1164–72. doi:10.1111/pme.12155.

Poncelet, A., F. Gemenne, M. Martiniello, and H. Bousetta H. 2010. "A Country Made for Disasters: Environmental Vulnerability and Forced Migration in Bangladesh." In *Environment, Forced Migration and Social Vulnerability*, edited by T. Afifi and Jäger, 211–22. Berlin, Heidelberg: Springer *Berlin Heidelberg.* doi:10.1007/978-3-642-12416-7_16.

Rademaker, M., K. Jans, C. Frattina Della Frattina, H. Rõõs, S. Slingerland, A. Borum, and L. van Schaik. 2016. *The Economics of Planetary Security Climate Change as an Economic Conflict Factor.* The Hague: The Hague Centre for Strategic Studies.https://hcss.nl/report/economics-planetary-security-climate-change-economic-conflict-factor.

Reed, M. S., and L. C. Stringer. 2016. *Land Degradation, Desertification and Climate Change.* London ; New York : Routledge. doi:10.4324/9780203071151.

Rodney, N. C., and C. J. Mulligan. 2014. "A Biocultural Study of the Effects of Maternal Stress on Mother and Newborn Health in the Democratic Republic of Congo." *American Journal of Physical Anthropology* 155 (2):200–9. doi:10.1002/ajpa.22568.

Sastry, N. 2007. *Tracing the Effects of Hurricane Katrina on the Population of New Orleans.* Santa Monica, CA: Rand Corporation. https://www.rand.org/pubs/working_papers/WR483.html.

Sastry, N., and J. Gregory. 2014. "The Location of Displaced New Orleans Residents in the Year after Hurricane Katrina." *Demography* 51 (3):753–75. doi:10.1007/s13524-014-0284-y.

Scheelbeek, P. F. D., F. A. Bird, H. L. Tuomisto, R. Green, F. B. Harris, E. J. M. Joy, Z. Chalabi et al. 2018. "Effect of Environmental Changes on Vegetable and Legume Yields and Nutritional Quality." *Proceedings of the National Academy of Sciences of the USA.* 115 (26):6804–9. doi:10.1073/pnas.1800442115.

Scheffran, J. 2012. *Climate Change, Human Security and Violent Conflict : Challenges for Societal Stability.* New York: Springer.

Schlenker, W., and M. J. Roberts. 2009. "Nonlinear Temperature Effects Indicate Severe Damages to U.S. Crop Yields under Climate Change." *Proceedings of the National Academy of Sciences of the USA* 106 (37):15594–98. doi:10.1073/pnas.0906865106.

Seal, K. H., D. Bertenthal, C. R. Miner, S. Sen, and C. Marmar. 2007. "Bringing the War Back Home." *Archives of Internal Medicine* 167 (5):476. doi:10.1001/archinte.167.5.476.

Snyder, M. G. 2005. "It Didn't Begin with Katrina." *Shelterforce Online. Published September* 1, 2005. https://shelterforce.org/2005/09/01/it-didnt-begin-with-katrina-2/.

Spatz Widom, C., K. DuMont, and S. J. Czaja. 2007. "A Prospective Investigation of Major Depressive Disorder and Comorbidity in Abused and Neglected Children Grown Up." *Archives of General Psychiatry* 64 (1):49. doi:10.1001/archpsyc.64.1.49.

Subramanian, S. V., and I. Kawachi. 2004. "Income Inequality and Health: What Have We Learned So Far?" *Epidemiologic Reviews* 26 (1):78–91. doi:10.1093/epirev/mxh003.

Sullivan, M. M., and R. Rehm. 2005. "Mental Health of Undocumented Mexican Immigrants: A Review of the Literature." *Advances in Nursing Science* 28 (3):240–51. http://www.ncbi.nlm.nih.gov/pubmed/16106153.

Thabet, A. M., S. S. Thabet, and P. Vostanis. 2016. "The Relationship between War Trauma, PTSD, Depression, and Anxiety among Palestinian Children in the Gaza Strip." *Health Science Journal* 10 (5). doi:10.4172/1791-809X.1000100503.

Thabet, A. M., and P. Vostanis. 1999. "Post-Traumatic Stress Reactions in Children of War." *Journal of Child Psychology and Psychiatry* 40 (3):385–91. doi:10.1111/1469-7610.00456.

Thompson, R., R. Hornigold, L. Page, and T. Waite. 2018. "Associations between High Ambient Temperatures and Heat Waves with Mental Health Outcomes: A Systematic Review." *Public Health* 161:171–91. doi:10.1016/J.PUHE.2018.06.008.

Tir, J., and D. M. Stinnett. 2012. "Weathering Climate Change: Can Institutions Mitigate International Water Conflict?" *Journal of Peace Research* 49(1):211–25. doi:10.1177/0022343311427066.

Townsend, M., M. Mahoney, J. A. Jones, K. Ball, J. Salmon, and C. F. Finch. 2003. "Too Hot to Trot? Exploring Potential Links between Climate Change, Physical Activity and Health." *Journal of Science and Medicine in Sport* 6 (3):260–65. http://www.ncbi.nlm.nih.gov/pubmed/14609142.

Trautmann, S., J. Rehm, and H.-U. Wittchen. 2016. "The Economic Costs of Mental Disorders: Do Our Societies React Appropriately to the Burden of Mental Disorders? *EMBO Reports* 17 (9):1245–49. doi:10.15252/embr.201642951.

Von Korff, M., P. Crane, M. Lane, D. L. Miglioretti, G. Simon, K. Saunders, P. Stang, N. Brandenburg, and R. Kessler. 2005. "Chronic Spinal Pain and Physical–Mental Comorbidity in the United States: Results from the National Comorbidity Survey Replication." *Pain* 113 (3):331–39. doi:10.1016/j.pain.2004.11.010

Watts, N., M. Amann, N. Arnell, S. Ayeb-Karlsson, K. Belesova, H. Berry, T. Bouley et al. 2018. "The 2018 Report of the Lancet Countdown on Health and Climate Change: Shaping the Health of Nations for Centuries to Come." *Lancet* 392 (10163):2479–2514. doi:10.1016/S0140-6736(18)32594-7.

Wehner, M., D. Stone, H. Krishnan, K. Achuta Rao, and F. Castillo. 2016. "The Deadly Combination of Heat and Humidity in India and Pakistan in Summer 2015." *Bulletin of the American Meteorological Society* 97 (12):S81–S86. doi:10.1175/BAMS-D-16-0145.1.

Widom, C. S. 1999. "Posttraumatic Stress Disorder in Abused and Neglected Children Grown Up." *American Journal of Psychiatry* 156 (8):1223–9. doi:10.1176/ajp.156.8.1223.

Wiebe, K., H. Lotze-Campen, R. Sands, A. Tabeau, D. van der Mensbrugghe, A. Biewald, B. Bodirsky et al. 2015. "Climate Change Impacts on Agriculture in 2050 under a Range of Plausible Socioeconomic and Emissions Scenarios." *Environmental Research Letters* 10 (8):085010. doi:10.1088/1748-9326/10/8/085010.

Wright, L. D., J. P. M. Syvitski, and C. R. Nichols. 2019. "Sea Level Rise: Recent Trends and Future Projections." In *Tomorrow's Coasts: Complex and Impermanent*, edited by L. D. Wright and C. R. Nichols, 47–57. Cham: Springer. doi:10.1007/978-3-319-75453-6_3.

Zimmerman, F. J., and W. Katon. 2005. "Socioeconomic Status, Depression Disparities, and Financial Strain: What Lies Behind the Income-Depression Relationship?" *Health Economics* 14 (12):1197–1215. doi:10.1002/hec.1011.

CHAPTER 11

WORKER HEALTH

Miranda Dally and Lee S. Newman

Introduction

Workers are particularly susceptible to experiencing negative health impacts from climate change. Across a broad range of occupations, workers are affected by a multitude of climate-related exposures for longer durations and at greater intensities than the general public (Kiefer et al. 2016). Climate change will result in increasing prevalence, distribution, and severity of known **occupational hazards** spanning a variety of geographic regions and occupations (Schulte et al. 2016). Additionally, with the emergence of new industries in response to climate change, new unanticipated hazards are expected.

Fundamentally, climate change is a stress multiplier, putting pressure on vulnerable systems, populations, and regions. Climate change affects human health by compounding existing medical conditions and health threats and by placing new stresses on housing, food and water security, job security, and many determinants of stable livelihoods and safe workplaces. Furthermore, occupational exposures may be exacerbated by onerous non-work-related issues, such as inadequate housing and lack of air conditioning, which are simultaneously affected by climate exposures (Kiefer et al. 2016).

This chapter explores the hazards that workers will face due to climate change. These include increased ambient temperature, air pollution, ultraviolet exposure, extreme weather, vector-borne disease and expanded habitats, industrial transitions, and emerging industries. We explore adaptation considerations and strategies and the burden of climate change on worker health and the impact of poor worker health on society as whole.

Hazards

Increased Ambient Temperature

Increased ambient temperature is associated with an increased risk of mortality from heat illness and the exacerbation of underlying medical conditions (Sarofim et al. 2016; Schifano et al. 2012). Excessive heat exposure is a particular problem for working people because internal heat production adds to environmental heat exposure when strenuous work is carried out (Kjellstrom, Holmer, and Lemke 2009). For example, workers in outdoor occupations with high physical load, such as agriculture and construction, are most at risk for heat-related illnesses (Lundgren et al. 2013). Workers in these industries who are paid a piece-rate and those with poor economic conditions, with few or nonexistent bargaining possibilities, are also particularly vulnerable (Schulte et al. 2016). The human body is designed to maintain a core body temperature of 37°C (98.6°F). To maintain this temperature, heat dissipation occurs through dry heat loss (radiation and convection) and evaporative heat loss (sweating). The evaporation of sweat is extremely effective and therefore becomes more and more critical with increasing environmental

KEY CONCEPTS

- Workers are one of the populations most susceptible to experiencing the effects of climate change. They are affected by climate-related exposures for longer durations and at greater intensities than the general public.

- There is a need to develop comprehensive adaptation and response strategies addressing multiple stakeholders: the individual worker, employer, and public health agencies.

- The burden climate change has placed on workers not only affects the individual's health; it causes economic hardship, and indirectly affects families, employers, and society overall.

temperature; however, sweating imposes the greatest strain on the body and can lead to dehydration. Individuals have varying abilities to tolerate heat stress and it is increasingly recognized that social determinants and personal characteristics affect individual vulnerability. Additionally, factors such as preexisting disease, clothing, age, gender, ability for heat acclimatization, level of physical activity, and body size can influence the health impact of heat stress (Lundgren et al. 2013). Occupational-related factors, such as the use of personal protective equipment, can add additional weight and heat burden to workers' bodies. Job requirements and demands coupled with a lack of heat safety protocols can inhibit the ability of workers to seek shade, hydration, and time for recovery. These issues are compounded especially in workers with already high heat loads, such as fire fighters, emergency response, construction, and agricultural workers. Heat illness ranges from minor to life threatening. Minor heat illnesses include heat cramps, which are intermittent and often occur because of electrolyte imbalances due to dehydration; heat edema, with swelling primarily in the feet and ankles; and prickly heat, which is an inflammatory disorder of the skin that results from the blockage of sweat glands. Heat syncope is a more severe illness in which a drop in cardiac output occurs, resulting in insufficient cerebral perfusion and loss of consciousness. Major heat illnesses include heat exhaustion and heatstroke. Symptoms of heat exhaustion include fatigue, generalized weakness, vertigo, nausea, and headache. These are often accompanied by total body salt and water depletion, and they occur when core body temperature is between 37°C and 40°C (98.6°F and 104°F). Heatstroke occurs when core body temperature is above 40°C. It is the most catastrophic heat illness, resulting in central nervous system dysfunction, liver injury, renal injury, and rhabdomyolysis, and multiorgan failure and ultimately can result in death (Marx and Rosen 2014).

Heat exposure can have other impacts on an individual's health. Heat exposure can exacerbate cardiovascular, respiratory, and renal disease, which can result in significant morbidity and mortality. Additionally, heat exposure may be implicated in emerging noninfectious occupational-related diseases. For example, there has been an epidemic of chronic kidney disease (CKD), which is not associated with the traditional risk factors of diabetes and hypertension disproportionately affecting young agricultural workers in hot environments (Johnson, Wesseling, and Newman 2019). In one study, sugarcane workers with normal kidney function were shown to experience recurrent subclinical kidney injury, associated with elevations in biomarkers of injury, suggesting that extreme physical work in high temperatures may be contributing factors (Figure 11.1) (Sorensen et al. 2019).

Increasing workplace temperatures are also associated with an increased risk of **occupational injuries**. Slips, trips, falls, wounds, lacerations, and amputations are the most commonly reported injuries under high heat exposure (Bonafede et al. 2016), likely due to slippery sweaty hands, foggy glasses, hot tools, and working faster to avoid the heat (Adam-Poupart et al. 2015). It has been shown that for each 1°C (1.8°F) increase in daily minimum temperature, the odds of workplace injury increased by 1 percent (McInnes et al. 2017), and another study showed that a 1°C increase in daily maximum temperature resulted in a 1.4 percent increase in work-related injury claims (Sheng et al. 2018). In more tropical climates, the odds of injury attributable to heat are even greater, with a 3% increase in recorded injury risk with each degree increase in daily average WBGT above 30 °C (Dally et al. 2020)

Air Pollution

Workplaces are an important source of exposure to many different types of air pollution such as PM_{10}, NO_2, and SO_2 with levels varying based on air conditioning use, proximity to roadways, and work environment (Pinault, van Donkelaar, and Martin 2017). It has been shown that an increase in NO_2 from the 25th to the 95th percentile was associated with a 1.30 (95

CLINICAL CORRELATES 11.1 CONSTRUCTION WORKERS AND HEAT STRESS

The construction industry comprises approximately 8 percent of workers in America the United States representing up to twelve million employees (Ringen et al. 2018). Hazards are related to job activities but also include exposure to severe weather conditions, such as extreme heat. Construction workers such as roofers and road workers are thirteen times more likely to die from heat-related illness than other professions (Acharya, Boggess, and Zhang 2018; Gubernot, Anderson, and Hunting 2015), and increasing amounts of work-related compensation claims have been associated with warming temperatures (Xiang et al. 2014). Globally, there is a paucity of policies and regulations to protect workers during high-peak seasons (Acharya, Boggess, and Zhang 2018). Heat acclimatization, optimizing work-rest cycles, heat minimizing clothing, adequate food and hydration, and access to climate-controlled environments are strategies to minimize heat-related illness. Some companies have begun to protect workers through anti-heat stress clothing uniforms (Chan et al. 2016) or through dedicated educational programs on the risks of heat illness for workers (El-Shafei et al. 2018). Policies and regulations that support public health not only protect worker health but can optimize worker productivity and advance health equity in an era of climate change.

Construction workers are vulnerable to heat stress representing an opportunity for policy development to protect public health, optimize worker conditions, and maximize productivity.

CLINICAL CORRELATES 11.2 COCOA FARMERS IN AFRICA

Turning cocoa beans into edible chocolate is a labor-intensive process. Cocoa is quite sensitive to weather events with specific periods of plant vulnerability and close surveillance needed for optimal harvesting. Climate change is challenging cocoa yields, particularly in West African countries, Indonesia, and South America. Drought, heat, soil nutrients, pest infestation, weeds, vector-borne diseases, extreme rainfall, wildfires, and deforestation influence production. Many rural farmers rely on rainfall for irrigation causing uncertainty in crop production. Farmers identified extremely high temperatures, stormy rainfall, or delay in rainfall as detrimental to cocoa production (Oyekale 2019).

Cocoa farming is threatened by extremes in precipitation, heat, pest infestation, and deforestation, and cocoa farmers also are affected by climate-sensitive conditions: infectious diseases, heat stress, and ocular abnormalities.

percent CI: 1.24, 1.37) increase in odds of occupational injury, whereas an increase in PM_{10} from the 25th to the 95th percentile resulted in an increase of 1.15 (95 percent CI: 1.11, 1.18), regardless of industry (Schifano et al. 2019). The same study showed the lagged effect of exposure to occupational air pollution on work-related injury was short (two to three days) during the hot season, suggesting that air pollution exposure causes acute neuropsychological effects, such as inattention, which could explain the increase in work-related injury (Sunyer et al. 2017).

Although all workers are at risk of air pollution exposure, whether it be indoor or outdoor, certain occupations are more at risk for **occupational illness** caused by pollutant exposure due to the nature of their work. For example, the average exposure to NO_2 in professional motorcyclists was shown to be 106.77 ± 20.17 ug/m³/h compared to 14.18 ± 3.69 ug/m³/h in office workers, placing the motorcyclists at higher risk for asthma, reduced heart rate variability, myocardial infarction, disruption in thyroid function, and development of otitis media(Carvalho et al. 2018). In traffic police, increases in PM_{10}, NO_2, and SO_2 have been shown to be associated with hyperuricemia (Tang et al. 2019), which can lead to elevated incidence of several diseases such as hypertension, cerebrovascular stroke, and chronic kidney disease (Galán et al.2018; Kamei et al. 2017; Shrivastav et al. 2016). To compound occupational exposure, outdoor workers engaging in physical exertion have increased respiratory rates and are

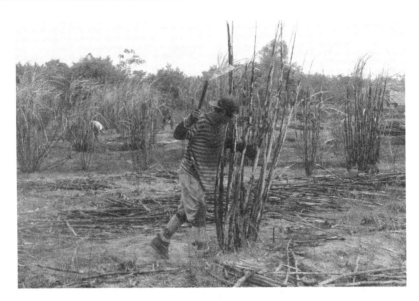

Figure 11.1   Guatemalan sugarcane field being harvested. Workers are in the field for approximately eight hours per day manually cutting sugarcane with a machete. Cut cane is then stacked and collected by workers. Conditions are hot and humid where daily maximum wet-bulb globe temperatures (WBGTs) can range from 29°C to 36°C (84°F to 96.8°F)
Source: Photo credit: Amanda Walker.

therefore especially at risk for health effects from inhaled pollutants due to increased total exposure to poor air. Physical exertion outdoors during ozone periods has been shown to increase cumulative exposure, resulting in respiratory tract inflammation as well as short-term, reversible decreases in lung function (Kinney 2008). Additionally, there is a potential for air pollution to exacerbate risk for both the incidence and severity of infectious disease, such as SARS-CoV-19 (Zhu et al. 2020 and Meo et al. 2020), placing workers with high air pollution exposure at greater risk of respiratory tract associated viral infections.

One disproportionately exposed and vulnerable group of workers are wildland firefighters. Because of the nature of the shift work and residence in fire camps, these workers are subjected to frequent exposure to severely unhealthy air containing polycyclic aromatic hydrocarbons, carbon monoxide, benzene, aldehydes, and fine particulate matter (Groot et al. 2019). In North America, arid conditions due to climate change are fueling more frequent and prolonged wild-fire events (Wuebbles et al. 2017). Research shows that exposure to wildfire smoke is related to negative respiratory health effects (Reid et al. 2016) with acute declines in lung function measures across a work shift (Betchley et al. 1997; Jacquin et al. 2011). Levoglucosan is a biomarker for wood smoke exposure and high levels of levoglucosan in the urine have been shown to be highly correlated with regional fires (Migliaccio et al. 2009). One study found that wildland firefighters in the defined high-levoglucosan exposure group had a mean forced expiratory volume in 1 s (FEV_1) decline of 0.23 L cross-shift compared to a decline of 0.02 L in the low-levoglucosan exposure group (Gaughan et al. 2014), with FEV_1 remaining declined (-0.28 L) three months after the end of the season compared to baseline (Jacquin et al. 2011). In addition to respiratory morbidity, wildland firefighting has mental health impacts, with the prevalence of posttraumatic stress symptoms of 10–20 percent among firefighters responding to major disasters (Leykin, Lahad, and Bonneh 2013; McFarlane 1988).

Air pollution and climate change are also drivers of the increasing burden of allergic diseases, by influencing the environmental abundance of allergenic bioparticles and the release of allergenic proteins and biogenic adjuvants (Reinmuth-Selzle et al. 2017). Increasing levels of CO_2 can influence the beginning, duration, and intensity of pollination as well as the allergen content and allergenicity of pollen grains (Reinmuth-Selzle et al. 2017). For outdoor workers, increased respiratory rates result in increased respiratory inhalation of allergens, which can result in occupational asthma, one of the most frequent work-related diseases (D'Ovidio et al. 2016). Contact with allergens can also result in eye and skin irritation (D'Ovidio et al. 2016).

Occupational illnesses can be affected by air pollution in less obvious ways. Baker's asthma is the most common cause of occupational asthma with an annual incidence of disease upwards of ten cases per 1,000 bakery workers (Brant 2007). Baker's asthma is caused by the inhalation of α-amylase/trypsin inhibitors (ATIs) from wheat and other gluten-containing grains. The ATIs become aerosolized when the grains are ground to flour, putting bakers, confectioners, flour millers, and food processors at risk for exposure. It has been shown that nitration affects the allergenic potential of ATIs suggesting that climate change related increases in NO_2 could lead to an increase in cases of baker's asthma through the increase in nitration of ATIs (Reinmuth-Selzle et al. 2017).

Ultraviolet Exposure

The adverse health effects of exposure to solar radiation are mostly attributed to ultraviolet radiation (Grandi et al. 2016). Climate change increases ultraviolet (UV) radiation levels at ground by affecting the expected recovery of the stratospheric ozone depletion and by altering UV absorbing tropospheric gases, aerosols, and clouds in the atmosphere (Harari Arjona et al. 2016). UV radiations A, B, and C are all considered carcinogenic to humans, increasing the risk for basal cell carcinoma, nonmelanocytic cell carcinoma, and melanoma (Harari Arjona et al. 2016). In addition to cancer, UV exposure can damage eye structures, with long-term exposure to short-wavelength light contributing to age-related macular degeneration, which is the leading cause of vision loss in developed countries (Grandi et al. 2016). Occupational exposure to solar radiation is estimated to account for a large portion of overall lifetime UV dose (Grandi et al. 2016).

Although outdoor workers are often exposed to higher levels of solar radiation, there are some indoor activities that involve exposure through unshielded windows or other glass/transparent plastic barriers (Grandi et al. 2016). For example, a few studies have shown that airline pilots are at increased risk of damage to their eyes from work-related UV exposure (Schulte et al. 2016). As human activity and climate change affects stratospheric ozone layers, workers' UV exposure will continue to increase without proper interventions (Schulte et al. 2016).

Extreme Weather and Natural Disasters

Climate change increases the risk of events like storms, droughts, and floods (World Health Organization 2009). The frequency, intensity, duration, timing, and spatial extent of these extreme events are also modified by climate change (Contessa et al. 2016). Since 2000, the occurrence of these events has increased by 46 percent (Watts et al. 2018). The frequency of natural disasters such as earthquakes, volcanic eruptions, and tsunamis have also increased with the changing climate (Liu, Linde, and Sacks 2009; McGuire 2012). For example, southern Alaska has seen an increase in earthquake activity as a result of reduced load pressures from widespread melting of ice cover, and eruptions of Pavlof in Alaska have been associated with fluctuations in sea level (McGuire 2012).

The health of many different types of workers, such as emergency responders, health care and public health workers, disaster recovery workers, utility workers, hazmat responders, firefighters, police, social services, volunteers, and more, can be affected by extreme weather events and natural disasters. Workers responding to these events can be exposed to storm-downed trees and electrical hazards (Ochsner, Marshall, and Lefkowitz 2018), asbestos (Wickramatillake, Fernando, and Frank 2019), hydrogen sulfide (Wnek et al. 2017), respirable dust (Rando, Kwon, and Lefante 2014), and mold (Bloom et al. 2009; Johanning et al 2014). Foreign relief volunteers can also be exposed to bacteria and viruses for which they are not vaccinated nor immune (Bhandari and Pandey 2018). Because of the increasing frequency and intensity of these events, the need for such workers is increasing (Keim 2008), exposing more people to the risky conditions posed by these events (Kiefer et al. 2106).

Climate-related disasters may also force workers to remain at the worksite and prolong work hours, causing mental fatigue that can lead to increased risk of accidents (Schulte et al. 2016). From 1992 to 2006, a total of 307 workers died while responding to natural disasters. Of these casualties, eighty were workers with fatal injuries from engaging in fighting wildfires, seventy-two worker fatalities were from cleanup and reconstruction after hurricanes, and sixty-two worker deaths resulted from floods (Schulte et al. 2016). Extreme weather events and natural disasters also increase the risk of nonfatal work-related injuries. After Hurricane Sandy the risk of falls (RR: 1.30; 95 percent CI: 1.08-1.57), cut/pierce injuries (RR: 1.24; 95 percent CI: 1.09-1.40), struck-by injuries (RR: 1.17; 95 percent CI: 1.02-1.34), and overexertion (RR: 1.26; 95 percent CI: 1.10-1.44) all increased (Marshall et al. 2016). A survey of earthquake relief workers showed that the most common location of injuries included ankle-foot and hand-wrist (n = 61, 26.5 percent), followed by injuries in leg-knee-calf (n = 22, 9.6 percent), head-neck (4.9 percent), thoracic and abdominal region (2.6 percent), and lower back (3.9 percent) (Du et al. 2016).

One group of workers for whom extreme weather and natural disasters has a severe impact on safety, both directly and indirectly, is those working with ionizing radiation (Contessa et al. 2016). Workers in both nuclear power plants, as well as any radiological facility, are at increased risk of exposure to ionizing radiation due to these events. Extreme weather and natural disasters can cause damage to infrastructure (Kiefer et al. 2016), one example being the disaster at the Tokyo Electric Power Company's Fukushima Dai-ichi Nuclear Power Plant in March 2011. The accident at Fukushima was the result of an extreme external event: a massive earthquake trigged a tsunami that led to flooding and loss of both on- and off-site electrical power causing the loss of essential safety functions at the plant and leading to core damage and the release of radioactive materials (Contessa et al. 2016). All told, by the end of October 2012, almost 25,000 workers had been involved in the mitigation and other activities at Fukushima, with an additional few hundred emergency response workers initially responding to the accident (Contessa et al. 2016). Using Fukushima as an illustration, Contessa and colleagues have analyzed the potential for flood-related radiological releases from workplaces such as hospitals that have nuclear medicine units and brachytherapy units and sites that store radioactive waste. Such facilities often build their radiation sources and storage units underground, raising the potential for water intrusion and radioactive release during floods. They also describe the potential for wildfires to affect ventilation systems and radiation monitoring systems, jeopardizing workers and communities who work and live in the vicinity of nuclear facilities and radiation sources.

Occupations such as health care providers, firefighters, police, and those working in search-and-rescue or body recovery are at risk of a wide range of posttraumatic reactions ranging from subclinical emotional symptoms such as fear to clinical posttraumatic stress disorder (PTSD; Brooks, Rubin, and Greenberg 2018). These responses are likely due to exposures to traumatic events, high levels of work demand, work with disrupted communities and evacuee populations, and separation from home and loved ones (Benedek, Fullerton, and Ursano 2007). Estimates of PTSD in disaster response workers vary widely, ranging from 5 percent and 40 percent (Galea, Nandi, and Vlahov 2005). Regardless, studies suggest that the prevalence of PTSD among rescue workers is much higher than the general population (Berger et al. 2012). One study found that 17 percent of disaster response workers reported symptoms consistent with PTSD and that symptoms were associated with having been injured in the response and being disconnected from family and friends (Schenk et al. 2017). Given this, it is important for employers in occupations related to disaster response to have mental health resources available for their workforce, given the increasingly frequent severe weather events (Perkison et al. 2018).

Vector-Borne Diseases, Expanded Habitats, and Pests

Increased prevalence of vector-borne diseases among workers in diverse geographic areas are a concerning result of climate change. Lyme disease accounts for more than 75 percent of all reported vector-borne diseases in the United States (Rosenberg et al. 2019). The risk of contracting Lyme disease for outdoor workers is five times the risk of indoor workers (Schulte et al. 2016). Over the last twenty years, the United States has seen an expanding geographic area at risk for Lyme disease, with the number of U.S. counties at high risk for Lyme disease increasing by more than 320 percent in the northeastern states and more than 250 percent in the north central states (Kugeler et al. 2015), which puts more outdoor workers at risk.

In response to rapidly changing environmental conditions, the range and distribution of certain poisonous plants and fungi that outdoor workers are exposed to is changing. Additionally, it has been shown that plants are also becoming increasingly toxic. Urushiol is the oil-like compound found in poison ivy that can cause phytodermatitis, which is a severe allergic contact dermatitis. Approximately two out of three individuals demonstrate a sensitivity to urushiol (Ziska et al. 2007). Studies have shown that poison ivy's exposure to elevated levels of CO_2 results in not just increases in leaf area but a more toxic form of urushiol when compared to current levels of atmospheric CO_2 (Mohan et al. 2006; Ziska et al. 2007). Currently, exposure to poison ivy accounts for 90 percent of cases of phytodermatitis in North America, with foresters and other outdoor workers the primary victims (Sasseville 2008).

Changing ecological conditions are also increasing agriculturally relevant pest populations, including weeds, invasive species, and insect-borne disease, which is leading to an increased use of pesticides. There are three main pathways by which a worker can be exposed to pesticides: dermal, respiratory, and oral. Health effects of exposure to pesticides depends on the type of pesticide and ranges from skin and eye irritation to effects on the endocrine system or the nervous system (Gatto, Cabella, and Gherardi 2016). Exposure to certain pesticides have also been linked to cancer (Clark and Snedeker 2005; Dharmani and Jaga 2005). Although farmworkers seem like a logical work group for increased exposure, the occupation most at risk are nonagricultural pesticide applicators who are exposed on a more regular basis, because the application of pesticides is a central task to their job, compared to those in the agricultural sector when the application of pesticides is more typically seasonal (Curwin et al. 2005; Macfarlane et al. 2013; Sperati et al. 1999).

Industrial Transitions and Emerging Industries

One response to climate change has been the shift to renewable sources of energy production, with half of all new U.S. electrical capacity installations each year being from a renewable source (Mulloy et al. 2013). These renewable sources of energy include hydroelectric, biofuel, solar, and wind. Although it has been postulated that renewable energy will offer benefits to workers in the form of reduced occupational injury, illness, and death (Mulloy et al. 2013), there are no certain data confirming an improvement in occupational health and safety issues over traditional extracted fossil fuel production (Valenti et al. 2016). To understand how to best protect workers in energy industry employment, we must first examine each of the production methods and risks that they pose to workers, as summarized by Mulloy et al. (2013).

Hydroelectric

Hydroelectric energy production poses risks to workers in both the construction phase as well as the operational phase. Although the construction of hydroelectric dams involves excavation and earthmoving, fill and concrete operations, and steelworks, workers will face the potential of injuries from vehicle and heavy equipment operations, falls, crush injuries, welding, silica dust, noise, and ocular hazards. Workers in an operational facility will face the potential for chemical and metal exposures, electric shock, explosions, machinery entanglement, and drowning.

Biofuel

The biofuel industry employs scientists, agricultural workers, production engineers, and transport workers. In addition to the traditional, well-documented, hazards agricultural workers face, there is also the potential for exposure to acids, bases, and gasoline as well as fire, explosion, and electrical hazards. Less understood is the impact exposure to bioaerosols and nanomaterials will have on acute and chronic health conditions.

Solar

Solar energy is produced via photovoltaic devices. There are specific hazards associated with the manufacturing and development of photovoltaic devices, depending on the type, including, but not limited to, exposure to alloys of heavy metals with varying degrees of toxicity (copper, indium, gallium, selenium), hazardous gases (phosphine, diborane, ammonia, and silane), and transparent conducting oxides such as indium-tin-oxide, which has been linked to pulmonary alveolar proteinosis. Notably, the installation of solar panels combines three occupations with high morbidity and mortality: roofing, carpentry, and electrical work.

Wind

The known hazards for workers in the wind energy production industry are not unique. They include falls, fires, release of hazardous energy during maintenance, working around cranes, arc flash, electric shock, and thermal burn. In addition, manufacturing workers face machine-related hazards, electrical hazards, and exposure to harmful gases, vapors, and dust.

Migrant Workers and Climate Change

Climate change impacts, such as extreme weather events, sea level rise, soil degradation, and food and water scarcity, are strongly associated with human migration (Schulte et al. 2016). By 2050 it is estimated that between twenty-five million to one billion people will be displaced because of degraded environmental conditions (International Energy Agency 2017). In 2018 there were 28.2 million foreign-born workers in the U.S. labor force, making up 17 percent of the total (Bureau of Labor Statistics [BLS] 2019). This was up from approximately 15 percent in 2005. Although these workers made up 15 percent of the workforce in 2005, they accounted for 18 percent of all work-related fatalities, resulting in 960 foreign-born worker deaths (Orrenius and Zavodny 2009). Given the increase in the proportion of the workforce that is foreign born, and their increased risk of suffering a work-related fatality, it is not unreasonable to assume that these numbers will only continue to rise with influxes of climate-change migrants without proactive action to safeguard the health of all workers.

Globally, immigrants are at a far greater risk of being injured or killed on the job compared to native-born workers, regardless of the host country. Additionally, foreign-born workers are more likely than native-born workers to be employed in service occupations such as natural resource extraction, construction, maintenance occupations as well as production, transportation, and material moving occupations (BLS 2016), which are some of the occupations most affected by climate change. Compounding the inherent risks related to the labor sector, many foreign-born individuals are employed in precarious or insecure jobs, without employment contracts (Moyce and Schenker 2018). Because of this, these workers often accept the dangers and risks posed by these jobs without complaint, for fear of losing employment. Precarious employment is also associated with higher rates of poverty, wage theft, a lack of overtime pay, and no health or employment benefits (Hege 2015). Fewer than one third of the occupational injuries and illnesses experienced by immigrant workers are paid for by employer funded workers' compensation. The burden for paying for these illnesses and injuries falls on the family of the injured worker, furthering cycles of poverty. Not only does the family of the worker carry the cost of the injury, they then must deal with consequences of the worker being potentially unemployed and unable to find work.

Adaptation and Response

Climate **adaptation** refers to the changes in processes, practices, and structures in response to climate change. Decision-makers, including in the business and government sector, have the responsibility to adapt—to develop, implement, evaluate, and improve guidelines and standards to protect workers' health under a changing climate (D'Ovidio et al. 2016) (see case study: Agricultural Workers in Guatemala). Affected sectors must anticipate and be prepared to respond quickly and effectively to protect workers' lives from the disasters caused by climate change, such as extreme weather events, as well as respond to "slow disasters," such as heat exposure. A multisectorial approach and broad stakeholder participation are necessary to ensure that working men and women will be involved in the adaptation efforts (Kiefer et al. 2016). Countries with limited economic resources, low levels of technology, poor information, poor infrastructure, and unstable or weak institutions have little capacity to adapt and therefore, workers in these places are highly vulnerable (Valenti et al. 2016).

Despite current limitations in resource investment in worker health, one area where action can be immediately taken is within worker health and safety programs currently in place. Occupational health and safety professionals can assess training needs and develop training programs or add a climate change component to an existing safety and health training course (Kiefer et al. 2016). Understanding how climate change alters the nature of occupations can inform the updating of current health and safety trainings and should include recognition of hazards, egress and evacuation, use of personal protective equipment, activation of emergency response system, incident command, and skills specific to their response duties (McCarthy et al. 2018). Nearly all occupational spheres can benefit from performing a worker-health risk analysis.

Under a changing climate, it is necessary to implement a range of medical surveillance programs targeted toward at-risk occupations (Perkison et al. 2018). Although most climate-related surveillance work has largely focused on the population level using easily accessible data, this may not accurately identify workplace exposures (Chretien et al. 2009). One exception is the Emergency Response Health Monitoring and Surveillance (ERHMS) system. The ERHMS is a collaboration between National Institute for Occupational Safety and Health (NIOSH), federal agencies, state health departments, and unions with the express goal of monitoring emergency responder health and safety throughout the predeployment, deployment, and postdeployment phases of natural disaster response (Lin et al. 2009). As threats from climate change only continue to grow, similar systems must be created for a wider range of jobs and exposures.

CASE STUDY: AGRICULTURAL WORKERS IN GUATEMALA

Industries and companies are recognizing that climate change not only affects worker health but also business sustainability. One such example is Pantaleon, a large agribusiness headquartered in Guatemala. Acknowledging the global epidemic of chronic kidney disease of unknown cause (CKDu) (Glaser et al., 2016; Johnson et al. 2019), Pantaleon has implemented preemployment screening and midharvest surveillance of workers at risk for developing the disease, which has been associated with work that requires high energy expenditure under extremely hot conditions (Butler-Dawson et al. 2018, 2019; Johnson et al. 2019; Sorensen and Garcia-Trabanino 2019; Sorensen et al. 2019). In 2015, and again in 2017, they have updated their standards for acceptable measures of preemployment kidney function that would deem an individual fit for work based on the emerging literature linking preseason kidney function with development of CKDu (Butler-Dawson et al. 2018). These changes have resulted in a reduction of incidence CKDu throughout the years. Any individual who is identified at midseason with severe reductions in kidney function is deemed to have a work-related illness and is temporarily removed from the workforce or put on modified duty. During this time, they are monitored by occupational health and safety medical personnel. Investments have been made by the company in a water, rest, and shade program to help protect workers from both the development of CKDu and other heat-related injuries (Butler-Dawson et al. 2018). In addition, policies have been implemented so that dehydration is now a recognized and reported occupational injury among their workers.

Worker, Family, and Societal Burden

There is an overreliance on economic measures to determine the true impact climate change carries for workers, families, and societies (Whitmee et al. 2015). Regardless, there is a need to address the costs associated with (1) increased health care and workers' compensation due to increased and changing severity of work-related morbidity and mortality, (2) worksite and public health interventions to address the changing nature of work and work related hazards, (3) lost work days and lower productivity, and (4) worker well-being. Currently, the true burden of occupational and work-related diseases and injuries is mostly unknown and significantly underestimated (Schulte et al. 2016) making future impact projections difficult.

Increased Health Care and Workers' Compensation Costs

Not only will workers experience a greater likelihood of a work-related injury or illness due to climate change, but it has been shown that insurance payouts increase (Ma et al. 2019). Although from 2000 to 2014 occupational heat injuries accounted for 0.1 percent of claims in Australia, the cumulative cost accounted for 0.04 percent of all-cause claim costs (Xiang et al. 2018), suggesting that the increase in insurance payouts is a result of the increased number of claims. Currently, scant research has been conducted on the increased cost of claims; however, a study in Spain found that there are an estimated forty-two days per 1,000 workers lost in Spain annually due to temperature, with an annual economic burden of approximately 415 million U.S. dollars (Martinez-Solanas et al. 2018). A study in South Australia found every 1°C (1.8°F) increase over 33°C (91.4°F) was associated with a 41.6 percent increase in medical costs and 74.8 percent increase in days lost due to an occupational heat illness (Xiang et al. 2018). Additionally, a study in Guangzhou, China found that 4.1 percent of work-related injury insurance payouts were attributed to heat stress (Ma et al. 2019).

Worksite and Public Health Interventions

Public health responses to climate change will require a range of actions, from timely public health and medical advice, early warning and surveillance systems, and the assurance that

CASE STUDY: INDIA, RICE, AND HEAT

India is the world's second largest producer of rice, producing 168,500,000 tons of rice paddy in 2017 (Food and Agriculture Organization 2019). In the Assam state of India, rice paddy accounts for more than 70 percent of the agricultural sector (Sharma and Sharma 2015). Assam has been identified as the state within India that is most vulnerable to climate change (Mohan 2019). Currently, from May to October the average maximum WBGT is above 27.5 °C (81.5°F) in Assam (Otto et al. 2014) (Figure 11.2, left). Under climate change models, these monthly maxima are only expected to increase (Figure 11.2, right). If OSHA recommendations were followed, current production levels could be maintained only by either doubling the workforce or putting the current workforce at risk for heat stress.

health care and social systems are ready to act (Huang et al. 2013). Each of these responses carries its own economic burden, from continuing education for health care service providers to development and maintenance costs of surveillance systems. Little research has been done to examine the cost vs. benefit of public health adaptation strategies. This is made more difficult by the entanglement of worker specific responses within the broader set of societal strategies (Huang et al. 2013). For example, to address the changing diversity of workforces due to migration, health and safety trainings will need to be updated to incorporate things such as pictograms, illustrations, and hands-on exercises that can transcend cultural, educational, and linguistic differences (De Jesus-Rivas, Conlon, and Burns 2016).

In addition to the public health response, employers must also invest in protecting their workers, for example, by enacting modified work schedules during heat advisories. The Occupational Safety and Health Administration (OSHA) has established a screening tool to evaluate whether a heat stress situation may exist based on WBGT, workload, and work/rest regimen (OSHA 2017). Under these guidelines, a worker is at risk for heat stress if they are performing 50 percent to 75 percent of work above 27.5°C (81.5°F). Similarly, workers conducting very heavy work should not be doing any work when temperatures are above 28°C (82.4°F). Adherence to these guidelines are not without consequence, as they result in decreased work productivity (see Case Study: India, Rice, and Heat).

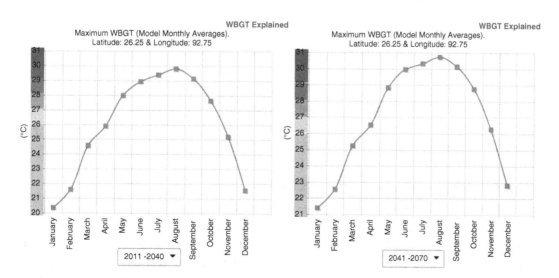

Figure 11.2   Monthly average WBGT projections based on NOAA model GFDL-esm2m for the Assam Region in India. Left: Years 2011–2040. Right: Years 2041–2070

Source: Data and image accessed from climatechip.org, August 2019 (Otto et al. 2014).

CLINICAL CORRELATES 11.3 MINE WORKER HEALTH FROM THE TRENCHES

Mining companies increasingly recognize climate change as disrupting infrastructure and operations, supply chains, and worker health via exposure to heat, floods, wildfires, food insecurity, and tropical diseases (Nelson and Schuchard 2011). Extreme heat is one area of concern in underground and open-pit mines. In one study of gold mine workers in Tanzania, 80 percent of miners had body temperatures above the recommended threshold (Meshi et al. 2018). Inhalation exposures from minerals like silica also risk chronic pulmonary disease (Haas, Cecala, and Hoebbel 2016). Companies have already begun to prepare by using scientific modeling for operations, developing technologies for water conservation, engineering robust structures against disasters, and incorporating climate change into company strategies and guidelines proactively (Nelson and Schuchard 2011).

Mining companies and nearby communities should adapt and build resilience now to protect mine workers and operations from climate stressors.

Under current climatic conditions, the OSHA guidelines are inadequate and in need of reconsideration as they do not accurately reflect current and future temperature exposures of outdoor workers. Currently there is no dedicated federal standard specifically addressing occupational heat exposure. Although NIOSH issued a revised Criteria Document in 2016 (NIOSH, 2016), OSHA has yet to develop an occupational exposure standard for heat and hot environments. With projections of temperature increases due to climate change to increase by an additional 3–5°C (5.4–9.0°F) by 2080, heavy work such as agriculture and construction will become very difficult during the hottest periods in densely populated areas and tropical countries in general (Kjellstrom et al. 2009). Regulatory bodies need to ensure proper protections for workers, and businesses must invest in ways to protect their workers so that jobs and productivity can be maintained without putting workers at undue risk.

One such investment is demonstrated by researchers who have recently translated the Water.Rest.Shade (WRS) program from OSHA into an intervention study among sugarcane harvesters in El Salvador (Bodin et al. 2016). Workers were supplied with a 3 L mounted water bladder with connected flexible tube and mouthpiece and access to 40 L coolers of water placed in the shade. Although preliminary findings showing that the intervention reduced dehydration while maintaining productivity are promising (Bodin et al. 2016), the study demonstrated additional issues such as feedback from the workers that the mounted water packs were cumbersome to use. Although the program was efficacious, the effectiveness at scale is questionable. More recently, a protocol that also provides sugarcane cutters with powdered electrolytes to add to drinking water has been shown to reduce the severity of rhabdomyolysis and to be well-accepted by workers during exertion in hot field conditions (Krisher et al. 2020). Regardless, any such interventions will require significant investment from businesses, ensuring acceptability from workers and business leaders alike. At a minimum, businesses should ensure that each worker has access to shade and clean water.

Lost Work Days and Lower Productivity

One of the more straightforward economic burdens to measure is productivity loss due to increasing temperature. One study found that a fourteen-day heat wave in 2013 cost the city of Nanjing, China approximately 400 million U.S. dollars in economic losses (Xia et al. 2018). A study in South Australia showed that between 2000 and 2014 there were 5,036 work days lost due to occupational heat-induced illness resulting in total medical expenditures of six million U.S. dollars (Xiang et al. 2018). In the United States it is estimated that 1.1 billion labor hours were lost between 2000 and 2017 due to increased heat exposure (Salas, Knappenberger, and Hess 2018). On a more micro level, investigations looking specifically at rice harvesters in

India have shown that there is a 0.6 percent reduction in direct work time (Li et al. 2016) and 5 percent reduction in work output of rice harvesters (Sahu, Sett, and Kjellstrom 2013) with increases in temperature. In our own research with Guatemalan sugarcane harvesters, we showed the cumulative effect of exposure to increased temperatures to be a reduction of 1.2 tons of harvested cane per worker over the work week (Dally et al. 2018).

Worker Well-Being

Currently, most occupational injury burden estimates do not adequately account for chronic disease caused or aggravated by work and often do not take into account the burden of disease that may result from all workplace exposures, whether acting alone, in combination with one another, or in conjunction with exposures from other life domains (Schulte et al. 2016). It has been established that impacts of climate change are disproportionately affecting the health of vulnerable populations and people in low- and middle- income countries (Watts et al. 2018), indicating that the health of the overall workforce could decline as a result of climate change. An analysis conducted in a Guatemalan agricultural cohort showed that individuals who came to work with preexisting health conditions experienced not only lower job performance but also greater job attrition, being twice as likely not to finish the harvest (Dally et al. 2018). Job loss can also mean loss of insurance, lack of access to prescriptions, and increases in poverty, all of which have health consequences. A study in 2015 showed that job loss was related to worse self-rated overall health among both men and women (Huijts et al. 2015). Specifically related to mental health, research has shown that a number of socioeconomic, sociodemographic, and social capital factors influence the mental health of workers experiencing job loss (Ziersch et al. 2014).

From 2000 to 2016 global labor capacity has decreased 5.3 percent because of temperature changes (Watts et al. 2018). In low- and middle-income countries that are dependent on manual labor, the health and welfare of workers are of paramount importance for sustained industrial growth (Krishnamurthy et al. 2017). Decreased agricultural production in major food producing regions will threaten food supplies worldwide (Janetos et al. 2017). Reductions in labor capacity will disproportionately affect developing countries (Lundgren et al. 2013) at a time when the global demand for agricultural production in developing countries will rise by an estimated 77 percent (Alexandratos and Bruinsma 2012). With agricultural workers at the bottom of the farm to table supply chain, what hurts the worker will hurt us all.

Figure 11.3 summarizes the relationship between climate change, worker health, and societal impacts.

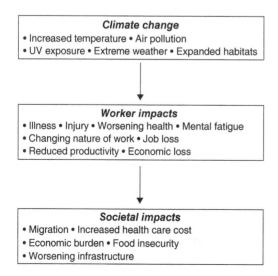

Figure 11.3   Multiple domains of burden of climate change-related impacts on worker health

CLINICAL CORRELATES 11.4 AGRICULTURAL WORKERS AND AIR POLLUTION

Ground ozone and particulate matter (PM) are both significant sources of air pollution. Ammonia and other pollutants related to agricultural production are precursors for PM contributing to rising global atmospheric levels ("How Can Climate Change" 2019). Climate-driven wildfire smoke also increases PM and ozone levels. These air pollutants influence respiratory health especially for susceptible individuals with asthma, chronic obstructive pulmonary disease, and bronchitis. Increased asthma prevalence in children living near livestock farms has been demonstrated with intense farming activities (Douglas et al. 2018). Air quality is also associated with worker productivity, as ground ozone decreases then productivity increases (Zivin and Neidell 2012).

Reducing emissions from agriculture would have a commensurate effect on PM concentrations (Pozzer et al. 2017) and potentially reduce health care utilization for workers, improve productivity, and reduce greenhouse gas emissions. Some rural areas have already offered incentives for renewable energy (solar) with positive feedback given by farmers (Kaya, Klepacka, and Florkowski 2019).

Protecting migrant and seasonal outdoor workers by evaluating emissions associated with farming activities and local air quality will be increasingly important with increasing food production demands.

Conclusions

In this chapter we have explored the workplace hazards that will be exacerbated by climate change as well as new hazards workers may face. Operating as a threat multiplier, climate change will put pressure on vulnerable worker populations. Increased heat, worsening air quality, extreme weather events and natural disasters, and increased exposures to diseases and pests will result in increased injuries, death, lost labor, economic poverty, and poor mental health of workers. Although there are many personal consequences suffered by workers with occupational injuries or illnesses, we must not lose sight of the impact these will have on their families, employers, and society overall.

Workers are thought of as the "climate canaries." (Roelofs and Wegman 2014) They are often subjected to higher exposure levels and for longer duration than the general public and lack the agency to control their exposures given the demands of their jobs. Unfortunately, workers are an overlooked population by U.S. researchers and federal agencies (Roelofs and Wegman 2014). Although research has begun to address the implications of climate change on worker health, much more is needed. Health and safety professionals, working in conjunction with employers, must understand climate risks, undertake assessments, and be prepared to respond as well as work to adapt in order to reduce the vulnerability of workers and increase their resilience to the impacts of climate change. Further research should assess the impact climate change has on deteriorating worker health and the economic and societal burden it will cause to motivate and inform solutions.

KEY TERMS

Adaptation: Changes in processes, practices, and structures in response to climate change.

Occupational hazard: Hazard experienced specifically in the workplace because of the worksite or the nature of the work.

Occupational illness: Chronic ailment or disease caused by work-related exposures.

Occupational injury: Physical—and potentially mental—harm resulting from work-related activities.

DISCUSSION QUESTIONS

The hierarchy of controls encompass (from most to least effective) physically removing the hazard (elimination), replacing the hazard with a safer option (substitution), isolating people from the hazard (engineering controls), changing the way people work or reducing the number of people allowed to be exposed to the hazard (administrative controls), protecting the worker with personal protective equipment (PPE), and providing workers with education regarding the hazard.

1. In this framework, in which ways can the hierarchy of controls be applied to address the hazards from climate change presented in this chapter?

2. What are the challenges of trying to apply the hierarchy of controls to hazards from climate change presented in this chapter?

3. If workers are one of the most susceptible to the effects of climate change, why are they an understudied population? What would be the benefits of studying workers? What are the challenges of using workers as a study population in research on climate change effects?

4. In this chapter we have suggested that simply measuring economic loss does not encompass the entire burden faced from climate change. What are the other ways in which climate-related harm to workers affects individual, families, employers, and society?

References

Acharya, P., B. Boggess, and K. Zhang. 2018. "Assessing Heat Stress and Health among Construction Workers in a Changing Climate: A Review." *International Journal of Environmental Research and Public Health* 15 (2):247. doi:10.3390/ijerph15020247.

Adam-Poupart, A., A. Smargiassi, M.-A. Busque, P. Duguay, M. Fournier, J. Zayed, and F. Labrèche. 2015. "Effect of Summer Outdoor Temperatures on Work-Related Injuries in Quebec (Canada)." *Occupational and Environmental Medicine* 72 (5):338–45.

Alexandratos, N., and J. Bruinsma. 2012. *World Agriculture towards 2030/2050: The 2012 Revision.* Rome: Food and Agriculture Organization.

Benedek, D. M., C. Fullerton, and R. J. Ursano. 2007. "First Responders: Mental Health Consequences of Natural and Human-Made Disasters for Public Health and Public Safety Workers." *Annual Review of Public Health* 28 (1):55–68.

Berger, W., E. S. F. Coutinho, I. Figueira, C. Marques-Portella, M. P. Luz, T. C. Neylan, C. R. Marmar, and M. V. Mendlowicz. 2012. "Rescuers at Risk: A Systematic Review and Meta-Regression Analysis of the Worldwide Current Prevalence and Correlates of PTSD in Rescue Workers." *Social Psychiatry and Psychiatric Epidemiology* 47 (6):1001–11.

Betchley, C., J. Q. Koenig, G. van Belle, H. Checkoway, and T. Reinhardt. 1997. "Pulmonary Function and Respiratory Symptoms in Forest Firefighters." *American Journal of Industrial Medicine* 31 (5):503–9.

Bhandari, D., and P. Pandey. 2018. "Health Problems while Working as a Volunteer or Humanitarian Aid Worker in Post-Earthquake Nepal." *Journal of the Nepal Medical Association* 56 (211):691–95.

Bloom, E., L. F. Grimsley, C. Pehrson, J. Lewis, and L. Larsson. 2009. "Molds and Mycotoxins in Dust from Water-Damaged Homes in New Orleans after Hurricane Katrina." *Indoor Air* 19 (2):153–8. doi: 10.1111/j.1600-0668.2008.00574.x.

Bodin, T., R. García-Trabanino, I. Weiss, E. Jarquín, J. Glaser, K. Jakobsson, R. A. I. Lucas, et al. 2016. "Intervention to Reduce Heat Stress and Improve Efficiency among Sugarcane Workers in El Salvador: Phase 1." *Occupational and Environmental Medicine* 73 (6):409–16.

Bonafede, M., A. Marinaccio, F. Asta, P. Schifano, P. Michelozzi, and S. Vecchi. 2016. "The Association between Extreme Weather Conditions and Work-Related Injuries and Diseases. A Systematic Review of Epidemiological Studies." *Annali dell'Istituto superiore di sanità* 52 (3):357–67.

Brant, A. 2007. "Baker's Asthma." *Current Opinion in Allergy and Clinical Immunology* 7 (2).

Brooks, S. K., G. J. Rubin, and N. Greenberg. 2018. "Traumatic Stress within Disaster-Exposed Occupations: Overview of the Literature and Suggestions for the Management of Traumatic Stress in the Workplace." *British Medical Bulletin* 129 (1):25–34.

Bureau of Labor Statistics. 2016. *Labor Force Characteristics of Foreign-Born Workers News Release. Published May* 19, 2016. https://www.bls.gov/news.release/archives/forbrn_05192016.htm.

Bureau of Labor Statistics. 2018. *Foreign-born workers: labor force characteristics—2018.* https://www.bls.gov/news.release/pdf/forbrn.pdf.

Butler-Dawson, J., L. Krisher, C. Asensio, A. Cruz, L. Tenney, D. Weitzenkamp, M. Dally, E. J. Asturias, and L. S. Newman. 2018. "Risk Factors for Declines in Kidney Function in Sugarcane Workers in Guatemala." *Journal of Occupational and Environmental Medicine* 60 (6):548–58.

Butler-Dawson, J., L. Krisher, H. Yoder, M. Dally, C. Sorensen, R. J. Johnson et al. 2019. "Evaluation of Heat Stress and Cumulative Incidence of Acute Kidney Injury in Sugarcane Workers in Guatemala." *International Archives of Occupational and Environmental Health* 92 (7):977–90.

Carvalho, R. B., M. F. Hornos Carneiro, F. Barbosa Jr., B. L. Batista, J. Simonetti, S. L. Amantéa, and C. R. Rhoden. 2018. "The Impact of Occupational Exposure yo Traffic-Related Air Pollution among Professional Motorcyclists from Porto Alegre, Brazil, and Its Association with Genetic and Oxidative Damage." *Environmental Science and Pollution Research* 25 (19):18620–31.

Chan, A. P., Y. P. Guo, F. K. Wong, Y. Li, S. Sun, and X. Han. 2016. "The Development of Anti-Heat Stress Clothing for Construction Workers in Hot and Humid Weather." *Ergonomics* 59 (4):479–95. doi:10.10 80/00140139.2015.1098733.

Chretien, J.-P., N. E. Tomich, J. C. Gaydos, and P. W. Kelley, 2009. "Real-Time Public Health Surveillance for Emergency Preparedness." *American Journal of Public Health* 99 (8):1360–3.

Clark, H. A., and S. M. Snedeker. 2005. "Critical Evaluation of the Cancer Risk of Dibromochloropropane (DBCP)." *Journal of Environmental Science And Health. Part C, Environmental Carcinogenesis & Ecotoxicology Reviews* 23 (2):215–60.

Contessa, G. M., C. Grandi, M. Scognamiglio, E. Genovese, and S. Sandri. 2016. "Climate Change and Safety at Work with Ionizing Radiations." *Annali dell'Istituto superiore di sanità* 52 (3):386–96.

Curwin, B. D., M. J. Hein, W. T. Sanderson, D. B. Barr, D. Heederik, S. J Reynolds, E. M. Ward, and M. C Alavanja. 2005. "Urinary and Hand Wipe Pesticide Levels among Farmers and Nonfarmers in Iowa." *Journal of Exposure Science & Environmental Epidemiology* 15 (6):500–8.

Dally, M., J. Butler-Dawson, L. Krisher, A. Monaghan, D. Weitzenkamp, C. Sorensen, R. J. Johnson et al. 2018. "The Impact of Heat and Impaired Kidney Function on Productivity of Guatemalan Sugarcane Workers." *PloS One* 13 (10):e0205181–e0205181.

Dally M, Butler-Dawson J, Sorensen CJ, Van Dyke M, James KA, Krisher L, Jaramillo D, Newman LS. Wet Bulb Globe Temperature and Recorded Occupational Injury Rates among Sugarcane Harvesters in Southwest Guatemala. Int J Environ Res Public Health. 2020 Nov 6;17(21):8195. doi: 10.3390/ijerph17218195. PMID: 33171945; PMCID: PMC7664243.

De Jesus-Rivas, M., H. A. Conlon, and C. Burns. 2016. "The Impact of Language and Culture Diversity in Occupational Safety." *Workplace Health & Safety* 64 (1):24–27.

Dharmani, C., and K. Jaga. 2005. "Epidemiology of Acute Organophosphate Poisoning in Hospital Emergency Patients." *Reviews on Environmental Health* 20:215–32.

Douglas, P., S. Robertson, R. Gay, A. L. Hansell, and T. W. Gant. 2018. "A Systematic Review of the Public Health Risks of Bioaerosols from Intensive Farming." *International Journal of Hygiene and Environmental Health* 221 (2):134–73. doi:10.1016/j.ijheh.2017.10.019.

D'Ovidio, M. C., I. Annesi-Maesano, G. D'Amato, and L. Cecchi 2016. "Climate Change and Occupational Allergies: An Overview on Biological Pollution, Exposure and Prevention." *Annali dell'Istituto superiore di sanità* 52 (3):406–14.

Du, F., J. Wu, J. Fan, R. Jiang, M. Gu, X. He, Z. Wang, and C. He. 2016. "Injuries Sustained by Earthquake Relief Workers: A Retrospective Analysis of 207 Relief Workers during Nepal Earthquake." *Scandinavian Journal of Trauma, Resuscitation and Emergency Medicine* 24:95. doi: 10.1186/s13049-016-0286-4.

El-Shafei, D. A., S. A. Bolbol, M. B. Awad Allah, and A. E. Abdelsalam. 2018. "Exertional Heat Illness: Knowledge and Behavior among Construction Workers." *Environmental Science and Pollution Research International* 25 (32):32269–76. doi:10.1007/s11356-018-3211-8.

Food and Agriculture Organization. 2019. *Countries by Commodity.* http://www.fao.org/faostat/en/#rankings/countries_by_commodity.

Galán, I., M. Goicoechea, B. Quiroga, N. Macías, A. Santos, M. S. García de Vinuesa, Ú. Verdalles et al. 2018. "Hyperuricemia Is Associated with Progression of Chronic Kidney Disease in Patients with Reduced Functioning Kidney Mass." *Nefrología (English Edition)* 38 (1):73–78.

Galea, S., A. Nandi, and D. Vlahov. 2005. "The Epidemiology of Post-Traumatic Stress Disorder after Disasters." *Epidemiologic Reviews* 27 (1):78–91.

Gatto, M. P., R. Cabella, and M. Gherardi. 2016. "Climate Change: The Potential Impact oOn Occupational Exposure to Pesticides." *Annali dell'Istituto superiore di sanità* 52 (3):374–85.

Gaughan, D. M., C. A. Piacitelli, B. T. Chen, B. F. Law, M. A. Virji, N. T. Edwards, P. L. Enright, et al. 2014. "Exposures and Cross-Shift Lung Function Declines in Wildland Firefighters." *Journal of Occupational and Environmental Hygiene* 11 (9):591–603.

Glaser, J., J. Lemery, B. Rajagopalan, H. F. Diaz, R. García-Trabanino, G. Taduri, M. Madero, et al. 2016. "Climate Change and the Emergent Epidemic of CKD from Heat Stress in Rural Communities: The Case for Heat Stress Nephropathy." *Clinical Journal of the American Society of Nephrology* 11 (8):1472–83.

Grandi, C., M. Borra, A. Militello, and A. Polichetti. 2016. "Impact of Climate Change on Occupational Exposure to Solar Radiation." *Annali dell'Istituto superiore di sanità* 52 (3):343–56.

Groot, E., A. Caturay, Y. Khan, and R. Copes. 2019. "A Systematic Review of the Health Impacts of Occupational Exposure to Wildland Fires." *International Journal of Occupational Medicine and Environmental Health* 32 (2):121–40.

Gubernot, D. M., G. B. Anderson, and K. L. Hunting. 2015. "Characterizing Occupational Heat-Related Mortality in the United States, 2000–2010: An Analysis using the Census of Fatal Occupational Injuries Database." *American Journal of Industrial Medicine* 58:203–11.

Haas, E. J., A. B. Cecala, and C. L. Hoebbel. 2016. "Using Dust Assessment Technology to Leverage Mine Site Manager-Worker Communication and Health Behavior: A Longitudinal Case Study." *Journal of Pprogressive Research in Social Sciences* 3 (1):154–67.

Harari Arjona, R., J. Piñeiros, M. Ayabaca, and F. H. Freire. 2016."Climate Change and Agricultural Workers' Health in Ecuador: Occupational Exposure to UV Radiation and Hot Environments. *Annali dell'Istituto superiore di sanità* 52 (3):368–73.

Hege, A. 2015. "Health Disparities of Latino Immigrant Workers in the United States." *International Journal of Migration, Health and Social Care* 11 (4):282–98.

"'How Can Climate Change Impact the Workplace and Worker Health?' Part 3: Air Pollution, Greenhouse Gases, and Cardiorespiratory Health." 2019. *Journal of Occupational and Environmental Medicine* 61 (10):e427–e428. doi:10.1097/JOM.0000000000001694.

Huang, C., A. G. Barnett, Z. Xu, C. Chu, X. Wang, L. R. Turner, and S. Tong. 2013. "Managing the Health Effects of Temperature in Response to Climate Change: Challenges Ahead." *Environmental Health Perspectives* 121 (4):415–9.

Huijts, T., A. Reeves, M. McKee, and D. Stuckler. 2015. "The Impacts of Job Loss and Job Recovery on Self-Rated Health: Testing the Mediating Role of Financial Strain and Income." *European Journal of Public Health* 25 (5):801–6.

International Energy Agency. 2017. *World Energy Outlook.* https://www.iea.org/weo2017.

Jacquin, L., P. Michelet, F.-X. Brocq, J.-G. Houel, X. Truchet, J.-P. Auffray, J.-P. Carpentier, and Y. Jammes 2011. "Short-Term Spirometric Changes in Wildland Firefighters." *American Journal of Industrial Medicine* 54 (11):819–25.

Janetos, A., C. Justice, M. Jahn, M. Obersteiner, J. W. Glauber, and M. William. 2017. *The Risks of Multiple Breadbasket Failures in the 21st Century: A Science Research Agenda.* Boston, MA: Boston University, Frederick S. Pardee Center for the Study of the Longer-Range Future.

Johanning, E., Pierre Auger, Philip R Morey, Chin S Yang, Ed Olmsted. 2014. "Review of Health Hazards and Prevention Measures for Response and Recovery Workers and Volunteers after Natural Disasters, Flooding, and Water Damage: Mold and Dampness." *Environmental Health and Preventive Medicine* 19 (2):93–99.

Johnson, R. J., C. Wesseling, and L. S. Newman. 2019. "Chronic Kidney Disease of Unknown Cause in Agricultural Communities." *New England Journal of Medicine* 380 (19):1843–52.

Kamei, K., T. Konta, A. Hirayama, K. Ichikawa, I. Kubota, S. Fujimoto, K. Iseki et al. 2017. "Associations Between Serum Uric Acid Levels and the Incidence of Nonfatal Stroke: A Nationwide Community-Based Cohort Study." *Clinical and Experimental Nephrology* 21 (3):497–503.

Kaya, O., A. M. Klepacka, and W. J. Florkowski. "Achieving Renewable Energy, Climate, and Air Quality Policy Goals: Rural Residential Investment in Solar Panel." *Journal of Environmental Management* 248:109309. doi:10.1016/j.jenvman.2019.109309.

Keim, M.E. 2008. "Building Human Resilience: The Role of Public Health Preparedness and Response as an Adaptation to Climate Change." *American Journal of Preventive Medicine* 35 (5):508–16.

Kiefer, M., J. Rodríguez-Guzmán, J. Watson, B. van Wendel de Joode, D. Mergler, and A. Soares da Silva. 2016. "Worker Health and Safety and Climate Change in the Americas: Issues and Research Needs." *Revista panamericana de salud publica (Pan American Journal of Public Health)* 40 (3):192–97.

Kinney, P. L. 2008. "Climate Change, Air Quality, and Human Health." *American Journal of Preventive Medicine* 35 (5):459–67.

Kjellstrom, T., I. Holmer, and B. Lemke. 2009. "Workplace Heat Stress, Health and Productivity—An Increasing Challenge for Low and Middle-Income Countries during Climate Change." *Global Health Action* 2:10.3402/gha.v2i0.2047.

Krishnamurthy, M., P. Ramalingam, K. Perumal, L. P. Kamalakannan, J. Chinnadurai, R. Shanmugam, K. Srinivasan, and V. Venugopal .2017. "Occupational Heat Stress Impacts on Health and Productivity in a Steel Industry in Southern India." *Safety and Health at Work* 8 (1):99–104.

Krisher L, Butler-Dawson J, Yoder H, Pilloni D, Dally M, Johnson EC, Jaramillo D, Cruz A, Asensio C, Newman LS. Electrolyte Beverage Intake to Promote Hydration and Maintain Kidney Function in Guatemalan Sugarcane Workers Laboring in Hot Conditions. J Occup Environ Med. 2020 Dec;62(12):e696-e703. doi: 10.1097/JOM.0000000000002033. PMID: 33003044; PMCID: PMC7720870.

Kugeler, K. J., G. M. Farley, J. D. Forrester, and P. S. Mead. 2015. "Geographic Distribution and Expansion of Human Lyme Disease, United States." *Emerging Infectious Diseases* 21 (8):1455–7.

Leykin, D., M. Lahad, and N. Bonneh. 2013. "Posttraumatic Symptoms and Posttraumatic Growth of Israeli Firefighters, at One Month Following the Carmel Fire Disaster." *Psychiatry Journal* 2013:274121–274121.

Li, X., K. H. Chow, Y. Zhu, and Y. Lin. 2016. "Evaluating the Impacts of High-Temperature Outdoor Working Environments on Construction Labor Productivity in China: A Case Study of Rebar Workers." *Building and Environment* 95:42–52.

Lin, S., M. Luo, R. J. Walker, X. Liu, S.-A. Hwang, and R. Chinery. 2009. "Extreme High Temperatures and Hospital Admissions for Respiratory and Cardiovascular Diseases." *Epidemiology* 20 (5):738–46.

Liu, C., A. T. Linde, and I. S. Sacks. 2009. "Slow Earthquakes Triggered by Typhoons." *Nature* 459 (7248):833–6.

Lundgren, K., K. Kuklane, C. Gao, and I. Holmér. 2013. "Effects of Heat Stress on Working Populations When Facing Climate Change." *Industrial Health* 51 (1):3–15.

Ma, R., S. Zhong, M. Morabito, S. Hajat, Z. Xu, Y. He, and J. Bao. 2019. "Estimation of Work-Related Injury and Economic Burden Attributable to Heat Stress in Guangzhou, China." *Science of the Total Environment* 666:147–54.

Macfarlane, E., R. Carey, T. Keegel, S. El-Zaemay, and L. Fritschi. 2013. "Dermal Exposure Associated with Occupational End Use of Pesticides and the Role of Protective Measures." *Safety and Health at Work* 4 (3):136–41.

Marshall, E. G., S.-E. Lu, Z. Shi, J. Swerdel, M. Borjan, and M. E. Lumia. 2016. "Work-Related Unintentional Injuries Associated with Hurricane Sandy in New Jersey." *Disaster Medicine and Public Health Preparedness* 10 (3):394-404. doi: 10.1017/dmp.2016.47. Epub 2016 Apr 15.

Martinez-Solanas, E., M. López-Ruiz, G. A Wellenius, A. Gasparrini, J. Sunyer, F. G. Benavides, and X. Basagaña. 2018. "Evaluation of the Impact of Ambient Temperatures on Occupational Injuries in Spain." *Environmental Health Perspectives* 126 (6):067002.

Marx, J., and P. Rosen. 2014. *Rosen's Emergency Medicine: Concepts and Clinical Practices*, 8th ed. 2014, *Philadelphia*, PA: Elsevier/Saunders.

McCarthy, R. B. et al. 2018. "How Can Climate Change Impact the Health of Workers? Part 1: Increased Ambient Temperature." *Journal of Occupational and Environmental Medicine* 60 (6):e288-e289.

McFarlane, A. C. 1988. "The Longitudinal Course of Posttraumatic Morbidity. The Range of Outcomes and Their Predictors." *Journal of Nervous and Mental Disease* 176 (1):30–9.

McGuire, B. 2012. *Waking the Giant : How a Changing Climate Triggers Earthquakes, Tsunamis, and Volcanoes.* Oxford: Oxford : Oxford University Press.

McInnes, J. A., M. Akram, E. M. MacFarlane, T. Keegel, M. R. Sim, and P. Smith. "Association between High Ambient Temperature and Acute Work-Related Injury: A Case-Crossover Analysis Using Workers' Compensation Claims Data." *Scandinavian Journal of Work, Environment & Health* 43 (1):86–94.

Meshi, E. B., S. S. Kishinhi, S. H. Mamuya, and M. G. Rusibamayila. 2018. "Thermal Exposure and Heat Illness Symptoms among Workers in Mara Gold Mine, Tanzania." *Annals of Global Health* 84 (3):360–8. doi:10.29024/aogh.2318.

Migliaccio, C. T., M. A. Bergauff, C. P. Palmer, F. Jessop, C. W. Noonan, and T. J. Ward. 2009. "Urinary Levoglucosan as a Biomarker of Wood Smoke Exposure: Observations in a Mouse Model and in Children." *Environmental Health Perspectives* 117 (1):74–79.

Mohan, D. 2019. *Climate Vulnerability Assessment for the Indian Himalayan Region using a Common Framework. Published July* 19, 2019. https://www.weadapt.org/knowledge-base/sdc-climate-change-environment-network/climate-vulnerability-assessment-for-the-indian-himalayan-region-using-a-common-framework.

Mohan, J. E., L. H. Ziska, W. H. Schlesinger, R. B. Thomas, R. C. Sicher, K. George, and J. S. Clark. 2006. "Biomass and Toxicity Responses of Poison Ivy (Toxicodendron Radicans) to Elevated Atmospheric CO2." *Proceedings of the National Academy of Sciences of the USA* 103 (24):9086–89.

Moyce, S. C., and M. Schenker. 2018. "Migrant Workers and Their Occupational Health and Safety." *Annual Review of Public Health* 39:351–65.

Mulloy, K. B., S. A. Sumner, C. Rose, G. A. Conway, S. J. Reynolds, M. E. Davidson, D. S. Heidel, and P. M. Layde. 2013. "Renewable Energy and Occupational Health and Safety Research Directions: A white paper from the Energy Summit, Denver Colorado, April 11–13, 2011." *American Journal of Industrial Medicine* 56 (11):1359–70.

Meo SA, Abukhalaf AA, Alomar AA, Alessa OM, Sami W, Klonoff DC. Effect of environmental pollutants PM-2.5, carbon monoxide, and ozone on the incidence and mortality of SARS-COV-2 infection in ten wildfire affected counties in California [published online ahead of print, 2020 Nov 25]. *Sci Total Environ.* 2020;757:143948. doi:10.1016/j.scitotenv.2020.143948

Nelson, J., and R. Schuchard R. 2011. *Adapting to Climate Change: A Guide for the Mining Industry.* New York: Business for Social Responsibility. https://www.bsr.org/reports/BSR_Climate_Adaptation_Issue_Brief_Mining.pdf

Navarro KM, Clark KA, Hardt DJ, Reid CE, Lahm PW, Domitrovich JW, Butler CR, Balmes JR. Wildland firefighter exposure to smoke and COVID-19: A new risk on the fire line. Sci Total Environ. 2020 Dec 11;760:144296. doi: 10.1016/j.scitotenv.2020.144296. Epub ahead of print. PMID: 33341613.

NIOSH [2016]. NIOSH criteria for a recommended standard: occupational exposure to heat and hot environments. By Jacklitsch B, Williams WJ, Musolin K, Coca A, Kim J-H, Turner N. Cincinnati, OH: U.S. Department of Health and Human Services, Centers for Disease Control and Prevention, National Institute for Occupational Safety and Health, DHHS (NIOSH) Publication 2016-106.

Occupational Safety and Health Administration. 2017. *OSHA Technical Manual Section III: Chapter 4 Heat Stress*. https://www.osha.gov/dts/osta/otm/otm_iii/otm_iii_4.html.

Ochsner, M. A.-O., E. G. Marshall, and D. Lefkowitz. 2018. "Trees Down, Hazards Abound: Observations and Lessons from Hurricane Sandy." *American Journal of Industrial Medicine* 61 (5):361-371.

Orrenius, P. M., and M. Zavodny. 2009. "Do Immigrants Work in Riskier Jobs?" *Demography* 46 (3):535–51.

Otto, M., B. Lemke, and T. Kjellstrom. 2014. *A Tool for the Estimation and Analysis of Local Climate and Population Heat Exposure*. ClimateCHIP. https://www.climatechip.org/sites/default/files/publications/141023%20software%20paper%20Otto%20Tech%20Rep%2014-3.pdf.

Oyekale, A. S. 2019. "Dataset on Cocoa Farmers' Agrochemical Handling Practices and Safety Compliance in Ahafo Ano North District, Ashanti Region, Ghana." *Data Brief* 27:104767. doi:10.1016/j.dib.2019.104767.

Perkison, W. B., G. D. Kearney, P. Saberi, T. Guidotti, R. McCarthy, M. Cook-Shimanek, M. A. Pensa, and I. Nabeel. 2018. "Responsibilities of the Occupational and Environmental Medicine Provider in the Treatment and Prevention of Climate Change-Related Health Problems." *Journal of Occupational and Environmental Medicine* 60 (2):e76–e81.

Pinault, A., A. van Donkelaar, and R. Martin. 2017. "Exposure to Fine Particulate Matter Air Pollution in Canada." *Health Reports* 28 (3):9–16.

Pozzer, A., A. P. Tsimpidi, V. A. Karydis, A. de Meij, and J. Lelieveld. 2017. "Impact of Agricultural Emission Reductions on Fine-Particulate Matter and Public Health." *Atmospheric Chemistry and Physics* 17:12813–26, https://doi.org/10.5194/acp-17-12813-2017.

Rando, R. J., C. W. Kwon, and J. J. Lefante. 2014. "Exposures to Thoracic Particulate Matter, Endotoxin, and Glucan during Post-Hurricane Katrina Restoration Work, New Orleans 2005–2012." *Journal of Occupational and Environmental Hygiene* 11 (1):9–18.

Reid, C. E., M. Brauer, F. H. Johnston, M. Jerrett, J. R. Balmes, and C. T Elliott. 2016. "Critical Review of Health Impacts of Wildfire Smoke Exposure." *Environmental Health Perspectives* 124 (9):1334–43.

Reinmuth-Selzle, K., C. J. Kampf, K. Lucas, N. Lang-Yona, J. Fröhlich-Nowoisky, M. Shiraiwa, P. S. J. Lakey et al. 2017. "Air Pollution and Climate Change Effects on Allergies in the Anthropocene: Abundance, Interaction, and Modification of Allergens and Adjuvants." *Environmental Science & Technology* 51 (8):4119–41.

Ringen, K., X. S. Dong, L. M. Goldenhar, and C. T. Cain. 2018. "Construction Safety and Health in the USA: Lessons from a Decade of Turmoil." *Annals of Work Exposures and Health* 62 (suppl 1):S25–S33. doi:10.1093/annweh/wxy069.

Roelofs, C., and D. Wegman. 2014. "Workers: The Climate Canaries." *American Journal of Public Health* 104 (10):1799–1801.

Rosenberg, R., N. P. Lindsey, M. Fischer, C. J. Gregory, A. F. Hinckley, P. S. Mead, G. Paz-Bailey et al. 2018. "Vital Signs: Trends in Reported Vectorborne Disease Cases—United States and Territories, 2004–2016." *MMWR. Morbidity and Mortality Weekly Report* 67 (17):496–501.

Sahu, S., M. Sett, and T. Kjellstrom. 2013. "Heat Exposure, Cardiovascular Stress and Work Productivity in Rice Harvesters in India: Implications for a Climate Change Future." *Industrial Health* 51 (4):424–31.

Salas, R. N., P. Knappenberger, and J. Hess. 2018. *2018 Lancet Countdown on Health and Climate Change Brief for the United States of America*. London: Lancet Countdown.

Sarofim, M. C., S. Saha, M. D. Hawkins, D. M. Mills, J. Hess, R. Horton, P. Kinney, J. Schwartz, and A. St. Juliana. 2016. "Temperature-Related Death and Illness. In *The Impacts of Climate Change on Human Health in the United States: A Scientific Assessment*, edited by A. Crimmins, J. Balbus, J. L. Gamble, C. B. Beard, J. E. Bell, D. Dodgen, R. J. Eisen et al., 43–68. Washington, DC: U.S. Global Change Research Program.

Sasseville, D. 2008. "Occupational Contact Dermatitis." *Allergy, Asthma, and Clinical Immunology* 4 (2):59–65.

Schenk, E. J., J. Yuan, L. D. Martel, G.-Q. Shi, K. Han, and X. Gao. 2017. "Risk Factors for Long-Term Post-Traumatic Stress Disorder among Medical Rescue Workers Appointed to the 2008 Wenchuan Earthquake Response in China." *Disasters* 41 (4):788–802. doi: 10.1111/disa.12222.

Schifano, P., F. Asta, A. Marinaccio, M. Bonafede, M. Davoli, and P. Michelozzi. 2019. "Do Exposure to Outdoor Temperatures, NO_2 and PM_{10} Affect the Work-Related Injuries Risk? A Case-Crossover Study in Three Italian Cities, 2001–2010." *BMJ Open* 9 (8):e023119–e023119.

Schifano, P., M. Leone, M. De Sario, F. de'Donato, A. M. Bargagli, D. D'Ippoliti, C. Marino, and P. Michelozzi. 2012. "Changes in the Effects of Heat on Mortality among the Elderly from 1998–2010: Results from a Multicenter Time Series Study in Italy." *Environmental Health* 11 (1):58.

Schulte, P. A., A. Bhattacharya, C. R. Butler, H. K. Chun, B. Jacklitsch, T. Jacobs, M. Kiefer et al. 2016. "Advancing the Framework for Considering the Effects of Climate Change on Worker Safety and Health." *Journal of Occupational and Environmental Hygiene* 13 (11):847–65.

Sharma, B. K., and S. H. Sharma. 2015. "Status of Rice Production in Assam, Indian." *Rice Research: Open Access* 3 (4):e121.

Sheng, R., C. Li, Q. Wang, L. Yang, J. Bao, K. Wang, R. Ma, and C.Gao et al. 2018. "Does Hot Weather Affect Work-Related Injury? A Case-Crossover Study in Guangzhou, China." *International Journal of Hygiene and Environmental Health* 221 (3):423–28.

Shrivastav, C., M. Kaur, M. L. Suhalka, S. Sharma, and A. Basu. 2016. "Hyperuricaemia–A Potential Indicator to Diagnose the Risk of Essential Hypertension." *Journal of Clinical and Diagnostic Research* 10 (3):CC01–CC3.

Sorensen, C., and R. Garcia-Trabanino. 2019. "A New Era of Climate Medicine—Addressing Heat-Triggered Renal Disease." *New England Journal of Medicine* 381 (8):693–96.

Sorensen, C. J., J. Butler-Dawson, M. Dally, L. Krisher, B. R. Griffin, R. J. Johnson, J. Lemery et al. 2019. "Risk Factors and Mechanisms Underlying Cross-Shift Decline in Kidney Function in Guatemalan Sugarcane Workers." *Journal of Occupational and Environmental Medicine* 61 (3):239–50.

Sperati, A., E. Rapiti, L. Settimi, A. Quercia, B. Terenzoni, and F. Forastiere. 1999. "Mortality among Male Licensed Pesticide Users and Their Wives." *American Journal of Industrial Medicine* 36 (1):142–46.

Sunyer, J., E. Suades-González, R. García-Esteban, I. Rivas, J. Pujol, M. Alvarez-Pedrerol, J. Forns, X. Querol, and X. Basagaña. 2017. "Traffic-Related Air Pollution and Attention in Primary School Children: Short-Term Association." *Epidemiology* 28 (2):181–89.

Tang, Y.-X., M. S Bloom, Z. M. Qian, E. Liu, D. R. Jansson, M. G. Vaughn, H.-L. Lin et al. 2019. "Association between Ambient Air Pollution and Hyperuricemia in Traffic Police Officers in China: A Cohort Study." *International Journal of Environmental Health Research*, 2019 Jun 11:1–9.

Valenti, A., D. Gagliardi, G. Fortuna, and S. Iavicoli. 2016. "Towards a Greener Labour Market: Occupational Health and Safety Implications." *Annali dell'Istituto superiore di sanità* 52 (3):415–23.

Watts, N., M. Amann, S. Ayeb-Karlsson, K. Belesova, T. Bouley, M. Boykoff, P. Byass et al. 2018. "The Lancet Countdown on Health and Climate Change: From 25 Years of Inaction to a Global Transformation for Public Health." *Lancet* 391 (10120):581–630.

Whitmee, S., A. Haines, C. Beyrer, F. Boltz, A. G. Capon, B. F. de Souza Dias, A. Ezeh et al. 2015. "Safeguarding Human Health in the Anthropocene Epoch: Report of the Rockefeller Foundation–Lancet Commission on Planetary Health." *Lancet* 386 (10007):1973–2028.

Wickramatillake, B. A., M. A. Fernando, and A. L. Frank. 2019. "Prevalence of Asbestos-Related Disease among Workers in Sri Lanka." *Annals of Global Health* 85 (1):108.

Wnek, S., M. Berg, S. Skelton, L. Lemond, and P. Goad. 2017. "Hazards after the Storm: Floodwater Drainage Pump Stations and Exposure to Hydrogen Sulfide." *Journal of Occupational and Environmental Hygiene* 14 (4):D39–D48.

World Health Organization. 2009. *Protecting Health from Climate Change*. Geneva: WHO.

Wuebbles, D., D. W. Fahey, K. A. Hibbard, D. J. Dokken, B. C. Stewart, and T. K. Maycock, eds. 2017. *Climate Science Special Report: Fourth National Climate Assessment, Vol. 1*. Washington, DC, U.S. Global Change Research Program.

Xia, Y., Y. Li, D. Guan, D. Mendoza Tinoco, J. Xia, Z. Yan, J. Yang; Q. Liu, and H. Huo. 2018. "Assessment of the Economic Impacts Of Heat Waves: A Case Study of Nanjing, China." *Journal of Cleaner Production* 171:811–19.

Xiang, J., P. Bi, D. Pisaniello, A. Hansen, and T. Sullivan. 2014. "Association between High Temperature and Work-Related Injuries in Adelaide, South Australia, 2001–2010." *Occupational and Environmental Medicine* 71:246–52.

Xiang, J., A. Hansen, D. Pisaniello, K. Dear, and P. Bi. 2018. "Correlates of Occupational Heat-Induced Illness Costs: Case Study of South Australia 2000 to 2014." *Journal of Occupational and Environmental Medicine* 60 (9):e463–e469.

Ziersch, A. M., F. Baum, R. J. Woodman, L. Newman, and G. Jolley. 2014. "A Longitudinal Study of the Mental Health Impacts of Job Loss: The Role of Socioeconomic, Sociodemographic, and Social Capital Factors." *Journal of Occupational and Environmental Medicine* 56 (7):714–20.

Zivin, J. G., and M. Neidell. 2012. "The Impact of Pollution on Worker Productivity." *American Economic Review* 102:3652–3673.

Ziska, L. H., R. C. Sicher, K. George, and J. E. Mohan. 2007. "Rising Atmospheric Carbon Dioxide and Potential Impacts on the Growth and Toxicity of Poison Ivy (*Toxicodendron radicans*). *Weed Science* 55 (4):288–92.

Zhu Y, Xie J, Huang F, Cao L. Association between short-term exposure to air pollution and COVID-19 infection: Evidence from China. Sci Total Environ. 2020 Jul 20;727:138704. doi: 10.1016/j.scitotenv.2020.138704. Epub 2020 Apr 15. PMID: 32315904; PMCID: PMC7159846.

CHAPTER 12

WOMEN'S HEALTH AND CLIMATE CHANGE: THE IMPACT OF GENDER

Tracy A. Cushing and Cecilia J. Sorensen

Introduction

As stated by the United Nations Framework Convention on Climate Change (UNFCCC) (United Nations 2017), women face unique risks from, and experience a greater burden of, climate change health impacts. To address these unique needs, the United Nations has developed a gender action plan for climate change, recognizing the role of gender in the physiologic and psychological health effects of climate change, as well as in disaster response, socioeconomic factors, migration patterns, and the integral role of women in future climate change mitigation.

Climate change is a risk multiplier for gender-based health disparities. Women have unique health needs, placing them at specific risk of suffering from climate-sensitive diseases (World Health Organization [WHO] 2014). Compounding these biologic vulnerabilities are cultural constructs, which amplify risk on a regional scale. This effect is greatest in societies where women have lower socioeconomic and political status (WHO 2002). Globally, a total of 1.3 billion people in the developing world live in poverty, and 70 percent of those are women (WHO 2002). Yet although the interactions between gender-based social discrimination, economics, and climate change threaten to amplify gender-based health disparities, women's integral social roles and potential for agency afford opportunities for promoting solutions to sustainability, disaster risk reduction, and health threats. Understanding the unique effects of climate change on women's health is the first step toward ensuring that policies move beyond traditional separations of health, gender, and environment to embrace proactive and gender-based solutions to protecting women's health and mobilizing their vast social potential in mitigating and adapting to the effects of climate change.

Direct Health Impacts of Climate Change on Women

Climate change affects health directly and indirectly through a multitude of mechanisms, including heat, poor air quality, extreme weather events, decreased food security, reduced water quality, and meteorologic changes that alter vector-borne disease epidemiology (Crimmins et al. 2016). The health risks associated with these exposure pathways are mediated through physiologic, cultural, and socioeconomic vulnerabilities, which differ substantially between men and women. A lack of gender-disaggregated health data restricts conclusive understanding of thresholds of exposure for harm from environmental pollutants, as well as for pregnant women and children. The resulting lack of gender-specific data may result in a lack of awareness by local, national, and even global decision-makers and health care personnel as to the unique needs and responses of women in dealing with the health effects of climate change (United Nations 2017).

KEY CONCEPTS

- Women suffer unique impacts from climate change because of their specific physiologic needs throughout the life cycle.

- Cultural and religiously based gender roles place women and girls at higher risk of morbidity and mortality during and after climate-related natural disasters.

- Women and girls are at increased risk of physical and sexual violence in the wake of natural disasters.

- Pregnant women have specific metabolic needs and undergo physiologic changes that place them and their offspring at particular risk of climate-related health effects.

- Women should be active participants in climate change adaptation and mitigation strategies, as they are often the people most affected by daily water procurement strategies, cooking fuel emissions exposure, and clean/renewable energy strategies.

CLINICAL CORRELATES 12.1 CLIMATE CHANGE AND THE UNIQUE PHYSIOLOGY OF PREGNANCY

As temperatures rise and heat waves increase in frequency, pregnant women are at increased risk of preeclampsia, gestational hypertension, and preterm delivery (Basu et al. 2017; Poursafa, Keikha, and Kelishadi 2015; Zheng et al. 2018). Poor indoor air quality from cook stoves and biomass fuels impair maternal cardiopulmonary health reducing placental function and causing poor fetal development (Arinola et al. 2018). Increased caloric demands during pregnancy and nursing will be constrained by climate-related food shortages and macronutrient deficiencies. Pregnant women have greater susceptibility to vector-borne diseases because of hormonally induced changes that result in increased peripheral blood flow, heat production, and chemo-attractants that result in higher rates of infection, and a reduced immune response with overall increases viremia and parasitemia—all leading to poor fetal outcomes (Paixão et al. 2018).

Metabolic and physiologic changes of pregnancy place women at greater risk of climate-related health risks and pregnancy complications.

Temperature

Rising annual global temperatures have become the norm rather than the exception, and climate change-fueled heat waves produce a variety of harmful health effects, many of which disproportionately affect women, resulting in their greater morbidity and mortality during heat waves (Neumayer and Plümper 2007; Schifano et al. 2009). Extreme heat events are responsible for the greatest number of weather-related fatalities in the United States (National Oceanic and Atmospheric Administration [NOAA] n.d.). Women have higher observed mortality during some heat waves whereas men appear more susceptible during others, particularly when social isolation is a factor in heat deaths (Duncan 2006; NOAA n.d.). Women have been observed to be at greater risk of death during and after large heat wave events (NOAA n.d.), both due to direct effects of heat on female physiology, as well as indirect effects of unequal resource distribution in the aftermath of such an event (United Nations 2017). Women are susceptible to the effects of rising temperatures and heat waves because of unique physiologic characteristics such as a higher working metabolic rate, reduced heat dissipation through sweating, and less effective radiative cooling due to greater subcutaneous adipose tissue, all of which predispose them to heat-related illness (Duncan 2006). Culturally prescribed garments and coverings may also limit evaporative cooling, further exacerbating the effects of heat waves.

Heat stress is particularly harmful during pregnancy: heat increases the incidence of adverse reproductive outcomes such as preterm delivery (Kuehn and McCormick 2017), congenital defects (Van Zutphen et al. 2012), gestational hypertension, low birth weight (Strand, Barnett, and Tong 2011), and **preeclampsia** (Makhseed et al. 1999; Van Zutphen et al. 2012), particularly in young mothers (Balbus and Malina 2009). Heat increases production of vasoactive substances that affect blood pressure, increase blood viscosity, and endothelial cell function, all of which may alter placental blood flow and increase propensity for hypertensive crises and stillbirth (Ha et al. 2017). Hyperthermia is teratogenic (harmful to developing fetuses), disrupting the normal sequence of gene activity during organogenesis (Van Zutphen et al. 2012), leading to early fetal demise and birth defects (Wells 2002). Pregnant women have a reduced ability to thermoregulate, making them more susceptible to rising temperatures (Wells 2002). The effects of heat stress are worsened in areas without access to shade, shelter, or cooling, usually in areas that also have barriers to health care access as well as prenatal care. Provision of cooling systems such as air conditioning or reflective roofing surfaces for maternity hospital wards has been shown to reduce the need for neonatal intensive care (Kakkad et al. 2014).

Air Quality

Globally, air quality is worsening in part because of emissions from ongoing fossil fuel combustion, as well as household biomass burning in many poor countries that disproportionately affects women, who spend much of their time in the home (Beggs and Bambrick 2005; WHO 2016). Levels of particulate matter as a marker of air pollution increased 8 percent globally from 2008 to 2013 (WHO 2016). It has been estimated that about 2.5 million women and children die annually as a consequence of exposures to indoor air pollution (Duncan 2006), as traditional biomass burning releases carbon monoxide, carbon dioxide, hydrocarbons, and particulate matter. Some countries such as India have seen a 150 percent rise in air pollution-related deaths during the past two decades (Health Effects Institute 2018), and there are well-studied relationships between episodes of severe air pollution and mortality (Dockery, et al. 1993; Pope et al. 1995; Samet et al. 2000; Zanobetti, A. et al.,2003). Although air pollution affects everyone, women have both a unique exposure pathway as the primary users of household biomass indoors and an associated increased burden of cardiovascular and respiratory disease from indoor air pollution (Chen et al. 2005). Half the global population relies on biomass fuels for heat and cooking, resulting in increased rates of chronic obstructive pulmonary disease, respiratory infections, and childhood respiratory infections and lung carcinoma (Behera, Chakrabarti, and Khanduja 2001; Liu et al. 2007). Outdoors, during episodes of high ambient air pollution, women suffer greater deposition of inhaled particles (Beggs and Bambrick 2006; Kim and Hu 1998) and have increased deaths from cardiopulmonary disease in the aftermath of severe air pollution episodes (Samet et al. 2000).

Poor air quality has been correlated with adverse reproductive outcomes such as stillbirth, congenital defects, intrauterine growth retardation, and low birth weight (Glinianaia et al. 2004; Gouveia, Bremner, and Novaes 2004; Pope et al. 2010; Šrám et al. 2005; Watts et al. 2017), though causation has been difficult to prove. Air pollution can both directly affect fetal health by passage through the placenta as well as indirectly through impaired maternal cardiovascular

CLINICAL CORRELATES 12.2 AIR QUALITY AND WHO'S COOKING?

Cook stoves and heating elements that use biofuels produce particulate matter, carbon monoxide, and hydrocarbons. Approximately half of the global population uses this type of fuel for domestic use, causing poor indoor air quality and contributing to diseases such as chronic obstructive pulmonary disease, childhood pneumonia, and lung cancer (Liu et al. 2007). As women are both largely responsible for cooking in many communities and spend a greater percentage of time indoors, they are at increased risk of exposure to these toxins, in addition to being more susceptible to their effects (Chen et al. 2005).

It is important to involve women in the development and utilization of clean energy sources for cooking and in using new technology, such as biogas systems, which can then be burned on low-pressure gas burners for cooking and illumination (World Health Organization 2014). However, the simple invention of new technology does not guarantee its use. A program in India called Project Surya offers incentives for the purchase of these safer stoves via innovative loans to female heads of households. Stoves are monitored for usage via a metric that translates use into tons of decreased carbon emission, for which users are then compensated for each ton. One area of India measured a 40 percent reduction in black carbon emissions after program implementation (Ramanathan et al. 2017), highlighting the importance and effectiveness of incorporating and supporting the participation of women at all levels of climate change policy mitigation and response.

As women spend a significant proportion of time being exposed to indoor air pollution from biomass fuel, they are important stakeholders in the invention, implementation, and utilization of new and clean fuel technologies, as they stand to gain most in health benefits from decreased pollution.

health, resulting in reduced placental function (Dockery et al.; Watts et al. 2017). As critical decision makers in household fuel choices and consumption, women form an integral part of strategies to reduce biomass use and to utilize other sources of fuel. Better access to clean-burning cook stoves reduces exposure to particulate matter and other inhalants, reducing health risks (Wilkinson et al. 2009).

Climate-Related Disasters and Forced Migration

Globally, there is increasing frequency of climate-related disasters including hurricanes, wildfires, and flooding (Wilkinson, et al. 2009). During such disasters, women suffer disproportionate mortality (Kuehn and McCormick 2017) and female survivors experience decreased life expectancy (Duncan 2006). The ability to migrate during a disaster is complicated by health status, literacy level, the presence of any communication barriers in language or dialect, and economic status. When women have unequal access to basic social goods, their relative mortality during disasters is increased (Lucas et al. 2015; Moosa and Tuana 2014). Women may be homebound caring for children and the elderly and may be restricted from immediate escape during a disaster. Baseline levels of dietary deficiencies for women of all ages can lead to worsened outcomes and increased vulnerability to the effects of disasters; this includes the physical ability to escape a disaster, as well as resiliency in the face of water and food shortages in the aftermath of a disaster (Cannon, Twigg, and Rowell 2003; Chowdhury et al. 1993; Dankelman 2008; Rahman 2013). Pregnant women who deliver in the time period following disasters are at greater risk of complications such as preeclampsia and delivery of low birth weight infants (Tong, Zotti, and Hsia 2011).

Forced migration and repeated short distance moves are especially significant in health outcomes for poorer people, as well as for groups such as women (Norris et al. 2002). The impacts are amplified when women have lower socioeconomic status in their communities (Kennedy and King 2014), worsened by disproportionate job loss and slower economic recovery for women after disasters (Tobin-Gurley, Peek, and Loomis 2010). As women have fewer employment opportunities, they may be unable to migrate into areas with better economic viability, and thus become "trapped" or unable to migrate. Women who do migrate are still faced with caring for young children and the elderly, in transit or in an unfamiliar new setting. Forced migration is both physiologically and psychologically stressful, leading to poor health outcomes, worsened by lack of health services, shelter, and sanitation during migration events (Adanu and Johnson 2009; Tobin-Gurley et al. 2010).

Although there is a dearth of statistical data on women and the poor post disaster, or on rates of sexual violence in the aftermath of climate-related disasters and during migration, the International Federation of the Red Cross *World Disaster Report* (IFRC 2007) states "women and girls are at high risk of sexual violence, sexual exploitation, and abuse, trafficking, and domestic violence in disasters." During such events, women and girls are at higher risk of physical and sexual abuse as well as intimate partner violence (Crimmins et al. 2016) and human trafficking (Adanu and Johnson 2009) and have a greater incidence of mood disorders such as depression and anxiety (Norris et al. 2002; United Nations Division for the Advancement of Women 2001). There has been a growing recognition of **transactional sex** as a response to forced migration and food shortages: different than traditional sex work, there is a transactional nature to this relationship based on the need for post-disaster resources such as food, fuel wood, and transportation (Stoebenau et al. 2016). Particularly documented in sub-Saharan Africa (Dunkle et al. 2010; Stoebenau et al. 2016), there is evidence of transactional sex around the globe, and it is anticipated to increase in response to decreasing resources in post-disaster settings (Willis 2013). This phenomenon was initially described through HIV public health mitigation efforts in Africa (McCoy et al. 2014), particularly around Lake Victoria, where sex is exchanged for food and transport in the fishing economy (Dunkle et al. 2010; Nathenson et al. 2017). As there are anticipated shortages of food, water, shelter, and resources in the face of climate change-fueled disasters and global warming, there is an increasingly urgent need to study the long-term health, morbidity and mortality of women and men who are engaged in transactional sex and who may be victims of climate migration and violence. Although women and girls are a particularly vulnerable population, groups involved in transactional sex can include the elderly, adolescents, women with disabilities, and single women, all of whom often have fewer resources from which to draw support, assistance, and protection and thus are at greatest risk for abuse.

Food Insecurity

As rising temperatures and shifting rainfall impair crop, livestock, and fishery yields, there is increasing food insecurity around the world (Food and Agriculture Organization [FAO] 2019; Myers et al. 2017). Globally, women suffer from higher rates of anemia and malnutrition at baseline and are sensitive to climate-driven food insecurity because of increased nutritional needs during menstruation, pregnancy, and nursing. Nutritional scarcity can be further exacerbated by cultural practices that prioritize feeding of men and children over women, worsening neonatal outcomes in pregnancy including intrauterine growth restriction and perinatal mortality (FAO 2019). Anemia is associated with cognitive impairments including poor attention span, diminished working memory, and poor educational outcomes (Jáuregui-Lobera 2014), as well as increased sensitivity to toxicological exposures (Chen et al. 2005), and iron deficiency anemia increases risk of maternal mortality in childbirth by as much as 20 percent (FAO 2001).

Women produce between 60 and 80 percent of all food in low-income countries, making food scarcity both a health issue and an economic issue, as climate conditions negatively affect agricultural yields, further decreasing women's access to food as well as their economic productivity (Knochel, Dotin, and Hamburger 1974). As they often lack ownership of the lands they farm, with even fewer in possession of documentation of land ownership, most women farmers suffer both direct effects of food scarcity and loss of economic livelihood (Knochel et al. 1974).

Water Scarcity

Fresh water resources are strained globally, with areas of increasing scarcity near areas of large population density. As many as 1.7 billion people currently lack access to an adequate fresh water supply (Cassela 2019), resulting in a large global burden of disease from unsafe water, poor sanitation, and limited hygiene (World Resources Institute 2019). As the number of people living in water-stressed areas increases, its scarcity leads to myriad effects. It is estimated that a family of five individuals needs 100 liters of water per day, weighing 100 kg (WHO 2014), and women are largely responsible for procurement and usage of household water. In some regions carrying water may use up to 85 percent of a woman's daily energy intake (Duncan 2006). As water availability changes, women may be forced to seek water from both geographically and biologically more dangerous sources. As they spend increasing time searching for and transporting water, women and girls have less time to spend on other activities of livelihood, with reduced opportunity for education and other pursuits, while simultaneously increasing their exposure to environmental stressors like heat-related illness (Birch, Meleis, and Wachter 2012; Jayasumana, Gunatilake, and Senanayake 2014; Shiva and Jalees 2005) or to dehydration, which results in decreased uterine blood flow during pregnancy and is associated with preterm labor (Kuehn and McCormick 2017). Reliance on biologically tainted water can result in both disease transmission and direct toxin ingestion (Duncan 2006), worsened by water shortages that restrict its use for hygiene. Cultural restrictions prioritizing the needs of men and children place women at greatest risk from the sequelae of water shortages.

Infectious Diseases and Vector-Borne Illness

Increasing global temperatures and changes in vector habitat range and location have resulted in the changing, often increasing prevalence of vector-borne diseases such as malaria, dengue fever, and Zika virus, among others. As women are the primary household members responsible for water procurement, they are often around standing water sources and other areas that can place them in close contact with mosquito breeding sites. Pregnant women are particularly susceptible to mosquito-borne illnesses: because of higher CO_2 production during pregnancy (CO_2 is a chemo-attractant for mosquitos) as well as increased peripheral blood flow, pregnant women are more prone to mosquito bites and are thus at higher risk of contracting vector borne illnesses (Lindsay et al. 2019; Mbonye, Neema, and Magnussen 2005). Human breath acts as a chemo-attractant for mosquitos to locate hosts; pregnancy increases forced vital capacity and forced expiratory volume (Grindheim et al. 2012), further increasing the risk of mosquito bites. Once infected, pregnant women are at greater risk of complications and severity of illness; their risk of severe malaria is three times higher than that of infected nonpregnant women (McMichael et al. 2008; Petersen et al. 2016), whereas dengue virus is associated with an increased risk of intrauterine growth restriction, **eclampsia**, and cesarean delivery (Pouliot et al. 2010). There is a diminished immune response during pregnancy because of hormonally induced changes in immunologic function; this results in a higher intensity of parasitemia when infected with malaria (Lindsay et al. 2019; Mbonye et al. 2005). Zika virus, which carries devastating fetal effects including microcephaly, central nervous system malformations, and impaired cognitive development (Petersen et al. 2016), has recently been increasing in prevalence. For women, infection while pregnant can result in anemia and increased risk of hemorrhagic complications during delivery (Petersen et al. 2016). Limited or total lack of access to prenatal and obstetrical care further worsens pregnancy and birth outcomes in this setting.

CLINICAL CORRELATES 12.3 SOCIAL AND CULTURAL ROLES OF WOMEN DURING AND AFTER CLIMATE-INDUCED DISASTERS

Women suffer disproportionate mortality in natural disasters (Kuehn and McCormick 2017), their adaptive capacity curtailed by being homebound and/or caring for children and the elderly. They may lack the physical resources to escape a disaster (lack of notification, transportation, inability to drive), or remain in place because of family members who cannot leave. Culturally and socially established clothing or garments may hinder movement and increase risk of heat illness in hot climates. The traditional women's role of water procurement in many parts of the world results in greater time spent carrying and walking to water sources in times of drought. Finally, migration and trapped populations (from displacement) after natural disasters leads to increased risk of physical and sexual violence, as well as exposure to human trafficking (Adanu and Johnson 2009).

Social and cultural factors can lead to lack of mobility in disasters, increased risk of environmental illness, and increased household labor focused on water procurement.

The Role of Women and Gender in Climate Change Policy and Planning

Although climate change, gender inequality, and poverty are increasingly recognized as global problems, achieving the integration of data collection, policies, and implementation necessary to make progress in solving these interrelated issues has proven challenging. A comprehensive assessment of women's assets and vulnerabilities is foundational to any adaptation or development project, including disaster risk reduction, transportation, finance, communication, water management, agriculture, and health. Such assessments not only provide a more in-depth understanding of the effects of climate change but also reveal the political, physical, and socio-economic reasons why women may suffer effects disproportionately, and thereby create opportunities for effective intervention.

The UNFCCC has recognized **gender mainstreaming** as integral to the success of meeting all climate change targets and in increasing the effectiveness of societal interventions. Because of their vital role in almost all aspects of community and household responses to climate change, the participation and inclusion of women has been shown to increase cooperation across political and social boundaries as well as to broaden responsiveness to individual and social needs in climate action plans (McMichael et al. 2008; Moosa, and Tuana 2014; Watts et al. 2017), all of which improve sustainable outcomes. An integrative policy approach must include engagement and communication with women and girls throughout society at all levels. For example, although there are energy-related indicators in the United Nations Sustainable Development Goals (SDGs) (related to household use of biomass fuels), there are no health-related indicators in the energy or climate goals (United Nations 2017). Unless there is explicit linking to the health effects of these other goals, there will be ongoing data disaggregation, inefficiencies, poorly or insufficiently designed policy changes, and communication barriers among the agencies tasked with solving these problems.

Recently, some advances have been made within UNFCCC and the United Nations International Strategy for Disaster Reduction (UNISDR). UNFCCC decision 21/CP.22 (2017) (United Nations 2017) calls for a "gender action plan" to incorporate a gendered perspective in all elements of mitigation, adaptation, capacity, technology, and finance. Although the plan offers an encouraging framework for action, it remains lacking in measurable indicators of progress and systematic integrative procedures. The **Sendai Framework**, an international covenant adopted in 2015 to establish common goals and standards for disaster risk reduction, formalizes climate change as a disaster-risk multiplier to women and recognizes women as important stakeholders in risk reduction (Aitsi-Selmi and Murray 2015; Chan and Murray 2017; Clarke et al. 2018). Furthermore, it calls on adopters to "prepare, review and periodically update preparedness policies, plans, and programmes with the involvement of all relevant institutions, considering climate change scenarios and their impact, and to facilitate the participation of all sectors and stakeholders" (United Nations 2015). Measurable accountability is fundamental to the framework, which contains thirty-eight indicators to track progress in implementing seven targets. The ultimate goal is to reduce disaster mortality and damage to critical infrastructure and economies, through increased multihazard early warning systems, improved national and local mitigation strategies, and enhanced international cooperation. Its goals require participation of *all* stakeholders and recognize women's roles as powerful agents of social change within that framework. Women should be empowered as key stakeholders at the outset of any project, with the understanding that combining scientific data and community knowledge will yield better results (Kratzer 2016).

In order to engage women and girls in participation, there must be understanding of the gender-specific threats of climate change and investment in education regarding the public health, medical, and social effects of climate change as well as policies and programs to mitigate or adapt to climate change. Investment in women's education, especially regarding climate change-related skills and capacity building, will foster leadership and strengthen resilience. In addition, there must be collection of high-quality, gender-disaggregated data in order to better understand climate-gender health associations and to assist in the development of community-based interventions using gender-specific predictive modeling. Ultimately, women's health outcomes and economic prosperity can serve as surrogate markers for development, disaster risk reduction, and climate adaptation, and these should be used as indicators for project and policy success.

Summary

Although gender has been increasingly factored into climate change projects and policy, progress has been slow in reducing gender-based health disparities and in mobilizing women as a vast social resource for climate change mitigation, adaptation, and disaster risk reduction and management (Sorensen et al. 2018). Compliance with the monitoring processes advocated by the United Nations SDGs and the Sendai Framework are critical to address the complex interactions among poverty, gender-based social discrimination, and climate change that may amplify gender-based health disparities (Sorensen et al. 2018). Women's unique social roles within families, groups, and societies at large afford opportunities for promoting effective solutions to combat climate change through sustainability, disaster risk reduction, and health threat mitigation. Recognition of this unique role, combined with high-level political engagement globally, is necessary to assure policies and programs embrace proactive and gender-based solutions that protect women's health and mobilize their vast social potential, starting with the collection of gender disaggregated public health data, because "access to information is critical to successful disaster risk management. You cannot manage what you cannot measure" (United Nations Office for Disaster Risk Reduction n.d.).

DISCUSSION QUESTIONS

1. Why is gender an important factor in data collection and policymaking related to climate change?

2. What are some of the unique aspects of female physiology that affect women's response to rising temperatures, food shortages, water shortages, and vector-borne illnesses?

3. What are some social factors that contribute to women's risk of immediate and long-term health effects of climate disasters?

KEY TERMS

Gender mainstreaming: The concept of integrating a gendered perspective into policy design, process, planning, implementation, and evaluation to promote equality between women and men.

Preeclampsia/Eclampsia: Complications of pregnancy including high blood pressure and protein loss in urine that may eventually lead to seizures and death for both mother and baby without prompt intervention.

Sendai Framework: An international covenant adopted in 2015 to establish common goals and standards for disaster risk reduction.

Transactional sex: A sexual relationship formed as a response to forced migration and food shortages based on the need for resources such as food, fuel wood, and transportation.

References

Adanu, R. M., and T. R. Johnson. 2009. "Migration and Women's Health." *International Journal of Gynecology & Obstetrics* 106 (2):179–81.

Aitsi-Selmi, A., and V. Murray. 2015. "The Sendai Framework: Disaster Risk Reduction through a Health Lens." *Bulletin of the World Health Organization* 93 (6):362.

Arinola, G. O., A. Dutta, O. Oluwole, and C. O. Olopade. 2018. "Household Air Pollution, Levels of Micronutrients and Heavy Metals in Cord and Maternal Blood, and Pregnancy Outcomes." *International Journal of Environmental Research and Public Health* 15 (12):2891. doi:10.3390/ijerph15122891.

Balbus, J. M., and C. Malina. 2009. "Identifying Vulnerable Subpopulations for Climate Change Health Effects in the United States." *Journal of Occupational and Environmental Medicine* 51 (1):33–7.

Basu, R., H. Chen, D. K. Li, and L. A. Avalos. 2017. "The Impact of Maternal Factors on the Association between Temperature and Preterm Delivery." *Environmental Research* 154:109–114. doi:10.1016/j.envres.2016.12.017.

Beggs, P. J., and H. J. Bambrick. 2005. "Is the Global Rise of Asthma an Early Impact of Anthropogenic Climate Change?" *Environmental Health Perspectives* 113 (8):915–9.

Beggs, P. J., and H. J. Bambrick. 2006. "Is the Global Rise of Asthma an Early Impact of Anthropogenic Climate Change?" *Ciência & Saúde Coletiva* 11 (3):745–52.

Behera, D., T. Chakrabarti, and K. L. Khanduja. 2001. "Effect of Exposure to Domestic Cooking Fuels on Bronchial Asthma." *Indian Journal of Chest Diseases & Allied Sciences* 43 (1):27–31.

Birch, E. L., A. Meleis, and S. Wachter. 2012. "The Urban Water Transition: Why We Must Address the New Reality of Urbanization, Women, Water, and Sanitation in Sustainable Development." *wH2O: The Journal of Gender and Water* 1 (1):1.

Cannon, T., J. Twigg, and J. Rowell. 2003. *Social Vulnerability, Sustainable Livelihoods and Disasters.* London: Department for International Development .

Cassela, C. 2019. "Nearly 25 Percent of the World's Population Faces a Water Crisis, and We Can't Ignore It." *ScienceAlert. August* 7, 2019. https://www.sciencealert.com/17-countries-are-facing-extreme-water-stress-and-they-hold-a-quarter-of-the-world-s-population.

Chan, E. Y. Y., and V. Murray. 2017. "What Are the Health Research Needs for the Sendai Framework?" *Lancet* 390 (10106):e35–e36.

Chen, L. H., S. F. Knutsen, D. Shavlik, W. L. Beeson, F. Petersen, M. Ghamsary, and D. Abbey. 2005. "The Association between Fatal Coronary Heart Disease and Ambient Particulate Air Pollution: Are Females at Greater Risk?" *Environmental Health Perspectives* 113 (12):1723.

Chowdhury, A. M. R., A. U. Bhuyia, A. Y. Choudhury, and R. Sen. 1993. "The Bangladesh Cyclone of 1991: Why So Many People Died." *Disasters* 17 (4):291–304.

Clarke, L., K. Blanchard, R. Maini, A. Radu, N. Eltinay, Z. Zaidi, and V. Murray. 2018. "Knowing What We Know—Reflections on the Development of Technical Guidance for Loss Data for the Sendai Framework for Disaster Risk Reduction. *PLoS Curr* Aug 2;10:ecurrents.dis.537bd80d1037a2ffde67d66c604d2a78.

Crimmins, A., J. Balbus, J. L. Gamble, C. B. Beard, J. E. Bell, D. Dodgen, R. J. Eisen et al., eds. *The Impacts of Climate Change on Human Health in the United States: A Scientific Assessment.* Washington, DC: U.S. Global Change Research Program.

Dankelman, I., K. Alam, W. B. Ahmed, Y. D. Gueye, N. Fatema, and R. Mensah-Kutin. 2008. *Gender, Climate Change and Human Security: Lessons from Bangladesh, Ghana and Senegal.* Brooklyn, NY: Women's Environment and Development Organization (WEDO); Accra, Ghana: ABANTU for Development; Dhaka: ActionAid Bangladesh; Dakar, Senegal: ENDA.

Dockery, D. W., C. A. Pope, X. Xu, J. D. Spengler, J. H. Ware, M. E. Fay, B. G. Ferris, Jr., and F. E. Speizer. 1993. "An Association between Air Pollution and Mortality in Six U.S. Cities." *New England Journal of Medicine* 329 (24):1753–9.

Duncan, K. 2006. *Global Climate Change, Air Pollution, and Women's Health. WIT Transactions on Ecology and the Environment, 99.* Southampton, UK: WIT Press.

Dunkle, K. L., G. M. Wingood, C. M. Camp, and R. J. DiClemente. 2010. "Economically Motivated Relationships and Transactional Sex among Unmarried African American and White Women: Results from a U.S. National Telephone Survey." *Public Health Reports* 125 (suppl 4):90–100.

Food and Agricultural Organization. 2001. *Gender and Nutrition.* Rome: FAO.

Food and Agriculture Organization. 2019. *The State of Food Security and Nutrition in the World.* Rome: FAO. http://www.fao.org/state-of-food-security-nutrition/en/.

Glinianaia, S. V., J. Rankin, R. Bell, T. Pless-Mulloli, and D. Howel. 2004. "Particulate Air Pollution and Fetal Health: A Systematic Review of the Epidemiologic Evidence." *Epidemiology* 15 (1):36–45.

Gouveia, N., S. A. Bremner, and H. M. Novaes. 2004. "Association between Ambient Air Pollution and Birth Weight in Sao Paulo, Brazil." *Journal of Epidemiology and Community Health* 58 (1):11–7.

Grindheim, G., K. Toska, M.-E. Estensen, and L. A. Rosseland. 2012. "Changes In Pulmonary Function during Pregnancy: A Longitudinal Cohort Study." *BJOG* 119 (1):94–101.

Ha, S., D. Liu, Y. Zhu, S. S. Kim, S. Sherman, K. L. Grantz, and P. Mendola. 2017. "Ambient Temperature and Stillbirth: A Multi-Center Retrospective Cohort Study." *Environmental Health Perspectives* 125(6).

Health Effects Institute. 2018. *Burden of Disease Attributable to Major Air Pollution Sources in India.* Boston, MA: HEI. https://www.healtheffects.org/publication/gbd-air-pollution-india.

International Federation of the Red Cross. 2007. *World Disasters Report: Focus on Discrimination.* Geneva: IFRC. http://www.ifrc.org/PageFiles/99876/2007/WDR2007-English.pdf.

Jáuregui-Lobera, I. 2014. "Iron Deficiency and Cognitive Functions." *Neuropsychiatric disease and treatment* 10:2087.

Jayasumana, C., S. Gunatilake, and P. Senanayake. 2014. "Glyphosate, Hard Water and Nephrotoxic Metals: Are They the Culprits Behind the Epidemic of Chronic Kidney Disease of Unknown Etiology in Sri Lanka?" *International Journal of Environmental Research and Public Health* 11 (2):2125–47.

Kakkad, K., M. L. Barzaga, S. Wallenstein, G. S. Azhar, and P. E. Sheffield. 2014. "Neonates in Ahmedabad, India, during the 2010 Heat Wave: A Climate Change Adaptation Study." *Journal of Environmental and Public Health* 2014:946875. doi: 10.1155/2014/946875.

Kennedy, J., and L. King. 2014. "The Political Economy of Farmers' Suicides In India: Indebted Cash-Crop Farmers with Marginal Landholdings Explain State-Level Variation in Suicide Rates." *Global Health* 10: article 16.

Kim, C. S., and S. C. Hu. 1998. "Regional Deposition of Inhaled Particles in Human Lungs: Comparison between Men and Women." *Journal of Applied Physiology* 84 (6):1834–44.

Knochel, J. P., L. N. Dotin, and R. J. Hamburger. 1974. "Heat Stress, Exercise, and Muscle Injury: Effects on Urate Metabolism and Renal Function." *Annals of Internal Medicine* 81 (3):321–28.

Kratzer, S., and V. Le Masson. 2016. "*Ten Things to Know: Gender Equality and Achieving Climate Goals in Climate and Development Knowledge Network*." Africa Portal. https://www.africaportal.org/publications/10-things-to-know-gender-equality-and-achieving-climate-goals.

Kuehn, L., and S. McCormick. 2017. "Heat Exposure and Maternal Health in the Face of Climate Change." *International Journal of Environmental Research and Public Health* 14 (8):853.

Lindsay, S., J. Ansell, C. Selman, V. Cox, K. Hamilton, and G. Walraven. 2000. "Effect of Pregnancy on Exposure to Malaria Mosquitoes." *Lancet* 355 (9219):1972.

Liu, S., Y. Zhou, X. Wang, D. Wang, J.n Lu, J. Zheng, N. Zhong, and P. Ran. 2007. "Biomass Fuels Are the Probable Risk Factor for Chronic Obstructive Pulmonary Disease in Rural South China." *Thorax* 62 (10):889–97.

Lucas, R. A., T. Bodin, R. García-Trabanino, C. Wesseling, J. Glaser, I. Weiss, E. Jarquin, K. Jakobsson, and D. H. Wegman. 2015. "Heat Stress and Workload Associated with Sugarcane Cutting—An Excessively Strenuous Occupation!" *Extreme Physiology & Medicine* 4 (suppl 1): A23.

Makhseed, M. A., V. M. Musini, M. A. Ahmed, and R. A. Monem. 1999. "Influence of Seasonal Variation on Pregnancy-induced Hypertension and/or Preeclampsia." *Australian and New Zealand Journal of Obstetrics and Gynaecology* 39 (2):196–99.

Mbonye, A. K., S. Neema, and P. Magnussen. 2005. "Preventing Malaria in Pregnancy: A Study of Perceptions and Policy Implications in Mukono District, Uganda." *Health Policy and Planning* 21 (1):17–26.

McCoy, S. I., L. J. Ralph, P. F. Njau, M. M. Msolla, and N. S. Padian. 2014. "Food Insecurity, Socioeconomic Status, and HIV-Related Risk Behavior among Women in Farming Households in Tanzania." *AIDS Behavior* 18 (7):1224–36.

McMichael, A. J., P. Wilkinson, R. S. Kovats, S. Pattenden, S. Hajat, B. Armstrong, N. Vajanapoom, et al. 2008. "International Study of Temperature, Heat and Urban Mortality: The 'ISOTHURM' Project." *International Journal of Epidemiology* 37 (5):1121–31.

Moosa, C. S., and N. Tuana. 2014. "Mapping a Research Agenda Concerning Gender and Climate Change: A Review of the Literature." *Hypatia* 29 (3):677–94.

Myers, S. S., M. R Smith, S. Guth, C. D. Golden, B. Vaitla, N. D. Mueller, A. D. Dangour, and P. Huybers. 2017. "Climate Change and Global Food Systems: Potential Impacts on Food Security and Undernutrition." *Annual Review of Public Health* 38:259–77.

Nathenson, P., S. Slater, P. Higdon, C. Aldinger, and E. Ostheimer. 2017. "No Sex for Fish: Empowering Women to Promote Health and Economic Opportunity in a Localized Place in Kenya." *Health Promotion International* 32 (5):800–7.

Neumayer, E., and T. Plümper 2007. "The Gendered Nature of Natural Disasters: The Impact of the Gender Gap in Life Expectancy 1981–2002." *Annals of the Association of American Geographers* 97:551–66.

National Oceanic and Atmospheric Administration. n.d. "Weather-Related Fatality and Injury Statistics." https://www.weather.gov/hazstat/.

Norris, F. H., M. J. Friedman, P. J. Watson, C. M. Byrne, E. Diaz, and K. Kaniasty. 2002. "60,000 Disaster Victims Speak: Part I. An Empirical Review of the Empirical Literature, 1981–2001." *Psychiatry: Interpersonal and Biological Processes* 65 (3):207-239.

Paixão, E. S., M. G. Teixeira, M. D. C. N. Costa, M. L. Barreto, and L. C. Rodrigues. 2018. "Symptomatic Dengue during Pregnancy and Congenital Neurologic Malformations." *Emerging Infectious Diseases* 24 (9):1748–50. doi:10.3201/eid2409.170361.

Petersen, L. R., D. J. Jamieson, A. M. Powers, and M. A. Honein. 2016. "Zika Virus." *New England Journal of Medicine* 374 (16):1552–63.

Pope, C. A., III, M. J. Thun, M. M. Namboodiri, D. W. Dockery, J. S. Evans, F. E. Speizer, and C. W. Heath Jr. 1995. "Particulate Air Pollution as a Predictor of Mortality in a Prospective Study of U.S. Adults." *American Journal of Respiratory and Critical Care Medicine* 151 (3 Pt 1):669–74.

Pope, D. P., V. Mishra, L. Thompson, A. R. Siddiqui, E. A. Rehfuess, M. Weber, and N. G. Bruce. 2010. "Risk of Low Birth Weight and Stillbirth Associated with Indoor Air Pollution from Solid Fuel Use in Developing Countries." *Epidemiologic Reviews* 32 (1):70–81.

Pouliot, S. H., X. Xiong, E. Harville, V. Paz-Soldan, K. M. Tomashek, G. Breart, and P. Buekens. 2010. "Maternal Dengue and Pregnancy Outcomes: A Systematic Review." *Obstetrical & Gynecological Survey* 65 (2):107–18.

Rahman, M. S. 2013. "Climate Change, Disaster and Gender Vulnerability: A Study on Two Divisions of Bangladesh." *American Journal of Human Ecology* 2 (2):72–82.

Poursafa, P., M. Keikha, and R. Kelishadi. 2015. "Systematic Review on Adverse Birth Outcomes of Climate Change." *Journal of Research in Medical Sciences* 20 (4):397–402.

Ramanathan, T., N. Ramanathan, J. Mohanty, I. H. Rehman, E. Graham, and V. Ramanathan. 2017. "Wireless Sensors Linked to Climate Financing for Globally Affordable Clean Cooking." *Nature Climate Change* 7 (1):44–47.

Samet, J. M., F. Dominici, F. C. Curriero, I. Coursac, and S. L. Zeger. 2000. "Fine Particulate Air Pollution and Mortality in 20 U.S. Cities, 1987–1994." *New England Journal of Medicine* 343 (24):1742–9.

Schifano, P., G. Cappai, M. De Sario, P. Michelozzi, C. Marino, A. M. Bargagli, and C. A. Perucci. 2009. "Susceptibility to Heat Wave-Related Mortality: A Follow-Up Study of a Cohort of Elderly in Rome." *Environmental Health* 8:50.

Shiva, V., and K. Jalees. 2005. *Water & Women: A Report by Research Foundation for Science, Technology, and Ecology for National Commission for Women.* New Delhi: Navdanya/RFSTE.

Sorensen, C., V. Murray, J. Lemery, and J. Balbus. 2018. "Climate Change and Women's Health: Impacts and Policy Directions." *PLoS Medicine* 15 (7):e1002603.

Šrám, R. J., B. Binková, J. Dejmek, and M. Bobak. 2005. "Ambient Air Pollution and Pregnancy Outcomes: A Review of the Literature." *Environmental Health Perspectives* 113 (4):375.

Stoebenau, K., L. Heise, J. Wamoyi, and N. Bobrova. 2016. "Revisiting the Understanding of 'Transactional Sex' in Sub-Saharan Africa: A Review and Synthesis of the Literature." *Social Science & Medicine* 168:186–97.

Strand, L. B., A. G. Barnett, and S. Tong. 2011. "The Influence of Season and Ambient Temperature on Birth Outcomes: A Review of the Epidemiological Literature." *Environmental Research* 111 (3):451–62.

Tobin-Gurley, J., L. Peek, and J. Loomis. 2010. "Displaced Single Mothers in the Aftermath of Hurricane Katrina: Resource Needs and Resource Acquisition." *International Journal of Mass Emergencies and Disasters* 28 (2):170–206.

Tong, V. T., M. E. Zotti, and J. Hsia. 2011. "Impact of the Red River Catastrophic Flood on Women Giving Birth in North Dakota, 1994–2000." *Maternal and Child Health Journal* 15 (3):281–88.

United Nations. 2015. *Sendai Framework for Disaster Risk Reduction 2015–2030*. Geneva: UNISDR. http://www.unisdr.org/files/43291_sendaiframeworkfordrren.pdf.

United Nations Division for the Advancement of Women. 2001. *Environmental Management and the Mitigation of Natural Disasters: A Gender Perspective. Ankara*, Turkey: UN.

United Nations Framework Convention on Climate Change. 2017. *Introduction to Gender and Climate Change*. https://unfccc.int/topics/gender/the-big-picture/introduction-to-gender-and-climate-change.

United Nations Office for Disaster Risk Reduction. 2019. "Disaster Statistics." https://undrr.org/publication/global-assessment-report-disaster-risk-reduction-2019.

Van Zutphen, A. R., S. Lin, B. A. Fletcher, and S.-A. Hwang. 2012. "A Population-Based Case–Control Study of Extreme Summer Temperature and Birth Defects." *Environmental Health Perspectives* 120 (10):1443.

Watts, N., M. Amann, S. Ayeb-Karlsson, K. Belesova, T. Bouley, M. Boykoff, P. Byass et al. 2018. "The Lancet Countdown on Health and Climate Change: From 25 Years of Inaction to a Global Transformation for Public Health." *Lancet* 391 (10120):581–630.

Wells, J. C. 2002. "Thermal Environment and Human Birth Weight." *Journal of Theoretical Biology* 214 (3):413–25.

Wilkinson, P., K. R. Smith, M. Davies, H. Adair, B. G. Armstrong, M. Barrett, and N. Bruce. 2009. "Public Health Benefits of Strategies to Reduce Greenhouse-Gas Emissions: Household Energy." *Lancet* 374 (9705):1917–29.

Willis, B. 2013. "The Global Public Health Burden of Sex Work: A Call for Research." *Lancet Global Health* 1 (2):e68.

World Health Organization. 2002. *The World Health Report 2002: Reducing Risks, Promoting Healthy Life*. Geneva: WHO.

World Health Organization. 2014. *Gender, Climate Change, and Health*. Geneva: WHO.https://www.who.int/globalchange/GenderClimateChangeHealthfinal.pdf.

World Health Organization. 2016. *Ambient Air Pollution: A Global Assessment of Exposure and Disease Burden*. Geneva: WHO. https://apps.who.int/iris/bitstream/handle/10665/250141/9789241511353-eng.pdf?sequence=1.

World Resources Institute. 2019. "Release: Updated Global Water Risk Atlas Reveals Top Water-Stressed Countries and States." *April 6, 2019*. https://www.wri.org/news/2019/08/release-updated-global-water-risk-atlas-reveals-top-water-stressed-countries-and-states.

Zanobetti, A., J. Schwartz, E. Samoli, A. Gryparis, G. Touloumi, J. Peacock, R. H. Anderson, et al. 2003. "The Temporal Pattern of Respiratory and Heart Disease Mortality in Response to Air Pollution." *Environmental Health Perspectives* 111 (9):1188–93.

Zheng, X., W. Zhang, C. Lu, D. Norbäck, and Q. Deng. 2018. "An Epidemiological Assessment of the Effect of Ambient Temperature on the Incidence of Preterm Births: Identifying Windows of Susceptibility during Pregnancy." *Journal of Thermal Biology* 74:201–07. doi:10.1016/j.jtherbio.2018.04.001.

CHAPTER 13

CLIMATE MODELING FOR HEALTH IMPACTS

Kristopher B. Karnauskas

Greenhouse Gases and Radiative Forcing

The global carbon cycle is changing, and that change is accelerating. Humanity emitted about 10 gigatons (Gt) of carbon into the atmosphere from fossil fuel use in 2018, equivalent to 37 Gt of CO_2 (Friedlingstein et al. 2019). These were the global **emissions**, as quantified by an international team of dozens of credentialed scientists and engineers representing governmental and academic institutions, with relatively small uncertainty (±5 percent). It is a couple of percentage points higher than in 2017, which was a couple of percentage points higher than in 2016. Another annual number that we know quite well is the amount by which the global **concentration** of atmospheric CO_2 has increased. In 2018, the concentration of CO_2 in Earth's atmosphere grew by about 3 parts per million (ppm), which is three times the annual growth rate in 1970.

Emissions and concentration are obviously linked, but it is worth appreciating their distinction, where the former is the amount deposited each year and the latter is the account balance. The strength of the greenhouse effect (described later) at a given time is a function of the composition of the global atmosphere at that time, so the total *concentration* of **greenhouse gases** (e.g., 411.44 ppm of CO_2 in 2019) is what the physical climate system responds primarily to. If annual CO_2 emissions were as high as they are but constant year after year, the CO_2 concentration might increase linearly. However, emissions themselves are steadily increasing; hence the concentration is growing exponentially.

The amount by which the atmospheric CO_2 concentration has increased since the beginning of the industrial revolution is not unprecedented. Both the rise in CO_2 concentration over the past 150 years due to anthropogenic emissions and the increases in CO_2 that occur at the termination of a glacial cycle are approximately 100 ppm. The pace of the recent rise in CO_2 concentration, however, is indeed unprecedented in the history of Earth's climate. If one lines up the beginning of the previous two deglaciations (roughly 137,000 and 15,000 years ago) with the year 1851, we can see just how rapidly CO_2 concentration is rising today compared to quite some pivotal climatic shifts in Earth's history (Figure 13.1). During the last two deglaciations, CO_2 concentrations rose by 80 ppm in somewhere between 6,000 and 10,000 years, whereas recent anthropogenic emissions drove CO_2 upward by the same amount in just 150 years (1851–2000). We are conducting a massive, uncontrolled physics experiment on planet Earth. At the present rate of increase (2.5 ppm per year), the next 80 ppm should be added in as little as thirty years.

It is not a coincidence that human activities are emitting CO_2 into the atmosphere and the concentration of CO_2 in the atmosphere is increasing. Apart, they are highly uncontroversial facts both within and outside of the scientific community. However, there are a couple of **attribution** ("cause and effect") cases that must be

KEY CONCEPTS

- Atmospheric concentrations of greenhouse gases are higher today than any time in at least the past million years, which is rigorously proven to be a result of human activities.

- Rising concentrations of greenhouse gases lead to a net energy imbalance in Earth's climate (primarily by reducing how much heat escapes), requiring an increase in global average temperature.

- Global climate models (GCMs) are computerized representations of the laws of physics that govern how the atmosphere, ocean, and other features of the climate system operate and interact.

- GCMs enable us to attribute the observed global warming over the past century to greenhouse gas forcing and to predict future warming (and other changes in the climate such as rainfall) given assumptions about future rates of greenhouse gas emissions.

- Climate modeling for global change science is an international collaboration; considering the dozens of GCMs developed and run at institutions around the world enables quantification of uncertainties in future climate change projections.

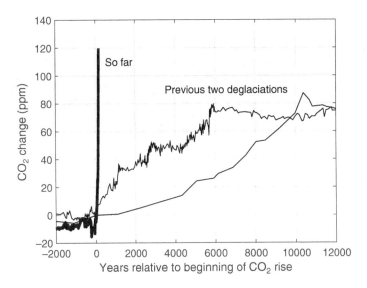

Figure 13.1   Three segments of the full CO_2 concentration (ppm) record shifted such that the beginning of the CO_2 rises associated with the previous two deglaciations and the modern era begin at coordinates (0,0) on the graph. This enables direct comparison of both the amount and rates of change associated with these three time periods. The last and next-to-last deglaciations were taken to start at years −15,410 and −136,900, respectively, and the modern era is aligned such that the year 1851 is at zero on the time axis.
Source: Kris Karnauskas, *Physical Oceanography and Climate*, 2020, © Kris Karnauskas 2020, published by Cambridge University Press, reproduced with permission.

made in order to bring them together, and although science has made them very well, they are the usual sources of confusion and contention among those whose expertise and life's work may lie outside of the field of climate science. The first is whether CO_2 is rising at the measured rates *because* of human activities. Earth's climate has, after all, changed in the distant past— including the atmospheric CO_2 concentration. For an ironclad case, we must go beyond simply correlation, which—as is often cited—doesn't prove causation.

The field of geochemistry has developed an extraordinary tool for detecting the fingerprint of fossil fuel combustion: isotopic fractionation. When humans engage in fossil fuel combustion, we are burning plant matter that has been buried in layers beneath the surface of the Earth and has become fossilized (Figure 13.2). When those plants were living and photosynthesizing, they were fixing carbon in the form of atmospheric CO_2. However, not all carbon atoms are the same. There are three naturally occurring carbon isotopes, which differ only in how many neutrons are present (as all isotopes do). Carbon–12 (^{12}C) and carbon–13 (^{13}C) are stable, meaning they do not decay radioactively like carbon–14 (^{14}C). When plants photosynthesize, they may use either ^{12}C or ^{13}C, but their physiology is able to discriminate between isotopes and they strongly prefer the lighter isotope, ^{12}C. Tracking the ratio of one isotope to the other in the atmosphere (^{13}C/^{12}C or simply δ^{13}C) thus enables us to determine *why* CO_2 started rising as rapidly as it did in the nineteenth century. By extracting long ice cores from the Antarctic ice sheet and examining air bubbles trapped inside of them, we have detected a precipitous drop in atmospheric δ^{13}C (higher ^{12}C relative to ^{13}C), which happens to be timed very well with the increase in *total* atmospheric CO_2 concentration, confirming that the modern rise in CO_2 is attributable to fossil fuel combustion (Francey et al. 1999; Rubino et al. 2013). Have anthropogenic emissions been *enough* to account for the atmospheric concentration passing 400 ppm in 2015? Unfortunately, we have emitted way more than enough to account for that. Had all of the CO_2 emitted into the atmosphere *stayed* in the atmosphere rather than some being absorbed by the ocean and land, we would have met the 400–ppm milestone about twenty years earlier (Denman and Brasseur 2007). About half of the CO_2 emitted by fossil fuel combustion so far has already been drawn out of the atmosphere, and that burden has been shared about evenly between the ocean and terrestrial biosphere.

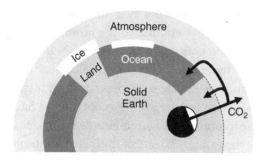

Figure 13.2   Illustration of carbon reservoirs and components of earth's climate system, including the atmosphere, ocean, cryosphere, and solid earth

Source: Kris Karnauskas, *Physical Oceanography and Climate*, 2020, © Kris Karnauskas 2020, published by Cambridge University Press, reproduced with permission.

Note: Black arrows represent anthropogenic carbon dioxide emissions, indicated as a flux from the solid Earth into the atmosphere, and subsequent fluxes of anthropogenic CO_2 from the atmosphere to the terrestrial biosphere and ocean.

The other question of attribution concerns whether the increasing concentration of CO_2 (which is definitely due to human activities) is in fact causing the climate changes that we have been observing. Even when one accepts that the global average surface temperature on Earth has risen by about 1.3°C (2.4°F) over the last century, firmly establishing cause and effect entails some basic understanding of the expected thermodynamic response of the climate system to increasing greenhouse gas concentrations. Building those laws into comprehensive Earth system models, we may show that the actual CO_2 emissions indeed account for the observed warming. The laws of thermodynamics in fact *require* the climate to warm when additional molecules of CO_2 are added to the atmosphere. CO_2 is regarded a greenhouse gas because of how it interacts with thermal radiation attempting to pass through it. Consider one molecule of CO_2 as comprised of three marbles (two oxygen atoms and one carbon in the middle) connected by two springs (covalent bonds); there are several ways for such a contraption to bend, wiggle, and vibrate. Like other greenhouse gases, including methane, nitrous oxide, and water vapor, the geometry of these molecules is well suited to intercepting thermal radiation, converting it to kinetic energy (i.e., raising their own temperature), and reemitting that thermal radiation at a rate proportional to their temperature to the fourth power (à la Stefan-Boltzmann Law).

A greenhouse is therefore not a bad analogy for this process; solar radiation passes through these molecules in the atmosphere to heat the surface (like sunlight passing through glass walls), but most of the thermal radiation emitted by the surface is intercepted by greenhouse gases on its way out and returned to the atmosphere. If Earth's atmosphere contained no greenhouse gases whatsoever, its equilibrium temperature would be a miserable −18°C. It is perhaps obvious that greenhouse gases are not just lining the floor; they are generally mixed throughout the lower layer of the atmosphere (called the **troposphere**). So, when greenhouse gases absorb and reemit thermal radiation, the fraction of that reemitted energy that is escaping to space has been reemitted on average by molecules with a *lower* temperature than that of the surface because they reside in a colder part of the atmosphere! It is both the radiative properties of greenhouse gases *and* their vertical distribution in the troposphere that allow them to reduce the amount of thermal radiation escaping to space. Because they do not change the amount of incoming energy (solar radiation), the incoming radiation in the presence of greenhouse gases exceeds the outgoing radiation. Given such a net energy imbalance, the fundamental laws of thermodynamics for a closed system guarantee that a new equilibrium will be reached after the temperature increases until the outgoing energy (thermal radiation escaping to space) exactly balances the incoming energy (solar radiation). With the presence of greenhouse gases in Earth's atmosphere, such equilibrium is (or was) achieved with Earth's average surface temperature set at about 15°C (59°F).

Today, we are maintaining a perpetual *disequilibrium* between the incoming and outgoing energy because each additional molecule of a greenhouse gas emitted to the atmosphere by human activity ensures that more of the thermal radiation emitted by Earth's surface is intercepted in the atmosphere and re–radiated at a lower temperature. This energy imbalance currently amounts to a **radiative forcing** of $1-2$ W/m^2, and meanwhile we witness the guaranteed consequence of an upward trend in global average surface temperature. Recent studies have unambiguously detected the fingerprints of radiative forcing in measurements of the *decreasing* trend of thermal radiation escaping to space (Harries et al. 2001) and of the *increasing* trend of thermal radiation reaching Earth's surface (Feldman et al. 2015). The greenhouse effect works, and we are making it stronger. As the greenhouse effect and the laws of thermodynamics in general are quite well known, they constitute an important function within the models that are discussed in the next section, and which we use both to attribute past changes in climate and to project future changes given various assumptions about how much CO_2 will be emitted throughout the remainder of this century.

What Is a Global Climate Model?

There are many pathways and manifestations of climate change in the real world, both past and future. In most cases, there is a common tool that is used for projecting the future impacts and regional expressions of climate change: **global climate models** (GCM)—that is, comprehensive models of the global climate system that incorporate the atmosphere *and* ocean, as well as other realms of the Earth system like the cryosphere (including sea ice, ice sheets, snow, and glaciers) and even the biosphere to a varying extent. The latest generations of GCMs are actually *combinations* of atmospheric general circulation models (AGCMs), ocean general circulation models (OGCMs), and other submodels, like ones that predict how ice sheets and fields of sea ice change and how terrestrial vegetation responds to climate (Figure 13.3). GCMs are also useful for investigating climate variations of the recent past, as certain experiments can be designed to estimate how much *natural* variability we might expect to see in various aspects of the climate system, and to attribute observed long-term changes in the climate to particular forcings. Those experiments will be discussed here as well.

What is a GCM? To the newcomer, the answer can take a while to sink in, particularly because of how tempting it is to conflate climate models with climate observations. In the most general sense of the word, *observations* of the natural world have led us to theories that explain in a universal sense how it all works. Think of Newton's *Principia* of 1687. He observed the proverbial apple falling from the tree, and following much more careful observation and consideration, the laws of classical mechanics, gravitation, etc. were developed. Most of the equations and other theoretical material comprising physics textbooks were inspired at some point in time by a set of such observations that made someone ask "why?" The various models (of the atmosphere, ocean, etc.) that make up a complete GCM are merely the laws of physics that govern those realms of the climate system, all packed into a computer program that solves those equations at every location on Earth and on any date (past or future) that is of interest to the researcher. Notice that the "observations" that were important in the development of GCMs were actually important in the development of their precursors—the laws of physics. GCMs are *not* observations of climate change. Climate change is the thing we want to diagnose and predict with GCMs, so observations *of* climate change are not fed into GCMs, and for some very good reasons that will become clear as we explore how GCM experiments are conceived. To summarize, GCMs are large collections of equations whose outputs have an impact on each other's inputs, and we know those equations largely because of systematic observations of the natural world—they are then translated from mathematical notation into computer code.

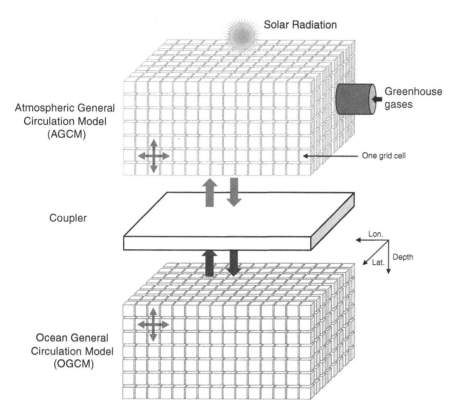

Figure 13.3 Anatomy of a GCM as a coupled model including component models representing the global atmosphere (AGCM), global ocean (OGCM), and other components such as ice and the terrestrial and/or marine biosphere (not pictured). The component models discretize their global realm with finite-sized grid cells whose size is a function of model resolution. Grid cells must communicate with each other (transparent arrows), and a coupler serves to exchange information (forcing) between the component models. Typical prescriptions during coupled GCM experiments include solar radiation and the concentration of greenhouse gases.

Source: Kris Karnauskas, *Physical Oceanography and Climate,* 2020, © Kris Karnauskas 2020, published by Cambridge University Press, reproduced with permission.

Given this general description of GCMs, you may be wondering why we need supercomputers the size of large classrooms to run climate simulations with them. The answer has less to do with the number of equations that constitute a GCM and more with how big Earth is and how far out the end of the twenty-first century still is (a conventional time frame to predict using GCMs). If you imagine all of the equations in a meteorology textbook, plus all the equations from books that similarly describe the behavior of the ocean, sea ice, ice sheets, and terrestrial biosphere, you can now imagine how simulating the time evolution of the climate system actually means solving those equations *everywhere!* It may also be obvious that those equations at one location cannot just be considered in isolation from neighboring locations, nor can a single time step be simulated in isolation of all of the previous times. It gets complicated and expensive, but fortunately there is some compromise that takes place by approximating "everywhere" with a reasonable number of volumes connected to one another.

GCMs divide the world into three-dimensional volumes called **grid cells**. If it is decided that each grid cell in the *atmosphere* component of the GCM is 0.5° latitude by 0.5° longitude by 100 meters in height, then we end up with about thirty million grid cells for the troposphere alone. Such numbers define the **resolution** of the GCM. In reality, a GCM's resolution can be different in different regions, depending on what the modeler thinks is going to be important to resolve in greater detail. For example, the atmospheric component of GCMs (or AGCMs) usually have finer vertical resolution packed into the lower altitudes of the troposphere to better resolve the detailed interactions with the surface. In addition, many OGCMs have "stretched" resolution such that grid cells are smaller (~0.2° latitude) but more numerous within a few degrees of the equator, and finer vertical resolution (1–10 m) in the upper ocean. The former is in recognition of how important the coupled dynamics in the deep tropics are in determining the evolution of the global climate system (e.g., **El Niño**). Finally, an important component of a GCM known as the "coupler" translates everything that is happening within the AGCM that matters to the ocean into a direct *input* (also referred to as forcing) to the ocean model (solar radiation, surface winds, etc.). At the same time, the coupler must also round up all of the variables from the OGCM that should affect the atmosphere and pass it along as forcing along the bottom of the AGCM. So, a GCM is truly a set of multiple submodels, each of which are responsible for simulating their own jurisdiction within Earth's climate, but exchanging information frequently along the way so that the overall climate evolution is determined by their *coupled* interaction—just like in the real world. Because GCMs are *coupled* models, there is no way to guarantee that the basic climatology that emerges in such simulations is perfect. Each model has mean state **biases**, meaning a little too much rainfall here, not enough there, this part of the ocean is too windy, or not enough low cloud cover over there. GCM biases are acceptable within reason and generally do not prevent us from using them to make predictions of *change*, but it is still the ambition of model developers to reduce biases with each new generation of GCMs.

The amount of computer time required for a GCM to complete a simulation is known as "wall clock" time—how long the climate modeler will actually have to wait for an experiment to finish and obtain the results. Wall clock time depends on many characteristics of the GCM and the experimental design including the spatial resolution and number of years to be simulated. The wall clock time also depends on the computer! Drawing on the comparison between the size of a supercomputer and a large classroom, a supercomputer is not unlike a classroom full of students, each with their own basic calculator. The supercomputer takes the whole Earth full of grid cells as defined by the modeler, splits it up into a number of tiles (similar to broad, rectangular regions), and assigns each tile to an individual processor to work on—a computing strategy known as **parallel processing**. The large number of calculations needed just for a single time step in the model simulation is thereby shared across a large number of processors that work on them simultaneously. When the first time step is finished (say 0 UTC [coordinated universal time] on January 1, 1900), all of the processors move on to the next time step (6:00 UTC), solve the equations for each grid cell in their assigned segment of the world, and so on. Eventually, 0 UTC on January 1, 2000 is reached and *voilà*, a retrospective simulation of last century has finished. For modern GCMs running on state-of-the-art supercomputers, such a simulation might take several days if not weeks or more, depending on the aforementioned characteristics of the GCM and experimental design and how many other climate modelers you are sharing the computer with.

Global Climate Models and Global Change Science

Although running a one–off GCM experiment for an esoteric problem might be a relatively solitary pursuit achievable by a single or small group of climate scientists, climate modeling for the purpose of global change science is a truly collaborative and international enterprise. There are dozens of GCMs that have been developed and are run on supercomputers at various research, academic, and governmental institutions around the world. Major centers in the United States, for example, include the National Oceanic and Atmospheric Administration (NOAA) Geophysical Fluid Dynamics Laboratory (GFDL), National Center for Atmospheric Research (NCAR), and the NASA Goddard Institute for Space Sciences (GISS). To put it mildly, these are incredibly sophisticated computer models, and *within* each of these institutions are large and diverse teams of climate scientists (as well as computer scientists, data scientists, and engineers) whose full-time jobs are to work on a single *component* of the full GCM (such as the AGCM or the coupler).

When it comes time to conduct the climate change experiments that inform the assessment reports issued periodically by the Intergovernmental Panel on Climate Change (IPCC), a special team must be assembled to coordinate *across* institutions. This coordinating effort is called the Coupled Model Intercomparison Project (CMIP). Just as the latest Assessment Report of the IPCC was AR5 (IPCC 2013), the most recent CMIP was CMIP5. The coordination achieved by CMIP is essential to ensure that, although each of the international modeling institutions may have its own GCM(s), the experiments are being conducted in a consistent manner. In other words, each GCM simulation uses the same prescribed historical greenhouse gas forcing, the same time periods being simulated, and the same assumptions about possible *future* CO_2 concentrations. The latter of course, depends critically on how society evolves in the coming decades, but at least the same **representative concentration pathways** (**RCPs**) are simulated by each model. This coordination and controlling for as many confounding variables as possible lead to a uniformity of experiments that enables teams of IPCC authors to merge the results from all models into one picture, ensuring that any differences between results from different institutions must be the result of their *models themselves* being different, not, say, because they used different historical records of nitrous oxide concentration.

Each time a new IPCC assessment report is on the horizon (every 5–7 years), several types of GCM experiments are conducted under the auspices of CMIP. GCM simulations in which the radiative forcing (greenhouse gases, volcanic aerosols, solar radiation) are held constant for a thousand years or more are known as **control experiments**. Control experiments yield insight into how much the climate system varies without any perturbation by humans or other external factors, which is important to know when determining whether a trend is undoubtedly due to radiative forcing or might just be a perfectly natural wiggle. **Attribution experiments** are two otherwise–identical GCM simulations conducted with and without "something," where that something is usually one or more of the anthropogenic forcings. These are counterfactual experiments from which we can estimate how the past century of climate would have unfolded *without* fossil fuel combustion simply by keeping the atmospheric CO_2 concentration set at its preindustrial level. Here's why observations of climate change (beyond the *forcing* like CO_2 concentration) are not just fed into the models! Because one of these GCM simulations represents the model's best attempt to reproduce the historical changes in global average temperature (and other changes mediated by warming) and the other excludes the greenhouse gases, we can *compare* both of them with the observational records and soundly establish attribution—we *cannot* explain the observed global warming unless we include the effect of greenhouse gases (Figure 13.4). It is not just a natural wiggle or due to some other natural forcing like volcanic aerosols or variations in the solar radiation emitted by the sun. We humans are responsible for the rise in greenhouse gases, which explains the observed warming; therefore we are responsible for the observed warming—we have now come full circle.

Finally, **future experiments** are conducted by running GCMs from the present to the year 2100 (or beyond) and introducing additional CO_2 into the atmosphere according to an assumption of how much humans will continue emitting the gases over that interval. This is where the coordinating role of CMIP is especially crucial for efforts to provide useful predictions for policymakers via IPCC. Rather than allowing every nation or modeling institution to use its own projection of CO_2 emissions, which is highly dependent on assumptions about population, technology, energy policy, international relations, national politics, etc., a set of four RCPs were agreed upon by CMIP and IPCC stakeholders, and each modeling center conducted GCM experiments using those RCPs so that, again, all of the model results could literally be combined onto a single graph and enable us to judge not only the consensus predictions but

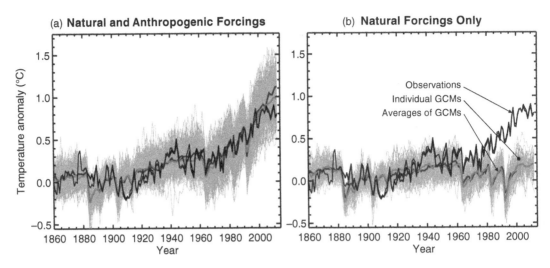

Figure 13.4   Historical simulations by ensembles of GCMs of the CMIP3 and CMIP5 generation of global mean surface temperature (°C) with natural (e.g., volcanic) and anthropogenic (e.g., greenhouse gases) forcings (a). The plot in (b) is the same except that only natural forcings were included in the model simulations, thus attributing the observed temperature change to anthropogenic forcings.
Note: Three different observational records are shown in thick black lines. Individual model simulations are shown in thin light gray lines, and the multimodel averages are indicated by thick dark gray lines.
Source: Adapted from IPCC AR5 WG1, Figure 10.1 (IPCC 2013) and reproduced from Kris Karnauskas, *Physical Oceanography and Climate*, 2020, © Kris Karnauskas 2020, published by Cambridge University Press, with permission.

the range of uncertainty. The most severe RCP is RCP8.5 (where 8.5 refers to 8.5 W/m² of radiative forcing due to the climatic energy imbalance at year 2100). RCPs of lesser end-of-century radiative forcing lie somewhere below RCP8.5: RCP6 and RCP4.5 may still be reasonable scenarios, whereas RCP2.6 sits so close to the year 2019 concentration by 2100 that one can only imagine the severity of policy changes required for it to be plausible. In most peer-reviewed studies considering future climate changes, and in the fifth IPCC assessment report itself, the most common comparison is between RCP8.5 and RCP4.5 as something of a comparison between unmitigated or "business-as-usual" versus "policy-mitigated emissions" scenarios, although even the term business as usual makes strong (and actively debated) assumptions about just what that means and of what we as a global society are capable.

Although it has been the norm to express the results of future experiments by GCMs as the change of a variable (such as rainfall) at a specific future time horizon (such as 2070) given a specified forcing scenario (such as RCP4.5) and perhaps compare that result with those from RCP8.5 simulations, a clever alternative is growing in popularity as a way to make GCM results more relevant to ongoing international climate policy discussions such as the 2°C target associated with the Paris Agreement. Rather than a *time horizon*, results can be portrayed for a particular *global warming threshold*. For example, the resulting illustration might be a map of the rainfall change that we expect if and when global average surface temperature reaches 2°C (3.6°F), which can be compared with the change expected for 1.5°C and 3°C (2.7°F and 37.4°F) to weigh the costs and benefits of meeting such targets through mitigation strategies. Although this might not satisfy the stakeholder who *is* interested in a particular time period, when averaging multiple models (as is usually the case in climate modeling for global change science), it does have the clear advantage of removing the confounding factor that every GCM might have a different **climate sensitivity**. If a GCM developed and run by NOAA GFDL reached 2°C global warming by 2030 under RCP8.5 forcing, but the one at NASA GISS didn't reach a global warming of 2°C under the same forcing until 2070, does it make sense to pull out the climate at year 2050 to compare between both models? Again, it depends on whether the stakeholder using the GCM results is interested in adaptation measures that must be in place by 2050 or understanding the climate impacts that can be expected, given different levels of global warming.

All of the coordination by CMIP and IPCC to ensure uniformity across climate change simulations carried out at modeling institutions around the world has paid off, especially in terms of our ability to characterize the uncertainties in future climate change predictions. If the world only had one GCM, and we ran only one future experiment once, we would be in a situation even worse than having uncertainty: We would not even know what the uncertainty is. Although there are probably many segments of computer code that may be shared between GCMs or at least descended from a common ancestor, each GCM is a little different from the others. As you may suspect, the attributes they share in common are the aspects of the climate system we understand the best (i.e., basic thermodynamics and force balances driving the wind and ocean currents), and where they differ the most are in those aspects that are either difficult to simulate or are heavily **parameterized** because we cannot explicitly resolve them. Examples of the latter include clouds and rainfall, as well as turbulence in the atmosphere and ocean). Simply put, they are driven by processes occurring at spatial (or temporal) scales smaller than the GCM's grid cells, so each model development team employs its own approaches and innovations to represent them since they could matter in the global or long-term sense. These challenges, either to our scientific understanding of the climate system or to our technical capabilities to run models of high enough resolution, has led to a useful diversity of GCMs. The same prescribed CO_2 forcing in thirty different GCMs leads to thirty different simulations of the future evolution of Earth's climate. We refer to this spread as the **scientific uncertainty** associated with GCM simulations. Climate scientists who gather observations and attempt to understand the essential nature of how the system works are working very hard to reduce this source of uncertainty with each successive generation of GCMs.

If the scientific uncertainty is essentially the *spread* about the average of model results for the same RCP, the **societal uncertainty** is the opposite—the difference between the average results associated with different RCPs. In other words, even if we had perfect GCMs, they would still predict different outcomes for different assumptions about future CO_2 emissions. No matter how hard we try, we will always have a considerable amount of societal uncertainty. The final major source of uncertainty is only recently becoming widely recognized as a substantial gap in our understanding of uncertainties. As each *coupled* GCM simulation steps forward in time from one year to the next, it is free to evolve its own **internal variability** (Figure 13.5). In other words, an enormous El Niño event might happen in the winter of 2059 in one GCM, but there is no reason such an event should occur in that year in any other model simulation. This is because the only thing being prescribed in such simulations is the CO_2 forcing, and El Niño events are not *forced* by gradually trending CO_2 concentration. At regional scales, internal variability can be a significant impediment to identifying anthropogenic trends compared to when quantities such as surface temperature are averaged over the entire globe.

The framework described here clearly places GCM experiments in the class of **boundary value problems**. The key constraint on the model solution is the *boundary* forcing, or in this case the amount of radiative forcing present. The key constraint of such GCM experiments as those described is *not* the initial state of the climate system—that is what short-term weather forecasts rely on. In fact, running so many GCMs so many times, each with ever-so-slightly different **initial conditions**, is the idea behind the new wave of large **ensembles**. When an ensemble of simulations by the *same* model is run on the *same* supercomputer, where the only difference is minute changes in the weather on the first day of the model simulation, that is enough of a butterfly effect that each simulation (even by the same model, on the same supercomputer) will evolve completely differently in terms of *internal* climate variability. This is analogous to diagnostic tests (e.g., blood tests) in a clinical setting; taking a sample on a few different days (and a few different times of the day) averages out the random effects that may obfuscate the underlying problem—what the patient was recently exposed to, what they just

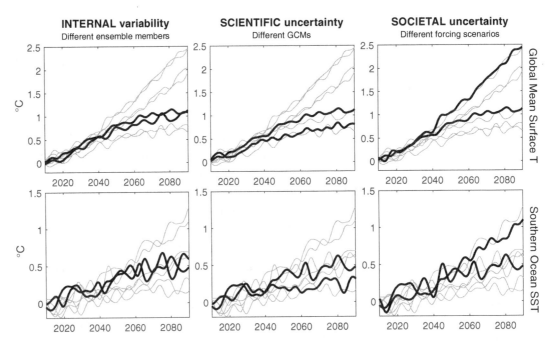

Figure 13.5 Schematic illustration of the major sources of uncertainty in future climate projections by GCMs. Top row for global mean surface temperature, bottom row for southern ocean sea surface temperature. The same eight simulations are repeated across each row (2 GCMs, 2 RCPs, 2 ensemble members). The first column highlights uncertainty due to internal variability by contrasting two ensemble members of the same GCM and subject to the same future radiative forcing scenario (RCP4.5). The only difference between ensemble members is the initial conditions (weather on day one of the experiment). The second column highlights scientific uncertainty by comparing two different GCMs subject to the same forcing scenario (RCP4.5). The third column highlights societal uncertainty by contrasting projections by the same GCM but under two different forcing scenarios (RCP4.5 and RCP8.5).
Source: Kris Karnauskas, *Physical Oceanography and Climate*, 2020, © Kris Karnauskas 2020, published by Cambridge University Press, reproduced with permission.

ate, or how much they slept the night before. So, too, in climate modeling, averaging an ensemble of experiments allows us to tease out what all of these seemingly different predictions actually have in common—that is, the inherent response to anthropogenic forcing.

Summary and Closing Remarks

In this chapter, we examined the scientific case—from physics to empirical evidence—attributing observed climate change to human activities. Greenhouse gases in the atmosphere are more abundant today than any time in at least the past million years, which is rigorously proven to be a result of human activities. This relatively abrupt shift in the composition of Earth's atmosphere has led to a net energy imbalance in Earth's climate (primarily by reducing how much heat escapes), requiring an increase in global average temperature—which we have indeed witnessed. We then delved into the mechanics of global climate models, which are a vitally important tool in the international enterprise of global change science, including efforts to understand the specific manifestations of climate change that may impact human health. GCMs are computerized renditions of the laws of physics that govern how the atmosphere, ocean, and other features of the climate system operate and interact. They enable us to attribute the observed global warming over the past century to **greenhouse gas** forcing, and to predict future changes in the climate given assumptions about future rates of greenhouse gas emissions. Climate modeling for global change science is an international collaboration; considering the dozens of GCMs developed and run at institutions around the world enables rigorous quantification of uncertainties in future climate change projections. Just like in a clinical setting, uncertainty may be inevitable, but knowledge of the uncertainties is helpful in making an informed decision.

For better or worse, the GCMs described in this chapter have been quite accurate in their future projections of global temperature change thus far, especially when accounting for the fact that our assumptions of future CO_2 emissions are always imperfect (Hausfather et al. 2019). Therefore, the predicted climate impacts described here are both serious and credible. Other studies have established that the imprint of anthropogenic radiative forcing on global climate will be detectable for thousands of years (Clark et al. 2016) because of the natural lags built into the ocean, and that with every year that passes before emissions begin to decline, the path to limiting global warming to 1.5°C (2.7°F) or even 2°C becomes less likely or feasible. Climate change and its growing influence on human health represents one of the grand challenges of our generation, and it will take more than just scientists working alone to solve it. A broader understanding of GCMs including how to interpret their results and uncertainties *across* these disciplines will lead to a deeper and more reliable diagnosis of the climate impacts on human health.

DISCUSSION QUESTIONS

1. Identify two lines of scientific evidence that support the notion that increasing concentrations of greenhouse gases in the atmosphere are causing the observed warming since the nineteenth century. Which line do you think makes a stronger case, and why?

2. Say you are interested in a future prediction of the change in a physical climate variable of relevance to health (e.g., temperature, humidity, rainfall). Compare the pros and cons of expressing this prediction as a function of time horizon (e.g., 2050) depending on emissions scenario (RCP4.5 or RCP8.5), or as a function of global warming threshold (e.g., 1.5°C or 2°C). What is more useful from a health outcome perspective, and does it depend on the particular health or social context?

3. Identify one disease or negative health outcome that is believed to be mediated in some way by climate. What is the spatial scale of predictions you would need for them to inform stakeholders interested in the future prevalence of that disease?

4. Compare and contrast the blend of uncertainties between GCM future projections of Arctic sea ice and ocean pH. For the latter, you will need to consult the Summary for Policymakers (Figure SPM.7) of the Fifth Assessment Report of the IPCC, available online at https://www.ipcc.ch/assessment-report/ar5/. Which projection has greater scientific uncertainty? Which has greater societal uncertainty relative to scientific uncertainty?

KEY TERMS

Attribution: The process of proving that a response is actually a direct result of a forcing, beyond simply observing a correlation between cause and effect. For example, see **attribution experiment**.

Attribution experiment: In the context of climate modeling, an attribution experiment is one in which a known forcing agent is withheld to determine the degree to which the result is a direct result of that forcing agent. For example, using a GCM to simulate the twentieth century with and without the observed increase in CO_2 concentration—the latter experiment not resulting in global warming attributes the global warming to the CO_2 increase.

Bias: In the context of GCMs, a bias is a discrepancy between today's climate as simulated by the GCM and that observed in real data (*in situ* measurements, satellite observations, etc.). A typical GCM bias might be that India does not receive enough rainfall or that the eastern Pacific Ocean is too cold. Some GCM biases are systemic (i.e., common across most of the GCMs from around the world) or vary enough from GCM to GCM that they effectively cancel out in the ensemble average of GCMs.

Boundary value problem: A model experiment in which the results will be strongly influenced by factors external to (or literally at the boundaries of) the system being modeled. This is the case in future climate change experiments (see **Future experiment**). For example, consider a GCM simulation of the period 2020 through 2100. The result in the year 2050 will be a function of the greenhouse gas concentrations at that point, rather than whatever the *initial* weather was on January 1, 2020. The opposite of a boundary value problem is an initial value problem. A five-day weather forecast is an initial value problem because the weather a few days from now is determined by how weather systems that are present right now continue to evolve; global concentrations of greenhouse gases will not change very much in that time frame.

Climate sensitivity: How strongly the global climate system responds to a given amount of forcing (see **Radiative forcing**). For example, how much will the global average surface temperature rise if the concentration of CO_2 in the atmosphere is doubled? Different GCMs have slightly different climate sensitivities. For example, given the same future greenhouse gas forcing scenario (say, RCP8.5), one GCM might reach 2°C of global warming by 2050 whereas another GCM has only warmed by 1.7°C at that point in the experiment (and doesn't reach 2°C until 2065). The first GCM in this example has the higher climate sensitivity. See **Representative concentration pathways**.

Concentration: The amount of a substance present in the medium, for example, carbon dioxide of methane in the atmosphere, usually expressed as parts per million. Contrast this definition to the closely related **Emissions**.

Control experiment: A "long" GCM simulation (typically simulating a time period of 1,000 years or more) in which greenhouse gas concentrations (and other facts such as solar output) are held constant. Year-to-year and even decade-to-decade climate fluctuations can still arise in such GCM simulations due to the internal dynamics of the climate system (i.e., ocean–atmosphere interaction) and due to random weather ("noise"), but there are no "external" influences (such as humans) on the climate that would lead to robust long-term trends. Control experiments can be used to determine how large an externally forced trend (in a different experiment) should be in order to be "detectable" amid the background, natural climate variability.

El Niño: A natural climate phenomenon in which the temperature of the surface of the eastern equatorial Pacific Ocean warms by a few degrees Celsius. El Niño is the warm phase of a cycle between abnormally warm and cold conditions in this region; the cold phase is called La Niña. This cycle is somewhat cyclical, but still irregular enough (with a period of 2–7 years) to be a challenge to predict more than a few months in advance. The broader cycle, referred to as El Niño–Southern Oscillation (ENSO), is entirely a result of internal climate dynamics—a manifestation of *coupled* ocean-atmosphere interactions.

Emissions: The amount of a substance added to the medium in a given time period. In the context of climate change, emissions refers to the amount of greenhouse gases added to the atmosphere per year (e.g., ~19 Gt of C per year). The relationship with concentration in terms of climate change mitigation strategies is important; for example, reduction of emissions does not necessarily lead to a decline in concentration.

Ensemble: In the context of climate modeling, an ensemble is a group of different GCMs that have conducted an otherwise identical experiment. Their results can be averaged to produce a multimodel ensemble mean; their spread or variance is a measure of the scientific uncertainty associated with that prediction. An ensemble may also be composed of an experiment conducted several times by a *single* GCM conducting an experiment several times, identical in every way except for the weather on the first day of the experiment (i.e., the **initial conditions**). In that case, the ensemble mean can be used to isolate the true forced response (according to that GCM) whereas the variance likely represents internal variability.

Future experiment: GCM experiments that simulate a future period of time (say, out to the year 2100) given a prescribed scenario of future greenhouse gas scenarios (see **representative concentration pathways**). These are, mathematically speaking, boundary value problems because the initial conditions (weather) on the first day of the experiment is essentially "forgotten" by the GCM after just a very short time into the experiment—perhaps after a few weeks. Such experiments are conducted by dozens of GCMs around the world; the collection of output from those GCMs constitutes an international ensemble of results whose average and spread can be examined to understand the various uncertainties.

Global climate model: A computerized representation of the laws of physics that govern how the atmosphere, ocean, and other features of the climate system operate and interact.

Greenhouse gas: Atmospheric constituents such as CO_2, methane, etc. whose molecular geometry render them particularly effective at intercepting thermal radiation (emitted by the surface of Earth) and reemitting it to the atmosphere rather than allowing it to escape into space. Rising concentrations of greenhouse gases lead to a net energy imbalance in Earth's climate, requiring an increase in global average temperature (hence the widely used term *greenhouse effect*).

Grid cell: The basic unit of space in a GCM. GCMs divide the global climate system into a large number of discrete cells, and the governing equations of the atmosphere, ocean, etc. are all solved for within each of these grid cells. The size of a grid cell is a function of the GCMs resolution and can vary from GCM to GCM depending on scientific objective and/or computer resources available.

Initial conditions: In the context of climate modeling, the particular state of the climate system at the first time step of a GCM simulation. In other words, the weather. In weather forecasting, initial conditions are crucially important; in general, the better we know the state of the atmosphere *now*, the better our forecast of the weather in forty-eight hours will be. In climate modeling, the initial conditions are long forgotten before the time period attempting to be predicted (decades in the future). In fact, it is becoming commonplace for GCM experiments to be run many times with extremely slight random noise added to the initial conditions to *ensure* that the initial conditions are not influencing the long-range climate change projection.

Internal variability: Loosely synonymous with *natural* climate variability, internal variability refers to the fluctuations in climate that are not driven by changes in *external* forcing agents such as greenhouse gases, volcanic eruptions, and solar output. Internal climate variability arises in the real world and in GCMs due to the coupled interactions between the atmosphere, ocean and other realms of the Earth system. El Niño (or ENSO) is a prime example of internal climate variability. Internal variability is relevant to climate change, particularly in efforts of detection and attribution, as internal variability introduces a source of noise that can obfuscate externally forced trends such as those arising due to increasing concentrations of greenhouse gases.

Parallel processing: The computation strategy often employed in climate modeling wherein the world is split into a number of tiles (each tile containing many grid cells), and the equation solving within those tiles is distributed across a number of individual computer processors. Parallel processing significantly speeds up a GCM experiment that needs to simulate a long time period (say, 2006 through 2100) at a reasonable spatial resolution.

Parameterization: The implementation of a real physical process in the climate system into a GCM without directly simulating that physical process. Rather, the process is implemented by way of its relationship with other *parameters* that *are* more confidently solved for by the GCM. A classic example for GCMs is clouds; one puffy cloud might be too small for a GCM to resolve, but we know the conditions in which different types of clouds are likely to form. Small-scale mixing and turbulence in both the atmosphere and ocean are also parameterized; they are surely important process in climate dynamics, but we do not know enough about them yet and/or do not have enough computer power to directly simulate them in global simulations.

Radiative forcing: The planetary energy imbalance (incoming minus outgoing) due to a particular forcing agent. Some anthropogenic forcings can result in a negative radiative forcing, such as aerosols (as they reflect incoming solar radiation). Anthropogenic greenhouse gas forcing currently amounts to a net 1–2 W/m^2 of radiative forcing.

Representative concentration pathway: Future trajectories of **greenhouse gas concentrations** (out to 2100) that may be used as forcing for GCM future experiments. Four RCPs are widely used in climate modeling for global change science; RCP2.6, RCP4.5, RCP6.0, and RCP8.5. The number following RCP indicates the radiative forcing (in W/m^2) at 2100.

Resolution: In the context of GCMs, the size of a grid cell. A "higher resolution" GCM has smaller grid cells and, consequently, more of them (so as to completely cover the planet). Higher resolution requires exponentially greater computer resources but may enable smaller-scale (and potentially important) physical processes to be directly simulated rather than relying heavily on parameterizations.

Scientific uncertainty: In the context of GCMs, the uncertainty due to imperfect scientific knowledge of the physics of the climate system (manifest as imperfect GCMs). The scientific uncertainty associated with future experiments is generally characterized by the *spread* among an ensemble of GCM results. Each GCM may be subject to the same assumptions about future greenhouse gas forcing, yet each GCM yielded slightly different results.

Societal uncertainty: In the context of future experiments, the uncertainty due to the fact that we cannot predict exactly how much greenhouse gases will continue to increase over the course of this century. Even if there was no scientific uncertainty, societal uncertainty would be inevitable. Societal uncertainty is built into the enterprise of climate modeling for global change by simulating four different RCPs—to account for a wide range of possible futures in terms of population, economics, technology, policy, etc.

Troposphere: The lowest layer of the atmosphere, in which the air temperature decreases with height. The depth of the troposphere is roughly 11 km on average, but with considerable geographical and seasonal variation. The boundary between the troposphere the next layer above, the stratosphere, is called the tropopause; above this altitude, temperature begins to increase with height.

References

Clark, P. U., J. D. Shakun, S. A. Marcott, A. C. Mix, M. Eby, S. Kulp, A. Levermann et al. 2016. "Consequences of Twenty-First-Century Policy for Multi-Millennial Climate and Sea-Level Change." *Nature Climate Change* 6:360–69.

Denman, K. L. and G. Brasseur. 2007. "Couplings between Changes in the Climate System and Biogeochemistry." In *Climate Change 2007: The Physical Science Basis edited by S. Solomon, D. Qin, M. Manning, M. Marquis, K. Avery, M. M. B. Tignor, H. L. Miller, and Z. L. Chen*, 499–587. Cambridge: Cambridge University Press.

Feldman, D. R., W. D. Collins, P. J. Gero, M. S. Torn, E. J. Mlawer, and T. R. Shippert. 2015. "Observational Determination of Surface Radiative Forcing by CO_2 from 2000 to 2010." *Nature* 519:339–43.

Francey, R. J., C. E. Allison, D. M. Etheridge, C. M. Trudinger, I. G. Enting, M. Leuenberger, R. L. Langenfelds, E. Michel, and L. P. Steele. 1999. "A 1000-Year High Precision Record of $\delta^{13}C$ in Atmospheric CO_2." *Tellus B* 51:170–93.

Friedlingstein, P., M. W. Jones, M. O'Sullivan, R. M. Andrew, J. Hauck, G. P. Peters, W. Peters et al. 2019. "Global Carbon Budget 2019." *Earth System Science Data* 11:1783–1838.

Harries, J. E., H. E. Brindley, P. J. Sagoo, and R. J. Bantges. 2001. "Increases in Greenhouse Forcing Inferred from the Outgoing Longwave Radiation Spectra of the Earth in 1970 and 1997." *Nature* 410:355–57.

Hausfather, Z., H. F. Drake, T. Abbott, and G. A. Schmidt 2019. "Evaluating the Performance of Past Climate Model Projections." *Geophysical Research Letters* https://doi.org/10.1029/2019GL085378.

Intergovernmental Panel on Climate Change. 2013. *Climate Change 2013: The Physical Science Basis.* Working Group I Contribution to the Fifth Assessment Report of the Intergovernmental Panel on Climate Change. Cambridge: Cambridge University Press.

Karnauskas, K. 2020. *Physical Oceanography and Climate.* Cambridge: Cambridge University Press.

Rubino, M., D. M. Etheridge, C. M. Trudinger, C. E. Allison, M. O. Battle, R. L. Langenfelds, L. P. Steele et al. 2013. "A Revised 1000 Year Atmospheric $\delta^{13}C$–CO_2 Record from Law Dome and South Pole, Antarctica." *Journal of Geophysical Research Atmospheres* 118:8482–99.

CHAPTER 14

CLIMATE AND HEALTH VULNERABILITY ASSESSMENTS: NEW APPROACHES AND TOOLS FOR ADAPTATION PLANNING

Peter Berry, Kristie L. Ebi, Rebekka Schnitter, Louise Aubin, and Sherilee Harper

Introduction

It is widely recognized that climate change poses major threats to the health of populations around the globe; many impacts are already being observed and scientists have begun attributing some health outcomes directly to warming (Ebi et al. 2017). Public health officials face the dual tasks of protecting health from the impacts of a rapidly warming climate while promoting the health co-benefits of expanding **adaptation** and greenhouse gas (GHG) mitigation measures developed and implemented in other sectors.

Health authorities must quickly scale up efforts to close the health adaptation gap at the individual, community, and **health systems** levels. Health systems include the organizations, people, and actions whose primary intent is to promote, restore, or maintain health (World Health Organization [WHO] 2007). Health adaptation means adjusting planning, policies, and programs by government and civil society partners to respond to current impacts and to prepare for future risks. Current efforts to protect populations are well below needed actions to prevent or reduce impacts that can be avoided and to cope with those residual effects that cannot (Martinez and Berry 2018; Haines and Ebi 2019). The costs to society, and to those most vulnerable to the impacts of ineffective health adaptation, will continue to grow. **Vulnerability** refers to the "degree to which a system is susceptible to, or unable to cope with, adverse effects of climate change, including climate variability and extremes" (Intergovernmental Panel on Climate Change [IPCC] 2001, p. 995). Decision-makers require the best scientific advice and information to chart the path forward toward resilient and sustainable health systems, including identification of innovative measures needed to understand and prepare for more severe and possibly compounding effects of future climate change, including tipping points and shock events that have no historical precedent (Berry et al. 2018).

Scientists and public health authorities have been examining climate change impacts on health and developing the needed methods and tools, including risk assessment guidance, for over two decades. The use of climate change and **health vulnerability and adaptation assessments** (V&As) to inform adaptation decision-making from local to national levels has steadily increased and guidance for conducting these studies has evolved as health authorities have learned from their experiences. This chapter builds upon and references the evolution of this topic in recent years by highlighting how V&A application and guidance has evolved and by discussing lessons learned and future opportunities for supporting health adaptation efforts moving forward.

KEY CONCEPTS

- As climate change increases threats to human health and well-being, public health officials require information about growing risks to individuals, vulnerabilities faced by specific groups, impacts on **health systems,** and effective and inclusive **adaptation** measures.

- Climate change and **health vulnerability and adaptation assessments** provide needed information, including Indigenous knowledge, to develop strategies, policies, and measures to reduce the current burden of disease and the risks of much more severe adverse health outcomes.

- The findings of assessments can help public health officials and community leaders estimate the human and **health system** costs of climate change and allocate scarce resources toward preparing for the future.

- As the first and last line of defense for protecting health from climate change, **health systems** and services can be vulnerable to impacts and should be resilient to future warming. New tools and methods for conducting assessments afford the opportunity to guide the transition of **health systems** to a climate resilient and sustainable future.

- The **health vulnerability and adaptation assessment** process can support efforts to engage the public and mobilize community and regional decision-makers to protect health from climate change, including through actions outside the health sector.

The Role of Vulnerability and Adaptation Assessments in Preparing for Climate Change Impacts on Health

Knowledge of climate change impacts on health, vulnerabilities facing specific populations, and adaptation options to prepare communities and individuals has increased (Haines and Ebi 2019; WHO 2018; Smith et al. 2014; Crimmins et al. 2016; Watts et al. 2018). Yet important information and data gaps still exist that are greater around some health outcomes and their drivers (e.g., mental health, conflict, food security) and for some regions (e.g., Africa). Many subnational and national health authorities are beginning to take actions to plan for climate change impacts, including mainstreaming adaptation considerations into regular policies and programs (Haines and Ebi 2019; Ebi et al. 2019).

The development of climate-resilient health systems, and targeted adaptation measures, requires robust evidence of current and future health risks. This is because of the complexity of drivers responsible for direct and indirect health impacts of climate variability and change over different temporal scales. In addition, the growing pace of climate change, and concomitant risks of very severe health outcomes if physiological or societal thresholds are crossed, means that incremental efforts to prepare individuals, communities and health systems are no longer adequate. WHO provided guidance to health authorities on building climate resilient health systems by identifying components and indicators related to the building blocks of health systems that should be the focus of adaptation efforts when preparing for climate change impacts (WHO 2015a). Priority areas of focus to strengthen health systems and prepare communities include (Ebi et al. 2019):

- Equipping the health workforce with needed information and tools to protect their own health when disasters occur, and help their clients prevent health impacts, or treat them when they occur

- Improving the effectiveness of service delivery, for example, during and after climate-related hazards like severe storms

- Providing adequate financing to support adaptation efforts

- Integrating considerations of impacts from current climate variability and future climate change into actions to maintain, upgrade or build and site new health infrastructure, like hospitals and clinics (e.g., medical clinics in areas of permafrost melt or flood risk)

- Development of health information systems (e.g., monitoring and surveillance systems/ syndromic surveillance systems) linked to other sources of information (e.g., meteorologic information) to aid in preparation efforts

- Evaluating the effectiveness of adaptation options to support iterative improvements to actions to protect health

CLINICAL CORRELATES 14.1 INTERDISCIPLINARY COLLABORATION TO ASSESS THE HEALTH IMPACTS OF CLIMATE CHANGE EFFECTS ON FOOD INSECURITY

Access to a diverse diet, adequate in both quantity and quality of food, is foundational for an individual's health and well-being. Indeed, much evidence suggests linkages between food insecurity and adverse health outcomes, such as issues related to birth outcomes and maternal health, child development, chronic diseases, and mental health and emotional well-being (Vozoris and Tarasuk 2003; Li et al. 2016; McIntyre et al. 2017). It has also been suggested that individuals that experience some level of food insecurity are higher cost users of the health system (Tarasuk et al. 2015).

Climate change impacts are becoming an increasing stressor for food systems (Nelson et al. 2016) with risks for human health (Schnitter and Berry 2019). The way climate-related impacts travel through the food system and affect the critical dimensions of food security to influence human health are complex (Schnitter and Berry 2019). The interdependent nature of food systems suggests that the disruption of one activity can impact the effective operation of other components in the systems. Additional determinants of food security and human health further compound the complexity of the issue as such determinants themselves can be challenged or exacerbated by climate-related impacts.

The relationship between food systems, food security, climate change and human health is dynamic and complex. This nexus represents an interdisciplinary problem that requires cross-sectoral collaboration to assess and understand risks and for the effective development of adaptation actions. A new framework illustrates this complexity, highlighting the need for collaboration among food system actors and stakeholders.

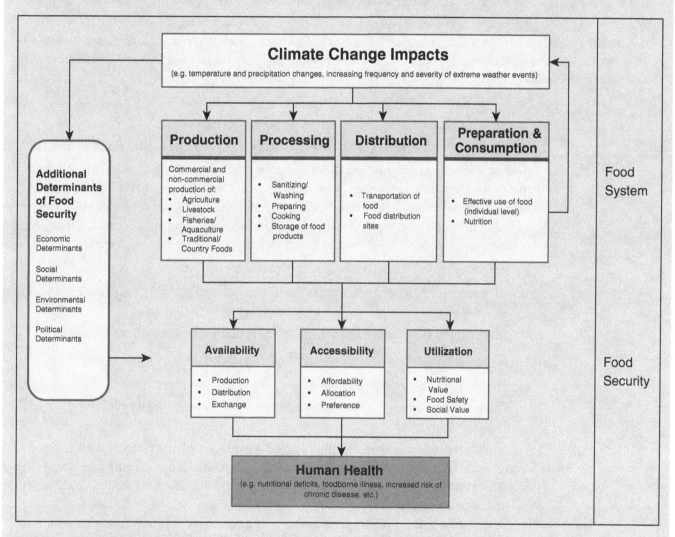

Figure 14.1   Food security, climate change, and human health nexus framework
Source: Schnitter and Berry (2019).

Climate change and health vulnerability and adaptation assessments are useful in illustrating particular characteristics and variations in social, political, economic and environmental factors among urban, rural, coastal, northern and Indigenous communities, along with associated vulnerabilities in food systems. Such information is critical to inform the development of adaptation strategies by health sector decision makers and those in related sectors, but have widely been left out of V&As, to date (Schnitter and Berry 2019).

Assessing risks to the health of populations from the impacts of climate change on food security faces significant challenges because of the large number of direct and indirect drivers of vulnerability in multiple sectors related to food production, processing, distribution and consumption. Efforts to assess climate change impacts on food security and health benefit from:

- Including stakeholders from all food system sectors – for example, transportation, agriculture, water, health, environmental conservation, natural resources, urban planning, trade, social programs, Indigenous partners and policy and regulation all play a role in the food system (Schnitter and Berry 2019)

- Examining and respecting the unique characteristics of Indigenous food systems and the linkages to the health and well-being of Indigenous peoples and communities

- Consideration for social and health equity to ensure that adaptation actions do not ignore or inadvertently advance root causes of food insecurity

Investigating the nexus of food security, climate change, and human health can provide useful information for vulnerability and adaptation assessments and equip decision makers within and outside of the health sector with information needed to protect health.

What Are the Benefits of Vulnerability and Adaptation Assessments?

As a core activity in utilizing health information systems in efforts to protect health from climate change, health authorities should undertake V&As (WHO 2015). These assessments provide information to public health officials from local to national levels on major categories of health risks to inform development of adaptation plans tailored to specific jurisdictions and populations (WHO 2013). These categories include (Campbell-Lendrum et al. 2015):

- The direct physical effects of extreme heat and thermal stress

- Climate change-related alterations in the frequency, intensity, and duration of other extreme weather events (e.g., floods, droughts, and windstorms)

- Infectious diseases transmitted by water, food, vectors, or zoonotic reservoirs

- Air quality impacts (e.g., wildfires, ground-level ozone, pollens)

- Nutrition and food security impacts

- Indirect effects through climate-induced economic dislocation and environmental decline (e.g., mental health)

Through development of Health National Adaptation Plans (HNAPs) countries can use V&A results to outline strategic goals and concrete activities for preparing for climate change impacts. HNAPs can be integrated into a country's broader National Adaptation Plan as the health sector contribution (WHO 2014).

As the need to ramp up adaptation efforts becomes more urgent, V&As are useful in helping health authorities raise awareness of threats to health and of needed adaptations. They also contribute to building capacity within organizations (e.g., climate and health data integration and analysis) and provide opportunities to engage with a range of partners within and outside of the health sector to understand existing vulnerabilities faced by individuals, communities, and health systems (Campbell-Lendrum et al. 2015). With broad enough consultation they can also provide useful information for decision-makers in other sectors important for shaping health outcomes (e.g., transportation, conservation, water, energy, agriculture, land use planning) and guide their efforts to maximize the health co-benefits of adaptation and GHG mitigation actions they undertake. Such efforts have enormous potential to benefit population health and help counterbalance the effects of climate change (Watts et al. 2018).

CLINICAL CORRELATES 14.2 APPLYING ASSESSMENT FINDINGS TO PROTECT HEALTH IN THE REGION OF PEEL, ONTARIO

The Region of Peel Public Health unit in Ontario, Canada undertook a vulnerability and adaptation assessment in 2012 with support from Health Canada (Buse, Aubin, and Pajot 2012). Peel Region is located immediately west of the City of Toronto, has a population of 1.3 million residents, and is growing rapidly. Using the WHO assessment guidance (WHO 2013), the study sought to identify indicators of current and future vulnerability to climate change health impacts along with populations most at risk, based on capacity to adapt (personal communication, Louise Aubin). The assessment found that climate change could increase health risks related to morbidity and mortality from extreme weather and natural hazards, respiratory and cardiovascular conditions due to impacts on air quality, temperature-related morbidity and mortality, impacts on food and water quality, and the possible spread of vector-borne diseases. It was concluded that climate change may worsen existing health inequalities in the region and that existing health programs and services alone would be inadequate to manage future risks to the population (personal communication, Louise Aubin).

Decision-makers in Peel Region are using the V&A results to inform a number of public health interventions. Working in partnership with a number of agencies, the results are being used to increase climate resilience among the population by developing an interactive geographic information system-based tool that will identify the best areas to plant trees to most effectively reduce the urban heat island affecting communities. The tool integrates information on twelve benefits of community greening through tree planting (e.g., reduced air pollution; improved surface water quality and quantity; enhanced natural heritage; increased social equity; improved physical health) to identify priority areas for planting. The results of the assessment have also been used to inform existing heat warning systems and enhance urgent response planning to assist in transitioning from business as usual operations to responding to events. Peel Public Health is currently completing a second assessment study based upon recent population census information for the region (personal communication, Louise Aubin). The assessment has resulted in increased capacity and understanding of the scope of the issues and public health staff working with new partners such as forestry departments.

Local level V&As can provide rigorous information to support immediate actions to protect population health from climate change.

With the recognition of the severe and growing risks to health from climate change, greater actions are underway to monitor and evaluate global efforts to prepare populations and health systems for future impacts and improve health outcomes associated with current hazards. For example, the WHO undertakes biannual surveys of national health authorities on their climate change and health adaptation efforts, including the conduct of assessments, and reports results in the WHO/United Nations Framework Convention on Climate Change (UNFCCC) Climate and Health Country Profiles (WHO 2018), https://www.who.int/globalchange/resources/countries/en/

In addition, the Lancet Countdown on Health and Climate Change (http://www.lancet-countdown.org/) launched a process in 2015 to regularly track and evaluate global efforts to tackle climate change threats to health. Annual reports present data on forty-one indicators related to climate change impacts, exposures, and vulnerability; adaptation, planning and resilience for health; mitigation actions and health co-benefits; finance and economics; and public and political engagement (Watts et al. 2018). Vulnerability and adaptation assessments make important contributions to building this global evidence base of the understanding of climate change impacts on health. This evidence base can be used for health adaptation planning as well as by decision-makers outside of the health sector for considerations around optimal pathways and levels of effort to reduce GHGs. The number of national V&As has increased greatly over the last decade with ninety-two countries in all regions of the world having completed at least one as of 2018 (Berry et al. 2018) (Figure 14.2).

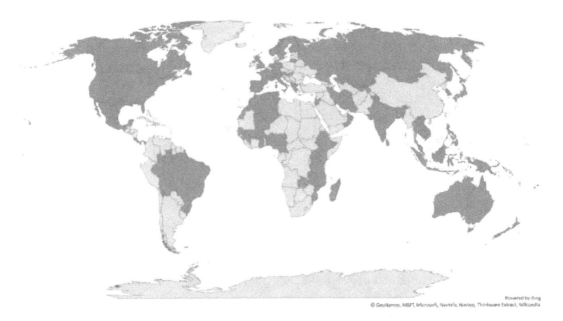

Figure 14.2   Countries that have completed a climate change and health vulnerability and adaptation assessment

Source: Berry et al. (2018).

Note: Not visible on the map: Antigua and Barbuda, Barbados, Brunei, Cook Islands, Dominica, Federated States of Micronesia, Fiji, Grenada, Kiribati, Maldives, Malta, Marshall Islands, Nauru, Niue, Palau, Samoa, Solomon Islands, St. Lucia, Timor-Leste, Tonga, Tuvalu, and Vanuatu.

Methods for Undertaking a Vulnerability and Adaptation Assessment

In 2003, the WHO developed the first technical guidance document for use by health authorities to conduct V&As (WHO 2003). Based on feedback from users and a consultative process in 2010, WHO and the Pan American Health Organization (PAHO) developed new guidance on conducting assessments. That guidance document, *Protecting Health from Climate Change: Vulnerability and Adaptation Assessment* (WHO 2013), is currently made available by WHO and includes a number of case studies. Table 14.1 presents its five steps for conducting a V&A.

Table 14.1   Five Steps for Undertaking a Climate Change and Health Vulnerability and Adaptation Assessment

Assessment Step	Activity
1. Framing and scoping the assessment	• Define the geographical range and health outcomes of interest • Identify the questions to be addressed and steps to be used • Identify the policy context for the assessment • Establish a project team and a management plan • Establish a stakeholder process • Develop a communications plan

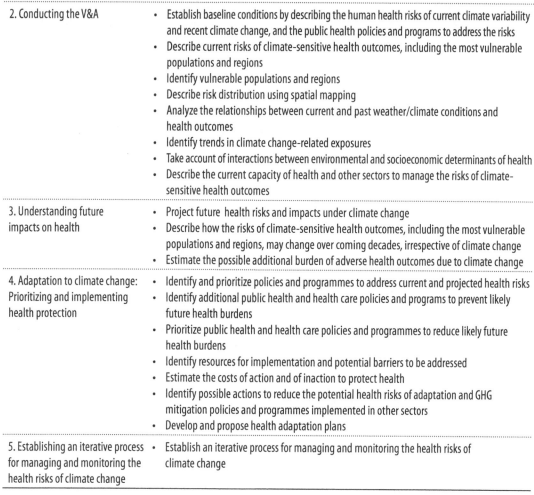

2. Conducting the V&A	• Establish baseline conditions by describing the human health risks of current climate variability and recent climate change, and the public health policies and programs to address the risks
	• Describe current risks of climate-sensitive health outcomes, including the most vulnerable populations and regions
	• Identify vulnerable populations and regions
	• Describe risk distribution using spatial mapping
	• Analyze the relationships between current and past weather/climate conditions and health outcomes
	• Identify trends in climate change-related exposures
	• Take account of interactions between environmental and socioeconomic determinants of health
	• Describe the current capacity of health and other sectors to manage the risks of climate-sensitive health outcomes
3. Understanding future impacts on health	• Project future health risks and impacts under climate change
	• Describe how the risks of climate-sensitive health outcomes, including the most vulnerable populations and regions, may change over coming decades, irrespective of climate change
	• Estimate the possible additional burden of adverse health outcomes due to climate change
4. Adaptation to climate change: Prioritizing and implementing health protection	• Identify and prioritize policies and programmes to address current and projected health risks
	• Identify additional public health and health care policies and programs to prevent likely future health burdens
	• Prioritize public health and health care policies and programmes to reduce likely future health burdens
	• Identify resources for implementation and potential barriers to be addressed
	• Estimate the costs of action and of inaction to protect health
	• Identify possible actions to reduce the potential health risks of adaptation and GHG mitigation policies and programmes implemented in other sectors
	• Develop and propose health adaptation plans
5. Establishing an iterative process for managing and monitoring the health risks of climate change	• Establish an iterative process for managing and monitoring the health risks of climate change

Source: WHO (2013).

As health authorities have taken strides toward mainstreaming climate change into health sector planning, they require more thematic and region-specific information and data to assess current and future risks and to help develop cost-effective adaptation measures targeted toward specific health programs and infrastructures (Berry et al. 2018). New guidance, tools, and approaches have become available that can be used to supplement application of the WHO/PAHO steps and to expand the scope of such investigations to the full health system. Some of these include, for example:

• Guidance for quantifying health impacts associated with climate change (Campbell-Lendrum and Woodruff 2007)

• Technical assessment guidelines for health authorities in Ontario, Canada, including case studies of health adaptation and multisectoral collaboration, a vulnerabilities assessment checklist, and an assessment workbook with fillable worksheets that can be used to obtain and analyze needed data and information (Ebi et al. 2016), http://www.health.gov.on.ca /en/common/ministry/publications/reports/climate_change_toolkit/climate_change _toolkit.aspx

• Guidance for countries to assess risks and invest in climate-resilient health systems (World Bank 2018), http://documents.worldbank.org/curated/en/552631515568426482/ A-country-based-approach-for-assessing-risks-and-investing-in-climate-smart-health-systems

- Guidance for assessing and preparing health facilities, like hospitals and clinics, for the impacts of climate change (Canadian Coalition for Green Health Care 2016; National Oceanic and Atmospheric Administration 2016; PAHO/WHO, 2016)

- Methods for stress testing health facilities and systems to gauge resilience to future climate change impacts (Ebi et al. 2018)

- Methods for projecting climate-related disease burdens (Hess et al. 2015)

- Shared Socioeconomic Pathways (SSPs) to help understand implications of different scenarios for climate change adaptation (including in the health sector) and GHG mitigation activities (Sellers and Ebi 2017)

CLINICAL CORRELATES 14.3 STRESS TESTING HEALTH SYSTEMS TO PREPARE FOR CLIMATE CHANGE IMPACTS

Health systems and health facilities are vital for efforts to address climate change impacts on health because of the important contributions they can make to reduce the rate of climate change through GHG mitigation measures and in protecting people from impacts when they occur. Health systems are vulnerable to a range of climate change hazards, including related shocks and stresses that can exceed tipping points in response capabilities (Ebi et al. 2018). In 2015, the capacity of Vanuatu's health system to respond to tropical cyclone Pam was significantly affected by destruction of health care infrastructure, low numbers of health care personnel, and challenges in accessing needed resources and funds (Government of Vanuatu 2015; WHO 2015).

Most V&As have focused on a narrow range of health outcomes related to climate change that are based on current risks; an examination of climate events outside the range of historical experience, which can affect the effectiveness and sustainability of health system functioning, is often absent (Ebi et al. 2018). Health authorities can investigate the climate resilience of health systems through **"health system stress testing,"** one or more of the building blocks identified by WHO as critical for adapting to climate change. By examining existing data and information related to current and projected exposures and capacities, and undertaking a tabletop or visioning exercise with key stakeholders, the stress test exercise can identify key vulnerabilities from climate change impacts and effective adaptation options (Ebi et al. 2018). For example, the resilience of core functions of health systems such as the ability to deliver services, or maintain access to health care facilities and supply chains, can be investigated with questions such as:

- To what extent do temperature, precipitation, other weather variables, and sea level rise affect the ability of health systems to deliver services?

- Have extreme weather and climate events affected access to health care systems in the past? How important was the disruption?

- Have extreme weather and climate events affected supply chains? How important was the disruption?

- Are mechanisms in place to mobilize resources (financial and human) during and after extreme weather and climate events?

Climate stress testing the health system can provide information that will supplement and extend the analysis of a V&A and provide a fuller picture of the vulnerability of a community to the health impacts of climate change.

The Path Forward: Lessons Learned and Opportunities for Undertaking Future Vulnerability and Adaptation Assessments

Although most guidance for conducting V&As includes a step to evaluate and monitor the assessment process and the effectiveness of actions taken to protect health (WHO/PAHO 2013; Ebi et al. 2016; Centers for Disease Control and Prevention [CDC] 2019b), there are few published papers reporting such results (Fox et al. 2019; Haines and Ebi 2019). Wheeler and Watts (2018) suggested that the U.S. Climate-Ready States and Cities Initiative (CRSCI) https://www.cdc.gov/climateandhealth/climate_ready.htm and the supporting Building Resilience Against Climate Effects (BRACE) Framework (CDC, 2019a) provides an excellent approach for health adaptation to climate change, utilizing an iterative risk management cycle. One study that evaluated the CRSCI/BRACE program, including the assessment tools, expertise and information exchange mechanisms developed for sixteen states and two cities, indicated that it was successful in building the capacity of health authorities to prepare for climate change. Participating jurisdictions benefited through the development of practice-informed guidance on quantitative risk assessment methods and new networks for information sharing, which ultimately increased understanding of climate change risks to health in the various jurisdictions, including for vulnerable populations (Sheehan et al. 2017). Opportunities for enhancing these efforts included greater knowledge of climate modeling tools and how they can be used to project future disease burdens for assessment purposes (Sheehan et al. 2017).

Another study used the Core Functions and Essential Services (CFES) structure that highlights ten essential core public health functions, which the CDC has drawn upon to inform its Climate and Health Program, and then examined progress in the last ten years toward implementing a public health approach to climate change (Fox et al. 2019). The authors suggested that the most substantial progress has been made in the monitoring and assessment of climate change risks to health. New tools, methods, data (e.g., climate services, vulnerability indices), and risk assessment frameworks have been developed and are being used by public health officials to evaluate current and potential climate change impacts. However, although the health sector role in broader efforts to build climate resiliency is growing, there are few studies on the effectiveness of health adaptations and insufficient strides have been made in communicating climate change risks to partners (Fox et al. 2019). Opportunities exist to strengthen these areas and iteratively manage health risks through regular evaluation and communication to the public and stakeholders; these features are key aspects of the climate change and health assessment process (Hess and Ebi 2016; WHO 2013).

A review of the first phase (2008–2013) of health adaptation projects in thirteen countries (Albania, Barbados, Bhutan, China, Fiji, Jordan, Kazakhstan, Kenya, Kyrgyzstan, Philippines, Russian Federation, Tajikistan, and Uzbekistan) highlighted the utility of undertaking V&As and identified a number of important success factors relevant to the conduct of, or use of, information provided by them (Ebi and del Barrio 2017):

- Representatives from targeted communities should participate fully in project implementation.

- Multisector collaboration, particularly between the meteorologic department and the ministry of health, is essential to be successful.

- Climate adaptation planning should be mainstreamed into health systems and the overall national adaptation planning processes.

- Projects are more successful when they have the requisite capacity (e.g., training, human and financial resources) in climate change and health for implementation before they begin. It is important to spend time and resources before, or at the very beginning of projects, to build capacity and stakeholder engagement.

- Indicators for monitoring and evaluation are required to support project implementation.

As practitioners learn more about data requirements, new methods of analysis, effective stakeholder engagement, prioritizing adaptations, and communicating study results by undertaking V&As, these studies will become more robust and make even greater contributions to efforts to prepare populations for climate change impacts on health.

Assessing New Risks to Health

Many climate change impacts on health are already common to public health officials (Ebi et al. 2019) and are the subject of established environmental health surveillance, assessment, and health protection measures (e.g., air pollution, water pollution, infectious diseases, food safety). However, climate warming may present risks that are new to a specific jurisdiction (e.g., health risks from algal blooms, exotic vector-borne diseases) or derived from climate hazards historically so infrequent as to not have established risk management measures for protecting health in place (e.g., wildfire smoke from distant fires). As the evidence base of climate change impacts on health grows, including understanding of these new or indirect risks, health authorities will be able to use V&As to target these health outcomes for investigation and resilience planning.

For example, limited understanding of the impacts of climate change on mental health has meant that many assessments have excluded examination of these risks (Hayes and Poland 2018). However, opportunities exist to develop strategies for rigorous monitoring and surveillance of mental health indicators of a changing climate that capture not only negative impacts and disorders but also posttraumatic growth and emotional resilience that can result from disasters (Hayes and Poland 2018). Such indicators may be used in V&As to understand whether threats to mental health are increasing from climate change in a community, region, or country. They would include both direct impacts from extreme weather events and less direct ones arising when hazards compromise economic activities or social supports available to individuals, or from greater awareness of existential threats facing people from a warming planet (i.e., climate despair) (Hayes and Poland 2018). Table 14.2 presents indicators and research methods that may be used to support V&As that include examination of the mental health impacts of climate-related extreme weather events.

The Role of Indigenous Knowledge in Climate Change and Health Vulnerability and Adaptation Assessments

The health impacts of climate change are not equitably distributed. For instance, Indigenous peoples are particularly sensitive to climate change-related health impacts (Ford 2012). This is due, in part, to their inhabiting geographies that are often particularly exposed to climate change impacts (Adger et al. 2014; Olsson et al. 2014), and their relationship with and dependence upon the environment for health and well-being (Cunsolo Willox et al. 2013b; Harper et al. 2015), as well as existing health inequities rooted in historical and ongoing processes of colonization (Delormier et al. 2017; Greenwood, De Leeuw and Lindsay 2018; King, Smith and Gracey 2009). Climate change has already had an impact on Indigenous peoples' physical, emotional, spiritual, and psychological health and wellness, with documented impacts on heat-related morbidity and mortality; unintentional injury and death; food-borne, water-borne, and vector-borne disease; mental health and wellness; and health service provision (Berrang-Ford et al. 2012; Cunsolo Willox et al. 2013a; Furgal and Seguin 2006; Green and

Table 14.2 Indicators and Research Methods for Examining the Mental Health Impacts of Climate-Related Extreme Weather Events

Climate Hazard	Populations of Concern	Potential Mental Health Outcomes	Indicators and Measurement Tools
Extreme weather event (flood, hurricane, drought, mudslides, etc.)	- Gender (Female) - Sex (Female, particularly pregnant women) - Age (children, infants, seniors) - Race and ethnicity (non-Caucasian, nonwhite) - Immigrants - People with preexisting health conditions - People with low-socioeconomic status - The under- and noninsured (health care and home insurance) - The underhoused and homeless - Outdoor laborers - First responders - People that do not speak the predominant language or have other communication barriers - People that are newly immigrated	- Posttraumatic stress disorder (PTSD) - Depression (including major depressive disorders) - Anxiety - Suicidal ideation - Aggression - Substance abuse and addiction - Violence - Survivor guilt - Vicarious trauma - Altruism - Compassion - Posttraumatic growth - Other	- Surveys - Self-report surveys of general health. Consider using: General Health Questionnaire (GHQ) - Self-report surveys of mental illness and mental problems. Consider using any, or a combination of: • Disaster-PAST; the Generalized Anxiety Disorder Scale (GAD-7); the Post-Traumatic Stress Disorder Checklist (PCL); The Center for Epidemiologic Studies Depression Scale (CES-D); the Kessler Psychological Distress Scale (K6) - Self-report surveys of affirmative mental health. Consider using: • Stress-Related Growth Scale (SRGS); Post-Traumatic Growth Index (PTGI); Benefit Finding Scale (BFS) • Patient records • Monitor emergency department visits after extreme weather events for an increase in patients reporting mental health problems or illness. • Review of new prescription use for mental health and behavioral disorders after an extreme weather event • Interviews - Interviews with primary care physicians and mental health care providers about any surges in patients reporting mental health issues following extreme weather events. - Interviews with people who experienced an extreme weather event about their perceptions regarding their mental health related to the extreme weather event.

Source: Adapted from Hayes and Poland (2018).

Minchin 2014; Harper et al. 2015; Hofmeijer et al. 2013; Jaakkola, Juntunen and Näkkäläjärvi 2018; Parkinson and Evengård 2009; Zavaleta et al. 2018).

In the face of these climate-health challenges, Indigenous peoples are actively taking climate change action, providing valuable insight and leadership in climate change adaptation and mitigation strategies (David-Chavez and Gavin 2018; Watt-Cloutier 2015). Indigenous knowledge (IK) has underpinned the success of these efforts. The IPCC defines IK as the "understandings, skills, and philosophies developed by societies with long histories of interaction with their natural surroundings. It is passed on from generation to generation, flexible, and adaptive in changing conditions, and increasingly challenged in the context of contemporary climate change" (Abram et al. 2019).

What Can Indigenous Knowledge Bring to Health Vulnerability and Adaptation Assessments?

The added value that IK brings to climate change assessments is increasingly recognized, including by the Inter-Agency Support Group on Indigenous Issues in 2007, the International Work Group for Indigenous Affairs in 2008 in preparation for the World Conference on Climate Change in 2009, and UNESCO in 2015 (Broto et al. 2019). IK can serve health V&As in three critical ways:

• *Observations:* IK is a rigorous and rich form of evidence that should be used to understand how climate change is impacting health (Broto et al. 2019; Crate et al. 2019).

- *Responses:* Indigenous peoples are already responding to climate change impacts on health—responses that are often underpinned by IK—and, thus, V&As can build from these responses and lessons learned (UNFCCC 2013; Crate et al. 2019).

- *Decision-making:* Utilizing IK in climate health decision-making requires the meaningful engagement of Indigenous peoples and their organizations, enabling the incorporation of relevant priorities and local context into adaptation and mitigation (Green, Niall and Morrison 2012; Crate et al. 2019).

How Can Indigenous Knowledge Be Included in Health Vulnerability and Adaptation Assessments?

Climate change and health vulnerability and adaptation assessments can utilize both IK and western science, or be entirely based on IK, depending on the context of the assessment. A number of conceptual frameworks are available to guide meaningful and rigorous use of IK and western science. Common among these frameworks is recognition that IK must not be reduced to data that are palatable to, and become subsumed within, western frameworks of understanding; rather, effective and meaningful integration requires an appreciation that understanding and responding to complex challenges is enriched through contrasting perspectives offered by diverse ways of knowing. For instance, "Two-Eyed Seeing," developed by Mi'kmaw Elders, entails "learning to see from one eye with the strengths of Indigenous knowledges and ways of knowing, and from the other eye with the strengths of western knowledges and ways of knowing, and to using both these eyes together, for the benefit of all" (Bartlett et al. 2012, p. 335). Valuing difference and contradiction over the integration of diverse perspectives, Two-Eyed Seeing encourages "a weaving back and forth" between diverse ways of knowing to reach understandings that would not be possible through "one eye" alone (Bartlett et al. 2012).

What Constitutes Meaningful Inclusion of IK?

To achieve effective utilization of IK in V&As, meaningful engagement—beyond consultation—is required. Indigenous peoples and their organizations should be included in the entire assessment process. Assessments that involve Indigenous-led processes are inherently grounded in IK, values, and experiences (David-Chavez and Gavin 2018; Tengö et al. 2017). Assessment processes and products should be accessible to Indigenous peoples and their organizations and be relevant and reported in the context of concerns or interests identified and defined by Indigenous peoples (David-Chavez and Gavin 2018). Indigenous-led approaches enable the assessment to go beyond secondhand interpretations of IK by non-Indigenous individuals. Although it is critical to engage Indigenous peoples and IK in assessments, it is important to acknowledge the intellectual property of IK (David-Chavez and Gavin 2018). Indigenous-led approaches can help ensure that the use of IK is protected and validated by Indigenous peoples themselves and not appropriated by non-Indigenous peoples, which upholds the principles of the United Nations Declaration on the Rights of Indigenous Peoples (Broto et al. 2019). Finally, given this central role that Indigenous peoples and their organizations can play in the assessment, Indigenous contributions should be recognized and credited in the final products, publications, and other outputs (David-Chavez and Gavin 2018). These products must be accessible, in forms that enable mutual comprehension among all assessment actors (Tengö et al., 2017). Finally, a strength-based approach should guide the work, neither portraying Indigenous peoples as "victims" of climate change nor as "heroic" groups whose IK can be taken, appropriated, and harnessed for finding solutions elsewhere (Broto et al. 2019; Ford et al. 2016; Roosvall and Tegelberg 2013). The Climate and Traditional Knowledges Workgroup (CTKW) created *Guidelines for Considering*

Traditional Knowledges in Climate Change Initiatives, which outlines actions for agencies, researchers, and Indigenous knowledge holders (CTKW, 2014).

Summary

Health sector officials from local to national levels recognize climate change as a dangerous and growing threat to health—perhaps the greatest this century (Watts et al. 2015)—and many are ramping up efforts to prepare populations, communities, and health systems for future impacts. The growing pace of climate change, and concomitant risks of very severe health outcomes if physiological or societal thresholds are crossed, means that incremental efforts to prepare individuals, communities and health systems are no longer adequate. Led by WHO, new methods and guidance for understanding climate change risks to health and vulnerabilities faced by specific populations, and for developing and evaluating adaptation plans and measures, have been developed and have evolved over the last two decades. Recognition of the importance of health systems and services in the fight against climate change impacts has meant increased attention on efforts to understand vulnerabilities faced by systems, for example, health facilities like hospitals and clinics, and on efforts to increase their climate resiliency and sustainability (Health Care Without Harm 2018).

Unprecedented opportunities exist to improve the knowledge base used for climate change and health adaptation efforts through V&As by utilizing new guidance (e.g., health facility resiliency checklists), frameworks (e.g., food security, climate change and health), tools (e.g., health system stress testing), and by including the perspectives and voices of Indigenous people and of those where sex, gender, and identity factors, such as age, ethnicity, income, ability, and geographic location, intersect in ways that contribute to individuals experiencing differences in health risks, health services, and health outcomes (Rudolph, Gould, and Berko 2015; Canadian Institutes of Health Research 2018; Friel 2019). Considering the effects of existing power dynamics, health equity, and related sex and gender factors in V&As is important to avoid overlooking unique risks and to ensure adaptation and resiliency efforts do not inadvertently perpetuate existing inequities and inequalities.

The transition to promoting climate resilient individuals, communities, and health systems must accelerate, given increasing risks posed by climate change, including the threat of catastrophic health outcomes. The information from V&As will continue to improve if they focus on practical issues faced by health decision-makers, foster sustained partnerships based upon continued learning and improvement, are informed by new methods and analysis (e.g., benefit-cost assessment), and utilize innovative tools such as citizen science and artificial intelligence (Moss et al. 2019).

DISCUSSION QUESTIONS

1. It is important to conduct broad consultations when conducting health vulnerability and adaptation assessments, within and outside of the health sector. Provide an explanation of why this is and create a list of stakeholders that could be engaged in a V&A.

2. List the broad categories of climate-related health risks that are important to consider in a V&A, including climate hazards that can affect health systems. What types of data would be beneficial for assessing these health risks?

3. How can V&As integrate Indigenous knowledge to improve understanding of health risks and vulnerabilities and support adaptation and resiliency building efforts?

KEY TERMS

Adaptation: According to the Intergovernmental Panel on Climate Change, adaptation is the process of adjustment to actual or expected climate and its effects. In human systems, adaptation seeks to moderate or avoid harm or exploit beneficial opportunities. In some natural systems, human intervention may facilitate adjustment to expected climate and its effects.

Health system: According to the WHO, a health system consists of all organizations, people, and actions whose primary intent is to promote, restore, or maintain health. This includes efforts to influence determinants of health as well as more direct health-improving activities.

Health system stress testing: Focusing on climate-related hypothetical scenarios, the effective operations of the health system are assessed and approaches for managing acute and chronic climate events are developed. Such exercises increase the capacity of health systems and related sectors to adapt and respond to climate-related shocks and challenges.

Health vulnerability and adaptation assessments: Allow local, regional, and national levels of government to understand climate change-related health risks, identify populations that are most at risk, recognize vulnerabilities in the health system, and inform effective and inclusive adaptation actions and response measures.

Vulnerability: According to the Intergovernmental Panel on Climate Change, vulnerability is the degree to which a system is susceptible to, or unable to cope with, adverse effects of climate change, including climate variability and extremes. Vulnerability is a function of the character, magnitude, and rate of climate variation to which a system is exposed, its sensitivity, and its adaptive capacity.

References

Abram, N., J.-P. Gattuso, A. Prakash, L. Cheng, M. P. Chidichimo, S. Crate, H. Enomoto et al. 2019. "Framing and Context of the Report." In *IPCC Special Report on the Ocean and Cryosphere in a Changing Climate*, edited by H.-O. Pörtner, D. C. Roberts, V. Masson-Delmotte, P. Zhai, M. Tignor, E. Poloczanska, K. Mintenbeck et al., 73–129. Geneva: IPCC.

Adger, W. N., J. M. Pulhin, J. Barnett, G. D. Dabelko, G. K. Hovelsrud, M. Levy, Ú. Oswald Spring, and C. H. Vogel. 2014. "Human Security." In *Climate Change 2014: Impacts, Adaptation, and Vulnerability. Part A: Global and Sectoral Aspects. Contribution of Working Group II to the Fifth Assessment Report of the Intergovernmental Panel on Climate Change*, edited by C. B. Field, V. R. Barros, D. J. Dokken, K. J. Mach, M. D. Mastrandrea, T. E. Bilir, M. Chatterjee et al, 755–91. Cambridge, UK and New York: Cambridge University Press.

Bartlett, C., M. Marshall, and A. Marshall. 2012. "Two-Eyed Seeing and Other Lessons Learned within a Co-Learning Journey of Bringing Together Indigenous and Mainstream Knowledges and Ways of Knowing." *Journal of Environmental Studies and Sciences* 2 (4):331–40.

Berrang-Ford, L., K. Dingle, J. D. Ford, C. Lee, S. Lwasa, D. B. Namanya, J. Henderson, A. Llanos, C. Carcamo, and V. Edge. 2012. "Vulnerability of Indigenous Health to Climate Change: A Case Study of Uganda's Batwa Pygmies." *Social Science & Medicine* 75 (6):1067–77. https://doi.org/10.1016/j.socscimed.2012.04.016.

Berry, P., P. M. Enright, J. Shumake-Guillemot, E. V. Prats, and D. Campbell-Lendrum. 2018. "Assessing Health Vulnerability and Adaptation to Climate Change: A Review of International Progress." *International Journal of Environmental Research and Public Health* 15:2626. doi:10.3390/ijerph15122626.

Broto, V. C., T. Mustonen, J. Petzold, G. Pecl, S. Harper, and T. A. Benjaminsen. 2019. *Discussion Paper: Indigenous Knowledge and Local Knowledge*. Durban, South Africa: IPCC WGII LAM1 Meeting.

Buse, C., L. Aubin, and M. Pajot. 2012. "Report on Health Vulnerability to Climate Change: Assessing Exposure, Sensitivity and Adaptive Capacity in the Region of Peel; Mississauga, ON" (unpublished report).

Campbell-Lendrum, D., and R. Woodruff. 2007. *Climate Change: Quantifying the Health Impact of Climate Change at National and Local Levels*. Geneva, Switzerland: World Health Organization.

Campbell-Lendrum, D., J. Guillemot, and K. Ebi. 2015. "Chapter 10: Climate Change and Health Vulnerability Assessments." In *Global Climate Change and Human Health: From Science to Practice*, edited by G. Luber and J. Lemery. San Francisco, CA: Jossey-Bass.

Canadian Coalition for Green Health Care. 2016. "Health Care & Climate Change Resiliency." https://greenhealthcare.ca/climate-change/resiliency/.

Canadian Institutes of Health Research. 2018. "How CIHR Is Supporting the Integration of SGBA." http://www.cihr-irsc.gc.ca/e/50837.html.

Centers for Disease Control and Prevention. 2019a. "CDC's Building Resilience Against Climate Effects (BRACE) Framework." https://www.cdc.gov/climateandhealth/BRACE.htm.

Centers for Disease Control and Prevention. 2019b. Climate Change and Health: Climate-Ready States and Cities Initiative. https://www.cdc.gov/climateandhealth/climate_ready.htm.

Chambers, S. N., and J. A. Tabor. 2018. "Remotely Identifying Potential Vector Habitat in Areas of Refugee and Displaced Person Populations due to the Syrian Civil War." *Geospatial Health* 13 (2):10.4081/gh.2018.670. doi:10.4081/gh.2018.670.

Climate and Traditional Knowledges Workgroup (CTKW). 2014. "Guidelines for Considering Traditional Knowledges in Climate Change Initiatives." http://climatetkw.wordpress.com/.

Crate, S., W. Cheung, B. Glavovic, S. Harper, H. J. Combes, M. Ell Kanayuk, B. Orlove et al. 2019. "Indigenous Knowledge and Local Knowledge in Ocean and Cryosphere Change." In *IPCC Special Report on Oceans and Cryosphere in a Changing Climate*, edited by H.-O. Pörtner, D. C. Roberts, V. Masson-Delmotte, P. Zhai, M. Tignor, E. Poloczanska, *K. Mintenbeck et al. Geneva: IPCC*.

Crimmins, A., J. Balbus, J. L. Gamble, C. B. Beard, J. E. Bell, D. Dodgen, R. J. Eisen et al., eds. 2016. *The Impacts of Climate Change on Human Health in the United States: A Scientific Assessment.* Washington, DC: U.S. Global Change Research Program. http://dx.doi.org/10.7930/J0R49NQX.

Cunsolo Willox, A., S. L. Harper, J. D. Ford, V. L. Edge, K. Landman, K. Houle, S. Blake, and C. Wolfrey. 2013. "Climate Change and Mental Health: An Exploratory Case Study from Rigolet, Nunatsiavut, Canada." *Climatic Change* 121 (2):255–70. https://doi.org/10.1007/s10584-013-0875-4.

Cunsolo Willox, A, S. L. Harper, Edge, V. L. Edge, K. Landman, K. Houle, J. D. Ford, and Rigolet Inuit Community Government. 2013. "The Land Enriches the Soul: On Climatic and Environmental Change, Affect, and Emotional Health and Well-Being in Rigolet, Nunatsiavut, Canada." *Emotion, Space and Society* 6 (1): 14–24. https://doi.org/10.1016/j.emospa.2011.08.005.

David-Chavez, D. M., and M. C. Gavin. 2018. "A Global Assessment of Indigenous Community Engagement in Climate Research." *Environmental Research Letters* 13 (12)"123005. https://doi.org/10.1088/1748-9326/aaf300.

Delormier, T., K. Horn-Miller, A. M. McComber, and K. Marquis. 2017. "Reclaiming Food Security in the Mohawk Community of Kahnawà ke through Haudenosaunee Responsibilities." *Maternal & Child Nutrition* 13 (S3):e12556. https://doi.org/10.1111/mcn.12556.

Ebi, K. L., P. Berry, C. Boyer, K. Hayes, P. M. Enright, S. Sellers, and J. J. Hess. 2018a. "Stress Testing the Capacity of Health Systems to Manage Climate Change-Related Shocks and Stresses." *International Journal of Environmental Research and Public Health* 15:2370.

Ebi, K. L., C. Boyer, K. J. Bowen, H. Frumkin, and J. Hess. 2018b. "Monitoring and Evaluation Indicators for Climate Change-Related Health Impacts, Risks, Adaptation, and Resilience." *International Journal of Environmental Research and Public Health* 15:1943.

Ebi, K. L., J. Paterson, A. Yusa, V. Anderson, and P. Berry. 2016. *Climate Change and Health Vulnerability Assessment Guidelines for the Province of Ontario; Report Developed for the Ministry of Health and Long-Term Care; Ministry of Health and Long-Term Care*, Toronto, ON, Canada.

Ebi, K. L., and M. Otmani del Barrio. 2017. "Lessons Learned on Health Adaptation to Climate Variability and Change: Experiences across Low- And Middle-Income Countries." *Environmental Health Perspectives* 125:065001.

Ebi, K. L., P. Berry, K. J. Bowen, D. Campbell-Lendrum, G. Cissé, J. Hess, N. Ogden, and R. Schnitter. 2019. *Health System Adaptation to Climate Variability and Change.* https://cdn.gca.org/assets/2019-12/HealthSystemAdaptationToClimateVariabilityandChange.pdf.

Ebi, K. L., N. H. Ogden, J. C. Semenza, and A. Woodward. 2017. "Detecting and Attributing Health Burdens to Climate Change." *Environmental Health Perspectives* 125 (8):085004.

Ford, J. D. 2012. "Indigenous Health and Climate Change." *American Journal of Public Health* 102 (7):1260–66. https://doi.org/10.2105/AJPH.2012.300752.

Ford, J. D., L. Cameron, J. Rubis, M. Maillet, D. Nakashima, A. C. Willox, and T. Pearce. 2016. "Including Indigenous Knowledge and Experience in IPCC Assessment Reports." *Nature Climate Change* 6 (4):349–53. https://doi.org/10.1038/nclimate2954.

Fox, M., C. Zuidema, B. Bauman, T. Burke, and M. Sheehan, M. 2019. "Integrating Public Health into Climate Change Policy and Planning: State of Practice Update." *International Journal of Environmental Research and Public Health* 16 (18):3232. https://doi.org/10.3390/ijerph16183232. https://www.mdpi.com/1660-4601/16/18/3232.

Friel, S. 2019. *Climate Change and the People's Health.* New York: Oxford University Press.

Furgal, C., and J. Seguin. 2006. "Climate Change, Health, and Vulnerability in Canadian Northern Aboriginal Communities." *Environmental Health Perspective,* 114 (12):1964–70.

Gostin, L. O., I. Abubakar, R. Guerra, S. F. Rashid, E. A. Friedman, and Z. Jakab. 2019. "WHO Takes Action to Promote the Health of Refugees and Migrants." *Lancet* 393 (10185):2016–18. doi:10.1016/S0140-6736(19)31051-7.

Government of Vanuatu. 2015. *Second Phase Harmonized Assessment Report Vanuatu: Tropical Cyclone Pam.* Port Vila, Vanuatu: Government of Vanuatu.

Green, D., and L. Minchin. 2014. "Living on Climate-Changed Country: Indigenous Health, Well-Being and Climate Change in Remote Australian Communities." *EcoHealth* 11 (2):263–72. https://doi.org/10.1007/s10393-013-0892-9.

Green, D., S. Niall, and J. Morrison. 2012. "Bridging the Gap between Theory and Practice in Climate Change Vulnerability Assessments for Remote Indigenous Communities in Northern Australia." *Local Environment* 17 (3):295–315. https://doi.org/10.1080/13549839.2012.665857.

Greenwood, M., S. De Leeuw, and N. M. Lindsay. 2018. *Determinants of Indigenous Peoples' Health: Beyond the Social,* 2nd ed. Toronto, Ontario: Canadian Scholars.

Haines, A., and K. Ebi. 2019. "The Imperative for Climate Action to Protect Health." *New England Journal of Medicine* 380:263–73. doi: 10.1056/NEJMra1807873.

Harper, S. L., V. L. Edge, J. Ford, A. C. Willox, M. Wood, IHACC Research Team, RICG, and S. A. McEwen. 2015. "Climate-Sensitive Health Priorities in Nunatsiavut, Canada." *BMC Public Health* 15 (1). https://doi.org/10.1186/s12889-015-1874-3.

Hayes, K., and B. Poland. 2018. "Addressing Mental Health in a Changing Climate: Incorporating Mental Health Indicators into Climate Change and Health Vulnerability and Adaptation Assessments." *International Journal of Environmental Research and Public Health* 15:1806.

Health Care Without Harm. 2018. *Safe Haven: Protecting Lives and Margins with Climate-Smart Health Care.* Reston, VA: HCWH. https://noharm-uscanada.org/sites/default/files/documents-files/5146/Safe_haven.pdf.

Hofmeijer, I., J. D. Ford, L. Berrang-Ford, C. Zavaleta, C. Carcamo, E. Llanos, C. Carcamo et al. 2013. "Community Vulnerability to the Health Effects of Climate Change among Indigenous Populations in the Peruvian Amazon: A Case Study from Panaillo and Nuevo Progreso." *Mitigation and Adaptation Strategies for Global Change* 18 (7):957–78. https://doi.org/10.1007/s11027-012-9402-6.

Hess, J. J., and K. L. Ebi. 2016. "Iterative Management of Heat Early Warning Systems in a Changing Climate." *Annals of the New York Academy of Sciences* 1382 (1):21–30.

Hess, J. J., S. Saha, P. J. Schramm, K. C. Conlon, C. K. Uejio, and G. Luber. 2015. *Projecting Climate-Related Disease Burden: A Guide for Health Departments. Climate and Health Technical Report Series.* Atlanta, GA: Climate and Health Program, Centers for Disease Control and Prevention. https://www.cdc.gov/climateandhealth/docs/ProjectingClimateRelatedDiseaseBurden_508.pdf.

Intergovernmental Panel on Climate Change. 2001. *Climate Change 2001: Impacts, Adaptation snd Vulnerability, Contribution of Working Group II to the Third Assessment Report of the Intergovernmental Panel on Climate Change,* edited by J. J. McCarthy, O. F. Canziani, N. A. Leary, D. J. Dokken and K. S. White. Cambridge, UK, and New York Cambridge University Press. https://www.ipcc.ch/site/assets/uploads/2018/03/WGII_TAR_full_report-2.pdf.

Jaakkola, J. J. K., S. Juntunen, and K. Näkkäläjärvi. 2018. "The Holistic Effects of Climate Change on the Culture, Well-Being, and Health of the Saami, the Only Indigenous People in the European Union." *Current Environmental Health Reports* 5 (4):401–17. https://doi.org/10.1007/s40572-018-0211-2.

King, M., A. Smith, and M. Gracey. 2009. "Indigenous Health Part 2: The Underlying Causes of the Health Gap." *Lancet* 374 (9683):76–85. https://doi.org/10.1016/S0140-6736(09)60827-8.

Li, N., N. Dachner, V. Tarasuk, R. Zhang, M. Kurrein, T. Harris, S. Gustin, and D. Rasal. 2016. *Priority Health Equity Indicators for British Columbia: Household Food Insecurity Indicator Report.* Vancouver, BC: Provincial Health Services Authority and PROOF. https://proof.utoronto.ca/wp-content/uploads/2016/08/1186-PHS-Priority-health-equity-indicators-WEB.pdf.

Martinez, G. S., and P. Berry. 2018. "The Adaptation Health Gap: A Global Overview." In *UNEP 2018. The Adaptation Gap Report 2018,* 29–37. Nairobi, Kenya: United Nations Environment Programme.

Moss, R. H., S. Avery, K. Baja, M. Burkett, A. M. Chischilly, J. Dell, P. A. Fleming, K. Geil et al. 2019. "Evaluating Knowledge to Support Climate Action: A Framework for Sustained Assessment. Report of an Independent Advisory Committee on Applied Climate Assessment." *Weather, Climate and Society* 11 (3):465–87.

National Oceanic and Atmospheric Administration. 2016. *U.S. Climate Resilience Toolkit.* https://toolkit.climate.gov/topics/human-health/building-climate-resilience-health-sector.

Olsson, L., M. Opondo, P. Tschakert, A. Agrawal, S. H. Eriksen, S. Ma, L. N. Perch, and S. A. Zakieldeen. 2014. "Livelihoods and Poverty." In *Climate Change 2014: Impacts, Adaptation, and Vulnerability. Part A: Global and Sectoral Aspects. Contribution of Working Group II to the Fifth Assessment Report of the Intergovernmental Panel on Climate Change*, edited by C. B. Field, V. R. Barros, D. J. Dokken, K. J. Mach, M. D. Mastrandrea, T. E. Bilir, M. Chatterjee et al., 793–832. Cambridge, UK and New York: Cambridge University Press.

Pan American Health Organization; World Health Organization. 2016. *SMART Hospitals Toolkit.* https://www.paho.org/disasters/index.php?option=com_content&view=article&id=1742:smart-hospitals-toolkit&Itemid=1248&lang=en.

Parkinson, A. J., and B. Evengård. 2009. "Climate Change, Its Impact on Human Health in the Arctic and the Public Health Response to Threats of Emerging Infectious Diseases." *Global Health Action* 2:1–3. https://doi.org/10.3402/gha.v2i0.2075.

Roosvall, A., and M. Tegelberg, M. 2013. "Framing Climate Change and Indigenous Peoples: Intermediaries of Urgency, Spirituality and De-Nationalization." *International Communication Gazette* 75 (4):392–409. https://doi.org/10.1177/1748048513482265.

Rudolph, L., S. Gould, and J. Berko. 2015. *Climate Change,* Health and Equity: *Opportunities for Action.* Oakland, CA. Public Health Institute.

Salman, I. S., A. Vural, A. Unver, and S. Saçar. 2014. "Cutaneous Leishmaniasis Cases in Nizip, Turkey after the Syrian Civil War." *Mikrobiyoloji Bülteni* 48 (1):106–13.

Schnitter, R., and P. Berry. 2019. "The Climate Change, Food Security and Human Health Nexus in Canada: A Framework to Protect Population Health" *Int. J. Environ. Res. Public Health* 16 (14):2531. https://doi.org/10.3390/ijerph16142531.

Sellers, S., and K. L. Ebi. 2017. "Climate Change and Health under the Shared Socioeconomic Pathway Framework." *International Journal of Environmental Research and Public Health* 15:3.

Sheehan, M. D., M. A. Fox, C. Kaye, and B. Resnick. 2017. "Integrating Health into Local Climate Response: Lessons from the U.S. CDC Climate-Ready States and Cities Initiative." *Environmental Health Perspectives* 125 (9):094501.

Smith, R. K., A. Woodward, D. Campbell-Lendrum, D. D. Chadee, Y. Honda, Q. Liu, J. M. Olwoch, B. Revich, and R. Sauerborn. 2014. "Human Health: Impacts, Adaptation, and Co-Benefits." In *Climate Change 2014: Impacts, Adaptation, and Vulnerability. Part A: Global and Sectoral Aspects. Contribution of Working Group II to the Fifth Assessment Report of the Intergovernmental Panel on Climate Change*, edited by C. B. Field, V. R. Barros, D. J. Dokken, K. J. Mach, M. D. Mastrandrea, T. E. Bilir, M. Chatterjee et al., 709–54. Cambridge, UK; New York: Cambridge University Press. https://www.ipcc.ch/site/assets/uploads/2018/02/WGIIAR5-Chap11_FINAL.pdf.

Tengö, M., R. Hill, P. Malmer, C. M. Raymond, M. Spierenburg, F. Danielsen, T. Elmqvist, and C. Folke. 2017. "Weaving Knowledge Systems in IPBES, CBD and Beyond—Lessons Learned for Sustainability." *Current Opinion in Environmental Sustainability* 26–27:17–25. https://doi.org/10.1016/j.cosust.2016.12.005.

United Nations Framework Convention on Climate Change. 2013. *Best Practices and Available Tools for the Use oOf Indigenous and Traditional Knowledge and Practices for Adaptation, and the Application of Gender Sensitive Approaches and Tools for Understanding and Assessing Impacts, Vulnerability and Adaptation to Climate Change.* Bonn: United Nations. https://unfccc.int/resource/docs/2013/tp/11.pdf.

United Nations High Commissioner for Refugees. 2019. "Figures at a Glance." *Updated June 19, 2019.* Accessed March 19, 2020. https://www.unhcr.org/en-us/figures-at-a-glance.html.

Watt-Cloutier, S. 2015. *The Right to Be Cold: One Woman's Story of Protecting Her Culture, the Arctic and the Whole Planet.* Toronto, ON: Penguin.

Watts, N., W. N. Adger, P. Agnolucci, J. Blackstock, P. Byass, W. Cai, S. Chaytor et al. 2015. "Health and Climate Change: Policy Responses to Protect Public Health." *Lancet* 386:861–1914.

Watts, N., M. Amann, S. Ayeb-Karlsson, K. Belesova, T. Bouley, M. Boykoff, P. Byass et al. 2018. "The Lancet Countdown on Health and Climate Change: From 25 Years of Inaction to a Global Transformation for Public Health." *Lancet* 391:581–630.

Wheeler, N., and N. Watts. 2018. "Climate Change: From Science to Practice." *Current Environmental Health Reports* 5 (1):170–8.

Wollina, U., A. Koch, C. Guarneri, G. Tchernev, and T. Lotti. 2018. "Cutaneous Leishmaniasis—A Case Series from Dresden." *Open Access Macedonian Journal of Medical Sciences* 6 (1):89–92. doi:10.3889/oamjms.2018.028.

World Bank; World Meteorological Organization; World Health Organization. 2018. *Madagascar: Climate Change and Health Diagnostic—Risks and Opportunities for Climate-Smart Health and Nutrition Investment*. Washington, DC: World Bank. http://documents.worldbank.org/curated/en/936661516004441146/pdf/121945-12-1-2018-11-21-5-WorldBankMadagascarClimateChange andHealthDiagnosticJan.pdf.

World Health Organization; World Meteorological Organization; Health Canada; United Nations Environment Programme. 2003. *Methods of Assessing Human Health Vulnerability and Public Health Adaptation to Climate Change*. Copenhagen, Denmark: WHO.

World Health Organization. 2007. *Everybody's Business: Strengthening Health Systems to Improve Health Outcomes—WHO's Framework for Action*. Geneva: WHO. https://www.who.int/healthsystems/strategy/everybodys_business.pdf.

World Health Organization. 2013. *Protecting Health from Climate Change: Vulnerability and Adaptation Assessment*. Geneva: WHO. http://www.who.int/iris/handle/10665/104200.

World Health Organization. 2014. *WHO Guidance to Protect Health from Climate Change through Health Adaptation Planning*. Geneva: WHO. http://apps.who.int/iris/bitstream/handle/10665/137383/9789241508001_eng.pdf?sequence=1&isAllowed=y.

World Health Organization. 2015a. *Operational Framework for Building Climate Resilient Health Systems*. Geneva: WHO. http://apps.who.int/iris/bitstream/10665/189951/1/9789241565073_eng.pdf?ua=1.

World Health Organization. 2015b. *Tropical Cyclone Pam: Vanuatu—Health Cluster Bulletin #4*. Manila, Philippines: World Health Organization Western Pacific Regional Office.

World Health Organization. 2018. *WHO UNFCCC Climate Health Country Profile Project—Monitoring Health Impacts of Climate Change and Progress in Building Climate Resilient Health Systems*. Geneva: WHO. http://www.who.int/globalchange/resources/countries/en/.

Zavaleta, C., L. Berrang-Ford, J. Ford, A. Llanos-Cuentas, C. Cárcamo, N. A. Ross, G. Lancha et al. (2018). "Multiple Non-Climatic Drivers of Food Insecurity Reinforce Climate Change Maladaptation Trajectories among Peruvian Indigenous Shawi in the Amazon." *PLoS ONE* 13(10):1–30. https://doi.org/10.1371/journal.pone.0205714.

CHAPTER 15

CLIMATE CHANGE HEALTH IMPACT PROJECTIONS: LOOKING INTO THE FUTURE

Nikhil A. Ranadive and Jeremy J. Hess

The potential adverse health impacts of climate change have been a topic of discussion ever since Arrhrenius (1896) broached the question of whether the earth would warm as a result of fossil fuel combustion in 1896. Yet up through 1991, when Longstreth wrote the first modern commentary on the topic in the health literature, the concerns were explored qualitatively. Our understanding of the relationships between atmospheric processes and human health impacts was too limited to quantify impacts, leading investigators to express their work in the form of cautionary narratives rather than testable propositions. Our ability to conceptually model the possible impacts still far outpaced our ability to model the impacts mathematically.

During the 1990s, the field of environmental health made significant progress toward quantifying the likely health impacts of environmental changes at a range of scales. In its broadest sense, this process is termed **health impact assessment (HIA),** and the first consensus statement regarding how such estimates should be made was published in 1999 (European Centre for Health Policy 1999). Generally, HIAs are aimed at quantifying and, where possible, improving the human health impacts resulting from policies and decisions made outside of the health sector (such as whether and how to invest in large infrastructure projects). A mix of quantitative and qualitative methods (Lock 2000) have continued to evolve in recent years.

The methodological advances that helped advance HIAs spurred hopes that similar methods might be used to quantify climate change health impacts. Climate change is, after all, the result of a specific set of policies and practices related to energy, travel, food production, and land use, with alternatives that can be stipulated and studied using methods similar to those applied in HIAs. As climate health impacts began to manifest and increasing rates, public health experts became increasingly concerned that such health impacts would become the dominant global health challenge of the twenty-first century (Chan 2007). Practitioners also expressed a need for **projections** that could be used in comparative risk assessments (Campbell-Lendrum and Woodruff 2006), wherein estimates of health impacts attributable to various exposures could be compared across settings to help prioritize policies and other public health interventions.

Early on, it was not clear whether existing epidemiological methods could achieve such projections. In 2001, McMichael outlined three roles for epidemiologists in relation to climate change: first, to conduct retrospective analyses of associations between climate-sensitive environmental exposures and health

KEY CONCEPTS

- Climate change health impact projections are modeled, scenario-based estimates of the health impacts associated with climatic change. They are a special case of health impact assessment.

- Climate change health impact projections are not predictions but projections—estimates of likely impacts associated with a stipulated set of conditions, typically scenarios of greenhouse gas emissions.

- Health impact projections use retrospectively derived exposure-outcome associations from epidemiological studies. Some associations are better studied than others.

- Some exposure-outcome pathways are relatively direct (e.g., heat and heat-related illness) whereas others are less so (e.g., rainfall patterns, forage abundance, rodent population size, and the zoonosis hantavirus pulmonary syndrome). Generally, more direct pathways are easier to model.

- The alternative scenario against which comparisons are made is called the counterfactual. Counterfactuals in climate change health impact projection studies are based on different scenarios of greenhouse gas emissions and may also include other variables such as adaptation, economic growth, and demographic change.

outcomes; second, to pursue surveillance for current public health impacts highly likely to be attributable to climate change; and third, to develop scenario-based health risk assessments of projected climate change health impacts (McMichael 2001). He was careful to note the interplay between the first priority, retrospective analyses to derive exposure-outcome associations, and the third, health impact projection, as projections are predicated on the ability to quantify these relationships. He also noted that the third task, conducting scenario-based health risk assessments, was perhaps the least familiar of the three.

In the years that followed, the number of papers devoted to each steadily increased, and several health impact projections were published, notably a global projection done by McMichael and colleagues (2004) at the World Health Organization. The requirements for pursuing climate change health impact projections—topical fluency (i.e., familiarity with climate change and public health), access to global circulation model outputs to use as exposure data, access to relevant exposure-outcome associations, and fluency with the modeling and mapping approaches required to produce projections—are now relatively common in many public health settings. The field has recently experienced a significant expansion in projection efforts, fueled partly out of a recognized need to perform quantitative risk assessment and partly out of the increasingly available technical expertise and available input data for models.

The field is currently in a state of flux. Health impact projections have become more commonplace, and there have been some important advances, including a recent step-by-step tutorial on how to conduct climate change health impact projections using R statistical software (Vicedo-Cabrera, Sera, and Gasparrini 2019). However, obstacles remain, and there is no expert consensus on how to address various methodological challenges, for example, how to uniformly express disease burdens, how to approach other sociodemographic variables, and whether and how to include adaptation into the projections. This chapter is an introduction to these issues and a modest attempt to begin filling that gap. After a conceptual overview of climate change health impact projections and related topics, we review the different approaches that have been used, consider important concerns identified to date, and discuss frontiers in conducting and using climate change health impact projections.

A Conceptual Overview of Climate Change Health Impact Projections

Fundamentally, a climate change health impact projection is a modeled, scenario-based estimate of the health impacts associated with climatic change. Although not all climate change health impacts will be adverse, most impact projections have focused on adverse health impacts, for two reasons. First, salutary changes are of less concern in preparedness and planning efforts but adverse impacts are a priority. Second, taken in sum, the health impacts of climate change are expected to be adverse, so the focus has been on identifying and quantifying novel and expanded population health risks. Climate change health impact projections may focus on drivers of adverse health impacts (the distribution of exposures that serve as risk factors in the causal pathway) or extend the analysis to the outcomes themselves (Confalonieri et al. 2007); either way, they aim to quantify components of the causal pathway linking environmental variables and human health impacts on a population basis. The process is depicted in Figure 15.1, which shows regional trends in heat and cold-related mortality under different climate change **scenarios** (Gasparrini et al. 2017).

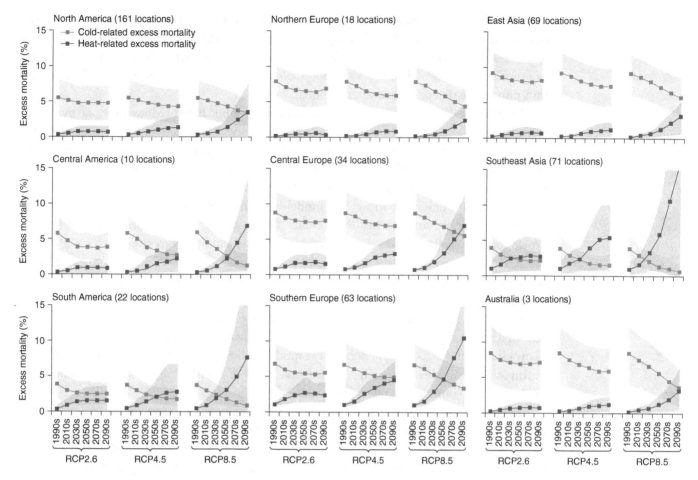

Figure 15.1 Global trends and heat and cold-related mortality projected under three climate change scenarios, ranging from mild warming (RCP2.6) to extreme warming (RCP8.5)

Source: Gasparrini et al. (2017). Reprinted with permission from Elsevier.

The remainder of this section is devoted to unpacking the definition to gain additional insights into the process, starting with the fundamental nature of the approach: modeling.

Modeling

Models are representations that "[mimic] relevant features of the situation being studied" (Bender 2000). Models, particularly mathematical models that use equations to represent either theoretical dynamics or observations, are central to scientific inquiry. They allow for characterization of systems and their components and for exploration of system behavior as various parameters are manipulated, including experimentation that may not be feasible for practical or ethical reasons or future-based situations.

Models are fundamental tools in studying climate change and its potential impacts. In particular, **global circulation models (GCMs)**, complex mathematical models of the Earth's atmosphere and oceans that include many atmospheric and terrestrial layers divided up into thousands of three-dimensional gridded spaces, are used to study the likely environmental impacts of shifts in greenhouse gas (GHG) emissions, such as changes in temperature, precipitation, and sea level. These changes can be used as health-relevant exposures themselves if there is a direct relationship between the exposure and health outcomes (e.g., ambient temperature and heat-related illness). They can also be used to generate indirect estimates of how health-relevant exposures may shift (e.g., warming, combined with changes in precipitation, can result in prolonged drought with potentially significant consequences for food supply and thus nutritional outcomes in certain regions).

Models of a different sort are also fundamental to public health. Modeling done by climate scientists is relatively rare in public health, but statistical (typically regression) modeling to estimate associations between observed exposures and outcomes is quite common. Again, such modeling can be used to describe relatively direct relationships between an environmental exposure and a health outcome, or it can be used to identify controlling factors in the indirect relationships described above. The modeling often used to examine associations between environmental exposures and health outcomes, results of which are used to drive health impact projections, typically involves time-series analyses and Poisson regressions, which allows for linear and nonlinear associations and can include lagged effects. While the statistics used in these analyses are complex, there are accessible online tutorials and R packages that can make such analyses more accessible (Gasparrini 2011).

In order to situate our discussion of climate change health impact projections, it is important first to briefly discuss some general aspects of mathematical models, of which there are many kinds (Bender 2000). In general, these models exhibit a wide range of approaches depending on the situation being studied and the conventions of the particular discipline. Some major distinctions are outlined in Table 15.1.

Importantly, models can be combined such that results from one model can be used to drive another. This combination can be used to expand the scope (i.e., the range of factors considered) or scale (i.e., spatial and temporal dimensions) of the effort. Models can be linked together in a chain, with outputs from one model (e.g., a GCM generating outputs for air temperature) generating inputs for another (e.g., an air pollution model linking temperature with atmospheric chemical processes to estimate air pollution formation) that is then linked to a third (e.g., a model linking air pollution exposure to health outcomes). Models can also be nested, with outputs from a model at a relatively coarse scale (e.g., global, with estimates at 50 km² resolution) used as boundary inputs for a model that works at a relatively granular scale (e.g., local, with estimates at a 4 km² resolution), thus generating estimations over different scales while reducing computational requirements. Climate change health impact projections are all combination models, as they include GCM projections of data from possible climate futures and modeled estimates of associations between environmental exposures and health outcomes.

Although models can be powerful tools, they are by nature subject to a number of limitations, all of which ultimately undermine their validity to some degree. Perhaps most important, models are based either on historical observations or theory (though some

Table 15.1 Some Simple Binary Classifications of Mathematical Models

Linear: Employ linear equations exclusively	Nonlinear: Employ nonlinear equations or a mix of the two
Static (also equilibrium): Time invariant, typically not allowing for interactions among variables over time	Dynamic: Include an element of time, and often allowing for interactions among variables over time
Discrete: Treat objects in the model separately	Continuous: Describe collective behavior of objects in model
Deterministic: Inputs and outputs expressed as point estimates	Probabilistic: Use probability distributions for inputs and outputs
Deductive: Based on theory	Inductive: Based on empirical observations

theoretical models incorporate significant empirical elements). Models based on historical observations, by definition, cannot account for observations outside the historical data set on which they are based and thus are fundamentally inadequate for predicting, hedging against, and taking advantage of extreme and rare events (e.g., the "turkey problem"; Taleb 2012). Theoretical models are relatively untested and therefore may not describe the systems under study as well as users would like. Regardless of whether models are based on data or theory, another significant limitation is that, as simplifications, they may misrepresent system behaviors deriving from factors that are not included among the model's components. While this concern can be addressed to an extent through sensitivity testing, there are fundamental uncertainties involved in modeling that are inherently difficult to characterize fully.

We move next to issues related to generating the GCM outputs used in health impact projections, then to considerations of exposure-outcome association modeling, after which we finally return to the topic of modeling climate-sensitive health impacts.

The Role of GCM Projections

In the climate change literature, the word *projections* has a very specific meaning. The Intergovernmental Panel on Climate Change (IPCC) defines a *climate projection* as "the simulated response of the climate system to a scenario of future emission or concentration of GHGs and aerosols, generally derived from climate models" (Matthews et al. 2018). Elaborating on this, the IPCC notes that "climate projections are distinguished from climate predictions by their dependence on the emission/concentration/radiative forcing scenario used, which is in turn based on assumptions concerning, for example, future socioeconomic and technological developments that may or may not be realized" (Matthews et al. 2018). Predictions, in contrast, are attempts to generate best estimates of future states, usually starting with current conditions. Weather forecasts, for instance, are near- and medium-term predictions of the weather for a specified location. Predictions or forecasts are not dependent on scenarios (put differently, no scenarios are made explicit in predictions, because they would contain no new forcing (e.g., changes in GHG concentrations in the atmosphere); the underlying drivers in the model remain unchanged).

The Role of Scenarios

As the preceding paragraph makes clear, projections are based on scenarios, which are essentially alternate storylines for future states that include information about important drivers of the processes being projected. The scenarios used to project global climate change have been determined by the IPCC, which first released scenarios (named IS92) in 1992; in 1996, these scenarios were revisited with an updated knowledge base, and the IPCC Special Report on Emissions Scenarios (IPCC SRES) was published in 2000 (Nakicenovic et al. 2000). As noted in the SRES Summary for Policymakers:

> Future greenhouse gas (GHG) emissions are the product of very complex dynamic systems, determined by driving forces such as demographic development, socio-economic development, and technological change. Their future evolution is highly uncertain. Scenarios are alternative images of how the future might unfold and are an appropriate tool with which to analyse how driving forces may influence future emission outcomes and to assess the associated uncertainties. (Nakicenovic et al. 2000)

The SRES scenarios encapsulated storylines for global development and cooperation regarding climate change mitigation, coupled with changes in emissions. They were categorized using a taxonomy and nomenclature, with scenario families being the largest class and the four families named A1, A2, B1, B2; scenario families were subdivided into groups, with group members having "similar demographic, societal, economic and technical-change storylines" (Baede, van der Linden, and Verbruggen 2007). The scenarios were representations of various development trajectories and were divided based on the degree of economic versus environmental focus (A scenario family versus B scenario family) and global versus regional development (1 scenario family versus 2 scenario family). From each group, one scenario was considered illustrative, or representative of the general storyline; these scenarios (the A1B, A2, B1, B2 scenarios from the SRES) were most commonly used in projection studies. The SRES scenarios were used to generate projections for the IPCC's Third and Fourth Assessment Reports.

The scenarios were updated again before the IPCC's Fifth Assessment Report and reoriented to focus primarily on the radiative forcings (energy imbalances) driving climate change. The new scenarios are referred to as **representative concentration pathways (RCPs)**, and there are four: RCP8.5, RCP6, RCP4.5, and RCP2.6. The numbers identifying each of the RCPs refer to the magnitude of the energy imbalance (measured in watts per square meter) in the scenario in the year 2100; the RCPs roughly correspond with year 2100 atmospheric carbon dioxide concentrations of about 490 parts per million (ppm), 650 ppm, 850 ppm, and 1,370 ppm, respectively (van Vuuren et al. 2011). In addition to quantifying forcing, the RCPs also quantify rates of emissions and concentrations of each of the major greenhouse gas concentrations. Data for each of the scenarios, which are meant to minimize duplication of modelers' efforts and facilitate interdisciplinary science, include baseline and historical emissions data and projected emissions and concentration data going forward to 2100, subdivided into cells measuring half a degree of latitude and longitude (Wayne 2013). The RCP scenarios are freely available for download.

It is important to note that IPCC scenarios used to project climate change health impacts were in fact devised to provide inputs into GCMs, which then project changes in the climate. These scenarios, particularly the RCP scenarios, are entirely silent in regard to changes over time in the many other factors and social systems known to affect population health, commonly called the social determinants of health (Marmot and Wilkinson 1998) However, modeling studies have increasingly used the **shared socioeconomic pathways (SSPs)**, a set of future scenarios that capture plausible trends in socioeconomic and environmental conditions over the twenty-first century (O'Neill et al. 2014). As shown in Figure 15.2, the RCPs and SSPs can be used in combination to capture uncertainty in future climate, environmental, and socioeconomic outcomes (Ebi et al. 2014; O'Neill et al. 2014).

Characterization of Projected Exposures

The principal exposures of interest in climate change health impact projections are taken from GCM projections using different RCPs, sometimes in combination with SSPs. The output from these projections is gridded, with grid cells roughly 100 km on a side in the mid-latitudes, and produced at various time steps. There are numerous issues in translating GCM outputs into exposures relevant for health modeling, including spatial and temporal scale and what downscaling approaches (intermediate models for going from the relatively coarse scale of a GCM's primary output to more refined spatial and temporal estimates). The issues attending these questions are complex and have been reviewed extensively in the literature. A thorough discussion is beyond the scope of this chapter but Carbone (2014) has conducted an excellent review.

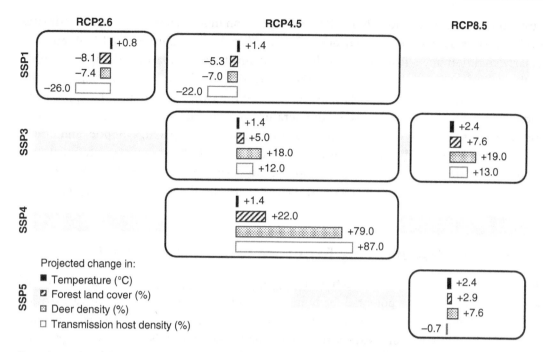

Figure 15.2   Projected changes in drivers for Lyme disease risk in Europe by the 2050s under different climate change (i.e., RCP) scenarios and plausible socioeconomic pathways, including SSP1 (a sustainable future), SSP3 (a future with low economic growth and environmental degradation), SSP4 (a future with socioeconomic and political inequality), and SSP5 (a fossil-fueled based future)

Source: From Li, Gilbert, Vanwambeke, Yu, Purse, and Harrison (2019), reproduced with permission from *Environmental Health Perspectives.*

The question of how exposures are quantified for health impact modeling deserves further attention. Most climate change health impact projections to date have used what is commonly termed the **delta method**, which refers to the exposure that is being projected and how it was derived. Gosling, McGregor, and Lowe (2009) refer to the application of the delta method to projection of health impacts from changes in temperature associated with climate change, highlighting that the exposure is a change in mean temperature, with the delta being expressed as the anomaly between the two:

> A mean climate warming [is applied] to the observed present-day climate to create a temperature projection time series that can be applied to the observed present temperature-mortality relationship. The degree of climate warming is calculated as the difference between the future period and present period mean temperatures, as estimated by climate models, to give a temperature anomaly. (Gosling et al. 2009)

The term *delta method* was coined by Déqué (2007), and a thorough analysis of many studies using the delta method was done by Gosling et al. in 2007. Gosling and colleagues developed a modified delta method in which projected changes in both mean temperature and temperature variability are included in the exposure of future populations and demonstrated that the combination of these two shifts is likely to result in greater heat-related mortality compared with projections of increased mean temperature alone.

Note that the reference baseline (e.g., "present period mean temperatures," in the preceding quotation), is a **counterfactual.** Explicit identification of the counterfactual(s) being evaluated in a modeling study, and assurance that the various aspects of the counterfactual(s) (e.g., population, GHG concentrations, etc.) are consistent is essential.

The exposure-outcome associations used in the delta method (and modified approaches) are modeled inputs, commonly developed from retrospective analyses using various regression techniques (Bender 2009). Poisson regression models, used to generate estimates of relative risks associated with various exposures (Frome and Checkoway 1985), are particularly common in environmental health for certain statistical reasons, though a number of other approaches may be more appropriate depending on the nature of the exposure and the outcome and the stipulated relationship between the two. For example, the approaches used to study the relationship between temperature and associated health outcomes include descriptive, case control, case only, case crossover, time series, spatial, synoptic, and others (Basu and Samet 2002; Huang et al. 2011). Basu and Samet (2002) have suggested that case crossover and time series are the most appropriate designs for studying heat–health relationships because of the short duration of the exposure and the brief lag between exposure and outcome.

Choosing and Quantifying Exposure–Outcome Associations

Climate change health impact projections focus on various path-dependent factors known or hypothesized to affect the potential for human health impacts from climate change. A wide array of health impacts are known to be climate sensitive, ranging from injuries like blunt and penetrating trauma commonly experienced in extreme weather events, to many vector-borne and zoonotic diseases, foodborne and waterborne illnesses, depression, and other mental health concerns (Watts et al. 2018). In many cases, the pathways leading from environmental conditions to human exposure to actual morbidity and mortality are remarkably complex (Portier et al. 2010), and there is substantial variation in the relationships across locations and populations.

The easiest pathways to model are the ones that are most direct (the ones with the shortest and least complex causal pathways) and the most consistent (pathways with physiological mechanisms that are consistent across populations and in which mediation by socio-economic development is minimal or relatively easily quantified). Cholera's sensitivity to weather and climate variability is well established, for instance, but the relationship between environmental variables like precipitation and cholera outbreaks is mediated by a wide range of factors from governance to socioeconomic status and thus varies markedly by setting (Murray et al. 2012). Given that these factors modify the relationship between precipitation and cholera, they need to be included in any modeling of this pathway as well, if the modeling effort is to be applied to a wide range of settings. If the modeling is not meant to be generalizable but is focused instead on a specific population and setting where circumstances can be assumed to be relatively stable for the period under investigation, then a more straightforward statistical estimate of the relationship may be sufficient.

Other considerations are also important, such as how well exposures can be characterized in both the retrospective analyses and the GCM projections. For instance, levels of airborne pollutants such as particulate matter can be measured at monitoring stations, and these measurements can serve as proxies for population-level exposure to the same species at a larger spatial scale with some degree of confidence (Miller et al. 2007). Similarly, temperature measured at one location is frequently used as a proxy for temperature exposure across a larger area (Green et al. 2010). In both cases, the assumption of scalability can facilitate health impact projection, though it is important to recognize that this simplification may come with drawbacks, such as exposure misclassification. For instance, while temperature measurements obtained from airport weather stations can facilitate health impact projection at the city level, this method may fail to capture temperature variability experienced at the neighborhood level. Assumptions regarding extrapolation of exposure may mask significant variability in actual exposures at the individual level, obscuring dynamics that may be significant for public health action (see, for example, Basagaña et al. 2013 for a discussion related to particulate air pollution, and Kuras et al. 2017 for a discussion related to heat).

Despite this concern, acute heat illness serves as a good example of a direct and relatively consistent pathway, wherein the environmental condition of ambient warmth (e.g., maximum daily temperature) can be clearly correlated with a population health outcome (e.g., the incidence of emergency department visits for acute heat illnesses such as heat exhaustion and heatstroke). As populations can be acclimatized to different baseline levels of heat exposure, the relationship is not always consistent across different settings, though the overall relationship between temperature and heat illness tends to be similar even if specifics vary within a certain range (Ye et al. 2012). For this reason, heat-related health impacts have been the most commonly projected climate change health impact (Huang et al. 2012).

Projecting Health Impacts of Extreme Weather Events

Extreme weather events impose a substantial burden of disease. The ways through which extreme weather events affect human health are complex, interrelated, and context dependent. In the direct wake of extreme weather, the need for medical services to treat injury increases. Secondary impacts, including human displacement, infectious disease, and loss of shelter and clean water, soon follow. However, the extent to which a particular event may affect an area depends on many factors that include ecosystem characteristics, health infrastructure, demographics, and the wealth of that region (Davis et al. 2010). In many settings, the direct impacts are much smaller than the indirect effects resulting from infrastructure damage, migration, and disruptions after the event. This complex, variable, and long causal pathway makes modeling the health impacts of disasters difficult. Nonlinear, dynamic approaches are often more appropriate for modeling associated health impacts (Berariu et al. 2015). Regardless of the modeling platform, vulnerability factors (e.g., socioeconomic status, age, etc.) are fundamental to include in the causal pathway in projecting climate change health impacts from disasters (Mechler and Bouwer 2015). Projections of health impacts from hydrometeorologic and climatic disasters have been relatively rare as a result of these challenges. The model outputs are most likely to be useful from a policy and advocacy perspective, acting as narratives to highlight the likely impacts of climate change on disaster health risks (Nissan and Conway 2018). Medical service agencies are an essential component of adaptive management of climate change disaster impacts, and projections can serve as a useful tool for anticipating and managing risk. As models to predict impacts of extreme weather events improve, the medical community must take these risks to life and longevity seriously and prepare accordingly.

Comparisons and the Counterfactual

Climate change health impact projections commonly take a few different forms depending on the scenarios projected. By definition, investigators include projected future climatic conditions in their models, but otherwise there is no consistent guidance regarding whether investigators should also project shifts in population demographics and sensitivity to the exposures being analyzed. For instance, because we can be most confident about the validity of recently observed relationships, should we restrict projections to recently derived exposure-outcome associations and apply them to present-day populations without attempting to include adaptation? Or because we are often projecting far into the future, should we project population differences in resilience (ability to resist the deforming impact of an exposure) when trying to determine health impacts?

These questions refer to counterfactuals, or hypothetical explorations of what might have happened if initial conditions had been as stipulated (Balke and Pearl 2011). Ultimately the team projecting the health impacts, often in consultation with stakeholders for the modeling effort, will be responsible for answering these questions, though the research community may come together to generate a consensus regarding these and other pressing questions (e.g., using the Delphi method; Adler and Ziglio1996) regarding climate change health impact projection methods.

When considering these issues, it is also important to note that many exposure-outcome associations used in climate change health impact projections are expressions of relative risk (RR), for example, RR of mortality associated with one temperature relative to another during a specific period of time, or RR of mortality associated with an extreme weather event compared with mortality risk during a nonevent baseline period. In these instances, the counterfactual is a population without the exposure of interest. However, in climate change health impact projections, this assumption generally does not hold, as the exposure develops over a sufficiently long period that other, significant changes in the population, many of which may affect the exposure–outcome association, will have occurred.

This is an important limitation of static models, which project impacts at a particular point in time without allowing for dynamic consideration of important feedbacks. For instance, socioeconomic development is known to be a major driver of population health status, and vice versa. Climate change is expected to have adverse impacts on population health status and thus to impede development over time, but it is not clear whether it might be more strategic to invest in development generally or mitigate climate change to protect health in low- and middle-income countries. Preliminary work using dynamic modeling techniques suggests that investment in development is likely to have a higher return in the short and medium terms, though climate change mitigation will have a more significant impact on population health several decades hence (Tol, Ebi, and Yohe 2007).

Merging Data Streams in the Climate Change Health Impact Model

As noted, several approaches have been used to project health impacts associated with climate change, all of which use GCM outputs to generate estimates of future exposures. The approach used to link these outputs with health outputs must accommodate the nature of climate change health impacts, which are expected to be not only significant but also "nonlinear, region specific, and time dependent" (Chan et al. 1999). Ideally, the projection modeling effort would accommodate these dynamics.

To date, however, the approach used to project health effects appears to have depended more on the usual approach in the investigator's discipline than on some of these other considerations. For instance, economists have tended to use economic models that estimate costs associated with climate change health impacts; in these models, which are typically inductive, nonlinear, continuous, and deterministic and can be dynamic or static, use health impacts as part of an overall estimating equation of damages to a local or world economy (Bosello, Roson, and Tol 2006). Ultimately, the approach used should accommodate the dynamics of the system being modeled.

Climate Change Health Impact Projections in the Health Literature

The number of studies projecting climate change health impacts has substantially increased over the past decade, particularly within the past five years. Investigators have focused on a wide range of health exposures and outcomes, including heat and associated impacts (Chen et al. 2018; Gasparrini et al. 2017; Guo et al. 2018; Onozuka et al. 2019), air quality and respiratory disease (Achakulwisut et al. 2019; Chen et al. 2018; Neumann et al. 2019; Wang et al. 2019), vector-borne diseases such as dengue, malaria, and Lyme disease (Hundessa et al. 2018; Li et al. 2019; Lippi et al. 2019; Liu-Helmersson, Rocklöv, Sewe, and Brännström 2019; Liu-Helmersson, Brännström, Sewe, Semenza, and Rocklöv 2019; Ryan et al. 2019; Sarkar et al. 2019; Stevens et al. 2019), and diet and nutrition (Beach et al. 2019; Colombo et al. 2020; Liu et al. 2018). A handful of studies have used projections not only for the purpose of generating estimates of disease burdens but as a means to the end of exploring uncertainty resulting from methodological choices and data constraints and thereby to clarify further research priorities (Kolstad and Johansson 2011; Wu et al. 2014).

Although approaches have varied, generally these investigators used linear, deterministic, static models calibrated to a particular future point in time to generate their estimates. Their models are empirical, in the sense that they involve higher-order abstractions from observed relationships that are simplified using general equations and assumptions regarding the future scenarios being projected. They all use some form of the delta method, though differences between future and present-day temperature are not necessarily the exposures that are projected; sometimes temperature shifts are used to drive air quality changes, and sometimes other exposures, such as changes in relative humidity, drive other ecological changes relevant to health, such as the relative abundance of ticks that can transmit Lyme disease (Ogden et al. 2014).

Investigators modeling climate change health impacts must answer a number of questions in the course of their modeling efforts, including:

- What are the model's scope and scale?
- What populations will be included? Will the analysis be stratified?
- What exposure factor(s) will be included in the response function?
- How will impacts be expressed?
- Will the model include adaptation? If so, how?
- How will uncertainty be considered and assessed?

Analysts have increasingly accounted for complex scenarios. For instance, models routinely account for future adaptation (Díaz et al. 2019; Guo et al. 2018; Huynen and Martens 2015; Wang et al. 2018; Zhang et al. 2018), demographic and population changes (Ahmadalipour et al. 2019; Guo et al. 2018; Liu-Helmersson, Brännström, Sewe, Semenza, and Rocklöv 2019), and plausible socioeconomic scenarios (Lee et al. 2018; Liu-Helmersson, Brännström, Sewe, Semenza, and Rocklöv 2019; Sun et al. 2019; Zhang et al. 2018). To date, analysts have taken a wide range of approaches to these considerations. The variability in methods for modeling adaptation is a significant source of uncertainty, perhaps greater than the uncertainty inherent in emissions and climate modeling (Gosling et al. 2017). Taken together, this has limited the comparability of results, even for the same general exposures and health outcomes (Huang et al. 2011), though it has likely also made the results more valid for specific locations and anticipated circumstances. Clarification of best practices regarding health impact projections, stratified by exposure and health outcome, will be an important next step in the evolution of climate change health impact projections science.

Work that better clarifies the relationships between environmental exposures and health impacts, McMichael's first task, will also be important to improving the utility of climate change health impact projections. Recent work has identified this as one of the primary sources of uncertainty in health impact projections (Kolstad and Johansson 2011; Wu et al. 2014). Because of the complexity of many exposure-outcome pathways, their diversity across settings, and our incomplete understanding of the specific dynamics in many cases, many pathways are oversimplifications. The equations used to summarize observed relationships, particularly in areas that are not well studied, are subject to confounding and other potential sources of bias and should be viewed as such. Moreover, unless the underlying pathways have been extensively researched, it is important to note that the relationships described in exposure-outcome pathways may not always be explicitly causal. Determining causality in environmental health is a difficult task that often requires various forms of evidence, including observational and experimental studies, and satisfies evidentiary criteria that can help distinguish correlation from causation (Hill 1965). In some cases, the exposure-outcome associations modeled in climate change health impact projections are, strictly speaking, correlations that are strongly suspected to represent causal relationships, an important caveat to keep in mind.

Characterization of Risk

Risk characterization and assessment are important because it funnels into risk communication, policymaking, and intervention prioritization. Climate change health impact projections have employed several approaches to characterizing risk and expressing its magnitude relative to other public health threats. Many studies express outcomes in terms of an increase in counts per unit time, for example, the number of excess deaths per day from a given exposure anticipated in a given setting at a given point in time assuming a particular emissions scenario. Some of these risk estimates are stratified, often by age or other demographic factors.

Some studies also characterize relative risks, for example, in comparison with population risk in some baseline period or in some other referent population. Some studies also explicitly link their risk estimates, for example, excess cases of acute asthma exacerbations due to elevated ozone concentrations that require a visit to the emergency department, to metrics such as **disability adjusted life years (DALYs)** that allow for comparative risk assessment (Longfield et al. 2013). Several investigators have recommended that DALYs are the appropriate metric for climate change health impact projections for this reason (Xun et al. 2010; Zhang, Bi, and Hiller 2007). One challenge with using DALYs, however, is that valuation metrics have not been assigned to all of the outcomes that may be of interest; another is that valuation is context dependent and heavily influenced by per capita incomes and other contextual factors. Despite these issues, the comparability that use of DALYs allows can confer significant advantage on studies that are able to employ this metric from a policymaking perspective.

Frontiers in Climate Change Health Impact Projection

Although the future is fraught with uncertainty, we can speculate about potential innovations in the science of climate change health impact projections. Several developments are likely.

First, we are likely to see a continued expansion of climate change health impacts modeling as the techniques become more familiar, expertise in the public health community develops, there is increased demand for such modeled impacts among a broader range of stakeholders, and we see additional advances in climate change health impact attribution studies and increased effectiveness in decadal-scale climate projections (Anderson et al. 2019). Related to this, it is likely that models will be integrated into planning efforts in certain jurisdictions in order to guide adaptation planning and that these models will be continuously updated using principles of **adaptive management** (Ebi 2011; Hess, McDowell, and Luber 2012; Petkova, Morita, and Kinney 2014), a framework that uses regularly updated models to facilitate management of complex systems subject with multiple stakeholders (Holling 1978; National Research Council 2004). There are early examples of heat projections being used in this way (Li et al. 2016; Li et al. 2018; Martinez et al. 2018; Petkova et al. 2017). Using climate change health impact projections in this way is likely to become more common as models become more adept at projecting medium-term impacts and can be revised as surveillance evidence accumulates.

Second, the range of projected health impacts is likely to broaden as we learn more about historical relationships between weather, climate variability, climate change, and health. This increased breadth will likely include further quantitative projections of health impacts in areas like undernutrition, which has received increasing attention of late (Beach et al. 2019; Smith and Myers 2018), and expanded analyses to include nutritional impacts associated with ocean acidification and other food system stressors. Projections of health impacts specific to particular regions are also likely to emerge. We may also be able to project impacts related to weather extremes, particularly as our ability to attribute health impacts to climate change improves (Anderson et al. 2019; Ebi et al. 2017), and to events with conditional probabilities, for example, failure of a sewage treatment plant in the setting of an extreme precipitation event or power outage during a severe heat wave.

Third, our projections will likely become more refined as we continue to deepen our understanding of factors affecting the central relationships we project, as we bring additional data resources to our efforts, and as our near-term forecasting models improve. As we learn more about factors that amplify or blunt certain exposures, for example, how neighborhood microclimates may affect ambient temperatures at a granular level, and about factors that modify the effects of exposure in susceptible populations, such as air conditioning prevalence and electricity prices, we will be able to make more refined projections that take these factors into account.

Fourth, we will likely see incorporation of alternative modeling techniques to characterize health impacts. These techniques may include approaches that accommodate dynamic factors and feedbacks within the systems being modeled (Luke and Stamatakis 2012) or allow for more realistic characterization of novel scenarios through the development of virtual worlds populated with agents operating based on various predetermined principles (Hartemink et al. 2015; Mellor et al. 2016). Incorporating novel approaches such as these will likely make it even more difficult to compare health impacts across studies but will also likely improve the ability to approximate some relationships of interest.

Finally, as public health invests more heavily in climate change health impact projections and they are used more widely, it is likely that there will be additional efforts to clarify best practices regarding modeling choices. Such efforts are already underway in regard to modeling of the health co-benefits of climate change mitigation activities (Chang et al. 2017; Gao et al. 2018), and Vicedo-Cabrera's recent development of a tutorial for projecting climate change health impacts is a significant step in this direction (Vicedo-Cabrera et al. 2019). Accommodating the wide range of exposures, health outcomes, and spatial and temporal scales at which projections are done will be challenging, but systematically addressing several central modeling issues could significantly clarify research priorities and improve the applicability of projections.

CLINICAL CORRELATES 15.1 CLINICAL INSIGHTS INTO CAUSAL PATHWAYS

Climate is, by definition, a thirty-year average, and climate change health impact projections necessarily focus on timelines that are out of sync with real-time clinical management decisions. This does not mean that clinicians have no role in developing climate change health impact projections. Clinicians, with their pathophysiological perspective, can be invaluable in developing the causal pathways used for climate change health impact projections. Take heat, for example. Many have focused on ambient temperature, an exogenous exposure, as the principal driver of risk for heat-related illnesses such as heat exhaustion and heatstroke and for exacerbations of chronic disease caused by the stress of extreme heat exposure. A physiological perspective, however, also highlights the importance of endogenous heat (e.g., from metabolic work) in an individual's overall heat load. Total heat load, a combination of endogenous and exogenous heat exposure, is the exposure of interest, and endogenous heat load varies most among younger, overall healthy individuals working and playing in hot conditions. Incorporating endogenous heat exposure into the causal pathways linking heat with health can substantially affect exposure assignment and produce markedly assessment of risk. For example, a study of heat exposure in Brisbane, Australia, highlighted the role of work in increasing heat exposure for younger people later in the century and, using years of life lost (YLL), a measure of premature mortality comparing age of death against predicted life expectancy, demonstrated that the overall burden in terms of lost years of productive life is much, much higher under a changed climate than previously thought (Huang et al. 2012).

This paper, produced by a clinician, was hailed for its use of a different metric, YLL, to highlight how climate change is likely to substantially affect the burden of disease in a way that examining mortality alone does not suggest (Kinney 2012).

CLINICAL CORRELATES 15.2 CLINICAL PRACTICE AND ADAPTIVE MANAGEMENT

Clinicians are important stakeholders in adaptation planning and projective assessment. They are in a unique position to see the impacts of climate-sensitive diseases on a case-by-case basis and may play an active role in surveillance, as well as in providing invaluable feedback to the health policy process. One application of this model is the detection and treatment of climate-sensitive infectious diseases. For example, Lyme disease is expanding its range because of changing environmental and climatic patterns (Li et al. 2019; McPherson et al. 2017; Monaghan et al. 2015). This has significant implications for prevention, diagnosis, and management (Fielding et al. 2016). Clinicians practicing within known and newly expanding Lyme regions may choose to change their practice of testing and treating, and provide feedback to affect regional practice recommendations.

Clinicians are stakeholders in adaptation planning and must respond in an active way by analyzing their management practices and feeding this information back to the level of policymaking institutions.

CLINICAL CORRELATES 15.3 CLIMATE CHANGE AND HUMAN HEALTH LITERATURE PORTAL AND LESSON PLANS

The National Institutes of Environmental Health Sciences (NIEHS) manages a literature portal that for key health impact studies from around the world. It features user-friendly search filters tailored for climate exposure, geographic location, health impact, model or methodology, model timescale, resource type, year published, and special topics (such as communication, climate justice, policy, research gaps, adaptation, economic impact). Further information can be found at https://tools.niehs.nih.gov/cchhl/index.cfm.

NIEHS also provides free climate change and human health lesson plans targeted for high school, secondary school, and graduate or professional school students. The modules integrate scientific evidence from the National Climate Assessment and challenge students on complex system process thinking by integrating health impacts knowledge on vulnerable populations. Lessons can be retrieved at https://www.niehs.nih.gov/health/scied/teachers/cchh/index.cfm.

Easily accessible resources help students and researchers develop critical thinking skills and apply current evidence on health impacts of climate change to projects.

Summary

In a relatively brief period, the public health community has moved from being limited to qualitative risk assessments of the health impacts of climate change to being able to quantify some likely impacts. These projections are made using global circulation models, emissions scenarios, and models linking environmental exposures and health impacts. To date, most projections made by public health scientists have used the delta method to project a relatively narrow set of impacts at fixed points in the future. The projections use a wide variety of methods and rely on many assumptions, and many have ignored complex issues related to adaptation and dynamic feedbacks in the systems being modeled. Those that have incorporated adaptation have used a range of approaches. Nevertheless, the projections to date have given us some sense of the order of magnitude of health impacts we might expect from climate change, and there is increasing sophistication in projecting impacts for which there is substantial reason for concern and extensive epidemiologic evidence, such as heat. Climate change health impact projection efforts are becoming more and more common, a trend that is likely to continue. In the future, it is likely that such modeling efforts will become more refined and will be applied to a wider range of settings and a broader suite of health impacts. An expert consensus regarding best practices may emerge.

DISCUSSION QUESTIONS

1. What is the difference between a prediction and a projection?

2. What factors can affect the validity of a climate change health impact projection?

3. What issues should one consider before applying climate change health impacts projected for one region to another geographical area?

4. List some of the ways in which risk is characterized and quantified (i.e., the metrics that are used to express risk) in climate change health impact projections.

5. What should practitioners know about climate change health impact projections, and how might they incorporate them into their practice?

KEY TERMS

Adaptive management: A framework that uses regularly updated models to facilitate iterative management of complex systems subjects with multiple stakeholders (Holling 1978; National Research Council 2004).

Counterfactual: Hypothetical exploration of what might have happened if initial conditions had been as stipulated (Balke and Pearl 2011).

Delta method: A commonly used method to create a temperature projection time series that relies on mean climate warming applied to the observed present-day climate (Gosling et al. 2009).

Disability adjusted life years (DALYs): A measure of disease burden that incorporates both years of life lost due to premature mortality and years lost due to disability (WHO n.d.).

Global circulation model: Complex mathematical models of the Earth's atmosphere and oceans that are used to study the likely environmental impacts of shifts in greenhouse gas emissions, such as changes in temperature, precipitation, and sea level.

Health impact assessment: A combination of procedures, methods, and tools by which a policy, project, or hazard may be judged as to its potential effects on the health of a population and the distribution of those effects within the population (WHO 1999).

Model: A representation that "[mimics] relevant features of the situation being studied" (Bender 2000).

Projection: Defined by the Intergovernmental Panel on Climate Change as the "response of the climate system to emission or concentration scenarios of GHGs and aerosols, or radiative forcing scenarios, often based upon simulations by climate models" (Baede, van der Linden, and Verbruggen 2007).

Representative concentration pathways (RCPs): Climate change and greenhouse gas emission scenarios adopted by the IPCC (van Vuuren et al. 2011).

Scenarios: Alternate images or storylines for future states that include details relevant to the processes being projected.

Shared socioeconomic pathways (SSPs): A set of future scenarios that capture plausible trends in socioeconomic and environmental conditions over the twenty-first century (O'Neill et al. 2014).

References

Achakulwisut, P., S. C. Anenberg, J. E. Neumann, S. L. Penn, N. Weiss, A. Crimmins, N. Fann et al. 2019. "Effects of Increasing Aridity on Ambient Dust and Public Health in the U.S. Southwest under Climate Change." *Geohealth* 3:127–44.

Adler, M., and E. Ziglio. 1996. *Gazing into the Oracle: The Delphi Method and Its Application to Social Policy and Public Health*. London: Jessica Kingsley Publishers.

Ahmadalipour, A., H. Moradkhani, A. Castelletti, and N. Magliocca. 2019. "Future Drought Risk in Africa: Integrating Vulnerability, Climate Change, and Population Growth." *Science of the Total Environment* 662:672–86.

Anderson, G. B., E. A. Barnes, M. L. Bell, and F. Dominici. 2019. "The Future of Climate Epidemiology: Opportunities for Advancing Health Research in the Context of Climate Change." *American Journal of Epidemiology* 188:866–72.

Arrhenius, S. 1896. "XXXI. On the Influence of Carbonic Acid in the Air upon the Temperature of the Ground." *The London, Edinburgh, and Dublin Philosophical Magazine and Journal of Science* 41:237–76.

Baede, A., P. van der Linden, and A. Verbruggen. 2007. *Annex II: Glossary to the IPCC Fourth Assessment Report: Climate Change 2007*. Geneva: Intergovernmental Panel on Climate Change.

Balke, A., and J. Pearl. 2011. "Probabilistic evaluation of counterfactual queries." https://cloudfront. escholarship.org/dist/prd/content/qt6vh9k0cf/qt6vh9k0cf.pdf.

Basagaña, X., I. Aguilera, M. Rivera, D. Agis, M. Foraster, J. Marrugat, R. Elosua, and N. Künzli. 2013. "Measurement Error in Epidemiologic Studies of Air Pollution Based on Land-Use Regression Models." *American Journal of Epidemiology* 178:1342–46.

Basu, R., and J. M. Samet. 2002. "Relation between Elevated Ambient Temperature and Mortality: A Review of the Epidemiologic Evidence." *Epidemiologic Reviews* 24:190–202.

Beach, R. H., T. B. Sulser, A. Crimmins, N. Cenacchi, J. Cole, N. K. Fukagawa, D. Mason-D'Croz et al. 2018. "Combining the Effects of Increased Atmospheric Carbon Dioxide on Protein, Iron, and Zinc Availability and Projected Climate Change on Global Diets: A Modelling Study." *Lancet Planet Health* 3:e307–e317.

Bender, E. A. 2000. *An Introduction to Mathematical Modeling*. North Chelmsford, MA: Courier Corporation.

Bender, R. 2009. "Introduction to the Use of Regression Models in Epidemiology." In *Cancer Epidemiology*, edited by M. Verma, 179–95. Totowa, NJ: Humana Press.

Berariu, R., C. Fikar, M. Gronalt, and P. Hirsch. 2015. "Understanding the Impact of Cascade Effects of Natural Disasters on Disaster Relief Operations." *International Journal of Disaster Risk Reduction* 12:350–56.

Bosello, F., R. Roson, and R. S. J. Tol. 2006. "Economy-Wide Estimates of the Implications of Climate Change: Human Health." *Ecological Economics* 58:579–91.

Campbell-Lendrum, D., and R. Woodruff. 2006. "Comparative Risk Assessment of the Burden of Disease from Climate Change." *Environmental Health Perspectives* 114:1935–41.

Carbone, G. J. 2014. "Managing Climate Change Scenarios for Societal Impact Studies." *Physical Geography* 35:22–49.

Chan, M. 2007. "Climate Change And Health: Preparing for Unprecedented Challenges. Statement by WHO Director-General Dr Margaret Chan."

Chan, N. Y., K. L. Ebi, F. Smith, T. F. Wilson, and A. E. Smith. 1999. "An Integrated Assessment Framework for Climate Change and Infectious Diseases." *Environmental Health Perspectives* 107:329–37.

Chang, K. M., J. J. Hess, J. M. Balbus, J. J. Buonocore, D. A. Cleveland, M. L. Grabow, R. Neff et al. 2017. "Ancillary Health Effects Of Climate Mitigation Scenarios As Drivers Of Policy Uptake: A Review Of Air Quality, Transportation And Diet Co-Benefits Modeling Studies. *Environmental Research Letters* 12:113001.

Chen, K., A. M. Fiore, R. Chen, L. Jiang, B. Jones, A. Schneider, A. Peters et al. 2018. "Future Ozone-Related Acute Excess Mortality under Climate and Population Change Scenarios in China: A Modeling Study." *PLoS Medicine* 15:e1002598.

Colombo, S. M., T. F. M. Rodgers, M. L. Diamond, R. P. Bazinet, and M. T. Arts. 2020. "Projected Declines in Global DHA Availability for Human Consumption as a Result of Global Warming." *Ambio* 49:865–80. doi:10.1007/s13280-019-01234-6.

Confalonieri, U., B. Menne, R. Akhtar, K. L. Ebi, M. Hauengue, R. S. Kovats, B. Revich et al. 2007. "Human Health." In *Climate Change 2007: Impacts, Adaptation and Vulnerability Contribution of Working Group II to the Fourth Assessment Report of the Intergovernmental Panel on Climate Change*, edited by M. L. Parry, O. F. Canziani, J. P. Palutikof, P. J. Van der Linden, and C. E. Hanson, 391–431. Cambridge: Cambridge University Press.

Davis, J. R., S. Wilson, A. Brock-Martin, S. Glover, and E. R. Svendsen. 2010. "The Impact of Disasters on Populations with Health and Health Care Disparities." *Disaster Medicine and Public Health Preparedness* 4:30–38.

Déqué, M. 2007. "Frequency of Precipitation and Temperature Extremes over France in an Anthropogenic Scenario: Model Results and Statistical Correction According to Observed Values." *Global and Planetary Change* 57:16–26.

Díaz, J., M. Sáez, R. Carmona, I. J. Mirón, M. A. Barceló, M. Y. Luna, and C. Linares. 2019. "Mortality Attributable to High Temperatures over the 2021–2050 and 2051–2100 Time Horizons in Spain: Adaptation and Economic Estimate." *Environmental Research* 172:475–85.

Ebi, K. L. 2011. "Overview: Adaptive Management for the Health Risks of Climate Change." In *Climate Change Adaptation in Developed Nations: From Theory to Practice*, edited by J. D. Ford and L. Berrang-Ford, 121–31. Dordrecht: Springer Netherlands.

Ebi, K. L., S. Hallegatte, T. Kram, N. W. Arnell, T. R. Carter, J. Edmonds, E. Kriegler et al. 2014. "A New Scenario Framework for Climate Change Research: Background, Process, and Future Directions." *Climatic Change* 122:363–72.

Ebi, K. L., N. H. Ogden, J. C. Semenza, and A. Woodward. 2017. "Detecting and Attributing Health Burdens to Climate Change." *Environmental Health Perspectives* 125:085004.

European Centre for Health Policy. 1999. *Health Impact Assessment: Main Concepts and Suggested Approach. Gothenburg Census Paper.* Brussels: ECHP.

Fielding, G., M. McPherson, P. Hansen-Ketchum, D. MacDougall, H. Beltrami, and J. Dunn. 2016. "Climate Change Projections and Public Health Systems: Building Evidence-Informed Connections." *One Health* 2:152–54.

Frome, E. L., and H. Checkoway. 1985. "Use of Poisson Regression Models in Estimating Incidence Rates and Ratios." *American Journal of Epidemiology* 121:309–23.

Gao, J., S. Kovats, S. Vardoulakis, P. Wilkinson, A. Woodward, J. Li, S. Gu et al. 2018. "Public Health Co-Benefits of Greenhouse Gas Emissions Reduction: A Systematic Review." *Science of the Total Environment* 627:388–402.

Gasparrini, A. 2011. "Distributed Lag Linear and Non-Linear Models in R: The Package dlnm." *Journal of Statistical Software* 43:1–20.

Gasparrini, A., Y. Guo, F. Sera, A. M. Vicedo-Cabrera, V. Huber, S. Tong, M. D. Z. S. Coehlo et al. 2017. "Projections of Temperature-Related Excess Mortality Under Climate Change Scenarios." *Lancet Planetary Health.* 1:e360–e367.

Gosling, S. N., D. M. Hondula, A. Bunker, D. Ibarreta, J. Liu, X. Zhang, et al. 2017. "Adaptation to Climate Change: A Comparative Analysis of Modeling Methods for Heat-Related Mortality." *Environmental Health Perspectives* 125:087008.

Gosling, S. N., G. R. McGregor, and J. A. Lowe. 2009. "Climate Change and Heat-Related Mortality in Six Cities Part 2: Climate Model Evaluation and Projected Impacts from Changes in the Mean and Variability of Temperature with Climate Change." *International Journal of Biometeorology* 53 (1):31–51. doi:10.1007/s00484-008-0189-9.

Gosling, S. N., G. R. McGregor, and A. Paldy. 2007. "Climate Change and Heat-Related Mortality in Six Cities Part 1: Model Construction and Validation." *International Journal of Biometeorology* 51:525–40.

Green, R. S., R. Basu, B. Malig, R. Broadwin, J. J. Kim, and B. Ostro. 2010. "The Effect of Temperature on Hospital Admissions in Nine California Counties." *International Journal of Public Health.* 55 (2):113–121. doi:10.1007/s00038-009-0076-0.

Guo, Y., A. Gasparrini, S. Li, F. Sera, A. M. Vicedo-Cabrera, M. Coelho, P. H. N. Saldiva et al. 2018. "Quantifying Excess Deaths Related to Heatwaves under Climate Change Scenarios: A Multicountry Time Series Modelling Study." *PLoS Medicine* 15:e1002629.

Hartemink, N., S. O. Vanwambeke, B. V. Purse, M. Gilbert, and H. Van Dyck. 2015. "Towards a Resource-Based Habitat Approach for Spatial Modelling of Vector-Borne Disease Risks." *Biological Reviews of the Cambridge Philosophical Society* 90:1151–62.

Hess, J. J., J. Z. McDowell, and G. Luber. 2012. "Integrating Climate Change Adaptation into Public Health Practice: Using Adaptive Management to Increase Adaptive Capacity and Build Resilience." *Environmental Health Perspectives* 120:171–79.

Hill, A. B. 1965. "The Environment and Disease: Association or Causation?" *Proceedings of the Royal Society of Medicine* 58 (5):295–300. doi:10.1177/003591576505800503.

Holling, C. S. 1978. *Adaptive Environmental Assessment and Management.* Chichester, UK: John Wiley & Sons.

Huang, C., A. G. Barnett, X. Wang, and S. Tong. 2012. "The Impact of Temperature on Years of Life Lost in Brisbane, Australia." *Nature Climate Change* 2:265–70.

Huang, C., A. G. Barnett, X. Wang, P. Vaneckova, G. FitzGerald, and S. Tong. 2011. "Projecting Future Heat-Related Mortality under Climate Change Scenarios: A Systematic Review." *Environmental Health Perspectives* 119 (12):1681–90. doi:10.1289/ehp.1103456.

Hundessa, S., G. Williams, S. Li, D. L. Liu, W. Cao, H. Ren, J. Guo et al. 2018. "Projecting Potential Spatial and Temporal Changes in the Distribution of Plasmodium Vivax and Plasmodium Falciparum Malaria in China with Climate Change." *Science of the Total Environment* 627:1285–93.

Huynen, M. M. T. E., and P. Martens. 2015. "Climate Change Effects on Heat- and Cold-Related Mortality in the Netherlands: A Scenario-Based Integrated Environmental Health Impact Assessment." *International Journal of Environmental Research and Public Health* 12:13295–320.

Kinney, P. L. 2012. "Health: A New Measure of Health Effects." *Nature Climate Change* 2:233–34.

Kolstad, E. W., and K. A. Johansson. 2011. "Uncertainties Associated with Quantifying Climate Change Impacts on Human Health: A Case Study for Diarrhea." *Environmental Health Perspectives* 119:299–305.

Kuras, E. R., M. B. Richardson, M. M. Calkins, K. L. Ebi, J. J. Hess, K. W. Kintziger, M. A. Jagger et al. 2017. "Opportunities and Challenges for Personal Heat Exposure Research." *Environmental Health Perspectives* 125:085001.

Lee, J. Y., E. Kim, W.-S. Lee, Y. Chae, and H. Kim. 2018. "Projection of Future Mortality Due to Temperature and Population Changes under Representative Concentration Pathways and Shared Socioeconomic Pathways." *International Journal of Environmental Research and Public Health* 15. doi:10.3390/ijerph15040822.

Li, S., L. Gilbert, S. O. Vanwambeke, J. Yu, B. V. Purse, and P. A. Harrison. 2019. "Lyme Disease Risks in Europe under Multiple Uncertain Drivers of Change." *Environmental Health Perspectives* 127:67010.

Li, T., R. M. Horton, D. A. Bader, M. Zhou, X. Liang, J. Ban, Q. Sun, and P. L. Kinney. 2016. "Aging Will Amplify the Heat-Related Mortality Risk under a Changing Climate: Projection for the Elderly in Beijing, China." *Scientific Reports* 6:28161.

Li, Y., T. Ren, P. L. Kinney, A. Joyner, and W. Zhang. 2018. "Projecting Future Climate Change Impacts on Heat-Related Mortality in Large Urban Areas in China." *Environmental Research* 163: 171–85.

Lippi, C. A., A. M. Stewart-Ibarra, M. E. F. B. Loor, J. E. D. Zambrano, N. A. E. Lopez, J. K. Blackburn, and S. J. Ryan. 2019. "Geographic Shifts in *Aedes aegypti* Habitat Suitability in Ecuador Using Larval Surveillance Data and Ecological Niche Modeling: Implications of Climate Change for Public Health Vector Control." *PLoS Neglected Tropical Diseases* 13:e0007322.

Liu, B., P. Martre, F. Ewert, J. R. Porter, A. J. Challinor, C. Müller, A. C. Ruane et al. 2018. "Global Wheat Production with 1.5 and 2.0°C above Pre-Industrial Warming." *Global Change Biology* doi:10.1111/gcb.14542.

Liu-Helmersson, J., Å. Brännström, M. O. Sewe, J. C. Semenza, and J. Rocklöv. 2019. "Estimating Past, Present, and Future Trends in the Global Distribution and Abundance of the Arbovirus Vector *Aedes aegypti* Under Climate Change Scenarios." *Frontiers in Public Health* 7:148.

Liu-Helmersson, J., J. Rocklöv, M. Sewe, and Å. Brännström. 2019. "Climate Change May Enable *Aedes aegypti* Infestation in Major European Cities by 2100." *Environmental Research* 172:693–99.

Lock, K. 2000. "Health Impact Assessment." *BMJ* 320:1395–98.

Longfield, K., B. Smith, R. Gray, L. Ngamkitpaiboon, and N. Vielot. 2013. "Putting Health Metrics into Practice: Using the Disability-Adjusted Life Year for Strategic Decision Making." *BMC Public Health* 13 (suppl 2):S2.

Longstreth, J. 1991. "Anticipated Public Health Consequences of Global Climate Change." *Environmental Health Perspectives* 96:139–44.

Luke, D. A., and K. A. Stamatakis. 2012. "Systems Science Methods in Public Health: Dynamics, Networks, and Agents." *Annual Review of Public Health* 33:357–76.

Marmot, M., and R. Wilkinson. 1998. *Social Determinants of Health*. New York: Oxford University Press.

Martinez, G. S., J. Diaz, H. Hooyberghs, D. Lauwaet, K. De Ridder, C. Linares C, et al. 2018. "Heat and Health in Antwerp under Climate Change: Projected Impacts and Implications for Prevention." *Environment International* 111:135–43.

Matthews, J. B. R. 2018. "Annex I: Glossary." In *Global Warming of 1.5°C. An IPCC Special Report on the Impacts of Global Warming of 1.5°C above Pre-Industrial Levels and Related Global Greenhouse Gas Emission Pathways, in the Context of Strengthening the Global Response to the Threat of Climate Change, Sustainable Development, and Efforts to Eradicate Poverty*, edited by V. Masson-Delmotte, P. Zhai, H.-O. Pörtner, D. Roberts, J. Skea, P. R. Shukla, A. Pirani, W. Moufouma-Okia et al. Geneva: Intergovernmental Panel on Climate Change.

McMichael, A. J. 2001. "Global Environmental Change as 'Risk Factor': Can Epidemiology Cope?" *American Journal of Public Health* 91:1172–74.

McMichael, A., D. Campbell-Lendrum, S. Kovats, S. Edwards, P. Wilkinson, T. Wilson, R. Nicholls, et al. 2004. "Global Climate Change." In *Comparative Quantification of Health Risks*, edited by M. Ezzati, A. Lopez, A. Rodgers, and C. Murray. Geneva: World Health Organization.

McPherson, M., A. García-García, F. J. Cuesta-Valero, H. Beltrami, P. Hansen-Ketchum, D. MacDougall, and N. H. Ogden. 2017. "Expansion of the Lyme Disease Vector Ixodes Scapularis in Canada Inferred from CMIP5 Climate Projections." *Environmental Health Perspectives* 125:057008.

Mechler, R., and L. M. Bouwer. 2015. "Understanding Trends and Projections of Disaster Losses and Climate Change: Is Vulnerability the Missing Link?" *Climatic Change.* 133:23–35.

Mellor, J. E., K. Levy, J. Zimmerman, M. Elliott, J. Bartram, E. Carlton, T. Clasen et al. 2016. "Planning for Climate Change: The Need for Mechanistic Systems-Based Approaches to Study Climate Change Impacts on Diarrheal Diseases." *Science of the Total Environment* 548–549:82–90.

Miller, K. A., D. S. Siscovick, L. Sheppard, K. Shepherd, J. H. Sullivan, G. L. Anderson, and J. D. Kaufman. 2007. "Long-Term Exposure to Air Pollution and Incidence of Cardiovascular Events in Women." *New England Journal of Medicine* 356:447–58.

Monaghan, A. J., S. M. Moore, K. M. Sampson, C. B. Beard, and R. J. Eisen. 2015. "Climate Change Influences on the Annual Onset of Lyme Disease in the United States." *Ticks and Tick-borne Diseases* 6:615–22.

Murray, V., G. McBean, M. Bhatt, S. Borsch, T. S. Cheong, W. F. Erian, S. Lhosa et al. 2012. "Case Studies." In *Managing the Risks of Extreme Events and Disasters to Advance Climate Change Adaptation. A Special Report of Working Groups I and II of the Intergovernmental Panel on Climate Change (IPCC)*, edited by C. B. Field, V. Barros, T. F. Stocker, D. Qin, D. J. Dokken, K .L. Ebi, M. D. Mastrandrea et al., 487–542. Cambridge, UK, and New York: Cambridge University Press. doi:10.1017/cbo9781139177245.012.

Nakicenovic, N., J. Alcamo, A. Grubler, K. Riahi, R. A. Roehrl, H.-H. Rogner et al. 2000. *Special Report on Emissions Scenarios (SRES), A Special Report of Working Group III of the Intergovernmental Panel on Climate Change.* Cambridge: Cambridge University Press.

National Research Council, Division on Earth and Life Studies, Ocean Studies Board, Water Science and Technology Board, Committee to Assess the U.S. Army Corps of Engineers Methods of Analysis and Peer Review for Water Resources Project Planning, Panel on Adaptive Management for Resource Stewardship. 2004. *Adaptive Management for Water Resources Project Planning.* Washington, DC: National Academies Press.

Neumann, J. E., S. C. Anenberg, K. R. Weinberger, M. Amend, S. Gulati, A. Crimmins, H. Roman, N. Fann, and P. L. Kinney. 2019. "Estimates of Present and Future Asthma Emergency Department Visits Associated with Exposure to Oak, Birch, and Grass Pollen in the United States." *Geohealth* 3:11–27.

Nissan, H., and D. Conway. 2018. "From Advocacy to Action: Projecting the Health Impacts of Climate Change." *PLoS Medicine* 15:e1002624.

Ogden, N. H., M. Radojevic, X. Wu, V. R. Duvvuri, P. A. Leighton, and J. Wu. 2014. "Estimated Effects of Projected Climate Change on the Basic Reproductive Number of the Lyme Disease Vector Ixodes Scapularis." *Environmental Health Perspectives* 122:631–38.

O'Neill, B. C., E. Kriegler, K. Riahi, K. L. Ebi, S. Hallegatte, T. R. Carter, R. Mathur, and D. P. van Vuuren. 2014. "A New Scenario Framework for Climate Change Research: The Concept of Shared Socioeconomic Pathways." *Climatic Change* 122:387–400.

Onozuka, D., A. Gasparrini, F. Sera, M. Hashizume, Y. Honda. 2019. "Future Projections of Temperature-Related Excess Out-of-Hospital Cardiac Arrest under Climate Change Scenarios in Japan." *Science of the Total Environment* 682:333–39.

Petkova, E. P., H. Morita, and P. L. Kinney. 2014. "Health Impacts of Heat in a Changing Climate: How Can Emerging Science Inform Urban Adaptation Planning?" *Current Epidemiology Reports* 1:67–74.

Petkova, E. P., J. K. Vink, R. M. Horton, A. Gasparrini, D. A. Bader, J. D. Francis, and P. L. Kinney. 2017. "Towards More Comprehensive Projections of Urban Heat-Related Mortality: Estimates for New York City under Multiple Population, Adaptation, and Climate Scenarios." *Environmental Health Perspectives* 125:47–55.

Portier, C. J., K. Thigpen-Tart, S. R. Carter, C. H. Dilworth, A. E. Grambsch, J. Gohlke, J. Hess, et al. 2010. *A Human Health Perspective on Climate Change.* Research Triangle Park, NC: Environmental Health Perspectives, National Institute of Environmental Health Sciences.

Ryan, S. J., C. J. Carlson, E. A. Mordecai, and L. R. Johnson. 2019. "Global Expansion and Redistribution of Aedes-Borne Virus Transmission Risk with Climate Change." *PLoS Neglected Tropical Diseases* 13:e0007213.

Sarkar, S., V. Gangare, P. Singh, and R. C. Dhiman. 2019. "Shift in Potential Malaria Transmission Areas in India, Using the Fuzzy-Based Climate Suitability Malaria Transmission (FCSMT) Model under Changing Climatic Conditions." *International Journal of Environmental Research and Public Health* 16. doi:10.3390/ijerph16183474.

Smith, M. R., and S. S. Myers. 2018. "Impact of Anthropogenic CO2 Emissions on Global Human Nutrition." *Nature Climate Change* 8:834–39.

Stevens, L. K., K. N. Kolivras, Y. Hong, V. A. Thomas, J. B. Campbell, and S. P. Prisley. 2019. "Future Lyme Disease Risk in the South-Eastern United States Based on Projected Land Cover." *Geospatial Health* 14. doi:10.4081/gh.2019.751.

Sun, Q. H., R. M. Horton, D. A. Bader, B. Jones, L. Zhou, and T. T. Li. 2019. "Projections of Temperature-Related Non-accidental Mortality in Nanjing, China." *Biomedical and Environmental Sciences* 32:134–39.

Taleb, N. N. 2012. *Antifragile: Things That Gain from Disorder.* New York: Random House.

Tol, R. S. J., K. L. Ebi, and G. W. Yohe. 2007. "Infectious Disease, Development, and Climate Change: A Scenario Analysis." *Environment and Development Economics* 12:687–706.

van Vuuren, D. P., J. Edmonds, M. Kainuma, K. Riahi, A. Thomson, K. Hibbard, G. C. Hurtt et al. 2011. "The Representative Concentration Pathways: An Overview." *Climatic Change* 109:5.

Vicedo-Cabrera, A. M., F. Sera, and A. Gasparrini. 2019. "Hands-on Tutorial on a Modeling Framework for Projections of Climate Change Impacts on Health." *Epidemiology* 30:321–29.

Wang, Q., J. Wang, J. Zhou, J. Ban, and T. Li. 2019. "Estimation of PM2·5-Associated Disease Burden in China in 2020 and 2030 Using Population and Air Quality Scenarios: A Modelling Study." *Lancet Planetary Health* 3:e71–e80.

Wang, Y., F. Nordio, J. Nairn, A. Zanobetti, and J. D. Schwartz. 2018. "Accounting for Adaptation and Intensity in Projecting Heat Wave-Related Mortality." *Environmental Research* 161:464–71.

Watts, N., M. Amann, N. Arnell, S. Ayeb-Karlsson, K. Belesova, H. Berry, T. Bouley et al. 2018. "The 2018 Report of the Lancet Countdown on Health and Climate Change: Shaping the Health of Nations for Centuries to Come." *Lancet* 392:2479–2514.

Wayne, G. P. 2013. "The Beginner's Guide to Representative Concentration Pathways." *Skeptical Science*. https://www.skepticalscience.com/rcp.php.

World Health Organization. 1999. Health Impact Assessment as a Tool for Intersectoral Health Policy. Bonn, Germany: WHO European Centre for Environment and Health/European Centre for Health Policy.

World Health Organization. n.d. "Metrics: Disability-Adjusted Life Year (DALY)." https://www.who.int/healthinfo/global_burden_disease/metrics_daly/en/.

Wu, J., Y. Zhou, Y. Gao, J. S. Fu, B. A. Johnson, C. Huang, Y.-M. Kim, and Y. Liu. 2014. "Estimation and Uncertainty Analysis of Impacts of Future Heat Waves on Mortality in the Eastern United States." *Environmental Health Perspectives* 122:10–16.

Xun, W. W., A. E. Khan, E. Michael, and P. Vineis. 2010. "Climate Change Epidemiology: Methodological Challenges." *International Journal of Public Health* 55:85–96.

Ye, X., R. Wolff, W. Yu, P. Vaneckova, X. Pan, and S. Tong. 2012. "Ambient Temperature and Morbidity: A Review of Epidemiological Evidence." *Environmental Health Perspectives* 120:19–28.

Zhang, B., G. Li, Y. Ma, and X. Pan. 2018. "Projection of Temperature-Related Mortality due to Cardiovascular Disease in Beijing under Different Climate Change, Population, and Adaptation Scenarios." *Environmental Research* 162:152–59.

Zhang, Y., P. Bi, and J. E. Hiller. 2007. "Climate Change and Disability–Adjusted Life Years." *Journal of Environmental Health* 70:32–38.

CHAPTER 16

PROTECTING ENVIRONMENTAL JUSTICE COMMUNITIES FROM THE DETRIMENTAL IMPACTS OF CLIMATE CHANGE

Cecilia Martinez and Nicky Sheats

Introduction

The problems posed by environmental risks to the health and livelihoods of communities across the globe are daunting. Even as we develop more sophisticated scientific methods for understanding their scope and magnitude, our efforts are seemingly unable to keep pace with the increasing range and complexity of emerging environmental hazards. The era of climate change has caused researchers, civil society organizations, and governments across the globe to focus on research and strategies that will reduce the harmful societal impacts caused by this global threat.

In the United States, the important question of how climate change impacts are distributed across communities in the context of historical environmental inequalities should also be of concern in climate assessment and planning. Many communities are already experiencing the effects of climate-related events like sea level changes and extreme weather, which are exacerbating public health risks in many significant ways. Although the impacts experienced by communities in the United States are different from those of the global South, the nation is by no means immune to the problem of inequality within its borders. In some cases, detrimental impacts on these communities have reached crisis conditions. This chapter offers an introduction to the importance of rooting climate and public health research in an examination of inequality in our society. Using an **environmental justice** (EJ) framework, we discuss several important climate change-related impacts that disproportionately affect Indigenous communities, communities Of Color and low-income communities, that is, EJ communities, and demonstrate why incorporating a structural approach to addressing climate and public health is required.

Climate Resiliency and Environmental Justice

Even with our best science, precise predictions about how and to what extent climate change will affect different communities are extremely difficult. We do know that environmental changes are occurring and that their impacts on people and communities do not occur in isolation; they are also determined to a great extent by existing social, political, economic, and environmental conditions (Intergovernmental Panel on Climate Change 2014). Acknowledgment of these uncertainties and complexities in the science of climate change has resulted in the development of a policy and planning framework built on the concept of **climate resiliency**, which intends to enhance the capacity of communities to prepare for and protect against impacts associated with climate-related events. Moreover, absent full and complete predictive knowledge about the scope and magnitude of these occurrences and their impacts, climate resiliency also focuses on increasing

KEY CONCEPTS

- Indigenous communities, communities Of Color, and low-income communities may be more vulnerable to the detrimental impacts of climate change at least in part because of structural inequalities in our society rooted in race and income.

- Climate change policy should explicitly address environmental justice and equity because if it does not it may perpetuate or exacerbate those inequalities that currently exist in our society which are based on race and income.

- Policy must be developed that addresses the problem of cumulative impacts in general and in the context of the need for climate change resiliency and mitigation.

community capacity for effective and timely recovery (O'Brien et al. 2004; Smit and Wandel 2006). In this chapter, we use the term resiliency interchangeably with the word adaptation. Climate resiliency is interdisciplinary in nature, and draws significantly from the fields of planning, public health and disaster management. In disaster management, **vulnerability** is defined as the "diminished capacity to anticipate, cope with, resist and recover from the impact of hazards" (International Federation of Red Cross and Red Crescent Societies n.d.).

Two general questions frame an analysis of vulnerability: What is the scope and intensity of the threat? What are the factors that create the condition of vulnerability? These two questions are also critically important in the EJ field. An important methodological problem is that vulnerability can be conceptualized in different and sometimes competing ways. As O'Brien et al. (2004) suggest, there are two general frameworks of vulnerability in climate change research, each with significantly different methodological approaches to resiliency research and planning. The first is defined as an **end point approach**, whereby vulnerability is essentially viewed as the impacts that result from the added effects of climate changes. This approach uses projections from climate modeling and from these projections estimates impacts on individuals with existing health predispositions. Community vulnerabilities are understood as the aggregate of individual vulnerabilities. In this approach, existing health conditions are the baseline for assessment, and climate-related impacts are measured as the additional risks to the baseline presented by climate events. Although this approach has some analytical merit, it does not easily integrate issues of existing inequality, and therefore from an EJ perspective can be viewed as useful but also contains a significant risk of being incomplete.

A second vulnerability framework that more easily incorporates EJ concerns is identified by O'Brien et al. (2004) as the **starting point approach**. Environmental, structural, and social processes of marginalization and inequalities that contribute to existing unequal distributions of risk are included in this approach, which also takes the underlying causes and contexts of climate vulnerability into account to avoid underestimating the magnitude (large), scope (social and environmental) and urgency (high) of climate change. The starting point approach corresponds to an EJ framework for understanding climate change. Climate impacts should not be divorced from the legacy of pollution and environmental harms already experienced by communities. To exclude or discount these harms in climate resiliency planning and research at a minimum presents incomplete analysis of vulnerability and, more significantly, may reinforce and exacerbate patterns of inequality. Understanding the social geography of vulnerability in climate and public health is as essential as understanding pathways of exposure. As Cutter (2006) notes, "The underlying dimensions of a place, including its social institutions, construct and define risks . . . Hazards and risks, then, are more than just the probability of occurrence of an extreme event. They include the underlying factors that contribute to risks in the first place."

From an EJ perspective, the fundamental problem of vulnerability is that communities live with existing physical and social challenges, which are compounded by climate change events. The challenges of building equitable climate-resilient communities emanate from the fact that vulnerability is determined by both individual-based and structural-based risk factors. As the research and practice of resilient communities continues to advance, EJ is critical to a full examination of the challenges and opportunities for an equitable, climate-resilient future. Fortunately, a significant body of research on environmental inequality and its causes has been developed over the past thirty years, including studies examining how and to what extent race, poverty, and institutional structures and practices are determinant factors in creating such conditions.

In the next sections, we provide examples of how EJ research can be integrated into climate change and public health analyses, planning, and project implementation, to illustrate how enhancing climate resiliency can also help address EJ concerns and inequality.

Cumulative Impacts, Environmental Justice, and Climate Change

A disproportionate number of polluting facilities are often located in EJ communities, and the issue of **cumulative impacts** focuses on how to address the effects of multiple pollutants from multiple sources (Morello-Frosch et al. 2011; California Environmental Protection Agency [EPA] 2010; Bullard et al. 2007; Mohai and Saha 2007). The current system of environmental protection does not effectively regulate the dangerous mixture of multiple toxins that often occurs in EJ neighborhoods, partly because it attempts to control pollution by establishing individual standards for each pollutant that do not account for their cumulative concentrations or effects (California EPA 2010; National Environmental Justice Advisory Council 2004; Environmental Protection Agency 2003). Another important aspect of cumulative impacts is social vulnerabilities that all too frequently exist in communities Of Color and low-income communities, including a lack of access to fresh food, a lack of planned open space, poor public infrastructure, health disparities, racial discrimination, poverty, and crime (Morello-Frosch et al. 2011). When these social vulnerabilities are combined with pollution from multiple facilities, conditions conducive to the production of harmful health impacts are created. Keeping all of the aforementioned factors in mind, a good working definition for cumulative impacts is the health risks and impacts caused by multiple pollutants, usually emitted by multiple sources of pollution in a community, and their interactions with each other and any social vulnerabilities that exist in the community (California EPA 2010; National Environmental Justice Council 2004; Environmental Protection Agency 2003).

Health disparities can both contribute to and be a result of cumulative impacts. Multiple polluting facilities that overburden communities with pollution may contribute to health disparities that consistently plague Indigenous communities, communities Of Color, and low-income communities in the United States (National Center for Health Statistics 2013; Morello- Frosch et al. 2011; Adler and Rehkopf 2008; Waldron 2007; Dressler, Oths, and Gravlee 2005; Spalter-Roth, Rowenthal, and Rubio 2005; Mensah et al. 2005). EJ research has investigated these disproportionate or unequal exposures to pollution, which can include a range of hazards from poor air quality to brownfields and toxic waste sites to unequal regulatory enforcement (Cutter 2006; Agyeman, Bullard, and Evans 2003; Mohai, Pellow, and Timmons 2009; Pearsall and Pearce 2010; Bullard and Wright 2009; Tsosie 2007). The EJ research and advocacy community has had a long-standing call to address the methodological shortcomings (Brulle and Pellow 2005; Corburn 2002) in both our legal system and in conventional research.

A high level of cumulative impacts can make EJ communities especially vulnerable to detrimental impacts from climate change. For example, communities with a significant number of polluting facilities can be at higher risk of toxic contamination left behind by receding storm surge waters. This risk may be more widespread in EJ communities where the risk of flooding can be intensified due to poor infrastructure. If cumulative impacts in a community include health disparities and a relative lack of access to high-quality health care (Little-Blanton and Hoffman 2005; Spalter-Roth et al. 2005; Williams and Rucker 2000), then community residents may also become especially vulnerable to climate change–related heat stress, increases in air pollution and elevations in the risk of vector borne disease.

Communities need community-level adaptation plans to protect them from climate change and if they have a high level of cumulative impacts, and no existing adequate cumulative impacts policy, then the adaptation plans should also address cumulative impacts. More specifically, that part of the adaptation plan that concerns construction when recovering from extreme weather events should include the following elements: (1) determine if the structure being rebuilt will emit significant amounts of pollution; (2) determine if the structure is being rebuilt in an EJ community with a high level of existing cumulative impacts; and (3) do not rebuild a polluting structure in an EJ community already suffering from high levels of cumulative impacts until existing pollution is reduced, or at least a strategy is in place to do so.

An effective and coherent cumulative impacts policy will make communities healthier in general and also protect against climate change. If this type of policy does not exist then the community level adaptation plan should also address cumulative impacts.

CLINICAL CORRELATES 16.1 CLIMATE CHANGE AND INCARCERATED POPULATIONS

There are 2.3 million individuals incarcerated in the United States (698 per 100,000 residents) primarily in federal prisons and jails, state prisons, local jails, immigration detention centers, territorial prisons, and youth confinement (Sawyer and Wagner 2020). Chronic diseases including mental health conditions, aging prisoners, and medications increase risk for heat-related illness for inmates and correctional facilities employees in an era of global warming. Lack of air conditioning and old correctional facilities contribute further to vulnerability in this population. At least thirteen states in southern latitudes lack universal policies for air conditioning (Jones 2019). Climate-driven extreme weather events (wildfires, hurricanes, floods) threaten infrastructure directly and indirectly via power outages (Mrkusic and Gross 2018). These events can influence acute on chronic disease exacerbations or cause primary heat illness/heatstroke.

Key recommendations to address heat stress in American prisons and jails (Professor Daniel Holt, MA, JD, Sabin Center for Climate Change Law; Holt 2015) include:

- Reduce the size of the incarcerated population
- Reduce inmates' and correctional officers' susceptibility to heat stress
- Phase out the most vulnerable facilities
- Retrofit adaptable facilities by maximizing passive cooling
- Build sustainable, adapted, and resilient facilities
- Require adequate cooling of private facilities
- Collaborate and cooperate

Correctional facilities ought to adapt and build resilience against extreme heat and climate disasters that threaten the health of millions of susceptible inmates and correctional officers.

Air Quality, Environmental Justice, and Climate Change

An extensive body of research exists on the human health effects of air pollution. Major air pollutants of concern include ozone, particulate matter, sulfur dioxide, nitrogen oxides, and volatile organic compounds (Tagaris et al. 2010; Ebi and McGregor 2008), with particulate matter and ozone of priority concern (Caiazzo et al. 2013; Tagaris et al. 2010). Studies estimate that air pollution-related deaths will increase in approximately two thirds of U.S. states by 2050 due to changes in climate (Tagaris et al. 2009, 2010). Increased carbon dioxide levels can result in longer pollen production seasons for ragweed and other aeroallergenic plants, which could cause an increase in allergic reactions and asthma episodes (Luber et al. 2014). Ozone can exacerbate allergic conditions, and both ozone and particulate matter have been connected to reduced lung function and asthma (Tagaris et al. 2009, 2010; Ebi and McGregor 2008; Knowlton et al. 2004; Kinney 1999; Brunekreef et al. 1997; Schwartz et al. 1993; Pope 1989). Although these conditions are a concern to a wide range of populations, asthma is also an EJ issue because it disproportionately affects children Of Color (Akinbami et al. 2014Zahran et al. 2018).

From an EJ framework, the ultimate question is what impact climate change has on the distributional burden of air pollution-related illness and mortality among different communities across the nation (Ebi and McGregor 2008). Several investigations have found that EJ communities are already disproportionately exposed to airborne pollutants (California EPA 2010; Ash et al. 2009; Pastor et al. 2005; Pastor, Sadd, and Morello-Frosch 2004; Houston, Ong, and Winer 2004; Jarrett et al. 2001; Wernette and Nieves 1992). Given these existing disproportionate exposures, the prospect of increased levels of air pollution due to climate change is particularly troubling for EJ communities. This is one reason that some EJ advocates and researchers maintain that climate change policy should address greenhouse gas co-pollutants such as particulate matter, as well as particulate matter and ozone precursors, that are simultaneously emitted with greenhouse gases (Sheats 2017; Boyce and Pastor 2012; Environmental Justice and Science Initiative 2010; Kaswan 2008; Sheats et al. 2008). By doing so climate change mitigation policy could help reduce disproportionate pollution burdens in EJ communities. If climate change policy does not address preexisting pollution inequalities, it runs the risk of perpetuating or exacerbating them.

CLINICAL CORRELATES 16.2 ASTHMA DISPARITIES IN ENVIRONMENTAL HEALTH

The Centers for Disease Control and Prevention report that asthma prevalence in the United States is 7.7 percent, with the percent increasing to 10.8% percent for those below the poverty threshold (CDC 2020). The death rate per million is 9.5 for non-Hispanic Whites compared with 21.8 for non-Hispanic Blacks and 11.3 for non-Hispanic American Indian and Alaskan Natives. Children aged less than eighteen years had 546,013 emergency department visits, 80,235 hospitalizations and 2,446,609 physician office visits for asthma in 2016. Deteriorating air quality due to climate change is a concerning threat to children in environmental justice communities. Air pollution, pollen, and mold are just three common contributors. Clinicians, regulators, public health officials, and housing authorities must come together to address this large and vulnerable population.

Deteriorating air quality threatens to increase rates of respiratory illness, especially in children and among those in environmental justice communities.

Heat Waves, Environmental Justice, and Climate Change

The impacts of climate change on weather patterns, especially the incidence of extreme heat days and heat waves, have been extensively studied (National Aeronautics and Space Administration 2010). People with preexisting cardiovascular, respiratory and cerebrovascular disease are especially vulnerable to heat-related stress, exacerbations of a variety of illnesses and even premature death (Basu 2009). The incidence of these illnesses is not uniform; however, a number of studies have found that race and socioeconomic status are important variables in contributing to the vulnerability to heat stress for a variety of underlying reasons (Cooney 2011; Uejio et al. 2011; Balbus and Molina 2009; Basu 2009; Harlan et al. 2006; O'Neill, Zanobetti, and Schwartz 2003; Curriero et al. 2002; Klinenberg 2003; Whitman et al., 1997; Greenberg et al. 1983).

Urban physical infrastructures can amplify the health impacts of extreme heat known as the **urban heat island (UHI) effect**. The UHI effect occurs as urban built environment materials absorb and re-radiate heat, resulting in elevated surface and air temperatures. Surfaces (roofs, roads, and sidewalks) can be up to 18–27°F warmer than surrounding areas during the daytime, and 9–18°F higher at nighttime (Environmental Protection Agency 2008). Urban air temperatures can range from 2 to 10°F higher than in neighboring rural and suburban areas (Berdahl and Bretz 1997). Nighttime temperature increases have been linked to increased deaths, particularly among the elderly and the socially isolated (Environmental Protection Agency 2008). The UHI effect can also be responsible for an estimated 5 to 10 percent of peak electricity demand (Hewitt, Mackres, and Shickman 2014; Akbari 2005). Increased electrical demand for cooling increases the need for additional generating capacity from peak-load generating units, which are generally among the least efficient power plants, further increasing air pollutant and greenhouse gas emissions.

Although research on the racial determinants of heat-related morbidity and mortality is relatively small, there are indications that Blacks (Uejio et al. 2011; Basu 2009; O'Neill et al. 2003; Curriero et al. 2002; Klinenberg 2003; Whitman et al. 1997; Greenberg et al. 1983), people of low and moderate income (Balbus and Molina 2009; Basu 2009; Harlan et al. 2006; O'Neill et al. 2003; Curriero et al. 2002; Klinenberg 2003), as well as Latinos (Uejio et al. 2011; Harlan et al. 2006) are particularly vulnerable to heat stress. Research has found income disparities to be an important variable of heat stress vulnerability due to higher exposure rates (Harlan et al. 2006), limited material resources (Balbus and Molina 2009; Harlan et al. 2006; Klinenberg 2003; Greenberg et al. 1983), and limited social capital for coping (Harlan et al. 2006; Klinenberg 2003). For example, in New York City, a strong correlation between income and the use of air conditioning, an obvious mechanism to combat high temperatures, was found to have implications for low-income communities (New York City Department of Health and Mental Hygiene 2007). Inadequate access to air conditioning may also be a factor in the disproportionate risk of mortality due to heat stress faced by Blacks (O'Neill, Zanobetti, and Schwartz 2005).

Another contributing factor to heat stress is the problem of social isolation and inadequate neighborhood infrastructures (O'Neill, Zanobetti, and Schwartz 2003; Klinenberg 2003). Disparities in physical and social capital investment and the creation of historically poor neighborhoods should be taken into account in estimating differences in vulnerability (Williams and Collins 2001; Committee on Public Health Strategies to Improve Health 2011). The effects of past racial segregation practices also mean that people Of Color are more likely than Whites to live in poor-quality housing, which pose a greater risk of exposure to conditions that can contribute to heat and other health risks such as indoor allergens (Committee on Public Health Strategies to Improve Health 2011). This inequality is evident in that approximately 40 to 45 percent of Black, Latino, and native individuals live in poor neighborhoods (Braverman, Egerter, and Mockenhaupt 2011; National Environmental Justice Advisory Council 2004).

Physical, economic, and social infrastructures are important variables in climate resiliency because they can and do affect the capacity for sustaining strong social networks. Klinenberg (2003) examined an African-American Chicago neighborhood that had a high mortality rate during the city's lethal 1995 heat wave and concluded that poor infrastructure helped to create conditions that foster social isolation among its residents. The legacy of historic discriminatory practices such as redlining, the unequal impacts of public infrastructure investments such as the engineering of highway systems through neighborhoods Of Color, and the disparities in the siting of Not In My Back Yard (NIMBY) industries have created a pattern of unequal neighborhood capacities. Where people live, and the condition of their neighborhoods is not only a consequence of the private real estate market but a product of unequal public housing subsidies and urban development programs as well. The infrastructure of today's cities was built with massive public and private investments and guided by planning models and public decisions that reproduced and reinforced segregation and inequality. Public health must now contend with the environmental and EJ impacts of this historical inequality (Braverman et al. 2011).

The higher heat mortality risk experienced by Blacks may in part be due to living in dispro-portionate numbers in older and substandard housing (Jacobs 2011) that may increase heat exposure and constrain heat mitigation efforts (Uejio et al. 2011). Racial discrimination could play a role in confining relatively more Blacks to this substandard housing. Several studies also produced evidence that Latinos living in Phoenix may be more vulnerable to or experience more heat stress. One investigation found more heat distress calls were made from neighbor-hoods with higher proportions of Latinos (and Blacks, the linguistically isolated, and renters) (Uejio et al. 2011) and another determined that low-income Latino neighborhoods experi-enced elevated levels of heat stress exposure (Harlan et al. 2006). We have suggested that heat stress vulnerability among these EJ communities is linked to societal problems such as the negative impacts of urban redevelopment, socioeconomic inequality, discrimination, and the urban heat island effect. To address community heat stress vulnerability in the context of these challenging issues, EJ advocates, urban planners, and health professionals will surely have to work closely together.

Extreme Weather Events and Environmental Justice

There are many EJ aspects connected to highly destructive extreme weather events. Racial and income disparities contribute to unequal impacts across communities when these events occur. These include disparities in community capacities for effective and safe evacuation; and recovery efforts (Fair Share Housing Center et al. 2014; Enterprise Community Partners 2013; Furman Center Moelis Institute 2013; Cutter et al. 2010; Bullard and Wright 2009; National Fair Housing Alliance 2006; Pastor et al. 2006). This discussion is drawn from the research and the experience the effects of Hurricane Katrina, Superstorm Sandy, and Hurricane Maria had on EJ communities.

Evacuation

A critical issue that has emerged is the unequal conditions and resources in emergency prepar-edness for EJ communities. Residents left stranded during Katrina were disproportionately Of Color and low income (Pastor et al. 2006), and various factors have been offered to explain this phenomenon. First, Blacks in New Orleans tend to be more reliant on public transit than Whites and thus access to transportation in emergency situations may be more limited, which leads to greater difficulty for evacuation (Pastor et al. 2006). Second, government warning sys-tems may not be as effective for people Of Color for several reasons: Pastor et al. have sug-gested that Blacks and Latinos may rely more on the use of meetings or social networks to obtain information than other populations, and the same may be true for immigrant popula-tions, rural populations, and Indigenous communities; and a higher level of distrust of govern-ment may exist among some segments of EJ communities (Pastor et al. 2006). In addition, low-income residents may face a lack of resources that leaves them both without the means to evacuate, and limited options for shelter (Pastor et al. 2006).

Impacts

For both Katrina and Sandy there is evidence that EJ communities suffered more physical and psychological harms post-storm than other communities (Enterprise Community Partners 2013; Logan 2006; Pastor et al. 2006). Several explanations have been offered: resource inequality and racial discrimination means that EJ communities are more likely to be located in flood-prone areas (Bullard and Wright 2009; Logan 2006; Pastor et al. 2006); and a higher percentage of residents of these communities may also live in substandard housing (Jacobs 2011) and are therefore vulnerable to greater damage (Uejio et al. 2011). Research has shown that posttraumatic stress disorder (PTSD) was a consequence of Hurricane Katrina possibly due to factors that included elevated stress due to forced relocation, difficulty in obtaining housing and employment, lack of access to basic necessities, and the impacts of community disruption and the dissolution of support networks (McLaughlin et al. 2011).

Recovery

Low-income and Of Color residents may have more difficulty recovering from extreme storms for a number of reasons, including limited income, intensification of existing poverty, limited savings, limited insurance, excessive pollution, health disparities, and racial discrimination (Bullard and Wright 2009; Pastor et al. 2006). At least one report found that recovery from Katrina was slower for Blacks relative to Whites even at similar income levels (Bullard and Wright 2009). One reason this could be true is the persistent problem of racial discrimination in housing, which can make it even more difficult for people Of Color to find housing in a market that has been reduced by the destructive force of an extreme weather event (Bullard and Wright 2009; National Fair Housing Alliance 2006). This also may be a reason that a smaller percentage of displaced Blacks were able to return to their community compared to displaced Whites (Bullard and Wright 2009). Difficulty obtaining loans and satisfactory insurance due at least in part to discrimination can also limit access to resources for residents Of Color to rebuild homes and businesses destroyed by an extreme weather event (Bullard and Wright 2009; Pastor et al. 2006).

There is some evidence from both Katrina and Sandy that low-income residents and residents Of Color have found it more difficult than White residents to access post-storm governmental services (Fair Share Housing et al. 2014; Bullard and Wright 2009). Federal Emergency Management Association services tend to focus on homeowners rather than renters and a higher percentage of renters tend to be low-income and Of Color (Samara 2014; Furman Center Moelis Institute 2013). After Katrina, a significant amount of public housing was destroyed or closed and not quickly rebuilt or reopened (Bullard and Wright; Logan 2006; National Fair Housing Alliance 2006), thus contributing to the difficulty of low-income residents finding post-storm housing. There are concerns that this public housing will never be fully replaced (Bullard and Wright). Businesses Of Color rooted in their own communities may also find it more difficult to recover, because of disproportionately high rates of displacement among their Of Color clientele (Bullard and Wright), as well as access to capital for rebuilding.

Language can present barriers to both the emergency response to (Pastor et al 2006) and recovery from (Fair Share Housing Center et al. 2014) severe storms, especially for the portion of the EJ population who are non-English speakers. This is particularly true if the government does not ensure that recovery information is fully and correctly translated into languages spoken in the community (Fair Share Housing Center et al.; Pastor et al.).

Hurricane Maria in Puerto Rico

The impacts of Maria on Puerto Rico are still being experienced. Puerto Rico, as an island, is highly vulnerable to climate change impacts; it has territorial political status (and is not a state); and its history has a unique sociohistorical context. All these factors have influenced recovery on the island.

Hurricane Maria landed on Puerto Rico in September 2017 and inflicted significant impacts on the island. For example, one study estimates the excess death toll at 2,975 six months after the storm (Santos-Burgoa et al. 2018). Three million residents were left in the dark for an extended period by the hurricane (Federal Emergency Management Agency 2018).

In addition, approximately 160,000 people left the island in the year after Maria (Centro 2018). One investigation stated, "This recent exodus represents one of the most significant historical movements of Puerto Ricans to the U.S. mainland in terms of both volume and duration" (Centro 2018).

The EJ context for Maria is different than that for Katrina and Sandy. As a U.S. territory with its own sociohistorical and racial context, the issue of equity in Puerto Rico is unique. On the mainland, the EJ question is: were Of Color communities treated differently than their White counterparts? In the case of Puerto Rico, a slightly different set of questions might be posed: what was the nature of the federal response? Was the island treated differently than states on the mainland in terms of emergency and recovery assistance? However, one similarity is clear: In both Puerto Rico and the mainland, there is evidence that class continues to have an effect on storm impacts, because Puerto Rico suffered higher mortality risks in economically challenged areas (Santos-Burgoa et al. 2018).

Indigenous Rights and Climate Change

There are approximately 565 federally recognized tribes within the United States, and numerous others whose recognition was either terminated or never acknowledged by the U.S. governmental process. The history of American Indian tribes and Indigenous peoples is unique and underscores how the complexities and intersectionalities of social and economic policies contribute to disproportionate climate change impacts. Indigenous history is also crucial in understanding the historical accumulation of social stressors that are background to human-induced climate change.

The experiential and traditional knowledge of Indigenous peoples has been transmitted orally from generation to generation (Ellen, Parkes, and Bicker 2000). Traditional Indigenous (or Ecological) Knowledge (TEK) is finally being acknowledged as legitimate and important to the bank of climate change information and data as it offers intricate and sophisticated information about environmental changes, including climate change (Doyle, Redsteer, and Eggers 2013; Weinhold 2010b; Cochran and Geller 2002; Ellen et al. 2000). Thus, TEK is being used as an important source of knowledge to understand and to develop strategies for addressing climate change.

Indigenous peoples and communities also pose a unique set of concerns with respect to climate change and public health. Environmental stressors such as climate change and loss of biodiversity are affecting Indigenous communities' ability to lead a subsistence existence, and also impacting cultural practices. In fact, some Indigenous communities have already had to relocate due to the effects of climate change. As climate change affects ecosystems, the extant knowledge base of Indigenous peoples is also threatened. For Indigenous communities, resiliency means using both TEK and mainstream knowledge to cope with the range of issues associated with climate change.

It is important that the present stressors associated with climate change be understood in the context of a history of traumas caused by social and political actions such as forced removal, forced assimilation, and cultural discrimination. The Indigenous experience is one of being the object of forced assimilationist and removal policies. Many tribal communities were relocated to entirely different regions and/or their sovereign rights were severely challenged. Duran and Duran (1995) explain that experiences of these types of societal-induced external stressors on Indigenous communities have resulted in a "soul wound" that continues in the community fabric from one generation to another. This concept of **historical trauma** is used to explain the generational consequences of traumatic experience, defined as a "cumulative trauma over both the lifespan and across generations that results from massive cataclysmic events" (Yellow

Horse 1999). Besides racism, these traumas can include loss of language and connection to the land, environmental deprivation, and spiritual, emotional, and mental disconnectedness. Being isolated from aspects of this historical identity is known to have harmful effects on Indigenous health.

Despite these traumas, tribal communities have continued to retain and revitalize cultural, linguistic, and livelihood practices that include hunting, fishing, and gathering (Lynn et al. 2013). Indigenous communities are rooted in place, and their way of life (food, medicine, ceremonies, and other cultural practices) is dependent on the quality of that environment (Whyte 2013). Environmental changes that affect the quality and character of the environment have significant implications for communities. The effects of climate change are already at a critical stage in many Indigenous communities, threatening to disrupt longstanding cultural practices.

CLINICAL CORRELATES 16.3 AMERICAN INDIAN AND ALASKA NATIVE HEALTH CHALLENGES

American Indians and Alaska Natives (AIANs) comprise 574 federally recognized Indian Nations and constitute roughly one percent of the U.S. population or 2.9 million people. AIANs are long recognized as having health disparities starting in childhood (Sarche and Spicer 2008) and propagating into adulthood with lower life expectancies compared with other racial and ethnic groups (Arias, Xu, and Jim 2014). They have higher rates of chronic diseases including diabetes and hypertension (Adakai et al. 2018; Cobb, Espey, and King 2014). Their cultural and historical backgrounds as well as their reliance on nature make many particularly vulnerable to environmental change and also sentinel observers to a changing climate. They continue to be vocal and active proponents of addressing environmental harms and opportunities (Norton-Smith et al. 2016).

AIANs and public health stakeholders have convened to implement culturally sensitive programs and interventions that address health issues. Efforts such as the Maniilaq Social Medicine Program combine partners in rural, underserved areas and academic settings to make health a right for American Indian and Alaska Natives (Trout, Kramer, and Fischer 2018). The program centers on primary care and structural determinants of health to address barriers to health. The Indian Health Service maintains an environmental sustainability program consisting of progress reports, educational materials, and green champions. Cultural values and a systems thinking approach also propel interdisciplinary environmental health collaboration on topics such as food systems and using plants for medicinal purposes in research (Isaac et al. 2018).

Culturally informed public health interventions, increased surveillance, and increased training for health professionals can help all committed to public health learn from both traditional practices and western science adapt during times of environmental strife.

Next Steps

To address climate change–related EJ issues identified in this chapter we offer the following recommendations for next steps:

1. Community-level climate change adaptation plans should be prepared for as many EJ communities as possible (see Pastor et al. 2006; Sheats 2014) with the understanding that (1) "community-level" is not meant to refer to a municipal government. The geographic scope of adaptation plans should reflect neighborhoods within municipalities, in order to speak to more local identities and dimensions of resilience; and (2) community residents, local community groups, and EJ organizations should play an integral role in creating and implementing community-level adaptation plans. This level of community involvement would require that residents, community groups, and EJ organizations have access to

sufficient resources to be equal partners with government in developing and implementing these plans.

2. Public policy and community-level adaptation or resiliency plans should address cumulative impacts. If rebuilding is necessary after an extreme weather event, a cumulative impacts policy should be in place before new industry is permitted in an already-polluted EJ community.

3. Climate change mitigation policy should address health-harming greenhouse gas co-pollutants, such as particulate matter and its precursors, as well as greenhouse gases. Special attention should be devoted to co-pollutants that affect EJ communities with high levels of **cumulative impacts**.

4. Public policy and community-level adaptation plans for Indigenous communities should address, but not be limited to, **historical trauma** and climate change impacts on subsistence living and cultural practices.

5. Public policy and community-level adaptation or resiliency plans that typically address evacuation, recovery and other issues associated with hazardous events should also address the factors that cause these events to have a disproportionate impact on EJ communities. Factors to address include (1) racial discrimination, particularly those types that may pose the greatest impediments to adaptation efforts such as housing and insurance discrimination—efforts should be made to ensure that these types of discrimination no longer exist or are at least minimized; (2) the gap in procuring government resources after hazardous events that appears to exist between residents of EJ communities and other communities; and (3) the resource gap that makes evacuation and recovery more difficult to achieve in EJ communities.

Summary

Indigenous communities, communities Of Color and low-income communities are especially vulnerable to the harmful impacts of climate change. There are specific issues surrounding climate change and protecting EJ communities, such as cumulative impacts and the conditions that combine to create them, which can make EJ communities especially climate vulnerable.

It is crucial that more research and resources, and more responsive methods, be developed to assess and mitigate the public health impacts of climate change on EJ communities. Effective public health planning can both lessen and make communities more resilient to the negative effects of climate change–related environmental impacts. We have already offered a set of recommendations addressing very specific and discrete issues. However, more broadly, in order to increase climate change related resiliency in EJ communities, it is imperative that the root causes of climate-related vulnerability are addressed. These include:

- Racial bias and discrimination

- Economic inequality

- Unequal political power and access

- Legacy pollution and **historical trauma**

- The impact of the climate change threat itself (through mitigation, prediction, and warning and preparedness)

- The capacity of EJ communities to withstand climate change related threats

Mitigating climate change and ensuring that EJ communities are resilient to the harmful impacts of climate change are obligations our society must meet.

DISCUSSION QUESTIONS

1. Explain the differences between a starting point approach and an end point approach, when defining climate vulnerability in EJ communities.

2. Describe some of the dimensions of climate vulnerability experienced by Indigenous communities.

3. What impact will climate change have on the distributional burden of air pollution-related illness and mortality among different communities across the nation?

KEY TERMS

Climate resiliency: The capacity of communities to prepare for, protect, and recover from the impacts associated with climate-related events.

Cumulative impacts: The health risks and impacts caused by multiple pollutants, usually emitted by multiple sources of pollution in a community, and their interactions with each other and any social vulnerabilities that exist in the community.

End point approach: An approach in which vulnerability is viewed as the impacts that result from the added effects of climate change influences, using projections from climate modeling. From these projections, impacts on individuals with existing health predispositions and vulnerabilities are estimated; community vulnerabilities are understood as the aggregate of individual vulnerabilities.

Environmental justice (EJ): The fair treatment and meaningful involvement of all people regardless of race, color, national origin, or income, with respect to the development, implementation, and enforcement of environmental laws, regulations, and policies (https://www.epa.gov/environmentaljustice).

Historical trauma: Cumulative trauma across both one person's lifespan and across generations, resulting from political, economic, and environmental stressors.

Starting point approach: A second vulnerability framework in which environmental and social processes are included, more easily incorporating environmental justice concerns; social and economic processes of marginalization and inequalities are diagnosed as the causes of climate vulnerability.

Urban heat island (UHI) effect: A phenomenon in which the higher thermal storage capacity of the urban environment combines with a relatively high concentration of local heat sources to increase temperatures relative to surrounding areas. The UHI effect results in both elevated surface and air temperatures; built environment materials re-radiates heat at night, raising nighttime temperatures.

Vulnerability: The susceptibility to harms and risks, which includes inequality of social, economic, and environmental conditions, in addition to individual health factors.

References and Further Reading

Adakai, M., M. Sandoval-Rosario, F. Xu, T. Aseret-Manygoats, M. Allison, K. J. Greenlund, K. l E. Barbour. 2018. "Health Disparities among American Indians/Alaska Natives—Arizona, 2017." *MMWR. Morbidity and Mortality Weekly Report* 67 (47):1314–18. doi:10.15585/mmwr.mm6747a4.

Adler, N. E., and D. H. Rehkopf. 2008. "US Disparities in Health: Descriptions, Causes, and Mechanisms." *Annual Review of Public Health* 29:235–52.

Agyeman J., R. Bullard, and B. Evans, eds. 2003. *Just Sustainabilities: Development in an Unequal World.* Cambridge, MA: MIT Press.

Akbari, H. 2005. *Energy Saving Potential and Air Quality Benefits of Urban Heat Island.* Berkeley, CA: Lawrence Berkeley National Laboratory.

Akinbami, L., J. Moorman, A. Simon, and K. Schoendorf. 2014. "Trends in Racial Disparities for Asthma Outcomes among Children 0 to 17 Years, 2001–2010." *Journal of Allergy and Clinical Immunology* 134:547–53.

Akinbami, L. J., J. E. Moorman, C. Bailey, H. Zahran, M. King, C. Johnson, and X. Liu. 2012. *Trends in Asthma Prevalence, Health Care Use and Mortality in the United States, 2001–2010.* NCHS data brief 94. Hyattsville, MD: National Center for Health Statistics.

Albrecht, G., G. Sartore, L. Connor, N. Higginbotham, S. Freeman, B. Kelly, and, G. Pollard. 2007. "Solastalgia: The Distress Caused by Environmental Change." *Australasian Psychiatry* 15 (S1):S95–S98. doi:10.1080/10398560701701288.

Arias, E., J. Xu, and M. A. Jim. 2014. "Period Life Tables for the Non-Hispanic American Indian and Alaska Native Population, 2007–2009." *American Journal of Public Health* 104 (suppl 3):S312–S319. doi:10.2105/AJPH.2013.301635.

Ash, M., J. Boyce, G. Chang, J. Scoggins, and M. Pastor. 2009. *Justice in the Air: Tracking Toxic Pollution from America's Industries and Companies to Our States, Cities, and Neighborhoods.* Amherst, MA: Political Economy Research Institute.

Balbus, J., and C. Molina. 2009. "Identifying Vulnerable Subpopulations for Climate Change Health Effects in the United States." *Journal of Occupational and Environmental Medicine* 51 (1):33–57.

Barringer, F. 2008. "Flooded Village Files Suit, Citing Corporate Link to Climate Change." *New York Times*, February 27. http://www.nytimes.com/2008/02/27/ us/27alaska.html.

Basu, R. 2009. "High Ambient Temperature and Mortality: A Review of Epidemiologic Studies from 2001 to 2008." *Environmental Health* 8 (1):40.

Berdahl, P., and S. Bretz. 1997. "Preliminary Survey of the Solar Reflectance of Cool Roofing Materials." *Energy and Buildings* 25:149–58.

Blanchard, W. 2008. "Deadliest U.S. Disaster: Top Fifty." Washington, DC: Federal Emergency Management Agency.

Boyce, J. K., and M. Pastor. 2012. *Cooling the Planet, Clearing the Air: Climate Policy, Carbon Pricing, and Co-Benefits.* Portland, OR: Economics for Equity and Environment.

Braverman, P. A., S. A. Egerter, and R. E. Mockenhaupt. 2011. "Broadening the Focus: The Need to Address the Social Determinants of Health." *American Journal of Preventive Medicine* 40:S4-S18.

Brulle, R. J., and D. N. Pellow, eds. 2005. *Power, Justice, and the Environment.* Cambridge, MA: MIT Press.

Brunekreef, B., and S. T. Holgate. 2002. "Air Pollution and Health." *Lancet* 360 (9341):133–42.

Brunekreef, B., N. A. Janssen, J. de Hartog, H. Harssema, M. Knape, and P. van Vliet. 1997. "Air Pollution from Truck Traffic and Lung Function in Children Living near Motorways." *Epidemiology* 8:298–303.

Bullard, R. D., P. Mohai, R. Saha, and B. Wright. 2007. *Toxic Wastes and Race at Twenty: 1987–2007.* Cleveland, OH: United Church of Christ.

Bullard, R. D., and B. Wright, eds. 2009. *Race and Environmental Justice after Hurricane Katrina: Struggles to Reclaim, Rebuild and Revitalize New Orleans and the Gulf Coast.* Boulder, CO: Westview Press.

Burritt, C., and B. K. Sullivan. 2012. "Hurricane Sandy Threatens $20 Billion in Economic Damage." *Bloomberg Business.* October 30. https://www.bloomberg.com/news/articles/2012-10-29/ hurricane-sandy-threatens-20-billion-in-u-s-economic-damage.

Caiazzo, F., A. Ashok, I. A. Waitz, S. H. L. Yim, and S. R. H. Barret. 2013. "Air Pollution and Early Deaths in the United States. Part 1: Quantifying the Impact of Major Sectors in 2005." *Atmospheric Environment* 79:198–208.

California Environmental Protection Agency. 2010. *Cumulative Impacts: Building a Scientific Foundation.* Sacramento, CA: Office of Environmental Health Hazard Assessment. http://oehha.ca.gov/ej/pdf/ CIReport123110.pdf.

Campbell-Lendrum, D., C. Corvalán, and M. Neira. 2007. "Global Climate Change: Implications for International Public Health Policy." *Bulletin of the World Health Organization* 85:161–244. https:// apps.who.int/iris/handle/10665/269855.

Centers for Disease Control and Prevention. 2012. "CDC Policy on Climate Change and Public Health." http://www.cdc.gov/climateandhealth/policy.htm.

Centers for Disease Control and Prevention. 2020. "Asthma." Updated March 24, 2020. Accessed April 6, 2020. https://www.cdc.gov/asthma/most_recent_national_asthma_data.htm.

Centro, Center for Puerto Rican Studies. 2018. *Puerto Rico, One Year after Hurricane Maria*. New York: Hunter College, City University of New York. https://centropr.hunter.cuny.edu/sites/default/files/data_briefs/Hurricane_maria_1YR.pdf.

Cobb, N., D. Espey, and J. King. 2014. "Health Behaviors and Risk Factors among American Indians and Alaska Natives, 2000–2010." *American Journal of Public Health* 104 (suppl 3):S481–S489. doi:10.2105/AJPH.2014.301879.

Cochran, P. L., and A. L Geller. 2002. "The Melting Ice Cellar: What Native Traditional Knowledge Is Teaching Us about Global Warming and Environmental Change." *American Journal of Public Health* 92 (9):1404–09.

Cochran, P., O. H. Huntington, C. Pungowiyi, S. Tom, F. S. Chapin III, H. P. Huntington, N. G. Maynard, and S. F. Trainor. 2013. "Indigenous Frameworks for Observing and Responding to Climate Change in Alaska." *Climatic Change* 120:557–67.

Committee on Public Health Strategies to Improve Health. 2011. *For the Public's Health: Revitalizing Law and Policy to Meet New Challenges*. Washington, DC: National Academies Press.

Confalonieri, U., B. Menne, R. Akhtar, K. Ebi, M. Hauengue, R. Kovats, B. Revich et al. 2008. "Human Health." In *Climate Change, 2007: Synthesis Report. Contribution of Working Groups I, II and III to the Fourth Assessment Report of the Intergovernmental Panel on Climate Change*, edited by M. L. Parry, O. F. Canziani, J. P. Palutikof, P. J. Van der Linden, and C. E. Hanson, 391–431. Cambridge: Cambridge University Press.

Cooney, C. M. 2011. "Preparing a People: Climate Change and Public Health." *Environmental Health Perspectives* 119:a166-a171.

Corburn, J. 2002. "Environmental Justice, Local Knowledge and Risk: The Discourse of a Community-Based Cumulative Exposure Assessment." *Environmental Management* 29:451–66.

Coto, D. 2018. "Report: Maria Had $43B impact on Puerto Rico's Economy." *AP News*. https://apnews.com/5e29ec136509469cb548e0f88cf1c815.

Curriero, F. C., K. S. Heiner, J. M. Samet, S. L. Zeger, L. Strug, and J. A. Patz. 2002. "Temperature and Mortality in Eleven Cities of the Eastern United States." *American Journal of Epidemiology* 155 (1):80–87.

Cutter, S. 2006. *Hazards, Vulnerability and Environmental Justice*. New York: Earthscan.

Cutter, S. L., E. T. Emrich, J. T. Mitchell, B. J. Boru, M. Gall, M. C. Schmidtlein, C. G. Burton, and G. Melton. 2010. "The Long Road Home: Race, Class, and Recovery from Hurricane Katrina." *Environment: Science and Policy for Sustain- able Development* 48 (2):8–20. doi:10.3200/ENVT.48.2.8–20.

Dockery, D. W., C. A. Pope, X. Xiping, J. D. Spengler, J. H. Ware, M. E. Fay, B. G. Ferris, and F. E. Speizer 1993. "An Association between Air Pollution and Mortality in Six U.S. Cities." *New England Journal of Medicine* 329:1753–59.

Doyle, J. T., M. H. Redsteer, and M. J. Eggers. 2013. "Exploring Effects of Climate Change on Northern Plains American Indian Health." *Climate Change* 120 (3):643–55. doi: 10.1007/s10584–013–0799-z.

Dressler, W. W., K. S. Oths, and C. C. Gravlee. 2005. "Race and Ethnicity in Public Health Research: Models to Explain Health Disparities." *Annual Review of Anthropology* 34:231–52.

Duran, E., and B. Duran. 1995. *Native American Postcolonial Psychology*. Albany: State University of New York Press.

Ebi, K. L., J. Balbus, P. L. Kinney, E. Lipp, D. Mills, M. S. O'Neill, and M. L. Wilson. 2009. "U.S. Funding Insufficient to Address the Human Health Impacts of and Public Health Responses to Climate Variability and Change." *Environmental Health Perspectives* 117:857–62.

Ebi, K., and G. McGregor. 2008. "Climate Change, Tropospheric Ozone and Particulate Matter, and Health Impacts." *Environmental Health Perspectives* 116:1449–55.

Ellen, R. P., P. Parkes, and A. Bicker, eds. 2000. *Indigenous Environmental Knowledge and Its Transformations: Critical Anthropological Perspectives*. Amsterdam: Gordon and Breach Publishing Group.

Enterprise Community Partners. 2013. "Hurricane Sandy: Housing Needs One Year Later." Research brief, October. Columbia, MD: ECP.

Environmental Justice and Science Initiative. 2010. "Letter on EPA Authority to Regulate Greenhouse Gases and Climate Change Co-Pollutant Policy." June 8, 2010.

Environmental Protection Agency. 2002. *Children's Environmental Health Disparities: Black and African American Children and Asthma*. Washington, DC: EPA. https://www.epa.gov/sites/production/files/2014-05/documents/hd_aa_asthma.pdf.

Environmental Protection Agency. 2003. *Framework for Cumulative Risk Assessment*. Washington, DC: Environmental Protection Agency.

Environmental Protection Agency. 2008. *Reducing Urban Heat Islands: Compendium of Strategies.* Washington, DC: Environmental Protection Agency. http://www.epa.gov/heatisld/resources/compendium.htm.

Environmental Protection Agency. 2019. "Environmental Justice." https://www.epa.gov/environmentaljustice.

Fair Share Housing Center, Housing and Community Development Network of New Jersey, Latino Action Network, and NAACP New Jersey State Conference. 2014. *The State of Sandy Recovery.* Cherry Hill, NJ: Fair Share Housing Center.

Federal Emergency Management Agency. 2018. *2017. Hurricane Season FEMA After-Action Report.* Washington, DC: FEMA. https://www.fema.gov/media-library-data/1531743865541-d16794d43d3082544435e1471da07880/2017FEMAHurricaneAAR.pdf.

Furman Center Moelis Institute for Affordable Housing Policy. 2013. *Sandy's Effects on Housing in New York City.* New York: Furman Center.

Garfin, G., G. Franco, H. Blanco, A. Comrie, P. Gonzalez, T. Piechota, R. Smyth, and R. Waskom. 2014. "Southwest." In *Climate Change Impacts in the United States: The Third National Climate Assessment,* edited by J. M. Melillo, T. C. Richmond, and G. W. Yohe, 462–86. Washington, DC: U.S. Global Change Research Program. doi:10.7930/J08G8HMN.

Greenberg, J. H., J. Bromberg, C. M. Reed, T. L. Gustafson, and R. A. Beauchamp. 1983. "The Epidemiology of Heat Related Deaths, Texas—1950, 1970–79, and 1980." *American Journal of Public Health* 73:805–807.

Harlan, S. L., A. J. Brazel, L. Prashad, W. L. Stefanov, and L. Larsen 2006. "Neighborhood Microclimates and Vulnerability to Heat Stress." *Social Science and Medicine* 63:2847–63.

Hewitt, V., E. Mackres, and K. Shickman. 2014. *Cool Policies for Cool Cities: Best Practices for Mitigating Urban Heat Islands in North American Cities.* Washington, DC: American Council for an Energy Efficient Economy.

Holt, D. W. 2015. "Heat in US Prisons and Jails: Corrections and the Challenge of Climate New York: Columbia Law School. https://web.law.columbia.edu/sites/default/files/microsites/climate-change/holt_-_heat_in_us_prisons_and_jails.pdf.

Houston, D., J. Wu, P. Ong, and A. Winer 2004. "Structural Disparities of Urban Traffic in Southern California: Implications for Vehicle Related Air Pollution Exposure in Minority and High Poverty Neighborhoods." *Journal of Urban Affairs* 26:565–92.

Interagency Climate Change Adaptation Task Force. 2011. *Federal Actions for a Climate Resilient Nation: Progress Report of the Interagency Climate Adaptation Task Force.* Washington, DC: Interagency Climate Change Adaptation Task Force.

International Federation of Red Cross and Red Crescent Societies. n.d. "What Is Vulnerability?" Geneva: International Federation of Red Cross and Red Crescent Societies. http://www.ifrc.org/en/what-we-do/disaster-management/about-disasters/ what-is-a-disaster/what-is-vulnerability/.

Intergovernmental Panel on Climate Change. 2007. *Climate Change, 2007: Synthesis Report. Contribution of Working Groups I, II and III to the Fourth Assessment Report of the Intergovernmental Panel on Climate Change,* edited by M. L. Parry, O. F. Canziani, J. P. Palutikof, P. J. van der Linden, and C. E. Hanson. Geneva, Switzerland: IPCC. http://www.ipcc.ch/ report/ar4/.

Intergovernmental Panel on Climate Change. 2014. *Fifth Assessment Report: Climate Change 2013.* Geneva: IPCC. http://www.ipcc.ch/report/ar5/.

Intergovernmental Panel on Climate Change. 2018. *Global Warming of 1.5°C. An IPCC Special Report on the Impacts of Global Warming of 1.5°C above Pre-Industrial Levels and Related Global Greenhouse Gas Emission Pathways, in the Context of Strengthening the Global Response to the Threat of Climate Change, Sustainable Development, and Efforts to Eradicate Poverty.* Geneva: IPCC.

Isaac, G., S. Finn, J. R. Joe, E. Hoover, J. P. Gone, C. Lefthand-Begay, and S. Hill. 2018. "Native American Perspectives on Health and Traditional Ecological Knowledge." *Environmental Health Perspectives* 126 (12):125002. doi:10.1289/EHP1944.

Jacob, C., T. McDaniels, and S. Hinch. 2010. "Indigenous Culture and Adaptation to Climate Change: Sockeye Salmon and the St'at'ime People." *Mitigation and Adaptation Strategies for Global Change* 15:859–76.

Jacobs. D. E. 2011. "Environmental Health Disparities in Housing." *American Journal of Public Health* 101:S115–22.

Jarrett, M., R. T. Burnett, P. Kanaroglou, J. Eyles, N. Finkelstein, C. Giovis, and J. R. Brook. 2001. "A GIS–Environmental Justice Analysis of Particulate Air Pollution in Hamilton, Canada." *Environment and Planning A* 33:955–73.

Jarrett, M., R. T. Burnett, R. Ma, C. A. Pope, D. Krewski, K. B. Newbold, G. Thurston, et al. 2005. "Spatial Analysis of Air Pollution and Mortality in Los Angeles." *Epidemiology* 16:727–36.

Jones, A. 2019. "Cruel and Unusual Punishment: When States Don't Provide Air Conditioning in Prison." June 18, 2019. Accessed April 1, 2020. https://www.prisonpolicy.org/blog/2019/06/18/air-conditioning/.

Kaswan, A. 2008. "Environmental Justice and Domestic Climate Change Policy." *Environmental Law Reporter* 38:10287–345.

King, M., A. Smith, and M. Gracey. 2009. "Indigenous Health Part 2: The Underlying Cause of the Health Gap." *Lancet* 374:75–85.

Kinney, P. L. 1999. "The Pulmonary Effects of Outdoor Ozone and Particle Air Pollution." *Seminars in Respiratory and Critical Care Medicine* 20:601–607.

Klinenberg, E. 2003. *Heat Wave: A Social Autopsy of Disaster.* Chicago: University of Chicago Press.

Knowlton, K., J. Rosenthal, C. Hogrefe, B. Lynn, S. Gaffin, R. Goldberg, C. Rosenzweig, et al. 2004. "Assessing Ozone-Related Health Impacts under a Changing Climate." *Environmental Health Perspectives* 112:1557–63.

Little-Blanton, M., and C. Hoffman. 2005. " The Role of Health Insurance Coverage in Reducing Racial/ Ethnic Disparities in Health Care." *Health Affairs* 24:398–408.

Logan, J. R. 2006. *The Impact of Katrina: Race and Class in Storm-Damaged Neighborhoods.* Providence, RI: Brown University.

Luber, G., K. Knowlton, J. Balbus, H. Frumkin, M. Hayden, J. Hess, M. McGeehin, et al. 2014. "Human Health." In *Climate Change Impacts in the United States: The Third National Climate Assessment*, edited by J. M. Melillo, T. C. Richmond, and G.W. Yohe, 220–56. Washington, DC: U.S. Global Change Research Program.

Lynn, K., J. Daigle, J. Hoffman, F. Lake, N. Michelle, D. Ranco, C. Viles, et al. 2013. "The Impacts of Climate Change on Tribal Traditional Foods." *Climatic Change* 120:545–56.

McLaughlin, K.A., P. Berglund, M. J. Gruber, R. C. Kessler, N. A. Sampson, and A. M. Zaslavsky. 2011. "Recovery from PTSD following Hurricane Katrina." *Depression and Anxiety* 28 (6):439–46. doi: 10.1002/da.20790.

Mensah, G. A., A. H. Mokdad, E. S. Ford, K. J. Greenlund, and J. B. Croft. 2005. "State of Disparities in Cardiovascular Health in the United States." *Circulation* 111:1233–41.

Minnesota Department of Natural Resources. 2008. "Natural Wild Rice in Minnesota." St. Paul: MDNR.

Mohai, P., D. Pellow, and R. Timmons. 2009. "Environmental Justice." *Annual Review of Environment and Resources* 34:405–30.

Mohai, P., and R. Saha. 2007. "Racial Inequality in the Distribution of Hazardous Waste: A National-Level Reassessment." *Social Problems* 54:343–70.

Morello-Frosch, R., M. Zuk, M. Jarrett, B. Shamasunder, and A. D. Kyle. 2011. "Understanding the Cumulative Impacts of Inequalities in Environmental Health: Implications for Policy." *Health Affairs* 30:879–87.

Mrkusic, M., and D. A. Gross. 2018. "Incarcerated People Remain Vulnerable to the Worst Ravages of a Warming World." Updated December 5, 2018. https://www.pbs.org/wgbh/nova/article/climate-change-mass-incarceration-prison/.

National Aeronautics and Space Administration. 2010. "Urban Heat Islands." https://earthobservatory.nasa.gov/images/47704/urban-heat-islands.

National Center for Health Statistics. 2013. *Health, United States, 2012: With Special Feature on Emergency Care.* Hyattsville, MD: NCHS.

National Congress of American Indians. n.d. "Housing and Infrastructure." Washington, DC: NCAI. http://www.ncai.org/policy-issues/economic-development-commerce/housing-infrastructure.

National Environmental Justice Advisory Council, Cumulative Risks/Impacts Work Group. 2004. *Ensuring Risk Reduction in Communities with Multiple Stressors: Environmental Justice and Cumulative Risks/Impacts.* Washington, DC: Environmental Protection Agency.

National Fair Housing Alliance. 2006. *Still No Home for the Holidays: A Report on the State of Housing and Housing Discrimination in the Gulf Coast Region.* Washington, DC: NFHA.

National Oceanic and Atmospheric Administration. 2015. "Sandy's Legacy: Improved Storm Surge Prediction Tools." http://www.regions.noaa.gov/north-atlantic/highlights/sandys-legacy-improved-storm-surge-prediction-tools/.

National Research Council. 2007. *Evaluating Progress of the US Climate Change Science Program: Methods and Preliminary Results.* Washington, DC: National Academies Press.

New Jersey Environmental Justice Alliance. 2018. *Responses to Questions Posed by the Board of Public Utilities Regarding New Jersey's Next Energy Master Plan,* prepared by Nicky Sheats. Available from the author.

New York City Department of Health and Mental Hygiene. 2007. "Air Conditioners in Home by High-Risk (DPHO) Neighborhood, 2007 (Unadjusted for Age)."

Norton-Smith, K., K. Lynn, K. Chief, K. Cozzetto, J. Donatuto, M. Hiza Redsteer, L. Kruger et al. 2016. *Climate Change and Indigenous Peoples: A Synthesis of Current Impacts and Experiences.* Gen. Tech. Rep. PNWGTR-944. Portland, OR: U.S. Department of Agriculture, Forest Service, Pacific Northwest Research Station.

O'Brien, K., S. Eriksen, A. Schjolden, and L. Nygaard. 2004. *What's in a Word? Conflicting Interpretations of Vulnerability in Climate Change Research.* Oslo, Norway: Center for International Climate and Environmental Research.

O'Neill, M. S., A. Zanobetti, and J. Schwartz. 2003. "Modifiers of the Temperature and Mortality Association in Seven US Cities." *American Journal of Epidemiology* 157:74–1082.

O'Neill, M. S., A. Zanobetti, and J. Schwartz. 2005. "Disparities by Race in Heat- Related Mortality in Four US Cities: The Role of Air Conditioning Prevalence." *Journal of Urban Health* 82:191–97.

Pastor, M., R. D. Bullard, J. K. Boyce, A. Fothergill, R. Morello-Frosch, and B. Wright. 2006. *In the Wake of the Storm: Environment, Disaster, and Race after Katrina.* New York: Russell Sage Foundation.

Pastor, M., R. Morello-Frosch, and J. L. Sadd. 2005. "The Air Is Always Cleaner on the Other Side: Race, Space, and Ambient Air Toxics Exposures in California." *Journal of Urban Affairs* 27:127–48. doi:10.1111/j.0735–2166.2005.00228.x.

Pastor, M., Jr., J. L. Sadd, and R. Morello-Frosch. 2004. "Waiting to Inhale: The Demographics of Toxic Air Release Facilities in 21st-Century California." *Social Science Quarterly* 85:420–40. doi:10.1111/j.0038–4941.2004.08502010.x.

Patz, J. A., M. A. McGeehin, S. M. Bernard, K. L. Ebi, P. L. Epstein, A. Grambsch, D. J. Gubler, et al. 2000. "The Potential Health Impacts of Climate Variability and Change for the United States: Executive Summary of the Report of the Health Sector of the U.S. National Assessment." *Environmental Health Perspectives* 108:367–76.

Pearsall, H., and J. Pearce. 2010. "Urban Sustainability and Environmental Justice: Evaluating the Linkages in Planning/Policy Discourse." *Local Environment* 15:569–80.

Plyer, A. 2016. "Facts for Features: Katrina Impact. Data Center." Published August 26, 2016. http://www.datacenterresearch.org/data-resources/katrina/facts-for-impact/.

Pope, A. 1989. "Respiratory Disease Associated with Community Air Pollution and a Steel Mill, Utah Valley." *American Journal of Public Health* 79:623–28.

Pope, C., R. T. Burnett, G. D. Thurston, M. J. Thun, E. E. Calle, D. Krewski, and J. Godleski. 2004. "Cardiovascular Mortality and Long-Term Exposure to Particulate Air Pollution, Epidemiological Evidence of General Pathophysiological Pathways of Disease." *Circulation* 109:71–77.

Pope, C. A., and D. W. Dockery. 2006. "Health Effects of Fine Particulate Air Pollution: Lines that Connect." *Journal of the Air and Waste Management Association* 56:709–42.

Reo, N. J., and A. Parker. 2013. "Rethinking Colonialism to Prepare for the Impacts of Rapid Environmental Change." In *Climate Change and Indigenous Peoples in the United States*, edited by J. K. Maldonado, C. Benedict, and T. Pandya, 163–74. New York: Springer.

Rosenzweig, C., and T. Wilbanks. 2010. "The State of Climate Change Vulnerability, Impacts, and Adaptation Research: Strengthening Knowledge Base and Community." *Climatic Change* 100 (May):103–106. doi:10.1007/s10584–010–9826–5.

Samara, T. R. 2014. *Rise Of the Renter Nation: Solutions to the Housing Affordability Crisis.* Brooklyn, NY: Homes for All Campaign of the Right to the City Alliance.

Sarche, M., and P. Spicer. 2008. "Poverty and Health Disparities for American Indian and Alaska Native Children: Current Knowledge and Future Prospects." *Annals of the New York Academy of Sciences* 1136:126–36. doi:10.1196/annals.1425.017.

Sawyer, W. and P. Wagner. 2020. "Mass Incarceration: The Whole Pie 2020." Updated March 24, 2020. Accessed April 1, 2020. https://www.prisonpolicy.org/reports/pie2020.html.

Schwartz, J., D. Slater, T. V. Larson, W. E. Pierson, and J. Q. Koenig. 1993. "Particulate Air Pollution and Emergency Room Visits for Asthma in Seattle." *American Review of Respiratory Disease* 147:826–31.

Sheats, N., T. Onyenaka, S. Gupta, V. Caffee, T. Carrington, K. Gaddy, and P. Montague. 2008. *An Environmental Justice Climate Change Policy for New Jersey.* Trenton: New Jersey Environmental Justice Alliance and Center for the Urban Environment.

Sheats, N. 2014. *Stakeholder Engagement Report: Environmental Justice, Climate Change Preparedness in New Jersey.* Trenton, NJ: New Jersey Climate Adaptation Alliance.

Sheats, N. 2017. "Achieving Emissions Reductions for Environmental Justice Communities through Climate Change Mitigation Policy, *William and Mary Environmental Law and Policy Review* 41 (2): 377–402. https://scholarship.law.wm.edu/wmelpr/vol41/iss2/3/.

Smit, B., and J. Wandel. 2006. "Adaptation, Adaptive Capacity and Vulnerability." *Global Environmental Change* 16:282–92.

Spalter-Roth, R., T. A. Rowenthal, and M. Rubio. 2005. *Race, Ethnicity, and the Health of Americans.* Washington, DC: Sydney S. Spivack Program in Applied Social Research and Social Policy, American Sociological Association. https://www.asanet.org/sites/default/files/savvy/images/research/docs/pdf/race_ethnicity_health.pdf.

Tagaris, K., L. Kuo-Jen, A. J. DeLucia, L. Deck, P. Amar, and A. G. Russell. 2010. "Sensitivity of Air Pollution–Induced Premature Mortality to Precursor Emissions under the Influence of Climate Change." *International Journal of Environmental Research and Public Health* 7:2222–37.

Targaris, E., K. J. Liao, A. J. Delucia, L. Deck, P. Amar, and A. G. Russell. 2009. "Potential Impact of Climate Change on Air Pollution-Related Human Health Effects." *Environment Science and Technology* 43:4979–88.

Trout, L., C. Kramer, and L. Fischer. 2018. "Social Medicine in Practice: Realizing the American Indian and Alaska Native Right to Health." *Health and Human Rights* 20 (2):19–30.

Tsosie, R. A. 2007. "Indigenous People and Environmental Justice: The Impact of Climate Change." *University of Colorado Law Review* 78:1625.

Uejio, C. K., O. V. Wilhelmi, J. S. Golden, D. M. Mills, S. P. Gulino, and J. P. Samenow. 2011. "Intra-Urban Societal Vulnerability to Extreme Heat: The Role of Heat Exposure and the Built Environment, Socioeconomics, and Neighborhood Stability." *Health and Place* 17:498–507.

United Nations News Centre. 2014. "One Year after Devastating Storm, UN Says Philippines 'Well on Road to Recovery.'" https://news.un.org/en/story/2014/11/483072-one-year-after-devastating-storm-un-says-philippines-well-road-recovery.

U.S. Army Corps of Engineers. 2009. *Alaska Baseline Erosion Assessment.* Anchorage: US Army Corps of Engineers. Alaska District.

Waldron, H. 2007. *Trends in Mortality Differentials and Life Expectancy for Male Social Security-Covered Workers, by Average Relative Earnings.* Washington, DC: U.S. Social Security Administration, Office of Research, Evaluation and Statistics.

Weinhold, B. 2010a. "Climate Change and Health: A Native American Perspective." *Environmental Health Perspectives* 118 (2):A64–65.

Weinhold, B. 2010b. "Health Disparities: Climate Change and Health: A Native American Perspective." *Environmental Health Perspectives* 118:a64-a65. http://dx.doi.org/10.1289/ehp.118-a64.

Wernette, D. R., and L. A. Nieves. 1992. "Breathing Polluted Air." *EPA Journal* 18:16.

Whitman, S., G. Good, E. R. Donoghue, N. Benbow, S. Wenyuan, and S. Mou. 1997. "Mortality in Chicago Attributed to the July 1995 Heat Wave." *American Journal of Public Health* 87:1515–18.

Whyte, K. P. 2013. "Justice Forward: Tribes, Climate Adaptation and Responsibility." *Climatic Change* 120:517–530. doi:10.1007/s10584–013–0743–2.

Williams, D. R., and C. Collins. 2001. "Racial Residential Segregation: A Fundamental Cause of Racial Disparities in Health." *Public Health Report* 226:404–16.

Williams, D. R., and T. D. Rucker. 2000. "Understanding and Addressing Racial Disparities in Health Care." *Health Care Financing Review* 21 (4):75–90.

World Health Organization. 2005. "Climate Change and Human Health." Fact sheet. http://www.who.int/globalchange/news/fsclimandhealth/en/.

World Health Organization. 2011. "The Social Dimensions of Climate Change, Discussion Draft." Geneva: WHO.

World Health Organization. 2014. "Climate Change and Health." Fact sheet 266. http://www.who.int/mediacentre/factsheets/fs266/en/.

Yellow Horse, M. 1999. "Oyate Ptayela: Rebuilding the Lakota Nation through Addressing Historical Trauma among Lakota Parents." In *Voices of First Nations People,* edited by H. Weaver, 109–26. Binghamton, NY: Haworth Press.

Zaffos, J. 2011. "Extreme Measures: The Push to Make Climate Research Relevant." *Daily Climate,* November 2. https://www.eurekareport.com.au/investment-news/extreme-measures-the-push-to-make-climate-research-relevant/89647.

Zahran, H. S., C. M. Bailey, S. A. Damon, P. L. Garbe, and P. N. Breysse. 2018. "Vital Signs: Asthma in Children—United States, 2001–2016." *MMWR. Morbidity and Mortality Weekly Report* 67 (5):149–55.

CHAPTER 17

CLIMATE CHANGE COMMUNICATION

Adam Corner, Chris Shaw, Stuart Capstick, and Nick Pidgeon

Introduction

While governments and campaigners have largely focused on the technological, economic, and political changes needed to reduce greenhouse gas emissions to avoid the worst impacts of climate change, less attention has been paid to engaging the public in the global response to climate change. What does it mean to live in a changing climate? How do public attitudes play into the global policy discourse on climate change? Are rapid emissions cuts possible without major social transformation, given the need for significant lifestyle change across a range of behaviors currently considered "normal" (in wealthy countries) or "aspirational" (in developing countries)?

The question of how members of the public engage with climate change and how to communicate with a range of public audiences more effectively, is increasingly important for the global goals of averting dangerous climate change and an increasingly central focus for social science researchers (Clarke, Corner, and Webster 2018; Corner and Clarke 2017; Höppner and Whitmarsh 2011; Oskamp 1995; Poortinga et al. 2019). The requirements to educate the public, to raise awareness, and to promote wider public participation, were formalized in the United Nations Paris Agreement of 2015.

Over the past two decades, a substantial literature has developed that has sought to better understand public perceptions of climate change, clarify conditions for **pro-environmental behavior** change, and develop **climate change communication** in ways that make the topic more comprehensible and personally relevant (Corner and Clarke 2017; Moser 2010; Steg and Vlek 2009). This task entails the communication of a global problem that is at once more abstract and less salient than many other social issues and yet also has the potential to lead to more serious and long-term implications than many of the previous challenges that humanity has faced (Moser 2010).

Many different sectors have a role to play in conveying the urgency and seriousness of climate change, and public health professionals have made the case for a concerted effort to communicate about climate change in terms of its health impacts and the health benefits of low-carbon behaviors and policies. Health professionals have the opportunity to bridge and translate the global, often abstract nature of climate change to the more tangible, personally relevant, and relatable territory of health outcomes and well-being.

This chapter aims to discuss some of the key considerations involved in effectively communicating with public audiences on climate change and the various ways in which climate change and health communication intersect. We first discuss research that has examined public understanding of climate change, as a basis for thinking about some of the principles that can be applied to ensure sound communication. We next examine some of the approaches that have been used to

KEY CONCEPTS

- Public engagement with climate change is critical to ensure an effective and society-wide response.

- People's views on climate change vary according to a range of sociodemographic factors, particularly in relation to their underlying values and worldviews.

- A focus on public health has the potential to draw attention to the personal relevance and wider significance of climate change.

- Health professionals can apply evidence-based principles for effective communication on climate change.

communicate about specific climate impacts, with a particular focus on heat events and flood risk. We then move on to consider some of the targeted research that has looked at ways of structuring communication about climate change from a health perspective.

Public Understanding of Climate Change and Principles of Climate Change Communication

Awareness of climate change is now almost universal, in developed nations and increasingly worldwide (Pidgeon 2012; Lee et al. 2015; Poortinga et al. 2019; Wike 2016). The meanings people attach to the idea of "climate change" vary immensely, however, leading to disagreements and disputes about climate change with which many of us are now familiar (Hulme 2009) and driving polarization around the issue in some English-speaking nations, in particular the United States (e.g., McCright and Dunlap 2011a, 2011b; Druckman and McGrath 2019).

The notion of "climate change" or "global warming" has been in the public domain since at least the late 1980s. Research into public understanding at that time emphasized the common misconceptions held by people, especially a confusion between weather and climate, and a conflation between climate change and the (largely unrelated) environmental problem of stratospheric ozone depletion (Kempton 1991, 1997; Bostrom et al. 1994). Research has shown that people's immediate associations with climate change often relate to remote and abstract imagery such as "melting ice" or "heat" and that climate change can be associated for some with "alarmist" imagery (such as concerning disaster or apocalyptic notions), or conversely for those with a skeptical viewpoint, that climate change constitutes a conspiracy theory (Lorenzoni et al. 2006; Smith and Leiserowitz 2012). Recent research suggests that there is a fairly narrow visual language associated with climate change—the ubiquitous polar bears and smokestacks familiar from nongovernmental organization (NGO) campaigns and digital media—and that this imagery often doesn't include human subjects (Wang et al. 2018).

Over the past quarter century, levels of concern about climate change have tended to rise and fall within the United States and worldwide: Figure 17.1 shows the proportion of the U.S. public who report they "personally worry" about global warming (Gallup 2019) over time. The noticeable decline in public concern about climate change that occurred in the late 2000s has been variously attributed to economic circumstances (Scruggs and Benegal 2012), cyclical patterns in public attention (Ratter, Philipp, and von Storch 2012), and the activities of

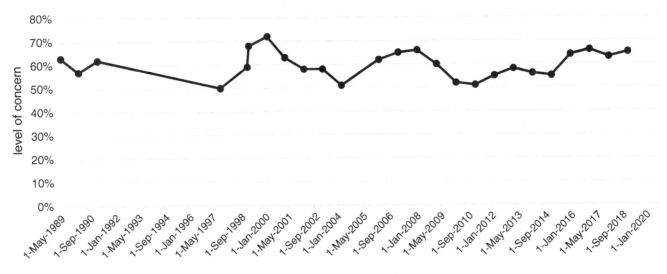

Figure 17.1 Change in concern about climate change over time

Note: Figure 17.1 shows the percentage of U.S. respondents responding that they worry "a great deal" or "a fair amount" about global warming over the time period 1989–2019. Data from U.S. Gallup polling (2019).

opinion-forming elites (Brulle, Carmichael, and Jenkins 2012). The signs are that, more recently, levels of awareness and concern have steadily risen in the United States, despite well-documented national political shifts. Leiserowitz et al. (2018) find that the proportion of the American public acknowledging climate change grew from around the 60 percent mark in 2010 to consistently above 70 percent from 2016 (the most recent figure in December 2018 being 73 percent). The proportion of U.S. respondents stating that they were "very worried" about climate change (the highest level of concern available to them to state) rose from around the 10 percent mark at the beginning of the 2010s to reach 29 percent by December 2018. Nevertheless, the United States as a nation still appears unusually doubtful about the basic facts of climate change, in comparison to many other parts of the world.

A wide range of research has established that people's perspectives on climate change are determined by a range of demographic, psychological, and cultural factors. Women express higher levels of overall concern about climate change than do men (Ballew et al. 2018; McCright 2010; Brody et al. 2008; O'Connor, Bord, and Fisher 1999). Levels of concern also vary with age: some research has viewed this in terms of an inverse linear relationship (e.g., Semenza, Ploubidis, and George 2011; Kellstedt, Zahran, and Vedlitz 2008) although others have suggested that those in the youngest and oldest age groups are less concerned overall than are middle-aged people (Upham et al. 2009; Capstick, Pidgeon, and Whitehead 2013). Studies also suggest that ethnicity plays a role in determining climate change attitudes: for example, Leiserowitz and Akerlof (2010) find that Hispanics and African-Americans often support a range of action on climate change at higher levels than did whites. Other U.S. studies have also noted that nonwhite research participants tend to be more concerned about climate change (Malka, Krosnick, and Langer 2009; Wood and Vedlitz 2007).

A growing body of research has demonstrated that people's values and political ideology are particularly important influences upon their perspectives on climate change and how communication about it is received (Kahan 2010). Particularly in the United States, climate change has become an increasingly politicized and partisan issue (McCright and Dunlap 2011a, 2011b) with longitudinal survey data showing a consistent gap between Democrat and Republican positions on the issue (Dunlap and McCright 2008).

In a related manner, a growing body of research has suggested that people's **cultural worldviews** underpin the ways in which they understand climate change (Bellamy and Hulme 2011; Kahan, Jenkins-Smith, and Braman 2011, 2012; Capstick and Pidgeon 2014a, 2014b; Leiserowitz 2006; Leiserowitz et al. 2010; Steg and Sievers 2000; Thompson and Rayner 1998; Thompson 2003; West, Bailey, and Winter 2010). For people holding a worldview in which collective organization and shared problem-solving are seen as desirable attributes for society (described as "egalitarians"), climate change tends to be an important matter of personal concern. By contrast, those with a cultural worldview that emphasizes freedom to act autonomously with few restrictions on personal choices (as is the case for "individualists") tend to downplay the importance or even reality of climate change.

A related strand of literature has applied social psychological insights into the different types of **values** that people typically hold and how these tend to be related to their attitudes toward climate change. A value is usually defined as a "guiding principle in the life of a person" (Schwartz 1992). Several decades of international research show that there are two broad categories of values, self-enhancing (or extrinsic) and self-transcending (or intrinsic). People who identify strongly with self-enhancing or extrinsic values (e.g., materialism, personal ambition) tend not to identify strongly with self-transcending or intrinsic values (e.g., benevolence, respect for the environment). With respect to people's likely degree of climate change engagement, people who hold self-transcendent values (especially pro-environmental values and high levels of altruism) are more likely to engage in sustainable behavior (Stern 2000), show higher concern about environmental risks like climate change (Slimak and Dietz 2006), perform specific actions such as recycling (Dunlap, Grieneeks, and Rokeach 1983), and support climate mitigation policies (Nilsson, von Borgstede, and Biel 2004).

Importantly for climate change communication, preexisting values and worldviews not only influence prior beliefs but also act as a perceptual filter for new information (Corner, Markowitz, and Pidgeon 2014). In an experimental setting, study participants presented with information about climate change by a putative expert on the subject offer different appraisals of whether they are trustworthy and knowledgeable, depending on the extent to which their own preconceptions match those of the expert (Kahan et al. 2011). Corner, Whitmarsh, and Xenias (2012) also highlight people's tendency to interpret information about climate change according to preexisting beliefs: study participants who already hold skeptical views about climate change are more likely to appraise information within a skeptical news article (i.e., one that casts doubt on climate change) as being convincing and reliable than would nonskeptics and vice versa. In research examining people's interpretations of the unusually cold weather across Europe in late 2009–2010, Capstick and Pidgeon (2014b) found those with skeptical viewpoints tend to interpret these events as evidence against climate change, whereas those more accepting of climate change tend to see the cold weather as a form of evidence supporting its existence.

There have been mixed findings concerning the extent to which people connect climate change and human health. More than ten years ago, Leiserowitz (2007) noted that not a single respondent in a U.S. survey sample of 673 adults spontaneously associated climate change and health impacts. Over a decade later, few North Americans can list specific climate-health impacts or who is at risk, even while viewing climate change as harmful to health (Hathaway and Maibach 2018). People's reference to climate-health risks often are not contextualized to personal or community health or understood in any detail (Cardwell and Elliott 2013).

Akerlof et al. (2010) and Leiserowitz (2007) recommend developing public health communication specifically to increase the salience of health risks from climate change. Cardwell and Elliott (2013) argue for reframing climate impacts from an "environmental issue" to a public health issue, to increase **public engagement** with climate change. Likewise, Petrovic, Madrigano, and Zaval (2014) propose that a reemphasis on the health benefits of reducing fossil fuel use has the potential to be more compelling than an emphasis on climate change mitigation, particularly for those of a conservative political orientation.

One point made repeatedly over the years, but nonetheless often overlooked, is that it is highly problematic to assume that public **skepticism** or lack of engagement derives principally from a lack of information or education on climate change. Certainly, research suggests that recognition of important facts, such as the high level of scientific consensus about the human causation of climate change, can exert a critical influence upon attitudes (Lewandowsky, Gignac, and Vaughan 2013). However, it is now clear that what has come to be termed the **information deficit model** of climate change communication—assuming that there is a "deficit" of knowledge that requires addressing—is inadequate to promote meaningful engagement with this topic (Moser and Dilling 2011).

There is now a strong evidence base that the ways in which we understand and respond to climate change intimately connect with our values and worldviews, and climate change communication may benefit from emphasizing certain values over others (Corner et al. 2014). There is a strong body of evidence that argues for "bigger-than-self" problems such as climate change, which require shared efforts to address, communication should affirm self-transcendent values that focus on commitment to a wider community to foster a durable and deeper sense of engagement (Crompton 2011).

This would seem to be congruent with community health promotion approaches (Hatcher, Allensworth, and Butterfoss 2010) emphasizing the needs and interdependencies of groups and the importance of social capital and community resilience for health (Poortinga 2012). This is a rather different message from those invoking economic incentives or self-interest to encourage action on climate change.

Messages emphasizing economic incentives may work in the short term but, in the long term, encouraging people to act out of self-interest, for what is essentially a common interest problem is counterproductive (Thøgersen and Crompton 2009; Evans et al. 2013). One study found that people at a gas station were more likely to get their tires checked when they were shown a message about the environmental benefits of correctly inflated tires, rather than the money they might save (Bolderdijk et al. 2013). Making low-carbon choices affordable is necessary, but not sufficient to catalyze behavior change (McLoughlin et al. 2019).

Images are powerful communication tools that have proven to be something of a sticking point for climate change communicators (Wang et al. 2018; O'Neill 2017) because climate change has been (until recently) something abstract and difficult to visualize. Typically "environmentalist" images of melting ice caps and polar bears can produce strong emotional reactions in some people but may also produce a feeling of powerlessness, as these sorts of images do not relate easily to people's lives (Manzo 2010; O'Neill and Nicholson-Cole 2009). Although images of vulnerable people (often children) from developing countries or a ravaged landscape may make climate change seem important, they can simultaneously lead to participants feeling unable to do anything about the problem (O'Neill et al. 2013). Other images, such as possible "energy futures" (e.g., electric cars or energy-efficient houses) were more successful in engendering a feeling of empowerment to act, yet successfully visualizing climate change is a critical area for future inquiry.

The absence of human stories is a persistent feature (Wang et al. 2018). One initiative has been developed explicitly to bridge the gap between research and practice on visual climate change communication and emphasize human visual stories: the Climate Visuals project (Corner, Webster, and Teriete 2015). Developed by Climate Outreach, the Climate Visuals project is a practitioner-focused initiative, centering on a set of principles for effective visual communication on climate change, based on empirical research in the United States, the United Kingdom, and Germany (see Figure 17.2).

The language of **uncertainty**—so central to scientists' vocabulary—is typically unfamiliar to members of the public and may generate the impression that the science of climate change is less well understood than it actually is (Budescu, Broomell, and Por 2009; Corbett and Durfee 2004). The everyday meaning of uncertainty is negative and is commonly equated with ignorance (Shome and Marx 2009). When people with initially different views about the seriousness of climate change are presented with conflicting or uncertain information about it, they tend to assimilate the information in different ways and may even become more polarized in their views than they were previously (Corner et al. 2012; Kahan et al. 2011).

It has been argued that communication about climate change should be reframed away from uncertainty and oriented toward **risk**—a concept that most people are more familiar with (Pidgeon and Fischhoff 2011). Risk is the language of the insurance, health, and national security sectors; the more the risks of climate change can be brought to life through mental models (e.g., practical examples of the risks of sea level rise), the more likely it is that people will respond to climate risks in a proactive way. In a handbook focused on communicating uncertainty in climate change messages more effectively, Corner et al. (2015) outline a number of principles including starting messages with what's *known* rather than with what's *unknown*, reframing uncertainty as risk, and emphasizing the scientific (and wider social) consensus on climate change.

Narratives have become increasingly common among climate communicators (Shaw and Corner 2017). There are many different ways of defining "narrative": in the context of

1. **Show "real people,"** not staged photo-ops. Discussion groups favored "authentic" images over staged photographs, which were seen as gimmicky or even manipulative.

2. **Tell new stories.** Familiar images are quickly and easily understood, but they also prompted cynicism and fatigue. Less familiar, thought-provoking images can help tell new stories about climate change, and remake the visual representation of climate change in the public mind.

3. **Show climate causes at scale.** When communicating the links between problematic individual behaviors and climate change, it is best to show for instance, a congested highway, rather than a single driver.

4. **Climate impacts are emotionally powerful.** Images of climate impacts can prompt a desire to respond, but because they are emotionally powerful, they can also be overwhelming. Coupling images of climate impacts with concrete behavioral actions may help overcome this.

5. **Show local (but serious) climate impacts.** When images of localized climate impacts show an individual person or group of people, with identifiable emotions, they are likely to be most powerful. It is also important to strike a balance, to show local, relatable impacts, and simultaneously avoid trivializing the issue.

6. **Be careful with protest imagery.** Images of "typical environmentalists" only resonated with people who already considered themselves activists and campaigners. Images showing people directly affected by climate change impacts were seen as more authentic and compelling.

7. **Understand your audience.** Reactions to climate imagery differ according to level of concern, skepticism, as well as political affiliations. For instance, images of distant climate impacts produced flatter emotional responses among those on the political right than the left, whereas solutions images produced positive emotions for both sides.

Figure 17.2   Seven principles for visual climate change communication
Source: Adapted from Climate Outreach (2004).

environmental science communication, we define narratives as stories that describe a problem, lay out its consequences and suggest solutions (Hermville 2016). Stories are also a way of building more sustainable and meaningful engagement with science (Corner and Clarke 2017; Shaw 2016). The use of narratives that connect climate change to personal experiences and concerns can help public audiences understand complex science, making it easier to remember and process (Bekker et al. 2013; Dahlstrom 2014; Kanouse et al. 2016; Winterbottom et al. 2008; Westerhoff and Robinson 2013).

A different way in which climate change narratives have been used is the conveying of apocalyptic futures, in movies such as *The Day After Tomorrow* that present a vision of a world devastated by inaction on climate change. Some research suggests that fear-inducing messages can prompt action among the public (e.g., Howell 2011; Lowe et al. 2006) and environmentalists (Veldman 2012), yet others argue that such messages can bring about "apocalypse fatigue" (Nordhaus and Shellenberger 2009). Messages of hope have been found to increase action in some cases (Ojala 2011) and reduce it in others by lowering risk perceptions (Hornsey and Fielding 2016). Although fear-based messages hold potential to change attitudes (Witte and Allen 2000), the impact of fear appeals is context and audience specific (Das, de Wit, and Stroebe 2003; Hoog, Stroebe, and de Wit 2005). Simply invoking fear without pointing to a means of attenuating it is unlikely to be an effective communication strategy (O'Neill and Nicholson-Cole 2009). Some of these key insights are condensed in a recent guide produced for the Intergovernmental Panel on Climate Change (IPCC) by Climate Outreach (Corner, Shaw, and Clarke 2018), which outlines a set of six recommendations (summarized in Figure 17.3).

1. **Be a confident communicator**

    Scientists are generally highly trusted. Use an authentic voice to communicate effectively with any audience.

2. **Talk about the real world, not abstract ideas**

    Although they define the science and policy discourse, the "big numbers" of climate change (global average temperature targets and concentrations of atmospheric carbon dioxide) don't relate to people's day-to-day experiences. Start your climate conversation on common ground, using clear language and examples audiences are familiar with.

3. **Connect with what matters to your audience**

    Research consistently shows that people's values and political views have a bigger influence on their attitudes about climate change than their level of scientific knowledge. Connect with widely shared public values, or points of local interest in communication and engagement so that your science will be heard.

4. **Tell a human story**

    Most people understand the world through anecdotes and stories, rather than statistics and graphs. Aim for a narrative structure and show the human face behind the science when presenting information to help tell a compelling story.

5. **Lead with what you know**

    Uncertainty is a feature of climate science that shouldn't be ignored or sidelined, but can become a major stumbling block in conversations with nonscientists. Focus on the knowns before the unknowns and emphasize the depth of scientific understanding before moving onto what is less established.

6. **Use the most effective visual communication**

    Choose images and graphs in an evidence-based way, along with verbal and written communication. The Climate Visuals project offers a useful set of tools for how to communicate effectively with visuals.

Figure 17.3   Six principles for IPCC authors to use in public engagement
Source: Adapted from Corner et al. (2018).

Communicating the Impacts of Climate Change

Experiencing extreme weather can affect people's concern about climate change as well as the level of support for policies and climate adaptation more widely (Demski et al. 2017; Renn 2011; November, Penelas, and Viot 2009; Spence et al. 2011; Capstick et al. 2013). It has also been argued, however, that for extreme weather events to influence views in these ways, such events must be directly attributed in a person's mind to climate change (Ogunbode et al. 2019). People's ability to effectively cope with such events via personal resilience could itself undermine associated levels of concern about climate change or intentions to act on it (Ogunbode et al.).

Climate change can seem distant in space and time, uncertain, and prone to happen to other people—what has been termed its **"psychological distance"** (Spence, Poortinga, and

Pidgeon 2012)—which is often used to argue for communication that can heighten the immediacy of climate change, for example by drawing attention to local impacts. As climate change increasingly comes to be **framed** in urgent terms, these types of issue will be important to consider where **framing** communication, with respect to the types of response that are sought from people (Brügger et al. 2015).

The science of "attributing" weather events to climate change is progressing rapidly, allowing scientists to state with increasing confidence the extent to which a particular weather event was made more (or less) likely by climate change. Marshall (2014) cautions that there is a high risk of ill-designed messaging around extreme weather events backfiring, potentially leading to the reinforcement of existing cultural divides or promoting a backlash against communicators (for example, messages conveyed by environmentalists as "I told you so"). Yet, personal experience and real-life stories that can generate empathy, offering the prospect of communicating about climate change in new, powerful, and convincing ways.

Health professionals may also be concerned to communicate directly about the problems arising from extreme weather events, especially the additional risks to vulnerable populations. The elderly and people with chronic illnesses are among those most susceptible to health problems and increased mortality from periods of intense heat (Kovats and Hajat 2008; Semenza et al. 1999; Semenza et al. 1996), and so are among those most at risk from the consequences of climate change (McGeehin and Mirabelli 2001).

Commonly provided health advice designed to reduce the risks from heat events includes the avoidance of alcohol, reduction in physical activity, and regular hydration (Hajat, O'Connor, and Kosatsky 2010). However, the passive dissemination of advice through websites is unlikely to be effective, given that high-risk groups include those who are socially isolated or who may have a disability with a cognitive and/or behavioral component (Kovats and Ebi 2006). In their research Lane et al. (2013), for example, found that although most elderly people and caregivers understood the dangers of heat and the importance of age as a risk factor, nevertheless age was seen primarily as an issue for "other people."

Wolf et al. (2010) suggest that a successful communication strategy for preventing heat morbidity should include provision of advice to the general population, in combination with tailored messages for those especially vulnerable, for example, those over age seventy-five. Sampson et al. (2013) suggest that it is important for health practitioners to recognize the importance of cultural and economic factors that influence susceptibility to heat. For example, individuals may hold the view that having previously lived in a warmer climate lowers a person's vulnerability to heat events or may be constrained by economic circumstances leading to unwillingness to use air conditioning (Toloo et al. 2013).

CLINICAL CORRELATES 17.1 PROFESSIONAL SOCIETIES BACKING PATIENTS

Health professional organizations are adopting policies and resolutions to support climate justice. They are working to educate members on the intersection of climate and health and advocate for at-risk populations. In the past few years, the Nurses Climate Challenge is a national campaign by Alliance of Nurses for Healthy Environments and Health Care Without Harm to engage 50,000 health professionals by 2022 (Schenk, Cook, and Demorest 2020). The American College of Physicians (ACP) released a position paper with specific policy recommendations and action items for physicians working to reduce the harmful health effects of climate change (Crowley 2016). The American Academy of Pediatrics (AAP) has a Council on Environmental Health dedicated to local and national policy development and engagement (Council on Environmental Health 2015).

Health professional organizations are creating policies that educate and advocate for climate action to protect the youngest and oldest on the planet from increasing climatic threats.

Communicating Climate Change through a Focus on Public Health

When there are so many other challenges facing healthcare providers, why take on the problem of climate change as well? Writing in the *British Medical Journal* in 2013, Anthony Costello and colleagues of the Institute for Global Health argue that the implications of climate change for public health are "profoundly worrying" and that health practitioners "need to shout from the rooftops that climate change is a health problem" (Costello et al. 2013). They argue that those working in health cannot escape a responsibility for reducing carbon emissions any more than they can for alleviating poverty or reducing tobacco use.

Writing in the *Lancet's* series on Health and Climate Change in 2010, Prof. Mike Gill and Dr. Robin Stott are of the view that there is no group better placed than health professionals to spell out the importance of acting on climate change (Gill and Stott 2009). They argue that health practitioners have an important story to tell about the links between climate change and health, and possess the public trust needed that will help this to be heard, adding, "We must be innovative and imaginative in how we amplify the voice of health practitioners, and disseminate the message, its significance to us all, and its urgency, by using all our existing networks."

The 2018 *Lancet Countdown on Health and Climate Change* is also clear that there is a need to ensure "a widespread understanding of climate change as a central public health issue . . . with the health profession beginning to rise to this challenge." In 2019, the *Lancet Countdown* report affirms this position, arguing that "the life of every child born today will be affected by climate change. Without accelerated intervention, this new era will come to define the health of people at every stage of their lives" (Watts et al. 2019).

As early as 1993, Edward Maibach and his colleagues explored the overlap between public perceptions of climate change and its health impacts, and lessons from the public health sector for climate change communicators (Maibach 1993; Maibach, Roser-Renouf, and Leiserowitz 2008). The potential advantages of using a public health frame have since been stressed by a number of authors in recent years (we use the term "frame" or "framing" here to refer to the selection and/or emphasis of particular meanings within communication). Nisbet (2009) suggests that communication about climate change that connects to health problems already familiar and seen as important (e.g., heatstroke and asthma) can make the issue seem more personally relevant. A public health frame can make climate change seem more locally relevant, replacing distant imagery typically used in climate change communication (for example, remote Arctic regions) with more socially proximate neighborhoods and localities. Affirming the health benefits of taking action on climate change offers an engaging frame of reference that makes climate change seem more personally significant and relevant to people (Maibach et al. (2010). These findings are consistent with other work from both health and climate change communication research, that emphasizing a "gain" frame (focusing on the benefits of action, rather than the negative consequences of not acting) produces more positive attitudes toward taking action on climate change (Spence and Pidgeon 2010; Rothman et al. 2006).

Myers et al. (2012) tested different messages about climate change framed either as an environmental, public health, or national security risk, concluding that a public health framing of climate change has the potential to inspire hope in a way more consistent with support for taking action on climate change. Maibach et al. (2011) note that a public health frame offers the prospect of shifting the climate change debate from one based on environmental values to one based on public health values, which are more widely held irrespective of ideology and political outlook. Kotcher et al. (2018) found that informing people about the health implications of global warming increased public engagement with the issue and reduced differences in opinion across political lines.

As well as stressing the advantages of applying a health frame to promote engagement with climate change, health practitioners have also emphasized the co-benefits that acting on health can bring for climate change and vice versa. McMichael et al. (2009) argue that well-judged mitigation policies also have the advantage of bringing health gains, with benefits accrued from moving away from air-polluting energy generation, choosing transport methods that encourage physical activity and social contact, and changing carbon-intensive food choices. Maibach et al. (2011) argue that health practitioners should reinforce the point that taking action can result in a win-win situation. A health care analogy can be useful in helping people understand that we often consider it wise to act when there is widespread agreement on a subject, even if this is not unanimous: if 95 percent of the world's leading pediatricians were to agree that a child was seriously ill, most parents would likely act on their advice, rather than on that of the 5 percent who disagree.

Frumkin and McMichael (2008) and Maibach et al. (2008) have drawn attention to the use of **social marketing** in promoting health behaviors and to encourage appropriate responses to climate change at the personal and collective level. McKenzie-Mohr (2013) suggest the use of social marketing to foster sustainable, pro-environmental behaviors based on a five-stage approach: the selection of specific behaviors to be changed or promoted; identification of the barriers and benefits of behavior change; development of appropriate strategies; piloting of the strategy; and broad-scale implementation and evaluation, Despite evidence that social marketing techniques for behavior change can be successful (Gordon et al. 2006), some authors caution about its limitations as a strategy for climate change engagement. Corner and Randall (2011) argue that one cannot "sell" climate change in the same way commercial goods are sold and that motivating a proportional response to climate change (i.e., bringing about more than small-scale and piecemeal behavior change) requires engaging people at a deeper level than is possible with social marketing.

A number of researchers suggest that using tailored and targeted health communication can also be applied to communicating climate change, premised on the notion that specific messages resonate with particular audiences (Noar et al. 2011; McKenzie-Mohr 2000). Such a **segmentation** approach in the area of climate change has been developed by the Yale Project on Climate Change Communication, who make the case that climate change is perceived differently across six attitudinal groups, termed "Global Warming's Six Americas" (Leiserowitz et al. 2013; Maibach et al. 2011; Leiserowitz and Smith 2010). As a consequence of these different, yet coherent, ways of understanding climate change, they argue that public education and engagement strategies are most likely to be successful when tailored to these target audiences (Maibach et al. 2011). Specific strategies for engaging those who are already concerned about climate change include providing information about what kind of actions can be taken to limit climate change; for those who are least concerned about climate change (or may dispute its existence), information relating to how climate scientists know that climate change is real, or caused by humans, is more relevant (Roser-Renouf et al. 2014).

Bostrom, Böhm and O'Connor (2013) also argue that targeting and tailoring climate change communication makes sense, based on experience from health risk communication, while cautioning that direct evidence of the effectiveness of tailoring climate change communication remains elusive to date. Other researchers have adopted a variety of alternative approaches to dividing up publics to customize communication to particular groups (Agyeman et al. 2007; Featherstone et al. 2009; Rose, Dade, and Scott 2007).

As well as giving consideration to audience characteristics and the structure of communication, it is worth bearing in mind that health practitioners are themselves in a distinctive position with respect to being able to convey messages. As Frumkin and McMichael (2008) note, the health sector has an opportunity to demonstrate leadership on climate change because health professionals are seen as having moral authority, professional prestige, and a reputation for science-based analysis. Because of their special position, health professionals are well placed to motivate people toward appropriate personal actions and collective decisions and to provide guidance to industry and policymakers. Indeed, health professionals may be able to exert political influence in the area of climate change mitigation through clear messages about the substantial public health benefits that such policies can also bring. Even skeptical politicians convinced that global warming is a scientific fraud cannot ignore proposals that directly improve the health of their constituents (Bloomberg and Aggarwala 2008).

CLINICAL CORRELATES 17.2 CLIMATE ACTIVISM AND THE PHYSICIAN

Climate change communication is not a routine part of curriculum and training for most practicing clinicians. Time constraints and other barriers often slow engagement following training. Yet clinicians have many skills sets that easily translate to communicating complex topics such as climate change with broad audiences. They also have unique lenses in which to view problems as they emerge, particularly for socially and medically vulnerable populations. A few simple steps for communicating climate change with others includes connecting on common values, being solutions focused, describing rather than labeling, and delivering a disciplined message (ecoAmerica 2013). Such an approach is part of most doctors' communication skills, and can be delivered when discussing health conditions, breaking bad news, or motivational interviewing with patients at the bedside.

Clinicians are trusted messengers with unique written and oral skills that translate to various audiences including patients, policymakers, scientists, colleagues, and the public.

Summary

The communication of climate change can be approached in a number of different ways, with a range of decisions required as to how language, imagery, narratives, emotional content, and values are portrayed. Now that the impacts of climate change are manifesting for people across the world, climate change is becoming a more current and local issue, although careful consideration is needed to communicate appropriately in ways that do not alienate audiences. The structuring of communication in ways that emphasize the linkages between climate change and health offers a unique opportunity to engage people with the issue of climate change, in terms that may be more relatable. Health professionals are uniquely placed to present these messages to the public and decision-makers. Their position in society and ability to understand and translate science-based issues makes them well placed to support efforts to address and communicate about climate change. Framing climate change as a health issue may work for some audiences, yet it does not *always* engage *all* audiences most effectively. Further research to build the evidence base on climate-health communication in the United States and beyond will help ensure that the potential for health practitioners to become powerful evidence-based climate advocates can be realized.

DISCUSSION QUESTIONS

1. What role do values, worldviews, and political beliefs play in determining how people understand and respond to messages about climate change?

2. What are the best ways to communicate risk and uncertainty?

3. What are the most appropriate ways to communicate the personal relevance and urgency of climate change?

4. Why might it be advantageous to stress issues of public health when communicating about climate change?

KEY TERMS

Climate change communication: Material designed to inform, persuade, or engage about climate change, which may be delivered face to face or using a variety of media.

Cultural worldview: A preference for a particular type of social control and organization; for example, egalitarians emphasize equal status and collective problem-solving whereas individualists emphasize personal autonomy and economic freedom.

Frames, framing: The selection and emphasis of particular meanings in communication, for example, a "public health frame" in climate change communication stresses the relevance of public health to climate change.

Information deficit model: A common or default assumption in communication that the audience requires education, information, or facts in order to be engaged with a topic.

Narratives: Stories and meaning-making in communication, for example, through relating climate change to people's real-life experiences.

Pro-environmental behavior: Personal action that contributes to addressing climate change, such as reducing energy usage in the home.

Psychological distance: The perception of being disconnected from an issue such as climate change; psychological distance has four dimensions: temporal (distance in time), social (distance between oneself and others), spatial (geographical distance), and uncertainty (how certain it is that an event will happen).

Public engagement: The extent to which people are cognitively, affectively (emotionally), and behaviorally connected with a problem such as climate change.

Risk: The potential for consequences where something of value is at stake and where outcomes are uncertain.

Segmentation: The use of statistical techniques to group a population according to common characteristics.

Skepticism (with regard to climate change): The holding of doubts about the physical reality, human causation, or importance of climate change and/or concerning the ability of human action to effectively address it.

Social marketing: The application of principles from commercial marketing for socially desirable ends.

Uncertainty: The probability that a statement is (in)valid; the IPCC uses shorthand statements (such as "very likely") to equate to numerical probabilities (e.g. "very likely" corresponds to ">90 percent probability").

Value: In the psychology literature, a guiding principle in the life of a person.

References and Further Reading

Abrahamson, V., J. Wolf, I. Lorenzoni, B. Fenn, R. S. Kovats, P. Wilkinson, and R. Raine. 2009. "Perceptions of Heatwave Risks to Health: Interview-Based Study of Older People in London and Norwich, UK." *Journal of Public Health* 31 (1):119–26.

Agyeman, J., B. Doppelt, K. Lynn, and H. Hatic. 2007. "The Climate-Justice Link: Communicating Risk with Low-Income and Minority Audiences." In *Creating a Climate for Change*, edited by S. Moser and L. Dilling, 119–38. Cambridge, UK: Cambridge University Press.

Ahern, M., R. Kovats, P. Wilkinson, R. Few, and F. Matthies. 2005. "Global Health Impacts of Floods: Epidemiologic Evidence." *Epidemiologic Reviews* 27 (1):36–46.

Akerlof, K., R. DeBono, P. Berry, A. Leiserowitz, C. Roser-Renouf, K. L. Clarke, A. Rogaeva, M. Nisbet, M. Weathers, and E. W. Maibach. 2010. "Public Perceptions of Climate Change as a Human Health Risk: Surveys of the United States, Canada and Malta." *International Journal of Environmental Research and Public Health* 7 (6):2559–2606.

Anderegg, W., J. Prall, J. Harold, and S. Schneider. 2010. "Expert Credibility in Climate Change.: *Proceedings of the National Academy of Sciences of the USA* 107 (27):12107–9.

Ballew, M., J. Marlon, A. Leiserowitz, and E. Maibach. 2018. *Gender Differences in Public Understanding of Climate Change*. New Haven, CT: Yale Program on Climate Change Communication.

Bellamy, R., and M. Hulme. 2011. "Beyond the Tipping Point: Understanding Perceptions of Abrupt Climate Change and Their Implications." *Weather, Climate & Society* 3 (1):48–60.

Bekker, H. L., A. E. Winterbottom, P. Butow, A. J. Dillard, D. Feldman-Stewart, F. J. Fowler, M. L. Jibaja-Weiss, V. A. Shaffer, and R. J. Volk. 2013. "Do Personal Stories Make Patient Decision Aids More Effective? A Critical Review of Theory and Evidence." *BMC Medical Informatics and Decision Making* 13 (suppl 2):S9. doi: 10.1186/1472-6947-13-S2-S9.

Bloomberg, M., and R. Aggarwala. 2008. "Think Locally, Act Globally: How Curbing Global Warming Emissions Can Improve Local Public Health." *American Journal of Preventive Medicine* 35 (5):414–23.

Bolderdijk, J., L. Steg, E. Geller, P. Lehman, and T. Postmes. 2013. "Comparing the Effectiveness of Monetary versus Moral Motives in Environmental Campaigning." *Nature Climate Change* 3 (4):413–16.

Bostrom, A., G. Böhm, and R. O'Connor. 2013. "Targeting and Tailoring Climate Change Communications." *WIREs Climate Change* 4 (5):447–55.

Bostrom, A., M.. Granger-Morgan, B. Fischoff, and D. Read. 1994. "What Do People Know about Global Climate Change?" *Risk Analysis* 14 (6):959–70.

Brody, S., S. Zahran, A. Vedlitz, and H. Grover. 2008. "Examining the Relationship between Physical Vulnerability and Public Perceptions of Global Climate Change in the United States." *Environment and Behavior* 40 (1):72–95.

Brugger, A., S. Dessai, P. Devine-Wright, T. A. Morton, and N. Pidgeon. 2015. "Psychological Responses to the Proximity of Climate Change." *Nature Climate Change* 5 (12):1031–37.

Brulle, R., J. Carmichael, and J. Jenkins. 2012. "Shifting Public Opinion on Climate Change: An Empirical Assessment of Factors Influencing Concern over Climate Change in the US, 2002–2010." *Climatic Change* 114 (2):169–88.

Budescu, D., S. Broomell, and H. Por. 2009. "Improving Communication of Uncertainty in the Reports of the Intergovernmental Panel on Climate Change." *Psychological Science* 20 (3):299–308.

Capstick, S., N. Pidgeon, and M. Whitehead. 2013. *Public Perceptions of Climate Change in Wales: Summary Findings of a Survey of the Welsh Public Conducted during November and December 2012*. Cardiff: Climate Change Consortium of Wales.

Capstick, S., and N. Pidgeon. 2014a. "What *Is* Climate Change Skepticism? Examination of the Concept Using a Mixed Methods Study of the UK Public." *Global Environmental Change* 24:389–401.

Capstick, S., and N. Pidgeon. 2014b. "Public Perception of Cold Weather as Evidence for and against Climate Change." *Climatic Change* 122 (4):695–708.

Capstick, S., L. Whitmarsh, W. Poortinga, N. Pidgeon, and P. Upham. 2015. "International Trends in Public Perceptions of Climate Change over the Past Quarter Century." *WIREs: Climate Change* 6 (1):35–61.

Cardwell, F., and S. Elliott. 2013. "Making the Links: Do We Connect Climate Change with Health? A Qualitative Case Study from Canada." *BMC Public Health* 13 (1):208.

Chapman, D., B. Lickel, and M. Markowitz. 2017. "Reassessing Emotion in Climate Change Communication." *Nature Climate Change* 7:850–52.

Clarke, J., A. Corner, and R. Webster. 2018. *Public Engagement for a 1.5 °C World: Shifting Gear and Scaling up*. Oxford: Climate Outreach.

Climate Outreach. 2004. "The 7 Climate Visuals Principles." https://climatevisuals.org/7-climate-visuals-principles.

Coninck, H., A. Revi, M. Babiker, P. Bertoldi, M. Buckeridge, M. Cartwright, W. Dong, et al. 2018. "Chapter 4: Strengthening and Implementing the Global Response." In *Global Warming of 1.5°C. An IPCC Special Report on the Impacts of Global Warming of 1.5°C above Pre-Industrial Levels and Related Global Greenhouse Gas Emission Pathways, in the Context of Strengthening the Global Response to the Threat of Climate Change, Sustainable Development, and Efforts to Eradicate Poverty,* edited by V. Masson-Delmotte, P. Zhai, H.-O. Pörtner, D. Roberts, J. Skea, P. R. Shukla, A. Pirani, W. Moufouma-Okia et al. Geneva: Intergovernmental Panel on Climate Change. http://report.ipcc.ch/sr15/pdf/sr15_chapter4.pdf.

Corbett, J., and J. Durfee. 2004. "Testing Public (Un) Certainty of Science Media Representations of Global Warming." *Science Communication* 26 (2):129–51.

Corner, A., and J. Clarke. 2017. *Talking Climate: From Research to Practice in Public Engagement.* Cham: Springer International Publishing. doi: 10.1007/978-3-319-46744-3.

Corner, A., S. Lewandowsky, M. Phillips, and O. Roberts. 2015. *The Uncertainty Handbook.* Bristol: University of Bristol.

Corner, A., C. Shaw, and J. Clarke. 2018. *Principles for Effective Communication and Public Engagement on Climate Change: A Handbook for IPCC Authors.* Oxford: Climate Outreach. https://climateoutreach.org/resources/ipcc-communications-handbook/.

Corner, A., E. Markowitz, and N. Pidgeon. 2014. "Public Engagement with Climate Change: The Role of Human Values." *WIREs Climate Change* 5:411–22.

Corner, A., and A. Randall. 2011. "Selling Climate Change? The Limitations of Social Marketing as a Strategy for Climate Change Public Engagement." *Global Environmental Change* 21 (3):1005–14.

Corner, A., R. Webster, and C. Teriete. 2015. *Climate Visuals: Seven Principles for Visual Climate Change Communication.* Oxford, England: Climate Outreach.

Corner, A., L. Whitmarsh, and D. Xenias. 2012. "Uncertainty, Skepticism and Attitudes towards Climate Change: Biased Assimilation and Attitude Polarization." *Climatic Change* 114 (3–4):463–78.

Costello, A., H. Montgomery, and N. Watts. 2013. "Climate Change: The Challenge for Healthcare Professionals (Editorial)." *BMJ* 347:f6060, doi:10.1136/bmj.f606.

Council on Environmental Health. 2015. "Global Climate Change and Children's Health." *Pediatrics* 136 (5):992–97.

Crompton, T. 2010. *Common Cause: The Case for Working with Our Cultural Values.* Woking, UK: WWF-UK. https://assets.wwf.org.uk/downloads/common_cause_report.pdf.

Crompton, T. 2011. "Finding Cultural Values that Can Transform the Climate Change Debate." *Solutions* 2 (4):56–63.

Crowley, R. A. and Health, Public Policy Committee of the American College of Physicians. 2016. "Climate Change and Health: A Position Paper of the American College of Physicians." *Annals of Internal Medicine* 164 (9):608–10.

Dahlstrom, M. F. 2014. "Using Narratives and Storytelling to Communicate Science with Non-Expert Audiences." *Proceedings of the National Academy of Sciences of the USA* 11 (4):13614–20. doi: 10.1073/pnas.1320645111.

Das, E., J. de Wit, and W. Stroebe. 2003. "Fear Appeals Motivate Acceptance of Action Recommendations: Evidence for a Positive Bias in the Processing of Persuasive Messages." *Personality and Social Psychology Bulletin* 29 (5):650–64.

Demeritt, D., and S. Nobert. 2014. "Models of Best Practice in Flood Risk Communication and Management." *Environmental Hazards* 13 (4):313–28.

Demski, C. C., S. Capstick, N. Pidgeon, R. G. Sposato, and A. Spence. 2017. "Experience of Extreme Weather Affects Climate Change Mitigation and Adaptation Responses." *Climatic Change* 140 (2):149–64. https://doi.org/10.1007/s10584-016-1837-4.

Druckman, J. N., and M. C. McGrath. 2019. "The Evidence for Motivated Reasoning in Climate Change Preference Formation." *Nature Climate Change* 9:111–19.

Dunlap, R. E., J. K. Grieneeks, and M. Rokeach. 1983. "Human Values and Pro-Environmental Behavior." In *Energy and Material Resources: Attitudes, Values, and Public Policy,* edited by W. Conn. Boulder, CO, Westview.

Dunlap, R., and A. McCright. 2008. "A Widening Gap: Republican and Democratic Views on Climate Change." *Environment: Science and Policy for Sustainable Development* 50 (5):26–35.

ecoAmerica. 2013. *Communicating on Climate: 13 Steps and Guiding Principles.* https://ecoamerica.org/wp-content/uploads/2013/11/Communicating-on-Climate-13-steps_ecoAmerica.pdf.

Edwards, P., and I. Roberts. 2009. "Population Adiposity and Climate Change." *International Journal of Epidemiology* 38 (4):1137–40.

Engels, A., O. Hüther, M. Schäfer, and H. Held. 2013. "Public Climate-Change Skepticism, Energy Preferences and Political Participation." *Global Environmental Change* 23 (5):1018–27.

Evans, L., G. Maio, A. Corner, C. Hodgetts, S. Ahmed, and U. Hahn. 2013. "Self-Interest and Pro-Environmental Behavior." *Nature Climate Change* 3 (2):122–25.

Featherstone, H., E. Weitkamp, K. Ling, and F. Burnet. 2009. "Defining Issue-Based Publics for Public Engagement: Climate Change as a Case Study." *Public Understanding of Science* 18 (2):214–28.

Feinberg, M., and R. Willer. 2010. "Apocalypse Soon?: Dire Messages Reduce Belief in Global Warming by Contradicting Just-World Beliefs." *Psychological Science* 22 (1):34–38.

Feldman, L., and S. Hart. 2018. "Climate Change as a Polarizing Cue: Framing Effects on Public Support for Low-Carbon Energy Policies." *Global Environmental Change* 51:54–66.

Frumkin, H., and A. McMichael. 2008. "Climate Change and Public Health: Thinking, Communicating, Acting." *American Journal of Preventive Medicine* 35 (5):403–10.

Gallup. 2019. "Americans' Views on Global Warming, 2019." Gallup Online. https://news.gallup.com/poll/248030/americans-views-global-warming-2019-trends.aspx.

Ganten, D., A. Haines, and R. Souhami. 2010. "Health Co-Benefits of Policies to Tackle Climate Change." *Lancet* 376 (9755):1802–4.

Gill, M., and R. Stott. 2009. "Health Professionals Must Act to Tackle Climate Change." *Lancet* Published online November 25, 2009. doi:10.1016/S0140-6736(09)61830-4.

Gordon, R., L. McDermott, M. Stead, and K. Angus. 2006. "The Effectiveness of Social Marketing Interventions for Health Improvement: What's the Evidence?" *Public Health* 120 (12):1133–39.

Gustafson, A., P. Bergquist, A. Leiserowitz, and E. Maibach. 2019. "A Growing Majority of Americans Think Global Warming Is Happening and Are Worried." New Haven, CT: Yale Program on Climate Change Communication. https://climatecommunication.yale.edu/publications/a-growing-majority-of-americans-think-global-warming-is-happening-and-are-worried/.

Haines, A., R. Kovats, D. Campbell-Lendrum, and C. Corvalán. 2006. "Climate Change and Human Health: Impacts, Vulnerability and Public Health." *Public Health* 120 (7):585–96.

Hajat, S., M. O'Connor, and T. Kosatsky. 2010. "Health Effects of Hot Weather: From Awareness of Risk Factors to Effective Health Protection." *Lancet* 375 (9717):856–63.

Hart, P. S., and L. Feldman. 2018. "Would It Be Better to Not Talk about Climate Change? The Impact of Climate Change and Air Pollution Frames on Support for Regulating Power Plant Emissions." *Journal of Environmental Psychology* 60:1–8. doi: 10.1016/j.jenvp.2018.08.013.

Hatcher, M., D. Allensworth, and F. Butterfoss. 2010. "Promoting Community Health. In *Health Promotion Programs: From Theory to Practice*, edited by C. Fertman and D. Allensworth. San Francisco: Jossey-Bass.

Hathaway, J., and E. Maibach. 2018. "Health Implications of Climate Change: A Review of the Literature About the Perception of the Public and Health Professionals." *Current Environmental Health Reports* 5:197–204.

Hermville, L. 2016. "The Role of Narratives in Socio-Technical Transitions—Fukushima And The Energy Regimes of Japan, Germany, and the United Kingdom." *Energy Research and Social Science* (January):237–46.

Hirabayashi, Y., R. Mahendran, S. Koirala, L. Konoshima, D. Yamazaki, S. Watanabe, H. Kim, and S. Kanae. 2013. "Global Flood Risk under Climate Change." *Nature Climate Change* 3 (9):816–21.

Hobson, K., and S. Niemeyer. 2013. "'What Skeptics Believe': The Effects of Information and Deliberation on Climate Change Skepticism." *Public Understanding of Science* 22 (4):396–412.

Hoog, N., W. Stroebe, and J. de Wit. 2005. "The Impact of Fear Appeals on Processing and Acceptance of Action Recommendations." *Personality & Social Psychology Bulletin* 31:24–33.

Höppner, C., and L. Whitmarsh. 2011. "Public Engagement in Climate Action: Policy and Public Expectations." In *Engaging the Public with Climate Change: Communication and Behavior Change*, edited by L. Whitmarsh, S. O'Neill, and I. Lorenzoni. London: Earthscan.

Hornsey, M., and Fielding, K. 2016. "A Cautionary Note about Messages of Hope: Focusing on Progress in Reducing Carbon Emissions Weakens Mitigation Motivation." *Global Environmental Change* 39:26–34.

Howell, R. 2011. "Lights, Camera ... Action? Altered Attitudes and Behaviour in Response to the Climate Change Film *The Age of Stupid*." *Global Environmental Change* 21:177–187.

Hulme, M. 2009. *Why We Disagree about Climate Change*. Cambridge, UK: Cambridge University Press.

Intergovernmental Panel on Climate Change. 2013. "Summary for Policymakers." In *Climate Change 2013: The Physical Science Basis. Contribution of Working Group I to the Fifth Assessment Report of the Intergovernmental Panel on Climate Change*, edited by T. Stocker, D. Qin, G.-K. Plattner, M. Tignor, S. Allen, J. Boschung, A. Nauels et al. Cambridge, UK: Cambridge University Press.

Kahan, D. 2010. "Fixing the Communications Failure." *Nature* 463:296–97.

Kahan, D., H. Jenkins-Smith, and D. Braman. 2011. "Cultural Cognition of Scientific Consensus." *Journal of Risk Research* 14 (2):147–74.

Kahan, D., E. Peters, M. Wittlin, P. Slovic, L. Ouellette, D. Braman, and G. Mandel. 2012. "The Polarizing Impact of Science Literacy and Numeracy on Perceived Climate Change Risks." *Nature Climate Change* 2:732–35.

Kanouse, D. E., M. Schlesinger, D. Shaller, S. C. Martino, and L. Rybowski. 2016. "How Patient Comments Affect Consumers' Use of Physician Performance Measures." *Medical Care* 54:24–31. doi:10.1097/MLR.0000000000000443.

Kellstedt, P., S. Zahran, and A. Vedlitz. 2008. "Personal Efficacy, the Information Environment, and Attitudes toward Global Warming and Climate Change in the United States." *Risk Analysis* 28 (1):113–26.

Kempton, W. 1991. "Lay Perspectives on Global Climate Change." *Global Environmental Change* 1 (3):183–208.

Kempton, W. 1997. "How the Public Views Climate Change." *Environment* 39 (9):12–21.

Kosatsky, T., J. Dufresne, L. Richard, A. Renouf, N. Giannetti, J. Bourbeau, M. Julien, J. Braidy, and C. Sauve. 2009. "Heat Awareness and Response among Montreal Residents with Chronic Cardiac and Pulmonary Disease." *Canadian Journal of Public Health* 100:237–40.

Kotcher, J., E. Maibach, M. Montoro, and S. J. Hassol. 2018. "How Americans Respond to Information about Global Warming's Health Impacts: Evidence from a National Survey Experiment." *GeoHealth* 2. https://doi.org/10.1029/2018GH000154.

Kovats, R., and K. Ebi. 2006. "Heatwaves and Public Health in Europe." *European Journal of Public Health* 16 (6):592–99.

Kovats, R., and S. Hajat. 2008. "Heat Stress and Public Health: A Critical Review." *Annual Review of Public Health* 29:41–55.

Lane, K., K. Wheeler, K. Charles-Guzman, M. Ahmed, M. Blum, K. Gregory, G. Nathan, N. Clark, and T. Matte. 2013. "Extreme Heat Awareness and Protective Behaviors in New York City." *Journal of Urban Health* 91 (3):403–14.

Lee, T., E. Markowitz, P. Howe, C. Ko, and A. Leiserowitz. 2015. "Predictors of Public Climate Change Awareness and Risk Perception around the World." *Nature Climate Change* 27 July 2015. doi: 10.1038/NCLIMATE2728. http://sciencepolicy.colorado.edu/students/envs3173/lee2015.pdf

Leiserowitz, A. 2006. "Climate Change Risk Perception and Policy Preferences: The Role of Affect, Imagery, and Values." *Climatic Change* 77:45–72.

Leiserowitz, A. 2007. "Communicating the Risks of Global Warming: American Risk Perceptions, Affective Images, and Interpretive Communities." In *Creating a Climate for Change*, edited by S. Moser and L. Dilling. Cambridge, UK: Cambridge University Press.

Leiserowitz, A., and K. Akerlof. 2010. *Race, Ethnicity and Public Responses to Climate Change*. New Haven, CT: Yale Project on Climate Change Communication. https://climatecommunication.yale.edu/publications/race-ethnicity-and-public-responses-to-climate-change/.

Leiserowitz, A., Maibach, E., Roser-Renouf, C., Feinberg, G., and Howe, P. (2013). *Global Warming's Six Americas in September 2012*. Yale University and George Mason University. New Haven, CT: Yale Project on Climate Change Communication. https://climatecommunication.yale.edu/publications/global-warmings-six-americas-in-september-2012/.

Leiserowitz, A., E. Maibach, C. Roser-Renouf, and J. Hmielowski. 2011. *Politics & Global Warming: Democrats, Republicans, Independents, and the Tea Party*. New Haven, CT: Yale Project on Climate Change Communication. http://environment.yale.edu/climate/files/PoliticsGlobalWarming2011.pdf.

Leiserowitz, A., E. Maibach, C. Roser-Renouf, S. Rosenthal, M. Cutler, and J. Kotcher. 2018. *Climate Change in the American Mind: March 2018*. New Haven, CT: Yale Program on Climate Change Communication. https://climatecommunication.yale.edu/publications/climate-change-american-mind-march-2018/.

Leiserowitz, A., E. Maibach, C. Roser-Renouf, N. Smith, and E. Dawson. 2010. *Climate Change, Public Opinion and the Loss of Trust*. New Haven, CT: Yale Project on Climate Change Communication. http://environment.yale.edu/climate/publications/climategate-public-opinion-and-the-loss-of-trust.

Leiserowitz, A., and N. Smith. 2010. *Knowledge of Climate Change Across Global Warming's Six Americas*. New Haven, CT: Yale Project on Climate Change Communication. http://environment.yale.edu/climate-communication/files/Knowledge_Across_Six_Americas.pdf.

Lewandowsky, S., G. Gignac, and S. Vaughan. 2013. "The Pivotal Role of Perceived Scientific Consensus in Acceptance of Science." *Nature Climate Change* 3 (4):399–404.

Lichterman, J. 2000. "A 'Community as Resource' Strategy for Disaster Response." *Public Health Reports* 115 (2–3):262–65.

Lorenzoni, I., A. Leiserowitz, M. Doria, W. Poortinga, and N. Pidgeon. 2006. "Cross National Comparisons of Image Associations with 'Global Warming' and 'Climate Change' among Laypeople in the United States of America and Great Britain." *Journal of Risk Research* 9 (3):265–81.

Lowe, T., K. Brown, S. Dessai, M. de França Doria, K. Haynes, and K. Vincent. 2006. "Does Tomorrow Ever Come? Disaster Narrative and Public Perceptions of Climate Change." *Public Understanding of Science* 15 (4):435–57.

McLoughlin, N., A. Corner, J. Clarke, L. Whitmarsh, S. Capstick, and N. Nash. 2019. *Mainstreaming Low-Carbon Lifestyles*. Oxford: Climate Outreach.

McCright, A. 2010. "The Effects of Gender on Climate Change Knowledge and Concern in the American Public." *Population and Environment* 32 (1):66–87.

McCright, A. M., and R. E. Dunlap. 2011a. "Cool Dudes: The Denial of Climate Change among Conservative White Males in the United States." *Global Environmental Change* 21 (4):1163–72.

McCright, A., and R. Dunlap. 2011b. "The Politicization of Climate Change and Polarization in the American Public's Views of Global Warming, 2001–2010." *Sociological Quarterly* 52:155–94.

McGeehin, M., and M. Mirabelli. 2001. "The Potential Impacts of Climate Variability and Change on Temperature-Related Morbidity and Mortality in the United States." *Environmental Health Perspectives* 109 (suppl 2):185.

McKenzie-Mohr, D. 2000. "Promoting Sustainable Behavior: An Introduction to Community-Based Social Marketing." *Journal of Social Issues* 56 (3):543–54.

McKenzie-Mohr, D. 2013. *Fostering Sustainable Behavior: An Introduction to Community-Based Social Marketing*. Gabriola Island, BC: New Society Publishers.

McMichael, A., M. Neira, R. Bertollini, D. Campbell-Lendrum, and S. Hales. 2009. "Climate Change: A Time of Need and Opportunity for the Health Sector." *Lancet* 374:2123–25.

Maibach, E. 1993. "Social Marketing for the Environment: Using Information Campaigns to Promote Environmental Awareness and Behavior Change." *Health Promotion International* 8 (3):209–24.

Maibach, E., P. Baldwin, K. Akerlof, G. Diao, and M. Nisbet. 2010. "Reframing Climate Change as a Public Health Issue: An Exploratory Study of Public Reactions." *BMC Public Health* 10 (1):299.

Maibach, E., A. Leiserowitz, C. Roser-Renouf, and C. Mertz. 2011. "Identifying Like-Minded Audiences for Global Warming Public Engagement Campaigns: An Audience Segmentation Analysis and Tool Development." *PLoS One* 6 (3):e17571.

Maibach, E., C. Roser-Renouf, and A. Leiserowitz. 2008. "Communication and Marketing as Climate Change–Intervention Assets: A Public Health Perspective." *American Journal of Preventive Medicine* 35 (5):488–500.

Malka, A., J. Krosnick, and G. Langer. 2009. "The Association of Knowledge with Concern about Global Warming: Trusted Information Sources Shape Public Thinking." *Risk Analysis* 29 (5):633–47.

Manzo, K. 2010. "Beyond Polar Bears? Re-Envisioning Climate Change." *Meteorological Applications* 17 (2):196–208.

Markowitz, E., C. Hodge, and G. Harp. 2014. *Connecting on Climate: A Guide to Effective Climate Change Communication*. New York: Center for Research on Environmental Decisions; Washington, DC: ecoAmerica. www.connectingonclimate.org.

Marshall, G. 2014. *After the Floods: Communicating Climate Change around Extreme Weather*. Oxford: Climate Outreach Information Network.

Messling, L., A. Corner, J. Clarke, N. F. Pidgeon, C. Demski, and S. Capstick. 2015. *Communicating Flood Risks in a Changing Climate*. Oxford: Climate Outreach. https://climateoutreach.org/resources/communicating-flood-risks-in-a-changing-climate/.

Milly, P., R. Wetherald, K. Dunne, and T. Delworth. 2002. "Increasing Risk of Great Floods in a Changing Climate." *Nature* 415 (6871):514–17.

Mocker, V. 2012. "'Blue Valuing Green': Are Intrinsic Value Frames Better than Economic Arguments to Communicate Climate Change and Transport Policies to Conservative Audiences?" Master's thesis, Oxford University.

Moser, S. 2010. "Communicating Climate Change: History, Challenges, Process and Future Directions." *WIREs Climate Change* 1:31–53.

Moser, S.. and L. Dilling. 2011. "Communicating Climate Change: Closing the Science-Action Gap." In *Oxford Handbook of Climate Change and Society*, edited by R. Norgaard, D. Schlosberg, and J. Dryzek. Oxford: Oxford University Press.

Mossler, M. V., A. Bostrom, R. P. Kelly, K. M. Crosman, and P. Moy. 2017. "How Does Framing Affect Policy Support for Emissions Mitigation? Testing the Effects of Ocean Acidification and Other Carbon Emissions Frames." *Global Environmental Change* 45:63–78.

Myers, T. A., M. C. Nisbet, E. W. Maibach, and A. A. Leiserowitz. 2012. "A Public Health Frame Arouses Hopeful Emotions about Climate Change." *Climatic Change* 113 (3–4):1105–12.

National Academies of Sciences, Engineering, and Medicine. 2017. *Communicating Science Effectively: A Research Agenda.* Washington, DC: National Academies Press. doi: 10.17226/23674.

Nilsson, A., C. von Borgstede, and A. Biel. 2004. "Willingness to Accept Climate Change Strategies: The Effect of Values and Norms." *Journal of Environmental Psychology* 24 (3):267–77.

Nisbet, M. 2009. Communicating Climate Change: Why Frames Matter for Public Engagement." *Environment: Science and Policy for Sustainable Development* 51 (2):12–23.

Noar, S., N. Harrington, S. Van Stee, and R. Aldrich. 2011. "Tailored Health Communication to Change Lifestyle Behaviors." *American Journal of Lifestyle Medicine* 5 (2):112–22.

Nordhaus, T., and M. Shellenberger. 2009. "Apocalypse Fatigue: Losing the Public on Climate Change." *Yale Environment blog.* http://e360.yale.edu/feature/apocalypse_fatigue_losing_the_public_on_climate_change/2210/.

November, V., M. Penelas, and P. Viot. 2009. "When Flood Risk Transforms a Territory: The Lully Effect." *Geography* 94 (3):189–97.

O'Connor, R., R. Bord, and A. Fisher. 1999. "Risk Perceptions, General Environmental Beliefs, and Willingness to Address Climate Change." *Risk Analysis* 19 (3):461–71.

Ogunbode, C. A., C. Demski, S. B. Capstick, and R. G. Sposato. 2019. "Attribution Matters: Revisiting the Link between Extreme Weather Experience and Climate Change Mitigation Responses." *Global Environmental Change* 54:31–39. doi: 10.1016/j.gloenvcha.2018.11.005.

O'Neill, S. J. 2017. "Engaging with Climate Change Imagery." In *Oxford Encyclopedia of Climate Change Communication*, edited by M. C. Nisbit. Oxford, England: Oxford Research Encyclopedias.

O'Neill, S., M. Boykoff, S. Niemeyer, and S. Day. 2013. "On the Use of Imagery for Climate Change Engagement." *Global Environmental Change* 23 (2):413–21.

O'Neill, S., and S. Nicholson-Cole. 2009. "'Fear Won't Do It': Promoting Positive Engagement with Climate Change through Visual and Iconic Representations." *Science Communication* 30 (3):355–79.

Ojala, M. 2012. "Hope and Climate Change: The Importance of Hope for Environmental Engagement among Young People." *Environmental Education Research* 18 (5):625–42. doi: 10.1080/13504622.2011.637157.

Oskamp, S. 1995. "Applying Social Psychology to Avoid Ecological Disaster." *Journal of Social Issues* 51 (4):217–39.

O'Sullivan, J., R. Bradford, M. Bonaiuto, S. De Dominicis, P. Rotko, J. Aaltonen, K. Waylen, and S. Langan. 2012. "Enhancing Flood Resilience through Improved Risk Communications." *Natural Hazards & Earth System Sciences* 12:2271–82.

Parker, D., S. Priest, and S. Tapsell. 2009. "Understanding and Enhancing the Public's Behavioral Response to Flood Warning Information." *Meteorological Applications* 16 (1):103–14.

Patt, A. G., and E. U. Weber. 2014. "Perceptions and Communication Strategies for the Many Uncertainties Relevant for Climate Policy." *WIREs Climate Change* 5 (2):219–32.

Petrovic, N., J. Madrigano, and L. Zaval. 2014. "Motivating Mitigation: When Health Matters More than Climate Change. *Climatic Change* 126 (1–2):245–54.

Pidgeon, N. 2012. "Public Understanding of, and Attitudes to, Climate Change: UK and International Perspectives and Policy." *Climate Policy* 12 (suppl 1):S85–S106.

Pidgeon, N., and B. Fischhoff. 2011. "The Role of Social and Decision Sciences in Communicating Uncertain Climate Risks." *Nature Climate Change* 1 (1):35–41.

Poortinga, W. 2012. "Community Resilience and Health: The Role of Bonding, Bridging, and Linking Aspects of Social Capital." *Health & Place* 18 (2):286–95.

Poortinga, W., A. Spence, L. Whitmarsh, S. Capstick, and N. Pidgeon. 2011. "Uncertain Climate: An Investigation of Public Skepticism about Anthropogenic Climate Change." *Global Environmental Change* 21 (3):1015–24.

Poortinga, W., L. Whitmarsh, L. Steg, G. Böhm, and S. Fisher. 2019. "Climate Change Perceptions and Their Individual-Level Determinants: A Cross-European Analysis." *Global Environmental Change* 55:25–35., doi:10.1016/j.gloenvcha.2019.01.007.

Ratter, B., K. Philipp, and H. von Storch. 2012. "Between Hype and Decline: Recent Trends in Public Perception of Climate Change." *Environmental Science & Policy* 18:3–8.

Renn, O. 2011. "The Social Amplification/Attenuation of Risk Framework: Application to Climate Change." *WIREs Climate Change* 2 (2):154–69.

Rose, C., P. Dade, and J. Scott. 2007. *Research into Motivating Prospectors, Settlers and Pioneers to Change Behaviors that Affect Climate Emissions.* Campaign Strategy. http://www.campaignstrategy.org/articles/behaviourchange_climate.pdf.

Roser-Renouf, C., N. Stenhouse, J. Rolfe-Redding, E. Maibach, and A. Leiserowitz. 2014. "Engaging Diverse Audiences with Climate Change: Message Strategies for Global Warming's Six Americas." In

The Routledge Handbook of Environment and Communication, edited by A. Hanson and R. Cox. London: Routledge.

Rothman, A., R. Bartels, J. Wlaschin, and P. Salovey. 2006. "The Strategic Use of Gain and Loss-Framed Messages to Promote Healthy Behavior: How Theory Can Inform Practice." *Journal of Communication* 56:202–20.

Sampson, N., C. Gronlund, M. Buxton, L. Catalano, J. White-Newsome, K. Conlon, M. O'Neill, S. McCormick, and E. Parker. 2013. "Staying Cool in a Changing Climate: Reaching Vulnerable Populations during Heat Events." *Global Environmental Change* 23 (2):475–84.

Schenk, B., C. Cook, and S. Demorest. 2020. "Nurses Climate Challenge: Educating 50,0000 Health Professionals by 2022." Updated January 31, 2020. Accessed March 27, 2020. https://www.wsna.org/news/2020/nurses-climate-challenge.

Scheufele, D. 1999. "Framing as a Theory of Media Effects." *Journal of Communication* 4:103–22.

Schuldt, J., S. Konrath, and N. Schwarz. 2011. "Global Warming" or "Climate Change"? Whether the Planet Is Warming Depends on Question Wording." *Public Opinion Quarterly* 75 (1):115–24.

Schulz-Hardt, S., D. Frey, C. Luthgens, and S. Moscovici. 2000. "Biased Information Search in Group Decision Making." *Journal of Personality and Social Psychology* 78 (4):655–69.

Schwartz, S. 1992. "Universals in the Content and Structure of Values: Theoretical Advances and Empirical Tests in 20 Countries." *Advances in Experimental Social Psychology* 25:1–65.

Scruggs, L., and S. Benegal. 2012. "Declining Public Concern about Climate Change: Can We Blame the Great Recession?" *Global Environmental Change* 22 (2):505–15.

Semenza, J., J. McCullough, D. Flanders, M. McGeehin, and J. Lumpkin. 1999. "Excess Hospital Admissions during the 1995 Heat Wave in Chicago." *American Journal of Preventive Medicine* 16:269–77.

Semenza, J., G. Ploubidis, and L. George. 2011. "Climate Change and Climate Variability: Personal Motivation for Adaptation and Mitigation." *Environmental Health* 10 (1):46.

Semenza, J., C. Rubin, K. Falter, J. Selanikio, W. Flanders, H. Howe, and J. Wilhelm. 1996. "Heat-Related Deaths during the July 1995 Heat Wave in Chicago." *New England Journal of Medicine* 335 (2):84–90.

Shaw, C. 2016. *The Two Degrees Dangerous Limit for Climate Change. Public Understanding and Decision Making.* Abingdon: Routledge.

Shaw, C., and A. Corner. 2017. "Using a Narrative Workshop Methodology to Socialize the Climate Policy Debate: Lessons from Two Case Studies." *Energy Research and Social Science* 31:273–83.

Sheridan, S. C. 2007. "A Survey of Public Perception and Response to Heat Warnings Across Four North American Cities: An Evaluation of Municipal Effectiveness." *International Journal of Biometeorology* 52 (1):3–15.

Shome, D., and S. Marx. 2009. *The Psychology of Climate Change Communication: A Guide for Scientists, Journalists, Educators, Political Aides and the Interested Public.* New York: Center for Research on Environmental Decisions, Columbia University.

Slimak, M., and T. Dietz. 2006. "Personal Values, Beliefs, and Ecological Risk Perception." *Risk Analysis* 26:1689–1705.

Smith, N., and H. Joffe. 2013. "How the Public Engages with Global Warming: A Social Representations Approach." *Public Understanding of Science* 22 (1):16–32.

Smith, N., and A. Leiserowitz. 2012. "The Rise of Global Warming Skepticism: Exploring Affective Image Associations in the United States over Time." *Risk Analysis* 32 (6):1021–32.

Spence, A., and N. Pidgeon. 2010. "Framing and Communicating Climate Change: The Effects of Distance and Outcome Frame Manipulations." *Global Environmental Change* 20(4):656–67.

Spence, A., W. Poortinga, C. Butler, and N. Pidgeon. 2011. "Perceptions of Climate Change and Willingness to Save Energy Related to Flood Experience." *Nature Climate Change* 1:46–49.

Spence, A., W. Poortinga, and N. Pidgeon. 2012. "The Psychological Distance of Climate Change." *Risk Analysis* 32 (6):957–72.

Stanke, C., V. Murray, R. Amlôt, J. Nurse, and R. Williams. 2012. "The Effects of Flooding on Mental Health: Outcomes and Recommendations from a Review of the Literature." *PLoS Currents* 4.

Steg, L., and I. Sievers. 2000. "Cultural Theory and Individual Perceptions of Environmental Risks." *Environment and Behavior* 32 (2):250–69.

Steg, L., and C. Vlek. 2009. "Encouraging Pro-Environmental Behavior: An Integrative Review and Research Agenda." *Journal of Environmental Psychology* 29 (3):309–17.

Stern, P. C. 2000. "New Environmental Theories: Toward a Coherent Theory of Environmentally Significant Behavior." *Journal of Social Issues* 56 (3):407–24.

Stokes, L. C., and C. Warshaw. 2017. "Renewable Energy Policy Design and Framing Influence Public Support in the United States." *Nature Energy* 2:17107.

Thøgersen, J., and T. Crompton. 2009. "Simple And Painless? The Limitations of Spillover in Environmental Campaigning." *Journal of Consumer Policy* 32:141–63.

Thompson, M. 2003. "Cultural Theory, Climate Change and Clumsiness." *Economic and Political Weekly* 38 (48):5107–12.

Thompson, M., and S. Rayner. 1998. "Risk and Governance Part I: The Discourses of Climate Change." *Government and Opposition* 33 (2):139–66.

Toloo, G., G. FitzGerald, P. Aitken, K. Verrall, and S. Tong. 2013. "Evaluating the Effectiveness of Heat Warning Systems: Systematic Review of Epidemiological Evidence." *International Journal of Public Health* 58 (5):667–81.

UK Health Protection Agency. 2011. *The Effects of Flooding on Mental Health*. https://webarchive. nationalarchives.gov.uk/20140714102456/http://www.hpa.org.uk/webc/HPAwebFile/HPAweb_C/1317131767423.

Upham, P., L. Whitmarsh, W., Poortinga, K. Purdam, A. Darnton, C. McLachlan, and P. Devine-Wright. 2009. *Public Attitudes to Environmental Change: A Selective Review of Theory and Practice. A Research Synthesis for the Living with Environmental Change Programme, Research Councils UK*. Swindon: Economic and Social Research Council/Living with Environmental Change Programme.

Veldman, R. G. 2012. "Narrating the Environmental Apocalypse: How Imagining the End Facilitates Moral Reasoning among Environmental Activists." *Ethics & the Environment* 17 (1):1–23.

Walker, B. J. A., T. Kurz, and D. Russel. 2017. "Towards an Understanding of When Non-Climate Frames Can Generate Public Support for Climate Change Policy." *Environment and Behavior* 13916517713299. https://doi.org/10.1177/0013916517713299.

Wang, S., A. Corner, D. Chapman, and E. Markowitz. 2018. "Public Engagement with Climate Imagery in a Changing Digital Landscape." *WIREs Climate Change* 9:e509.

Watts, N., M. Amann, N. Arnell, S. Ayeb-Kaisson, K. Belesova, M. Boykoff, P. Byass et al. 2019. "The 2019 Report of the Lancet Countdown on Health and Climate Change: Ensuring that the Health of a Child Born Today Is Not Defined by a Changing Climate." *Lancet* 394 (10211):1836–78.

Webb, G. J., and G. Egger. 2013. "Obesity and Climate Change Can We Link the Two and Can We Deal with Both Together?" *American Journal of Lifestyle Medicine* https://doi.org/10.1177/1559827613502452.

Weber, E. U. 2006. "Experience-Based and Description-Based Perceptions of Long-Term Risk: Why Global Warming Does Not Scare Us (Yet)." *Climatic Change* 77:103–20.

Weber, E. U. 2010. "What Shapes Perceptions of Climate Change?" *WIREs Climate Change* 1 (3):332–42.

West, J., I. Bailey, and M. Winter. 2010. "Renewable Energy Policy and Public Perceptions of Renewable Energy: A Cultural Theory Approach." *Energy Policy* 38 (10):5739–48.

Westerhoff, L., and J. Robinson. 2013. *The Meanings of Climate Change: Exploring Narrative and Social Practice in the Quest for Transformation*. IRES Working Paper Series (2013-01). Vancouver: Centre for Interactive Research on Sustainability, University of British Columbia. https://circle.ubc.ca/handle/2429/44563.

Whitmarsh, L. 2009. "What's in a Name? Commonalities and Differences tn Public Understanding of 'Climate Change' and 'Global Warming.'" *Public Understanding of Science* 18:401–20.

Whitmarsh, L. 2011. "Skepticism and Uncertainty about Climate Change: Dimensions, Determinants and Change over Time." *Global Environmental Change* 21:690–700.

Wike, R. 2016. "What the World Thinks about Climate Change in 7 Charts." Pew Research Center. April 18, 2016. http://www.pewresearch.org/fact-tank/2016/04/18/what-the-world-thinks-about-climate-change-in-7-charts/.

Winterbottom, A., H. L. Bekker, M. Conner, and A. Mooney. 2008. "Does Narrative Information Bias Individuals' Decision Making?" *Social Science & Medicine*, 67 (12):2079–88. doi: 10.1016/j.socscimed.2008.09.037.

Witte, K., and M. Allen. 2000. "A Meta-Analysis of Fear Appeals: Implications for Effective Public Health Campaigns." *Health Education & Behavior* 27 (5):591–615.

Wolf, J., W. N. Adger, I. Lorenzoni, V. Abrahamson, and R. Raine. 2010. "Social Capital, Individual Responses to Heat Waves and Climate Change Adaptation: An Empirical Study of Two UK Cities." *Global Environmental Change* 20 (1):44–52.

Wood, B., and A. Vedlitz. 2007. "Issue Definition, Information Processing, and the Politics of Global Warming." *American Journal of Political Science* 51 (3):552–68.

CHAPTER 18

INTERNATIONAL PERSPECTIVE ON CLIMATE CHANGE ADAPTATION

Kristie L. Ebi

Introduction

Climate change is altering the mean and variability of temperature, precipitation, and other weather variables, and sea level rise is increasing the regions at risk of storm surges, flooding, and saltwater intrusion into freshwater (Intergovernmental Panel on Climate Change [IPCC] 2018). Impacts are already evident in many sectors and regions, with some species extinction, childhood mortality, and changing landscapes already attributed to climate change (IPCC 2018). Changing weather patterns are often not the only driver of harmful impacts but can exacerbate other stresses to significantly increase risks. Growing understanding of the breadth and depth of these multiple stresses means that climate change is an issue of global development and equity.

Adaptation and mitigation are the main policy approaches to manage the risks of climate change. The IPCC defines **adaptation** as:

> In human systems, the process of adjustment to actual or expected climate and its effects, in order to moderate harm or exploit beneficial opportunities. In natural systems, the process of adjustment to actual climate and its effects; human intervention may facilitate adjustment to expected climate. (IPCC 2012)

The importance of adaptation has increased over the last thirty years with the scientific understanding that the planet is committed to additional warming over the next few decades no matter the degree of success of mitigation activities (IPCC 2018; van Vuuren et al. 2011). Implementing a wide range of adaptation policies and measures is critical in the short term if human and natural systems are to successfully cope with the consequences of ongoing changes in the climate system, although it will not be possible to prevent all impacts. It is not just the changing weather patterns themselves that need to be adapted to but also the consequences of those changing patterns, such as increases in the geographic range of insects and other disease vectors leading to the possible spread of infectious diseases into new regions. Over the longer term, the magnitude and pattern of climate change risks will depend on the mix of adaptation and mitigation, with rapid and successful reductions in greenhouse gas emissions decreasing how much adaptation will be needed later this century (van Vuuren et al. 2011). Slower and less comprehensive mitigation will increase the likelihood of crossing thresholds that could result in dangerous impacts to human and natural systems.

Historical Perspective

National and international organizations began seriously considering the possible consequences for human and natural systems of increasing greenhouse gas

KEY CONCEPTS

- Adaptation is one of the main policy approaches for managing the risks of climate change. The framing of adaptation has changed over time, leading to a more nuanced understanding of the strategies, policies, and measures needed to increase resilience to the health risks of current and future climate variability and change.

- The health risks of climate change are a function of three factors: hazards created by climate change, such as changes in temperature, precipitation, and extreme weather and climate events, and the consequences for natural systems that have relevance for human health; the populations exposed to those hazards; and their associated individual and community vulnerabilities.

- Understanding the effectiveness of current public health and health care policies and programs is a first step in understanding what modifications are needed to address the risks of a changing climate.

- Many current health adaptation options focus on improving public health and health care functions. While these are critically important, they may not be sufficient to protect population health as the climate continues to change. Adaptive risk management is needed.

- The costs of health adaptation may be significant over coming decades.

emissions in the 1970s. For example, in 1970, the Massachusetts Institute of Technology convened a Study of Critical Environmental Problems (SCEP), focusing on environmental problems whose large, prevalent, and cumulative effects on ecological systems would have worldwide significance (SCEP 1970). The primary concerns were the effects of pollution on humans through changes in climate, ocean ecology, and large terrestrial ecosystems. Climatic effects included the increasing carbon dioxide (CO_2) content of the atmosphere, particle concentrations in the atmosphere, and emissions from subsonic and supersonic aircraft contaminating the troposphere and stratosphere. These topics, discussions, and conclusions highlight important historical perspectives that carry forward to today: climate change as an environmental (as opposed to a health) issue, with consequences possibly felt in the future, and reducing greenhouse gas emissions through mitigation as the key activity to avoid negative consequences.

This perspective is understandable in context of other environmental concerns starting in the 1960s. The publication of *Silent Spring* by Rachel Carson about the environmental hazards of pesticides, particularly on birds, helped launch the contemporary environmental movement (Carson 1962). The 1970s and 1980s saw new environmental issues arise, including stratospheric ozone and acid rain. Stratospheric ozone depletion went from an unknown issue in early 1970 to a multilateral environmental agreement in 1985 and an international treaty (Montreal Protocol on Substances the Deplete the Ozone Layer) in 1987 that led to successful reduction of the emissions of ozone-depleting chemicals (United Nations [UN] 2009). Throughout the 1970s and 1980s, there was ongoing scientific and policy debate about the effects of sulfur deposition ("acid rain") on ecosystem resources in the United States, resulting in Congress passing the Acid Precipitation Act of 1980, establishing an eighteen-year assessment and research program that successfully reduced the relevant emissions (Lackey and Blair 1997; Likens and Bormann 1974).

Lessons from these and similar environmental problems include that an agent (pesticides, chemicals that deplete ozone, sulfur compounds) can harm the environment; reducing the agent was relatively easy and successful, after overcoming initial resistance; and reduction led to improvements in the impacts of concern. In short, humans can create environmental problems, and humans can resolve these on fairly short time scales once there is the political commitment to do so. A key first step in managing the problem was risk identification (identifying which agent(s) of concern led to adverse impacts), followed by the scientific determination of a level of exposure that would result in "acceptable" risk (where acceptable was defined by regulators), usually in terms of risk to human health (Bernard and Ebi 2001). This approach (and its successes) informed later efforts to understand the impacts of and strategies to control climate change.

The framing under this approach is that impacts are directly related to emissions and the way to manage impacts is to reduce greenhouse gas emissions, with mitigation as the primary policy task. That perspective is reflected in the language in the United Nations Framework Convention on Climate Change (UNFCCC) and activities since its negotiation, underscoring the original intention that the treaty should focus on reducing the source of climate change (e.g., mitigation), rather than on adapting to the changes (Schipper 2006); even though the inherent inertia in the climate system means the Earth is committed to decades of climate change no matter the success of mitigation (e.g., there is a climate change commitment) (van Vuuren et al. 2011). Adaptive capacity in the Convention was considered to be an indicator of the extent to which societies could tolerate changes in climate, not a policy objective. Climate change policy during the 1990s and early 2000s was characterized by this tension between mitigation and adaptation. Increasing scientific understanding of the magnitude and pattern of climate change and the associated risks for human and natural systems altered this discourse to focus on how to promote adaptation and mitigation most effectively locally, nationally, and internationally, taking into consideration their interactions and trade-offs.

Climate change has moved from being considered primarily a pollution problem to a much more complex and nuanced worldwide challenge, involving questions not just about the costs of strategies, policies, and measures to control, prepare for, respond to, and recover from impacts but also about sustainable development, equity, and social justice.

As scientific understanding of climate change and its impacts has increased, so has the social construction of what impacts are unacceptable. The Framework Convention specified three criteria for avoiding what is termed *dangerous anthropogenic interference* with the climate system (UN 1992): time for ecosystems to adapt naturally, food production not to be threatened, and economic development enabled in a sustainable matter. However, these are not quantifiable criteria that can be measured and monitored (Burton, Chandani, and Dickinson 2011; Smith et al. 2009). Furthermore, although these criteria are clearly important, they are not the only possible impacts of climate change that could have large-scale consequences. For example, there are growing concerns about a wide range of other consequences that could be considered dangerous, including the availability of sufficient quantities of safe water in some regions, the impacts of changing patterns of extreme weather and climate events, changes in the geographic range and incidence of climate-sensitive health outcomes, melting of large ice sheets in Greenland, the Arctic, and Antarctica, sea level rise, and the acidification of the oceans (Smith et al. 2009).

The Copenhagen Accord in 2009 stated the "international scientific consensus" that a global mean surface temperature increase of 2°C (3.6°F) above preindustrial levels is the upper limit of what human societies could adapt to and that anything above that temperature would be dangerous (UN 2009). This was more a political than a scientific consensus. In 2015, the Paris Agreement (UN 2015) stated that:

> . . . enhancing the implementation of the Convention, including its objective, aims to strengthen the global response to the threat of climate change, in the context of sustainable development and efforts to eradicate poverty, including by: (a) Holding the increase in the global average temperature to well below 2°C above pre-industrial levels and pursuing efforts to limit the temperature increase to 1.5°C above pre-industrial levels, recognizing that this would significantly reduce the risks and impacts of climate change; (b) Increasing the ability to adapt to the adverse impacts of climate change and foster climate resilience and low greenhouse gas emissions development, in a manner that does not threaten food production; and (c) Making finance flows consistent with a pathway towards low greenhouse gas emissions and climate-resilient development.

The Intergovernmental Panel on Climate Change (IPCC) Special Report on Warming of 1.5°C concluded that (IPCC 2018):

> Warming from anthropogenic emissions from the pre-industrial period to the present will persist for centuries to millennia and will continue to cause further long-term changes in the climate system, such as sea level rise, with associated impacts (high confidence), but these emissions alone are unlikely to cause global warming of 1.5°C (medium confidence).

> Climate-related risks for natural and human systems are higher for global warming of 1.5°C than at present, but lower than at 2°C (high confidence). These risks depend on the magnitude and rate of warming, geographic location, levels of development and vulnerability, and on the choices and implementation of adaptation and mitigation options (high confidence).

International Framework for Adaptation

Research over the past thirty years on the impacts and projected risks of climate change led to a framework that the magnitude and pattern of possible human and natural system risks of climate change depend on the interaction of (IPCC 2012):

- The hazards created by changes in temperature, precipitation, and other weather variables and in sea level rise and ocean acidification

- The extent to which human and natural systems are exposed to these changes, including people and their livelihoods, infrastructure, economic, social, or cultural assets, environmental services and resources, etc.

- The **vulnerability** of these systems, where vulnerability is defined as the propensity or predisposition to be affected

Figure 18.1 illustrates this framework, focusing on extreme weather and climate events. The figure shows the three components of risk, highlighting that realized risk (e.g., impacts) can influence subsequent development, including through risk management and climate change adaptation, and that development is a driver of anthropogenic climate change, which influences the frequency and intensity of the hazards created by a changing climate.

This framework highlights that adaptation is understood to increase resilience by decreasing exposure or vulnerability.

An important issue this framing does not incorporate is the iterative nature of adaptation (Ebi 2011). Health policy- and decision-makers are generally concerned with managing risks over short time scales, often the next five to ten years. Because climate will continue to change for decades to centuries, adaptation needs to simultaneously consider short periods of importance for current decisions and how climate change over longer time scales could affect the robustness of these decisions, in an iterative cycle of assessment, implementation, monitoring, and evaluation (National Research Council 2009). It is important to consider whether choices made today are likely to be resilient under new and different weather patterns, how easily these choices could be modified to adjust to changing situations, and what the consequences might be for population health.

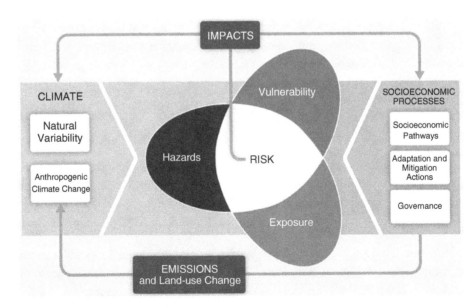

Figure 18.1   Framework for key drivers of climate-related risks
Source: IPCC (2014). Reproduced with permission from the Working Group II contribution to the IPCC Fifth Assessment report.

Assessing Adaptation Needs and Options

Public health has more than a century of experience with implementing policies and measures to reduce the burden of climate-related health outcomes. However, current programs were typically not designed to account for changes in the incidence, seasonality, and geographic range of these outcomes in a changing climate. Vulnerability and adaptation assessments can be conducted at any scale, from local to national, to identify strategies, policies, and measures for reducing the current and projected health risks due to climate change.

Vulnerability and adaptation assessments share similar features across sectors (Preston et al. 2011). Basic aims include identifying high priority health outcomes and vulnerable populations; identifying modifications to current and planned programs to address the additional risks of climate change; and identifying opportunities for new policies and measures to reduce burdens of climate-sensitive health outcomes. In most cases, an adaptation assessment builds on the results of a vulnerability assessment (Lindgren et al. 2001). This process is intended to characterize the present situation, including factors that increase or decrease vulnerability, such as population characteristics, disease burdens, functioning of health care systems, and effectiveness of programs to control the burden of health outcomes. Assuming that a vulnerability assessment identifies how the current burden of climate-related health outcomes could change with climate change over specific temporal and spatial scales, the main steps in conducting an adaptation assessment include (Ebi et al. 2013):

- Evaluating the effectiveness of policies and measures to reduce the current burden of climate-sensitive health outcomes

- Identifying adaptation options to manage the health risks of current and projected climate change

- Evaluating and prioritizing adaptation options

- Identifying human and financial resources needs and options to overcome possible barriers, constraints, and limits to implementation

- Developing monitoring and evaluation programs to facilitate continued effectiveness of policies and measures in a changing climate

In the United States, the Centers for Disease Control and Prevention developed the BRACE framework (Building Resilience Against Climate Effects) to facilitate risk management of the health risks of climate change, including using modeling to project risks, engaging all relevant stakeholders, and regularly updating models and risk management plans as new information because becomes available (Marinucci et al. 2014).

Identifying, prioritizing, and implementing strategies, policies, and measures to address the health risks of climate change must be based on an evaluation of the strengths and weaknesses of current policies and measures to address current climate variability and recent climate change (Ebi 2009; Frumkin et al. 2008; Jackson and Shields 2008). A first step in adaptation may be to enhance these programs to address current climate variability and change (Ebi 2011; Hess et al. 2012). Determining where populations are affected by currently climate variability can facilitate identifying the additional policies and measures needed now. At the same time, implementing options that address only current vulnerabilities may not be sufficient to protect against health risks from future and possibly more severe climate change (Ebi 2011; Hess et al. 2012).

Because a health ministry, nongovernmental organizations, and others may have individual or joint responsibility for programs designed to manage climate-sensitive health outcomes, representatives from all relevant organizations and institutions should be consulted to determine what is working well, what could be improved, and the capacity of the policies and measures to address possible increases in incidence or changes in the geographic range of the health outcome of concern (Lim et al. 2005). The observed increase in extreme weather and climate events means that organizations and agencies responsible for disaster risk management are important partners.

Awareness, motivation for action (at political, institutional, societal, and individual levels), human and financial resources, and institutional capacity are essential for any response to climate change (Ebi et al. 2013). Thus, national and local policymaking processes, institutions, and resources should be explicitly considered when conducting an adaptation assessment, as they influence the choices of which policies and measures to implement to address the current and future health risks of climate change (Bowen and Ebi 2015).

There is a significant need to evaluate the effectiveness of adaptation options to increase resilience to climate change (Bouzid, Hooper, and Hunter 2013; Hutton and Menne 2014). Studies are needed that conduct economic evaluations of the costs and benefits of adaptation options. The challenge is establishing frameworks and indicators for measuring costs and effectiveness over the short time period of a project when the goal is to facilitate individuals and societies preparing for and coping with climate change over decades and longer.

The number of national health vulnerability and adaptation assessments is growing (Berry et al. 2018), not all of which are quantitative. For example, an assessment for the Solomon Islands used a qualitative, participatory process to estimate the likelihood and consequences of health risks of climate change and to identify potential adaptation policies and measures to reduce and manage risks (Spickett and Katscherian 2014). Vector-borne and respiratory diseases were considered to be extreme risks. Adaptation actions were categorized as legislative or regulatory (e.g., regulate and enforce disease notification procedures), public education and communication, surveillance and monitoring (e.g., improving capacity, including laboratory capacity), ecosystem intervention (e.g., integrated vector management), infrastructure development (e.g., strengthening networks across sectors), technology or engineering (e.g., modifying building design), health intervention (e.g., training health professionals), and research and information (e.g., develop early warning systems). These vulnerability and adaptation assessments are beginning to be incorporated into national adaptation plans and policies.

CLINICAL CORRELATES 18.1 CRITICAL INFRASTRUCTURE IN THE SEYCHELLES

The Seychelles is a low-lying archipelago in the Indian Ocean, vulnerable to the impact of increasing heavy rainfalls and rising sea levels. In 2007, severe coastal flooding affected island infrastructure. With projections for similar events in the future, long-term adaptation initiatives emerged in partnerships with the University of Michigan and the United Nations Framework Convention on Climate Change, among a myriad of other island stakeholders (University of Michigan n.d.). As part of the project, a story map was created to illustrate sea level rise and storm surge risks to roads, ports, government buildings, sewerage systems, and water distribution (University of Michigan 2019). Specific adaptation measures included building retaining walls, sea walls, and vegetation planting.

Critical infrastructure along island coasts such as the Seychelles represents an opportunity to engage international partners to adapt and build resilience against sea level rise and storm surges.

NAPAs and NAPs

All countries that are signatories to the UNFCCC are required to submit regular National Communications covering their greenhouse gas emissions, climate change vulnerabilities, and adaptation and mitigation options to manage risks. Non-Annex I countries (a negotiated list of developing countries) submit National Communications (see http://unfccc.int/national_reports/non-annex_i_natcom/items/2979.php); many countries are working on their fourth such report. In addition, least developed countries (LDCs) developed National Adaptation Programmes of Action (**NAPAs**) to identify their most "urgent and immediate adaptation needs." These were submitted to the UNFCCC for possible funding from the Least Developed Country Fund. Urgent needs were defined as those for which further delay in implementation would increase vulnerability to climate change or increase adaptation costs at a later stage. Generally, staff within ministries of the environment conducted the assessments, using a top-down approach focused on impacts and consulting the relevant sectors only to verify information. Despite the limited involvement of ministries of health in developing the NAPAs, health is prioritized in nearly all of them. For example, among the Pacific island LDCs, Kiribati, Tuvalu, and Vanuatu ranked vector- and waterborne diseases as priority climate change risks to address in the short term. Unfortunately, limited funding was available to focus on the health concerns identified in the NAPAs.

Under the Cancun Adaptation Framework (UN 2010), a process was established to enable LDCs to formulate and implement National Adaptation Plans (NAPs) that build on the NAPAs but shift the focus toward identifying medium- and long-term adaptation needs, and strategies and policies to address these needs. Other countries have begun or are beginning to use this modality in their adaptation assessments.

Under the Paris Agreement (UN 2015), countries agreed to formulate and implement NAPs. The UNFCCC has a registry where countries can share their plans (UNFCCC 2020).

There is often a misperception that developed countries are taking the lead on adaptation because low- and middle-income countries are most at risk from climate change and have considerable human and financial resource constraints for implementing adaptation options. In fact, the UNFCCC has been funding adaptation projects under various funds since the late 1990s. For example, the Global Environment Facility funded three large regional adaptation projects in the Caribbean in the late 1990s and early 2000s: the Pacific Islands Climate Change Assistance Programme, 1997–2002: US$4 million; Caribbean Planning for Adaptation to Global Climate Change, 1998–2002: US$6.7 million; and Mainstreaming Adaptation to Climate Change in the Caribbean, 2004–2007: US$5.3 million (Nurse and Moore 2005). There has been similar funding in other highly vulnerable countries and regions. Lessons learned from the considerable expertise and experience gained in low- and middle-income countries on developing and implementing adaptation policies and measure could be helpful for all countries.

Adaptation Options

There are many schemes for categorizing adaptation options, including from the perspective of actors and their responsibilities (Ebi 2009); from the perspective of the types of actions (e.g., legislative, technical, educational, and behavioral/cultural; (McMichael et al. 2001); and from the perspective of the main public health functions, such as monitoring health status and diagnosing and investigating health problems (Frumkin et al. 2008). Because these categorizations are typically organized by health outcome, they may not be as effective to address the major concerns of the twenty-first century, including food and water security and extreme weather and climate events. For example, climate change can affect food security not just through malnutrition, but also through impacts on diarrheal diseases and malaria (World Bank 2008). Promoting food security requires considering the interactions of a range of issues that often cross departmental structures within ministries of health.

To reinforce the iterative nature of adaptation, strategies, policies, and measures to adapt to the health impacts of climate change can be categorized as incremental, transitional, and transformational actions (O'Brien et al. 2012). **Incremental adaptation** occurs when information on the risks of climate change is integrated into policies and measures, without changing underlying assumptions. This includes improving public health and health care services for climate-sensitive health outcomes, without necessarily considering the possible impacts of climate change. **Transitional adaptation** occurs with changes in underlying assumptions, including shifts in attitudes and perceptions. This includes vulnerability mapping, early warning systems, and other measures when they explicitly incorporate climate change. **Transformation** occurs with changes in social and other structures that mediate the construction of risk (Kates, Travis, and Wilbanks 2012). Although there is considerable interest in transformational adaptation, examples do not yet exist for health.

Incremental Adaptation: Improving Public Health Functions

Most health adaptation is focusing on improving public health functions, such as surveillance and interpretation of data related to the impacts of climate change, outbreak investigation and response, regulations, education, enhancing partnerships, and conducting research (Frumkin et al. 2008; Semenza and Menne 2009). Enhancing current programs is critical because the baseline health status of a population may be the most important predictor of health impacts in a changing climate and of the costs of adaptation and inaction (Pandey 2010). Reducing background rates of disease and injury can improve population resilience and minimize poor health outcomes from climate change. The design and implementation of incremental policy changes should be grounded in an understanding of the adequacy of existing policies and measures, and how their effectiveness could change under different scenarios of climate and socioeconomic change.

Surveillance is the core activity for identifying changes in the incidence and distribution of climate-sensitive diseases and the factors responsible (Last 2001). Surveillance programs are designed to keep local, regional, national, and global public health departments and ministries of health informed about the health status of the populations they serve and the real and potential problems they face (Wilson and Anker 2005). Surveillance involves systematically collecting data, including on risk factors and potential exposures that affect the incidence and distribution of a disease, and interpreting and distributing information to all relevant actors (including public health decision-makers, health care providers, and others) so that informed decisions can be taken.

Modifying or expanding current surveillance programs may be recommended in areas where changing weather patterns affect the incidence or facilitate the spread of infectious diseases. For example, because the risk of salmonella may increase with warmer ambient temperatures that favor the growth and spread of the bacteria (Kovats et al. 2004), enhancing salmonella control programs and improving measures to encourage adherence to proper food-handling guidelines can lower current and future disease burdens. Examples from Europe to address infectious disease risks under climate change include routine data analyses from mandatory notifications, pharmacy-based monitoring of prescription and nonprescription drug sale or health-related data preceding diagnosis, sentinel surveillance (collection and analysis of high-quality and accurate data at a geographic location; e.g., tick-borne encephalitis, Lyme borreliosis, etc.), and vector surveillance (Semenza and Menne 2009).

Transitional Adaptation

Transitional adaptation moves beyond a focus on reducing current adaptation deficits to explicitly incorporate climate change into the design of programs and measures, including how these options could increase population health resilience to climate change, and how climate change could alter the effectiveness of the options. Indicators of community functioning and connectedness are relevant because communities with high levels of social capital tend to be more successful in disseminating health and related messages, which often provides support to those in need (Ebi and Semenza 2008).

Some adaptation options being used or considered that are transitional when they incorporate climate change include:

- Vulnerability mapping
- Early warning systems
- **e-Health**

Vulnerability Mapping

Mapping the locations of populations particularly vulnerable to current climate variability and future climate change is increasingly being used in adaptation planning, spurred by the availability and use of geospatial data and remote sensing capabilities. Better understanding of where susceptible populations are located can help target adaptation activities, focusing services on the most sensitive and effectively using scarce public health resources. To enhance such mapping efforts, it would be beneficial to include indicators of the capacity of communities to cope with current and future changes in weather patterns.

For example, the European Centre for Disease Prevention and Control implemented a "European Environment and Epidemiology (E3) Network" (see http://E3geoportal.ecdc. europa.eu/) that links environmental, remotely sensed, demographic, epidemiologic, and other data sets for integrated analysis of environmental conditions related to infectious disease threats (Semenza et al. 2013). The network is facilitating identification of short-term events associated with environmental conditions that can improve and accelerate early warning and response activities; and identification of long-term trends that will build the evidence base for strategic public health policies and measures. The E3 network was used to identify the environmental profile of cases of locally acquired malaria (*Plasmodium vivax*) in 2009–2012 in Greece and to guide malaria control efforts in affected regions and in nonaffected regions whose characteristics suggested possible malaria transmission (Sudre et al. 2013). A model was developed to predict the suitability of areas that could support persistent malaria transmission; it included variables such as day- and nighttime land surface temperature, vegetation seasonal variations, altitude, land cover, and demographic indicators. Regions of concern were those with low elevation, elevated temperatures, and intensive, year-round irrigated agriculture with complex cultivation patterns. Based on this, recommendations were made of areas to implement spraying and other malaria control measures. This model could be used to determine what the consequences could be for malaria transmission of higher surface temperatures and changes in seasonal vegetation.

Vulnerability mapping carried out in other sectors of projected climate change impacts, such as flood zones (e.g., Hirabayashi et al. 2013), can provide helpful input for public health programs to increase resilience to (in this case) more extreme precipitation and flooding events.

Early Warning Systems

Disaster risk management has become more urgent with increases in the frequency and intensity of many extreme weather and climate events (IPCC 2018). An effective management option is an early warning system coupled with fine-scale understanding of where human and natural systems are particularly vulnerable. Early warning systems are being increasingly implemented in health and other sectors, as skill in seasonal forecasting has increased, and with increased sophistication in using these forecasts to warn populations of impeding risks and how to prepare and respond most effectively. Effective early warning systems take into consideration the range of factors that can drive risk and are developed in collaboration with end users (e.g.. Lowe, Ebi, and Forsberg 2011).

Much of the focus in the health sector has been on heat wave early warning systems. Components of effective early warning systems include forecasting weather conditions associated with increased morbidity or mortality, predicting possible health outcomes, identifying triggers of effective and timely response plans that target vulnerable populations, communicating risks and prevention responses, and evaluating and revising the system to increase effectiveness in a changing climate (e.g., Lowe et al., 2011). A review of heat wave early warning systems in the twelve European countries with such plans concluded that evaluations of the effectiveness of these systems is urgently needed to inform good practices, particularly understanding which action(s) increase resilience (Lowe et al. 2011). A 2012 review (Morabito et al. 2012) of the effectiveness of heat wave early warning systems or heat prevention activities to reduce heat-related mortality found that seven reported fewer deaths during heat waves after implementation of the system (Palecki, Changnon, and Kunkel 2001; Weisskopf et al. 2002; Ebi et al. 2004; Tan et al. 2007; Fouillet et al. 2008; Chau, Chan, and Woo 2009; Schifano et al. 2012).

Early warning systems also are being developed for vector-borne and foodborne infections using predictive models.

eHealth

eHealth and other emerging technologies offer opportunities to increase effectiveness of early warning and response systems and to better target adaptation options to those most at risk (Holmner et al. 2012). eHealth is not just telemedicine; it also includes activities such as home monitoring of vital parameters using mobile technology and electronic health surveillance systems. eHealth's international applications can be broadly categorized into the use of distance-spanning technology for health care and the use of electronic documentation of health services (e.g., electronic health records, surveillance systems). Possible examples for adaptation include telemedicine during disease outbreaks and extreme events, point-of-care diagnostic tools, strengthening of public health surveillance using mobile technologies, and promoting knowledge, awareness, and preparedness among the public, volunteers, and health workers.

CLINICAL CORRELATES 18.2 EHEALTH FOR GLOBAL HEALTH ACTION

Virtual eHealth is an emerging priority of the World Health Organization (WHO) and recognized as a way to support universal health care and resilient health systems (WHO 2016). It is used for virtual health care visits, remote diagnostics, and electronic documentation of health records and prescriptions (Holmner et al. 2012). Many view eHealth as a policy opportunity to reduce greenhouse gas emissions within the health sector, with promising evidence for being of cost-effectiveness across health systems (Elbert et al. 2014; Haines et al. 2009). Most recently, the coronavirus disease 2019 global pandemic brought new attention to the use of eHealth for public health response in outbreaks (Ohannessian, Duong, and Odone 2020).

eHealth not only connects patients and health professionals for routine visits but bridges communication and knowledge across continents during global health emergencies.

CLINICAL CORRELATES 18.3 ELECTRONIC HEALTH RECORDS AND DISASTER MANAGEMENT

Clinicians working in areas susceptible to climate change are on the front lines of detecting and treating climate-sensitive conditions. The practice of medicine in vulnerable, low-resource settings is complicated by the fact that health records rarely exist and paper records have the tendency to be destroyed and lost during disasters. Electronic health records have the potential to radically improve the way clinicians practice in disaster areas. Partners in Health, a nongovernmental organization working in Haiti, created an electronic health records system using open source software for their 500-bed hospital. The technology allowed for continuity in care and increased efficiency in the hospital and health system. In addition, these records are vital sources of real-time data that allows clinicians and public health officials to develop early warning systems and have an evidence-based approach for handling community-level problems related to climate change. The medical community should continue to advocate for extension of electronic health records as a means of increasing adaptive management of climate-related health issues.

Investing in medical information technology is a way to address issues related to continuity of care and disease surveillance in resource-poor environments.

Costs of Adaptation and/or of Inaction

The UNFCCC states that all countries have a common but differentiated responsibility with respect to climate change (UN 1992). One consequence is that developed countries have a responsibility to help developing countries adapt to climate change, within the context that developed countries are responsible for most of the cumulative greenhouse gases in the atmosphere. International negotiations on funding adaptation for low- and middle-income countries should be informed by the costs of inaction on climate change (e.g., the cost of impacts without adaptation or mitigation), the costs of impacts assuming various levels of adaptation (and mitigation for estimates later in the century), and the costs of impacts that could be expected to remain after adaptation and mitigation efforts. Increasing research is focusing on providing estimates of these costs.

Estimating the costs of climate impacts and associated responses includes considering immediate health sector response costs (additional medicine and costs of treatment) when an extreme weather event occurs, or an impact arises from changing weather trends (Ebi, Hess, and Watkiss 2017). Injuries, illnesses, deaths, and lost work time also lead to economic costs. Impacts on people's quality of life and well-being also occur, even if these are not captured in economic terms. Global estimates of the costs of treating future cases of adverse health outcomes due to climate change are in the range of billions of US dollars annually, with the largest burdens in low- and middle-income countries, particularly in Southeast Asia and Africa. National and regional studies extend these estimates.

Estimates of how worker productivity could be affected by increasing heat stress due to climate change, assuming current work practices, indicate that productivity has already declined during the hottest and wettest seasons in parts of Africa and Asia, with more than half of afternoon hours projected to be lost to the need for rest breaks in 2050 in Southeast Asia and up to a 20 percent loss in global productivity in 2100, assuming greenhouse gas emissions reductions under RCP4.5 (e.g., Kjellstrom, Holmer, and Lemke 2009; Kjellstrom et al. 2009; Kjellstrom, Lemke, and Otto 2013; Dunne, Stouffer, and John 2013).

CLINICAL CORRELATES 18.4 TRANSLATIONAL ADAPTIVE MANAGEMENT

Using emerging mobile technologies to crowdsource health information is an innovation that has the potential to create benefits in communities vulnerable to climate change. Public health crowdsourcing is a way of amassing information from the local community to build a larger picture of an emerging health threat. Examples include The GLOBE Program (globe. gov) launched an application to share scientific observations in countries around the world, to further empower public health research projects. Students in Maryland started the DustWatch application (dustapp.org) as an easily accessible early warning tool for dust storms. The Voices of Youth Maps Initiative in Haiti is another example of identifying changing environmental conditions favorable for infectious disease spread.

The health sector can continue to promote such technologies as an adaptive strategy for climate change. For example, communities may have advance warning of diarrheal outbreaks, contaminated water sources, dust storms, and heat warnings. Projects such as these foster social resilience while improving efficiency of resource use. Clinicians working in these areas can play a vital role in educating their patients to be aware of these tools, and even to identify and document risks.

Community investment and education using new technologies are crucial factors for building resilience to the impacts of climate change.

Co-benefits of Health Adaptation Strategies

Public health policies to address the health risks of climate change often have associated health co-benefits, with most co-benefits related to improvements in health associated with building social capital (e.g. improved mental health) and improving urban design (e.g. reduced obesity and cardiovascular disease) through increased physical activity, cooling spaces, and social connectivity (Cheng and Berry 2013). Risks could include, for example, exacerbating pollen allergies with increased urban green space.

Summary

Avoiding, preparing for, responding to, coping with, and recovering from the health risks of climate change requires urgent proactive international adaptation if projected impacts over the next few decades are to be significantly reduced. Because many locations worldwide face similar risks, or have experiences relevant to other regions, there are significant opportunities to work across regions and countries to understand lessons learned and best practices for designing, implementing, monitoring, and evaluating adaptation options. Conducting a vulnerability and adaptation assessment is an important first step in understanding the sources of health risks of current and future climate variability and change and identifying priority modifications of public health and health care policies and programs to increase effective and efficient adaptation. Within and outside the health sector, a wide range of options is available that can facilitate building resilience. Research needs include developing new international adaptation options to manage ever more complex and challenging risks and increasing understanding of how to implement iterative risk management approaches that explicitly incorporate climate change within the context of institutional structures in ministries of health. Failing to do so will leave populations ill prepared to manage what could be significant health risks, with morbidity, mortality, and their associated societal costs. The extent to which health impacts will occur depends in large part on public health and health care researchers and practitioners actively incorporating the risks of climate variability and change into all relevant activities.

DISCUSSION QUESTIONS

1. How has the framing of adaptation changed over time, and what difference does that framing make to when considering international adaptation strategies, policies, and measures?

2. What factors together are required to result in climate change risks?

3. What are some adaptation options for managing the infectious disease risks of changing weather patterns?

KEY TERMS

Adaptation: In human systems, the process of adjustment to actual or expected climate and its effects, in order to moderate harm or exploit beneficial opportunities. In natural systems, the process of adjustment to actual climate and its effects.

e-Health: The use of distance-spanning technology for health care and the use of electronic documentation of health services, including telemedicine, activities such as home monitoring of vital parameters using mobile technology, and electronic health surveillance systems.

Incremental adaptation: Occurs when information on the risks of climate change is integrated into policies and measures, without changing underlying assumptions. This includes improving public health and health care services for climate-relevant health outcomes, without necessarily considering the possible impacts of climate change.

National Adaptation Programmes of Action (NAPAs): Drafted by least developed countries (LDCs) to identify their most "urgent and immediate adaptation needs"—those for which further delay in implementation would increase vulnerability to climate change or increase adaptation costs at a later stage—and submitted to the UNFCCC for possible funding from the Least Developed Country Fund.

Transformation: Changes in social and other structures that mediate the construction of risk.

Transitional adaptation: Can occur with changes in underlying assumptions, including shifts in attitudes and perceptions. This includes vulnerability mapping, early warning systems, and other measures when they explicitly incorporate climate change.

Vulnerability: The propensity or predisposition to be adversely affected.

References

Bernard, S. M., and K. L. Ebi. 2001. "Comments on the Process and Product of the Health Impacts Assessment Component of the United States National Assessment of the Potential Consequences of Climate Variability and Change". *Environmental Health Perspectives* 109 (suppl 2):177–84.

Berry, P., P. M. Enright, J. Shumake-Guillemot, E. Villalobos Prats, and D. Campbell-Lendrum. 2018. *International Journal of Environmental Research and Public Health* 15:2626; doi:10.3390/ijerph15122626.

Bouzid, M., L. Hooper, and P. R. Hunter. 2013. "The Effectiveness of Public Interventions to Reduce the Health Impact of Climate Change: A Systematic Review of Systematic Reviews." *PLoS ONE* 8 (4):e62041.

Bowen, K., and K. L. Ebi. 2015. "Governing the Health Risks of Climate Change: Towards Multi-Sector Responses." *Current Opinion in Environmental Sustainability* 12: 80–85.

Burton, I., A. Chandani, and T. Dickinson. 2011. "UNFCCC Article 2 Revisited. European Capacity Building Initiative Background Paper."

Carson, R. 1962. *Silent Spring*. New York: Houghton Mifflin.

Chau, P. H., K. C. Chan, and J. Woo. 2009. "Hot Weather Warning Might Help to Reduce Elderly Mortality in Hong Kong." *International Journal of Biometeorology* 53 (5):461–8.

Cheng, J., and P. Berry. 2013. "Health Co-Benefits and Risks of Public Health Adaptation Strategies to Climate Change: A Review of Current Literature." *International Journal of Public Health* 58:305–11.

Dunne, J., R. Stouffer, and J. John. 2013. "Reductions in Labour Capacity from Heat Stress under Climate Warming." *Nature Climate Change* 3 (3):1–4.

Ebi, K. L. 2009. "Public Health Responses to the Risks of Climate Variability and Change in the United States." *Journal of Occupational and Environmental Medicine* 51:4–12.

Ebi, K. 2011. "Climate Change and Health Risks: Assessing and Responding to Them Through 'Adaptive Management.'" *Health Affairs (Millwood)* 30 (5):924–30.

Ebi, K., J. Hess, and P. Watkiss. 2017. "Health Risks and Costs of Climate Variability and Change. In *Disease Control Priorities*, 3rd ed., Vol. 7, *Injury Prevention and Environmental Health*, edited by C. N. Mock, R. Nugent, O. Kobusingye, and K. Smith. Washington, DC: World Bank.

Ebi, K. L., E. Lindgren, J. E. Suk, and J. C. Semenza. 2013. "Adaptation to the Infectious Disease Impacts of Climate Change." *Climatic Change* 118,:355–65. doi 10.1007/s10584-012-0648-5.

Ebi, K. L., and J. Semenza. 2008. "Community-Based Adaptation to the Health Impacts of Climate Change." *American Journal of Preventive Medicine* 35:501–7.

Ebi, K. L., T. J. Teisberg, L. S. Kalkstein, L. Robinson, and R. F. Weiher. 2004. "Heat Watch/Warning Systems Save Lives: Estimated Costs and Benefits for Philadelphia 1995–1998." *Bulletin of the American Meteorological Society (BAMS)* 85 (8):1067–73.

ecoAmerica. 2013. *Communicating on Climate: 13 Steps and Guiding Principles*. https://ecoamerica.org/wp-content/uploads/2013/11/Communicating-on-Climate-13-steps_ecoAmerica.pdf.

Elbert, N. J., H. van Os-Medendorp, W. van Renselaar, A. G. Ekeland, L. Hakkaart-van Roijen, H. Raat, T. E. C. Nijsten, and S. G. M. A. Pasmans. 2014. "Effectiveness and Cost-Effectiveness of Ehealth Interventions in Somatic Diseases: A Systematic Review of Systematic Reviews and Meta-Analyses." *Journal of Medical Internet Research* 16 (4):e110. doi:10.2196/jmir.2790.

Fouillet, A., G. Rey, V. Wagner, K. Laaidi, P. Empereur-Bissonnet, A. Le Tertre, P. Frayssinet et al. 2008. "Has the Impact of Heat Waves on Mortality Changed in France since the European Heat Wave of Summer 2003? A Study of the 2006 Heat Wave." *International Journal of Epidemiology* 37 (2):309–17.

Frumkin, H., J. Hess, G. Luber, J. Malilay, and M. McGeehin. 2008. "Climate Change: The Public Health Response." *American Journal of Public Health* 98 (3):435–45.

Haines, A., A. J. McMichael, K. R. Smith, I. Roberts, J. Woodcock, A. Markandya, B. G. Armstrong et al. 2009. "Public Health Benefits of Strategies to Reduce Greenhouse-Gas Emissions: Overview and Implications for Policy Makers." *Lancet* 374 (9707):2104–14. doi:10.1016/S0140-6736(09)61759-1.

Hess, J. J., J. Z. McDowell, and G. Luber. 2012. "Integrating Climate Change Adaptation into Public Health Practice: Using Adaptive Management to Increase Adaptive Capacity and Build Resilience." *Environmental Health Perspectives* 120:171–9.

Hirabayashi, Y., R. Mahendran, S. Koirala, L. Konoshima, D. Yamazaki, S. Watanabe, H. Kim, and S. Kanae. 2013. "Global Flood Risk under Climate Change." *Nature Climate Change* 3:816–21: doi: 10.1038/NCLIMATE1911.

Holmner, A., J. Rocklov, N. Ng, and M. Nilsson. 2012. "Climate Change and eHealth: A Promising Strategy for Health Sector Mitigation and Adaptation." *Global Health Action* 5:18428. http://dx.doi.org/10.3402/gha.v5i0.18428.

Hutton, G., and B. Menne. 2014. "Economic Evidence on the Health Impacts of Climate Change in Europe." *Environmental Health Insights* 8:43–52.

Intergovernmental Panel on Climate Change. 2012. "Summary for Policymakers." In *Managing the Risks of Extreme Events and Disasters to Advance Climate Change Adaptation. A Special Report of Working Groups I and II of the Intergovernmental Panel on Climate Change*, edited by C. B. Field, V. Barros, T. F. Stocker, D. Qin, D. J. Dokken, K. L. Ebi, M. Mastrandrea et al., 3–21. Cambridge, UK, and New York: Cambridge University Press.

Intergovernmental Panel on Climate Change. 2014. "Summary for Policymakers." In *Climate Change 2014: Impacts, Adaptation, and Vulnerability. Contribution of Working Group II to the Fifth Assessment Report of the Intergovernmental Panel on Climate Change*, edited by C. B. Field, V. R. Barros, D. J. Dokken, K. J. Mach, M. D. Mastrandrea, T. E. Bilir, M. Chatterjee et al., 1–32. Cambridge, UK and New York: Cambridge University Press.

Intergovernmental Panel on Climate Change. 2018. "Summary for Policymakers." *In Global Warming of 1.5°C. An IPCC Special Report on the Impacts of Global Warming of 1.5°C above Pre-Industrial Levels and Related Global Greenhouse Gas Emission Pathways, in the Context of Strengthening the Global*

Response to the Threat of Climate Change, Sustainable Development, and Efforts to Eradicate Poverty, edited by V. Masson-Delmotte, P. Zhai, H.-O. Pörtner, D. Roberts, J. Skea, P. R. Shukla, A. Pirani, W. Moufouma-Okia et al., 3–24. Geneva: Intergovernmental Panel on Climate Change.

Jackson, R., and K. N. Shields. 2008. "Preparing the U.S. Health Community for Climate Change." *Annual Reviews of Public Health* 29:57–73.

Kates, R. W., W. R. Travis, and T. J. Wilbanks. 2012. "Transformational Adaptation When Incremental Adaptations to Climate Change Are Insufficient." *Proceedings of the National Academies of Science* 109:7156–61.

Kjellstrom, T., I. Holmer, and B. Lemke. 2009a. "Workplace Heat Stress, Health and Productivity—An Increasing Challenge for Low and Middle-Income Countries During Climate Change." *Global Health Action* 2:10.3402/gha.v2i0.2047.

Kjellstrom, T., R. S. Kovats, S. J. Lloyd, T. Holt, and R. S. Tol. 2009b. "The Direct Impact of Climate Change on Regional Labor Productivity." *Archives of Environmental and Occupational Health* 64 (4):217–27.

Kjellstrom, T., B. Lemke, and M. Otto. 2013. "Mapping Occupational Heat Exposure and Effects in South-East Asia: Ongoing Time Trends 1980–2009 and Future Estimates to 2050." *Industrial Health* 51:56–67.

Kovats, R. S., S. Hajat, S. Edwards, K. L. Ebi, B. Menne, Collaborating Group. 2004. "The Effect of Temperature on Food Poisoning: A Time Series Analysis of Salmonellosis in 10 European Populations." *Epidemiology and Infection* 132:443–53.

Lackey, R. T., and R. L. Blair. 1997. "Science, Policy, and Acid Rain: Lessons Learned." *Renewable Resources Journal* 15:9–13.

Last, J. M. 2001. *A Dictionary of Epidemiology*, 4th ed. Oxford, UK: Oxford University Press.

Likens, G. E., and F. H. Bormann. 1974. "Acid Rain: A Serious Regional Environmental Problem." *Science* 184:1176–79.

Lim, B., E. Spanger-Siegfried, I. Burton, E. Malone, S. Huq, eds. 2005. *Adaptation Policy Frameworks for Climate Change*. Cambridge, UK: Cambridge University Press.

Lindgren, E., and R. Gustafson. 2001. "Tick-Borne Encephalitis in Sweden and Climate Change." *Lancet* 358 (9275):16–18.

Lowe, D., K. L. Ebi, and B. Forsberg. 2011. "Heatwave Early Warning Systems and Adaptation Advice to Reduce Human Health Consequences of Heatwaves." *International Journal of Environmental Research and Public Health* 8 (12):4623–48.

Marinucci, G. D., G. Luber, C. K. Uejio, S. Saha, and J. J. Hess. 2014. "Building Resilience against Climate Effects: A Novel Framework to Facilitate Climate Readiness in Public Health Agencies." *International Journal of Environmental Research and Public Health* 11:6433–58.

McMichael, M., A. Githeko, R. Akhtar, R. Carcavallo, D. Gubler, A. Haines, R. S. Kovats et al. 2001. "Human health." In *Climate Change 2001: Impacts, Adaptation, and Vulnerability. Contribution of Working Group II to the Third Assessment Report of the Intergovernmental Panel on Climate Change*, edited by J. J. McCarthy, O. F. Canziani, N. A. Leary, D. J. Dokken, and K. S. White, 452–85.. Cambridge, UK: Cambridge University Press.

Morabito, M., F. Profili, A. Crisci, P. Francesconi, G. F. Gensini, and S. Orlandini. 2012. "Heat-Related Mortality in the Florence Area (Italy) before and after the Exceptional 2003 Heat Wave in Europe: An Improved Public Health Response?" *International Journal of Biometeorology* 56:801–10.

National Research Council. 2009. *America's Climate Choices, Panel on Adapting to the Impacts of Climate Change*. Washington, DC: National Academies Press.

Nurse, L., and R. Moore. 2005. "Adaptation to Global Climate Change: An Urgent Requirement for Small Island Developing States.: *RECIEL* 14 (2):100–7.

O'Brien, K., M. Pelling, A. Patwardhan, S. Hallegatte, A. Maskrey, T. Oki, U. Oswald-Spring, T. Wilbanks, and P. Z. Yanda. 2012. "Toward a Sustainable and Resilient Future." In *Managing the Risks of Extreme Events and Disasters to Advance Climate Change Adaptation. A Special Report of Working Groups I and II of the Intergovernmental Panel on Climate Change*, edited by C. B. Field, V. Barros, T. F. Stocker, D. Qin, D. J. Dokken, K. L. Ebi, M. Mastrandrea et al., 437–86. Cambridge, UK, and New York: Cambridge University Press.

Ohannessian, R., T. A. Duong, and A. Odone. 2020. "Global Telemedicine Implementation and Integration within Health Systems to Fight the COVID-19 Pandemic: A Call to Action." JMIR Public Health and Surveillance 6 (2):e18810. doi:10.2196/18810.

Palecki, M. A., S. A. Changnon, and K. E. Kunkel. 2001. "Nature and Impacts of the July Heat Wave in the Midwestern United States: Learning from the Lessons of 1995." *Bulletin of the American Meteorological Society* 82:1353–67.

Pandey, K. 2010. *Costs of Adapting to Climate Change for Human Health in Developing Countries. Development and Climate Change Discussion Paper No. 11.* Washington, DC: World Bank. https://openknowledge.worldbank.org/handle/10986/27750.

Preston, B. L., E. J. Yuen, and R. M. Westaway. 2011. "Putting Vulnerability to Climate Change on the Map: A Review of Approaches, Benefits, and Risks." *Sustainability Science* 6:177–202. doi: 10.1007/s11625-011-0129-1

Schifano, P., M. Leone, M. De Sario, F. de'Donato, A. M. Bargagli, D. D'Ippoliti, C. Marino, and P. Michelozzi. 2012. "Changes in the Effects of Heat on Mortality among tThe Elderly from 1998–2010: Results from a Multicenter Time Series Study in Italy." *Environmental Health* 11:58. http://www.ehjournal.net/content/11/1/58.

Schipper, E. L. F. 2006. "The History of Adaptation in the UNFCCC Process." *RECIEL* 15:82–92.

Semenza, J. C., and B. Menne. 2009. "Climate Change and Infectious Diseases in Europe." *Lancet Infectious Diseases* 9:365–75.

Semenza, J. C., B. Sudre, T. Oni, J. E. Suk, and J. Giesecke. 2013. "Linking Environmental Drivers to Infectious Diseases: The European Environment and Epidemiology Network." *PLOS Neglected Tropical Diseases* 7 (7):e2323. doi:10.1371/journal.pntd.0002323

Smith, J. B., S. H. Schneider, M. Oppenheimer, G. W. Yohe, W. Hare, M. D.Mastrandrea, A. Patwardhan et al. 2009. "Assessing Dangerous Climate Change through an Update of the Intergovernmental Panel on Climate Change (IPCC) 'Reasons for Concern.'" *Proceedings of the National Academies of Science* 106:4133–7.

Spickett, J. T., and D. Katscherian. 2014. "Health Impacts of Climate Change in the Solomon Islands: An Assessment and Adaptation Action Plan." *Global Journal of Health Science* 6:261–73.

Study of Critical Environmental Problems. 1970. *Man's Impact on the Global Environment: Assessment and Recommendations for Action.* Cambridge, MA: MIT Press. http://mitpress.mit.edu/books/mans-impact-global-environment.

Sudre, B., M. Rossi, W. V. Bortel, K. Danis, A. Baka, N. Vakalis, and J. C. Semenza. 2013. "Mapping Environmental Suitability for Malaria Transmission, Greece." *Emerging Infectious Diseases* 19:784–6. http://dx.doi.org/10.3201/eid1905.120811.

Tan, J., Y. Zheng, G. Song, L. S. Kalkstein, A. J. Kalkstein, and X. Tang. 2007. "Heat Wave Impacts on Mortality in Shanghai, 1998 and 2003." *International Journal of Biometeorology* 51 (3):193–200.

United Nations. 1992. *United Nations Framework Conventions on Climate Change.* Document FCCC/INFORMAL/84, GE.05-62220 (E) 200705.

United Nations. 2009. *United Nations Framework Convention on Climate Change, Copenhagen Accord.* Document FCCC/CP/2009/L.7.

United Nations. 2010. "United Nations Framework Convention on Climate Change, Cancun Adaptation Framework." Document FCCC/CP/2010/7/Decision 1/CP.16. http://unfccc.int/adaptation/items/5852.php.

United Nations. 2015. "United Nations Framework Convention on Climate Change, The Paris Agreement." https://unfccc.int/process-and-meetings/the-paris-agreement/the-paris-agreement.

United Nations Framework Convention on Climate Change. 2020. "National Adaptation Plan." https://unfccc.int/topics/adaptation-and-resilience/workstreams/national-adaptation-plans.

University of Michigan. 2019. "Evaluating the Impacts of Sea-Level Rise and Storm Surges on the Seychelles' Critical Infrastructure." Accessed April 7, 2020. https://umich.maps.arcgis.com/apps/MapSeries/index.html?appid=529d197fc7374f9b9fcc40c6106baa6d#.

University of Michigan. n.d. "Improving Climate Resilience in the Seychelles: Evaluating the Impacts of Sea-Level Rise and Storm Surges on Seychelles' 'Critical Infrastructure.'" Accessed April 4, 2020. https://seas.umich.edu/academics/resources/capstone/improving_climate_resilience_seychelles_evaluating_impacts_sea_level.

van Vuuren, D. P., J. A. Edmonds, M. Kainuma, K. Riahi, and J. Weyant. 2011. "A Special Issue on the RCPs." *Climatic Change* 109:1–4. doi: 10.1007/s10584-011-0157-y.

Weisskopf, M. G., H. A. Anderson, S. Foldy, L. P. Hanrahan, K. Blair, and T. J. Török. 2002. "Heat Wave Morbidity and Mortality, Milwaukee, Wis, 1999 vs 1995: An Improved Response?" *American Journal of Public Health* 29 (5):830–3.

Wilson, M. L., and M. Anker. 2005. "Disease Surveillance in the Context of Climate Stressors: Needs and Opportunities." In *Integration of Public Health with Adaptation to Climate Change: Lessons Learned and New Directions,* edited by K. L. Ebi, J. Smith, and I. Burton, 191–214. London: Taylor & Francis.

World Bank. 2008. *Environmental Health and Child Survival; Epidemiology, Economics, Experiences.* Washington, DC: Economic and Health Sector, Environment Department, World Bank.

World Health Organization. 2016. *Global Diffusion of eHealth: Making Universal Health Coverage Achievable. Report of the Third Global Survey on eHealth.* Geneva: World Health Organization. License: CC BY-NC-SA 3.0 IGO.

CHAPTER 19

HEALTH CO-BENEFITS OF CLIMATE MITIGATION STRATEGIES

Elizabeth J. Carlton, Amber S. Khan, and Justin V. Remais

Introduction

Global efforts to address climate change will require ambitious and robust mitigation actions that reduce emissions of **climate-altering pollutants (CAPs)**. **Climate mitigation** policies will limit the adverse health consequences that accompany climate change, but many of those climate-health benefits will take decades to accrue. This is because reductions in CAPs today are not expected to yield discernable climate impacts until midcentury in most cases, and thus the health gains of limiting climate change will also accrue over this timeline (Intergovernmental Panel on Climate Change [IPCC] 2014b).

Mitigation measures also have the potential to yield direct, near-term health impacts. For example, a shift to low-carbon transportation can reduce CAPs from fossil fuel combustion and also reduce traffic-related air pollution and corresponding cardiovascular and respiratory illnesses (Figure 19.1). Health impacts that directly accrue from mitigation strategies are termed health **co-benefits**. Estimates of the potential co-benefits, as well as adverse impacts (termed here **co-harms**), of climate mitigation policies can further the justification for particular climate mitigation policies, and prevent unintended negative health consequences of climate action. Because health co-benefits of climate mitigation can accrue more rapidly than the health gains of limiting climate change, health co-benefits can help motivate cross-sector support for mitigation policy and prioritize no-regrets strategies that address both climate and public health priorities (Chang et al. 2017; Haines et al. 2009; McMichael et al. 2009). At the same time, if the health impacts of a mitigation strategy are found to be negative (i.e., expected to yield co-harms), this information can aid in deprioritizing such policies to prevent unintended adverse consequences of climate mitigation.

In 2014, the IPCC (Smith et al. 2014) assessed the current evidence for and the degree of confidence in four key domains in which mitigation policies can potentially impact health:

- *Energy systems.* Improvements in energy efficiency and transitioning to cleaner energy sources can reduce greenhouse gas emissions and the adverse health effects of co-emitted air pollution (degree of confidence: *very high*).

- *Transportation.* Transportation systems that promote **active transport** (e.g., walking and biking) and reduce use of combustion vehicles can reduce CAP emissions and traffic-related air pollution, improve physical activity, and lower obesity and noncommunicable disease burden (degree of confidence: *high*).

- *Food and agriculture.* Reduced consumption of animal products, particularly from ruminants (e.g., cattle) in regions where people eat meat-intensive diets, can reduce CAP emissions, improve cardiovascular health, and reduce colorectal cancer risk (degree of confidence: *medium*).

KEY CONCEPTS

- Climate mitigation policies, such as reducing emissions from transport-related fuel combustion, can have significant, direct impacts on health.

- These direct health effects of mitigation—positively termed "co-benefits"—represent public health benefits from mitigation policies in addition to benefits that result from reductions in the adverse impacts of climate change itself.

- Climate mitigation policies are generally expected to yield health co-benefits that accrue shortly after implementation, providing near-term public health benefits of climate mitigation policies.

- Quantitative assessment of the direct health impacts of mitigation can yield critical policy guidance, help build cross-sectoral support for climate mitigation policies, and avoid unintended adverse health effects.

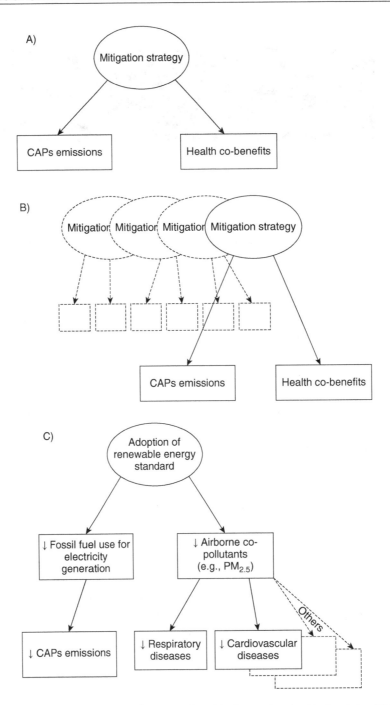

Figure 19.1   Schematics of climate and health benefits: accruing through implementation of a mitigation strategy (A); being evaluated alongside other strategies in a comparative co-benefit study (B); example of a mitigation strategy within the electricity generation sector being evaluated on the basis of its climate and health benefits (C). Not indicated here: additional, longer-term health benefits from averting climate change that accrue from reductions in CAP emissions

- *Reproductive health.* Mitigation measures to reduce population growth and corresponding energy use through improved access to reproductive health services can reduce population growth and corresponding energy use, as well as improve child and maternal health (degree of confidence: *medium*).

In this chapter, we discuss approaches for estimating co-benefits and co-harms, review current evidence for the expected health co-benefits among key sectors, evaluate current challenges, and summarize the implications of co-benefits for climate policy.

Climate Mitigation

Climate mitigation refers to efforts to reduce CAP concentrations through reductions in emissions and/or increases in carbon capture. This is distinct from climate **adaptation**, which is intended to lessen the impacts of climate change through measures to prepare populations for a changing climate, such as disaster preparedness and flood control.

When assessing the potential co-benefits of climate mitigation, it is helpful to understand the major sources of CAP emissions, which can be divided across five sectors. In 2010, the energy sector accounted for 35 percent of CAP emissions, primarily used for heating, cooling, and electricity (IPCC 2014a). Emissions from the agriculture, forestry, and land use sector (24 percent) include deforestation, methane emissions from ruminants and animal manure, and, to a lesser extent, emissions from rice paddies. In the industry sector (21 percent), iron, steel, and cement production are key drivers of emissions, as well as chemical, paper, aluminum, and fertilizer production. Transportation (14 percent) emissions are primarily through mobile source combustion. The industry and building sectors are key consumers of energy for heating, cooling, and electricity. When this energy use is assigned to the end-use sector, industry accounted for 32 percent of global CAP emissions in 2010, and buildings 19 percent (IPCC 2014a).

Efforts to reduce emissions in these sectors include measures to improve energy efficiency, reduce dependence on highly CAP-emitting coal-burning power plants, and transition to low-carbon energy sources.

Two of the strongest drivers of CAP emissions are population growth and economic development. This plays out in large regional variation in CAP emissions: low-income countries generated approximately 2 percent of CAP emissions in 2010, primarily due to agriculture and forestry, whereas upper middle- and high-income countries generated approximately 36 percent and 38 percent global CAP emissions, respectively, with the greatest emissions from the energy, transportation, and industry sectors (IPCC 2014a). Notably, global CAP emissions dipped following the 2007–2008 financial crisis but are on the rise again since 2017 (Jackson et al. 2018). These heterogeneities in emissions create opportunities and challenges for climate mitigation policymaking.

Climate mitigation policymaking requires collective action across a range of stakeholders. This is challenging as stakeholders differ sharply in their current and historical contributions to CAP emissions and also in the threats they face from climate inaction. Mitigation policymaking therefore involves core issues of equity, justice, and fairness (IPCC 2014a). It is also strongly influenced by how populations perceive long- and short-term risk. Assessments of the health co-benefits of climate mitigation policies can help identify areas where efforts to address the long-term effects of climate change intersect with near-term societal goals surrounding improvements in public health.

Estimating the Health Co-Benefits of Climate Mitigation

Modeling the Health Effects of Mitigation

Early work on the health co-benefits of mitigation approached the issue qualitatively, positing relationships between mitigation activities and health. These studies explored health co-benefits of strategies ranging from less polluting energy production (Aunan et al. 2006; Bell et al. 2008; Cifuentes et al. 2001; Walsh 2008), active transport (Rissel 2009; Roberts and Arnold 2007; Woodcock et al. 2007), changes in the built environment (Younger et al. 2008), reduced meat consumption (McMichael et al. 2007), and improved access to reproductive health services (Kippen, McCalman, and Wiseman 2010; Rao and Samarth 2010; Richards 2007; Stephenson, Newman, and Mayhew 2010; Stott 2010). More recently, a number of groups have taken up the challenge of generating *quantitative* estimates of co-benefits that could result from mitigation actions in a range of sectors and areas, including land transport (Maizlish et al. 2013; Xia et al. 2015), food and agriculture (Hallström et al. 2017; Springmann et al. 2016), built environment (MacNaughton et al. 2018), electric power generation (Partridge and Gamkhar 2012; Plachinski et al. 2014; Rafaj et al. 2013), short-lived CAPs (Anenberg et al. 2012; Sarofim, Waldhoff, and Anenberg 2017), and household energy (Freeman and Zerriffi 2014; Shen 2015). Such modeling analyses are valuable because they can demonstrate and compare which major mitigation policies have health benefits, as well as provide the means of estimating the cost savings associated with health impacts, which are essential for economic analyses of mitigation strategies (Chang et al. 2017).

Estimating the health co-benefits of mitigation strategies can be pursued using mathematical and statistical models that take several forms. Some use a comparative risk assessment approach (Woodcock, Givoni, and Morgan 2013; Xia et al. 2015); some incorporate complex mechanistic submodels (such as building physics models, e.g., Shindell et al. 2012; Wilkinson et al. 2009); others make use of macroeconomic approaches (Crawford-Brown et al. 2013; Jensen et al. 2013) or integrated assessment models (Rao et al. 2013; West, Fiore, and Horowitz 2012); and still others integrate detailed technological and behavioral elements (Macmillan et al. 2014). Despite these differences, models characterizing the health effects of mitigation policies generally share a common basic approach involving four steps: framework and scoping, impact assessment, valuation, and sensitivity/uncertainty analyses (Remais et al. 2014) (Figure 19.2).

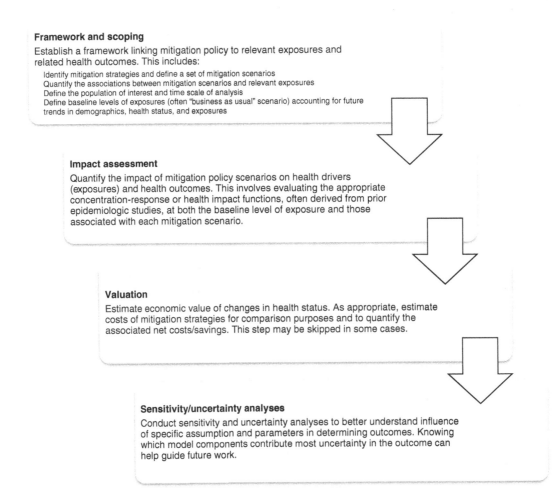

Framework and scoping

Establish a framework linking mitigation policy to relevant exposures and related health outcomes. This includes:
Identify mitigation strategies and define a set of mitigation scenarios
Quantify the associations between mitigation scenarios and relevant exposures
Define the population of interest and time scale of analysis
Define baseline levels of exposures (often "business as usual" scenario) accounting for future trends in demographics, health status, and exposures

Impact assessment

Quantify the impact of mitigation policy scenarios on health drivers (exposures) and health outcomes. This involves evaluating the appropriate concentration-response or health impact functions, often derived from prior epidemiologic studies, at both the baseline level of exposure and those associated with each mitigation scenario.

Valuation

Estimate economic value of changes in health status. As appropriate, estimate costs of mitigation strategies for comparison purposes and to quantify the associated net costs/savings. This step may be skipped in some cases.

Sensitivity/uncertainty analyses

Conduct sensitivity and uncertainty analyses to better understand influence of specific assumption and parameters in determining outcomes. Knowing which model components contribute most uncertainty in the outcome can help guide future work.

Figure 19.2   The key steps in estimating the health co-benefits of mitigation
Source: Adapted from Remais et al. (2014).
Note: Estimation of longer-term health benefits from averting climate change is not considered in this co-benefits estimation framework.

Estimation Challenges

Although dozens of health co-benefit studies have been conducted, there are several overlapping challenges that have been highlighted in recent reviews (Chang et al. 2017; Deng et al. 2018; Gao et al. 2018; Remais et al. 2014; Smith et al. 2016), summarized in Table 19.1. These include difficulties generating credible and comparable scenarios owing to uncertainties in future CAP emissions, particularly in rapidly developing countries that may dramatically increase their emissions in coming decades; challenges in estimating the uptake of mitigation strategies and policies; ethical and economically viable valuation of resulting gains in health, particularly those reducing premature mortality; and the evaluation of key modeling assumptions during estimation of co-benefits and the interpretation of their results (Chang et al. 2017; Gao et al. 2018; Garcia-Menendez et al. 2015; Macmillan et al. 2014; Remais et al. 2014; Rojas-Rueda et al. 2011). These challenges generate uncertainties (e.g., from assumptions related to future scenario demographics, technologies, and economies) that should be characterized during co-benefits analysis and should be reported alongside the estimated health impacts as overall uncertainty estimates.

Finally, it is worth noting that there are serious analytical consequences of compounding conservative assumptions in co-benefits analyses. Conservative assumptions that are routinely incorporated into co-benefits estimation include the exclusion of numerous health outcomes

Table 19.1 Elements of Health Co-Benefit Analyses, Including Those Involved in Analysis of Health Co-Benefits (Left Column) Associated with CAP Reductions, and Those Involved in Estimating CAP Reductions Associated with a Mitigation Policy (Right Column). Estimation of Longer-Term Health Benefits from Averting Climate Change Are Not Considered Here.

Health analysis	Mitigation analysis
Baseline characteristics • Demographic characteristics (e.g., population size, age distribution, socioeconomic status) • Baseline disease burden • Baseline distribution of exposure	*Baseline characteristics* • Demographic characteristics (e.g., population size, income) • Distribution of economic activity by sector • Distribution of fuel sources, land use patterns, energy technologies by sector
Scenario assumptions • Health-damaging pollutant(s) to include • Exposure model(s) (e.g., emission-dispersion) • Secular trends in disease • Counterfactual (or reference) exposure • Secular trends in exposure • Demographic trends	*Scenario assumptions* • CAPs to include • Emissions model(s) • Emission reduction per unit mitigation effort • Uptake of mitigation, both rate and coverage • Secular trends in emissions • Economic development and demographic trends • Trend in cooling aerosols
Model assumptions • Time-horizon • Age weighting • Time discounting • Exposure-response relationship(s) • Lags between exposure and outcome • Duration of health outcome/chronicity	*Model assumptions* • Time-horizon • Time discounting • Global warming potentials • Emission factors
Cross-cutting methodological issues • Valuation methodology (economic and cost-benefit analysis, multicriteria analysis) • Treatment of low probability high impact events • Treatment of uncertainty • Temporal and spatial resolution	

with potentially large effects; the exclusion of longer-term health benefits from averting climate change; the selection of lower, conservative ranges for model parameters; the partiality for including well-understood, short-term health effects over long-term sequelae; excluding potential "tail" events; and the unambitious implementation of mitigation strategies. These can lead to excessively conservative estimates of health co-benefits, and although they represent intentionally underestimated impacts that are meant to be interpreted as a lower bound, such results can have the unintended consequence of diminishing the estimated potential impact of mitigation policies and ultimately result in less effective climate change policy (Field et al. 2014).

Climate Mitigation Health Co-Benefits by Sector

Here, we review recent evidence for the expected health co-benefits resulting from mitigation actions within key sectors (Table 19.2).

Electricity and Energy Generation

Climate Impacts

The electricity and energy generation sector is the largest contributor to CAP emissions worldwide due to the combustion of fossil fuels, and growing global demand for heating, cooling and other uses of electrical power (IPCC 2014a). In the U.S., electric power generation accounted

Table 19.2   Summary of Sector, Mitigation Strategy, and Potential Health Co-Benefits of Mitigation Strategies. Longer-Term Health Benefits from Averting Climate Change Are Not Considered Here.

Sector and mitigation strategy	Health drivers	Potential health co-benefits
Electricity and Energy Generation		
Increased adoption of renewable energy	Reduced conventional air pollutants (PM, ozone, NOx)	Decreased cardiovascular morbidity and mortality; asthma and other respiratory diseases
Transportation		
Increased adoption of low-emission vehicles	Reduced conventional air pollutants	Decreased cardiovascular morbidity and mortality; asthma and other respiratory diseases
Increased active transport methods	Reduced conventional air pollutants	Decreased cardiovascular morbidity and mortality; asthma and other respiratory diseases
	Increased physical activity levels	Decreased obesity and diabetes risk; risk of dementia, depression, injury
	Decreased noise	Decreased hypertension, cardio-vascular disease, depression and sleep-related disorders
Food and Agriculture		
Reduced consumption of red meat and transition toward health diets	Reduced consumption of processed and red meats, saturated fats and dietary cholesterol	Decreased ischemic heart disease, stroke, colorectal cancers
	Reduction in overnutrition, increased consumption of fruits and vegetables.	Decreased diabetes, obesity, ischemic heart disease, stroke, colorectal cancers
Reproductive Health		
Increased access to family planning	Increased birth spacing Reduction in family size	Decreased maternal and child mortality Increased maternal education

for 35 percent of U.S. CAP emissions in 2018 (Environmental Protection Agency [EPA] 2019). This sector relies heavily on the combustion of fossil fuels, primarily coal and natural gas, although noncarbon energy sources such as wind, solar, hydropower, and nuclear are growing rapidly (Watts et al. 2018).

Health Impacts

A number of important co-pollutants detrimental to health accompany the CAP emissions of the electricity generation sector, including particulate matter (PM), sulfur dioxide (SO_2), nitrogen oxides (NO_x), and carbon monoxide (CO). These pollutants are a leading source of morbidity and mortality worldwide: in 2017, 3.4 million deaths globally were attributable to ambient particulate matter and ambient ozone pollution (Lancet 2018). Coal use alone accounts for approximately 16 percent of global air pollution-related premature mortality (Watts et al. 2018). Exposure to PM causes respiratory and cardiovascular deaths (e.g., Pope, Ezzati, and Dockery 2009), lung cancer (International Agency for Research on Cancer [IARC] 2018) and is linked to respiratory and cardiovascular morbidity including chronic obstructive pulmonary disease, asthma, and acute respiratory infections (Guarnieri and Balmes 2014; Lim et al. 2012). The energy generation sector can also contribute to ground-level ozone, which forms when NO_x (a primary pollutant produced by the energy sector) and volatile organic compounds react with sunlight. Like PM, ozone has been linked to a number of respiratory outcomes including asthma exacerbations and premature death (e.g., Anenberg et al. 2010; Bell et al. 2004; Nazare et al. 2013).

Health Co-Benefits of Mitigation Strategies

Decarbonization of the electricity generation sector is projected to substantially reduce CAP emissions while simultaneously improving human health (Chang et al. 2017; Gao et al. 2018) through reductions of co-pollutants, such as $PM_{2.5}$ and ozone. Prior studies describe consequent reductions in mortality and morbidity associated with reduced exposures to these pollutants (e.g., Anenberg et al. 2012; Markandya et al. 2009; Sarofim et al. 2017; Shindell et al. 2012). For example, a multisite study found that a policy reducing CO_2 emissions by 50 percent by 2050 would prevent 104, 542, and 1,492 years of life lost per million people in the European Union, China, and India, respectively (Markandya et al. 2009). A more ambitious policy modeled in Mexico, reducing CAP emissions by 77 percent relative to a baseline scenario, was estimated to avert nearly 3,000 deaths per year in the country (Crawford-Brown et al. 2012).

There are a range of available mitigation strategies for decarbonizing electricity generation, including: implementation of renewable portfolio standards (i.e., setting 50 percent of statewide electricity sales to renewables by 2030); market-based initiatives (i.e., carbon trading programs and carbon taxes); and setting CO_2 emissions standards for power plants (Driscoll et al. 2015). A key study of **renewable energy** technologies in California estimated that the net effect of renewable energy implementation in the state is expected to reduce overall emissions of criteria air pollutants and $PM_{2.5}$ concentrations, thus avoiding approximately 880 premature deaths per year in 2030 (Zapata, Muller, Kleeman 2013).

Carbon trading and carbon taxes provide market-based solutions that incentivize decarbonization and thus reductions in CAP emissions (Haites et al. 2018). Carbon trading programs, including the cap-and-trade approaches in California, the European Union, and some Canadian provinces, are examples of market-based strategies that set upper limits on the total emissions that can be released, allowing emitters to trade emissions credits ("carbon credits") from those that have not used their full allowance (Richardson, English, and Rudolph 2012).

A study in California found that this approach had larger net health co-benefits than policies that targeted specific sectors, such as transportation (Thompson et al. 2014). However, concerns have been raised surrounding the ways in which cap-and-trade approaches can inadvertently incentivize facilities to concentrate their emissions around lower-income communities as they pursue the purchase of offsets in other areas, creating emission "hotspots." As companies reduce emissions off site, and continue to emit within the lower-income communities in which they operate, potential health disparities can arise (California Air Resources Board 2018; Cushing et al. 2018).

Mitigation strategies that set CO_2 emission standards on power plants also hold promise for reducing CAP emissions and improving health outcomes. One study estimating the impact of CO_2 emission standards similar to the U.S. Clean Power Plan resulted in the largest reductions of co-pollutant emissions by 2020, including PM2.5 and ozone, and the greatest health co-benefits, when compared to scenarios with less stringent emission standards (Driscoll et al. 2015), resulting in health co-benefits of approximately $12 billion (95 percent confidence interval, $-15 billion to $51 billion) accounting for the cost of the policy implementation (Buonocore et al. 2016). Thus, power plant carbon standards hold potential as powerful mitigation tools with a marked impact on air quality and health.

Challenges, Uncertainties, and Future Directions

The energy sector is associated with a number of additional adverse environmental exposures, both from the emissions of harmful co-pollutants during energy generation and during oil and gas extraction. For example, burning coal generates mercury, a neurotoxin that can bioaccumulate in the food chain. Detrimental health effects have been associated with unconventional natural gas development (UNGD), also known as hydraulic fracturing or fracking (Adgate, Goldstein, and McKenzie 2014; Wilke and Freeman 2017) including asthma exacerbation (Rasmussen et al. 2016), adverse birth outcomes (Casey 2016; McKenzie et al. 2014), and effects associated with contaminated ground water (Rozell and Reaven 2012). Oil and gas extraction also presents considerable occupational risks as workers face high rates of occupational mortality (Mason et al. 2015). However, given the very large contribution of ambient air pollution to morbidity and mortality, the focus of health co-benefits studies in the energy sector has been on the impacts of mitigation on reductions to ambient air pollution, primarily PM and ozone, and the health sequelae of these reductions.

Although renewable energy adoption is growing, changing policy and practice in this sector is challenging. Renewable energy technology policies have been effective in driving recent adoption and growth of renewable energy, but ongoing support is needed (e.g., in the form of renewable energy quota obligations for states or cities, sufficiently high carbon prices to push for renewable energy adoption, regulatory stability etc.) to accelerate the integration of renewable energy technologies into future electricity systems (IPCC 2014a). The uptake of renewable energy sources for electricity generation is additionally complicated by the low cost of coal, particularly in developing countries (Markandya et al. 2009). Because no energy source is free of health impacts, it is important that co-benefits studies fully synthesize the downstream impacts of new policies to effectively protect public health and environmental quality.

Transportation

Climate Impacts

Transportation is an important source of CAP emissions globally as fossil fuels are burned to move passenger cars, light-duty trucks, ships, trains, and planes. Owing to economic development and global travel, transportation-sourced CAP emissions are rising faster than those of other sectors and are predicted to approximately double from 2010 to 2050 in the absence of mitigation policies, with rapid growth projected in low- and middle-income countries (LMICs) (IPCC 2014a). In the United States, the transportation sector accounted for 29 percent of CAP emissions in 2017 and they continue to grow steadily (EPA 2019). The majority of CAP emissions in this sector globally are due to road travel (72 percent of global transportation CAP emissions in 2010), including cars and freight vehicles (IPCC 2014a). Notably, there is great potential for mitigation to reduce emissions in this sector, through increased fuel efficiency, lower carbon emissions vehicles, and reducing carbon-intensive vehicle travel through public transportation and urban design.

Health Impacts

Transportation is a major source of morbidity and mortality through health risks including transportation-associated air pollution, traffic accidents and injuries, and chronic diseases associated with reductions in active transport. Worldwide, motorized road transport accidents are responsible for roughly 1.2 million deaths annually, with ten times as many people injured, leading to an estimated loss of 75.5 million disability-adjusted life years (GBD 2013 DALYs and HALE Collaborators et al. 2015) in 2010 (World Health Organization [WHO] 2015). Motor vehicles emit health-damaging air pollutants, including $PM_{2.5}$, VOCs, and oxides of nitrogen, which can lead to respiratory and cardiovascular illness. The transportation sector is estimated to be responsible for up to 50 percent of PM emissions across Organisation for Economic Co-operation and Development countries, yet it is LMICs that suffer higher burdens of disease from ambient air pollution (WHO 2019).

Additionally, reliance on passenger car transport can decrease physical activity and contribute to risks of obesity, diabetes, and depression (Grabow et al. 2012; Younger et al. 2008). Shifting away from personal motor vehicle travel toward active transport—for example, walking or bicycling—can increase physical activity, which has both mental and physical health benefits, including reduced risk of cardiovascular disease, colon cancer, diabetes, obesity, dementia, breast cancer, and depression (Woodcock et al. 2009; Younger et al. 2008). Motorized transportation is also a major source of noise pollution, which has been associated with higher rates of hypertension, cardiovascular disease, depression, sleep-related disorders, and inattention among children (Basner et al. 2014).

Health Co-Benefits of Mitigation Strategies

Estimates of the health co-benefits of mitigation policies targeting the transportation sector have primarily focused on mitigation policies to increase active transport (e.g., through investments in public transportation, walking, and cycling infrastructure) as well as policies promoting increased use of lower carbon-emitting motor vehicles.

Many studies have investigated hypothetical scenarios where personal automobiles are replaced with active transport, yielding significant health and economic benefits (Grabow et al. 2012; Lindsay, Macmillan, and Woodward 2011; Rojas-Rueda et al. 2011). These studies have primarily considered the combined impacts of active transport (and a corresponding reduction in vehicle miles traveled) on ambient air quality and associated health effects, traffic-related injuries, and physical activity. A consistent finding across studies is that the health benefits of increased physical activity from active transport generally outweigh those from improved air quality or fewer injuries (e.g., Grabow et al. 2012; Maizlish et al. 2013). For example, a shift of 5 percent of vehicle kilometers traveled to bicycling in New Zealand was estimated to reduce CAP emissions by 0.4 percent annually, as well as to prevent 116 deaths due to increases in physical activity and 6 deaths due to air pollution (Lindsay et al. 2011).

Co-benefits studies of active transport policies include establishing bikeshare programs (Rojas-Rueda et al. 2011), improving public transport options (Xia et al. 2015), and introducing congestion charges or similar pricing schemes to reduce personal vehicle use (Chang et al. 2017). A growing body of literature shows that active transport programs are most successful when they employ an integrated approach that provides safe infrastructure, such as sidewalks and protected bike lanes, land use planning that minimizes travel time and distance, advocacy and education (IPCC 2014a). Low-carbon transport system opportunities may be most beneficial in fast-growing, emerging economies, where infrastructure investments can help avoid future lock-in to carbon intensive modes (IPCC 2014a).

Several studies have estimated the health impacts of efforts to reduce vehicle emissions through increased adoption of lower carbon emission motor vehicles, such as fuel cell, gas-electric hybrids, and electric vehicles that lower CAP emissions per passenger mile traveled, with concurrent reductions in air pollutant emissions (Maizlish et al. 2013; Perez et al. 2015; Woodcock et al. 2009). Research focused on the San Francisco Bay Area found that low-carbon driving, including adoption of light-duty diesel, biofuel, gas-electric hybrid and electric vehicles, could potentially reduce CAP emissions in 2035 by 33.5 percent compared to a 2000 baseline of 27.9 million metric tons of CO_2 (Maizlish et al. 2013). Although increased adoption of **low-emission vehicles** reduces ambient air pollution, lowering air pollution-related morbidity and mortality, studies have generally found that increases in active transportation yield greater health effects than increases in use of low-emission vehicles (Maizlish et al. 2013; Woodcock et al. 2009).

Challenges, Uncertainties, and Future Directions

In spite of technological advances in vehicle efficiency and adoption of low-carbon transportation policies, growth in transport-associated CAP emissions has continued over the past decade (Watts et al. 2018). To spur the rapid adoption of carbon-reducing transportation policies, behavioral changes are needed such as purchasing low-carbon vehicles and avoiding short-distance driving (Watts et al. 2018; Woodcock et al. 2009). Suburban sprawl presents a particular challenge as low-density, spatially disconnected suburban and rural communities generate longer vehicle trips and commutes (Milner, Davies, and Wilkinson 2012), encourage greater dependency on private transport, and make it more difficult to implement effective public transit (WHO 2009).

There is uncertainty regarding the impact of active transportation policies on traffic-related injuries. Several studies have suggested injuries will increase as more people walk and cycle, highlighting the need for policies that address road safety (Perez et al. 2015; Rojas-Rueda et al. 2016; Woodcock et al. 2009). For example, an increase in active commuting time in the San Francisco Bay Area was estimated to contribute a 39 percent increase in the injury burden (Maizlish et al. 2013) and can result in larger intake of air pollutants during active commuting (Banerjee et al. 2012). Despite conflicting research assumptions and results, co-benefits studies have found that the health benefits of walking and cycling outweigh the risks, often by orders of magnitude (e.g., Lindsay et al. 2011; Otero, Nieuwenhuijsen, and Rojas-Rueda 2018; Rojas-Rueda et al. 2011; Woodcock et al. 2009).

CLINICAL CORRELATES 19.1 TRANSPORTATION FOR HEALTHY EMPLOYEES AND PATIENTS IN SEATTLE

Seattle Children's Hospital is investing in systemwide transportation changes to minimize noise and air pollution including greenhouse gas emissions. Employees reduced single occupancy vehicle transportation from 73 percent in 1995 to 38 percent in 2015 through an incentive program for transit, bicycling, walking, and carpooling (Practice Greenhealth n.d.). A Comprehensive Transportation Plan (Seattle Children's Comprehensive Transportation Plan n.d.) further outlines goals including a 2028 target of less than 30 percent of employees driving alone to work. Success is being measured by reduction in parking spots needed, estimated reduction of carbon emissions, and travel time on nearby streets. To minimize vehicle trips, Seattle Children's offers financial incentives for commuting, well-connected shuttle-to-transit systems, and bicycle programs. They are also investing in a $2 million bicycle and pedestrian project to improve safety and infrastructure in Northeast Seattle, further incentivizing alternative forms of transportation and public health.

Hospitals can lead in reducing single occupancy vehicle transportation through employee incentive programs and investing in community infrastructure development that promotes safe walking and bicycling.

CLINICAL CORRELATES 19.2 NEW YORK CITY PROTECTS CHILDREN WITH ANTI-IDLE LAWS

One-minute of automobile idling creates more carbon monoxide than three packs of cigarettes, with demonstrable environmental health effects on infants, young children, the elderly, and those with chronic diseases (Children's Environmental Health Center [CEHC] n.d.b). New York City passed an anti-idle law to protect these populations, limiting idling to one minute outside of schools and three minutes in the rest of New York City (Burgess, Peffers, and Silverman 2009). Fines are distributed for idling and financial incentives are given to report idling. This policy also intended to incentivize alternative transportation including biking and walking.

The CEHC creates free, downloadable infographics and materials for patients and family members highlighting environmental determinants of health and specific issues such as health harms of idling vehicles (CEHC n.d.a). A children's coloring book "Healthy World, Health You" encourages use of bikes and scooters instead of vehicles for transportation. Other pages focus on consuming plant-based snacks as part of health and to protect the planet. The pictures are paired with science pearls on air pollution, climate change, asthma, and other health conditions. A series of infographics use pictures, colors, and captions to emphasize co-benefits of policies in place.

Child-centered policies and educational materials help ensure children are engaged in healthy behaviors from an early age and are considered in policy development processes.

Food and Agriculture

Climate Impacts

The food and agriculture sector is a key source of global CAP emissions (IPCC 2014a) including methane, nitrous oxide, and carbon dioxide. Methane is released by ruminants, such as cows and sheep (also called enteric fermentation) and by methane-producing bacteria in flooded rice paddies during the breakdown of organic matter. Nitrous oxide is released during cultivation of crops and by manure and other fertilizers. Carbon dioxide is released during deforestation to provide land for crops and livestock, from farm equipment operation (e.g., tractors, irrigation systems), and during transportation of agricultural products. Livestock account for approximately 80 percent of the emissions from the food and agriculture sector, largely due to enteric fermentation and deforestation to provide additional land for ruminants and cultivation of feed crops (Food and Agriculture Organization 2006). Because of a combination of rising prosperity and population growth, demand for animal products is expected to rise through mid-century (Popkin 2006; Springmann et al. 2017).

Health Impacts

Estimates of food and agriculture sector health co-benefits focus primarily on the health impacts of reduced meat consumption and reduction in overnutrition. The consumption of red and processed meat has been linked to cardiovascular disease and certain cancers. The IARC has classified red meat as a probable human carcinogen based on evidence linking red meat consumption to colorectal cancer, and possibly pancreatic and prostate cancer (IARC 2018). IARC classifies processed meat (defined as meat that has been salted, cured, fermented, or smoked) as a carcinogen, linked to colorectal cancer, and possibly stomach cancer (IARC). However, the association between animal protein consumption and cardiovascular disease (from consumption of dietary cholesterol and saturated fat) has the greatest implications for population health. Ischemic heart disease and stroke are leading causes of death globally (GBD 2017 Causes of Death Collaborators 2018) and even modest increases in risk due to red meat consumption can have major impacts on population health. Overnutrition (excess caloric intake) is also linked to cardiovascular disease, as well as obesity and type 2 diabetes (Popkin 2006). Overnutrition is a global problem (Mendez, Monteiro, and Popkin 2005), and many countries face the dual burden of over- and undernutrition (Lim et al. 2012).

Health Co-benefits of Mitigation

Evaluations of health co-benefits of reduced food/agriculture sector CAP emissions have focused on the climate and health co-benefits of (1) mitigation measures focused on changing demand for high-CAP foods, primarily reducing red meat consumption; and (2) bringing diets in line with global recommendations (Chang et al. 2017). Technological changes can reduce emissions at the point of cultivation, via improved manure management and enhanced efficiency of livestock farming, but the reductions in emissions are modest and these interventions are not expected to yield meaningful health co-benefits (Friel et al. 2009; McMichael et al. 2007).

Several studies have estimated the health co-benefits and potential changes in CAP emissions from reductions in red meat consumption (e.g., Friel et al. 2009; Scarborough et al. 2012). The greatest health benefits and reductions in CAP emissions appear to come from efforts to replace meat and dairy consumption with the consumption of fruit and vegetables (Aston, Smith, and Powles 2012; Scarborough et al. 2012; Springmann et al. 2016).

Others have estimated the climate and health benefits of adopting healthier diets (Farchi et al. 2017; Hallström et al. 2017; Milner et al. 2015; Springmann et al. 2016). For example, if globally, diets were to conform with the 2003 World Health Organization dietary guidelines (WHO 2003) and constrain caloric intake to those needed for a health body weight by 2050, global mortality would decline 6–10 percent due to reductions in the consumption of meat, increased consumption of fruits and vegetables, and reductions in overweight and obesity, and food-related CAP emissions would decline 30–70 percent, compared to dietary projections for 2050 based on current consumption patterns (Springmann et al. 2016).

Challenges, Uncertainties, and Future Directions

One of the key challenges in this sector is how to reduce meat and total calorie consumption. One approach is to tax food commodities according to their emissions. For example, a commodity tax borne by consumers could yield a 9 percent reduction in food-related CAP emissions, primarily because of reduced consumption of beef and, to a lesser extent, milk, along with approximately 100,000 global deaths averted in 2020 (Springmann et al. 2017). Opinions vary regarding what levels of reduction in red meat consumption will be widely acceptable. In 2019, a global commission recommended a healthy diet include on average 14 g of red meat per day (approximately one tenth of a quarter pounder hamburger); this would require a global reduction in red meat consumption by 50 percent (Willett et al. 2019). Given that food is closely linked with cultural identity, adoption of recommended diets and policies to promote their adoption should be tailored to target populations.

Another key challenge is addressing diverse nutritional needs among global populations. Dietary habits vary by sex and region, and therefore associated dietary changes will vary by population, as will the expected changes in health (Farchi et al. 2017; Springmann et al. 2016; Willett et al. 2019). Accounting for regional variation in current dietary practices and access is important, because there are populations who are not meeting their basic dietary needs for total calories and micronutrients, with young children and pregnant women in low-income settings particularly vulnerable.

CLINICAL CORRELATES 19.3 HEALTH CARE INSTITUTIONS FOR FOOD SUSTAINABILITY

Health care institutions are recognizing the need to incorporate environmental sustainability in their food and nutrition operations. They are investing in sustainable food options for patients, employees, and visitors by purchasing local foods, reducing meat served, purchasing meat without routine antibiotics, offering fruit and vegetable prescription programs, and having onsite community supported agriculture (CSA) programs (Health Care Without Harm 2019). Medical centers are also becoming creative by having gardens open for patients and caregivers to grow produce and are launching mobile kitchens in partnership with dietitians and chefs to educate the public about healthy foods (Ohio State University n.d.). The Cool Food Pledge and Health Care Culinary Contest are two other opportunities offered by Health Care Without Harm and Practice Greenhealth to provide incentives for healthy food and environmental sustainability.

Health care institutions are addressing nutrition, health, food production, and greenhouse gas emissions through changes in food purchasing and education with employees and patients.

Reproductive Health and Other Areas

There are potential opportunities for health co-benefits (or co-harms) in addition to the aforementioned areas. Improved reproductive health and family planning access offer health co-benefits, because population growth acts in concert with economic, geopolitical, and other factors to affect global CAP emissions (O'Neill et al. 2010). Concurrently, health improvements in children and mothers can accompany reproductive health and family planning (Canning and Schultz 2012). Contraceptive access and family planning can improve birth spacing, reduce maternal and child mortality, and reduce high-risk births for women of very young maternal age (Cleland et al. 2012). Family planning can reduce the average number of births a woman may have in her lifetime, providing increased opportunities for women to obtain skills that raise lifetime productivity and earnings, and leave more resources for parents to invest per child in health, nutrition, and education (Canning and Schultz 2012). Birth spacing has an impact on neonatal and infant mortality, with the risk of dying decreasing with increasing birth interval lengths (Rutstein 2005).

These same changes in fertility can influence global CAP emissions. In a seminal analysis, the climate benefits of fulfilling the unmet need for family planning and reproductive health services in many countries was estimated to be substantial, amounting to more than 1 gigaton of carbon per year by 2050 as certain CAP emissions associated with energy use are proportionally driven by changes in population size (O'Neill et al. 2010). Still, substantial uncertainties remain. For one, reductions in fertility leading to slowed population growth may yield rising incomes per person, potentially offsetting CAP emissions reductions. Additionally, population affects CAP emissions via impacts on tropical deforestation, migration, and other effects; these interconnected dimensions of reproductive health co-benefits represent a significant research gap.

There are mitigation measures that could harm public health. Cultivation of biofuels could negatively impact health through increases in food prices, leading to potential co-harms (Christian 2010; Friel et al. 2009). Some strategies to restrict global warming to 1.5° C (2.7°F) involve carbon capture and storage (IPCC 2018), including through technologies currently under development with potential adverse health implications. The co-benefits estimation framework provides a useful tool for evaluating the health implications of these emerging technologies.

Challenges and Considerations

Climate health co-benefit analyses are ultimately intended to inform policy. Ensuring policy relevance requires matching the interventions explored in co-benefits models with real-world policy possibilities and administrative realities (Remais et al. 2014). Collaboration between scientists and policymakers is critical to developing credible mitigation scenarios (Dilling and Lemos 2011). This is particularly important as it relates to generating reasonable assumptions about the implementation of mitigation strategies, including the uptake of new technologies (e.g., **renewable energy** generation) or behaviors (e.g., choosing **active transportation**). Estimates of multiple **health co-benefits** across diverse **climate mitigation** policies ideally would be available to policymakers when they are weighing policy options (Remais et al. 2014). However, generating consistent, comparable results of co-benefits analyses to inform mitigation policy has been a challenge. Establishment and adoption of conventions for conducting and reporting results of co-benefits analyses would aid in assessing the validity of co-benefits estimates, and comparing the health impacts of different mitigation policies.

Another area in need of attention is the potential of mitigation measures to reduce or exacerbate health inequalities (Anderson et al. 2018; Chang et al. 2017; Cushing et al. 2018; Springmann et al. 2017). Approaching analyses through an equity lens can help identify populations that will reap the greatest gains and/or risks.

Summary

Climate mitigation policies have the potential to directly affect human health. It is possible to generate quantitative estimates of these health impacts using a four-step process starting with mapping a framework linking the policy to potential health outcomes, followed by estimating impacts, valuation of the health impacts and, lastly, conducting sensitivity analyses to evaluate the impact of different assumptions on estimates. A number of climate mitigation policies and actions are expected to have a large, net positive impact on health in the near term. Characterizing health co-benefits can help inform and motivate climate mitigation policies (IPCC 2014a). Co-benefit analysis provides an opportunity for epidemiology and public health to play an important role in global climate mitigation policymaking. There are indications that more optimal societal benefits can be achieved when diverse experts, constituencies, and stakeholders—including health scientists, health care providers, and public health practitioners—participate in tandem with policy makers in the design and push for a low-carbon economy (Haines et al. 2009). The extent to which these near-term health impacts influence mitigation policy depends on a combination of factors, including the perceived rigor of the co-benefits estimates, as well as the values and priorities of policymakers.

DISCUSSION QUESTIONS

1. Promoting access to contraception has been proposed as a climate mitigation policy. Describe how this could affect carbon emissions, and outline the potential health co-benefits (and/or co-harms) of such a policy.

2. Many scenarios to meet carbon emission reduction targets rely in part on carbon capture and storage technologies, many of which are still under development. What information would you want to know about these technologies to assess health co-benefits?

3. The health co-benefits of climate mitigation policies may not be distributed equally. Consider policies to improve access to public transport in an urban area. What populations might benefit most? Least? What policies could be adopted to increase the equitable distribution of co-benefits?

KEY TERMS

Active transport: The use of nonmotorized transportation forms, such as walking, cycling, or public transit.

Adaptation: Efforts to lessen the impacts of climate change through measures to prepare populations for a changing climate, such as disaster preparedness and flood control.

Climate-altering pollutants (CAPs): Pollutants that contribute to global warming, including carbon dioxide, methane, and nitrous oxides.

Climate mitigation: Efforts to reduce climate-altering pollutant concentrations through reductions in emissions and/or increases in carbon capture.

Co-benefits: The near-term health benefits that directly accrue from climate mitigation strategies.

Co-harms: Adverse health impacts of climate mitigation strategies.

Low-emission vehicles: Gas-alternative or gas-hybrid vehicles (e.g., fuel cell, gas-electric hybrids, electric vehicles) that lower CAP emissions per passenger mile traveled, with concurrent reductions in air pollutant emissions.

Renewable energy: Cleaner energy sources that include solar photovoltaic (PV) cells, wind turbines, and hydroelectric power.

References

Adgate, J. L., B. D. Goldstein, L. M. McKenzie. 2014. "Potential Public Health Hazards, Exposures and Health Effects from Unconventional Natural Gas Development." *Environmental Science and Technology* 48:8307–20.

Anderson, C. M., K. A. Kissel, C. B. Field, and K. J. Mach. 2018. "Climate Change Mitigation, Air Pollution, and Environmental Justice in California." *Environmental Science and Technology* 52:10829–38.

Anenberg, S. C., L. W. Horowitz, D. Q. Tong, and J. J. West. 2010. "An Estimate of the Global Burden of Anthropogenic Ozone and Fine Particulate Matter on Premature Human Mortality Using Atmospheric Modeling." *Environmental Health Perspectives* 118:1189–95.

Anenberg, S. C., J. Schwartz, D. Shindell, M. Amann, G. Faluvegi, Z. Klimont, G. Janssens-Maenhout et al. 2012. "Global Air Quality and Health Co-Benefits of Mitigating Near-Term Climate Change through Methane and Black Carbon Emission Controls." *Environmental Health Perspectives* 120:831–39.

Aston, L. M., J. N. Smith, and J. W. Powles. 2012. "Impact of a Reduced Red and Processed Meat Dietary Pattern on Disease Risks and Greenhouse Gas Emissions in the UK: A Modelling Study." *BMJ Open* 2.

Aunan, K., J. Fang, T. Hu, H. M. Seip, and H. Vennemo. 2006. "Climate Change and Air Quality—Measures with Co-Benefits in China." *Environmental Science and Technology* 40:4822–29.

Banerjee, R., S. M. Benson, D. H. Bouille, A. Brew-Hammond, A. Cherp, S. T. Coelho, L. Emberson et al. 2012. *Global Energy Assessment—Toward a Sustainable Future: Key Findings; Summary for Policymakers; Technical Summary.* Cambridge, UK: Cambridge University Press; Laxenburg, Austria: International Institute for Applied Systems Analysis.

Basner, M., W. Babisch, A. Davis, M. Brink, C. Clark, S. Janssen, and S. Stansfield. 2014. "Auditory and Non-Auditory Effects of Noise on Health." *Lancet* 383:1325–32.

Bell, M. L., D. L. Davis, L. A. Cifuentes, A. J. Krupnick, R. D. Morgenstern, and G. D. Thurston. 2008. "Ancillary Human Health Benefits of Improved Air Quality Resulting from Climate Change Mitigation." *Environmental Health: A Global Access Science Source* 7:41.

Bell, M. L., A. McDermott, S. L. Zeger, J. M. Samet, and F. Dominici. 2004. "Ozone and Short-Term Mortality in 95 US Urban Communities, 1987–2000." *JAMA* 292:2372–78.

Buonocore, J. J., K. F. Lambert, D. Burtraw, S. Sekar, and C. T. Driscoll. 2016. "An Analysis of Costs and Health Co-Benefits for a U.S. Power Plant Carbon Standard." *PLoS One* 11:e0156308.

Burgess, E., M. Peffers, and I. Silverman. 2009. "The Health, Environmental and Economic Impacts of Engine Idling in New York City." Environmental Defense Fund. https://www.edf.org/sites/default/files/9236_Idling_Nowhere_2009.pdf.

California Air Resources Board. 2018. "Public Hearing to Consider the Amendments to the California Cap on Greenhouse Gas Emissions and Market-Based Compliance Mechanisms." https://ww3.arb.ca.gov/regact/2018/capandtrade18/ct18fsor.pdf.

Canning, D., and T. P. Schultz. 2012. "The Economic Consequences of Reproductive Health and Family Planning." *Lancet* 380:165–71.

Casey, J. A., D. A. Savitz, S. G. Rasmussen, E. L. Ogburn, J. Pollak, D. G. Mercer, and B. S. Schwartz. 2016. "Unconventional Natural Gas Development and Birth Outcomes in Pennsylvania, USA." *Epidemiology* 27:163.

Chang, K. M., J. J. Hess, J. M. Balbus, J. J. Buonocore, D. A. Cleveland, M. L. Grabow, R. Neff et al. 2017. "Ancillary Health Effects of Climate Mitigation Scenarios as Drivers of Policy Uptake: A Review of Air Quality, Transportation and Diet Co-Benefits Modeling Studies." *Environmental Research Letters* 12.

Children's Environmental Health Center. n.d.a. "Educational Materials." Accessed March 28, 2020. https://icahn.mssm.edu/about/departments/environmental-public-health/cehc/information.

Children's Environmental Health Center. n.d.b. "Idling Vehicles." Accessed March 28, 2020. https://icahn.mssm.edu/files/ISMMS/Assets/Departments/Environmental%20Medicine%20and%20Public%20Health/CEHC/CEHCInfographics-IdlingVehicles.pdf.

Christian, P. 2010. "Impact of the Economic Crisis and Increase in Food Prices on Child Mortality: Exploring Nutritional Pathways." *Journal of Nutrition* 140:177S–181S.

Cifuentes, L., V. H. Borja-Aburto, N. Gouveia, G. Thurston, and D. L. Davis. 2001. "Assessing the Health Benefits of Urban Air Pollution Reductions Associated with Climate Change Mitigation (2000–2020): Santiago, Sao Paulo, Mexico City, and New York City." *Environmental Health Perspectives* 109 (suppl 3):419–25.

Cleland, J., A. Conde-Agudelo, H. Peterson, J. Ross, and A. Tsui. 2012. "Contraception and Health." *Lancet* 380:149–56.

Crawford-Brown, D., T. Barker, A. Anger, and O. Dessens. 2012. "Ozone and PM Related Health Co-Benefits of Climate Change Policies in Mexico." *Environmental Science and Policy* 17:33–40.

Crawford-Brown, D., P. C. Chen, H. C. Shi, and C. W. Chao. 2013. "Climate Change Air Toxic Co-Reduction in the Context of Macroeconomic Modelling." *Journal of Environmental Management* 125:1–6.

Cushing, L., D. Blaustein-Rejto, M. Wander, M. Pastor, J. Sadd, A. Zhu, and R. Morello-Frosch. 2018. "Carbon Trading, Co-Pollutants, and Environmental Equity: Evidence from California's Cap-and-Trade Program (2011–2015). *PLoS Medicine* 15:e1002604.

Deng, H.-M., Q.-M. Liang, L.-J. Liu, and L. D. Anadon. 2018. "Co-Benefits of Greenhouse Gas Mitigation: A Review and Classification by Type, Mitigation Sector, and Geography." *Environmental Research Letters* 12.

Dilling, L., and M. C. Lemos. 2011. "Creating Usable Science: Opportunities and Constraints for Climate Knowledge Use and Their Implications for Science Policy." *Global Environmental Change* 21:680–9.

Driscoll, C. T., J. J. Buonocore, J. I. Levy, K. F. Lambert, D. Burtraw, S. B. Reid et al. 2015. "US Power Plant Carbon Standards and Clean Air and Health Co-Benefits." *Nature Climate Change* 5:535.

Environmental Protection Agency. 2019. *Inventory of U.S. Greenhouse Gas Emissions and Sinks, 1990–2017.* Washington, DC: EPA.

Farchi, S., M. De Sario, E. Lapucci, M. Davoli, and P. Michelozzi. 2017. "Meat Consumption Reduction in Italian Regions: Health Co-Benefits and Decreases in GHG Emissions." *PLoS One* 12:e0182960.

Field, C. B., V. R. Barros, D. J. Dokken, K. J. Mach, M. D. Mastrandrea, T. E. Bilir, M. Chatterjee et al. 2014. "Summary for Policymakers." In *Climate Change 2014: Impacts, Adaptation, and Vulnerability. Contribution of Working Group II to the Fifth Assessment Report of the Intergovernmental Panel on Climate Change*, edited by C. B. Field, V. R. Barros, D. J. Dokken, K. J. Mach, M. D. Mastrandrea, T. E. Bilir, M. Chatterjee et al., 1–32. Cambridge, UK and New York: Cambridge University Press.

Food and Agriculture Organization. 2006. *Livestock's Long Shadow.* Rome: FAO.

Freeman, O. E., and H. Zerriffi. 2014. "How You Count Carbon Matters: Implications of Differing Cookstove Carbon Credit Methodologies for Climate and Development Co-Benefits." *Environmental Science and Technology* 48:14112–20.

Friel, S., A. D. Dangour, T. Garnett, K. Lock, Z. Chalabi, I. Roberts, A. Butler et al. 2009. "Public Health Benefits of Strategies to Reduce Greenhouse-Gas Emissions: Food and Agriculture." *Lancet* 374:2016–25.

Gao, J., S. Kovats, S. Vardoulakis, P. Wilkinson, A. Woodward, J. Li, S. Gu et al. 2018. "Public Health Co-Benefits of Greenhouse Gas Emissions Reduction: A Systematic Review." *Science of the Total Environment* 627:388–402.

Garcia-Menendez, S. R., R. K. Saari, E. Monier, and N. E. Selin. 2015. "U.S. Air Quality and Health Benefits from Avoided Climate Change under Greenhouse Gas Mitigation." *Environmental Science and Technology* 49:7580–8.

GBD 2017 Causes of Death Collaborators. 2018. "Global, Regional, and National Age-Sex-Specific Mortality for 282 Causes of Death in 195 Countries and Territories, 1980-2017: A Systematic Analysis for the Global Burden of Disease Study 2017." *Lancet* 392:1736–88.

GBD DALYs and HALE Collaborators, C. J. Murray, R. M. Barber, K. J. Foreman, A. Abbasoglu Ozgoren, F. Abd-Allah, S. F. Abera, V. Aboyans et al. 2015. "Global, Regional, and National Disability-Adjusted Life Years (DALYs) for 306 Diseases and Injuries and Healthy Life Expectancy (HALE) for 188 Countries, 1990–2013: Quantifying the Epidemiological Transition." *Lancet* 386:2145–91.

Grabow, M. L., S. N. Spak, T. Holloway, B. Stone, A. C. Mednick, and J. A. Patz. 2012. "Air Quality and Exercise-Related Health Benefits from Reduced Car Travel in the Midwestern United States." *Environmental Health Perspectives* 120:68–76.

Guarnieri, M., and J. R. Balmes. 2014. "Outdoor Air Pollution and Asthma." *Lancet* 383:1581–92.

Haines, A., A. J. McMichael, K. R. Smith, I. Roberts, J. Woodcock, A. Markandya, B. G. Armstrong et al. 2009. "Public Health Benefits of Strategies to Reduce Greenhouse-Gas Emissions: Overview and Implications for Policy Makers." *Lancet* 374:2104–14.

Haites, E., D. Maosheng, K. S. Gallagher, S. Mascher, E. Narassimhan, K. R. Richards, and M. Wakabayashi. 2018. "Experience with Carbon Taxes and Greenhouse Gas Emissions Trading Systems." *Duke Environmental Law & Policy Forum* 2018:109–82.

Hallström, E., Q. Gee, P. Scarborough, and D. A. Cleveland. 2017. "A Healthier US Diet Could Reduce Greenhouse Gas Emissions from Both the Food and Health Care Systems." *Climatic Change* 142:199–212.

Health Care Without Harm. 2019. "2019 Health Care Food Trends." November 13, 2019. Accessed March 24, 2020. https://medium.com/@HCWH/2019-health-care-food-trends-77994ade7fa8.

International Agency for Research on Cancer. 2018. *Consumption of Red Meat and Processed Meat.* IARC Monographs on the Evaluation of Carcinogenic Risks to Humans: Vol. 114. Lyon, France: IARC.

Intergovernmental Panel on Climate Change. 2014a. *Climate Change 2014: Impacts, Adaptation, and Vulnerability. Contribution of Working Group II to the Fifth Assessment Report of the Intergovernmental Panel on Climate Change,* edited by C. B. Field, V. R. Barros, D. J. Dokken, K. J. Mach, M. D. Mastrandrea, T. E. Bilir, M. Chatterjee et al. Cambridge, UK and New York: Cambridge University Press.

Intergovernmental Panel on Climate Change. 2014b. *Climate Change 2014: Synthesis Report. Contribution of Working Groups I, II and III to the Fifth Assessment Report of the Intergovernmental Panel on Climate Change,* edited by Core Writing Team, R. K. Pachauri, and L. A. Meyer. Geneva, Switzerland: IPCC.

Intergovernmental Panel on Climate Change 2018. *Global Warming of 1.5°C. An IPCC Special Report on the Impacts of Global Warming of 1.5°C above Pre-Industrial Levels and Related Global Greenhouse Gas Emission Pathways, in the Context of Strengthening the Global Response to the Threat of Climate Change, Sustainable Development, and Efforts to Eradicate Poverty,* edited by V. Masson-Delmotte, P. Zhai, H.-O. Pörtner, D. Roberts, J. Skea, P. R. Shukla, A. Pirani, W. Moufouma-Okia et al. Geneva: Intergovernmental Panel on Climate Change.

Jackson, Q. C. L., R. M. Andrew, J. G. Canadell, J. I. Korsbakken, Z. Liu, G. P. Peters, and B. Zheng. 2018. "Global Energy Growth Is Outpacing Decarbonization." *Environmental Research Letters* 13.

Jensen, H. T., M. R. Keogh-Brown, R. D. Smith, Z. Chalabi, A. D. Dangour, M. Davies, P. Edwards et al. 2013. "The Importance of Health Co-Benefits in Macroeconomic Assessments of UK Greenhouse Gas Emission Reduction Strategies." *Climatic Change* 121:223–37.

Kippen, R., J. McCalman, and J. Wiseman. 2010. "Climate Change and Population Policy: Towards a Just and Transformational Approach." *Journal of Public Health* 32:161–2.

Lancet. 2018. "Global, Regional, and National Comparative Risk Assessment of 84 Behavioural, Environmental and Occupational, and Metabolic Risks or Clusters of Risks for 195 Countries and Territories, 1990–2017: A Systematic Analysis for the Global Burden of Disease Study 2017." *Lancet* 392:1923–94.

Lim, S. S., T. Vos, A. D. Flaxman, G. Danaei, K. Shibuya, H. Adair-Rohani, M. A. AlMazroa et al. 2012. "A Comparative Risk Assessment of Burden of Disease and Injury Attributable to 67 Risk Factors and Risk Factor Clusters in 21 Regions, 1990–2010: A Systematic Analysis for the Global Burden of Disease Study 2010." *Lancet* 380:2224–60.

Lindsay, G., A. Macmillan, and A. Woodward. 2011. "Moving Urban Trips from Cars to Bicycles: Impact on Health and Emissions." *Australian and New Zealand Journal of Public Health* 35:54–60.

Macmillan, A., J. Connor, K. Witten, R. Kearns, D. Rees, and A. Woodward. 2014. "The Societal Costs and Benefits of Commuter Bicycling: Simulating the Effects of Specific Policies Using System Dynamics Modeling." *Environmental Health Perspectives* 122:335–44.

MacNaughton, P., X. Cao, J. Buonocore, J. Cedeno-Laurent, J. Spengler, A. Bernstein, and J. Allen. 2018. "Energy Savings, Emission Reductions, and Health Co-Benefits of the Green Building Movement." *Journal of Exposure Science & Environmental Epidemiology* 28:307.

Maizlish, N., J. Woodcock, S. Co, B. Ostro, A. Fanai, and D. Fairley. 2013. "Health Cobenefits and Transportation-Related Reductions in Greenhouse Gas Emissions in the San Francisco Bay Area." *American Journal of Public Health* 103:703–9.

Markandya, A., B. G. Armstrong, S. Hales, A. Chiabai, P. Criqui, S. Mima, C. Tonne, and P. Wilkinson. 2009. "Public Health Benefits of Strategies to Reduce Greenhouse-Gas Emissions: Low-Carbon Electricity Generation." *Lancet* 374:2006–15.

Mason, K. L., K. D. Retzer, R. Hill, J. M. Lincoln, Centers for Disease Control and Prevention. 2015. "Occupational Fatalities during the Oil And Gas Boom—United States, 2003–2013." *MMWR. Morbidity and Mortality Weekly Report* 64:551–4.

McKenzie, L. M., R. Guo, R. Z. Witter, D. A. Savitz, L. S. Newman, and J. L. Adgate. 2014. "Birth Outcomes and Maternal Residential Proximity to Natural Gas Development in Rural Colorado." *Environmental Health Perspectives* 122:412–17.

McMichael, A. J., M. Neira, R. Bertollini, D. Campbell-Lendrum, and S. Hales. 2009. "Climate Change: A Time of Need and Opportunity for the Health Sector." *Lancet* 374:2123–25.

McMichael, A. J., J. W. Powles, C. D. Butler, and R. Uauy. 2007. "Food, Livestock Production, Energy, Climate Change, and Health." *Lancet* 370:1253–63.

Mendez, M. A., C. A. Monteiro, and B. M. Popkin. 2005. "Overweight Exceeds Underweight among Women in Most Developing Countries." *American Journal of Clinical Nutrition* 81:714–21.

Milner, J., M. Davies, and P. Wilkinson. 2012. "Urban Energy, Carbon Management (Low Carbon Cities) and Co-Benefits for Human Health." *Current Opinion in Environmental Sustainability* 4:398–404.

Milner, J., R. Green, A. D. Dangour, A. Haines, Z. Chalabi, J. Spadaro, A. Markandya, and P. Wilkinson. 2015. "Health Effects of Adopting Low Greenhouse Gas Emission Diets in the UK." *BMJ Open* 5:e007364.

Nazare, J. A., J. Smith, A. L. Borel, N. Almeras, A. Tremblay, J. Bergeron, P. Poirier, and J.-P. Després. 2013. "Changes in Both Global Diet Quality and Physical Activity Level Synergistically Reduce Visceral Adiposity in Men with Features of Metabolic Syndrome." *Journal of Nutrition* 143:1074–83.

Ohio State University. n.d. "Sustainability at The Ohio State University Wexner Medical Center." Accessed April 2, 2020. https://wexnermedical.osu.edu/about-us/sustainability.

O'Neill, B. C., M. Dalton, R. Fuchs, L. Jiang, S. Pachauri, and K. Zigova. 2010. "Global Demographic Trends and Future Carbon Emissions." *Proceedings of the National Academy of Sciences of the USA* 107:17521–26.

Otero, I., M. J. Nieuwenhuijsen, and D. Rojas-Rueda. 2018. "Health Impacts of Bike Sharing Systems in Europe." *Environment International* 115:387–94.

Partridge, I., S. Gamkhar. 2012. "A Methodology for Estimating Health Benefits of Electricity Generation Using Renewable Technologies." *Environment International* 39:103–110.

Perez, L., S. Trueb, H. Cowie, M. P. Keuken, P. Mudu, M. S. Ragettli, et al. 2015. "Transport-Related Measures to Mitigate Climate Change in Basel, Switzerland: A Health-Effectiveness Comparison Study." *Environment International* 85:111–19.

Plachinski, S. D., T. Holloway, P. J. Meier, G. F. Nemet, A. Rrushaj, J. T. Oberman, et al. 2014. "Quantifying the Emissions and Air Quality Co-Benefits of Lower-Carbon Electricity Production." *Atmospheric Environment* 94:180–91.

Pope, C. A., III, M. Ezzati, and D. W. Dockery. 2009. "Fine-Particulate Air Pollution and Life Expectancy in the United States." *New England Journal of Medicine* 360:376–86.

Popkin, B. M. 2006. "Global Nutrition Dynamics: The World Is Shifting Rapidly toward a Diet Linked with Noncommunicable Diseases." *American Journal of Public Health* 84:289–98.

Practice Greenhealth. n.d. Accessed February 27, 2020. https://practicegreenhealth.org/tools-and-resources/seattle-childrens-hospital-employee-commuting.

Rafaj, P., W. Schöpp, P. Russ, C. Heyes, and M. Amann. 2013. "Co-Benefits of Post-2012 Global Climate Mitigation Policies." *Mitigation and Adaptation Strategies for Global Change* 18:801–24.

Rao, M., and A. Samarth. 2010. "Population Dynamics and Climate Change: Links and Issues for Development." *Journal of Public Health* 32:163–4.

Rao, S., S. Pachauri, F. Dentener, P. Kinney, Z. Klimont, K. Riahi, and W. Schoepp. 2013. "Better Air for Better Health: Forging Synergies in Policies for Energy Access, Climate Change and Air Pollution." *Global Environmental Change* 23:1122–30.

Rasmussen, S. G., E. L. Ogburn, M. McCormack, J. A. Casey, K. Bandeen-Roche, D. G. Mercer, and B. S. Schwartz. 2016. "Association between Unconventional Natural Gas Development in the Marcellus Shale and Asthma Exacerbations." *JAMA Internal Medicine* 176:1334–43.

Remais, J. V., J. J. Hess, K. L. Ebi, A. Markandya, J. M. Balbus, P. Wilkinson, A. Haines, and Z. Chalabi. 2014. "Estimating the Health Effects of Greenhouse Gas Mitigation Strategies: Addressing Parametric, Model, and Valuation Challenges." *Environmental Health Perspectives* 122:447–55.

Richards, T. 2007. "The Hitch Hiker's Guide to Population Growth and Climate Change." *BMJ* 335:374.

Richardson, M. J., P. English, and L. Rudolph. 2012. "A Health Impact Assessment of California's Proposed Cap-and-Trade Regulations." *American Journal of Public Health* 102:e52–58.

Rissel, C. E. 2009. "Active Travel: A Climate Change Mitigation Strategy with Co-Benefits For Health." *New South Wales Public Health Bulletin* 20:10–13.

Roberts, I., and E. Arnold. 2007. "Policy at the Crossroads: Climate Change and Injury Control." *Injury Prevention* 13:222–3.

Rojas-Rueda D., A. de Nazelle, M. Tainio, M. J. Nieuwenhuijsen. 2011. "The Health Risks and Benefits of Cycling in Urban Environments Compared with Car Use: Health Impact Assessment Study." *BMJ* 343:d4521.

Rojas-Rueda D., A. de Nazelle, Z. J. Andersen, C. Braun-Fahrlander, J. Bruha, H. Bruhova-Foltynova, H. Desqueyroux et al. 2016. "Health Impacts of Active Transportation in Europe." *PLoS One* 11:e0149990.

Rozell, D. J., and S. J. Reaven. 2012. "Water Pollution Risk Associated with Natural Gas Extraction from the Marcellus Shale." *Risk Analysis: An International Journal* 32:1382–93.

Rutstein, S. O. 2005. "Effects of Preceding Birth Intervals on Neonatal, Infant and Under-Five Years Mortality and Nutritional Status in Developing Countries: Evidence from the Demographic and Health Surveys." *International Journal of Gynaecology and Obstetrics* 89 (suppl 1):S7–S24.

Sarofim, M. C., S. T. Waldhoff, and S. C. Anenberg. 2017. "Valuing the Ozone-Related Health Benefits of Methane Emission Controls." *Environmental and Resource Economics* 66:45–63.

Scarborough, P., S. Allender, D. Clarke, K. Wickramasinghe, and M. Rayner. 2012. "Modelling the Health Impact of Environmentally Sustainable Dietary Scenarios in the UK." *European Journal of Clinical Nutrition* 66:710–15.

Seattle Children's Comprehensive Transportation Plan. n.d. Accessed March 27, 2020. http://www.nunes-ueno.com/uploads/7/2/7/2/72721009/childrens_ctp.pdf.

Shen, G. 2015. "Quantification of Emission Reduction Potentials of Primary Air Pollutants from Residential Solid Fuel Combustion by Adopting Cleaner Fuels in China." *Journal of Environmental Sciences* 37:1–7.

Shindell, D., J. C. Kuylenstierna, E. Vignati, R. van Dingenen, M. Amann, Z. Klimont, S. C. Anenberg et al. 2012. "Simultaneously Mitigating Near-Term Climate Change and Improving Human Health and Food Security." *Science* 335:183–9.

Smith, A. C., M. Holland, O. Korkeala, J. Warmington, D. Forster, H. ApSimon, T. Oxley et al. 2016. "Health and Environmental Co-Benefits and Conflicts of Actions to Meet UK Carbon Targets." *Climate Policy* 16:253–83.

Smith, K. R., A. Woodward, D. Campbell-Lendrum, D. D. Chadee, Y. Honda, Q. Liu, J. M. Olwoch, B. Revich, and R. Sauerborn. 2014. "Human Health: Impacts, Adaptation, and Co-Benefits." In *Climate Change 2014: Impacts, Adaptation, and Vulnerability. Contribution of Working Group II to the Fifth Assessment Report of the Intergovernmental Panel on Climate Change*, edited by C. B. Field, V. R. Barros, D. J. Dokken, K. J. Mach, M. D. Mastrandrea, T. E. Bilir, M. Chatterjee et al., 709–54. Cambridge, UK and New York: Cambridge University Press.

Springmann, M., H. C. Godfray, M. Rayner, P. Scarborough. 2016. "Analysis and Valuation of the Health and Climate Change Cobenefits of Dietary Change." *Proceedings of the National Academy of Sciences of the USA* 113:4146–51.

Springmann, M., D. Mason-D'Croz, S. Robinson, K. Wiebe, H. C. J. Godfray, M. Rayner M, et al. 2017. "Mitigation Potential and Global Health Impacts from Emissions Pricing of Food Commodities." *Nature Climate Change* 7:69–74.

Stephenson, J., K. Newman, and S. Mayhew. 2010. "Population Dynamics and Climate Change: What Are the Links?" *Journal of Public Health* 32:150–6.

Stott. R. 2010. "Population and Climate Change: Moving toward Gender Equality Is the Key." *Journal of Public Health* 32:159–60.

Thompson, T. M., S. Rausch, R. K. Saari, and N. E. Selin. 2014. "A Systems Approach to Evaluating the Air Quality Co-Benefits of US Carbon Policies." *Nature Climate Change* 4:917.

Walsh, M. P. 2008. "Ancillary Benefits for Climate Change Mitigation and Air Pollution Control in the World's Motor Vehicle Fleets." *Annual Review of Public Health* 29:1–9.

Watts, N., M. Amann, N. Arnell, S. Ayeb-Karlsson, K. Belesova, H. Berry, T. Bouley et al. 2018. "The Lancet Countdown on Health and Climate Change: Shaping the Health of Nations for Centuries to Come." *Lancet* 392:2479–2514.

West, J. J., A. M. Fiore, and L. W. Horowitz. 2012. "Scenarios of Methane Emission Reductions to 2030: Abatement Costs and Co-Benefits to Ozone Air Quality and Human Mortality." *Climatic Change* 114:441–61.

Wilke, R. A., and J. W. Freeman. 2017. "Potential Health Implications Related to Fracking." *JAMA* 318:1645–6.

Wilkinson, P., K. R. Smith, M. Davies, H. Adair, B. G. Armstrong, M. Barrett, N. Bruce et al. 2009. "Public Health Benefits of Strategies to Reduce Greenhouse-Gas Emissions: Household Energy." *Lancet* 374:1917–29.

Willett, W., J. Rockström, B. Loken, M. Springmann, T. Lang, S. Vermeulen, T. Garnett et al. 2019. "Food in the Anthropocene: The EAT-Lancet Commission on Healthy Diets from Sustainable Food Systems." *Lancet* 393:447–92.

Woodcock, J., D. Banister, P. Edwards, A. M. Prentice, and I. Roberts. 2007. "Energy and Transport." *Lancet* 370:1078–88.

Woodcock, J., P. Edwards, C. Tonne, B. G. Armstrong, O. Ashiru, D. Banister, S. Beevers et al. 2009. "Public Health Benefits of Strategies to Reduce Greenhouse-Gas Emissions: Urban Land Transport." *Lancet* 374:1930–43.

Woodcock, J., M. Givoni, and A. S. Morgan. 2013. "Health Impact Modelling of Active Travel Visions for England and Wales Using an Integrated Transport and Health Impact Modelling Tool (ITHIM)." *PLoS One* 8. https://doi.org/10.1371/journal.pone.0051462.

World Health Organization. 2003. *Diet, Nutrition and the Prevention of Chronic Diseases: Report of the Joint WHO/FAO Expert Consultation*. Geneva: WHO. https://www.who.int/dietphysicalactivity/publications/trs916/en/.

World Health Organization. 2009. *Healthy Transport in Developing Cities*. Geneva: WHO. https://www.who.int/heli/risks/urban/transportpolicybrief2010.pdf.

World Health Organization. 2015. *Summary: Global Status Report on Road Safety 2015*. Geneva: WHO. https://www.who.int/violence_injury_prevention/road_safety_status/2015/GSRRS2015_Summary_EN_final.pdf.

World Health Organization. 2019. *Ambient Air Pollution: Health Impacts*. Geneva: WHO. https://www.who.int/airpollution/ambient/health-impacts/en/.

Xia, T., M. Nitschke, Y. Zhang, P. Shah, S. Crabb, and A. Hansen. 2015. "Traffic-Related Air Pollution and Health Co-Benefits of Alternative Transport in Adelaide, South Australia." *Environment International* 74:281–90.

Younger, M., H. R. Morrow-Almeida, S. M. Vindigni, and A. L. Dannenberg. 2008. "The Built Environment, Climate Change, and Health: Opportunities for Co-Benefits." *American Journal of Preventive Medicine* 35:517–26.

Zapata, C., N. Muller, and M. J. Kleeman. 2013. "PM$_{2.5}$ Co-Benefits of Climate Change Legislation Part 1: California's AB 32." *Climatic Change* 117:377–97.

CHAPTER 20

INTERNATIONAL INSTITUTIONS AND GLOBAL GOVERNANCE ON CLIMATE CHANGE

Ambereen K. Shaffie

Introduction

Prior chapters examine climate change and its detrimental effects on human health as a **"risk multiplier"** (World Bank Group 2017a). This prompts several questions: what can be done to mitigate the **climate crisis**, who is doing it, and how can the medical field shape governance?

A climate-health governance structure should aim to be comprehensive, address all relevant sectors, and be inclusive. **Governance** is "the totality of political, organizational and administrative processes through which stakeholders, including governments, civil society and private-sector interest groups, articulate their interests, exercise their legal rights, make decisions, meet their obligations, and mediate their differences" (Swinburn et al. 2019). **Climate change** governance is the combined efforts of these actors to design policies that affect both **adaptation** and **mitigation** of climate impacts. (Hunter, Salzman, and Zaelke, 2015). Mitigation efforts in the health community can take various forms such as political action, financing, divestment, patient education, reforming procurement, participation in lawmaking processes, and social action. Governance structures also take various forms and can be found within other structures, including a public government body, a health institution such as a hospital, or a private sector partner.

This chapter's focus is on international governance structures addressing mitigation. Although not exhaustive, it introduces this complex topic by discussing institutions that govern approximately 80 percent of global emissions. The framework for mitigation governance is divided into three prongs:

(1) *Carbon-related strategies*

(2) *Energy policy* within carbon-related strategies. Energy policy falls into two categories: demand reduction (**energy efficiency** and energy conservation) and energy supply (renewable energy, etc)

(3) *Non-carbon related strategies*. This set of strategies encompasses a range of topics but the majority of focus is usually with short-lived climate pollutants.

Some governance structures address all three (e.g., the United Nations), some address either carbon or non-carbon related strategies, while others address an overlap (e.g., the Food and Agricultural Organization). In addition to carbon and non-carbon-related strategies explored here, significant emissions reductions can be achieved through the agriculture and land use sectors, which are not explored in depth in this chapter.

This chapter follows the three-part framework described here. The next section discusses challenges to creating an effective health-climate governance

KEY CONCEPTS

- The broad scientific consensus is that the world has approximately ten years to mitigate emissions to a sustainable level.

- An effective climate-health governance structure must be comprehensive, inclusive of actors that influence governance, and address all relevant sectors—buildings, transport, the cold chain, etc.

- Successful solutions to climate mitigation center on vulnerable populations as the most affected and key to implementation, as well as accounting for asymmetry of power and information.

- Power asymmetries in decision-making can be offset by developing a "right to healthy environment" framework, interdisciplinary communication strategies across broad stakeholders, and coalition-building.

- Governance structures dedicated to reducing energy emissions are crucial to overlapping climate-health goals.

- Sound energy policy must be given prominent attention by encouraging negative-emissions technologies and carbon capture and storage; prohibiting new CO_2-emitting technoogies; and committing to energy efficiency and renewable energy resources.

- Addressing short-lived climate pollutants (SLCPs) can mitigate 45 percent of global emissions in the near term, because SLCPs are hundreds of times more potent than CO_2 and remain in the atmosphere for a shorter period

KEY CONCEPTS *(CONTINUED)*

of time. However, governance
must simultaneously pursue
strategies for the reduction of
CO_2 reduction and SLCPs.

- Environmental problems do not
  progress linearly but rather
  implicate synergistic reactions
  and tipping points.

- Governance structures have not
  yet decoupled economic growth
  from continuous carbon
  emissions.

- The precautionary principle,
  polluter pays principle, and
  principle of common but
  differentiated responsibility are
  proven guides.

- A web of influencers with
  common foundational facts is
  important.

- Mechanisms within the Montreal
  Protocol that were the most
  impactful:

  ○ (1) using a science-policy
    framework, (2) building trust
    among industry, civil society
    and governments, (3) allowing
    developing countries to move
    according to their capabilities,
    (4) using an in-built funding
    mechanism to assist these
    developing countries in
    meeting obligations, and
    (5) employing a start-and-
    strengthen model

structure. The section that follows introduces several key international governance structures addressing climate, mitigation, and health. It categorizes organizations according to the framework, and discusses carbon-related strategies and energy, and highlights non-carbon strategies. The subsequent section provides an introduction to relevant international legal instruments relevant to the framework.

Challenges to Creating Effective Health-Climate Policies

Many governance structures rely on the assumption that environmental problems develop in a linear way, progressing steadily with a cause and consequence (Hunter et al. 2015). If a problem is linear with an identifiable cause, it is easier to develop a policy solution that addresses and prioritizes the cause. However, environmental problems actually progress in a nonlinear manner and are often the result of **"tipping points," synergistic reactions**, or **feedback loops**. (Hunter et al.; Steffen et al. 2018). A tipping point is a threshold "beyond which the impact may be many times greater than expected," such as the irreversible loss of ice sheets once the temperature and melting rate has reached a particular level which in turn triggers greater warming (Hunter et al.). Influential scientists and researchers explain that "the evidence from tipping points alone suggests that we are in a state of planetary emergency: both the risk and urgency of the situation are acute" (Lenton et al. 2019).

Synergistic reactions are ones where the combination of one or more factors leads to a drastically worse result than the effects of individual factors, such as human exposure to multiple harmful chemicals that produce unforeseen health effects, as in the case of DDT (dichlorodiphenyltrichloroethane). Feedback loops are a "cyclical process triggered by an environmental change that leads back to more change," such as when global warming melts ice caps, which in turn exposes darker land mass that absorbs more solar heat, which in turn triggers greater warming. Another example is ozone depletion, which increases ultraviolet radiation, which in turn suppresses the human immune system (Lenton et al. 2019). Thus environmental problems are a complex web of interrelated—but often unforeseen or unknown—causes and effects. Each of these strands links to many other strands, each of which are quite sensitive. One tipping point can lead to a cascade effect, triggering other tipping points.

Furthermore, the scientific process contains uncertainty (Hunter et al. 2015). Scientists test and retest hypotheses and draw limited, results-specific conclusions. These findings are used to confirm or deny an aspect of a scientific theory. Therefore, governance structures are better served by relying on broad scientific consensus and the **precautionary principle**. The precautionary principle prioritizes action over inertia while final scientific results are pending. It allows **policymakers** to act when there is a probability of significant threat to health and environment (Hunter et al.).

Another key challenge is the lack of power vulnerable populations face. The poorest and weakest populations are disproportionately affected by climate change and are often left to ruin, without the spotlight of government assistance, public outcry, or health care. Like other health issues, disparities and negative impacts are disproportionately borne by marginalized groups, particularly women, children, and communities of color. Although these populations are the most affected, they are also the most effective sources of solution and innovation. Therefore, an effective governance structure will fully account for these populations (United Nations Environment Programme [UNEP] 2019; World Bank Group 2017a; World Economic and Social Survey 2016).

Furthermore, climate-health challenges require coordinated action at both global and local levels, and across multiple sectors, which is difficult to maintain (Swinburn et al. 2019). Indeed, a "web of drivers," including political champions, heads of state, nongovernmental organizations (NGOs), civil society, industry, subject matter experts, scientists, interagency and multiagency national actors, and influential **multilateral** organizations, must agree on foundational facts and priorities in order to coordinate policy. Another critical factor is asymmetry in decision-making power among these actors (Swinburn et al.).

Although it is difficult for governance structures to design comprehensive policies that can effectively address climate-health issues, there are numerous ways to strengthen governance and ensure transparency and accountability in governance structures. These include developing a "right to healthy environment" framework, lobbying and advocacy, broad stakeholder engagement, interdisciplinary communication strategies across those same stakeholders, and coalition-building to name a few. The following is a sample of issues that a governance structure may consider when developing policy (Pearce 2014):

- Whether laws, policies, or obligations should be legally binding or aspirational
- Which stakeholders binding provisions should affect and how
- How to finance the policy or action and how to accommodate vulnerable populations
- How to implement climate-health goals, which targets to set, what baseline to compare targets to, and how to measure targets
- How to compensate stakeholders for damages caused by climate change
- How to deal with noncompliance

As governance structures in various settings develop law and policy addressing the **health–climate nexus**, there are several principles that can guide them, including but not limited to the following.

1. The **"polluter pays" principle**—the principle that polluters and users of natural resources bear the full environmental and social costs of their actions. The principle "integrates environmental protection and social costs by ensuring that the full environmental and social costs . . . are reflected in the ultimate market price for a good or service (Hunter et al. 2015, 485). The principle was first proposed by the Organisation for Economic Co-operation and Development (OECD) in 1972.

2. The **"precautionary" principle**—although scientific findings do not guarantee 100 percent certainty, and scientific developments evolve slowly, responses to environmental threats should move forward with all deliberate speed rather than embrace inertia until definite answers are found. Rather, policymakers can and should act when there is a significant probability of threat to health and environment.

3. The principle of **"common but differentiated responsibility"**—A foundational principle of environmental law aimed at facilitating fairness and cooperation between developed and developing nations. This principle is based on the premise that although all nations have the same responsibility to protect the environment and encourage sustainable development, their obligations to meet such responsibilities are nonetheless proportionate to their commensurate level of resources, capabilities, and advantages/disadvantages.

International Governance Structures Addressing Climate Mitigation

This section describes important governance structures related to mitigation and delves more deeply into the interplay among organizations using at least one key recent example. This serves as a brief introduction to the topic and should be updated continuously to remain useful to professionals.

The entities described here do not always place health at the center of their respective missions, but each has an impact on human health. The entities are categorized according to the climate mitigation governance framework discussed at the beginning of the chapter. Mitigation strategies fall into two categories: carbon-related strategies and non-carbon-related strategies. Within carbon-related strategies, energy demand reduction and energy supply policies are critical to mitigating climate.

Many structures fit into the intergovernmental organization known as the United Nations (UN). For example, the UN Framework Convention on Climate Change is governed under UN Environment, a program under the umbrella UN principal organ, the General Assembly. The **World Health Organization** and the **World Meteorological Organization** are both specialized agencies under a different UN principal organ, the Secretariat. (See Figure 20.1.)

The broad scientific consensus at the time of this text is that the world has approximately ten years to mitigate all emissions to a sustainable level (UNEP 2019). Whether structures are willing to adopt such a coordinated policy within the next ten years is unknown.

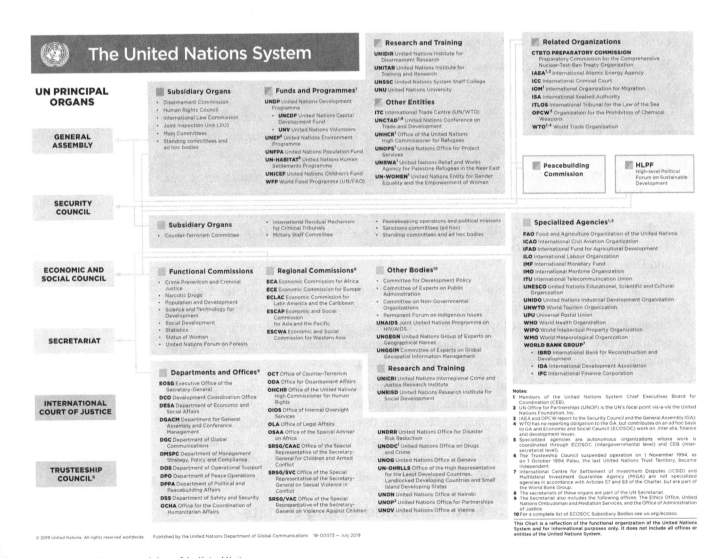

Figure 20.1 Organizational chart of the United Nations
Source: United Nations (2013).

Mitigation: Carbon-Related Strategies

Governance structures that address energy issues are critical to understanding and discussing climate mitigation. In the most widely read peer-reviewed scientific article of 2019, scientists determined that emissions from existing energy infrastructure completely surpass the carbon budget outlined by the Paris Agreement, and further, that committed energy infrastructure render achieving climate mitigation goals impossible (Tong et al. 2019). Committed infrastructure entails power plants already in the pipeline with some stage of funding or development, plus planned power plants not yet built. The entire **carbon budget** available to fall below the 1.5° mark set by Paris, based on the **Intergovernmental Panel on Climate Change**'s estimates, is between 420 and 580 gigatons of CO_2. If operated at current levels (a business-as-usual scenario) existing energy infrastructure will cumulatively emit 658 gigaton s of CO_2, with more than half of these emissions due to electricity alone (Tong et al.). China and the United States will represent 41 percent and 9 percent respectively of emissions resulting electricity sector infrastructure. If built, proposed power plants will emit another 188 gigatons of CO_2. If all proposed power plants are built, **total committed emissions** from existing and proposed energy infrastructure will exceed 846 gigatons of CO_2 (Tong et al.). Unless "compensated by negative-emissions technologies or by retrofitting with carbon capture and storage, 1.5°C (2.7°F) carbon budgets allow for no new emitting infrastructure and require substantial changes to the lifetime of operation of existing energy infrastructure" (Tong et al.).

Among other solutions, the article determines that mitigating energy-related **greenhouse gas (GHG)** emissions demands a **triple-policy energy mitigation strategy**: (1) "a transition to energy systems with net zero emissions by mid-century," (2) "global prohibition of all new CO_2-emitting devices (including many or most of the already-proposed fossil-fuel burning power plants), and (3) substantial reductions in the historical lifetimes and/or utilization rates of existing industry and electricity infrastructure" (Tong et al. 2019).

Reducing energy emissions requires both developing clean and renewable energy and reducing energy demand through measures such as increasing energy efficiency within all sectors (buildings, equipment, industry, transport, etc.). Therefore, although not directly related to health, the governance structures that are dedicated to reducing energy emissions are paramount to overlapping climate-health goals.

Energy Demand and Supply

International Energy Agency The International Energy Agency (IEA) is an international forum with a mission to produce analysis, data, and policy recommendations on sustainable energy. It is comprised of 29 industrialized member countries under the OECD and also engages key nonmembers, including Brazil, China, India, Indonesia, South Africa, Thailand, Singapore, Morocco, Mexico, and Chile. The IEA was established after the 1973 oil crisis to help its members respond to major oil supply disruptions. Though limited, its mandate has expanded over time to include analyzing key global energy trends and fostering multinational energy technology cooperation. Although critics including Oil Change International assert that the IEA's energy projections continue to assume widespread fossil fuel use, recently the IEA has begun to examine current and projected fossil fuel infrastructure in its energy technology perspectives and in its World Energy Outlook reports. In addition, it has been adding policy scenarios on deep decarbonization to influence policymakers. (IEA 2020, see, e.g., https://www.iea.org/events/iea-clean-energy-transitions-summit). As one of the first of many international forums to discuss and analyze energy trends, the IEA plays a unique role internationally in terms of mitigation of carbon-related emissions and advocating sound energy policies, including increasing adoption of renewable energy, and a strong focus on energy efficiency and energy technology cooperation among members to enable climate change mitigation. Although the criticisms are valid, it is a key organization upon which governance structures rely, and therefore is important has an impact upon health and climate.

International Renewable Energy Agency   The International Renewable Energy Agency (IRENA) is an intergovernmental organization comprised of 180 countries. It serves as a platform for cooperation and a repository of policy, technology, resource, and financial knowledge on renewable energy. IRENA promotes the adoption and sustainable use of all forms of renewable energy, including bioenergy, geothermal, hydropower, ocean, solar, and wind energy to support sustainable development, energy access, energy security, and low-carbon economic growth. IRENA plays an important role in climate change mitigation through increased adoption of renewable energy thus addressing adverse climate-health impacts indirectly through reduction in power-sector related greenhouse gas emissions.

World Bank   The World Bank is the primary UN agency responsible for development lending for infrastructure and thus for a significant percentage of energy (and thus carbon) related infrastructure. As of 2017 the World Bank estimates that only 15 percent of countries have policies centered on the health-climate nexus (World Bank Group 2017a). Although its focus on health is recent, the World Bank informs governance structures and as such, remains an important institution. The World Bank has only recently begun to introduce health-climate issues in its operations and strategies in multiple sectors (World Bank Group 2017a). For example, its health and climate directors authored a joint report with Health Care Without Harm on May 20, 2017, proposing a framework for health systems in every country. The report, *Climate-Smart Healthcare*, estimates that health care generates 5 percent of worldwide GHG emissions, or the CO2-equivalent of 2.6 billion metric tons of carbon dioxide (World Bank Group 2017b). A key finding of the report is that climate-smart strategies contribute to more efficient, lower-cost health systems.

World Meteorological Organization   The **World Meteorological Organization (WMO)** is one of the specialized agencies under the United Nations. It is the authoritative scientific voice within the United Nations on weather, climate, and water. It coordinates cooperation the National Meteorological and Hydrological Services of its 191 Member States and Territories and is essential to climate change adaptation. WMO's role in mitigation is related to its formation in 1988 along with the **UN Environment Programme** (UNEP) of the **Intergovernmental Panel on Climate Change** (IPCC), which is the authoritative body for assessing the science related to climate change. Thus any policies undertaken to mitigate climate change and adverse climate health impacts must follow the scientific consensus outlined by the IPCC. The WMO also issues scientific assessments of the **ozone layer**, which have identified various fluorinated gases ("F-gases") as highly potent greenhouse gases (discussed with short-lived climate pollutants and the **Kigali Amendment** later in the chapter). The WMO's role in forming the scientific foundation for mitigation of F-gases is also crucial.

Mitigation: Non-Carbon-Related Strategies and Short-Lived Climate Pollutants

This section covers governance structures that focus on non-carbon strategies. While reading this section, it is important to note that if business-as-usual scenarios continue, the world will exceed 4.2°C (7.6°F) warming from preindustrial levels to 2100. (Hu et al. 2013)

Short-lived climate pollutants (SLCPs)—methane, black carbon, hydrofluorocarbons, and tropospheric ozone—are very closely linked to public health concerns. SLCPs are

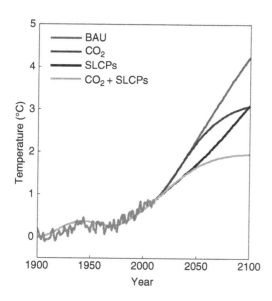

Figure 20.2   The combined effect of mitigating carbon dioxide in conjunction with aggressive SLCP mitigation

Source: Reprinted/adapted by permission from Springer Nature: Springer, Mitigation of short-lived climate pollutants slows sea-level rise by Aixue Hu, et. al. [COPYRIGHT] (2013).

thousands of times more potent than carbon dioxide. These emissions remain in the atmosphere for a much shorter time frame than carbon dioxide but are responsible for up to 45 percent of global emissions and contribute up to 40 percent of radiative forcing (Climate and Clean Air Coalition [CCAC] 2019d; (Hu et al. 2013). Carbon dioxide can remain in the atmosphere for approximately 500 years, while SLCPs have a lifetime ranging from one week (black carbon) to one decade (methane) (Hu et al.). Therefore, emissions reductions of SLCPs lead to a reduction in atmospheric concentrations in the immediate term (Hu et al.). Reducing SLCPs can reduce global warming by approximately 0.6°C (1°F), delaying the onset of 2° warming by several decades (Hu et al.). Importantly, although SLCP mitigation is more effective than CO_2-mitigation in the near term, by 2100 the CO_2 mitigation effect becomes paramount in achieving warming below 2 degrees Celsius (See Figure 20.2.) Solely mitigating SLCPs will cut warming to 3.5°C (6.3°F), whereas solely mitigating CO_2 will reduce warming by only 1.1°C (2°F). Neither strategy by itself is sufficient to achieve a below-2° target (Hu et al.). In terms of health co-benefits, mitigation of methane and black carbon alone can avoid ~2.4 million premature deaths and ~50 million tons of staple crop losses every year (Blackstock and Allen 2013). It is important to also note the differences in metrics related to both. Although SLCP mitigation can complement aggressive CO_2 mitigation, it is not an equivalent to near-term CO_2 reductions, in part because the relevant time frames become significant at different times (Blackstock and Allen). In fact metrics that calculate equivalence between SLCP and CO_2 mitigation could create "perverse incentives" to prioritize one strategy to the detriment of the other, thereby compromising the 2°C goal (Blackstock and Allen).

The combined effects of reducing SLCPs can slow the increase in global warming by as much as 0.6°C (1°F) by 2050 and prevent disastrous climate tipping points (CCAC 2019d; Hu, et al. 2013). Among the organizations listed in this chapter, the CCAC has made significant effort to link climate change and SLCPs to health. See Figure 20.3.

Climate and Clean Air Coalition

The CCAC is a voluntary multilateral coalition founded by UNEP and six member countries in 2012. Its mitigation strategies focus on long-term climate assessments, planning, and funding

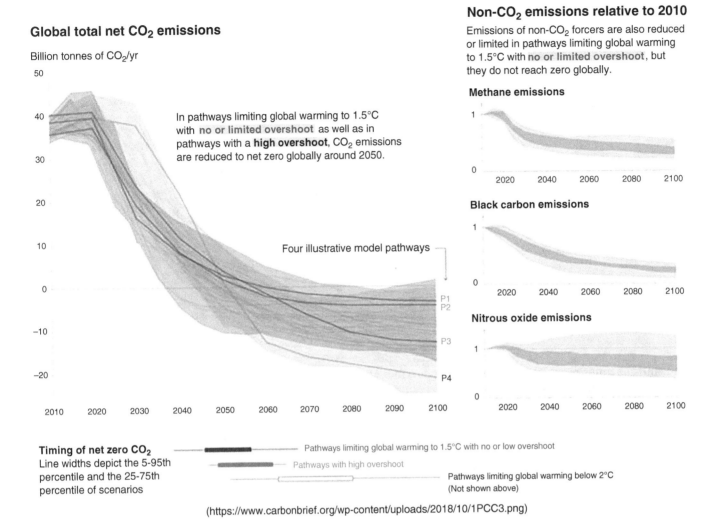

Figure 20.3 Combined mitigation of CO₂ and SLCPs are required to achieve Paris Agreement goals

Source: Policymakers. In: Global Warming of 1.5°C. An IPCC Special Report on the impacts of global warming of 1.5°C above pre-industrial levels and related global greenhouse gas emission pathways, in the context of strengthening the global response to the threat of climate change, sustainable development, and efforts to eradicate poverty [Masson-Delmotte, V., P. Zhai, H.-O. Pörtner, D. Roberts, J. Skea, P.R. Shukla, A. Pirani, W. Moufouma-Okia, C. Péan, R. Pidcock, S. Connors, J.B.R. Matthews, Y. Chen, X. Zhou, M.I. Gomis, E. Lonnoy, T. Maycock, M. Tignor, and T. Waterfield (eds.)]. In Press.

related to SLCP mitigation (CCAC 2019d). In 2019, the CCAC had 141 partners (including 66 countries), implemented actions in 110 countries and 22 regions, raised over $4 million toward SLCP mitigation, and helped develop and pass 8 new laws and 12 policies. (CCAC 2019b).

The CCAC targets black carbon, derived largely from inefficient fuel usage; hydrofluorocarbons, used primarily in refrigeration and air conditioners; and methane, which has multiple sources, the most prominent being natural gas systems and livestock production. The CCAC's initiatives target the following sectors: agriculture, brick production, cooling and refrigeration, heavy-duty vehicles, household energy, oil and gas, and waste. Within these sectors, the CCAC invests in near-term impacts such as technological changes and long-term impacts such as policy development and training. (CCAC 2019b). The CCAC's 2030 vision aligns with the Paris Agreement targets.

A key organizational goal is to deliver a 90 percent reduction in **hydrofluorocarbons (HFC)** emissions by 2050. Two primary vehicles for this goal are the HFC Initiative and the Efficient Cooling Initiative. The HFC Initiative works directly with manufacturers and consumers to promote HFC-alternative technologies. The Efficient Cooling Initiative, launched on May 5, 2019, aligns with the Kigali Amendment to the Montreal Protocol. The initiative promotes cooling efficiency policies and the phasedown of HFC-based targets that equipment efficiency can lead to 75 percent of HFC mitigation. Although the CCAC has been effective within its limited mandate and funding, the coalition recognizes the need to increase the scale of action. The IPCC Special Report on Global Warming led to the CCAC setting control measures to mitigate methane and HFCs beyond its initial targets, and to reduce black carbon by 60 percent (CCAC 2019a, 2019b, 2019d, 2020).

Food, Agriculture, and Land Use Structures

Land use is a significant contributor to reduction of global emissions and is explored extensively in Chapter 9 (Harper et al. 2018; (IPCC 2019). Because food production is "the dominant driver" of global land use and is closely tied to health, this section focuses on structures that cover food production and use (Harper et al.). Unfortunately, international governance structures compartmentalize food emissions sources, separating production from food processing, storage and transport, and consumption (Rosenzweig et al. 2020). These issues crosscut mitigation and adaptation, as well as carbon and non-carbon strategies.

The Food and Agriculture Organization (FAO) of the UN leads international efforts to eliminate hunger and reduce food insecurity through agriculture, forestry, and fishery practices. The FAO seeks to improve nutrition and access to food by developing initiatives to research and address underlying causes of food insecurity. It works with partners to develop and implement strategies and programs that address these causes, many of which are climate related. (See fao.org.)

The FAO has identified climate change as a threat to global food security and incorporated climate change into its reports and action items (FAO 2019e). Climate mitigation strategies focus on emission reductions in agriculture, livestock, the cold chain, carbon sequestration, and related practices (FAO 2019a, 2019b, 2019c). FAO's central mission is directly related to the health-climate nexus. The food supply chain creates around 13.7 billion metric tons of CO_2-equivalent of anthropogenic GHG emissions (Poore and Nemececk 2018). Further, sustainable cooling systems also produce the co-benefit of reducing food waste, which combats hunger and waste emissions while reducing the harmful HFCs produced by the cold chain. Increasing cold chain capacity in developing countries can save an estimated 200 million tons of food loss annually (FAO 2019d). Consider this when reviewing the discussion of HFCs later in the chapter.

A recent Meeting of the Parties to the Montreal Protocol held at the FAO Headquarters in November 2019 led to seventy-six parties signing the Rome Declaration. The declaration recognizes the importance of the Kigali Amendment in developing efficiency in the cold chain to phase down HFCs, while still prioritizing reduction in food waste (see Rome Declaration 2019). The FAO plays a key role in progress on these fronts. The recent report, *The State of Food and Agriculture*, prioritizes cooling solutions as an opportunity for growth not only in a reduction of food loss but also as a potential reduction point for emissions (FAO, 2019d). The report provides examples of actions the FAO has already taken, specifically in partnership with the European Bank for Reconstruction and Redevelopment (EBRD) to reduce food loss and waste and contribute to climate mitigation. In addition, the Finance Technology Transfer Center for Climate Change helps businesses adopt efficient measures developed through the FAO and EBRD collaboration (FAO 2019d).

Additional key structures include but are not limited to the following. The Warsaw Framework on Reducing Emissions from Deforestation and Forest Degradation (REDD+) was a landmark 2013 deal under the United Nations Framework Convention on Climate Change (UNFCCC) that addresses the forest sector, and the North America Climate Smart Agriculture

Alliance is a farmer-led platform for agricultural partners to trade best practices on climate-smart agriculture.

Multilateral and Bilateral Initiatives

The European Union (EU) is composed of twenty-seven countries, omitting the United Kingdom. The EU is a cooperative institution for European countries to encourage peace and economic growth (European Union n.d.). From 1990 to 2017 the EU has reduced its GHG emissions by 22 percent (European Commission 2018).

The EU often acts through the European Commission (EC), which develops and implements EU policies. (EC n.d.a, n.d.b). The EC has been aggressively working to reduce emissions since the turn of the century. (EC n.d.b). It established the European Climate Change Program (ECCP) in 2000 to identify policies and measures to cut GHG emissions in Europe. The ECCP initially focused on the EU meeting its target emission reductions under the Kyoto Protocol but has since evolved to include more specific and extensive opportunities and action on emission reduction. (EC n.d.a). The EC has adopted a target to achieve a climate-neutral economy by 2050 through decarbonization of Europe's energy supply, maximizing energy efficiency, halving energy consumption, and creating carbon sinks through sustainable agriculture and land use (EC 2018).

In 2018 the EC updated its 2030 Climate and Energy Framework. (EC 2018b). This Framework sets the following goals: to reduce GHG emissions by 40 percent from 1990 levels, to meet a binding renewable energy target of at least 32 percent of final energy consumption, and to increase energy efficiency by at least 32.5 percent (EC 2018b).

Additional relevant multilateral groups have formed or evolved to include countries, organizations and institutions focused on mitigation. The Group of 8 (G8) and the Major Economies Forum on Energy and Climate (MEF) are examples. MEF was launched by President Barack Obama in 2009 and includes seventeen of the largest global economies. MEF promotes cooperation between developed and developing economies to advance clean energy (U.S. Department of State 2009). Its most recent forum convened in 2016, prior to the succession of the Trump administration. MEF's action plans seek to increase solar energy, carbon capture, and energy efficiency.

In 2017, Canada, China, and the EU formed a replacement body, the Ministerial on Climate Action (MCA), with representatives from thirty-four major economies (Hajnal 2019). MCA held its third Ministerial in 2019 directed at UNFCCC challenges, implementation, and future ambitions (EC 2019). Ministers encouraged international cooperation, a shift from negotiation to implementation, financing emission reductions, implementation of current commitments, and updating of **nationally determined contributions (NDCs)** (Ministerial on Climate Action, 2019).

The G8 originally included France, Germany, Italy, the United Kingdom, Japan, the United States, Canada, and Russia. It held annual meetings to develop consensus around issues including climate change and global energy (Council on Foreign Relations 2014). The G8 is largely considered nonfunctional today and is overshadowed by the Group of 20 (G20), which was developed to include emerging economic powers (Center on International Cooperation n.d.). The most recent G20 Summit saw world leaders reach an agreement on climate change action despite sharp differences with the United States (European Council 2019). The agreement provides that nations explore "a wide range of clean technologies, pursue NDCs and encourage growth in cooling innovation in the private sector" (European Council 2019). The new declaration restated the United States' recent intent to withdraw from the Paris Agreement and to utilize all energy sources including advanced fossil fuels, further differentiating U.S. policy from that of its historical allies (European Council 2019).

The Arctic Council is an intergovernmental membership group consisting of the eight Arctic states (Canada, Denmark, Finland, Iceland, Norway, Russia, Sweden, and the United

States), and six organizations representing Arctic Indigenous Peoples (Arctic Council 2018). It was established in 1996 to promote cooperation on common issues the Arctic nations face (Arctic Council 1996). It operates through six Working Groups. The responsibilities of the Working Groups include monitoring the Arctic environment, providing scientific advice to governments, working to protect the Arctic environment, encouraging nations to reduce emissions, and working to advance sustainable development in the Arctic (Arctic Council 2018). Although the Arctic Council lacks enforcement powers and must rely upon the Arctic States and other entities to accomplish its goals, it has implemented numerous successful measures (Exner-Pirot et al. 2019).

Two successful mitigation measures are The Iqaluit Declaration and the Framework for Action on Enhanced Black Carbon and Methane Emissions Reductions (Arctic Council 2015). Most recently, the 2017 Fairbanks Declaration called for immediate action to mitigate climate change in light of Arctic warming and continued financing of mitigation projects through the Arctic Council Project Support Instrument, which funds the council (Arctic Council 2016, 2017). As of 2016, the Project Support Instrument allocated 25 percent of funds to mitigation projects and 20 percent to projects for energy efficiency, clean production, and SLCPs (Arctic Council 2016). Of the projects dedicated to mitigating SLCPs, twelve were either complete or nearing completion in 2016 (Arctic Council 2016).

The Evolving Role of the United States in International Climate Mitigation Governance

In 2016, President Barack Obama and President Xi Jinping of China met as representatives of the two nations that produce the most greenhouse gases and explicitly urged other countries to sign the Paris Agreement (White House 2016a). Partially due to this endorsement, 187 countries ultimately signed and **ratified** the Paris Agreement. (See Figure 20.4.) The iconic image of two of the largest contributors of GHG emissions cooperating despite political and historical differences was widely recognized as a catalyst for global momentum toward the Paris Agreement.

The Paris Agreement requires each party to establish a domestic plan of action set forth in Nationally Determined Contributions (NDCs). The Paris Agreement aims to limit the average global temperature increase to *below* 1.5 degrees Celsius above pre-industrial levels. The 1.5° "guardrail" was recognized as a level beyond which catastrophic climate impacts and tipping points would occur. The following year, the Obama administration acted as a strong proponent

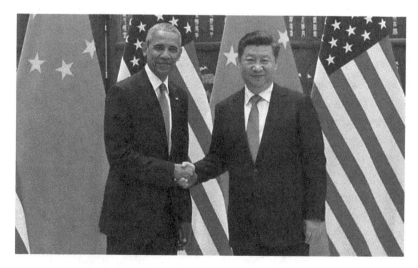

Figure 20.4   President Obama and President Xi shake hands ahead of the G20 Summit, shortly after pledging the United States and China would ratify the Paris Agreement and urging other nations to do the same

to amend the Montreal Protocol to phase out hydrofluorocarbons. Many environmentalists, advocates, scientists, and organizations lobbied regularly throughout his time in office until the message of HFCs mitigation eventually became adopted as White House policy. President Obama ended his eight-year term before the United States could ratify the treaty (White House 2016b).

Under the Obama Administration, the U.S. Global Change Research Program (USGCRP 2016) released *The Impacts of Climate Change on Human Health in the United States: A Scientific Assessment* in 2016. Developed by thirteen federal agencies, the assessment asserted that ongoing climate change risked human health in two main ways: first, "by changing the severity or frequency of health problems that are already affected by climate or weather factors; and second, by creating unprecedented or unanticipated health problems or health threats in places where they have not previously occurred" (USGCRP 2016). In addition, the USGCRP periodically releases the National Climate Assessment, a comprehensive report on climate change that directly informs the IPCC process.

Although science has historically informed U.S. government policy on the health-climate nexus, U.S. policy has recently begun to significantly shift. Donald Trump's administration has minimized the 2019 NCA and removed archived scientific climate research from government databases. The administration has also considered changing the methodology used in the NCA reports. The proposed changes would project potential climate change effects only to the year 2040 and abandon "worst case scenario" modeling. In addition, in 2019 President Trump formally withdrew the United States from the Paris Agreement. As the U.S. government shifted away from its prior strong environmental protection policies, state and local governance structures developed their own strong mitigation strategies. These state and local groups include the U.S. Climate Alliance; the We Are Still In coalition, which issued several commitments and set up a U.S. presence at the 2019 Conference of the Parties (COP); America's Pledge and the C40 Cities Climate Leadership Group.

Newly elected President Joseph R. Biden has instituted sweeping environmental reforms since taking office, which depart from the prior administration's priorities. The administration's stated goals are to achieve a carbon pollution-free power sector by 2035 and a net-zero emissions economy by 2050. One of President Biden's first acts in office was to re-join the Paris Agreement and review the standards lowered by the prior administration on clean air and water. On January 27, 2021 President Biden issued multiple executive orders, re-establishing the President's Council of Advisors on Science and Technology, with the aim to protect scientists from political interference. The January orders list numerous additional goals including: centering the climate crisis in national security and foreign policy considerations; initiating the development of U.S. NDC's; establishing a White House Office of Domestic Climate Policy and a National Climate Task Force with leaders from 21 federal agencies as part of a whole-of-government approach to climate; advancing conservation; and prioritizing environmental justice. At the time of this text, President Biden is set to host a Leader's Climate Summit on Earth Day, April 22, 2021 which could set the tone for domestic and global presence in the near future.

World Health Organization

The global public health authority, centered on the World Health Organization (WHO), has begun to integrate climate change risks within its framework. The WHO was formed in 1948 to direct and coordinate international health within the UN system. It identifies and addresses public health concerns by creating policy initiatives and programs to educate and support partners in executing health objectives. The WHO partners with institutions within the UN system, countries, international organizations, foundations, and research institutions. (See who.int.)

The WHO has historically focused on adaptation. However, it has recently begun to prioritize mitigation and the health-climate nexus by promoting relevant research and initiatives (WHO 2014). With respect to mitigation, WHO has partnered with UNEP and WMO to launch the global coalition on health, environment, and climate change in May 2018 (WHO 2018b). The WHO is working on a plan with the CCAC to improve air quality and hosted a Global Conference on Air Pollution and Health, which took place in November 2018. The conference put forth an action agenda calling for various measures, such as increased access to renewable energy to achieve a goal of reducing deaths from air pollution by two thirds in 2030 (WHO 2018a).

The WHO also worked with various partners, including the World Organization of Family Doctors Working Party on the Environment and the World Medical Association to create a special report on health and climate change for the UNFCCC COP24. The report provided recommendations for governments to maximize the health benefits of mitigating climate change. Recommendations include procurement policies for low-carbon supply chains and investment in renewable energy and efficiency in the health care sector. The report pointed to actions taken by other organizations, such as Health Care Without Harm (HCWH), and their work to achieve climate-smart health care (WHO 2018a).

Two key organizations in the global public health community exemplify NGOs that significantly influence governance structures. HCWH is a global organization dedicated to reducing the environmental footprint of health care institutions and practitioners. HCWH has offices in four continents and work with global partners and health care practitioners as well. It addresses waste management, greening buildings and medical equipment, and standards for purchasing of environmentally safe products. The Medical Society Consortium on Climate and Health (MSCCH) represents a consortium of medical associations within the United States, whose volunteer membership comprises over 50 percent of the practicing physicians in the United States.

NGOs and intergovernmental organizations can be a powerful, organized influence on health-climate governance, by lobbying state and local representatives, compiling action alerts and policy statements, educating patient populations and networks about the health-climate nexus, convening like-minded partners, developing curricula for crossover classes and textbooks, and using leadership positions from within health care institutions to advocate for climate actions such as greening hospital facilities (Hunter et al. 2015).

An Introduction to Legal Instruments Relevant to the Health-Climate Nexus

This section serves as a brief nonexclusive introduction to major international developments in this global consensus, while mentioning relevant subnational governance structures where possible. The emphasis on international law should not undermine the importance of other structures targeting emissions or other sectors but rather to give attention to structures that cover approximately 80 percent of emissions mitigation.

Efforts to build a meaningful regime to address climate change began in the late 1980s and led to the eventual adoption of the UNFCCC, the Kyoto Protocol, the Copenhagen Accord, the Paris Agreement, and the Kigali Amendment to the Montreal Protocol. These agreements contributed to a global consensus regarding mandatory reductions of greenhouse gas emissions.

Within these forums, climate clubs, minilateral efforts (e.g., CCAC), and alliances often form to influence governance (Nordhaus 2015; Keohane, Petsonk, and Hanafi 2017) (minilateralism involves efforts by subsets of countries that focus on specific topics or issues). Blocs or groups of countries with common interests can exert negotiation leverage by pooling political and other types of capital, thereby circumventing the power imbalances alluded to earlier in the chapter.

Mitigation: Both Carbon and Non-Carbon-Related Strategies

UNFCCC

In 1990, the United Nations first authorized an Intergovernmental Negotiating Committee on Climate to begin formal discussions of a climate regime. The United Nations Framework Convention on Climate Change (UNFCCC) was then adopted in May 1992 (UN 1992). The framework set nonbinding limits on countries and outlined how specific international treaties ("protocols" or "Agreements") could be negotiated to achieve the UNFCCC's objective to "stabilize greenhouse gas concentrations in the atmosphere at a level that would prevent dangerous anthropogenic interference with the climate system" (UN 1992). UNFCCC also refers to the UN Secretariat, which manages the convention and is now located in Bonn, Germany.

The general framework left out specific substantive commitments, frustrating many stakeholders (Hunter et al. 2015). This was in part because of divisions between developed and developing countries, divisions among developing countries, and tensions between the EU and the United States (Hunter et al. 2015). Several positive outcomes the UNFCCC produced include a strong institutional framework, a funding body (the Global Environmental Facility), provisions related to technology transfer, and the establishment of the COP to evaluate the convention implementation (Hunter et al. 2015). As previously mentioned, the IPCC also enhances and informs the UNFCCC's work.

Parties meet annually at the COP to discuss the range of activities related to treaty governance. Further, the COP is a mechanism to decide whether to adopt modifications or amendments. (Hunter et al. 2015). Stakeholders from industry, NGOs, advocacy groups, environmentalists, and interest groups regularly participate as official "Observers" at the COPs to understand and to participate in the proceedings. There are several helpful insider discussions of this process. (See, e.g., Hunter et al. 2015), and the section that appears later in this chapter, Climate Negotiations: What Is It Like to Be in the Room?)

The Kyoto Protocol and Post-Kyoto Negotiations

A 1995 IPCC report on the broad scientific consensus of human impacts on global climate precipitated the negotiations for The Kyoto Protocol (IPCC 2015). Kyoto was established in 1997 during the third meeting of the Conference of the Parties to the UNFCCC (COP3). The treaty placed mandatory obligations on thirty-seven industrialized nations to cut emissions to stabilize seven greenhouse gases. The Kyoto Protocol excluded developing countries from mandatory or numerical targets based on the premise that industrialization requires activities that produce emissions. The Kyoto Protocol also offered flexible mechanisms that could be used internationally to incentivize emission reductions across the board.

In 2001, the United States refused to ratify and formally withdrew from the Kyoto Protocol (Hunter et al. 2015); nevertheless most of the remaining parties ratified the treaty and agreed to cut emissions 5 percent below 1990 levels during the first reporting period (2008–2012). After withdrawing its support, the United States focused on voluntary domestic regulations. Criticisms of Kyoto pointed to elements such as significantly lowered ambition, exclusion of developing country commitments, the United States' (and later Canada's) reversal of participation. Two positive legacies of Kyoto were the European Community's adoption of significant mitigation targets, and a functional emissions trading system (Hunter et al. 2015).

Post-Kyoto negotiations centered on two goals: to cover a second commitment period (2013–2020), and to develop binding commitments that would include both the United States and developing countries (Hunter et al. 2015). The next major development in law and governance was the Copenhagen Accord in 2009. During the Copenhagen Summit that same year, a smaller group of countries (the United States, Brazil, South Africa, India, China) abruptly bypassed the democratic protocols of the UN and negotiated the accord in a smaller subgroup, pushing the agreement through as various political pressures mounted (Hunter et al. 2015). The resulting controversial and nonbinding agreement established voluntary targets to limit global average temperature increases to less than 2°C Celsius above preindustrial levels. Although this subgroup of parties circumvented established negotiation protocols and decorum, it did set forth enhanced actions on mitigation, adaptation (notably on deforestation and degradation [REDD]), technology transfer, and financing (the Green Climate Fund) (Hunter et al. 2015).

After the Copenhagen Accord, the Kyoto Protocol parties adopted the second phase of commitments, to extend from 2013–2020. In 2011 in Durban, South Africa, the UNFCCC Parties set a deadline to achieve a universal international climate agreement at the 2015 Paris negotiations.

The Paris Agreement

The first universal climate treaty was adopted by 195 nations in Paris in 2015. The Paris Agreement is a voluntary, non-legally binding agreement that seeks to limit global temperature rise to "well below 2 degrees Celsius" and to "pursue efforts toward 1.5 degrees Celsius." Under the agreement each country sets **Nationally Determined Contributions** (NDC's) or voluntary targets aimed toward achieving the 1.5° limits through reduction of GHG emissions. The targets include both mitigation and adaptation strategies. A "ratchet and review" mechanism within the Paris Agreement requires each country to assess its NDC progress every five years and then progressively increase goals.

The IPCC's 2015 report, as well as the Copenhagen Accord and Durban Framework, informed the foundation of the Paris Agreement. The IPCC report stated that the 2° guardrail was insufficient and unsustainable, and encouraged countries to aim for less than 1.5°C (2.7°F), or "as low as possible" (IPCC 2015). The Paris Agreement invited the IPCC to issue a special report on the impact of warming beyond 1.5°C, which was issued in 2018 (IPCC 2018) The 2018 Report identified disastrous climate impacts that "have already resulted in profound alterations to human and natural systems" (IPCC 2015). It also showed that those most affected lived in low and middle-income countries. The IPCC noted that overshooting the 1.5°C mark would cause malnutrition and a host of other negative health effects (IPCC 2015). The 1.5° C guardrail is widely adopted by scientists as crucial to avoid tipping points. Global temperatures have already warmed by around 1°C above preindustrial times, and most scientific reports indicate that the world is on track to reach a 4°C (7.2°F) increase by midcentury, unless much more rapid reduction efforts are urgently implemented.

There is still a scientific debate that the "1.5°C" mark lacks the nuanced understanding required to parse GHG emissions. However, the influence of the Paris Agreement is undeniable and most mitigation structures follow recommendations that are framed in terms of the 1.5° guardrail (Figure 20.5).

Mitigation: Non-Carbon-Related Strategies
The Montreal Protocol and Kigali Amendment

The Montreal Protocol is to date the most successful example of international cooperation in the history of both international law and environmental law. It also represents a model of good governance. It is the only treaty that boasts 100 percent compliance, and represents the potential for global cooperation on climate mitigation actions that produce health co-benefits.

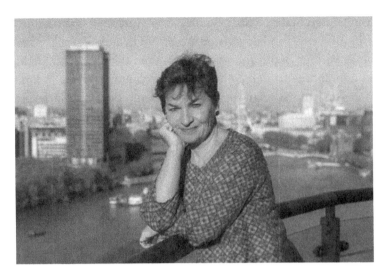

Figure 20.5   Christiana Figueres, former executive secretary of the UNFCCC from 2010–2015, gained international recognition and influene with her conviction that limiting climate change is both necessary and completely possible. She was instrumental in the adoption of Paris Agreement.

The 1987 Montreal Protocol bans the production and consumption of **chlorofluorocarbons (CFCs)** and other classes of chemicals that destroy the ozone layer and warm the climate. In 1973, scientists Frank Rowland and Mario Molina discovered that CFCs (toxic coolants and refrigerants) in the earth's atmosphere were in fact catalyzing ozone depletion. The earth's atmosphere contains two layers: the troposphere (12 km above the earth), and the stratosphere (from 12 km to 50 km above the earth). Ozone occurs naturally in both layers, but the highest concentration appears in the middle of the stratosphere and is commonly known as the "ozone layer." Its function is to absorb incoming UV-B radiation from the sun, which in turn depletes the **stratospheric ozone layer**, ideally at a rate that does not outstrip ozone regeneration. When the ozone layer is overdepleted, UV-B radiation cannot be absorbed effectively, causing a host of direct and indirect health impacts including skin cancer, cataracts, depression of immune systems, depletion of crops, and the disruption of important ecosystems (Hunter et al. 2015). In the ensuing fifteen years, additional scientists validated Rowland and Molina's hypothesis, confirming the drastic depletion of ozone above the Antarctic, the "ozone hole." This alarming discovery prompted twenty nations to sign the Vienna Convention on the Protection of the Ozone Layer in 1985, which established a framework for negotiating international regulations on ozone-depleting substances. Thereafter it took only eighteen months for the world to reach a binding agreement on CFCs through the Protocol to the Vienna Convention.

Several factors contributed to the Montreal Protocol's success, including (1) a science-policy framework; (2) trust among industry, civil society and governments;, (3) common but differentiated responsibility (allowing developing countries to phase out in a later time frame); (4) an internal funding mechanism to assist developing countries (the Multilateral Fund); (5) the precautionary principle; and (6) a start-and-strengthen model. By acting during an early period of scientific discovery (the precautionary principle), governments set a precedent for acting with urgency and understanding, allowing a continuous flow of information to inform the agreement implementation. The parties also created an expert, independent Technology and Economic Assessment Panel to continuously inform and update the Montreal Protocol parties on scientific and technical complexities.

Because the sectors and chemicals were clearly defined in the Protocol, manufacturers of CFCs could predict with certainty how, when, and in which sectors the phase-out would begin and work to meet the new demands of their industries. Industry players including DuPont were strongly convinced to advocate for the treaty in part because of these flexible measures, as well as their own desire to develop early alternatives and capture competitive market advantage.

Last, the Montreal Protocol relied upon a "start-and-strengthen" model of phasedown rather than an immediate complete phaseout, thereby boosting compliance as well as spurring innovation. Countries were given a reasonable time frame according to their capabilities to phase down, and industries had a chance to catch up. Once given the signal that laws would change, companies could concentrate on innovating new chemicals with little or no ozone-depleting potential, for use in the refrigeration and air conditioning sectors. In fact, industry rose to the occasion and kept on innovating, producing better products at a reasonable price, and taking advantage of the new demand for non-CFC chemicals.

As a result of the Montreal Protocol and the phaseout of CFCs, the ozone layer is expected to return to its 1980 levels within the next fifteen to twenty years, provided compliance continues. In addition, during the shift out of CFCs, alternatives were produced at more or less the same cost, the result being that today, CFCs are now virtually nonexistent.

The Kigali Amendment to the Montreal Protocol builds on the Montreal Protocol's more than thirty years of success. The amendment adds phasedown requirements on most HFCs, which are also used in cooling equipment and in insulating foams and some aerosols. Emissions from cooling equipment are growing faster than ever as global temperatures increase. Cooling emissions are expected to increase by 90 percent from 2017 levels by 2050, which will produce GHG emissions equivalent to one-third of all current emissions. (CCAC 2019c). HFCs are one of the fastest-growing greenhouse gases and are responsible for roughly 4 billion tons of CO_2 emissions every year (CCAC 2019c). Further, refrigeration management has been quantified as the number one intervention to achieve maximum climate mitigation (Hawken 2017). Refrigerant management can achieve a total reduction of 89.74 gigatons of CO_2. (Hawken 2017; see also Shah et al. 2015).

Several low-lying alone island nations were the first to call for the amendment and faced great resistance. However, negotiations continued for seven years. A key 2015 scientific report titled *Benefits of Leapfrogging to Superefficiency and Low Global Warming Potential Refrigerants in Room Air Conditioning* helped inform the negotiations (Shah et al. 2015). The report, authored by the Lawrence Berkeley National Laboratory (LBNL), articulated the growing problem of cooling energy demand. The LBNL report quantified for the first time the impact of improving energy efficiency (EE) in tandem with the HFC refrigerant phasedown, thereby doubling the benefits of either strategy alone, and directly led to the adoption of the Kigali Amendment and subsequent decisions on energy efficiency (Shah et al. 2015). This research was also influential because it formed a bridge between science and policy. The LBNL paper triggered the raising of $78 million in private philanthropic funds (in addition to government funding) toward the fast-start implementation of the Amendment. If implemented properly, in tandem with energy efficiency and carbon dioxide mitigation, the Amendment will be a significant step toward slowing the onset of IPCC-predicted catastrophic climate impacts. It will also be a significant step toward lowering global temperatures within the bounds of the Paris Agreement.

On October 15, 2016, after negotiating throughout the night and into the early hours of the morning, governments agreed that eliminating HFCs could avoid up to 0.5°C (1°F) of global warming and up to one full degree when combine with increasing equipment energy efficiency (UNEP 2016).

The Kigali Amendment, if timely implemented and adequately funded in tandem with energy efficiency, will also provide the world access to affordable, more efficient cooling. Industry is working to innovate and produce affordable, superefficient alternatives. Poor access to cooling efficiency is a critical health issue in the following ways: (1) it contributes to a lack of access to vaccines that must be developed and distributed at scale and which rely upon the cold chain; (2) it contributes to poor air quality which increases incidences of lung disease; and (3) it contributes to wide-scale heath deaths during longer, hotter summers which are increasingly common in a warming world. Extreme temperatures result in longer periods where cooling is critical to maintain health. These factors drive cooling demand ever higher, which increases electricity usage by exponential rates (see Shah et al. 2015). Indeed, most high ambient temperature countries face surges in cooling demands within the next ten years, saturating markets and households with appliances. By cutting loads on the grid during peak cooling times, countries will save their reserves and the environment billions of dollars in investments in added power plants. A 30 percent improvement in equipment efficiency of room air conditioners can save enough energy to avoid 2,500 500 MW power peak power plants by 2050 (each power plant requires about $1 billion in capital costs) (see Shah et al. 2015). Better, more efficient cooling ensures energy access for the poor, a more even distribution of savings and costs allocated to cooling, greater profits for utilities that avoid blackouts, and greater quality of life.

Climate Negotiations: What Is It Like to Be in the Room?

As referenced previously, negotiation groups and blocs form according to various circumstances. Groups may coalesce according to a common economic position, political clout, regional or political alliances, national interests, domestic climate-induced disasters, resource issues, security concerns, financial incentives, and multiple pressures (Nordhaus, 2015; Keohane et al. 2017). Each alliance or factor shifts according to and/or in response to changes in the positions of other countries and groups of countries. Alliances and strategic positions change often and can be obscure to outsiders. Revealing information from ongoing negotiations is at best frowned upon and at worst a diplomatic violation of mutual trusts, and compromises the integrity and reputation of an attendee. Negotiators typically say only what is necessary, and what is unsaid is often the most important element. Figure 20.6 and Figure 20.7 are both interesting real-world examples where an NGO documented the shifting political alliances within the Paris Agreement negotiations that took place in 2015.

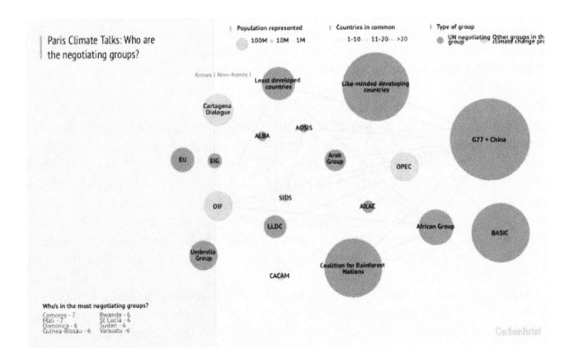

Figure 20.6   Negotiating groups at the Paris Climate Talks
Source: Pearce (2014).

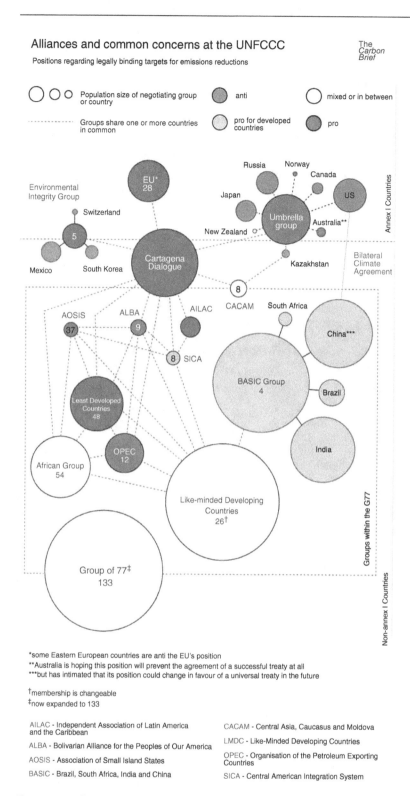

Alliances and common concerns at the UNFCCC

The Carbon Brief

Positions regarding legally binding targets for emissions reductions

Figure 20.7   Alliances at the 2014 UNFCCC Negotiations
Source: Pearce (2014).

Conclusion

Three questions introduced this chapter: what can be done to mitigate the climate crisis, who is doing it, and how can the medical field shape governance? The relevant parties influencing health-climate governance and mitigation are government and nongovernmental actors, from multilateral institutions to individuals, each of whom play a role in influencing governance through political action, financing, divestment, procurement, social action, policy advising, and lawmaking. Each governance structure should be tailored to solve a defined problem. There is no one model that will adequately address climate mitigation.

The cumulative contributions of many stakeholders have expanded the sophistication and reach of governance structures over climate, health, and mitigation. As noted, the broad scientific consensus is that the world has less than ten years to mitigate the climate crisis. Note that governance structures have not yet embraced a model that decouples economic growth from continuous carbon emissions. Therefore, there has never been a more opportune time to form a clear, robust global response. There has also never been a more opportune time to act on an individual level in coordination with the global consciousness and scientific consensus, whether one is a student, practitioner, teacher, or professional, to address the health climate nexus.

CLINICAL CORRELATES 20.1 BUILDING RESILIENCE AGAINST CLIMATE EFFECTS (BRACE)

The Centers for Disease Control and Prevention created the following five-step model for wide dissemination amongst local health departments to organize their adaptation planning:

Step 1 Anticipate climate impacts and assess vulnerabilities

Step 2 Project the disease burden

Step 3 Assess public health interventions

Step 4 Develop and implement a climate and health adaptation plan

Step 5 Evaluate impact and improve quality of activities

The process allows integration of data from multiple sources to best predict and respond to climate events. It also offers local health officials guidance for program development for their specific community. See https://www.cdc.gov/climateandhealth/BRACE.htm.

The BRACE Framework gives local public health agencies the guidance to build resilience with community stakeholders against short- and long-term climate threats.

DISCUSSION QUESTIONS

1. The energy sector is a significant climate-health problem and therefore is an important component of climate mitigation. Health systems are entrenched in an energy sector that will surpass the available carbon budget. Reducing carbon emissions to a level that avoids tipping points and synergistic reactions requires (1) eliminating fossil fuel reliance, (2) achieving net-zero emissions energy systems, and (3) active carbon removal. Is there reluctance within health professionals to focus on this issue, or are energy issues well understood by health professionals? Why or why not? What are coordinated strategies within hospitals and health care institutions to mitigate energy emissions? What would a strong, coordinated response to energy system transformation in the health community look like? What is one thing an individual can do to ensure that this happens?

2. Reflect on the climate negotiations for the Paris Agreement and Kigali Amendment, and how negotiation blocs or climate clubs form, evolve and re-form. What medical and health-related groups are present at current climate negotiations, formally or as members of the NGO community? Who should be at the table that is not already? If you were to attend the next negotiations and conduct a "side event" (an event held on the sidelines of the main negotiations,

usually a training seminar to bring parties up to date on an idea, technology, or latest research), what would be your central thesis and topic? Let us say you, as the representative of a major medical organization, were permitted to give a high-level statement from the floor of the negotiations. You have between five and ten minutes to construct remarks, which will be delivered in front of representatives (and likely ministers of environment or senior officials) from every country in the world, with attendant media coverage. What would you say in your high-level remarks? Write down the most critical health issue that demands an important policy position, in your opinion. Let us say you had the opportunity to draft the policy position, and the high-level remarks, of the influential country that if followed, would have significant impact in the "right direction"—according to you—on this position (such as the United States, India, or Brazil). Which country would it be, and what are your draft talking points?

3. There is no singular model for good governance of health-climate issues generally, or mitigation specifically. A one-size-fits-all approach to governance ignores the nuanced understanding and inclusivity that is a requirement of good governance. What are some methods or elements of good governance? Which of these elements needs to be cultivated in the climate-health governance structures?

KEY TERMS

Adaptation: The process of adjustment to climate-related changes that either are already in place or are anticipated in the future. One example is increasing a growing season of crops to increase yields.

Chlorofluorocarbon: A fluorinated gas (F-gas)—a potent greenhouse gas; a synthetic chemical capable of destroying the earth's atmosphere more quickly than it can naturally restore itself. These migrate into the upper atmosphere, break down and release chlorine and bromine ions, which catalyze the breakdown of the ozone molecules, and each ion can destroy thousands of ozone molecules. The Montreal Protocol successfully phased CFCs out of production and consumption

Climate change: Refers to the phenomenon of the climate warming at a rapid, unprecedented rate due to anthropogenic impacts.

Climate crisis: The anthropogenic impacts that have accelerated the earth's warming and environmental destruction to near catastrophic levels. This term is used to distinguish from changes in weather, temperature, or environment that have occur naturally over time.

Common but differentiated responsibilities: A foundational principle of environmental law aimed at facilitating fairness and cooperation between developed and developing nations. This principle is based on the premise that although all nations have the same responsibility to protect the environment and encourage sustainable development, their obligations to meet such responsibilities are nonetheless proportionate to their commensurate level of resources, capabilities, and advantages/disadvantages.

Energy efficiency: Reducing energy consumption by using less energy to perform the same task or attain the same level of output. This encompasses eliminating energy waste. This is distinguished from energy conservation, the concept of reducing energy consumption through minimizing energy-consuming activities, which requires changes in individual behavior. Examples of energy efficiency range from more energy-efficient light bulbs and air conditioners, to increasing insulation or installing better windows on a building, which increases the energy efficiency of the building envelope. (Energy Sage 2019)

Feedback loops: Feedback loops are a "cyclical process triggered by environmental change that leads back to more change," such as melting ice caps that in turn expose darker land mass absorbing more solar heat and triggering greater warming. Another example is ozone depletion, which increases ultraviolet radiation, which in turn suppresses the human immune system (Lenton et al. 2019).

Governance: The totality of "political, organizational and administrative processes through which stakeholders, including governments, NGOs, civil society and private-sector interest groups, articulate their interests, exercise their legal rights, make decisions, meet their obligations, and mediate their differences" (Swinburn et al. 2019)

Greenhouse gases (GHGs): Atmospheric constituents that accumulate in the atmosphere, trap heat, and create increasing warming in the atmosphere. Examples include carbon dioxide, water vapor, ozone, and methane.

Health–climate nexus: The impact of the climate crisis on human health and the intersection of the health and climate fields.

Hydrofluorocarbons (HFCs): A potent short-lived climate pollutant used in air conditioning, refrigeration, solvents, some foams such as fire extinguishing systems, and aerosols. As an SLCP it is orders of magnitude more potent than carbon dioxide and has a much shorter atmospheric lifetime. The Kigali Amendment to the Montreal Protocol, agreed to in 2016, specifically added HFCs to the list of gases to phase down.

Intergovernmental Panel on Climate Change (IPCC): Expert panel established in 1988 by the World Meteorological Organization (WMO) and the United Nations Environment Programme (UNEP) to summarize the state of the science on climate change, impacts, and policy response strategies. The group consists of over 2,500 international voluntary scientists who curate periodic assessment reports that are later reviewed by representatives of the member states of the United Nations, which in turn will either reject or accept them.

Kigali Amendment: The Kigali Amendment to the Montreal Protocol was adopted in 2016 to phase down the use of hydrofluorocarbons by cutting consumption and production. HFCs are a short-lived climate pollutant and as such, the drastic decrease of usage will lead to an immediate atmospheric effect. The Amendment was a significant step to reducing global warming by 0.5°C (1°F). When combined with increasing equipment energy efficiency, it is projected to remove *up to* 1°C (1.8°F) of warming from the earth's atmosphere. Because climate models project a 4°C (7.2°F) scenario, this intervention is a powerful step toward achieving the goals of the Paris Agreement.

Mitigation: Climate change mitigation includes efforts to reduce or prevent the emission of greenhouse gases such as encouraging renewable energy, phasing out fossil fuels, carbon capture and sequestration, increasing energy efficiency, changing consumer behavior, and a host of other activities.

Montreal Protocol: The Montreal Protocol is a multilateral environmental agreement that focuses on the reduction of ozone depleting substances (ODS). It does so by creating country-specific timetables for phasing out groups of ODS and has binding, time-targeted, measurable commitments.

Multilateral: A policy, proposal, or act that has been agreed upon by three or more parties. It is not limited to countries and also refers to multiple stakeholders in agreement. From a climate perspective, multilateral agreements are key to affecting temperature increases and greenhouse gas accumulation.

Nationally determined contributions (NDCs): The Paris Agreement requires that each country communicate the explicit ways in which they will reduce emissions and by how much; NDCs are a country's stated targets and timelines.

Ozone layer: Blanket of diffuse gases encircling the earth at a distance of 12 to 50 kilometers above the surface; also refers to three oxygen atoms (ozone, or O3) that concentrate there.

Paris Agreement Carbon Budget: The carbon budget available to fall below the 1.5° (2.7°F) mark set by Paris, based on the Intergovernmental Panel on Climate Change's estimates, is between 420 and 580 gigatons of CO_2.

Policymakers: Government actors who directly promulgate policies in public spaces, private actors who promulgate policies within their governance structures and influence public policy, and other nongovernmental actors that influence public policy through advocacy, research, activism, and lending subject matter expertise in formal and informal ways, such as advising multilateral negotiations.

Polluter Pays Principle: The principle that polluters and users of natural resources bear the full environmental and social costs of their actions, ensuring that a more complete picture of the cost is reflected in the ultimate market price for a good or service.

Precautionary principle: States that political, social, and economic responses to environmental threats should move forward with all deliberate speed rather than embrace inertia until definite scientific answers are found. Policymakers can and should act when there is a probability of threat to health and environment.

Ratification: In the context of the United Nations, ratification of treaties refers to the agreement by a country or state to be bound by a treaty. Ratification usually requires time for a country to gain domestic approval for the treaty and enact legislation that follows the treaties requirements. For example, the United States did not ratify the Kyoto Protocol and was thus not required to follow its principles.

Risk multiplier: A multiplier is an economic factor that when increased/changed causes increases/changes in many other variables. A cumulatively reinforcing induced interaction between one factor and multiple variables. Climate change is a risk multiplier to health; it is multiplying the risks not only associated with climate change-induced disasters and catastrophic effects but also those associated with health risks affected on multiple levels by climate change. For example, global warming causes water evaporation and extreme, unpredictable temperatures that affect food and water supplies, which can lead to malnutrition, diarrhea, heart and respiratory diseases, and waterborne or insect-transmitted diseases.

Short-lived climate pollutants (SLCPs): Pollutants that have shorter atmospheric lifetimes but are hundreds or thousands of times more potent than carbon dioxide in warming effects. The four key SLCPs are methane, HFCs, black carbon, and tropospheric ozone.

Stratospheric ozone layer: The layer of the earth's atmosphere that extends between 12 km and 50 km above the earth, as distinguished from the troposphere, which resides within the first 12 km above earth. The stratosphere contains the highest concentration of ozone, known as the "ozone layer." Its function is to protect the earth from harmful ultraviolet (UV-B) radiation, which in high concentrations has dire effects on human health.

Synergistic reaction: A reaction where the combination of one or more factors leads to a significantly worse result than the sole effect of individual factors, such as human exposure to multiple harmful chemicals that produce unforeseen health effects, as in the case of DDT.

Tipping point: A threshold beyond which the impact may be many times greater than expected, such as the irreversible loss of ice sheets once the temperature and melting rate has reached a particular level that in turn triggers greater warming. Leading scholars and researchers point to tipping points as an indicator that we are in an acute stage of climate crisis. Tipping points often have cascading effects—one leads to another and so on, triggering a systemic reaction that is unstoppable. Environmental problems are nonlinear with complex causes and effects and are often the result or cause of "tipping points," synergistic interactions, or feedback loops.

Total committed emissions from the energy sector: If operated at current levels (a business-as-usual scenario) existing energy infrastructure combined with emissions from all proposed power plants, total committed emissions will exceed 846 gigatons of CO_2.

Triple-policy energy mitigation strategy: To avoid tipping points and synergistic reactions requires simultaneously (1) shutting off fossil fuel reliance, (2) net-zero emissions energy systems, and (3) aggressive carbon-removal strategies.

UN Environment Programme (UNEP or UNE): UNEP is the leading global environmental authority that sets the global environmental agenda, advocates for the environment, and promotes the coherent implementation of the environmental dimension of sustainable development. A United Nations program under the General Assembly organ, UNEP has historically been one of the least funded of the funds or programs

World Health Organization (WHO): A specialized agency under the United Nations System, under the umbrella of the United Nations Economic and Social Council. Its primary role is to direct and coordinate international health within the UN system. Its main areas of work are in health systems, health through the life cycle, noncommunicable and communicable diseases; preparedness, surveillance, and response; and corporate services. They mostly work on climate adaptation, not mitigation.

World Meteorological Organization (WMO): An international body with 193 member states that falls under the umbrella of the United Nations. It provides international cooperation on weather, climate, hydrologic services, and other geophysical sciences among its member countries. Because WMO deals mostly with meteorology and thus weather or natural disasters, its activities are generally more relevant to climate adaptation. An exception is its ozone reports.

References and Further Reading

Arctic Council. 1996. "Declaration on the Establishment of the Arctic Council." September 19. https://oaarchive.arctic-council.org/bitstream/handle/11374/85/EDOCS-1752-v2-ACMMCA00_Ottawa_1996_Founding_Declaration.PDF?sequence=5&isAllowed=y.

Arctic Council. 2015. "Iqaluit Declaration." https://oaarchive.arctic-council.org/bitstream/handle/11374/662/EDOCS-2547-v1-ACMMCA09_Iqaluit_2015_Iqaluit_Declaration_formatted_brochure_low-res.PDF?sequence=6&isAllowed=y.

Arctic Council. 2016. "Update from the Nordic Environment Finance Corporation (NEFCO) on the Arctic Council Project Support Instrument (PSI)." https://oaarchive.arctic-council.org/bitstream/handle/11374/1741/EDOCS-3209-v1A-ACSAOUS202_Fairbanks_2016_InfoDoc3_NEFCO_Update_Report_PSI.pdf?sequence=1&isAllowed=y

Arctic Council. 2017. "Fairbanks Declaration." https://oaarchive.arctic-council.org/bitstream/handle/11374/1910/EDOCS-4339-v1-ACMMUS10_FAIRBANKS_2017_Fairbanks_Declaration_Brochure_Version_w_Layout.PDF?sequence=8&isAllowed=y.

Arctic Council. 2018. "The Arctic Council: A Backgrounder." September 13. https://arctic-council.org/index.php/en/about-us.

Blackstock, J. J., and M. R. Allen. 2013. *The Science and Policy of Short-Lived Climate Pollutants, Oxford Martin Policy Brief*. Oxford: Oxford Martin School.

Center on International Cooperation. n.d. "G8 and G20." https://cic.nyu.edu/topic/g8-and-g20.

Climate and Clean Air Coalition. 2019a. "About the Climate and Clean Air Coalition." www.ccacoalition.org/en/resources/about-climate-and-clean-air-coalition-infosheet.

Climate and Clean Air Coalition. 2019b. "Climate and Clean Air Coalition Annual Report 2018-2019." www.ccacoalition.org/en/resources/climate-clean-air-coalition-2018-2019-annual-report.

Climate and Clean Air Coalition. 2019c. "Countries Pledge Fast Action on Efficient Cooling." August 30, 2019. https://www.ccacoalition.org/en/news/countries-pledge-fast-action-efficient-cooling-big-win-clean-air-and-climate.

Climate and Clean Air Coalition. 2019d. "Why Act on Short-Lived Climate Pollutants." www.ccacoalition.org/en/resources/why-act-short-lived-climate-pollutants-infosheet.

Climate and Clean Air Coalition. 2020. "Assessment of Climate and Development Benefits of Efficient and Climate-Friendly Cooling." www.ccacoalition.org/en/resources/assessment-climate-and-development-benefits-efficient-and-climate-friendly-cooling.

Council on Foreign Relations. 2014. "The Group of Eight (G8) Industrialized Nations." https://www.cfr.org/backgrounder/group-eight-g8-industrialized-nations.

Council on Foreign Relations. 2019. "Report Card on International Cooperation 2018–2019." 2019. https://www.cfr.org/interactive/councilofcouncils/reportcard2019/#!/.

Ebi, K. L., J. J. Hess, and P. Watkiss. 2017. "Health Risks and Costs of Climate Variability and Change." In *Injury Prevention and Environmental Health*, 3d ed., edited by C. N. Mock, R. Nugent, O. Kobusingye, and K. R. Smith. Washington, DC: World Bank. https://www.ncbi.nlm.nih.gov/books/NBK525226/.

Energy Sage. 2019. "Energy Efficiency 101. What Is Energy Efficiency?" Updated September 23, 2019. https://www.energysage.com/energy-efficiency/101/.

European Commission. n.d.a. "About the European Commission." https://ec.europa.eu/info/about-european-commission_en.

European Commission. n.d.b. "European Climate Change Program." https://ec.europa.eu/clima/policies/eccp_en.

European Commission. 2018. "Our Vision for a Clean Planet for All." https://ec.europa.eu/clima/sites/clima/files/docs/pages/vision_1_emissions_en.pdf.

European Commission. 2019. "Commissioner Arias Cañete co-convenes third Ministerial on Climate Action (MoCA) in Brussels." https://ec.europa.eu/clima/news/commissioner-arias-ca%C3%B1ete-co-convenes-third-ministerial-climate-action-moca-brussels_en.

European Union. n.d. "Countries." https://europa.eu/european-union/about-eu/countries_en.

European Council. 2019. "G20 Osaka Leaders' Declaration." https://www.consilium.europa.eu/media/40124/final_g20_osaka_leaders_declaration.pdf.

Exner-Pirot, H., M. Ackrén, N. Loukacheva, H. Nicol, A. E. Nilsson, and J. Spence. 2019. "Form and Function: The Future of the Arctic Council." February 5. https://www.thearcticinstitute.org/form-function-future-arctic-council/

Food and Agriculture Organization. 2019a. *Climate-Smart Agriculture and the Sustainable Development Goals*. Rome: FAO. http://www.fao.org/publications/card/en/c/CA6043EN/.

Food and Agriculture Organization. 2019b. *FAO's Work on Climate Change: Fisheries and Aquaculture 2019*. Rome: FAO. http://www.fao.org/3/ca7166en/ca7166en.pdf.

Food and Agriculture Organization. 2019c. *Five Practical Actions Towards Low-Carbon Livestock*. Rome: FAO. http://www.fao.org/3/ca7089en/ca7089en.pdf.

Food and Agricultural Organization. 2019d. *The State of Food and Agriculture*. http://www.fao.org/3/ca6030en/ca6030en.pdf.

Food and Agriculture Organization. 2019e. *The State of Food Security and Nutrition in the World*." http://www.fao.org/3/ca5162en/ca5162en.pdf.

Haines, A., and K. Ebi. 2019. "The Imperative for Climate Action to Protect Health." *New England Journal of Medicine* 380:263–73. doi: 10.1056/NEJMra1807873.

Hajnal, P. I. 2019. *The G20: Evolution, Interrelationships, Documentation*, 2d ed. New York: Routledge.

Harper, A. B., T. Powell, P. M. Cox, J. House, C. Huntingford, T. M. Lenton, S. Sitch et al. 2018. "Land-Use Emissions Play a Critical Role in Land-Based Mitigation for Paris Climate Targets." *Nature Communications* 9:2938. doi: 10.1038/s41467-018-05340-z.

Hawken, P. 2017. *Drawdown: The Most Comprehensive Plan Ever Proposed to Reverse Global Warming*. San Francisco, CA: Project Drawdown. https://www.drawdown.org.

Hu, A., Y. Xu, C. Tebaldi, W. M. Washington, and V. Ramanathan. 2013. "Mitigation of Short-Lived Climate Pollutants Slows Sea-Level Rise." *Nature Climate Change* 3:730–34.

Hunter, D., J. E. Salzman, and D. Zaelke. 2015. *International Environmental Law and Policy*, 5th ed. St. Paul, MN: Foundation Press. https://faculty.westacademic.com/Book/Detail?id=3128.

International Energy Agency. 2019. "History: From Oil Security to Steering the World toward Secure and Sustainable Energy Transitions." December 2. https://www.iea.org/about/history.

International Energy Agency. 2020. "Building a 'Grand Coalition' to Bridge the Gap Between Energy and Climate Goals." February 12, 2020. https://www.iea.org/news/building-a-grand-coalition-to-bridge-the-gap-between-energy-and-climate-goals.

Intergovernmental Panel on Climate Change. 2015. *IPCC Second Assessment Climate Change*, Geneva: IPCC. https://www.ipcc.ch/site/assets/uploads/2018/06/2nd-assessment-en.pdf.

Intergovernmental Panel on Climate Change. 2018. *Global Warming of 1.5°C. An IPCC Special Report on the Impacts of Global Warming of 1.5°C above Pre-Industrial Levels and Related Global Greenhouse Gas Emission Pathways, in the Context of Strengthening the Global Response to the Threat of Climate Change, Sustainable Development, and Efforts to Eradicate Poverty*, edited by V. Masson-Delmotte, P. Zhai, H.-O. Pörtner, D. Roberts, J. Skea, P. R. Shukla, A. Pirani, W. Moufouma-Okia et al. Geneva: Intergovernmental Panel on Climate Change. https://www.ipcc.ch/sr15/.

Intergovernmental Panel on Climate Change. 2019. *Climate Change and Land: an IPCC Special Report on Climate Change, Desertification, Land Degradation, Sustainable Land Management, Food Security, and Greenhouse Gas Fluxes in Terrestrial Ecosystems*, edited by P. R. Shukla, J. Skea, E. Calvo Buendia, V. Masson-Delmotte, H.-O. Pörtner, D. C. Roberts, P. Zhai et al. Geneva: Intergovernmental Panel on Climate Change. https://www.ipcc.ch/srccl/.

Keohane, N., A. Petsonk, and A. Hanafi. 2017. "Toward a Club of Carbon Markets," *Climatic Change* 144:81–95.

Lenton, T., J. Rockström, O. Gaffney, S. Rahmstorf, K. Richardson, W. Steffen, and H. J. Schellnhuber. 2019. "Climate Tipping Points—Too Risky to Bet Against." *Nature* November 27, 2019. https://www.nature.com/articles/d41586-019-03595-0.

Lewis, P. B., and G. Coinu. 2019. "Climate Change, The Paris Agreement, and Subsidiarity." *John Marshall Law Review* 52: 320.

Meiro-Lorenzo, M., T. Bouley, G. Kleiman, P. L. Osewe, T. S. Rabie, R. M. Seifman, and H. Wang. 2017. *Climate Change and Health Approach and Action Plan*. Washington, DC: World Bank. http://documents.worldbank.org/curated/en/421451495428198858/Climate-change-and-health-approach-and-action-plan.

Ministerial on Climate Action. 2019. "Chairs' Summary." https://ec.europa.eu/clima/sites/clima/files/news/20190628_chairs_summary_en.pdf.

Nordhaus, W. 2015. "Climate Clubs: Overcoming Free-Riding in International Climate Policy." *American Economic Review* 105 (4):1339–70.

Pan American Health Organization. 2015. *Health in All Policies: Case Studies from the Region of the Americas.* Washington, DC: PAHO. https://www.paho.org/hq/dmdocuments/2015/HiAP-Case-Studies-from-the-Americas-ENG.pdf.

Pearce, R. 2014. "Infographic: Mapping Country Alliances at the International Climate Talks." December 10, 2014. https://www.carbonbrief.org/infographic-mapping-country-alliances-at-the-international-climate-talks.

Peters, T. 2018. "Cooling for All—the 18th Sustainable Development Goal." June 25, 2018. https://ccacoalition.org/en/blog/cooling-all---18th-sustainable-development-goal.

Project Drawdown. 2020. accessed February 1, 2020. A https://www.drawdown.org/solutions.

Poore, J., and T. Nemecek. 2018. "Reducing Food's Environmental Impacts through Producers and Consumers." *Science* 360 (6392):987–92.

Rome Declaration on the Contribution of the Montreal Protocol to Food Loss Reduction through Sustainable Cold Chain Development—Thirty-First Meeting of the Parties. November 8, 2019. https://ozone.unep.org/treaties/montreal-protocol/meetings/thirty-first-meeting-parties/decisions/annex-i-rome-declaration.

Rosenzweig, C., C. Mbow, L. G. Barioni, T. G. Benton, M. Herrero, M. Krishnapillai, E. T. Liwenga et al. 2020. "Climate Change Responses Benefit from a Global Food System Approach." *Nature Food* 1:94–97. https://doi.org/10.1038/s43016-020-0031-z.

Savaresi, A. 2016. "The Paris Agreement: A New Beginning?" *Journal of Energy & Natural Resources Law* 34 (1):16–26.

Shah, N., M. Wei, V. Letschert, an A. Phadke. 2015. *Benefits of Leapfrogging to Superefficiency and Low Global Warming Potential Refrigerants in Room Air Conditioning.* Berkeley, CA: Berkeley National Laboratory. https://ies.lbl.gov/sites/default/files/lbnl-1003671.pdf.

Steffen, W., J. Rockström, K. Richardson, T. M. Lenton, C. Folke, D. Liverman, C. P. Summerhayes et al. 2018. "Trajectories of the Earth System in the Anthropocene." *PNAS* 115 (33):8252–9.

Swinburn, B. A., V. I. Kraak, S. Allender, V. J. Atkins, P. I. Baker, J. R. Bogard, H. Brinsden et al. 2019. "The Global Syndemic of Obesity, Undernutrition, and Climate Change: *The Lancet* Commission Report." *Lancet* 393:791–846.

Tong, D, Q. Zhang, Y. Zheng, K. Caldeira, C. Shearer, C. Hong, Y. Qin, and S. J. Davis. 2019. "Committed Emissions from Existing Energy Infrastructure Jeopardize 1.5 Degree Celsius Climate Target." *Nature* 572:373–77.

United Nations. 1992. *United Nations Framework Convention on Climate Change.* https://unfccc.int/resource/docs/convkp/conveng.pdf.

United Nations. 2013. "The United Nations System." https://www.unfpa.org/sites/default/files/resource-pdf/UN%20system%20chart_11x17_color_2013.pdf.

United Nations. 2016. *World Economic and Social Survey 2016. Climate Change Resilience: An Opportunity for Reducing Inequalities.* New York: UN. https://www.un.org/development/desa/dpad/wp-content/uploads/sites/45/publication/WESS_2016_Report.pdf.

United Nations Development Programme. 2019. *Human Development Report 2019.* New York: UNDP. http://hdr.undp.org/sites/default/files/hdr2019.pdf.

United Nations Environment Programme. 2016. "The Kigali Amendment to the Montreal Protocol: Another Commitment to Stop Climate Change." https://www.unenvironment.org/news-and-stories/news/kigali-amendment-montreal-protocol-another-global-commitment-stop-climate.

United Nations Environment Programme. 2019. "Emissions Gap Report." https://wedocs.unep.org/bitstream/handle/20.500.11822/30797/EGR2019.pdf?sequence=1&isAllowed=y.

United Nations Framework Convention on Climate Change. 2013. "United Nations Framework Convention on Climate Change: A Visual Introduction." https://issuu.com/earthinbrackets/docs/unfcccenglish; see also: https://www.theclimategroup.org/sites/default/files/archive/files/UNFCCC_timeline.pdf.

United Nations Framework Convention on Climate Change. n.d.a. Kyoto Protocol Base Year Data (for the Second Commitment Period of the Kyoto Protocol). https://unfccc.int/process-and-meetings/transparency-and-reporting/reporting-and-review-under-the-kyoto-protocol/second-commitment-period/kyoto-protocol-base-year-data-for-the-second-commitment-period-of-the-kyoto-protocol

United Nations Framework Convention on Climate Change. n.d.b. "The Paris Agreement." https://unfccc.int/process-and-meetings/the-paris-agreement/the-paris-agreement

United Nations Framework Convention on Climate Change. n.d.c. "UNFCCC—25 Years of Effort and Achievement." https://unfccc.int/timeline/.

United Nations Industrial Development Organization. n.d. "The Montreal Protocol Evolves to Fight Climate Change." https://www.unido.org/our-focus/safeguarding-environment/implementation-multilateral-environmental-agreements/montreal-protocol/montreal-protocol-evolves-fight-climate-change

United Nations Office for the Coordination of Humanitarian Affairs. n.d.a. "Environmental Dimensions of Emergencies." https://www.unocha.org/themes/environmental-dimensions-emergencies

United Nations Office for the Coordination of Humanitarian Affairs. n.d.b. "Our Work." https://www.unocha.org/our-work.

United States Department of State. 2009. "Major Economies Forum on Energy and Climate." https://2009-2017.state.gov/e/oes/climate/mem/index.htm.

U.S. Global Change Research Program. 2016. "The Impacts of Climate Change on Human Health in the United States: A Scientific Assessment." https://health2016.globalchange.gov/.

White House. 2016a. "U.S.-China Joint Presidential Statement on Climate Change." https://obamawhitehouse.archives.gov/the-press-office/2016/03/31/us-china-joint-presidential-statement-climate-change

White House. 2016b. "Statement by the President on the Montreal Protocol." https://obamawhitehouse.archives.gov/the-press-office/2016/10/15/statement-president-montreal-protocol.

World Bank Group. 2017a. *Climate Change and Health Approach and Action Plan*. Washington, DC: World Bank.

World Bank Group. 2017b. *Climate-Smart Healthcare*. Washington, DC: World Bank.

World Health Organization. 2014. "WHO Guidance to Protect Health from Climate Change through Health Adaptation Planning." https://apps.who.int/iris/bitstream/handle/10665/137383/9789241508001_eng.pdf?sequence=1&isAllowed=y.

World Health Organization. 2018a. "COP24 Special Report: Health and Climate Change." https://www.who.int/globalchange/publications/COP24-report-health-climate-change/en/.

World Health Organization. 2018b. "Health, Environment and Climate Change Coalition." https://www.who.int/globalchange/coalition/en/.

CHAPTER 21

CLIMATE CHANGE AND THE RIGHT TO HEALTH

Alison Blaiklock, Carmel Williams, and Rhys Jones

Introduction

> The fight against climate change is fundamentally about human rights and securing justice for those suffering from its impact - vulnerable countries and communities that are least culpable for the problem. (Robinson 2018)

We all have human rights. The climate catastrophe is a serious threat to human rights and yet the ways we respond can bring great opportunities to fulfill people's rights, including the **right to health**, and achieve health equity. In this chapter we look at the impact of climate change on the right to health and other human rights and outline ways in which human rights can strengthen and extend useful current responses and develop new equitable ones.

What Are Human Rights?

Human rights are inspired by shared moral and ethical values and guaranteed by international law. Everyone is "born free and equal in dignity and rights" (United Nations 1948). Everyone, everywhere, has human rights, regardless of their nationality, place of residence, sex, ethnicity, disability, or any other status. Everyone should be treated with dignity and in ways that recognize our shared humanity—this is what underpins the compassion that is essential to healing and the solidarity essential to social justice (Williams, Blaiklock, and Hunt forthcoming)

International human rights law includes the fundamental commitments of states to treat all people with fairness and without discrimination and to enable everyone to enjoy all their human rights, including the right to health. The 1948 Universal Declaration of Human Rights was created in response to global outrage at the human suffering and atrocities of World War II. The world united to ensure that humankind would never again experience such loss of dignity and freedom. Unabated climate change poses such a threat. A rights-based approach provides an imperative to guide the process and actions to mitigate such disaster (Lemery, Williams, and Farmer 2014).

The rights described in the Universal Declaration of Human Rights have been enshrined in legally binding human rights treaties and covenants. These confer entitlements on people and impose obligations on governments, transnational corporations, organizations, and people including health workers whose roles and responsibilities affect others.

The climate emergency has an impact on many rights, including rights to life, health, food, water, sanitation, housing, education, an adequate standard of living, self-determination and so forth. Some groups are affected much more than others (see Chapters 14 and 16). It is terribly unjust that the countries and communities that have done least to cause climate change are worst affected and yet have the least economic and infrastructure resources to adapt (Patz et al. 2007; Levy and Patz 2015; Metcalfe 2015).

What Is the Right to Health?

The right to the highest attainable standard of physical and mental health (abbreviated to the right to health) is not a right to be healthy. It is, however, a right to personal and public health services and the underlying determinants of health such as potable water, sanitation, an adequate supply of nutrition, safe housing, and clean air. The right to health depends on people living in a healthy, safe, clean, and sustainable environment (Knox 2018).

The right to health is recognized in the Universal Declaration on Human Rights (United Nations 1948), the International Convention on Economic, Social and Cultural Rights (United Nations 1966), the United Nations Convention on the Rights of the Child (United Nations 1989), and other human rights treaties. It is in the Declaration on the Rights of Indigenous Peoples that established a universal framework of minimum standards for the survival, dignity, well-being, and rights of all **Indigenous peoples** (United Nations 2007). These agreements can be viewed online at the website of the United Nations High Commissioner for Human Rights (see www.ohchr.org).

The right to health is also in key international health agreements, including the World Health Organization (WHO) Constitution (World Health Organization 1946), the Alma Ata Declaration (World Health Organization 1979) and the Framework Convention on Tobacco Control (World Health Organization 2003).

The first multilateral environmental agreement to explicitly recognize human rights was the 2015 Paris Agreement (Conference of the Parties 2015). The right to health is among those specifically included in its preamble: "Parties should, when taking action to address climate change, respect, promote and consider their respective obligations on human rights, the right to health, the rights of indigenous peoples, local communities, migrants, children, persons with disabilities and people in vulnerable situations and the right to development, as well as gender equality, empowerment of women and intergenerational equity" (Conference of the Parties 2015).

Various international and regional human rights laws include obligations relating to the environment. These include obligations for governments to have legal and institutional frameworks that protect people against environmental harm, assess environmental impacts, inform the public, facilitate participation in environmental decision-making, provide access to remedies for harm, recognize additional obligations towards groups particularly vulnerable to environmental harm, and protect the rights of people striving for a safe, healthy, and sustainable environment (Knox 2013).

When a state ratifies a treaty, it agrees to be bound to it in international law. When states ratify a United Nations (UN) human rights treaty, they have to report regularly and have their progress reviewed by an expert committee. In 2000, the meaning of health rights entitlements was clarified by the UN Committee on Economic Social and Cultural Rights in **General Comment 14**, which was adopted by the UN state members. State obligations include the provision of primary health services such as maternal and child health and essential medicines, among many others. The General Comment allows for the impossibility of all states being able to meet the same standards of health care immediately. But it does specify that over time, there must be a gradual improvement in the provision of health care and in access to the underlying determinants of health, which is called **progressive realization of the right to health**. This means that when states report every four years to the Committee on their right to health achievements, they must demonstrate that health entitlements have improved—that there is greater realization of people's health rights (United Nations Committee on Economic Social and Cultural Rights 2000).

However, there are also rights to health obligations that the state must implement immediately. These include the fundamental human rights principle that all people are equal and must be treated with dignity and without discrimination. In practice, this means that no one can be denied access to health care on the basis of discrimination and all people have an equal right to participate in decisions about their own health. Principles of equality and nondiscrimination also mean that Indigenous people, people living remotely, people in poverty, people with disabilities, women, and children are entitled to the same access to health care and the same quality of water, sanitation, nutrition, clean air, and other public goods as everyone else. In order to achieve equality, the most disadvantaged people are entitled to have their rights to health prioritized.

General Comment 14 provided a basis for the UN Committee on Economic Social and Cultural Rights, UN Special Rapporteurs on the right to health, WHO, civil society organizations, academics, and many others to make the right to health easier to understand and use in developing, delivering, and evaluating services, programs, and policies that affect health. Considerable work has been done in identifying key features of the right to health in order to assist operationalizing the right (Williams et al. forthcoming). We use examples to illustrate these features in the section, Human Rights-Based Approaches to the Climate Crisis.

Three overlapping and mutually reinforcing approaches are often used to put the right to health into practice. These can be termed empowerment, policy, and judicial approaches (Williams et al. forthcoming).

- *Empowerment.* This happens when people know that they have a human rights entitlement to be treated fairly and with dignity, and they act individually or collectively with others to claim their rights.

- *Policy.* The right-to-health perspective is useful in the development, implementation and evaluation of health-related policies and programs. This approach goes through the usual policy and program processes (identifying problems, possible solutions and so forth) in ways that are informed by the right to health—for example, those who are most disadvantaged are prioritized and progress indicators are disaggregated into subpopulations.

- *Judicial.* Sometimes a judicial approach is taken. In the past few years, although access to legal redress varies within and between countries, there has been an exponential increase in the number of health-related rights cases being taken to court (Yamin 2014). Litigation can be used strategically alongside other approaches to change health-related laws, policies, and practices (Ezer and Patel 2018).

Climate Crisis Impacts on the Right to Health

The industrial revolution has led to the Anthropocene, the era in which human actions have become the main drivers of global environmental change. If human actions continue to overload the climate and other interlinked environmental systems that provide a "safe operating space" for humanity on the planet, then the results could be catastrophic for large parts of the world (Rockström et al. 2009).

Even small increases in global warming can harm health via associated changes in extreme weather events, heat waves, flooding, sea level rise, infectious and waterborne diseases, air quality, food and water security, sustainable development, migration, displacement, and working conditions. Yet the response to climate change could be this century's greatest opportunity to improve global health (Watts, Adger et al. 2015) with massive health gains to be made through actions to reduce greenhouse gas emissions, especially if global warming is kept below

1.5°C (2.7°F). Strengthening adaptation through climate-resilient health systems and achieving equitable access to the determinants of health mean the benefits can be even greater (World Health Organization 2018b).

Unjust Disparities

All people have an equal right to health. Yet the impacts of climate change are disproportionately borne by those in developing countries and marginalized communities everywhere (Smith et al. 2014). Poorer countries and countries whose greenhouse gas emissions are lower are first and worst affected. This is vividly seen in Figure 21.1, which compares countries' cumulative carbon dioxide emissions from 1950 to 2013 with five climate-sensitive health consequences.

Some groups of people—including Indigenous peoples, children, women, older people, people living with disabilities, people who are ill, poor people, people in climate-sensitive occupations, and people experiencing discrimination, marginalization, or living in unsafe environments—are especially vulnerable. Some are vulnerable in multiple ways. There is also growing recognition of intergenerational inequity and that the stability of the climate is entrusted to governments to keep it safe for future generations; it is unjust that those yet to be

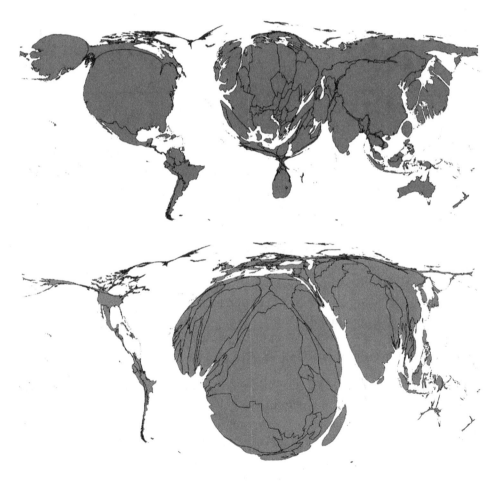

Figure 21.1   The climate gap: those who have emitted most and those affected first and worst

Note: Cartograms of countries' cumulative fossil CO_2 emissions 1950–2013 (upper map); compared with additional deaths attributable to climate change, from five climate-sensitive health consequences (undernutrition in children aged under five years, malaria, dengue, diarrheal disease in children, heat stress in elderly over sixty-five years) projected for 2030 (lower map). Based on the method of Patz et al. (2007), with data from the Climate Equity Reference Calculator Database via http://calculator.climateequityreference.org and Hales, Kovats, and Campbell-Lendrum 2014. Analysis by Scott Metcalfe, mapping by Mark Metcalfe. The publishers thank the *New Zealand Medical Journal* for permission to reproduce this figure

Source: Metcalfe (2015).

born face a worsening breakdown of the climate (World Health Organization 2014; Levy and Patz 2015; Metcalfe 2015; Watts, Amann èt al. 2019; Williams et al. forthcoming).

The impacts of the climate crisis on Indigenous peoples, children, and Small Island Developing States (SIDS) illustrate the disparities. For Indigenous peoples, despite the diversity of geographical, social, cultural, and political contexts, a range of common factors confer disproportionate risk from climate change. These include unique relationships with the natural environment, existing health inequities, socioeconomic deprivation, poor quality housing and infrastructure, climate impacts on customary food sources, and poor access to and quality of health care (Jones 2019). In many countries, the underlying causes of these factors are colonial systems, structures, and practices that marginalize and discriminate against Indigenous peoples. In addition, societal responses to climate change threaten to impact disproportionately on Indigenous communities and exacerbate existing social and health inequities (Jones et al. 2014). Human rights approaches offer mechanisms to ensure that the inequitable climate risks for Indigenous populations are addressed and that any adverse consequences of climate policies are avoided or mitigated.

For several reasons, the health of children, especially young or disadvantaged children, is at higher risk from climate change. Children depend on their families and adults for their care, well-being, and the environment in which they live and grow. When caregivers are affected by climate change, their children are affected. Children are rapidly developing and their physiology, anatomy, immunology, psychology, cognition, and behaviors may be affected by climate change in ways different to adults. They experience higher relative exposures to, for example, heat or air pollution, for their body size. Because they have more years of life ahead of them, they will have a greater proportionate exposure to a worsening climate and more time to acquire diseases with long latency periods (Ahdoot et al. 2015; Stanberry, Thomson, and James 2018; Watts, Amann et al. 2019).

Common causes of global child mortality and morbidity—malaria, respiratory diseases, diarrheal diseases, malnutrition, and communicable diseases—are expected to worsen with climate change (Ahdoot et al. 2015; Stanberry, Thomson, and James 2018; Watts, Amann et al. 2019). The breakdown of the climate affects children's access to education and other determinants (all of which are human rights) that underpin the foundations of lifelong health. However, equity-based climate action—for example, by increasing girls' access to affordable safe public and active transport—can improve health and equity (Hosking et al. 2011).

Although SIDS have made a tiny contribution to global greenhouse emissions, they are in the frontline of the climate crisis. They are uniquely vulnerable because of their small geographic area, exposure to extreme weather and climate events (including storms, floods, droughts, sea level rise, and salinization of water supplies and soil) and ocean acidification. Furthermore, their isolation, small populations, and limited resources and infrastructure compound these issues. Climate change affects people's health and well-being, livelihoods, societies, natural and culture heritage, and historic relationship with their lands and oceans and threatens their survival. SIDS also face the triple burden of climate change, communicable diseases, and noncommunicable diseases. The climate emergency acts as a risk multiplier, with increased frequency of disasters, changes in transmission of vector-borne, waterborne and other infectious diseases, psychosocial stress, the impact on other health determinants, especially food and water supplies, quality, and access, and so forth. Health services are vulnerable—for example, health centers and hospitals are often located in areas at risk from extreme weather events and sea level rise. SIDS have been among the strongest advocates for climate action and climate-resilient health systems (Kim, Costello, Campbell-Lendrum 2015; Leaders of the Pacific Islands Development Forum 2015; World Health Organization 2018a).

The states carrying the greatest burden of climate change often have limited financial, health care, and other resources. General Comment 14 has made the duties of international states and partners clear: subject to adequate resourcing, states are expected to offer financial and technical assistance to less well-resourced states to realize human rights. This has a direct bearing on climate change responses because states must ensure their actions in their own countries and elsewhere respect and protect human rights, including the right to health. Therefore, the right to health can be the basis on which less-resourced countries ask for international assistance to support climate change mitigation and adaptation.

Human Rights-Based Approaches to the Climate Crisis

Human rights provide mechanisms and processes through which the most vulnerable can be protected and human rights violators held to account. "Such procedures include information-sharing, grievance redress mechanisms, and the active participation of various participants including rights-holders in decision-making. These procedures can help guide iterative, participatory and accountable solutions, offering an avenue for equitable decision-making, including over rights conflicts" (Hall 2014). Use of these procedures constitutes a **human rights–based approach** (**HRBA**) to the climate crisis.

HRBAs explicitly assist governments to meet their internationally and nationally binding human rights obligations. But it is more than just this: an HRBA also empowers people to know and claim their rights. It provides people with knowledge and tools to challenge power imbalances or discriminatory practices. In this way, the state is held accountable for its human rights obligations. Key human rights principles and concepts are consistent across all human rights conventions. These include equality and nondiscrimination, participation, transparency, and accountability. Helpful guidance on HRBAs can be found on the United Nations Development Programme HRBA portal, https://hrbaportal.undg.org/.

Climate change can be examined using key features of the right to health. Here we draw on the work of various authors, some of whom published their work in a special climate justice edition of the *Health and Human Rights Journal* (www.hhrjournal.org) in June 2014, to describe these key features.

Identification of Relevant Laws, Norms, and Standards

The 1945 Charter of the United Nations, 1948 Universal Declaration on Human Rights, 1966 International Covenant on Economic Social and Cultural Rights, 1986 Declaration on the Right to Development, 1989 Declaration on the Rights of Indigenous Peoples, and other international human rights laws require states to act individually and together on climate change (United Nations 1945, 19 48, 1966, 1986, 2007). International law requires states to "take measures to mitigate climate change; to prevent negative human rights impacts; to ensure that all persons, particularly those in vulnerable situations, have adequate capacity to adapt to changing climactic conditions; and to regulate the private sector in order to mitigate its contribution to climate change and ensure respect for human rights (para. 54)" (Office of the United Nations High Commissioner for Human Rights 2016).

An HRBA places emphasis on ensuring an enabling legal and policy framework and environment. It requires an understanding of how laws and social or institutional practices affect the enjoyment of human rights (Yamin and Cantor 2014). In the context of the climate crisis and its impact on health, this involves examining domestic and international law, conventions, and climate change negotiations to determine whether enjoyment of the right to health is protected or, if not, whether there is a remedy for violations to rights. As with all other elements of this framework, such examination requires participation from diverse sectors to ensure protection is afforded to all people.

By 2019 more than 1,300 cases about climate change had been filed against governments and companies (de Wit, Quinton, and Meehan 2019). In 2015 a Dutch court ruled that the Dutch government's stance on climate change was illegal and ordered them to cut greenhouse gas emissions by at least 25 percent within five years relative to 1990 levels. The case came about when 886 Dutch citizens sued their government for violating human rights and climate change treaties (Walls 2018). In *Juliana v. United States* young plaintiffs have asserted that the U.S. federal government has violated children's constitutional rights to life, liberty, and property and failed to protect the atmosphere and other essential public trust resources for future generations (see the Our Children's Trust website, www.ourchildrenstrust.org). Public health experts, public health organizations, and doctors are among those who have filed supporting Amici Curiae briefs (Jacobs and Goho 2019).

Ensuring People's Fundamental Entitlements to Dignity, Equality, and Nondiscrimination

Health inequities, the unjust and avoidable inequalities in health (Commission on Social Determinants of Health 2008), often occur when people experience discrimination. The human rights principles of equality and nondiscrimination require responses to climate change impacts to be considered in terms of impacts on all people. But equality does not just mean people have equal opportunity to participate in planning; it also means ensuring an equality of achievement of human rights, so that all people will have the same degree of access to health care or the same quality of water and sanitation and nutrition. This frequently requires a greater level of resource commitment to communities that are now disadvantaged to achieve an equality of outcome. Health care services, information, and education for people at greater risk of climate-related diseases must increase proportionately to their risk.

In the aftermath of Hurricane Katrina in 2005, New Orleans residents were able to evacuate the devastated city only if they had access to private transport. In effect, this was an entirely discriminatory evacuation plan, which resulted in the poor and marginalized communities being stranded without adequate access to food or clean water, despite the fact that the authorities had several days' warning that the hurricane would hit the city (Carmalt 2014). The discriminatory suffering of these residents is a human rights violation that could have been avoided if authorities had engaged people in these communities to play an active role in the design of evacuation plans.

Similarly, health benefits from climate change responses should be equitable. Campaigns to increase active transport and reduce animal fat consumption benefit health and the climate. But the benefits might not be available to everyone unless policies and interventions are designed to promote the benefits specifically to those who are most disadvantaged (Jones et al. 2014). This might require use of different languages or media in the distribution of messages and prioritizing investment and interventions in disadvantaged communities. Another mitigation measure is taxation on the cost of carbon, intended to reduce emissions; but this usually increases the costs of goods and services, which in turn imposes a disproportionate financial burden on poor people.

New technologies that reduce emissions can also have negative impacts on people living in poverty. Electric car batteries and solar energy units contain heavy metals and toxic substances that create health hazards associated with their disposal. Most of this e-waste has been shipped to China or India for disposal, during which is it handled predominantly by poor women and children (McAllister, Magee, and Hale 2014). So although these technological solutions may help reduce emissions, they can often violate the right to health in the impoverished and marginalized communities that eke out a living from working in disposal areas. Special attention must be given to all climate change responses to check for equitable impacts through their entire life cycle.

Participation

People's active and informed participation is crucial to the achievement of human rights because it converts passive targets of policies and programs into active agents who demand their rights with respect to their own well-being (Yamin and Cantor 2014). Meaningful participation takes place when people who are at risk of rights violations actively pursue solutions to overcome their disadvantages and have their rights respected, protected, and fulfilled. In so doing, they hold the powerful to account. "In reality, effective participation (like access to information) is power" (Potts 2008).

True participation in climate change responses is not limited to just one phase of developing climate change plans; rather, participation extends through whole cycles from planning, to implementing adaptation or mitigation plans, determining indicators, monitoring, and adjusting the project in accordance with indicator feedback and other data, and holding those responsible for action (nationally and internationally) to account. Meaningful participation is not achieved simply by inviting representatives to state- or donor-funded climate change meetings, where the powerful and privileged set the agenda and control decision-making processes and outcomes. This has particular and urgent relevance to Indigenous peoples and those who are losing their land to climate change in small island states. In New Zealand, for example, meaningful participation and respect for Māori rights to self-determination require recognizing Māori knowledges and worldviews. Not only does this enable relevant and appropriate climate change strategies to protect Māori health, but their traditional ecological knowledge and expertise means they have much to contribute to developing and implementing effective, sustainable mitigation and adaptation strategies (Jones et al. 2014). Meaningful participation can thus be a win for all.

The Committee on the Rights of the Child has described climate change as one of the biggest threats to child health and one that exacerbates inequalities (United Nations Committee on the Rights of the Child 2013). Accordingly, child rights advocates have called for children's participation in global forums on climate change and lament children's absent voice and influence in declarations, while also noting the absence of other vulnerable and minority groups including women, Indigenous people, and people with disabilities (Gibbons 2014).

Accountability

Accountability means transparent, accessible, and effective monitoring of progress, reviewing what has been done, and, where necessary, taking remedial action (Williams and Hunt 2017). Human rights experts have called for urgent development and enforcement of strong mechanisms to hold states and others much more accountable for their contributions to climate change as well as their duties to protect human rights. Some suggestions include ensuring existing human rights mechanisms for accountability consider climate change, establishing public forums for debate, citizens' charters, litigation, grievance redress, and other new, independent mechanisms (Hunt and Khosla 2010; Hall 2014).

Under the United Nations Guiding Principles on Business and Human Rights, businesses must be accountable for their climate impacts and participate responsibly in climate mitigation and adaptation actions in ways that fully respect human rights. This includes remedial action for any harm they have done (Ruggie 2011). In the Philippines, the national human rights institution has taken a landmark inquiry into corporate accountability for climate change (Commission on Human Rights, Republic of the Philippines 2019).

In the face of inadequate responses to the climate emergency, health professionals are considering when civil disobedience is an ethical means to hold the powerful to public account and persuade governments to urgent action (Bennett et al. 2020).

International Assistance and Cooperation

There is an urgent need to substantially increase financing and support for climate resilient health systems, especially in the most climate vulnerable countries and communities. Rising greenhouse gas emissions demonstrate that people's human rights are impacted not only by what happens in the country they live in, but also by actions and omissions that occur in other countries. The Maastricht Principles make it clear that states have obligations under the United Nations Charter and other human rights treaties to respect, protect, and fulfill human rights both within their territories and extraterritorially (De Schutter 2012).

General Comment 14 includes the duties of states toward each other in matters imping- ing on the right to health. Resource-rich states have responsibilities toward the right to health of people in low-resource countries which in turn have a responsibility and entitle- ment to seek international assistance and cooperation. This means that in order to protect human rights, states must take whatever measures are possible to reduce emissions and to hold other states to account for their global warming activities. There are also specific inter- national obligations—for example, in times of disaster relief and humanitarian assistance, "Priority in the provision of international medical aid, distribution and management of resources, such as safe and potable water, food and medical supplies, and financial aid should be given to the most vulnerable or marginalized groups of the population" (United Nations Committee on Economic Social and Cultural Rights 2000, para. 40).

Respect, Protect, and Fulfill All Human Rights

Respecting the right to health involves ensuring that state action or inaction does not undermine health rights. States must take action to mitigate increased risks to health and ensure that eco- nomic development does not increase risks. For example, when Hurricane Katrina hit the city of New Orleans, over 1,800 people died, and many more lost their homes. Jean Carmalt claims the U.S. government "violated the obligation to respect health by building a shipping canal that sub- stantially increased the threat of flooding in New Orleans" (Carmalt 2014).

Protecting the right to health places an obligation on the state to ensure that third parties do not interfere with attainment of this right. States have a human rights responsibility to ensure that other parties, in their own countries and internationally, honor their climate agree- ments, especially regarding emissions. For example, the effects of war, nuclear testing and climate change has meant the small Pacific country of the Marshall Islands is increasingly dependent on imported food but the diet change has contributed to poor health. Ahlgren and colleagues write, "donors and the government should reexamine the content of food aid and ensure it is of sufficient quality to meet the right to health obligations" (Ahlgren, Yamada, and Wong 2014).

Fulfilling the right to health requires legislative and budgetary measures, services and facilities, including those pertaining to the underlying determinants of health, to meet people's increased climate change-related health demands. The state has an obligation to plan for these climate impacts in a way that is nondiscriminatory and results in equitable outcomes with disadvantaged communities receiving the same quality of health services, air, water, and nutri- tion as others. Less resourced countries where health systems are not equipped to tackle the increased demands arising from climate change have human rights responsibilities to seek international assistance, and high-income countries have human rights obligations to honor their commitments (Hunt and Khosla 2010).

States must ensure that proposed solutions to climate change do not damage human rights. The development of sustainable energy sources has often happened in the territories of Indigenous peoples without their free, prior, and informed consent and harmed their wellbeing. The UN Committee on the Elimination of Racial Discrimination has told Canada it is deeply concerned about the continuing violations of land rights of Indigenous peoples in Canada and that the government should halt construction of a large hydroelectric power dam in British Columbia that will cause irreversible destruction to Indigenous lands and subsistence (United Nations Committee on the Elimination of Racial Discrimination 2017; Amir 2018).

Progressive Realization

Because of resource constraints, states must work to ensure *progressive realization* of the right to health. Progress should not go backwards except in very exceptional circumstances. States must have national plans to address the impact of climate change on health. These should be developed out of meaningful engagement with communities, health professionals, Indigenous people, and others. They must make difficult decisions to ensure that those most vulnerable to climate change are prioritized, and include the sustained provision of health care and underlying determinants of health (for example, safe water, sanitation, and nutritious food) with indicators of progress and regular reviews.

Obligations of Immediate Effect

Obligations of equality and nondiscrimination should be implemented immediately. This requires that states plan for access to health-related services and facilities on a nondiscriminatory basis, especially for disadvantaged individuals, communities, and populations. "This means, for example, that a state has a core obligation to establish effective outreach programs for those living in poverty" (Hunt and Backman 2008). People living in malarial areas, for example, have the right to at least the same level of access to health services as those living in urban areas. This often requires plans to address an urgent scale-up of health services to poorer and more remote regions.

Available, Accessible, Acceptable, and Good Quality (AAAQ) Health Services, Goods, and Facilities

Climate change places increasing pressures on health care and adds to the urgency of the challenge to ensure that services are progressively available and accessible, as well as culturally appropriate, acceptable, and of good quality, especially for those who are most vulnerable. For example, as more people experience malaria or dengue fever, understaffed and remote health clinics that have irregular supplies of appropriate medicines will be under more strain to cope with additional patients. Increasing the numbers of health workers and strengthening other health system components can take several years or even longer to achieve. Therefore, planning health system responses to climate change has to begin immediately to be effective when needed, and in the countries that are most vulnerable, planning is urgent.

AAAQ also applies to the determinants of health. For example, if climate change causes failure of local crops, alternative sources of food must be made available in an area in ways that are affordable; accessible without discrimination to all (for example, to women- or child-headed households); obtainable from places that are physically accessible; supported with accessible information about its use; culturally acceptable; and are nutritious and safe to store, cook, and eat.

Strengthening Health Systems

Health services can uphold the right to health and minimize their climate impact through moving to sustainable and low-carbon health systems. Action can come with co-benefits: for example, holding more clinics closer to where patients live can reduce overall travel-related emissions and improve access (Watts, Adger et al. 2015; World Health Organization 2018b). WHO has developed an operational framework for building climate-resilient health systems (World Health Organization 2015). A right-to-health lens can be used in planning and implementing the framework to ensure that those who are most vulnerable are the first to benefit.

Summary

All people have a right to health regardless of their nationality, place of residence, sex, or socio-economic status. The impact of climate change on health will be significant to all people, but people whose health is already compromised and who have little access to appropriate and good-quality health care will suffer the most. Their right to health, which includes the right to health care and to the underlying determinants of health, will be further eroded unless urgent action is taken. Strengthening health systems in countries most vulnerable to climate change is a crucial element in the protection and fulfillment of health rights. So too is the empowerment of people living in at-risk situations, so that they have the knowledge and confidence to engage meaningfully in the domestic and international forums where decisions affecting their lives, livelihoods, and health, and those of their children, are being made.

In this chapter, we have used a right-to-health framework to explore what a human rights–based approach to climate change would incorporate. The key human rights principles of equality and nondiscrimination, participation, and accountability apply to each element of the framework to ensure all voices are heard, and states and others are held to account for their human rights obligations as the world addresses its health-threatening warmer future.

CLINICAL CORRELATES 21.1 PROTECTING VULNERABLE PEOPLE AGAINST CLIMATE CHANGE

That the vulnerable will bear the brunt of climate change health impacts is a recurring theme throughout this book. Climate change will act as a threat multiplier, worsening human security through environmental damage, population displacement, violent conflict, and poverty entrenchment. Clinicians will bear witness in both primary events (heat waves, extreme weather events, infectious disease outbreaks) and secondary events (disruption in health care services from the aforementioned). They will also be faced with changing disease patterns and increased rates of health problems as a result of the multifaceted impacts of climate change.

Adopting a rights-based approach to climate change begins by recognizing the obligations of states to respect, protect, and fulfill all human rights threatened by climate change. By invoking existing human rights constructs (laws, treaties, and international agreements), such an approach requires states to have a transparent and participatory process to determine a plan of mitigation and adaptation, addressing the rights of the most vulnerable people first.

Clinicians hold a powerful fulcrum to invoke a human rights approach to climate change and are uniquely positioned to work with policymakers, patients, families, and communities to bring a rights-based perspective to climate actions.

DISCUSSION QUESTIONS

1. Why are some groups and countries more vulnerable to the impacts of climate change on their health?
2. Why are vulnerable health systems disproportionately burdened by climate change?
3. Why does a human rights–based approach focus on getting health care to the most disadvantaged people?
4. How should global responsibilities for mitigation and adaptation be fairly shared between countries?

KEY TERMS

General Comment 14: Drafted by the Committee on Economic, Social and Cultural Rights to explain the meaning of the right to health; adopted by UN members in 2000.

Human rights: The entitlements everybody has, by virtue of being born, to live a life of equality and dignity.

Human rights–based approaches (HRBA): Explicitly assist governments to meet their internationally and nationally binding human rights obligations and empower people to know and claim their rights.

Indigenous: There is no universally recognized definition of Indigenous peoples; however key features include self-identification as Indigenous; historical continuity with precolonial and/or presettler societies; links to territories and surrounding natural resources; distinct social, economic, or political systems; and distinct language, culture, and beliefs (United Nations Permanent Forum on Indigenous Issues 2015).

Progressive realization of the right to health: A specific and continuing state obligation to move as expeditiously and effectively as possible toward the full realization of the right to health. Retrogressive measures are not permissible (health rights must not deteriorate), and states must prove any such measures were introduced only after the most careful consideration of all alternatives.

Right to health: Arising from the International Covenant on Economic, Social and Cultural Rights (Article 12) and spelled out in UN General Comment 14 that all people are entitled to the highest attainable standard of mental and physical health. This extends to timely and appropriate health care as well as access to the underlying determinants of health, such as access to safe and potable water and adequate sanitation, safe food, nutrition and housing, healthy occupational and environmental conditions, and health information.

References

Ahdoot, S., S. E. Pacheco, and Council On Environmental Health. 2015. "Global Climate Change and Children's Health." *Pediatrics* 136 (5):e1468–1484.

Ahlgren, I., S. Yamada, and A. Wong. 2014. "Rising Oceans, Climate Change, Food Aid, and Human Rights in the Marshall Islands." *Health and Human Rights* 16 (1):69–80.

Amir, N. 2018. "Letter from the Chair of the United Nations Committee on the Elimination of Racial Discrimination to the Permanent Representative of Canada to the United Nations Office Geneva, 14 December 2018." UN Doc. CERD/EWUAP/Canada-Site C dam/2018/JP/ks. Geneva: United Nations.

Bennett, H., A. Macmillan, R. Jones, A. Blaiklock, and J. McMillan. 2020. "Should Health Professionals Participate in Civil Disobedience in Response to the Climate Change Health Emergency?" *Lancet* 395 (10220):304–8.

Carmalt, J. 2014. "Prioritizing Health: A Human Rights Analysis of Disaster, Vulnerability, and Urbanization in New Orleans and Port-au-Prince." *Health and Human Rights* 16 (1):41–53.

Commission on Human Rights, Republic of the Philippines. 2019. "National Inquiry on Climate Change." Accessed December 3, 2019. http://chr.gov.ph/nicc-2/.

Commission on Social Determinants of Health. 2008. *Closing the Gap in a Generation: Health Equity through Action on the Social Determinants of Health. Final Report of the Commission on Social Determinants of Health.* Geneva: World Health Organization.

Conference of the Parties. 2015. "Adoption of the Paris Agreement, 21st Conference of the Parties, 12 December 2015." UN Doc. FCCC/CP/2015/L.9/Rev.1, United Nations.

De Schutter, O., A. Eide, A. Khalfan, M. A. Orellana, M. E. Salomon, and I. D. Seiderman. 2012. "Commentary to the Maastricht Principles on Extraterritorial Obligations of States in the Area of Economic, Social and Cultural Rights." *Human Rights Quarterly* 34:1084–1169.

de Wit, E., A. Quinton, and F. Meehan. 2019. "Climate Change Litigation Update." March 25, 2019. Accessed April 23 2019. https://www.nortonrosefulbright.com/en/knowledge/publications/848dafd1/climate-change-litigation-update#section2.

Ezer, T., and P. Patel. 2018. "Strategic Litigation to Advance Public Health." *Health and Human Rights* 20 (2):149–60.

Gibbons, E. D. 2014. "Climate Change, Children's Rights, and the Pursuit of Intergenerational Climate Justice." *Health and Human Rights* 16 (1):19–31.

Hales, S., S. Kovats, S. Lloyd, and D. Campbell-Lendrum, eds. 2014. *Quantitative Risk Assessment of the Effects of Climate Change on Selected Causes of Death, 2030s and 2050s*. Geneva: World Health Organization.

Hall, M. J. 2014. "Advancing Climate Justice and Right to Health through Procedural Rights." *Health and Human Rights* 16 (1) 8–18.

Hosking, J., R. Jones, T. Percival, N. Turner, and S. Ameratunga. 2011. "Climate Change: The Implications for Child Health in Australasia." *Journal of Paediatrics and Child Health* 47 (8):493–6.

Hunt, P., and G. Backman. 2008. "Health Systems and the Right to the Highest Attainable Standard of Health." *Health and Human Rights* 10 (1):81–92.

Hunt, P., and R. Khosla. 2010. "Climate Change and the Right to the Highest Attainable Standard of Health." In *Human Rights and Climate Change*, edited by S. Humphreys, 238–56. Cambridge: Cambridge University Press.

Jacobs, W. B., and S. A. Goho. 2019. *Brief of Amici Curiae Public Health Experts, Public Health Organizations in Support of Plaintiffs–Appellants Kelsey Cascadia Rose Juliana et al. v. United States of America et al No. 18-36082 in the United States Court of Appeals for the Ninth Circuit*. Filing date: 1 March 2019.

Jones, R. 2019. "Climate Change and Indigenous Health Promotion." *Global Health Promotion* 26 (3 suppl):73–81.

Jones, R., H. Bennett, G. Keating, and A. Blaiklock. 2014. "Climate Change and the Right to Health for Maori in Aotearoa/New Zealand." *Health and Human Rights* 16 (1):54–68.

Kim, R., A. Costello, and D. Campbell-Lendrum. 2015. "Climate Change and Health in Pacific Island States." *Bulletin of the World Health Organization* 93 (12):819.

Knox, J. H. 2013. *Report of the Independent Expert on the Issue of Human Rights Obligations Relating to the Enjoyment of a Safe, Clean, Healthy and Sustainable Environment, Mapping Report*. Human Rights Council. 30 December 2013. UN Doc. A/HRC/25/53. Geneva: United Nations Human Rights Council.

Knox, J. H. 2018. *Report of the Special Rapporteur on the Issue of Human Rights Obligations Relating to the Enjoyment of a Safe, Clean, Healthy and Sustainable Environment. Seventy-Third Session of the United Nations General Assembly*. 19 July 2018. UN Doc. A/73/188. New York: United Nations.

Leaders of the Pacific Islands Development Forum. 2015. *Suva Declaration on Climate Change, 4th September 2015*. Fiji: Pacific Islands Development Forum Secretariat.

Lemery, J., C. Williams, and P. Farmer. 2014. "Editorial: The Great Procrastination." *Health and Human Rights* 16 (1):1–3.

Levy, B. S., and J. A. Patz. 2015. "Climate Change, Human Rights, and Social Justice." *Annals of Global Health* 81 (3):310–22.

McAllister, L., A. Magee, and B. Hales. 2014. "Women, E-Waste, and Technological Solutions to Climate Change." *Health and Human Rights* 16 (1):166-176.

Metcalfe, S. 2015. "Fast, Fair Climate Action Crucial for Health and Equity." *New Zealand Medical Journal* 128 (1425):14–23.

Office of the United Nations High Commissioner for Human Rights. (2016). Analytical study on the relationship between climate change and the human right of everyone to the enjoyment of the highest attainable standard of physical and mental health. 6 May 2016. UN Doc. A/HRC/32/23. Geneva, United Nations Office of the High Commissioner for Human Rights.

Patz, J. A., H. K. Gibbs, J. A. Foley, J. V. Rogers, and K. R. Smith. 2007. "Climate Change and Global Health: Quantifying a Growing Ethical Crisis." *EcoHealth* 4 (4):397–405.

Potts, H. 2008. *Participation and the Right to the Highest Attainable Standard of Health*. Colchester: Human Rights Centre, University of Essex.

Robinson, M. 2018. *Climate Justice: Hope, Resilience, and the Fight for a Sustainable Future*. London: Bloomsbury Publishing.

Rockström, J., W. Steffen, K. Noone, A. Persson, F. S. Chapin, III, E. F. Lambin, T. M. Lenton et al. 2009. "A Safe Operating Space for Humanity." *Nature* 461 (7263):472–5.

Ruggie, J. 2011. *Guiding Principles on Business and Human Rights: Implementing the United Nations "Protect, Respect and Remedy" Framework*. UN Doc. HR/PUB/11/04. New York and Geneva: United Nations and Office of the United Nations High Commissioner for Human Rights.

Smith, R. K., A. Woodward, D. Campbell-Lendrum, D. D. Chadee, Y. Honda, Q. Liu, J. M. Olwoch, B. Revich, and R. Sauerborn. 2014. "Human Health: Impacts, Adaptation, and Co-Benefits." In *Climate Change 2014: Impacts, Adaptation, and Vulnerability. Part A: Global and Sectoral Aspects. Contribution of Working Group II to the Fifth Assessment Report of the Intergovernmental Panel on Climate Change*, edited by C. B. Field, V. R. Barros, D. J. Dokken, K. J. Mach, M. D. Mastrandrea, T. E.

Bilir, M. Chatterjee et al., 709–54. Cambridge, UK; New York: Cambridge University Press. https://www.ipcc.ch/site/assets/uploads/2018/02/WGIIAR5-Chap11_FINAL.pdf.

Stanberry, L. R., M. C. Thomson, and W. James. 2018. "Prioritizing the Needs of Children in a Changing Climate." *PLoS Medicine* 15 (7):e1002627.

United Nations. 1945. *Charter of the United Nations*, adopted 26 June 1945, entered into force 24 October 1945, as amended by GA Res 1991 (XVIII) 17 December 1963, entered into force 31 August 1965 (557 UNTS143); 2101 of 20 December 1965, entered into force 12 June 1968 (638 UNTS 308); and 2847 (XXVI) 20 December 1971, entered into force 24 September 1973. (892 UNTS 119). New York: United Nations.

United Nations. 1948. *Universal Declaration of Human Rights.* GA Resolution 217A (III), UN GAOR. Resolution 71, UN Document A/810. New York: United Nations.

United Nations. 1966. *International Covenant on Economic, Social and Cultural Rights (ICESR),* UN GA Resolution 2200 A (XXI), 16 December 1966. New York: United Nations.

United Nations. 1986. *United Nations General Assembly, Declaration on the Right to Development.* Resolution Adopted by the General Assembly, 4 December 1986, UN Doc. A/RES/41/128. New York: United Nations.

United Nations. 1989. *Convention on the Rights of the Child (CRC).* UN GA Resolution 44/25, 20 November 1989. New York: United Nations.

United Nations. 2007. *United Nations Declaration on the Rights of Indigenous Peoples (DRIP).* Resolution adopted by the General Assembly on 13 September 2007, UN Doc. A/RES/61/295. New York: United Nations.

United Nations Committee on Economic Social and Cultural Rights. 2000. *The Right to the Highest Attainable Standard of Health.* General comment No. 14 (Twenty Second Session). The right to the highest attainable standard of health. UN Doc. E/C.12/2000/4. Geneva: United Nations.

United Nations Committee on the Elimination of Racial Discrimination. 2017. *Concluding Observations on the Combined Twenty-First to Twenty-Third Periodic Reports of Canada, 13 September 2017.* UN Doc. CERD/C/CAN/CO/21-23. Geneva: United Nations.

United Nations Committee on the Rights of the Child. 2013. *General Comment No. 15. The Right of the Child to the Enjoyment of the Highest Attainable Standard of Health (Article 24).* 17 April 2013. UN Doc CRC/C/GC/15. Geneva: United Nations.

United Nations Permanent Forum on Indigenous Issues. 2015. *Who Are Indigenous Peoples?* 5th Session. Fact Sheet 1. New York: United Nations.

Walls, H. L. 2018. "Wicked Problems and a 'Wicked' Solution." *Globalization and Health* 14 (34).

Watts, N., M. Amann, N. Arnell, S. Ayeb-Karlsson, K. Belesova, M. Boykoff, P. Byass et al. 2019. "The 2019 Report of the Lancet Countdown on Health and Climate Change: Ensuring that the Health of a Child Born Today Is Not Defined by a Changing Climate." *Lancet* 394 (10211):1836–78.

Watts, N., W. N. Adger, P. Agnolucci, J. Blackstock, P. Byass, W. Cai, S. Chaytor et al. 2015. "Health and Climate Change: Policy Responses to Protect Public Health." *Lancet* 386 (10006):1861–1914.

Williams, C., A. Blaiklock, and P. Hunt. Forthcoming. "The Right to Health Supports Global Public Health." In *Oxford Textbook of Global Public Health*, edited by R. Detels, F. Baum, L. Li, and Q. A. Karim. Oxford: Oxford University Press.

Williams, C., and P. Hunt. 2017. "Neglecting Human Rights: Accountability, Data and Sustainable Development Goal 3." *International Journal of Human Rights* 21 (8):1114–43.

World Health Organization. 1946. *Constitution of the World Health Organization*, adopted by the International Health Conference, New York, 19 June to 22 July 1946, signed on 22 July 1946. Geneva: WHO.

World Health Organization. 1979. *Declaration of Alma-Ata*, adopted by the International Conference on Primary Health Care, 6-12 September, 1979.

World Health Organization. 2003. *WHO Framework Convention on Tobacco Control.* Geneva: WHO.

World Health Organization. 2014. *Gender, Climate Change and Health.* Geneva: WHO.

World Health Organization. 2015. *Operational Framework for Building Climate Resilient Health Systems.* Geneva: WHO.

World Health Organization. 2018a. *Climate Change and Health in Small Island Developing States. A WHO Special Initiative.* Geneva: WHO.

World Health Organization. 2018b. *COP24 Special Report: Health & Climate Change.* Geneva: WHO.

Yamin, A. E. 2014. "Editorial: Promoting Equity in Health: What Role for Courts?" *Health and Human Rights* 16 (2):1–9.

Yamin, A. E., and R. Cantor (2014). "Between Insurrectional Discourse and Operational Guidance: Challenges and Dilemmas in Implementing Human Rights-Based Approaches to Health." *Journal of Human Rights Practice* 6 (3):451–85.

CHAPTER 22

CLIMATE CHANGE AND DISASTER RISK REDUCTION

Virginia Murray, Debra Parkinson , and Ellen Bloomer

Overview

The recent synchronous adoption of landmark United Nations (UN) agreements—the **Sendai Framework for Disaster Risk Reduction**, **Sustainable Development Goals (SDGs)**, and Conference of the Parties (COP)21's **Paris Climate Conference**—has created a rare but significant opportunity to build coherence across different but overlapping international policy areas. The agreements represent a major turning point in the global efforts to tackle existing and future challenges in all countries.

The Sendai Framework was the first major agreement of the post-2015 development agenda and recognizes that each UN member state has the primary role to reduce disaster risk and enhance climate change adaptation but that responsibility should be shared with other stakeholders including local government, health professionals, emergency planners, business partners, and nongovernmental organizations. Specific emphasis is made on the need to support health care professionals to implement resilience-building measures and shift away from managing crises to proactively reducing risks of their occurrence.

Although many countries have underpinned capacities through the implementation of multihazard disaster risk management, the International Health Regulations (World Health Organization [WHO] 2005), and health system strengthening, many other communities and countries remain highly vulnerable to emergencies and disasters. The ability to achieve optimal health outcomes has been hindered by fragmented approaches to different types of hazards, an overemphasis on reacting to events instead of preventing and preparing properly, and gaps in coordination across the entire health system and between health and other sectors. In view of current and emerging risks to public health, such as climate change, and the need for effective utilization and management of resources, there is a need to consolidate contemporary approaches and practice in the conceptual frame or paradigm of "health emergency and disaster risk management" (Health EDRM).

Health EDRM provides a common language and an adaptable approach that can be applied by all actors in health and other sectors who are working to reduce health risks and consequences and to improve health outcomes and well-being for communities at risk of emergencies and disasters in different contexts, including in fragile, low-resource, and high-resource settings. Health EDRM emphasizes assessing, communicating, and reducing risks across the continuum of prevention, preparedness, response, and recovery and building the resilience of communities, countries, and health systems. Health EDRM is derived from the disciplines of risk management, emergency management, epidemic preparedness and response, and health systems strengthening. It is fully consistent with and helps to align policies

KEY CONCEPTS

- "Disasters, many of which are exacerbated by climate change and which are increasing in frequency and intensity, significantly impede progress towards sustainable development" (United Nations International Strategy for Disaster Reduction 2015b).

- The role of the Sendai Framework for Disaster Risk Reduction 2015–2030 and its coherence with the Sustainable Development Goals and the Paris Climate Agreement enables climate change adaptation and disaster risk reduction.

- By implementing the Sendai Framework disaster risk reduction strategies, actions can lead to improving resilience to climate change and extreme events and other disasters by identifying local vulnerabilities, tracking health impacts from extreme events related to climate change, and enhancing planning, preparedness, response, and recovery.

- Health professionals (particularly those working in public health) can actively engage with these frameworks and provide vital roles, including leadership, in the climate change and disaster risk reduction domain and thus enhance public health practitioners' and clinicians' involvement in outreach toward developing strategies to prepare for those health-harming effects that cannot be avoided.

and actions for health security, disaster risk reduction, humanitarian action, climate change, and sustainable development.

This chapter demonstrates how public health practitioners' and clinicians' involvement can engage actively and provide leadership that will assist the successful implementation of the recently adopted UN frameworks, particularly the Sendai Framework for Disaster Risk Reduction, to improve climate change readiness.

Climate-Related Disasters and Their Impacts

The global increase of natural disasters such as riverine flooding, cyclonic winds, storms, droughts, and heat waves is related to climate change as depicted in Figure 22.1 (Thomas and López 2015). In this regard, climate change acts as a "force multiplier," exacerbating many of the world's global health challenges (Thomas and Lopez 2015; Patz et al. 2014).

A disaster is defined as:

a serious disruption of the functioning of a community or a society at any scale due to hazardous events interacting with conditions of exposure, vulnerability and capacity, leading to one or more of the following: human, material, economic and environmental losses and impacts. (United Nations International Strategy for Disaster Reduction [UNISDR] 2017)

Disasters may be human induced (e.g., armed conflict, environmental degradation, industrial) or natural (e.g., flood, earthquake, drought, volcano). Globally, the commonest emergencies are transportation crashes, floods, cyclones/windstorms, infectious disease outbreaks, industrial accidents, and earthquakes (International Federation of Red Cross and Red Crescent Societies [IFRCRC] 2016). Any type of disaster, however, can interrupt essential services, such as the provision of health care services, electricity, water, sewage/waste removal,

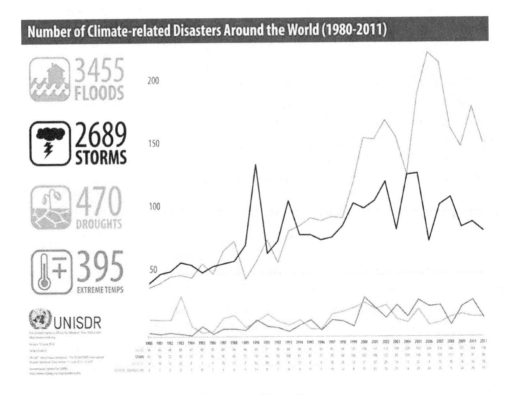

Figure 22.1   Increasing frequency of climate-related disasters around the world
Source: United Nations International Strategy for Disaster Reduction (2015a).

transportation, and communications, seriously affecting the health, social, and economic networks of local communities and countries long after the disaster has struck (UNISDR 2017).

Disasters often result in significant impacts on people's health and well-being, including the loss of lives. However, deaths, injuries, diseases, disabilities, psychosocial problems, and other health-related impacts can be avoided or reduced by effective risk management measures involving health and other sectors (World Conference on Disaster Risk Reduction [WCDRR] 2014). Approximately 190 million people are directly affected annually by emergencies due to natural and technological hazards, with over 77,000 deaths (IFRCRC 2016). A further 172 million are affected by conflict (Centre for Research on the Epidemiology of Disasters 2013). From 2012 to 2017, WHO recorded more than 1,200 communicable disease outbreaks, including those due to new or reemerging infectious diseases in 168 countries. Then in 2018 alone, another 352 communicable disease events, including Middle East respiratory syndrome (MERS) and Ebola, were tracked by WHO (WHO 2018).

Risk is differentially distributed between and within countries. For example, in 2017 many parts of the Indian subcontinent were affected by monsoonal flooding, with the most serious flooding occurring in mid-August in eastern Nepal, northern Bangladesh, and nearby northern India (World Meteorological Organization [WMO] 2017). More than 1,200 deaths were reported in India, Bangladesh, and Nepal, and more than 40 million people were displaced or otherwise affected. WHO indicated that in Bangladesh alone, more than 13,000 cases of waterborne diseases and respiratory infections were reported during three weeks in August, and extensive damage was reported to public health facilities in Nepal (WMO).

Vulnerable groups of individuals and communities require special attention during and after a disaster (WCDRR 2014). Those who experience disaster may suffer from ill health and harm against their person and property (e.g., loss of household possessions, livestock).

Women as well as underserved groups experience greater difficulty surviving and recovering from disasters due to discrimination and gender inequality (Bolin 2007; Fothergill, Maestas, and Darlington 1999; Baker and Cormier 2014). For example, differences in legal status (such as regarding land rights), lack of access to education, less mobility (due to family obligations), and economic insecurity all render women particularly vulnerable to the repercussions of disasters.

Figure 22.2 illustrates the impacts disasters have had between 2000 and 2012 in terms of numbers affected, damages, and mortality. In 2015 alone, from 346 reported disasters linked to natural hazards, there were an estimated 22,500 deaths, 100 million affected, and over $66 billion economic damages (UNISDR 2015a). Furthermore, although these data refer to large-scale disasters, there are many smaller-scale hazardous events, emergencies, and disasters that affect communities, their health, and livelihoods.

The 2015 United Nations Landmark Agreements

In 2015, several landmark UN agreements were adopted by the international community: the Sendai Framework for Disaster Risk Reduction (2015–2030), the Sustainable Development Goals (SDGs), and the Paris Climate Agreement. A brief description of each of these frameworks is as follows.

Description of 2015 UN Landmark Agreements

- The Sendai Framework for Disaster Risk Reduction (SFDRR) 2015–2030 was endorsed by the UN General Assembly and adopted by 187 countries at the third World Conference for Disaster Risk Reduction in Sendai, Japan. It puts health at the center of global disaster risk reduction policy and advocates for action to reduce disaster risks for the next fifteen years.

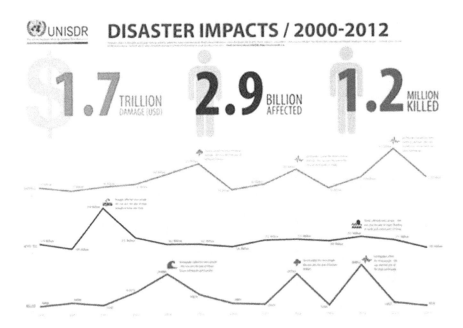

Figure 22.2 Summary of disaster impacts 2000–2012
Source: UNISDR (2015a).

It is a voluntary, nonbinding agreement with seven global targets, aimed at the reduction of disaster risk and losses in lives, livelihoods, and health (UNISDR 2015b).

- The Sustainable Development Goals represent seventeen aspirational "Global Goals" with 169 targets between them, including the universal call to action to end poverty, protect the planet from climate change, and ensure that all people enjoy peace and prosperity. Target 3.d of the Health Goal is to "strengthen the capacity of all countries, in particular developing countries, for early warning, risk reduction and management of national and global health risks" (United Nations 2015a).

- The international political response to climate change that began at the Rio Earth Summit in 1992 was complemented with the adoption of the Paris Climate Conference in November 2015. The Paris Climate Change Agreement aims to achieve a legally binding and universal agreement on climate and keeping global warming below 2°C (3.6°F) (United Nations 2015b).

As illustrated in Figure 22.3, many of these agreements have been borne out of previous incarnations showing the international engagement at the UN for the development of these frameworks.

Yet, the synchronous adoption of multiple international agreements in 2015 is somewhat unprecedented and has helped to both create momentum as well as the unique opportunity to coordinate and build coherence across overlapping policy areas (Dickinson et al. 2016; Murray et al. 2017).

Taken together, the UN agreements make for a more complete resilience agenda; building resilience requires action spanning development, humanitarian, climate, and disaster risk reduction areas (Murray et al. 2017). Ensuring coherence between them will serve to strengthen attention to existing risk fragility and resilience frameworks for multihazard assessments and help develop a dynamic, local, preventive, and adaptive urban governance system at the global, national, and local levels (Murray et al.). Specific emphasis is made on the need to support health care professionals to implement resilience-building measures and proactively reduce the risks of disasters, rather than exclusively focussing on the management of crises (UNISDR 2015b).

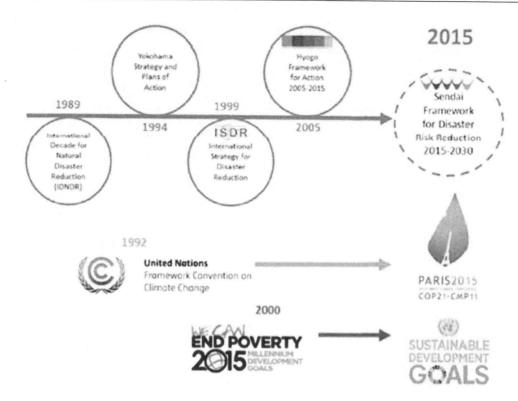

Figure 22.3   International commitments to the 2015 UN Landmark Agreement of Sendai Framework, SDGs, and the Climate Change Agreement
Source: Reproduced with permission from the Launch of the 2015 Global Assessment Report on Disaster Risk Reduction by Andrew Maskrey, 2015, Geneva, Switzerland: UNISDR.

The Sendai Framework for Disaster Risk Reduction

The rest of this chapter focuses mainly on the Sendai Framework for Disaster Risk Reduction and how it applies to the delivery of public health practitioners' and clinicians' involvement in outreach toward developing strategies to prepare for those health-harming effects of climate change that cannot be avoided.

The Sendai Framework aims to reinforce the shift in policy and practice of governments and stakeholders from managing disasters and other events to managing disaster risk (UNISDR 2015b). Rather than focusing exclusively on the response to emergencies, it recognizes that by reducing and managing conditions of hazard, exposure, and vulnerability—while building the capacity of communities and countries for prevention, preparedness, response, and recovery—losses and impacts from disasters can be effectively alleviated (UNISDR 2015b). Biological hazards such as epidemics and pandemics are also addressed in addition to natural hazards as a key area of focus for disaster risk management.

By 2030, the framework calls for:

The substantial reduction of disaster risk and losses in lives, livelihoods and health and in the economic, physical, social, cultural and environmental assets of persons, businesses, communities and countries. (UNSIDR 2015b)

It specifically advocates for an all-of-society disaster risk management approach, which increases leadership, participation, and risk awareness among marginalized groups including women, children and youth, persons with disabilities, older persons, Indigenous peoples, and migrants (UNISDR 2015b).

The Sendai Framework also states the need to strengthen disaster risk governance in the management of disaster risk by:

> build[ing] awareness and knowledge of disaster risk through sharing and dissemination of non-sensitive disaster risk information and data, contribute to and coordinate reports on local and national disaster risk, coordinate public awareness campaigns on disaster risk, facilitate and support local multisectoral cooperation (e.g. among local governments) and contribute to the determination of and reporting on national and local disaster risk management plans and all policies relevant for disaster risk management. These responsibilities should be established through laws, regulations, standards and procedures. (UNISDR 2015b, para 27g)

Health features as a core theme throughout the framework. Four of the seven Sendai Framework global targets have direct links to health focusing on reducing mortality, enhancing population well-being, improving early warning, and promoting the safety of health facilities and hospitals.

Global Targets of the Sendai Framework for Disaster Risk Reduction 2015–2030

The Sendai Framework states in paragraph 18 that to support the assessment of global progress in achieving the outcome and goal of the present framework, seven global targets have been agreed (UNISDR 2015b):

1. Substantially reduce global disaster mortality by 2030, aiming to lower the average per 100,000 global mortality rate in the decade 2020–2030 compared to the period 2005–2015;

2. Substantially reduce the number of affected people globally by 2030, aiming to lower the average global figure per 100,000 in the decade 2020–2030 compared to the period 2005–2015;

3. Reduce direct disaster economic loss in relation to global gross domestic product (GDP) by 2030;

4. Substantially reduce disaster damage to critical infrastructure and disruption of basic services, among them health and educational facilities, including through developing their resilience by 2030;

5. Substantially increase the number of countries with national and local disaster risk reduction strategies by 2020;

6. Substantially enhance international cooperation to developing countries through adequate and sustainable support to complement their national actions for implementation of the present Framework by 2030;

7. Substantially increase the availability of and access to multihazard early warning systems and disaster risk information and assessments to people by 2030.

The Sendai Framework also places strong emphasis on resilient health systems by the integration of disaster risk management into health care provision at all levels and by the development of the capacity of health workers in understanding disaster risk and applying and implementing disaster risk approaches in health work (Aitsi-Selmi and Murray 2016). Public Health England has reviewed and reported on its work to implement the Sendai Framework and linking this as appropriate to climate change adaptation (PHE 2017). National health and care systems can be strengthened by promoting and enhancing the training capacities in the field of disaster medicine and by supporting and training community health groups in disaster risk reduction approaches in health programs.

WHO's Role in the Implementation of the Sendai Framework

The World Health Organization (WHO) works with a wide range of partners to improve health outcomes for people at risk of emergencies and disasters, including resources globally for public health. For example, the WHO provides support for increasing country and community capacities in health and other sectors to manage the health risks associated with emergencies and disasters. This is done in several ways including the WHO's commitment to supporting emergency and disaster risk management for health (WHO 2017a). The WHO provides support globally to countries for a wide range of threats to public health, including infectious disease outbreaks, unsafe food and water, chemical and radiation contamination, natural and technological hazards, wars and other societal conflicts, and the health consequences of climate change. To help meet these and other challenges, countries are encouraged to strengthen their capacities for emergency risk management incorporating measures for prevention, mitigation, preparedness, response and recovery. To enable this, in 2011 the WHO developed a partnership to build a WHO Thematic Platform for Health Emergency and Disaster Risk Management. There are several outputs from this platform and they include:

- **The WHO Disaster Risk Management for Health Fact Sheets** (WHO 2017b). These advocacy materials are an introduction for health workers engaged in disaster risk management and for multisectoral partners to consider how to integrate health into their disaster risk management strategies. The overview places disaster risk management in the context of multisectoral action and focuses on the generic elements of disaster risk management, including potential hazards, vulnerabilities of a population, and capacities, which apply across the various health domains. The accompanying fact sheets identify key points for consideration within several essential health domains. However, importantly, all health domains are interlinked; each fact sheet should therefore be considered as part of the entire set and in conjunction with the overview. These fact sheets address all hazards including natural, biological, technological, and societal hazards, especially those associated with climate change, and provide reminders of those populations whose health is put at risk by these events. Examples of hazards include:

  - Natural: earthquake, landslide, tsunami, cyclones, extreme temperatures, floods, or droughts

  - Biological: disease outbreaks including human, animal, and plant epidemics and pandemics

  - Technological: chemical and radiological agent release, explosions, transport and infrastructure failures

  - Societal: conflict, stampedes, acts of terrorism, migration, and humanitarian emergencies

Of note, emergencies and disasters may cause ill health directly or through the disruption of health systems, facilities, and services, leaving many without access to health care in times of emergency. Such events can affect basic infrastructure such as water, food, power supplies, and communication.

- **The WHO Thematic Platform for Health Emergency and Disaster Risk Management Research Group** (WHO 2017c). The health disaster research community should engage in the Health EDRM to provide relevant evidence to support and maximize the global disaster risk reduction effort. These efforts will be taken forward through the WHO Thematic Platform in Health-EDRM Research Group, which was established in September 2016, and aims to coordinate activity, promote information-sharing, develop partnerships, provide technical advice, and facilitate the generation of robust and scientific health research to support the implementation of the Sendai Framework and related global agendas. Public health professionals' and clinical practitioners' colleagues may be interested in engaging with this research platform (Chan and Murray 2017; Lo et al. 2017; Kayano et al. 2019).

- **The WHO Health and Emergency and Disaster Risk Reduction Framework** was launched in May 2019 at the Global Platform for Disaster Risk Reduction and shared at the World Health Assembly in May 2019. Published on the WHO website in August 2019, the Health Emergency and Disaster Risk Management Framework addresses *Reducing health risks and consequences of emergencies for community and country resilience and health security, universal health coverage and sustainable development.* The vision of WHO's Health EDRM is to build the highest possible standard of health and well-being for all people who are at risk of emergencies, and stronger community and country resilience, health security, universal health coverage, and sustainable development. It is expected that Health EDRM will encourage countries and communities to have stronger capacities and systems across health and other sectors resulting in the reduction of the health risks and consequences associated with all types of emergencies and disasters. In summary the principles of WHO's Health EDRM Framework includes:

  - Comprehensive emergency management (across prevention, preparedness, response, and recovery)

  - All-hazards approach

  - Inclusive, people- and community-centered approach

  - Multisectoral and multidisciplinary collaboration

  - Integration of Health EDRM with health system strengthening

  - Ethical considerations

  The components of Health EDRM include policies, strategies and legislation, planning and coordination, health and related services, health infrastructure and logistics, community capacities for Health EDRM human resources, information and knowledge management, risk communications, financial resources, and monitoring and evaluation.

  WHO's Framework provides the scaffolding to link together many other regulations and frameworks including the International Health Regulations (2007) (WHO 2016a), joint external evaluation tool (JEE) (WHO 2016b), and the R&D blueprint for action to prevent epidemics (WHO 2016c).

Roles and Responsibilities of Health Care Professionals in Implementing the Sendai Framework for Climate Change Adaptation

The Sendai Framework for Disaster Risk Reduction 2015–2030 states:

> To enhance the resilience of national health systems, including by integrating disaster risk management into primary, secondary and tertiary health care, especially at the local level; developing the capacity of health workers in understanding disaster risk and applying and implementing disaster risk reduction approaches in health work; promoting and enhancing the training capacities in the field of disaster medicine; and supporting and training community health groups in disaster risk reduction approaches in health programmes, in collaboration with other sectors, as well as in the implementation of the International Health Regulations (2005) of the World Health Organization. (UNISDR 2015b, para 30I)

This call to action offers a major opportunity for health workers, particularly public health practitioners' and clinical professionals' involvement in outreach toward developing strategies to prepare for those health-harming effects that cannot be avoided, to engage at all levels of disaster preparedness, including risk assessment and multidisciplinary management strategies at all system levels, which are critical to the delivery of effective responses to the short-, medium-, and long-term health and care needs of a disaster-stricken population.

With their technical skills and knowledge of epidemiology, physiology, pharmacology, cultural-familial structures, and psychosocial issues, health professionals can actively contribute in disaster preparedness programs, as well as during disasters. Public health practitioners and clinical professionals, as global citizens and team members can advocate for a significant strategic and leadership role in coordinating and leading health and social disciplines, government bodies, community groups, and nongovernmental agencies, including humanitarian organizations.

However, many public health practitioners and clinical professionals across the world do not possess the knowledge, skills, and abilities that they will need to be able to participate in a timely and appropriate manner during a disaster response. This issue has significant implications for health care systems to mount effective response and recovery initiatives and this chapter helps to fill this gap.

CLINICAL CORRELATES 22.1 DOMESTIC VIOLENCE AND DISASTER

Disaster and drought—exacerbated by climate change—increase violence against women (Austin 2016; Campbell and Jones 2016; Enarson and Chakrabarti 2009; Fothergill 2008; Houghton 2010; Parkinson 2019; Schumacher et al. 2010; Whittenbury 2013). Research has posited that with the loss of "institutions of the state, the workplace, and the home, men feel their hegemony is in crisis" (Austin 2008) and that the experience may "provoke attempts to restore a dominant masculinity" (Connell 2005). Men's violence against their partners may be new in the relationship or exacerbated in frequency or intensity after disasters (Parkinson 2019). Sympathies tend to lie with traumatized men, their "heroism" or postdisaster trauma fostering a community more willing to excuse their violence (Anastario, Shehab, and Lawry 2009; Parkinson and Zara 2013).

Gender roles before an emergency become even more stereotyped in the aftermath, in some cases reverting to traditional roles of decades earlier. Susannah Hoffman writes, "Men launched into command and took action . . . Women further fell unwittingly into old habits of compliance" (Hoffman 1998). The association between stringent gender stereotypes and domestic violence is known (Our Watch, ANROWS, and VicHealth 2015).

The disaster context means women are less likely to report domestic violence out of feelings of loyalty and concern for traumatized partners or children. There are perceptions that their needs are less important than others in the crisis and there are frequently inadequate responses from community, health, and legal professionals when women do seek help. During the Black Saturday bushfires in Australia (2009), there was a documented increase of domestic violence against women, with little attention to the problem in both emergency planning and response (Parkinson, Lancaster, and Stewart 2011).

The subsequent Australian Government's Gender and Emergency Management Guidelines outline a number of strategies to address this issue, including improving data collection and information; educating emergency and health personnel on the dynamics of domestic violence in disasters to understand the risk; and identifying strategies to prevent and respond to domestic violence, especially in relation to changed environments postdisaster (Parkinson, Duncan, and Joyce 2017).

Summary

2015 was the year during which several notable UN agreements were adopted and included the Sendai Framework for Disaster Risk Reduction, Sustainable Development Goals, and COP21's Paris Climate Conference. The policy areas pertaining to the frameworks are closely interrelated. For example, climate mitigation and adaptation strategies may contribute to reducing the frequency of disasters, which in turn supports sustainable development.

Disasters can result in significant impacts on people's health and well-being, including the loss of many lives. However, deaths, injuries, diseases, disabilities, psychosocial problems, and other health-related impacts can be avoided or reduced by effective risk management measures.

This chapter has demonstrated how public health practitioners' and clinicians' involvement in outreach toward developing strategies to prepare for those health-harming effects that cannot be avoided can both engage actively and provide leadership that will assist the successful implementation of the recently adopted UN frameworks, particularly the Sendai Framework for Disaster Risk Reduction.

DISCUSSION QUESTIONS

1. Summarize the outcome of the 2015 UN Agreements, particularly the Sendai Framework for Disaster Risk Reduction 2015–2030, that are particularly relevant for you in your role in public health practitioners' and clinicians' involvement outreach toward developing strategies to prepare for those health-harming effects that cannot be avoided

2. Public health practitioners' and clinicians' involvement in outreach toward developing strategies to prepare for those health-harming effects that cannot be avoided should be encouraged by being part of the agreed local, national, regional, and global mechanisms to address all the needs for public health professionals and clinical practitioners from disaster preparedness for understanding risk to effective response and to "Build Back Better" in recovery, rehabilitation, and reconstruction. How can you help to implement this?

3. Consider reflecting on a recent disaster and how you would plan to implement the priorities for action within the Sendai Framework to reduce the impact of a future similar disaster.

KEY TERMS

Paris Climate Agreement: An international treaty created among attendees of the 2015 United Nations Climate Change conference in Paris, France, aimed at reducing the emission of gases responsible for global warming.

Sendai Framework for Disaster Risk Reduction: An international covenant adopted in 2015 by the United Nations to establish common goals and standards for disaster risk reduction.

Sustainable Development Goals (SDGs): Seventeen aspirational goals for global well-being, created by the United Nations in 2015. Example targets include ending poverty and protecting the planet from climate change.

References

Aitsi-Selmi, A., and V. Murray. 2016. "Protecting the Health and Wellbeing of Populations from Disaster: Health and Health Care in The Sendai Framework for Disaster Risk Reduction 2015–2030." *Prehospital and Disaster Medicine* 31 (1):74–78.

Anastario, M., N. Shehab, and L. Lawry. (2009). "Increased Gender-Based Violence among Women Internally Displaced in Mississippi Two Years Post-Hurricane Katrina." *Disaster Medicine and Public Health Preparedness* 3 (1):18–26.

Austin, D. W. 2008. "Hyper-Masculinity and Disaster: Gender Role Construction in the Wake of Hurricane Katrina." Paper presented at the American Sociological Association Annual Meeting, Boston, MA.

Austin, D. 2016. "Hyper-Masculinity and Disaster: The Reconstruction of Hegemonic Masculinity in the Wake of Calamity." In *Men, Masculinities and Disaster*, edited by E. Enarson and B. Pease, 45–55. London: Routledge.

Baker, L. R., and L. A. Cormier. 2014. *Disasters and Vulnerable Populations: Evidence-Based Practice for the Helping Professions.* New York: Springer.

Bolin, B. 2007. "Race, Class, Ethnicity, and Disaster Vulnerability." In *Handbook of Disaster Research*, edited by H. Rodríguez, E. L. Quarantelli, and R. R. Dynes, 113–29. New York: Springer.

Campbell, L., and S. Jones. 2016. "An Innovative Response to Family Violence After the Canterbury Earthquake Events: Canterbury Family Violence Collaboration's Achievements, Successes, and Challenges." *Australian Journal of Disaster and Trauma Studies* 20 (People in Disasters special issue):89–100.

Chan, E. Y. Y., and V. Murray. 2017. "What Are the Health Research Needs of Sendai Framework?" *Lancet* 390 (10106): e35–e36. http://dx.doi.org/10.1016/S0140-6736(17)31670-7.

Centre for Research on the Epidemiology of Disasters. 2013. *People Affected by Conflict—Humanitarian Needs in Numbers, 2013.* Brussels: CRED. https://reliefweb.int/report/world/people-affected-conflict-humanitarian-needs-numbers-2013.

Connell, R. W. 2005. *Masculinities*, 2d ed. Berkeley and Los Angeles: University of California Press.

Dickinson, C., A. Aitsi-Selmi, P. Basabe, C. Wannous, and V. Murray. 2016. "Global Community of Disaster Risk Reduction Scientists and Decision Makers Endorse a Science and Technology Partnership to Support the Implementation of the Sendai Framework for Disaster Risk Reduction 2015–2030." *International Journal of Disaster Risk Science* 7 (1):108–9. https://link.springer.com/article/10.1007/s13753-016-0080-y.

Enarson, E., and P. Chakrabarti, eds. 2009. *Women, Gender and Disaster: Global Issues and Initiatives.* Thousand Oaks, CA: Sage.

Endericks, T. 2015. *Public Health for Mass Gatherings: Key Considerations*, 2d ed. Geneva: World Health Organization. https://apps.who.int/iris/bitstream/handle/10665/162109/WHO_HSE_GCR_2015.5_eng.pdf;jsessionid=C986329AA44C2CAE751F5ACCB415B33E?sequence=1.

Fothergill, A. 2008. "Domestic Violence after Disaster: Voices from the 1997 Grand Forks Flood." In *Women and Disasters: From Theory to Practice*, edited by B. D. Phillips and B. H. Morrow, 131–54. International Research Committee on Disasters.

Hoffman, S. 1998. "Eve and Adam among the Embers: Gender Patterns after the Oakland Berkeley Firestorm." In *The Gendered Terrain of Disaster: Through Women's Eyes*, edited by E. Enarson and B. H. Morrow, 55–61. London: Praeger.

Houghton, R. 2010. *Domestic Violence and Disasters: A Fact Sheet for Agencies.* Wellington, New Zealand: Massey University.

International Federation of Red Cross and Red Crescent Societies. 2016. *World Disasters Report: Resilience: Saving Lives Today, Investing for Tomorrow.* Geneva: IFRC. https://www.ifrc.org/Global/Documents/Secretariat/201610/WDR%202016-FINAL_web.pdf.

Kayano, R., E. Y. Chan, V. Murray, J. Abrahams, and S. L. Barber. 2019. "WHO Thematic Platform for Health Emergency and Disaster Risk Management Research Network (TPRN): Report of the Kobe Expert Meeting." *International Journal of Environmental Research and Public Health* 16 (7):E1232. doi: 10.3390/ijerph16071232. https://www.mdpi.com/1660-4601/16/7/1232.

Lo, S. T. T., E. Y. Y. Chan, G. K. W. Chan, V. Murray, J. Abrahams, A. Ardalan, R. Kayano et al. 2017. "Health Emergency and Disaster Risk Management (Health-EDRM): Developing the Research Field within the Sendai Framework Paradigm." *International Journal of Disaster Risk Science* 8:145–49. doi:10.1007/s13753-017-0122-0.

Murray, V., R. Maini, L. Clarke, and N. Eltinay. 2017. *Coherence between the Sendai Framework, the SDGs, the Climate Agreement, New Urban Agenda and World Humanitarian Summit and the Role of Science in Their Implementation.* Paris: International Council for Science; Integrated Research on Disaster Risk. http://www.irdrinternational.org/2017/05/12/irdr-published-5-policy-briefs-for-2017-global-platform-for-drr/.

Parkinson, D. 2019. "Investigating the Increase in Domestic Violence Post Disaster: An Australian Case Study." *Journal of Interpersonal Violence* 34 (11):2333–62.

Parkinson, D., A. Duncan, and K. Joyce. 2017. *National Gender and Emergency Management Guidelines.* Gender & Disaster Pod. https://knowledge.aidr.org.au/resources/ajem-jan-2017-national-gender-and-emergency-management-guidelines/.

Parkinson, D., C. Lancaster, and A. Stewart. 2011. "A Numbers Game: Women and Disaster." *Health Promotion Journal of Australia* 22 (3):42–45.

Parkinson, D., and C. Zara. 2013. "The Hidden Disaster: Violence in the aftermath of Natural Disaster." *Australian Journal of Emergency Management* 28 (2): 28–35.

Patz, J. A., H. Frumkin, T. Holloway, D. J. Vimont, and A. Haines. 2014. "Climate Change: Challenges and Opportunities for Global Health." *JAMA* 312 (15):1565–80.

Public Health England. 2017. *PHE and the Sendai Framework for Disaster Risk Reduction 2015–2030: A Review.* London: PHE. https://assets.publishing.service.gov.uk/government/uploads/system/uploads/attachment_data/file/653164/PHE_and_the_Sendai_Framework.pdf.

Our Watch, Australia's National Research Organisation for Women's Safety (ANROWS) and VicHealth. 2015. *Change the Story: A Shared Framework for the Primary Prevention of Violence against Women and Their Children in Australia.* Melbourne, Australia: Our Watch. https://www.ourwatch.org.au/resource/change-the-story-a-shared-framework-for-the-primary-prevention-of-violence-against-women-and-their-children-in-australia/.

Schumacher, J., S. Coffey, F. Norris, M. Tracy, K. Clements, and S. Galea. 2010. "Intimate Partner Violence and Hurricane Katrina: Predictors and Associated Mental Health Outcomes." *Violence and Victims* 25 (5):588–603.

Thomas, V., and R. López. 2015. *Global Increase in Climate Related Disasters.* Manila: Asian Development Bank. https://www.adb.org/publications/global-increase-in-climate-related-disasters.

United Nations International Strategy for Disaster Reduction. 2017. *Terminology.* Geneva: UNISDR. https://www.preventionweb.net/publications/view/51748.

United Nations International Strategy for Disaster Reduction. 2015a. *2015 Disasters in Numbers.* Geneva: UNISDR. http://www.unisdr.org/files/47804_2015disastertrendsinfographic.pdf.

United Nations International Strategy for Disaster Reduction. 2015b. *Sendai Framework for Disaster Risk Reduction 2015–2030.* Geneva: UNISDR. http://www.preventionweb.net/files/43291_sendaiframeworkfordrren.pdf.

United Nations. 2015a. *Transforming Our World: The 2030 Agenda for Sustainable Development.* http://www.preventionweb.net/publications/view/45418.

United Nations. 2015b. *Paris Agreement.* http://www.preventionweb.net/publications/view/49265.

World Conference on Disaster Risk Reduction. 2014. *Health and Disasters.* http://www.wcdrr.org/uploads/HEALTH.pdf.

Whittenbury, K. 2013. "Climate Change, Women's Health, Wellbeing and Experiences of Gender Based Violence in Australia." In *Research, Action and Policy : Addressing the Gendered Impacts of Climate Change*, edited by M. Alston and K. Whittenbury, 207–21. Dordrecht: Springer.

World Health Organization. 2016a. *International Health Regulations (2005)*, 3rd ed. Geneva: WHO. https://www.who.int/publications/i/item/9789241580496.

World Health Organization. 2016b. *Joint External Evaluation Tool (JEE): International Health Regulations (2005).* Geneva: WHO. http://apps.who.int/iris/bitstream/10665/204368/1/9789241510172_eng.pdf?ua=1.

World Health Organization. 2016c. *An R&D Blueprint for Action to Prevent Epidemics.* Geneva: WHO. https://www.who.int/blueprint/what/improving-coordination/workstream_5_document_on_financing.pdf.

World Health Organization. 2017a. "Health Emergency and Disaster Risk Management." Geneva: WHO. http://www.who.int/hac/techguidance/preparedness/en/.

World Health Organization. 2017b. "Health Emergency and Disaster Risk Management Fact Sheets." Geneva: WHO. http://www.who.int/hac/techguidance/preparedness/factsheets/en/.

World Health Organization. 2017c. *WHO Statement to the 2017 Global Platform for Disaster Risk Reduction.* Geneva: WHO. http://www.unisdr.org/files/globalplatform/whostatementfinal24may.pdf.

World Health Organization. 2018. "Disease Outbreaks by Year (2018)." Geneva: WHO. https://www.who.int/csr/don/archive/year/2018/en/.

World Meteorological Organization. :2017 Is Set to Be in Top Three Hottest Years, with Record-Breaking Extreme Weather." Press Release. Published November 6, 2017. Accessed June 9, 2019. https://public.wmo.int/en/media/press-release/2017-set-be-top-three-hottest-years-record-breaking-extreme-weather.

CHAPTER 23

CLIMATE CHANGE AND FORCED MIGRATION

Craig Spencer, Amit Chandra, and Micaela Y. Arthur

Introduction

Human migration defines human history, shaping the rise and fall of civilizations across the planet. The decision to migrate is complex and can stem from a desire to explore new opportunities or to escape difficult situations. Climate change, migration, and health are inextricably linked. Climate change directly affects health and also drives migration, which in turn has an impact on health (see Figure 23.1).

The world currently faces a global **forced migration** crisis of unprecedented proportion. Political instability, conflict, and economic stagnation have led to the forced displacement of hundreds of millions of people, and currently, at the time of writing of this chapter, nearly seventy million people are living in a state of displacement (United Nations High Commissioner for Refugees [UNHCR] n.d.). The majority of displacement occurs in lower-income countries, where poverty and weak social protection systems drive forced migration.

Over the coming decades, climate change will move from exacerbating the causes of migration to becoming a direct cause itself (Benko 2017). Families will increasingly be forced from their homes, communities, and countries by climate change-induced food insecurity, water scarcity, land degradation, **extreme weather events**, conflict over resources, and public health emergencies. By 2050, climate change is projected to lead to the forced displacement of over 143 million people in sub-Saharan Africa, Latin America, and South Asia alone (Rigaud et al. 2018). *Beyond taking action to prevent climate change, the global public health community must prepare to meet the humanitarian and long-term needs of a growing population of forcibly displaced communities for whom returning home is not an option.*

This chapter discusses the public health implications of forced migration caused or exacerbated by climate change. Forced migration has serious health consequences for the migrants, their communities, and the systems that serve them. Before exploring the connections between climate, migration, and health, it is important to understand a few key concepts related to migration. Individuals, families, and communities move in three primary ways: forced migration, **voluntary migration**, and **relocation** (see Figure 23.2). The alternative to migration is to stay and adapt to changes in the environment, social structures, economy, or politics.

Forced migration can be further viewed through the status of the migrants themselves. Those who have been forced from their homes and have crossed an international border are legally defined as **refugees** and protected by the 1951 United Nations Convention and 1967 Protocol Relating to the Status of Refugees. Migrants who have been forced from their homes and have not crossed an international border are considered **internally displaced persons (IDP)** and remain under the jurisdiction of their own national governments. Later in the chapter we discuss how this status relates to access to high-quality health care services.

KEY CONCEPTS

- Climate change is an important contributor to migration, in particular forced migration. Projected future climate change will likely exacerbate this impact.

- Climate change will affect internal and international migration worldwide, regardless of a country's economic status.

- There is significant uncertainty related to the applicability of prevailing legal protections to climate change migrants.

- The mechanisms by which climate change affects migration vary by geographic, cultural, political, and social context and are not completely understood. These include, but are not limited to food security, water availability, land availability, extreme climate events, and disease patterns.

- Climate change will have a pronounced negative impact on the health of migrants, which must be considered by policies and response systems (including those lead by national governments and the international community, e.g., United Nations agencies like the World Health Organization, United Nations High Commissioner for Refugees, and the International Organization for Migration).

Planetary Context:
Political Economy
Climate Change
Health
Migration

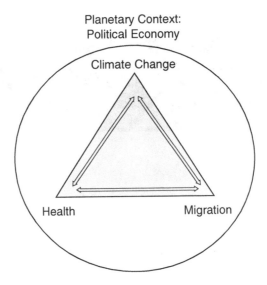

Figure 23.1 Context of climate change, health, and migration
Source: Adapted from Schütte et al. (2018).

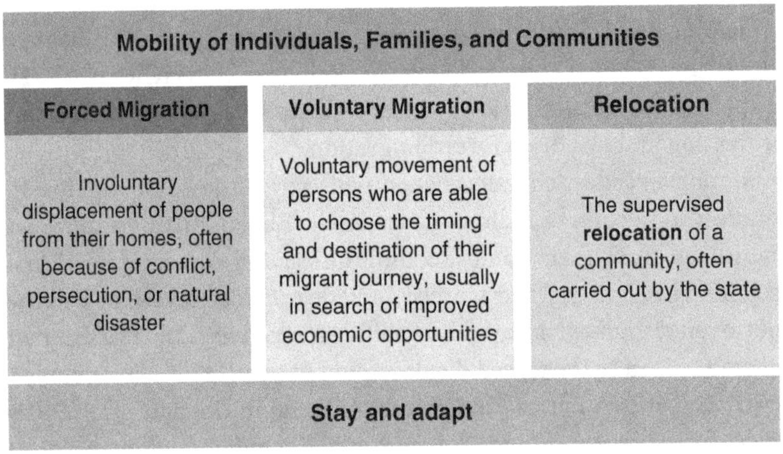

Mobility of Individuals, Families, and Communities
Forced Migration
Involuntary displacement of people from their homes, often because of conflict, persecution, or natural disaster
Voluntary Migration
Voluntary movement of persons who are able to choose the timing and destination of their migrant journey, usually in search of improved economic opportunities
Relocation
The supervised **relocation** of a community, often carried out by the state
Stay and adapt

Figure 23.2 Mobility of individuals, families, and communities
Source: Adapted from Advisory Group on Climate Change and Human Mobility (2015).

There are numerous reasons why individuals or families may be forced from their homes. The drivers of forced migration are multifaceted and intertwined in complexity and causation (see Table 23.1). The likelihood of migration increases as more of these driving factors emerge within a community or for an individual. Although this chapter focuses on forced migration caused or exacerbated by climate change, migrants are affected by multiple drivers of migration. These multiple drivers make it difficult to pinpoint one dominant reason why an individual migrates. The reality of ongoing climate change, its outsized impact on vulnerable populations, and its known role as a significant driver of forced migration means that climate change will continue to play a large role in forced migration in the future.

In this chapter, we discuss four case studies that examine different drivers of climate change that result in forced migration. The Lake Chad Basin crisis demonstrates the importance of water security by looking at the role of water in poverty, conflict, and regional stability. We discuss land availability in the small island nation of the Marshall Islands and its vulnerability to a rising sea and extreme weather events. Extreme weather events are again discussed in the case study of Bangladesh to understand recurrent natural disasters as a driver of

Table 23.1 Drivers of Forced Migration

Drivers of Migration	Examples
Political	Conflict and insecurity Weak state institutions Persecution and marginalization
Economic	Lack of employment Cost of living
Demographic	Population size and density Disease prevalence (e.g., outbreaks)
Environmental	Land and water security Land productivity Habitability
Social	Obligations to family Existing social network Pursuit of education

Source: Adapted from Government Office for Science (2011).

migration. The final case study links climate change with infectious diseases, linking climate mediated rural-urban migration with the 2019 dengue outbreak.

The Decision to Migrate

Individuals experiencing political, economic, and environmental hardships face a difficult choice: stay in their homes and attempt to adapt to the changing environment or migrate to a new community or country. Both lead down roads with uncertain futures. The relative weight between these options depends on the individual's specific situation and broader socioeconomic context. Ongoing armed conflict may prevent migration, for example, if any form of travel could be more dangerous than remaining in place. Extreme poverty creates another barrier, since travel is risky and requires significant resources (Black et al. 2011).

Figure 23.3 shows a simple model of how climate change affects decision-making systems and changes the factors leading to a decision on local adaption versus migration. On the macro-level, climate affects social, political, and economic drivers of migration. Environmental degradation leads to decreased incomes, conflict over increasingly scarce resources (e.g., water), and disruption of traditional coping mechanisms. Household, or micro level, factors determine how an individual or family responds. A household may decide to migrate based on

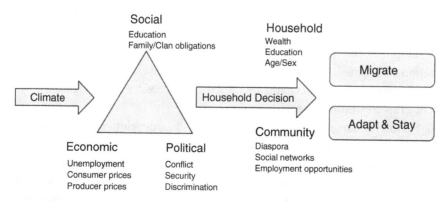

Figure 23.3   Drivers of household migration
Source: Adapted from Government Office for Science (2011).

their access to resources for travel, perceived opportunities for employment, and connections to friends and family outside their home community.

Climate Change and Migration: A Geographic Perspective

Although climate change is a global phenomenon, the most profound impacts will disproportionately affect poor, vulnerable, and marginalized individuals and communities. Communities and countries with greater resources, stronger institutions, and the motivation to adapt to climate change are able to make investments to dampen or delay the impact of climate change (e.g., massive seawalls planned for New York City) (U.S. Army Corps of Engineers n.d.). Individuals and families with greater resources have the ability to improve their home infrastructure, change their type or location of employment, or move elsewhere before climate change noticeably affects their daily lives, whereas poor families may not have the resources to invest in early modes of adaptation. Even within economically developed contexts, the largest impact of climate change will be felt by vulnerable populations, including the poor and members of marginalized communities.

Certain populations, including ethnic minorities and low-income groups, are at higher risk of exposure to the negative health impacts of climate change because of their greater likelihood of living in risk-prone areas (areas of low-lying land, poor infrastructure, and/or higher air pollution). According to the U.S. Climate and Health Assessment, minority groups and poor families already experience a greater incidence of chronic diseases, including cardiovascular disease, diabetes, and asthma/chronic obstructive pulmonary disease, all of which can be further exacerbated by climate change (U.S. Global Change Research Program 2016). Further, these groups are less likely to have access to medical care and may face greater barriers in obtaining quality medications. As a result, they may experience more complications and a higher likelihood of disease-related death. This is true for asthma, a disease related to air pollution and the negative impacts of climate change. In the United States, the mortality rate for asthma is nearly three times higher for blacks than whites. Similarly, research shows that air pollution exposure during pregnancy increases the risk of low birth weight and that pregnant women who are of low socioeconomic status or have asthma are more vulnerable to the effects of air pollution (Westergaard et al. 2017). For these communities, migration to areas with better air quality is an adaptation strategy to mitigate the health impacts on their families; however, this option may not be possible due to a myriad of factors.

Another issue that will have a disproportionate impact on vulnerable communities is "climate gentrification." This term is used to describe the increased desirability of areas more resilient to the effects of climate change, the very areas identified as more desirable by the vulnerable communities described here. Whereas many of these areas had previously been inhabited by less-affluent populations, they are now in higher demand and are becoming more costly, a trend that is likely to increase with the impacts of climate change. Miami-Dade county in Florida exemplifies this phenomenon, where a recent study demonstrated that homes at higher elevation are appreciating faster than those closer to sea level (Keenan, Hill, and Gumber 2018). There are currently no mechanisms in place to protect vulnerable communities from displacement caused by climate gentrification.

Although climate change will force populations within developed countries (high-income settings) to move—especially communities along vulnerable coastline—this will likely be overshadowed by the number of people attempting to migrate toward developed countries in search of refuge from the impact of climate change in their own low- or middle-income countries. The greatest impacts of climate change—including temperature rise, changing weather patterns, water insecurity, and desertification—will be most profoundly felt in the same places that are currently the poorest and least resilient. A growing body of research demonstrates that climate change has already led to an increase in migration and the number of asylum claims in the European Union, a trend that is projected to grow as temperatures rise (Missirian and Schlenker 2017).

International Frameworks and Conventions Governing Forced Migrant Protection

As mentioned previously, "refugee" is an internationally recognized status given to people who have been forced to leave their country to escape war, persecution, or natural disaster. The 1951 Refugee Convention and its 1967 Protocol clarify the rights of refugees and the legal obligations of the 148 states that are signatories to one or both of these instruments. In addition to prohibiting countries from expelling refugees or forcing them to return to their home countries, these instruments stipulate that host countries should provide registration documents, free access to local courts, and a pathway to naturalization and assimilation. There are 145 state signatories of the 1951 Convention and 146 of the 1967 Protocol. The United States is a signatory only of the 1967 Protocol, not the original convention. The stipulations are monitored by the UNHCR, but the only formal enforcement mechanism is by referral to the UN International Court of Justice in The Hague, Netherlands.

Although the convention does not have a specific article related to refugee health, Article 23 stipulates parity with citizens relating to access to "public relief and assistance." Additionally, the convention does not define a specific category of "climate refugees" or "environmental migrants." The lack of clarity related to both health and environmental push factors, coupled with the convention's weak enforcement mechanism, leads to significant uncertainty around the applicability of prevailing legal protections to climate migrants. Climate factors are nevertheless tightly linked to other proximal factors that cause forced migration, including drought, famine, armed conflict, economic collapse following an extreme weather event, and more.

The 70th World Health Assembly in May 2019 endorsed a resolution on Promoting the Health of Refugees and Migrants. Although not legally binding, the action plan urges member states to promote the framework of priorities and guiding principles outlined in Figure 23.4. Key aspects of this resolution include avoiding discrimination based on health conditions, improving migrant access to health services, and promoting gender equality.

In 2018, United Nations member states developed the Global Compact for Safe, Orderly and Regular Migration (GCM) to respond to contemporary challenges in international migration. Although this cooperation framework does not propose new legal protections for climate migrants, it is the first major migration policy agreement to recognize environmental degradation and climate change as significant drivers of migration. There has also been a growing focus on the intersection of climate change and migration at the International Organization for Migration's (IOM) Migration, Environment and Climate Change (MECC) division.

While there are more refugees in 2020 than in any prior decade, the number of IDPs is far greater but much harder to measure as they have not crossed an international border. The only legal instrument to protect IDPs is the **Kampala Convention**, ratified in 2012 and agreed upon in 2009 at the African Union Convention for the Protection and Assistance of Internally Displaced Persons in Africa. The Kampala Convention is legally binding, but is restricted to the African Union; no other region of the world has legal protectionary measures in place for IDPs (Brookings Institute 2013). Article 4 of the convention calls for protection of all people from "arbitrary displacement" resulting from discrimination, conflict, and natural disasters (including climate change).

Promoting the Health of Refugees and Migrants

Guiding Principles	Priorities
The right to the enjoyment of the highest attainable standard of physical and mental health Equality and nondiscrimination Equitable access to health services People-centered, refugee- and migrant- and gender-sensitive health systems Nonrestrictive health practices based on health conditions Whole-of-government and whole-of-society approaches Participation and social inclusion of refugees and migrants Partnership and cooperation	Advocate mainstreaming refugee and migrant health in the global, regional, and country agendas and contingency planning Promote refugee- and migrant-sensitive health policies, legal and social protection, and program interventions Enhance capacity to address the social determinants of health Strengthen health monitoring and health information systems Accelerate progress towards achieving the Sustainable Development Goals including universal health coverage Reduce mortality and morbidity among refugees and migrants through short- and long-term public health interventions Protect and improve the health and well-being of women, children, and adolescents living in refugee and migrant settings Promote continuity and quality of care Develop, reinforce, and implement occupational health safety measures Promote gender equality and empower refugee and migrant women and girls Support measures to improve communication and counter xenophobia Strengthen partnerships, intersectoral, intercountry, and interagency coordination and collaboration mechanisms

Figure 23.4   Principles and priorities to promote the health of refugees and migrants
Source: Adapted from WHO (2019).

Climate Change Risks and Forced Migration

Food Security

Food security means that people have adequate access to food in terms of both quality and quantity (Food and Agriculture Organization [FAO] 2019). This includes availability, access, utilization, and source stability of nutritious food necessary in order to live a productive life. Inadequate food security results in hunger, malnutrition, and economic hardship in affected regions. In rural areas, insufficient economic opportunities limit the ability of households to earn nonfarm income, making these communities more vulnerable to climate mediated shocks (droughts, floods, etc.). This is a major driver of migration in lower income countries (Laborde et al. 2017). Food insecurity, coupled with poverty, has also been shown to drive conflict, which itself further drives migration. According to the World Food Programme, the number of people fleeing their home country increases by 0.4 percent with each year of ongoing conflict, and by 1.9 percent with each percentage increase in food insecurity (World Food Programme 2017).

Climate change is a major contributing factor to food insecurity. Extreme weather events, which are increasing in severity and intensity, along with rising global temperatures, destroy crops and agricultural infrastructure. Changing weather patterns leading to drought or excessive precipitation also threaten rural livelihoods. Without mitigating actions, regions affected by these phenomena face both decreased food production and decreased food availability in the years following the event. Even gradual changes in regional climates affect the availability of water and the agricultural productivity of the land over time.

According to the Food and Agriculture Organization's 2019 report on the State of Food Security, the number of people around the world facing food insecurity is rising despite the gains made over the Millennium Development Goals era. The report estimates that over 26 percent of the world's 2018 population was moderately or severely food insecure, with 149 million children stunted and persistently high levels of maternal anemia (FAO 2019). Stunting, measured by height for age, is an indication of chronic undernutrition. Stunting can result from poor maternal nutrition, frequent childhood illnesses, inadequate nutrition quality and quantity during the first years of life, and inappropriate infant and young child feeding practices. Maternal malnutrition leading to maternal anemia (inadequate red blood cells or blood hemoglobin content) can lead to low birth weight infants and also reduces the ability of mothers to provide infants with adequate nutrition. Stunted children and adults face higher mortality from infectious diseases, a higher incidence of noncommunicable diseases, lower educational attainment, and lower incomes as adults.

Water Availability

It is no coincidence that our earliest civilizations were centered around water and that many of the world's largest cities today are built on rivers, lakes, and oceans. Access to reliable and clean water is essential to human society, not only for drinking but also for agriculture, transport, health, and hygiene. Inadequate access to and utilization of clean water are major contributors to childhood diarrhea, the second leading cause of mortality in children under five (Centers for Disease Control and Prevention 2015).

It is estimated that the number of people without reliable access to clean drinking water is at least 1.8 billion (United Nations Children's Fund and World Health Organization 2017). With the global population expected to reach over nine billion by 2050, there is growing pressure on existing water resources for personal use, with greater demand from agricultural and industrial sectors, coupled with increased water pollution (UN Department of Economic and Social Affairs 2011). Compounding the increase in demand, climate change will alter the availability of fresh water and threaten water security. Considering the impact of climate change in this context raises the likelihood of conflict, instability, and crisis over water in the future. Climate change is projected to increase the severity, frequency, and intensity of extreme weather events including heavy rainfall and hurricanes which can result in flooding and contamination of fresh water resources. In September 2019, for example, sea surge over twenty feet from Hurricane Dorian in the low-lying Bahamas contaminated cisterns used to collect rainwater, leaving thousands of people without this most basic resource.

As global temperatures rise, arid and semi-arid regions will be more susceptible to drought risk, further exacerbating water insecurity and contributing to poor health due to inadequate sanitation and hygiene. A special report by the Intergovernmental Panel on Climate Change (IPCC) estimates that around one billion people living in dry environments, especially in the Mediterranean and southern Africa, will be affected by increasing water scarcity (Hoegh-Guldberg, Jacob, and Taylor 2018).

A lack of water is a factor in the decision to migrate, either temporarily or permanently. In this way, water security can act as both a "push" factor (forcing people to leave an area or region with low water availability) and also a "pull" factor (attracting people to areas where water is more abundant). A 2018 report by the FAO found that "water insecurity, especially when coupled with a high level of temperature, causing water evaporation, undermines the livelihood systems of those affected and induces migration" (Wrathal et al. 2018).

Many modern examples exist that demonstrate the impact of water scarcity on migration. The 2016 World Water Development Report found that water scarcity, secondary to drought and groundwater depletion, contributed to increased rural to urban migration in the Middle

East (UNESCO World Water Assessment Programme 2016). It also showed how water availability was one of the key driving factors in the decision to migrate across multiple countries in Asia, most notably in Bangladesh. A 2018 report from IOM's Displacement Tracking Matrix demonstrated how a severe drought in Afghanistan has affected millions and forced tens of thousands to flee their homes in search of stable water sources near rivers and cities (IOM 2018).

Although it is difficult to measure the exact impact water security has on an individual or family's decision to migrate, it is clear that lack of access to water increases the potential for migration. Research shows that water and climatic conditions may have played a role in provoking Syria's civil war and the resultant refugee exodus, two intertwined drivers that often inform the decision or need to migrate (Kelley et al. 2015).

CLINICAL CORRELATES 23.1 LAKE CHAD BASIN CASE STUDY

Lake Chad is a freshwater lake in west central Africa and one of the largest lakes on the continent. Over twenty-five million people in Cameroon, Chad, Niger, and Nigeria rely heavily on Lake Chad's resources for their livelihoods, yet the region is experiencing a protracted crisis caused by multiple factors. In the past decade, violence and conflict combined with decreased water availability has contributed to massive population displacement, with over 4.2 million people forcibly displaced (International Organization for Migration 2019). One of the greatest factors has been decreased water availability secondary to the profound shrinking of Lake Chad. In the past fifty years, Lake Chad has lost 90 percent of its surface water, leading to increased water insecurity for those who rely on the lake for agriculture, fisheries, and livestock.

Although there are numerous factors contributing to the decreasing size of Lake Chad—including increased population and poor irrigation practices, rising temperatures, and unpredictable precipitation exacerbated by climate change have likewise been implicated in playing a significant role.

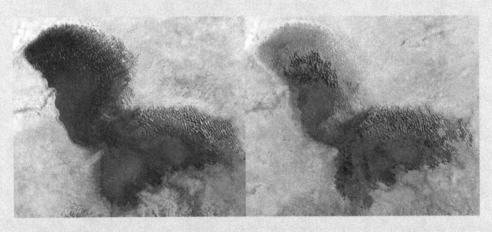

Lake Chad in 1973 (left) and 2017 (right)
Source: NASA Earth Observatory.

Land Availability: Sea Level Rise and Desertification

The loss of land suitable for agriculture and habitation is a driver of **forced migration**, especially in areas of the world where the population relies heavily on subsistence farming or has few resources to adapt to changing conditions. Among the greatest threats to land availability are sea level rise and desertification, both caused wholly or in part by climate change.

As the oceans warm and glaciers melt, sea level is expected to rise, putting coastal populations at risk around the world. The majority of the world's largest cities are on coasts, which coupled with increased rural-urban migration, means that a significant percentage of the world's population is vulnerable to sea level rise (Neumann et al. 2015). Especially vulnerable are places like Bangladesh, where a large population lives in low-lying areas. It is estimated that by 2050, as much as 17 percent of the country may be lost to rising sea levels, forcibly displacing twenty million people and further driving migration into the overpopulated capital, Dhaka (Rahman 2012). Whereas large coastal population centers in wealthier countries may be able to prevent or delay the impact of sea level rise with infrastructure and mitigation projects, many places like Bangladesh do not have similar resources. For people living in these already vulnerable areas, migration will be the only option.

For many island nations, such as Kiribati in the Pacific, climate change and sea level rise threatens their very existence. These low-lying atolls may be uninhabitable in as little as thirty years and they have already planned migration strategies into their governmental action programs (Government of Kiribati n.d.; IPCC 2014). Other island nations such as the Marshall Islands and the Maldives face similar threats and are outlining adaptation and migration strategies before their homes become inhabitable. These strategies—including elevated causeways, land reclamation, and protection of freshwater aquifers—are in reality only temporary fixes in the face of unrelenting sea level rise.

In addition to sea level rise, desertification caused by climate change will also play a role in forced migration in coming years. A report by the Intergovernmental Panel on Climate Change estimated that 500 million people are at risk of being displaced by desertification (IPCC 2019). Like sea level rise, desertification will have the most impact on the world's poor and vulnerable. Desertification is defined as land degradation in "drylands," the water scarce areas which make up 40 percent of the world's surface and host nearly two billion people (United Nations Convention to Combat Desertification n.d.). As global temperatures rise and drought-prone areas expand in arid and semiarid environments, the impact of desertification on livelihoods and migration will become more pronounced. Desertification reduces the amount of arable land available for farming and can lower agricultural yields, in turn decreasing food security. If extended over a greater area or time period, widespread famine can result, which has historically acted as a major driver of migration toward areas with better food availability.

CLINICAL CORRELATES 23.2 MARSHALL ISLANDS

The Marshall Islands are located in the Pacific Ocean and spread across numerous low-lying atolls. They are home to over 50,000 people whose homes are at severe risk because of the impact of climate change. Much of the land in the Marshall Islands is under two meters in elevation, making it sensitive to sea level rise. Extreme weather events are also a climate change risk there, causing higher tides and more frequent storms, threatening the integrity of freshwater supplies on the islands. Recent modeling predicts that most of the atolls in the Marshall Islands may be uninhabitable by the mid-twenty-first century (Storlazzi et al. 2018).

Extreme Climate Events

Extreme climate events can drive migration and negatively affect health through their effect on food security, water availability, and land availability. They can also be independent drivers of migration and poor health as a direct result of the devastation they cause to personal property and local infrastructure. Extreme weather events include cyclones, hurricanes, drought, and flooding that occur with a frequency, duration, or intensity that would not normally be predicted by past observations. According to the IPCC, "when a pattern of extreme weather persists for some time, such as a season, it may be classed as an extreme climate event, especially if it yields an average or total that is itself extreme" (IPCC n.d.).

CLINICAL CORRELATES 23.3 BANGLADESH

Bangladesh is a low-lying coastal country that is home to the largest river delta (Ganges) in the world. Over recent decades, climate change has increased the frequency and severity of cyclones and has shifted the intensity and timing of the annual monsoon season (Rigaud et al. 2018). These changes have had the dual effect of exacerbating flooding and prolonging drought conditions, threatening food security in this populous region, as well as the risks to sanitation and enteric disease.

Irregular rainfall also increases the risk of landslides. Heavy rainfall in Chittagong, Bangladesh in 2007 caused landslides affecting over 2,500 families and killing 137 people; the majority of the affected population had migrated to the area following a cyclone in 1991 and the deforestation caused by their settlement also contributed to the landslide (Alam 2016).

Infectious Disease

There is ample research suggesting that rising temperatures will increase infectious disease outbreaks caused by waterborne, arthropod, and other vectors (Martens et al. 1995). A shifting seasonality and geographic range for many diseases, including malaria, Lyme disease, and dengue, means that more people will be susceptible to these and other illnesses. To highlight the impact of changing weather on disease impacts, a 2019 study in *Nature* showed that the intensity of disease activity increased in the wake of the strong 2015–2016 El Niño event, including an outbreak of plague in the United States and a cholera outbreak in Tanzania (Anyamba et al. 2019). Some have even theorized that the 2014–2016 Ebola outbreak in West Africa may have also been related to climate change-mediated deforestation and human-animal interactions (Omoleke, Mohammed, and Saidu 2016). As rural populations move to cities and humans are forced into new environments in closer contact with animal populations, the likelihood of further disease outbreaks and transmission increases.

ASIA DENGUE OUTBREAK CASE STUDY

Between 1970 and 2020, the world has seen a thirty-fold increase in the incidence of dengue fever. Seventy percent of people who are at risk for dengue infection reside in the Asia-Pacific region. In 2019, Asia experienced a surge in dengue fever infections. The Philippines declared an epidemic, Thailand's case rate doubled between 2018 and 2019, and Bangladesh experienced its worst outbreak in history. Climate change is leading to longer breeding periods for *Aedes aegypti* mosquitoes, the vector that transmits dengue virus from human to human. It also shortens the incubation time the virus needs before it can be spread from an infected person to a healthy one. Migration further perpetuates these cycles as rapid and unplanned urbanization, poor living conditions, and inadequate sanitation all increase potential breeding grounds for mosquitoes (Rashid 2019).

Although it is clear that the most vulnerable communities will be disproportionately affected by the impact of climate change, there has been little action taken to mitigate potential infectious disease outbreaks arising from the interaction of health and migration in the midst of a changing climate. Although it can be assumed that people in need of health services secondary to climate change will migrate to seek medical care, many may not have the resources to do so.

Summary

Climate and environmental change are powerful drivers of forced migration. Forced migration in turn strains already overburdened health systems, disrupts livelihoods, and exacerbates human suffering and vulnerability. In addition to climate factors, there are numerous other proximate causes, including political instability, economic collapse, and other intervening factors related to forced migration. These often interact with each other along with other risk factors including poverty, age, gender, political context, conflict, education, and social networks.

In the absence of a framework of action, governments, international organizations (primarily IOM and UNHCR), and global civil society organizations are now evaluating the best ways to respond to changing human settlement patterns associated with accelerating climate change. This will involve first minimizing the push factors that drive migration through local mitigation efforts and humanitarian assistance. Improving government coordination around cross-border migration can improve safety, security, and opportunities for those who choose to migrate. Finally, governments can facilitate the planned relocation of communities where the local environment is no longer viable.

Through its impacts on food security, water availability, land availability, extreme weather events, and infectious diseases, climate change has profound impacts on a person's decision to migrate. As climate change accelerates over the coming decades, it threatens to roll back hard-fought human development gains and spawn new waves of forced migration. Although the effects will be global, poor and vulnerable groups in lower-income countries will suffer the most. The challenge facing these countries, with the support of the global community, will be to prevent, mitigate, and adapt to climate change in order to protect their citizens and prevent profound economic and social disruption.

Online Resources

Doctors without Borders—Global Refugee and Migration Crisis: https://www.doctors withoutborders.org/refugees

International Organization for Migration—Migration, Environment and Climate Change (MECC) Division: https://www.iom.int/migration-and-climate-change

Migration Policy Institute—Climate Change Site: https://www.migrationpolicy.org/topics/climate-change

DISCUSSION QUESTIONS

1. What role does climate change play in migration, both voluntary and forced?

2. Who are the major international stakeholders involved in migration issues and what are they doing to prevent and mitigate climate change mediated forced migration?

3. How does the status of a forced migrant influence their ability to access high-quality health care services? Consider how climate change may complicate health access within national boundaries and across borders.

4. Consider Figure 23.3 and the influence of climate change on drivers of migration. How may each driver be uniquely affected by climate change? How are these drivers linked to health in determining long-term outcomes for individuals, families, and communities?

5. What challenges will the international community face when addressing the health effects of climate-mediated forced migration?

KEY TERMS

Extreme climate events: Occur when the exacerbation of extreme weather events lasts for a prolonged period of time, for example, a season.

Extreme weather events: Cyclones, hurricanes, drought, or flooding of a frequency, duration, or intensity that would not normally be predicted by past observations.

Forced migration: The involuntary displacement of people from their homes, usually due to conflict, persecution, or natural disasters.

Internally displaced persons (IDP): Migrants forced from their homes who have not crossed an international border and remain under the jurisdiction of their own national governments.

Kampala Convention: A legally binding instrument, restricted for use within the African Union, designed to protect internally displaced persons.

Refugees: Migrants forced from their homes who have crossed an international border. They are legally defined and protected by the 1951 United Nations Convention Relating to the Status of Refugees and the related 1967 Protocol.

Relocation: The action of moving a community to another place, often organized and carried out by the national government.

Voluntary migration: The voluntary movement of persons who are able to choose the timing and destination of their migrant journey, usually in search of improved economic opportunities.

References

Advisory Group on Climate Change and Human Mobility COP 20 Lima, Peru. 2015. *Human Mobility in the Context of Climate Change.* https://www.unhcr.org/en-my/54942dde9.pdf.

Alam, E. 2016. "Adaptation Actions, Migration and Disaster Vulnerability of Bangladeshi Coastal Communities." Middle East Institute. https://www.mei.edu/publications/adaptation-actions-migration-and-disaster-vulnerability-bangladeshi-coastal

Anyamba, A., J.-P. Chretien, S. P. Britch, R. Soebiyanto, J. Small, R. Jepsen, B. M. Forshey et al. 2019. "Global Disease Outbreaks Associated with the 2015–2016 El Niño Event." *Scientific Reports* 9:1930. https://doi.org/10.1038/s41598-018-38034-z.

Benko, J. 2017. "How a Warming Planet Drives Human Migration." *New York Times*, April 19, 2017. https://www.nytimes.com/2017/04/19/magazine/how-a-warming-planet-drives-human-migration.html

Black, R., S. R. G. Bennett, S. M. Thomas, and J. R. Beddington. 2011. "Migration as Adaptation." *Nature* 478 (7370):447–49. https://doi.org/10.1038/478477a.

Brookings Institute. 2013. *Climate Change and Internal Displacement.* Washington, DC: Brookings Institute. https://www.brookings.edu/wp-content/uploads/2016/06/Climate-Change-and-Internal-Displacement-October-10-2014.pdf.

Centers for Disease Control and Prevention. 2015. "Global Diarrhea Burden | Global Water, Sanitation and Hygiene | Healthy Water Fact Sheet." Last reviewed December 17, 2015. https://www.cdc.gov/healthywater/global/diarrhea-burden.html

Feed the Future. 2018. *Global Food Security Strategy: Ethiopia Country Plan.* https://www.feedthefuture.gov/resource/global-food-security-strategy-gfss-ethiopia-country-plan/.

Food and Agriculture Organization. 2019. *The State of Food Security and Nutrition in the World.* Rome: FAO. http://www.fao.org/state-of-food-security-nutrition/en/.

Government of Kiribati. n.d. "Relocation | Climate Change." http://www.climate.gov.ki/category/action/relocation/.

Government Office for Science: London. 2011. *Foresight: Migration and Global Environmental Change.* https://assets.publishing.service.gov.uk/government/uploads/system/uploads/attachment_data/file/287717/11-1116-migration-and-global-environmental-change.pdf.

Hoegh-Guldberg, O., D. Jacob, and M. Taylor. 2018. "Impacts of 1.5°C of Global Warming on Natural and Human Systems." In *Global Warming of 1.5°C. An IPCC Special Report on the Impacts of Global Warming of 1.5°C above Pre-Industrial Levels and Related Global Greenhouse Gas Emission Pathways, in the Context of Strengthening the Global Response to the Threat of Climate Change, Sustainable Development, and Efforts to Eradicate Poverty*, edited by V. Masson-Delmotte, P. Zhai, H.-O. Pörtner, D. Roberts, J. Skea, P. R. Shukla, A. Pirani, W. Moufouma-Okia et al., 175–311. Geneva: Intergovernmental Panel on Climate Change.

Intergovernmental Panel on Climate Change. 2014. *Climate Change 2014: Synthesis Report.* Geneva: IPCC.

Intergovernmental Panel on Climate Change. 2019. *Special Report on Climate Change, Desertification, Land Degradation, Sustainable Land Management, Food Security, and Greenhouse Gas Fluxes in Terrestrial Ecosystems.* Geneva: IPCC.

Intergovernmental Panel on Climate Change. n.d. "IPCC DDC Glossary." Accessed May 3, 2019. http://www.ipcc-data.org/guidelines/pages/glossary/glossary_e.html.

International Organization for Migration. 2018. "Displacement Tracking Matrix: Afghanistan September 2018." https://afghanistan.iom.int/reports/displacement-tracking-matrix.

International Organization for Migration. 2019. "New Report Outlines Displacement, Human Mobility Figures in Lake Chad Basin." March 22, 2019. Accessed June 20, 2020. https://www.iom.int/news/new-report-outlines-displacement-human-mobility-figures-lake-chad-basin.

Keenan, J. M., T. Hill, and A. Gumber. 2018. "Climate Gentrification: From Theory to Empiricism in Miami-Dade County, Florida." *Environmental Research Letters* 13 (5):054001. https://doi.org/10.1088/1748-9326/aabb32.

Kelley, C. P., S. Mohtadi, M. A. Cane, R. Seager, and Y. Kushnir. 2015. "Climate Change in the Fertile Crescent and Implications of the Recent Syrian Drought." *Proceedings of the National Academy of Sciences of the USA* 112 (11):3241–246. https://doi.org/10.1073/pnas.1421533112.

Laborde, D., L. Bizikova, T. Lallemant, and C. Smaller. 2017. *What Is the Link between Hunger and Migration?* Winnipeg, Manitoba: International Institute of Sustainable Development; Washington, DC: International Food Policy Research Institute. https://www.iisd.org/sites/default/files/publications/link-between-hunger-migration.pdf.

Martens, W., T. Jetten, J. Rotmans, and L. Niessen. 1995. "Climate Change and Vector-Borne Diseases: A Global Modelling Perspective." *Global Environmental Change* 5 (3):195–209. https://doi.org/10.1016/0959-3780(95)00051-O.

Missirian, A., and W. Schlenker. 2017. "Asylum Applications Respond to Temperature Fluctuations." *Science* 358 (6370):1610–14. https://doi.org/10.1126/science.aao0432.

Neumann, B., A. T. Vafeidis, J. Zimmermann, and R. J. Nicholls. 2015. "Future Coastal Population Growth and Exposure to Sea-Level Rise and Coastal Flooding—A Global Assessment." *PLoS One* 10 (3):e0118571. doi: 10.1371/journal.pone.0118571.

Omoleke, S. A., I. Mohammed, and Y. Saidu. 2016. "Ebola Viral Disease in West Africa: A Threat to Global Health, Economy and Political Stability." *Journal of Public Health in Africa* 7 (1). https://doi.org/10.4081/jphia.2016.534.

Rahman, A. A. 2012. "Regional Cooperation to Combat Climate Change: The Way Forward." Bangladesh Centre for Advanced Studies. http://www.bcas.net/article-full-desc.php?article_id=11.

Rashid, M. 2019. "Climate Change and Asia's Deadly Dengue Fever Outbreaks." United Nations Development Programme. https://www.asia-pacific.undp.org/content/rbap/en/home/blog/2019/climate-change-and-asias-deadly-dengue-fever-outbreaks.html.

Rigaud, K. K., A. de Sherbinin, B. Jones, J. Bergmann, V. Clement, K. Ober, J. Schewe et al. 2018. *Groundswell: Preparing for Internal Climate Migration.* Washington, DC: World Bank. https://openknowledge.worldbank.org/handle/10986/29461.

Schütte, S., F. Gemenne, M. Zaman, A. Flahault, and A. Depoux. 2018. "Connecting Planetary Health, Climate Change, and Migration." *Lancet Planetary Health* 2 (2):e58–e59. https://doi.org/10.1016/S2542-5196(18)30004-4.

Storlazzi, C. D., S. B. Gingerich, A. van Dongeren, O. M. Cheriton, P. W. Swarzenski, E. Quataert, C. I. Voss et al. 2018. "Most Atolls Will Be Uninhabitable by the Mid-21st Century Because of Sea-Level Rise Exacerbating Wave-Driven Flooding." *Science Advances* 4 (4):eaap9741. https://doi.org/10.1126/sciadv.aap9741.

UNESCO World Water Assessment Programme. 2016. *World Water Development Report 2016: Water and Jobs.* https://unesdoc.unesco.org/ark:/48223/pf0000243938.

United Nations Convention to Combat Desertification. n.d. *Migration and Desertification.* Paris: UNCCD.

United Nations Children's Fund and World Health Organization. 2017. *Progress on Drinking Water, Sanitation, and Hygiene.* Geneva: WHO.

United Nations Department of Economic and Social Affairs. 2011. *World Economic and Social Survey 2011: The Great Green Technological Transformation*. Geneva: UNDESA. https://www.un.org/development/desa/publications/world-economic-and-social-survey-2011-the-great-green-technological-transformation.html.

United Nations High Commissioner for Refugees. n.d. "Figures at a Glance." Geneva: UNHCR. https://www.unhcr.org/figures-at-a-glance.html.

U.S. Army Corps of Engineers. n.d. "South Shore of Staten Island Costal Storm Risk Management Feasibility Study." https://www.nan.usace.army.mil/Missions/Civil-Works/Projects-in-New-York/South-Shore-of-Staten-Island/.

U.S. Global Change Research Program. 2016. *The Impacts of Climate Change on Human Health in the United States*. Washington, DC: USGCRP.

Westergaard N., U. Gehring, R. Slama, and M. Pedersen. 2017. "Ambient Air Pollution and Low Birth Weight—Are Some Women More Vulnerable than Others?" *Environment International Journal* 104:146–54. https://www.ncbi.nlm.nih.gov/pubmed/28390661.

World Health Organization. 2019. *Promoting the Health of Refugees and Migrants Draft Global Action Plan, 2019–2023*. Report by the Director-General. Geneva: WHO.

World Food Programme. 2017. *At the Root of Exodus: Food Security Conflict and International Migration*. Rome: WFP.

Wrathal, D. J., J. Van Den Hoek, A. Walters, and A. Devenish. 2018. *Water Stress and Human Migration: A Global, Georeferenced Review of Empirical Research*. Rome: Food and Agriculture Organization.

CHAPTER 24

VALUING CLIMATE CHANGE IMPACTS ON HUMAN HEALTH

Allison Crimmins

Introduction: Why Do We Value the Climate Change Impacts on Human Health?

Economic value is determined by choices, specifically what one is willing to give up to gain something else or to protect the things we value. As an absolute number, economic value is more of a theoretical construct, as what one is willing to give up will differ for each person and often at different times within a person's life. This may be more relevant for the health sector than for economic valuation of impacts in sectors measuring goods or services, such as infrastructure or energy. Is there anything more important, and more difficult to quantify, than your health? Some may argue we should refrain from attempting to put a dollar sign on our health at all.

Why then do we undertake the valuation of health impacts from climate change (or other environmental threats for that matter)? Because many public policies that address threats to our health call for economic evidence to justify decisions, including the decision of whether to institute a policy and at what stringency the policy should be written. Furthermore, climate change impacts on our health impose a cost to human society beyond the harder-to-quantify effects of individual pain, suffering, and premature death. We value the economic impacts of climate change on health to assign the importance we give to it and thus the importance we give to protecting it.

Economic Valuation: How Do We Value the Climate Change Impacts on Human Health?

Evaluating economic impacts is crucial to understanding risk from climate change. Adverse health effects attributed to climate change can have many economic and social consequences, including (Chestnut 1999):

- Direct medical costs: These include costs of treating health impacts to the affected individual or family, whether out of pocket or paid by public health care or insurance.

- Lost work or school: The loss of productivity can be monetized using lost wages or cost of sick-pay to a business. Loss of school hours can reflect loss of future earnings.

- Increased care-giving costs: Such costs are accrued if an affected individual has a reduced ability to do chores or requires caregiving or other services not included in medical costs.

KEY CONCEPTS

- Economic valuation is crucial to the process of making informed decisions about protecting human health and addressing climate change.

- Quantification of climate-related costs to health is challenging. Advancements in modeling capabilities have led to a growing body of studies that define relationships between climate change and health outcomes to estimate future benefits and costs.

- Economic damages associated with climate change impacts on human health in the United States are very large; global mitigation actions could save thousands of lives and hundreds of billions of dollars each year by the end of the century.

- Other opportunity costs: Time spent on other everyday activities, including the enjoyment of leisure, recreation, or social contact, may be given up or reduced to focus on an illness or disability. Other social costs include pain or discomfort, anxiety or additional mental health effects from physical impairment, and worry or inconvenience to family and friends.

To properly account for health costs to society (or conversely, the benefits of measures to prevent adverse health effects), the value of all these impacts (or the value of reducing these impacts) must be measured. Valuing such costs, however, becomes more difficult as one progresses through the preceding list; few measures go beyond an estimation of the first two types of costs. In addition, spending devoted to the consequences listed above may result in important impacts on human health and well-being by reducing resources available for future preventative health measures or resiliency (Balbus et al. 2016).

Health Impact Functions

Economic policy analysis is not a crystal ball; it will never reveal which specific individual on which specific date will become ill or die under one scenario or another. While the outcome of keen interest to someone may be the impact of climate change on their personal health, the impact evaluated in epidemiological studies is how an environmental threat alters the risk of any one individual experiencing a health effect. In other words, what is valued is the change in the *probability* of adverse health outcomes.

Epidemiologists typically estimate **relative risk**, or the ratio of the probability of an exposed group of people experiencing an adverse health outcome in relation to the probability of that outcome in an unexposed group. Relative risk values above one imply greater risk to the exposed group, less than one lower risk, and values of exactly one imply no more or less risk than the unexposed or reference group. A **dose-, exposure-,** or **concentration-response function** is the relative risk of adverse health outcomes at various exposure levels (e.g., concentration of an environmental pollutant). For instance, if a person in an exposed population is expected to experience a simple, linear 10 percent increase in relative risk of an adverse health outcome for every 1°C (1.8°F) increase in global average surface temperature, then exposure can be calculated by multiplying the exposure-response function (relative risk of 1.1 per 1°C increase) by the expected temperature change under the scenario of interest. Such response functions, when combined with estimates of baseline changes in population and incidence rates, can be used to construct a **health impact function.** Finally, the health impact function can be multiplied by the cost of health consequences to estimate economic damages (see Figure 24.1). How does one measure the cost of health consequences (bold outlined box in the

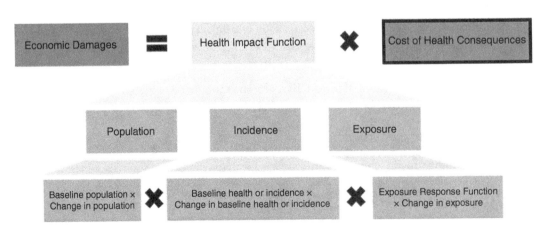

Figure 24.1 Calculating economic damages of health impacts associated with a change in environmental exposure

figure) or, more relevant to policy analysis, the benefits of avoiding health risks? The rest of this section focuses on this last element.

Benefit-Cost vs. Cost-Effectiveness Analyses

Economic analysis is crucial to informing sound environmental policies because it provides policy makers with the ability to systematically assess consequences of various actions (Environmental Protection Agency 2010b). The official guidance to federal agencies on economic analyses related to regulatory actions is the Office of Management and Budget (OMB) Circular A4, required reading for students of policy analysis and the source for much of the information in this section.

Policy analysts often have a better idea of the cost of a proposed policy than they do the benefits; the benefits of improved health or avoided health effects are difficult to evaluate because they are not items bought or sold in markets. These may be evaluated using **Benefit-Cost Analysis (BCA)** or **Cost-Effectiveness Analysis (CEA)**.

Benefit-cost analyses are used when both the benefits and the costs can be expressed in monetary terms. Estimating the size of net benefits (*not* the ratio of benefits to costs) allows the analyst to consider which alternative policy—including a no-policy option—provides the largest benefit to society. But if benefits and costs cannot be monetized, BCA is less effective, and CEA may be used to evaluate policy options. CEA can be used to determine which alternative policy most efficiently uses available resources to achieve a given goal.

Benefit Estimates

There are a number of ways to estimate the economic value of environmental improvements that protect health or what a person is willing to give up to avoid health impacts. The first method is **Cost-of-Illness (COI)**, which simply measures the medical costs and lost income of a health effect. Although COI is easily understood and data on hospitalization costs and wages are readily available, it is a conservative estimate of the full extent of welfare impacts caused by a health effect.

Another method is **Willingness-to-Pay (WTP)**, or its rough inverse **Willingness-to-Accept (WTA)**. WTP is what an individual would pay to avoid a health impact; WTA is the least amount of payment an individual would accept to experience the health impact (Environmental Protection Agency 2010a). A person's WTP or WTA may be revealed by their choices or actions or stated in response to a hypothetical situation. A person may reveal their preferences, for example, by demonstrating what they are willing to pay for extra safety features in a car or what they are willing to be paid to work a dangerous job. A person's stated preferences may also be discovered by asking them how much they are willing to pay to avoid an incremental increase in risk.

Monetizing Mortality and Morbidity

When the health impact being measured is mortality, it is important to remember that no one is placing a macabre dollar sign on any one person's life or death. There is no WTA value for certain death, nor WTP to ensure survival. Instead, a person's WTP for a small change in the risk of death is used to calculate the **Value of a Statistical Life (VSL)**. Even the term is misleading, as this metric should be thought of more as "value of mortality risk."

Estimating VSL comes with controversies and caveats. There is wide variation in published values and debate on whether the mode of death (e.g., sudden or accidental versus the dread associated with a chronic disease like cancer), a person's age (more accurately, years left to live), or income should be considered in the calculation. Even the economic status of a person's country of origin may be a factor as resource-poor countries have more competing needs for each dollar. And, of course, there are limitations to how well COI, WTP, WTA, or other forms of economic valuation can capture the real benefits to society of avoiding health impacts. Valuing mortality risk changes for children is particularly difficult, as a parent's personal preferences may not be the same as a child's and children rarely earn wages or make purchases that reveal their preferences.

The reason for controversy over any specific VSL estimate is that if it is too low, the benefits of policy actions that protect human health may be undervalued. If it is too high, too much money may be spent on policy actions for which benefits have been overvalued. Despite the caveats, there are estimates of VSL in the United States from several federal agencies. The Environmental Protection Agency (EPA) recommends for benefit analyses the use of $7.4 million (in $2006), to be adjusted for inflation and income growth to the year of study (EPA 2018). Thus in the analyses described in section 4 below, VSLs are adjusted to $10.0 million for the baseline year of 2015, $12.4 million in 2050, and $15.2 million in 2090.

When the health impact of interest is morbidity rather than mortality, there are a number of additional measures to use in estimating health benefits. For example, a **Quality-Adjusted Life Year (QALY)** evaluates both the quantity (years of life remaining) and quality of life (state of health). In doing so, it values the young, who have more years of life to live, more than the old. But the QALY assumes the amount someone is willing to pay for additional years of life does not depend on the fraction of one's lifespan those years represent. For instance, what one would be willing to accept for the loss of one year of life may be different if that person knew they were going to live five more years or fifty more years; QALY does not capture that preference.

Related to the QALY is the **Disability-Adjusted Life Years (DALY)**, which measures not just the benefits of an intervention to protect health but the overall disease burden over the course of one's lifespan. In measuring the health impacts of an environmental threat, it combines the years of life lost (YLL) and years of life living with a disease or disability (YLD), using weighted values to represent thousands of diseases and disabilities (World Health Organization 2013). This measure can account for short-term and chronic health effects, as it multiplies the weighted burden of the condition by the years spent experiencing that condition to calculate YLD.

Discounting

Discounting is an important consideration when estimating future impacts of climate change, particularly because the costs and the benefits of climate action (and inaction) may not occur at the same time (Roberts 2012; Stavins 2007; Stokey and Zeckhauser 1978; Teitenberg and Lewis 2009). Consumption is more expensive in the present than the future. You can think of this in terms of buying a hamburger when you are young and have little or no income versus buying a hamburger later in life, when, it is hoped, you do. Even if the cost of the hamburger goes up a bit over the years, the impact to your wallet as an older adult is less painful. Similarly, we tend to value benefits in the near term higher than benefits in the long term. If offered $1 today versus $2 next year, you would likely choose the $1 today, whether because you have immediate need, or plan to invest it, or don't trust the offer. Put more crudely, people in the future will be richer than they are today and more capable of dealing with the impacts of climate change because every additional dollar (marginal consumption) has less value than it does today. Thus, it is appropriate to adjust economic estimates to reflect timing, with benefits and costs that occur farther in the future more discounted than those that occur in the near term.

As with VSL, there is an active debate about the correct level of discounting, as the discount factor chosen will likewise factor into estimates of benefits and costs and therefore decisions about policies. Confounding this is that climate change itself has an important impact on economic growth and resources (Diffenbaugh and Burke 2019) and the inertia of the Earth system means choices made about emissions today have long-lasting effects far into the future. Some of these climate impacts may be irreversible within a time frame of relevance to humanity (Collins et al. 2013; Kopp et al. 2017).

The U.S. government recommends providing benefit and cost estimates using both a 3 percent and 7 percent discount adjustment. The 3 percent represents the "social rate of time preference," or the return on long-term government debt (e.g., Treasury notes); the 7 percent represents the average rate of return on private capital. However, recent evidence suggests long-term interest rates have come down since these values were calculated (Council on Economic Advisors 2017). This finding supports lower discount adjustments, such as 2 percent for the lower rate. Discounting both health benefits and health costs is appropriate in both BCA and CEA, though some argue that the discount rate for health benefits should not be the same as for economic benefits (Viscusi 1995; Weinstein 1990).

Economic Models: Projecting Future Climate Damages

Challenges

A 2015 review of literature on climate-related health damages in Europe states, "We found that the evidence base on the health economics of climate change is scarce, incomplete, and inconsistent" (Martinez, William, and Yu 2015). Although this assessment may have improved over the last few years with recent literature, it is still not far off the mark. Valuing climate-related costs to health, or benefits of avoiding climate impacts on health, comes with a number of challenges, especially when attempting to project future costs (Crimmins et al. 2016a).

The ability to quantify health impacts depends on having reliable, long-term incidence data and a clear understanding of how climate change, among the many other factors driving changes in human health, affects these outcomes. Health effects rarely happen in isolation and impacts can be cumulative or nonlinear, especially if repeated exposures lead to chronic conditions or reduced resiliency. Further confounding matters are decisions over how to account for future adaptation to climate change (which could lessen impacts) and the uncertain potential for low-probability high-impact outcomes (Weitzman 2009).

Despite the growing field of research on economic damages associated with health impacts of climate change, results from many studies cannot be compared "apples to apples" due to methodological choice of inputs, scenarios (both climatological and socioeconomic), metrics, or assumptions of values like VSL, income elasticity, or discount rate. That said, an ever-growing number of tools and studies are becoming available to better characterize health risks from climate change.

Modeling Approaches

Even beyond the health sector, it is no small task to attempt to estimate economic costs of climate change. Since the 1980s, cost-benefit **integrated assessment models (IAMs)** have been used primarily to develop damage functions. These functions connect an additional unit of greenhouse gas emitted to the resultant change in global average temperature, and that change in temperature to the resultant climate damages. Aggregate damage functions that can relate a future change in temperature to social damages allows for the calculation, when discounted, of the net present-day **social cost of carbon (SCC** or **SC-CO2)**. An Interagency Working Group (IWG) (2010) was formed to calculate the SCC in 2009 and used three IAMs, named DICE (Nordhaus 1992, 2010), PAGE (Hope 2006), and FUND (Tol 1995). These models aggregate estimated damages across multiple sectors (not just health) to calculate total social costs. Although all three are simplified models by nature, DICE and PAGE do not specify categories of climate damages; FUND reports fifteen categories, including cardiovascular, respiratory, and vector-borne diseases; morbidity; diarrhea;[1] and migration (Tol 1996). The IWG reported the first SCC estimates in 2010 and provided several updates, the most recent in 2016 (IWG 2016), before being disbanded by an Executive Order of the Trump administration in 2017. The 2016 report provided a central estimate of SCC in 2015 of $36; this means that, assuming a 3 percent discount rate, the global social costs of emitting each additional metric ton of CO_2 in 2015 is $36.[2] This value nearly doubles by 2050, so that emissions of each additional metric ton of CO_2 cost society $69 by midcentury. More recent studies have resulted in a range of SCC values, many much larger.

Instead of the more top-down style of estimating damages using IAMs (e.g., by deriving a function to approximate all damages associated with each extra ton of emissions), recent research collaborations have attempted to evaluate climate impacts using a bottom-up approach, aggregating costs estimated separately within individual sectors. Advancements in modeling capabilities have led to a growing body of studies that use relationships between observed socioeconomic outcomes (e.g., premature deaths, hospitalizations, costs of adaptation) and changes in climate variables to estimate future impacts of climate change (Hsiang et al. 2017; Müller et al. 2017). These econometric methods (i.e., use of statistical relationships) have allowed for modeling of impacts in sectors that IAMs either omitted or lumped into corrections for "intangible" impacts, such as health, migration, crime, or conflict. Advancements in process-based sectoral models, which provide detailed projections of physical and socioeconomic changes within a single sector (e.g., agricultural yields; Houser et al. 2015; Rosenzweig et al. 2014), can be more computationally intensive than IAMs or econometric models but have the benefit of better representing meteorologic impacts at a more disaggregated or downscaled geographical scale, which may be more useful to, for instance, public health officials. And if standardized to use the same modeling framework, costs estimated from either econometric or process-based models across multiple sectors can be compared to one another (Diaz and Moore 2017). All of the examples presented in the following section describe one such modeling collaboration called Climate Change Impacts and Risk Analysis (CIRA), which represents an internally consistent, bottom-up modeling approach.

CLINICAL CORRELATES 24.1 HEALTH-RELATED COSTS FROM CLIMATE CHANGE

Climate-sensitive events contribute to deaths, costly hospitalizations, and emergency department visits. Limaye et al. (2019) studied ten climate-sensitive events that occurred in 2012 across eleven states and found more than $10 billion in health-related costs, the majority coming from outright mortality. As climate events progress in coming years, further research should consider the wide-ranging effects on human health including medication costs, lost wages, and health care utilization. Other cost considerations include use of supplies and environmental impacts within health care facilities. Understanding this broader range of cost estimates may also assist policymakers and health care systems in discussing and advancing climate action plans.

More than $10 billion was spent on health care costs related to ten climate-sensitive events in the United States over one year highlighting the need for continued attention to health care utilization as an opportunity to reduce costs, build climate resilience, and support health.

---

[1] In the Tol (1995) study, the value of a human life is assumed to equal $250,000 + (175x the per capita income in the region).

[2] In 2015, an estimated 34.8 billion metric tons of CO_2 was emitted globally; using the central SCC estimate with a 3 percent discount rate for 2015 of $36/metric ton of CO_2, this would result in a cost to society of $1.25 trillion.

Examples of Health Damage Estimates from Climate Change

CIRA (EPA 2018a) results have been chosen as an example to present here because, although there are several other coordinated, internally consistent multisector modeling frameworks (Martinich et al. 2018), CIRA explores a greater range of distinct health impacts. Physical and economic damages in each sectoral analysis described in this section can be compared to one another because they use consistent inputs and assumptions (EPA 2017a) but should not be directly compared to health results in other modeling frameworks without understanding the differences in methodologies.

CIRA results describe the costs to the United States under two global mitigation scenarios (defined in Chapter 1), a very high emissions scenario (representative concentration pathway [RCP]8.5) and a moderate emissions scenario (RCP4.5), to illustrate potential impacts and damages of alternative future climates. Importantly, CIRA does not estimate costs of reducing greenhouse gas emissions nor the health benefits associated with reductions in other air pollutants (see Chapter 19) and so is not a BCA or CEA.

Although a consistent framework allows for comparison across sectors (e.g., how large are the impacts from extreme heat mortality compared to premature deaths associated with ozone?), it would not be entirely accurate to add up all the health damages and claim the sum to be the total health impacts to the United States from climate change (Martinich and Crimmins 2019). This is because there are many health impacts and economic costs not captured within the analyses. For instance, the extreme temperatures analysis evaluates mortality but not morbidity impacts such as hospitalizations, cardiorespiratory illnesses, or pregnancy complications (Kim, Lee, and Rossin-Slater 2019; Konkel 2019). Climate change has many impacts on mental health and well-being (Dodgen et al. 2016)—particularly following extreme weather events like storms, floods, and drought (Ebi et al. 2018; Limaye et al. 2019), after contracting disease (Nolan, Hause, and Murray 2012), or where economic impacts are high (Hayes et al. 2018; Obradovich et al. 2018). However, mental health consequences are not captured either as their own outcome or as a metric within the related health impact sector analyses. And there are some other important health sectors not covered at all, such as impacts of climate change on Lyme disease (Adrion et al. 2015; Mac da Silva, and Sander 2019)[3] or indoor air quality impacts from mold after flooding. Also not quantified here are the significant impacts climate change has on the health care system (e.g., impacts on hospitals, nursing homes, or other medical facilities; costs of evacuations or continued service during extreme events; rising costs of insurance; reduced access to future health care services) nor the health impacts that occur outside the United States that may result in costs to the United States (Smith et al. 2018) (e.g., health impacts to military personnel serving overseas, outbreaks of diseases that require international response). Thus, the impacts presented here likely greatly underestimate the actual economic cost of climate change on health in the United States. Research is ongoing to fill in these gaps.

Unless otherwise noted, the CIRA damages reported here are in 2015 dollars for the years 2050 and 2090, under the very high (RCP8.5) and moderate (RCP4.5) scenarios, compared to a baseline of 1986–2005 (EPA 2017a).

---

[3] Using different methods than CIRA, Limaye et al. (2019) estimated economic damages from Lyme disease in Michigan in 2012 to be $8 million in 2018 dollars. Other recent studies quantified the national burden of Lyme disease to be between $712 million and $1.3 billion annually (Adrion et al. 2015; Mac, da Silva, and Sander 2019)

CLINICAL CORRELATES 24.2 MENTAL HEALTH IMPACTS ARE OFTEN LEFT OUT OF DAMAGE ESTIMATES

Climate change has many impacts on mental health and well-being, ranging from minimal stress to clinical disorders, such as anxiety, depression, posttraumatic stress, and suicidal thoughts (Dodgen et al. 2016). Climate change and extreme weather events can affect mental health directly; for instance, individuals whose households experienced a flood or risk of flood report higher levels of depression and anxiety, persisting several years after the event (Ebi et al. 2018). But indirect mental health impacts can also be experienced when adverse health outcomes occur. For example, clinical depression has been observed in patients suffering from West Nile virus, a disease expected to increase with climate change (Nolan, Hause, and Murray 2012). Furthermore, socioeconomic status is a determinant of well-being, and people living in poverty or with low socioeconomic status are some of the most vulnerable to climate related health impacts. Undermining the determinants of mental health can therefore exacerbate social inequalities (Hayes et al. 2018).

Mental health is commonly affected by climate-related events and should be a high priority for clinicians considering climate health impacts.

Extreme Temperatures

Climate change will result in more extremely hot days and fewer extremely cold days (Vose et al. 2017). The resulting increase in premature deaths from more frequent extremely hot days is projected to outweigh the decrease in premature deaths from reductions in extremely cold days (Sarofim et al. 2016). The analysis used in CIRA examines forty-nine cities in the contiguous United States, accounting for approximately one third of the total population (Mills et al. 2014). Under RCP8.5, the net increase in projected temperature-related deaths is approximately 3,400 deaths per year in 2050 and 9,300 deaths per year in 2090. In comparison, RCP4.5 avoids nearly 800 deaths (24 percent) each year by 2050 and more than 5,400 deaths (58 percent) each year by 2090. Most cities with large heat-related mortality increases in recent years are in the Northeast and the Midwest; these cities are projected to see greater future increases in mortality than most southern cities.

Damages from increases in heat-related deaths are projected to be $43 billion each year by 2050 and $140 billion each year by 2090, under RCP8.5. Under RCP4.5, damages are reduced to $32 billion each year in 2050 and $60 billion each year by 2090. As a sensitivity analysis, CIRA also assumed a future in which the health-adaptive response in all forty-nine cities was similar to that seen in Dallas today (e.g., from widely available air conditioning or physiological adaptation). By assuming everyone demonstrates this high level of adaptive capacity, approximately half of the premature deaths were avoided. Although it is reasonable to expect some level of adaptation to reduce the health effects of increasing extreme heat, adaptation responses are rarely perfectly timed and managed; health damages from extreme heat mortality most likely fall somewhere between these bounding values (Ebi et al. 2018).

When exposed to high temperatures, workers face elevated risk for health impacts (e.g., heatstroke and heat exhaustion), safety concerns (especially if fatigued or dizzy), and lost productivity from the need to take more frequent breaks or to stop work entirely (Gamble et al. 2016). Occupations where workers are doing physical labor, work outside, or occupy buildings without climate control (e.g., agriculture, construction, utilities, and manufacturing) are particularly risky (Graff Zivin and Neidell 2014). Under RCP8.5, almost 1.9 billion lost labor hours are projected each year by 2090 due to unsuitable working conditions. Losses are

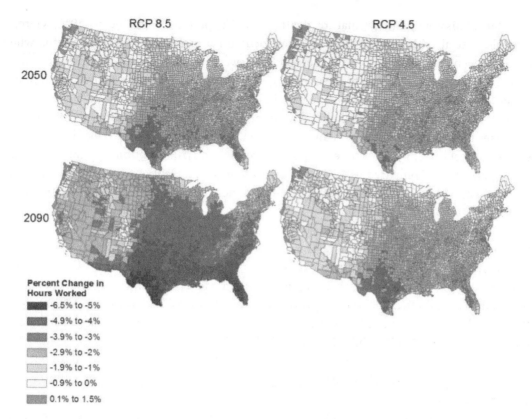

Figure 24.2   Projected labor changes due to extreme temperatures

Source: EPA (2017a); Graff Ziven and Niedell (2014).

Note: Estimates represent projected percent change in annual hours worked in 2050 and 2090 from the 2003–2007 reference period at the county level for industries that are at high risk because of extreme temperatures (e.g., construction, agricultural work). Values represent five-year averaged results across five global climate models under two emissions scenarios, RCP4.5 and RCP8.5, and are normalized by the high-risk working population within each county. Costs associated with these changes in labor hours can be estimated by adjusting the Bureau of Labor Statistics' estimated average wage in 2005 for high risk labor categories (Bureau of Labor Statistics 2017) and calculating to 2100 using an index reflecting projected changes in gross domestic product (GDP) per capita given real 2015 GDP and population.

particularly large in the Midwest (0.40 billion labor hours annually) and the Southeast (0.57 billion labor hours annually), where estimated work hours losses of up to 6.5 percent are estimated for counties in Texas and Florida (Figure 24.2). A separate study using similar methods also found high productivity losses in the Southeast region (3.1 percent) by the end of the century because of changes in heat and humidity (Gordon 2014).

Loss of labor hours result in lost wages, which is one of the costliest impacts of climate change. In 2050, lost wages from extreme temperatures (both hot and cold) are projected to be $35 billion each year under RCP4.5 and $44 billion each year under RCP8.5. By 2090, these damages increase to $80 billion each year under RCP4.5 and $160 billion each year under RCP8.5. More than a third of the national loss under RCP8.5 in 2090 is projected to occur in the Southeast ($47 billion annually). The difference between RCP8.5 and RCP4.5 represent a savings of nearly $9.0 billion in annual wages in 2050 and nearly $75 billion in 2090.

Air Quality

Climate change is expected to result in weather conditions that are increasingly conducive to high concentrations of ground-level ozone over many parts of the United States (Fann et al. 2016). Ozone harms human health through respiratory and cardiovascular pathways, resulting in additional reported acute respiratory symptoms, missed school and work days, hospital admissions, and premature deaths (see Chapter 5) (Fann et al. 2015; Garcia-Menendez et al. 2015). The CIRA analyses focus on mortality in summer months when ozone concentrations tend to be higher. By 2090, warming temperatures lead to seasonal-average ozone increases of up to 5 parts per billion (ppb) in some parts of the United States under RCP8.5. This effect is often referred to as the "climate penalty" (Wu et al. 2008) because climate change can make attaining national air quality standards more difficult. Increases in ozone from climate change are projected to result in an additional 790 premature deaths each year by 2050 under RCP8.5, increasing to 1,700 additional premature deaths annually by 2090. Compared to RCP8.5, RCP4.5 reduces mortality impacts by avoiding 240 deaths by 2050 and 500 deaths by 2090. Projected increases in premature deaths are largest in the Midwest and Northeast.

These projected ozone-related deaths result in national damages under RCP8.5 of $9.8 billion each year by 2050 and $26 billion each year by 2090. Under RCP4.5, annual costs of premature deaths are projected to be $6.9 billion in 2050 and $18 billion in 2090. Though not included in the economic valuation, morbidity impacts from climate-driven changes in ozone are also significant. For example, projections under RCP8.5 estimate that, by 2090, there will be an additional 1,700 elderly people admitted to the hospital each year for respiratory issues, 1.2 million children between six and eighteen years old experiencing exacerbated asthma symptoms each year, 2.8 million days with minor restricted activity for adults, and nearly one million days of missed school for children across the country each year (EPA 2017b).

Climate-driven changes in meteorologic patterns will also have an impact on particulate matter concentrations throughout the United States. There is clear consensus that wildfires and smoke-associated particulate matter will continue to increase because of climate change (Nolte et al. 2018). Wildfire exposure modeled in CIRA suggest that tens of millions of people will be exposed to wildfire smoke under either emissions scenario, though three million more people are exposed to wildfire smoke in 2050 under RCP8.5 compared to RCP4.5, and nearly ten million more people are exposed in 2090 under RCP8.5 compared to RCP4.5 (Mills et al. 2018). Of those ten million people avoiding exposure to wildfire smoke each year under RCP4.5, nearly one million are young children and 1.7 million are older adults.

Modeling work is still underway for non-wildfire particulates, as it is difficult to quantify a direct net climate signal. Projections suggest that climate change could result in small (less than ±1.0 µg m-3) but regionally varying shifts in fine particulate matter ($PM_{2.5}$) over the next century under both emissions scenarios. However, even small changes in $PM_{2.5}$ in urban areas can yield large numbers of premature deaths as well as serious chronic and acute health effects, including lung cancer, chronic obstructive pulmonary disease, cardiovascular disease, and asthma development and exacerbation. Older adults are particularly sensitive to short-term particle exposure, with a higher risk of hospitalization and death (Bell and Dominici 2008; Sacks et al. 2011).

Climate change is also expected to have impacts on fine ($PM_{2.5}$) and coarse ($PM_{2.5-10}$) dust, with associated health damages (Achakulwisut et al. 2019). One study of four states in the southwestern United States projected severe, multidecadal droughts due to human-caused climate change. By the end of the century, these droughts are projected to result in a 57 percent increase in fine and 38 percent increase in coarse dust particles, which are already major contributors to air pollution in this region due to abundant deserts and drylands. Under RCP8.5, higher levels of fine dust lead to a 220 percent increase in mortality (1,900 deaths/year) and a 350 percent increase in hospitalizations (2,200 admissions/year) by 2090 compared to the

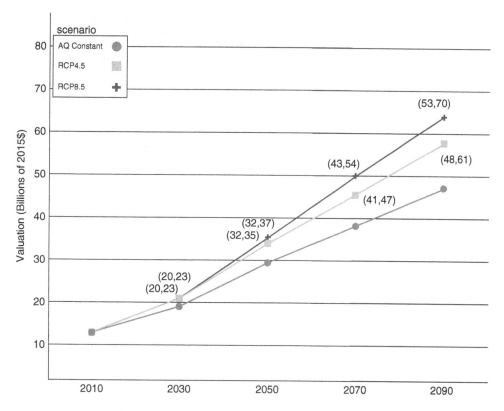

Figure 24.3   Annual economic damages of health impacts related to dust exposure

Source: Achakulwisut et al. (2018).

Note: Projected health-related damages due to climate-induced increases in fine and coarse dust exposure for 2010, 2030, 2050, 2070, and 2090 for Arizona, Colorado, New Mexico, and Utah. Damages are summed across the following mortality and morbidity endpoints: fine-dust-attributable all-cause mortality and cardiovascular, acute myocardial infarction, and respiratory hospital admissions; and coarse dust-attributable cardiovascular mortality and asthma emergency department visits. The parentheses display the lowest and highest estimates based on the modelling range. The "AQ constant" scenario is calculated using 1988–2005 fine dust concentrations combined with projected population and baseline incidence rates but without projected climate impacts.

baseline year (2010).[4] The majority of these mortality estimates come from cardiopulmonary-related deaths for adults aged seventy-five years and older. Coarse dust levels lead to increases in cardiovascular mortality and asthma emergency department visits of 210 percent (970 deaths/year) and 90 percent (1,500 visits/year), respectively, by the end of the century. The highest incidence rates of mortalities and asthma emergency room visits from coarse dust are found in older adults and children.

Dust-related health damages are estimated to be approximately $13 billion/year (in 2015 dollars) in the reference year 2010 (Figure 24.3). Under RCP8.5, additional damages of $22 billion/year in 2050 and $47 billion/year in 2090 are estimated. Projected dust-related mortality and morbidity burdens in 2090 are 60 percent higher under RCP8.5 than RCP4.5. Under the lower emissions scenario, 110 and 420 premature deaths could be avoided each year by 2050 and 2090, respectively, avoiding annual economic damages of $1.6 billion by 2050 and $6.4 billion by 2090 compared to the high emissions scenario. Despite this sectoral analysis covering only four states, dust-related health impacts are ranked fourth costliest within all the CIRA sectors, demonstrating the immensity of damages associated with climate change-air quality impacts.

---

[4] The historical reference burdens are estimated using 2010 population and baseline incidence rates combined with 1988–2005 dust concentrations.

Although health threats from airborne allergens (aeroallergens) are often less severe than those associated with ozone or particulate matter, climate change is also projected to increase pollen-related health outcomes (Anenberg et al. 2017; Neumann et al. 2018). Oak and birch pollen in the spring currently account for 25,000–50,000 pollen-related asthma emergency department visits annually, roughly two thirds of which are among children. Grass pollen in the summer currently accounts for less than 10,000 cases. Climate change increases pollen season length, which is projected to increase those emergency department visits by 14 percent (>10,000 additional cases/year) under RCP8.5 and 8 percent (>6,000 additional cases/year) under RCP4.5 by the end of the century. Grass pollen production, which is more sensitive to changes in climatic conditions, is a primary contributor to this increase in health effects, particularly in the Northeast, Midwest, and Southern Great Plains regions.

The projected excess burden from climate-related health impacts of aeroallergens in 2050 is $2.5 million annually for RCP4.5 and $3.0 million annually for RCP8.5 (on top of increases projected in 2050 and 2100 because of nonclimate factors like population).[5] By 2090, damages increase to $3.0 million annually for RCP4.5 and $5.2 million for RCP8.5. These estimates do not include the substantial costs of medication, other health care utilization, or lost school or work days. The large size of the over-the-counter allergy medication market nationally (e.g., annual sales over $6.8 billion and more than 735 million medications units sold in 2016; Johnsen 2017) suggests even a small increase in allergen-related health outcomes could amount to a large economic effect. A 2007 study by Nathan found allergic rhinitis from all causes (including pollen, mold, animal dander, or dust) results in 3.5 million lost workdays and 2 million lost schooldays annually, which translates to current annual costs of lost productivity from allergic rhinitis of over $0.5 billion per year.[6]

Food, Water, and Vector-Borne Health Risks

Though the links between climate change impacts and increased exposure to food-, water-, and vector-borne illnesses are well known (Crimmins et al. 2016b), research quantifying economic damages from these health effects is limited. In the CIRA framework, only West Nile virus and the recreational damages associated with closed beaches due to harmful algal blooms are evaluated, omitting many other health effects.

Warming temperatures are expected to continue to increase incidence of West Nile virus across the United States (Beard et al. 2016). Approximately 1 percent of people infected with West Nile virus contract West Nile neuroinvasive disease (WNND), though more severe syndromes mean that nearly half of reported cases are neuroinvasive (Centers for Disease Control and Prevention 2016; Lindsey et al. 2015). Patients with WNND are projected to more than double in the United States by 2050, increasing by 1,000 cases each year

---

[5] The cost of a pollen-related emergency department visit is estimated at $490, adjusted for inflation, in $2015 dollars.

[6] This estimation applied a median wage rate of $106 and cost of a lost school day of $75 (based on the probability that a parent will have to stay home from work to care for the child, not the lost educational development of the child).

under RCP4.5 and 1,300 cases each year under RCP8.5 (Hahn et al. 2015). By 2090, an additional 1,700 and 3,300 cases each year are projected under RCP4.5 and RCP8.5, respectively (Belova et al. 2017). The Southeast is expected to experience more than 1,100 additional cases in 2090 under RCP8.5. The total national costs associated with these increases are $0.87 billion each year under RCP4.5 and $1.1 billion each year under RCP8.5 in 2050. Damages increase in 2090 to $1.8 billion each year under RCP4.5 and $3.3 billion each year under RCP8.5.[7]

Warming temperatures and changes in precipitation are projected to increase the occurrence of harmful algal blooms in many U.S. watersheds (Trtanj et al. 2016). Nearly half of all disease outbreaks linked to recreational freshwater in 2009 and 2010 were due to exposure to cyanotoxins (Hilborn et al. 2014). Climate change is projected to lead to an additional full month of the year where harmful algal concentrations in lakes and other freshwater bodies are above a recommended public health threshold (World Health Organization 1999)[8] in 2090 under RCP8.5; this period is halved under RCP4.5 (Chapra et al. 2017). The resulting losses to reservoir recreation in the contiguous United States are estimated to be $71 million each year under RCP4.5 and $82 million each year under RCP8.5 by 2050. These damages increase to $130 million each year under RCP4.5 and $250 million each year under RCP8.5 by 2090. These costs, which are estimated in CIRA only for freshwater recreational reservoirs, do not include potential health effects and thus greatly underestimate total damages from harmful algal blooms. For instance, a separate study of the health costs associated with coastal harmful algal blooms experienced by just six Florida counties in 2012 estimated $557 million in annual damages (in 2018 dollars) associated with digestive and respiratory disease (Hoagland et al. 2014; Limaye et al. 2019).

Summary and Regional Variations

A clear finding from these examples is that the severe health outcomes and large economic damages projected in future years are reduced under the more moderate emissions scenario. By the end of this century, thousands of lives could be saved and hundreds of billions of dollars in health-related economic benefits gained each year under RCP4.5 compared to RCP8.5 (Ebi et al. 2018), demonstrating the significant benefit that global greenhouse gas mitigation would have on the health of Americans. Similar to economic damages estimated using other methodologies (Gordon 2014; Jones et al. 2018; Marsha et al. 2016; Oleson et al. 2015; O'Neill et al.; Tebaldi and Wehner 2016), annual health impacts and costs are roughly halved under RCP4.5 in many of the sectors (Table 24.1; Figure 24.4).

---

[7] A mortality rate of 6.5 percent for WNND cases was used to calculate costs of premature deaths; non-fatal outcomes were assigned a cost of $41,391 to reflect incurred hospital charges for patients with meningitis, encephalitis, or acute flaccid paralysis syndrome.

[8] 100,000 cells/ml is a threshold determined by the World Health Organization to represent very high risk of short or long-term adverse health effects

Table 24.1   Projected Annual Physical Health Effects and Associated Economic Damages of Climate Change in 2090

		Health Outcomes			Economic Damages (in millions undiscounted $2015)	
		RCP4.5	RCP8.5		RCP4.5	RCP8.5
Extreme Temperatures	Number of premature deaths (adaptation not shown)	3,900 (2,400 to 7,400)	9,300 (5,400 to 13,000)	Income-adjusted VSL[9]	$59,000 ($37,000 to $110,000)	$140,000 ($82,000 to $200,000)
Labor	Lost labor hours (millions)	970 (620 to 1,500)	1,900 (1,000 to 2,700)	Lost wages (scaled by economic growth)	$80,000 ($52,000 to $120,000)	$160,000 ($87,000 to $220,000)
Ozone	Number of premature deaths (morbidity not shown)	1,200 (630 to 1,700)	1,700 (920 to 2,500)	Income-adjusted VSL	$18,000 ($1,600 to $51,000)	$26,000 (−$2,200 to $78,000)
Wildfire Smoke Exposure (Mills et al. 2018)	Number of people exposed to wildfire smoke (millions)	27.10	36.80	Not calculated	-	-
Fine and Coarse Dust (Achakulwisut et al. 2019)	Number of premature deaths (morbidity not shown)	3,800 (3,300 to 4,300)	4,200 (3,700 to 4,900)	Income-adjusted VSL	$54,000 ($49,000 to $61,000)	$60,000 ($47,000 to $70,000)
Aeroallergens (Neumann et al. 2018)	Asthma Emergency Department Visits (oak, birch, grass)	6,100 (2,200 to 11,000)	11,000 (4,000 to 20,000)	Cost per visit	$3.0 ($1.1 to $5.5)	$5.2 ($1.9 to $9.6)
West Nile Virus	Number of cases (WNND)	1,700 (1,200 to 2,400)	3,300 (2,000 to 4,600)	Income-adjusted VSL/ hospital costs	$1,800 ($1,200 to $2,500)	$3,300 ($2,000 to $4,700)
Harmful Algal Blooms	Number of days above 100k cells/ml	9 (2.7 to 15)	15 (6.5 to 24)	Lost consumer surplus	$110 ($54 to $230)	$200 ($130 to $390)
Total Annual Costs of CIRA Health Impacts[10]					$213,000 ($141,000 to $345,000)	$390,000 ($216,000 to $573,000)

Source: EPA (2017b).

These national estimates hide important regional variations across different health impacts (Martinich and Crimmins 2019). Ozone and aeroallergen impacts are greatest in the Midwest and Northeast; extreme temperature mortality and labor productivity impacts are severe in the Southeast; large dust impacts are projected in the Southwest, wildfire exposure and increased cases of West Nile virus are expected in the Northwest. Outside the CIRA framework, health impacts associated with hurricane and coastal flooding are projected to increase along the coasts,[11] including Hawaii, Puerto Rico, the Virgin Islands, and Guam (Gould et al. 2018; Keener et al. 2018), with very high associated economic damages (Fleming et al. 2018). Away from the coasts, health impacts are projected to occur from increasingly frequent and more severe inland flooding (Wobus et al. 2017) and drought (Wehner et al. 2017). There are no regions of the United States that escape some mix of adverse health impacts and associated economic damages from climate change.

[9] VSLs are adjusted to account for GDP and income growth such that adjusted income VSL is $10.0 million for the baseline year of 2015, $12.4 million in 2050, and $15.2 million in 2090

[10] As noted extensively throughout this chapter, there are many health impacts and economic costs not captured or only partially captured in the CIRA project; thus it is not accurate to assume these values to be the total sum of annual health damages projected for the United States in 2090. These values are very likely immensely underestimated.

[11] Limaye et al. (2019) estimated health costs associated with the 2012 Hurricane Sandy in New Jersey and New York to be greater than $3 billion (in 2018 dollars).

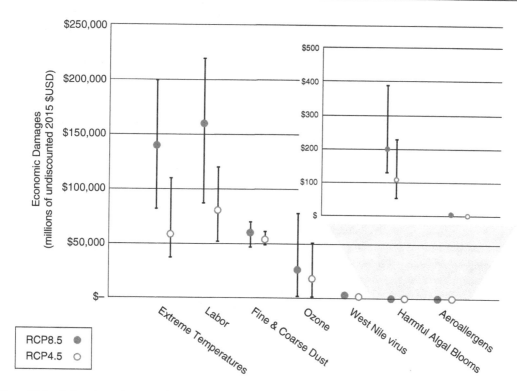

Figure 24.4 Projected annual economic damages from CIRA health impact sectors under two scenarios

Source: Adapted from Martinich and Crimmins (2019).

Note: Projected annual economic damages in the United States in 2090 are shown under RCP8.5 (filled circle) and RCP4.5 (open circle) for seven climate-related health impacts. Values are in millions of undiscounted 2015 dollars; data shown in Table 24.1. The inset provides a separate y-axis scale for harmful algal blooms and aeroallergens.

CLINICAL CORRELATES 24.3 SUPERSTORM SANDY

Superstorm Sandy devastated the New York metropolitan area in 2012. With its 14-foot storm surge, it disrupted basic patient care, hospital staffing, power supplies, and nutrition services throughout the region. The storms caused closure of four hospitals in New York City and New Jersey, including the primary safety-net tertiary care hospital in Manhattan for uninsured and underinsured patients. One emergency department was closed for eighteen months and 500 of its health care providers went elsewhere to work (Health Care Without Harm 2018). A large increase in health care utilization, including emergency department visits and hospitalizations, was demonstrated following the storm (McQuade et al. 2018).

As seen during Superstorm Sandy, closure of safety-net hospitals has rippling effects on patients having to seek care elsewhere: increased demands at surrounding hospitals, extended employment disruptions for health care workers, and expenses for recovery and as lost revenue.

CLINICAL CORRELATES 24.4 MORTALITY IN PUERTO RICO FROM HURRICANE MARIA

On September 20, 2017, hurricane Maria struck Puerto Rico just two weeks after hurricane Irma, causing a humanitarian crisis and nearly $100 billion dollars in damages (National Centers for Environmental Information 2019). By that December, the official death toll from the hurricane was reported at sixty-four people. This number was widely regarded as well below the actual attributable mortality, as each disaster-related death in Puerto Rico had to be confirmed by medical officials, who were themselves without power and relying on an unreliable system of paper records (Salas, Knappenberger, and Hess 2018).

Even with ample warnings, mortality rates increase after such extreme events because of lack of electricity, potable water and safe food, communication and transportation infrastructure, and access to adequate health care (Gould et al. 2018). In fact, the death toll in Puerto Rico grew by an estimated 1700% percent in the three months following Maria's landfall (Shultz et al. 2018). Several estimates of mortality have since been published. A study released in 2018 estimated 1,139 excess deaths in Puerto Rico between September and December 2017 (Santos-Lozada and Howard 2018). Another by researchers at the George Washington University's Milken Institute of Public Health, University of Puerto Rico, and John Hopkins University estimated 2,975 excess deaths (Santos-Burgoa et al. 2018), a number also cited by the National Oceanic and Atmospheric Administration (National Centers for Environmental Information 2019). A third group of researchers used door-to-door surveys to estimate a mean of 4,645 excess deaths (Kishore et al. 2018). Although difficult to attribute to just hurricane Maria, another study found a 26 percent increase in suicides in the first six months post-landfall (Ramphal 2018) and evidence from social media suggests a 17 percent increase in the number of Puerto Ricans migrating to the mainland United States in the year after Maria because of hardships from the hurricane (Alexander, Zagheni, and Polimis 2019). Indirect or long-term health impacts, such as those resulting from lost agricultural yields, injuries and illnesses during rebuilding, lost resiliency to future events, or morbidity from mental health conditions may never be fully quantified. Lack of consistent public health impact data makes it difficult to estimate the full extent of damages associated with this extreme event.

Summary

Assessing the benefits and costs of health improvements and damages is crucial to the process of making informed decisions about protecting human health and addressing climate change. Climate-related health impact valuation continues to be a growing field, with new modeling capabilities leading to frequent advancements in our estimates of climate damages to health. Despite a limited set of internally consistent economic studies and gaps in the health sectors where climate impacts have been estimated, it is evident that damages to the United States are projected to be very large, especially without global mitigation actions.

DISCUSSION QUESTIONS

1. What are the pros and cons of different ways of measuring benefits and costs?

2. What other health costs were not included in the examples described in the chapter?

3. What makes economic damages of certain health sectors (e.g., from extreme temperatures or increased ozone) greater than other sectors (e.g., aeroallergens)?

4. This chapter primarily reported national estimates of climate-related health damages. How do you think these damages would differ by state or region? What communities would face unique costs?

5. How does the valuation of climate change impacts on human health consider (or fail to consider) environmental justice?

KEY TERMS

Benefit-Cost Analysis (BCA): An analysis that compares the costs and benefits of an action in monetary terms.

Cost-effectiveness analysis (CEA): An analysis that determines which alternative most efficiently uses available resources (monetary or not) to achieve a given goal.

Cost-of-illness (COI): A measure of the costs resulting from a disease or condition (or the monetary expression of total burden of disease), including the direct medical and nonmedical costs, lost productivity, and other costs to society.

Dose-, exposure-, or **concentration response function:** The **relative risk** of adverse health outcomes at various dose, exposure, or concentration levels.

Health impact function: Equation used to estimate the number of health outcomes (e.g., mortality or morbidity events) in a population associated with a given exposure.

Integrated assessment model (IAM): Computer modeling frameworks that link human behaviors (e.g., population characteristics, economic development, emissions of greenhouse gases, etc.) with physical earth dynamics (e.g., atmosphere-ocean interactions, carbon storage in the biosphere, etc.) to inform environmental policy.

Quality-adjusted life year (QALY) and **disability-adjusted life year (DALY):** Metrics used for measuring morbidity benefits or costs; see chapter text for detailed explanations.

Relative risk: The probability of an exposed group of people experiencing an adverse health outcome in relation to the probability of that outcome in an unexposed group.

Social cost of carbon (SCC): A measure of the net present value to the global society of emitting one additional unit of CO_2.

Value of a statistical life (VSL): A calculation of the value of a small change in the risk of death, better termed "value of mortality risk."

Willingness-to-pay (WTP) or **willingness-to-accept (WTA):** WTP is what an individual would pay to avoid a health impact; WTA is the least amount of payment an individual would accept to experience the health impact.

References

Achakulwisut, P., S. C. Anenberg, J. E. Neumann, S. L. Penn, N. Weiss, A. Crimmins, N. Fann et al. 2019. "Effects of Increasing Aridity on Ambient Dust and Public Health in the U.S. Southwest under Climate Change." *GeoHealth* Published April 5, 2019. https://doi.org/10.1029/2019GH000187.

Adrion, E. R., J. Aucott, K. W. Lemke, and J. P. Weiner. 2015. "Health Care Costs, Utilization and Patterns of Care Following Lyme Disease." *PLoS ONE* 10 (2):e0116767. https://doi.org/10.1371/journal.pone.0116767.

Alexander, M., E. Zagheni, and K. Polimis. (2019). "The Impact of Hurricane Maria on Out-Migration From Puerto Rico: Evidence from Facebook Data." January 28, 2019. https://doi.org/10.31235/osf.io/39s6c.

Anenberg, S. C., K. R. Weinberger, H. Roman, J. E. Neumann, A. Crimmins, N. Fann, J. Martinich, and P. L. Kinney. 2017. "Impacts of Oak Pollen on Allergic Asthma in the United States and Potential Influence of Future Climate Change." *GeoHealth* 1. doi:10.1002/2017GH000055.

Balbus, J., A. Crimmins, J. L. Gamble, D. R. Easterling, K. E. Kunkel, S. Saha, and M. C. Sarofim. 2016. "Introduction: Climate Change and Human Health." In *The Impacts of Climate Change on Human Health in the United States: A Scientific Assessment*, 25–42. Washington, DC: U.S. Global Change Research Program. http://dx.doi.org/10.7930/J0VX0DFW.

Beard, C. B., R. J. Eisen, C. M. Barker, J. F. Garofalo, M. Hahn, M. Hayden, A. J. Monaghan, N. H. Ogden, and P. J. Schramm. 2016. " Vector-Borne Diseases." In *The Impacts of Climate Change on Human Health in the United States: A Scientific Assessment*, 129–56. Washington, DC: U.S. Global Change Research Program. http://dx.doi.org/10.7930/J0765C7V.

Bell, M. L., and F. Dominici. 2008. "Effect Modification by Community Characteristics on the Short-Term Effects of Ozone Exposure and Mortality in 98 US Communities." *American Journal of Epidemiology* 167:986–97. doi:10.1093/aje/kwm396.

Belova, A., D. Mills, R. Hall, A. S. Juliana, A. Crimmins, C. Barker, and R. Jones. 2017. "Impacts of Increasing Temperature on the Future Incidence of West Nile Neuroinvasive Disease in the United States." *American Journal of Climate Change* 6:166–216. https://doi.org/10.4236/ajcc.2017.61010.

Bureau of Labor Statistics. 2017. "Quarterly Census of Employment and Wages." https://www.bls.gov/cew/publications/employment-and-wages-annual-averages/2017/home.htm.

Centers for Disease Control and Prevention. 2016. "West Nile Virus Statistics and Maps." https://www.cdc.gov/westnile/statsmaps/index.html.

Chapra, S. C., B. Boehlert, C. Fant, V. J. Bierman, J. Henderson, D. Mills, D. M. L. Mas et al. 2017. "Climate Change Impacts on Harmful Algal Blooms in U.S. Freshwaters: A Screening-Level Assessment." *Environmental Science and Technology* 51 (16):8933–43. doi:10.1021/acs.est.7b01498.

Chestnut, L. G. 1999. "Air Quality Valuation Model v3." Stratus Consulting.

Collins, M., R. Knutti, J. Arblaster, J.-L. Dufresne, T. Fichefet, P. Friedlingstein, X. Gao et al. 2013. "Long-Term Climate Change: Projections, Commitments and Irreversibility." In *Climate Change 2013: The Physical Science Basis. Contribution of Working Group I to the Fifth Assessment Report of the Intergovernmental Panel on Climate Change*, edited by T. F. Stocker, D. Qin, G.-K. Plattner, M. Tignor, S. K. Allen, J. Boschung, A. Nauels et al., 1029–1136. Cambridge and New York: Cambridge University Press.

Council on Economic Advisors. 2017. *Discounting for Public Policy: Theory and Evidence on the Merits of Updating the Discount Rate. Issue Brief of The White House.* https://obamawhitehouse.archives.gov/sites/default/files/page/files/201701_cea_discounting_issue_brief.pdf.

Crimmins, A., J. Balbus, J. L. Gamble, D. R. Easterling, K. L. Ebi, J. Hess, K. E. Kunkel, D. M. Mills, and M. C. Sarofim. 2016a. "Appendix 1: Technical Support Document: Modeling Future Climate Impacts on Human Health." In *The Impacts of Climate Change on Human Health in the United States: A Scientific Assessment*, 287–300. Washington, DC: U.S. Global Change Research Program. http://dx.doi.org/10.7930/J0KH0K83.

Crimmins, A., J. Balbus, J. L. Gamble, C. B. Beard, J. E. Bell, D. Dodgen, R. J. Eisen et al., eds. 2016b. *The Impacts of Climate Change on Human Health in the United States: A Scientific Assessment.* Washington, DC: U.S. Global Change Research Program. http://dx.doi.org/10.7930/J0R49NQX.

Diaz, D., and F. Moore. 2017. *Valuing Potential Climate Impacts: A Review of Current Limitations and the Research Frontier.* Report# 3002011885. Palo Alto, CA: Electric Power Research Institute.

Diffenbaugh, N., and M. Burke. 2019. "Global Warming Has Increased Global Economic Inequality." *Proceedings of the National Academy of Sciences of the USA* 116 (20):9808–13.

Dodgen, D., D. Donato, N. Kelly, A. La Greca, J. Morganstein, J. Reser, J. Ruzek et al. 2016. " Mental Health and Well-Being." In *The Impacts of Climate Change on Human Health in the United States: A Scientific Assessment*, 217–46. Washington, DC: U.S. Global Change Research Program. http://dx.doi.org/10.7930/J0TX3C9H.

Ebi, K. L., J. M. Balbus, G. Luber, A. Bole, A. Crimmins, G. Glass, S. Saha et al. 2018. "Human Health." In *Impacts, Risks, and Adaptation in the United States: Fourth National Climate Assessment, Vol. II*, edited by D. R. Reidmiller, C. W. Avery, D. R. Easterling, K. E. Kunkel, K. L. M. Lewis, T. K. Maycock, and B. C. Stewart, 539–71. Washington, DC: U.S. Global Change Research Program. doi: 10.7930/NCA4.2018.CH14.

Environmental Protection Agency. 2010a. *Guidelines for Preparing Economic Analyses. Appendix A Economic Theory.* Washington, DC: EPA. https://www.epa.gov/sites/production/files/2017-09/documents/ee-0568-21.pdf.

Environmental Protection Agency. 2010b. *Guidelines for Preparing Economic Analyses. Chapter 7 Analyzing Benefits.* Washington, DC: EPA. https://www.epa.gov/sites/production/files/2017-09/documents/ee-0568-07.pdf.

Environmental Protection Agency. 2017a. *Multi-Model Framework for Quantitative Sectoral Impacts Analysis: A Technical Report for the Fourth National Climate Assessment.* EPA 430-R-17-001. Washington, DC: EPA.

Environmental Protection Agency. 2017b. *Technical Appendix for Multi-Model Framework for Quantitative Sectoral Impacts Analysis: A Technical Report for the Fourth National Climate Assessment.* EPA 430-R-17-001. Washington, DC: EPA.

Environmental Protection Agency. 2018a. "Climate Change in the United States: Benefits of Action." Updated November 2018. https://www.epa.gov/cira.

Environmental Protection Agency. 2018b. "Mortality Risk Valuation." Updated February 2018. https://www.epa.gov/environmental-economics/mortality-risk-valuation.

Fann, N., T. Brennan, P. Dolwick, J. L. Gamble, V. Ilacqua, L. Kolb, C. G. Nolte, T. L. Spero, and L. Ziska. 2016. "Air Quality Impacts." In *The Impacts of Climate Change on Human Health in the United States: A Scientific Assessment*, 69–98. Washington, DC: U.S. Global Change Research Program. http://dx.doi.org/10.7930/J0GQ6VP.

Fann, N., C. G. Nolte, P. Dolwick, T. L. Spero, A. Curry Brown, S. Phillips, and S. Anenberg. 2015. "The Geographic Distribution and Economic Value of Climate Change-Related Ozone Health Impacts in the United States in 2030." *Journal of the Air & Waste Management Association* 65:570–80. http://dx.doi.org/10.1080/10962247.2014.996270.

Fleming, E., J. Payne, W. Sweet, M. Craghan, J. Haines, J. F. Hart, H. Stiller, and A. Sutton-Grier. 2018.: "Coastal Effects." In *Impacts, Risks, and Adaptation in the United States: Fourth National Climate Assessment, Vol. II*, edited by D. R. Reidmiller, C. W. Avery, D. R. Easterling, K. E. Kunkel, K. L. M. Lewis, T. K. Maycock, and B. C. Stewart, 322–52. Washington, DC: U.S. Global Change Research Program. doi: 10.7930/NCA4.2018.CH8.

Gamble, J. L., J. Balbus, M. Berger, K. Bouye, V. Campbell, K. Chief, K. Conlon et al. 2016. " Populations of Concern." *The Impacts of Climate Change on Human Health in the United States: A Scientific Assessment*, 247–86. Washington, DC: U.S. Global Change Research Program. doi: 10.7930/J0Q81B0T.

Garcia-Menendez, F., R. K. Saari, E. Monier, and N. E. Selin. 2015. "U.S. Air Quality and Health Benefits from Avoided Climate Change under Greenhouse Gas Mitigation." *Environmental Science and Technology* 49:7580–8. doi:10.1021/acs.est.5b01324.

Gordon, K. 2014. *Risky Business: The Economic Risks of Climate Change in the United States. A Climate Risk Assessment for the United States*, edited by M. Lewis and J. Rogers. New York: Risky Business Project. http://riskybusiness.org/site/assets/uploads/2015/09/RiskyBusiness_Report_WEB_09_08_14.pdf.

Gould, W. A., E. L. Díaz, N. L. Álvarez-Berríos, F. Aponte-González, W. Archibald, J. H. Bowden, L. Carrubba et al. 2018. "U.S. Caribbean." In *Impacts, Risks, and Adaptation in the United States: Fourth National Climate Assessment, Vol. II*, edited by D. R. Reidmiller, C. W. Avery, D. R. Easterling, K. E. Kunkel, K. L. M. Lewis, T. K. Maycock, and B. C. Stewart, 809–71. Washington, DC: U.S. Global Change Research Program. doi:10.7930/NCA4.2018.CH20

Graff Zivin, J., and M. Neidell. 2014. "Temperature and the Allocation of Time: Implications for Climate Change." *Journal of Labor Economics* 32:1–26. doi:10.1086/671766.

Hahn, M. B., A. J. Monaghan, M. H. Hayden, R. J. Eisen, M. J. Delorey, N. P. Lindsey, R. S. Nasci, and M. Fischer. 2015. "Meteorological Conditions Associated with Increased Incidence of West Nile Virus Disease in the United States, 2004–2012." *American Journal of Tropical Medicine and Hygiene* 92 (5):1013–22. doi:10.4269/ajtmh.14- 0737

Hayes, K., G. Blashki, J. Wiseman, S. Burke, and L. Reifels. 2018. "Climate Change and Mental Health: Risks, Impacts and Priority Actions." *International Journal of Mental Health Systems* 12:28 https://doi.org/10.1186/s13033-018-0210-6.

Health Care Without Harm. 2018. "Safe Haven in the Storm." Reston, VA: HCWH. https://noharm-uscanada.org/safehaven.

Hilborn, E. D., V. A. Roberts, L. Backer, E. DeConno, J. S. Egan, J. B. Hyde, D. C. Nicholas et al. 2014. "Algal Bloom–Associated Disease Outbreaks among Users of Freshwater Lakes—United States, 2009–2010." *MMWR. Morbidity and Mortality Weekly Report* 63:11–15. http://www.cdc.gov/mmwr/preview/mmwrhtml/mm6301a3.htm.

Hoagland, P., D. Jin, A. Beet, B. Kirkpatrick, A. Reich, S. Ullmann, L. E. Fleming, and G. Kirkpatrick. 2014. "The Human Health Effects of Florida Red Tide (FRT) Blooms: An Expanded Analysis." *Environment International* 68:144–53. https://doi.org/10.1016/j.envint.2014.03.016.

Hope, C. W. 2006. "The Marginal Impact of CO2 from PAGE2002: An Integrated Assessment Model Incorporating the IPCC's Five Reasons for Concern." *The Integrated Assessment Journal* 6 (1):19–56.

Houser, T., S. Hsiang, R. Kopp, K. Larsen, M. Delgado, A. Jina, M. Mastrandrea et al. 2015. *Economic Risks of Climate Change: An American Prospectus*. New York: Columbia University Press.

Hsiang, S., R. Kopp, A. Jina, J. Rising, M. Delgado, S. Mohan, D. J. Rasmussen et al. 2017. "Estimating Economic Damage from Climate Change in the United States." *Science* 356 (6345):1362–69. doi:10.1126/science.aal4369.

Interagency Working Group on Social Cost of Carbon, United States Government. 2010. *Technical Support Document: Social Cost of Carbon for Regulatory Impact Analysis Under Executive Order 12866*. https://obamawhitehouse.archives.gov/sites/default/files/omb/inforeg/for-agencies/Social-Cost-of-Carbon-for-RIA.pdf.

Interagency Working Group on Social Cost of Greenhouse Gases, United States Government. 2016. Technical Support Document: *Technical Update of the Social Cost of Carbon for Regulatory Impact Analysis Under Executive Order 12866*. https://www.epa.gov/sites/production/files/2016-12/documents/sc_co2_tsd_august_2016.pdf.

Johnsen, M. 2017. "Record-Breaking Heat, Precipitation Make Allergy Medications More Important." *Drugstore News*, March 2017, 16.

Jones, B., C. Tebaldi, B. C. O'Neill, K. Oleson, and J. Gao, 2018: "Avoiding Population Exposure to Heat-Related Extremes: Demographic Change vs Climate Change." *Climatic Change* 146 (3):423–37. doi:10.1007/s10584-017-2133-7.

Keener, V., D. Helweg, S. Asam, S. Balwani, M. Burkett, C. Fletcher, T. Giambelluca et al. 2018. "Hawai'i and U.S.-Affiliated Pacific Islands." In *Impacts, Risks, and Adaptation in the United States: Fourth*

National Climate Assessment, Vol. II, edited by D. R. Reidmiller, C. W. Avery, D. R. Easterling, K. E. Kunkel, K. L. M. Lewis, T. K. Maycock, and B. C. Stewart, 1242–1308. Washington, DC: U.S. Global Change Research Program. doi:10.7930/NCA4.2018.CH27.

Kim, J., A. Lee, and M. Rossin-Slater. 2019. *What to Expect When It Gets Hotter: The Impacts of Prenatal Exposure to Extreme Heat on Maternal and Infant Health. NBER Working Paper No. 26384.* Cambridge, MA: National Bureau for Economic Research. https://www.nber.org/papers/w26384.

Kishore, N., D. Marqués, A. Mahmud, M. V. Kiang, I. Rodriguez, A. Fuller, P. Ebner et al. 2018. "Mortality in Puerto Rico after Hurricane Maria." *New England Journal of Medicine* 379 (2):162–70. http://www.nejm.org/doi/10.1056/NEJMsa1803972.

Konkel, L. 2019. "Taking the Heat: Potential Fetal Health Effects of Hot Temperatures." *Environmental Health Perspectives.* 127:10. https://doi.org/10.1289/EHP6221.

Kopp, R. E., K. Hayhoe, D. R. Easterling, T. Hall, R. Horton, K. E. Kunkel, and A. N. LeGrande. 2017. "Potential Surprises—Compound Extremes and Tipping Elements." In *Climate Science Special Report: Fourth National Climate Assessment, Vol. I*, edited by D. J. Wuebbles, D. W. Fahey, K. A. Hibbard, D. J. Dokken, B. C. Stewart, and T. K. Maycock. 411–29. Washington, DC: U.S. Global Change Research Program. doi: 10.7930/J0GB227J.

Limaye, V. S., W. Max., J. Constible, and K. Knowlton. 2019. "Estimating the Health-Related Costs of 10 Climate-Sensitive U.S. Events during 2012." *GeoHealth* 3 (9):245–65. https://doi.org/10.1029/2019GH000202.

Lindsey, N. P., J. A. Lehman, E. Staples, and M. Fischer. 2015. "West Nile Virus and Other Nationally Notifiable Arboviral Diseases—United States, 2014." *MMWR. Morbidity and Mortality Weekly Report* 64:929–34.

Mac, S., S. R. da Silva, and B. Sander. 2019. "The Economic Burden of Lyme Disease and the Cost-Effectiveness of Lyme Disease Interventions: A Scoping Review." *PLoS One* 14 (1):e0210280. https://doi.org/10.1371/journal.pone.0210280.

Marsha, A., S. R. Sain, M. J. Heaton, A. J. Monaghan, and O. V. Wilhelmi. 2016. "Influences of Climatic and Population Changes on Heat-Related Mortality in Houston, Texas, USA." *Climatic Change* 146:471–85. doi:10.1007/s10584-016-1775-1.

Martinich, J., and A. Crimmins. 2019. "Climate Damages and Adaptation Potential across Diverse Sectors of the United States." *Nature Climate Change* 9:397–404. https://www.nature.com/articles/s41558-019-0444-6.

Martinich, J., B. J. DeAngelo, D. Diaz, B. Ekwurzel, G. Franco, C. Frisch, J. McFarland, and B. O'Neill. 2018. "Reducing Risks through Emissions Mitigation." In *Impacts, Risks, and Adaptation in the United States: Fourth National Climate Assessment, Vol. II*, edited by D. R. Reidmiller, C. W. Avery, D. R. Easterling, K. E. Kunkel, K. L. M. Lewis, T. K. Maycock, and B. C. Stewart, 1346–86. Washington, DC: U.S. Global Change Research Program. doi: 10.7930/NCA4.2018.CH29.

Martinez, G. S., E. William, and S. S. Yu. 2015. "The Economics of Health Damage and Adaptation to Climate Change in Europe: A Review of the Conventional and Grey Literature." *Climate* 3:522–41.

McQuade, L., B. Merriman, M. Lyford, B. Nadler, S. Desai, R. Miller, and S. Mallette. 2018. "Emergency Department and Inpatient Health Care Services Utilization by the Elderly Population: Hurricane Sandy in the State of New Jersey." *Disaster Medicine and Public Health Preparedness* 12 (6):730–8.

Mills, D., R. Jones, C. Wobus, J. Ekstrom, L. Jantarasami, A. St. Juliana, A. Crimmins. 2018. "Projecting Age-Stratified Risk of Exposure to Inland Flooding and Wildfire Smoke in the United States under Two Climate Scenarios." *Environmental Health Perspectives* 126(4):047007.

Mills, D., J. Schwartz, M. Lee, M. Sarofim, R. Jones, M. Lawson, M. Duckworth, and L. Deck. 2014. "Climate Change Impacts on Extreme Temperature Mortality in Select Metropolitan Areas in the United States." *Climatic Change* doi: 10.1007/s10584-014-1154-8.

Müller, C., J. Elliott, J. Chryssanthacopoulos, A. Arneth, J. Balkovic, P. Ciais, D. Deryng et al. 2017. "Global Gridded Crop Model Evaluation: Benchmarking, Skills, Deficiencies and Implications." *Geoscientific Model Development* 10 (4):1403–22. doi:10.5194/gmd-10-1403-2017.

Nathan, R. A. 2007. "The Burden of Allergic Rhinitis." *Allergy and Asthma Proceedings* 28:3–9.

National Centers for Environmental Information. 2019. "U.S. Billion-Dollar Weather and Climate Disasters." Updated July 2019. Accessed September 3, 2019. https://www.ncdc.noaa.gov/billions/summary-stats.

Neumann, J. E., S. C. Anenberg, K. R. Weinberger, M. Amend, S. Gulati, A. Crimmins, H. Roman, N. Fann, and P. L. Kinney. 2018. "Estimates of Present and Future Asthma Emergency Department Visits Associated with Exposure to Oak, Birch, and Grass Pollen in the United States." *GeoHealth* 3 (1):11–27.

Nolan, M. S., A. M. Hause, and K. O. Murray. 2012. "Findings of Long-Term Depression up to 8 Years Post Infection from West Nile Virus." *Journal of Clinical Psychology* 68:801–8. doi:10.1002/jclp.21871.

Nolte, C. G., P. D. Dolwick, N. Fann, L. W. Horowitz, V. Naik, R. W. Pinder, T. L. Spero, D. A. Winner, and L. H. Ziska., 2018. "Air Quality." In *Impacts, Risks, and Adaptation in the United States: Fourth National Climate Assessment, Vol. II*, edited by D. R. Reidmiller, C. W. Avery, D. R. Easterling, K. E. Kunkel, K. L. M. Lewis, T. K. Maycock, and B. C. Stewart, 512–38. Washington, DC: U.S. Global Change Research Program. doi: 10.7930/NCA4.2018.CH13.

Nordhaus, W. D. 1992. "An Optimal Transition Path for Controlling Greenhouse Gases. *Science* 258 (5086):1315–19.

Nordhaus, W. D. 2010. "Economic Aspects of Global Warming in a Post-Copenhagen Environment." *Proceedings of the National Academy of Sciences of the USA* 107 (26):11721–26.

Obradovich, N., R. Migliorinic, M. P. Paulus, and I. Rahwana. 2018. "Empirical Evidence of Mental Health Risks Posed by Climate Change." *Proceedings of the National Academy of Sciences of the USA* 115 (43):10953–8.

Office of Management and Budget. 2003. *Regulatory Analysis. Circular A4.* https://www.whitehouse.gov/sites/whitehouse.gov/files/omb/circulars/A4/a-4.pdf.

Oleson, K. W., G. B. Anderson, B. Jones, S. A. McGinnis, and B. Sanderson. 2015. "Avoided Climate Impacts of Urban and Rural Heat and Cold Waves over the U.S. Using Large Climate Model Ensembles for RCP8.5 and RCP4.5." *Climatic Change* 146 (3–4):377–92. doi:10.1007/s10584-015-1504-1.

O'Neill, B. C., J. M. Done, A. Gettelman, P. Lawrence, F. Lehner, J.-F. Lamarque, L. Lin et al. 2017. "The Benefits of Reduced Anthropogenic Climate changE (BRACE): A Synthesis." *Climatic Change* doi:10.1007/s10584-017-2009-x.

Ramphal, L. 2018. "Medical and Psychosocial Needs of the Puerto Rican People after Hurricane Maria." *Proceedings (Baylor University. Medical Center)* 31 (3):294–6. http://www.ncbi.nlm.nih.gov/pubmed/29904291.

Roberts, D. 2012. "Discount Rates: A Boring Thing You Should Know About (with Otters!). *Grist,* September 24 2012. https://grist.org/article/discount-rates-a-boring-thing-you-should-know-about-with-otters/.

Rosenzweig, C., J. Elliott, D. Deryng, A. C. Ruane, C. Müller, A. Arneth, K. J. Boote et al. 2014. "Assessing Agricultural Risks of Climate Change in the 21st Century in a Global Gridded Crop Model Intercomparison." *Proceedings of the National Academy of Sciences of the USA* 111 (9):3268–73. doi:10.1073/pnas.1222463110.

Sacks, J. D., L. W. Stanek, T. J. Luben, D. O. Johns, B. J. Buckley, J. S. Brown, and M. Ross., 2011. "Particulate Matter–Induced Health Effects: Who Is Susceptible?" *Environmental Health Perspectives* 119:446–54. doi: 10.1289/ehp.1002255.

Salas, R. N., P. Knappenberger, and J. J. Hess. 2018. *2018 Lancet Countdown on Health and Climate Change Brief for the United States of America. Lancet Countdown U.S. Brief.* London: Lancet Countdown.

Santos-Burgoa, C., J. Sandberg, E. Suárez, A. Goldman-Hawes, S. Zeger, A. Garcia-Meza, and C. M. Pérez. 2018. "Differential and Persistent Risk of Excess Mortality from Hurricane Maria in Puerto Rico: A Time-Series Analysis." *Lancet Planetary Health* 2:e478–88.

Santos-Lozada, A. R., and J. T. Howard. 2018. "Use of Death Counts from Vital Statistics to Calculate Excess Deaths in Puerto Rico Following Hurricane Maria." *JAMA* 320:14.

Sarofim, M. C., S. Saha, M. D. Hawkins, D. M. Mills, J. Hess, R. Horton, P. Kinney, J. Schwartz, and A. St. Juliana. 2016. "Temperature Related Death and Illness. "In *The Impacts of Climate Change on Human Health in the United States: A Scientific Assessment*, 43–68. Washington, DC: U.S. Global Change Research Program. doi: 10.7930/J0MG7MDX.

Shultz, J. M., J. P. Kossin, J. M. Shepherd, J. M. Ransdell, R. Walshe, I. Kelman, and S. Galea. 2018. "Risk, Health Consequences, and Response Challenges for Small-Island-Based Populations: Observations from the 2017 Atlantic Hurricane Season." *Disaster Medicine and Public Health Preparedness* 1–13. doi:10.1017/dmp.2018.28.

Smith, J. B., M. Muth, A. Alpert, J. L. Buizer, J. Cook, A. Dave, J. Furlow et al. 2018. "Climate Effects on U.S. International Interests." In *Impacts, Risks, and Adaptation in the United States: Fourth National Climate Assessment, Vol. II*, edited by D. R. Reidmiller, C. W. Avery, D. R. Easterling, K. E. Kunkel, K. L. M. Lewis, T. K. Maycock, and B. C. Stewart, 604–37. Washington, DC: U.S. Global Change Research Program. doi: 10.7930/NCA4.2018.CH16.

Stavins, R. 2007. *Environmental Economics. NBER Working Paper 13574.* Cambridge, MA: National Bureau of Economic Research.

Stokey, E., and R. Zeckhauser. 1978. *A Primer for Policy Analysis.* New York: W.W. Norton.

Tebaldi, C., and M. F. Wehner. 2016. "Benefits of Mitigation for Future Heat Extremes under RCP4.5 Compared to RCP8.5." *Climatic Change* First online, 1–13. doi:10.1007/s10584-016-1605-5.

Teitenberg, T., and L. Lewis. 2009. *Environmental & Natural Resource Economics*, 8th ed. Boston, MA: Pearson Education Inc.

Tol, R. S. J. 1995. "The Damage Costs of Climate Change toward More Comprehensive Calculations." *Environmental & Resource Economics* 5 (4):353–74.

Tol, R. S. J. 1996. "The Damage Costs of Climate Change toward a Dynamic Representation." *Ecological Economics* 19:67–90. https://pdfs.semanticscholar.org/6d37/c4fb0aa012cea0606fffd97 0874f1f09e099.pdf.

Trtanj, J., L. Jantarasami, J. Brunkard, T. Collier, J. Jacobs, E. Lipp, S. McLellan et al. 2016. "Climate Impacts on Water-Related Illness." In *The Impacts of Climate Change on Human Health in the United States: A Scientific Assessment*, 157–88. Washington, DC: U.S. Global Change Research Program. http://dx.doi.org/10.7930/J03F4MH.

Viscusi, W. K. 1995. "Discounting Health Effects for Medical Decisions." In *Valuing Health Care: Costs, Benefits, and Effectiveness of Pharmaceuticals and Medical Technologies*, edited by F. A. Sloan, 125–47. New York: Cambridge University Press.

Vose, R. S., D. R. Easterling, K. E. Kunkel, A. N. LeGrande, and M. F. Wehner. 2017. "Temperature Changes in the United States." In *Climate Science Special Report: Fourth National Climate Assessment, Vol. I*, edited by D. J. Wuebbles, D. W. Fahey, K. A. Hibbard, D. J. Dokken, B. C. Stewart, and T. K. Maycock, 185–206. Washington, DC: U.S. Global Change Research Program. doi: 10.7930/J0N29V45.

Wehner, M. F., J. R. Arnold, T. Knutson, K. E. Kunkel, and A. N. LeGrande. 2017. "Droughts, Floods, and Wildfires." In *Climate Science Special Report: Fourth National Climate Assessment, Vol. I*, edited by D. J. Wuebbles, D. W. Fahey, K. A. Hibbard, D. J. Dokken, B. C. Stewart, and T. K. Maycock, 231–56. Washington, DC: U.S. Global Change Research Program. doi: 10.7930/J0CJ8BNN.

Weinstein, M. C. 1990. "Principles of Cost-Effective Resource Allocation in Health Care Organizations." *International Journal of Technology Assessment in Health Care* 6 (1):93–103.

Weitzman, M. L. 2009. "On Modeling and Interpreting the Economics of Catastrophic Climate Change." *Review of Economics and Statistics* 91 (1):1–19.

Wobus, C., E. D. Gutmann, R. Jones, M. Rissing, N. Mizukami, M. Lorie, H. Mahoney et al. 2017. "Climate Change Impacts on Flood Risk and Asset Damages within Mapped 100-Year Floodplains of the Contiguous United States." *National Hazards and Earth Systems Sciences* 17:2199–2211.

World Health Organization. 1999. *Toxic Cyanobacteria in Water: A Guide to Their Public Health Consequences, Monitoring and Management*. London: E & FN Spon. http://www.who.int/water_sanitation_health/resourcesquality/toxcyanobacteria.pdf?ua=1.

World Health Organization. 2013. *WHO Methods and Data Sources for Global Burden of Disease Estimates 2000–2011*. Global Health Estimates Technical Paper WHO/HIS/HSI/GHE/2013.4. Geneva: WHO. https://www.who.int/healthinfo/statistics/GlobalDALYmethods_2000_2011.pdf.

Wu, S., L. J. Mickley, E. M. Leibensperger, D. J. Jacob, D. Rind, and D. G. Streets. 2008. "Effects of 2000–2050 Global Change on Ozone Air Quality in the United States." *Journal of Geophysical Research* 113:D06302. doi:10.1029/2007JD008917.

CHAPTER 25

HEALTH CARE SYSTEM RESILIENCE

Caitlin S. Rublee, Emilie Calvello Hynes, and John M. Balbus

Introduction

Climate-related extreme weather events have major direct impacts on health care facilities, patient care, and sectors relied upon by health care such as transportation, food, energy, water, information technology, and communications (Health Care Without Harm 2018). Climate-related disasters also significantly affect the human resources required to support service delivery; high-quality direct patient care, essential laboratory services, and environmental services rely on various skilled professionals who are affected as individuals and community members by climate-related disasters (Kabene et al. 2006). In addition to essential medical services, health care facilities provide critical nonmedical resources to communities in the wake of disasters; hospitals can become default providers of shelter, food, water, energy, and sanitation when community access is disrupted (Berkowitz et al. 2018; Doran et al. 2016; Gray and Hebert, 2006; Swerdel et al. 2016; Texas Hospital Association 2018).

Health care facilities may undergo forced evacuation and closure during and after extreme weather events, resulting in direct mortality and indirect postclosure morbidity and mortality (Sternberg, Lee, and Huard, 2004; U.S. Department of Health and Human Services, 2014; Willoughby et al. 2017). For example, Hurricane Maria caused a 62% increase in the Puerto Rican mortality rate and almost 3,000 excess deaths (Kishore et al. 2018; Santos-Burgoa et al. 2018). At least one third of those deaths were attributable to delayed or interrupted health care as a result of closures. Similar effects are documented elsewhere (Bell et al. 2018; Gray and Hebert, 2006; Issa et al. 2018; Thomas et al. 2012). According to the Pan American Health Organization (PAHO), every hospital disabled because of disasters in Latin America and the Caribbean leaves an estimated 200,000 people without services, often for months to years (PAHO 2014). Populations with disabilities, chronic diseases, low socioeconomic status, some racial and ethnic minorities, and older adults are especially vulnerable to adverse health consequence as a result of loss of access to health care (U.S. Global Change Research Program [USGCRP] 2016). Furthermore, disproportionate loss of access to services can further exacerbate health disparities. (Davis et al. 2010; Hutchins et al. 2018).

A number of international, national, and nongovernmental organizations recognize this imminent threat to health by the loss of health care facilities and are developing frameworks and guidance to assist decision-makers with clear steps to enhance resilience. This chapter reviews these conceptual frameworks and guidelines, beginning with definitions of terms and an overview of climate-related hazards to health care delivery. The chapter concludes with a set of case studies, emphasis on health system disparities, and a discussion of ongoing research needs to answer critical questions.

KEY CONCEPTS

- Extreme weather events impair health service delivery through damage to health care facilities and their supporting infrastructure.

- The disruption of access to health care services may result in significantly more deaths and illnesses than the direct impacts of the events.

- Guidance and initiatives for increasing health care facility resilience are available for low-, middle-, and high-income countries.

- Increased climate-related extreme weather events create an urgent need for climate-smart health care to support communities and healthy populations.

Table 25.1   Definitions of Concepts Relevant to Health Care System Impacts and Preparedness

Key Term	Definition
Exposure	Contact between a person [or health care facility] and one or more biological, psychosocial, chemical, or physical stressors, including stressors affected by climate change (USGCRP 2016)
Sensitivity	The degree to which people or communities are affected, either adversely or beneficially, by climate variability or change (USGCRP 2016)
Adaptive capacity	The ability of communities, institutions, or people to adjust to potential hazards, to take advantage of opportunities, or to respond to consequences (USGCRP 2016)
Resilience (climate context)	The ability of a system and its component parts to anticipate, absorb, accommodate, or recover from the effects of a hazardous event in a timely and efficient manner, including through ensuring the preservation, restoration, or improvement of its essential basic structures and functions (Intergovernmental Panel on Climate Change [IPCC] 2012)
Disaster resilience	The ability of countries, communities, and households to manage change, by maintaining or transforming living standards in the face of shocks or stresses—such as earthquakes, drought, or violent conflict— without compromising their long-term prospects (Department for International Development 2011)
Health care system resilience	Capacity of the system itself to cope with and manage health risks in a way that the essential functions, identity, and structure of health systems are maintained (WHO 2015)
Climate-resilient health system	Capable to anticipate, respond to, cope with, recover from and adapt to climate-related shocks and stress, so as to bring sustained improvements in population health, despite an unstable climate (WHO 2015)

Definitions

Various definitions of **resilience** have been used by different scientific disciplines and policy communities (Table 25.1). In simplified terms, resilience involves an individual, community, or system's ability to absorb a shock or stress and maintain functionality. The World Health Organization (WHO) defines resilience as decreased vulnerability with increased adaptive capacity and improved choices and opportunities that transform outcomes (WHO 2015) (Figure 25.1). Health system resilience is prioritized when addressing health effects of climate related stressors. **Vulnerability** is composed of exposure, sensitivity, and adaptive capacity (USGCRP 2016) and the term can be applied to individuals, populations, and health care systems. During a climate stressor, individual or population-level vulnerability determines health outcomes and impacts. These effects are seen across a range of domains such as mental health effects, chronic disease exacerbation, vector-borne and diarrheal diseases, and acute traumatic injuries. Similarly, health system vulnerability determines operationality of health facilities during climate events and the ability to provide ongoing emergent and longitudinal care (Figure 25.1).

Impacts of Extreme Weather Events on Health Care Systems

Extreme weather events, such as tropical cyclones, wildfires, flooding, heat waves, and droughts, are increasing in frequency, severity, and duration because of climate change (Table 25.2) (USGCRP 2018). These events already have caused a significant financial impact; from 2004 to 2013 in the United States, there was an estimated $392 billion in losses from hurricanes, $78 billion due to heat waves and droughts, and $76 billion from severe storms, tornadoes, and flooding (USGCRP 2016). In 2019, there were fourteen extreme weather events in the United States that each led to more than a billion dollars in damages, response, and recovery, totaling more than $45 billion in 2019 alone (National Centers for Environmental Information [NCEI], 2020).

Health impacts from extreme weather events can be classified as either direct or indirect (Banwell et al. 2018; WHO 2015). Direct impacts occur when humans are exposed to a climate

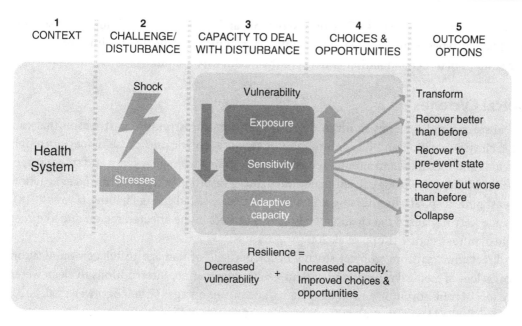

Figure 25.1   World Health Organization conceptual framework for resilience
WHO (2015). Used with permission.

Table 25.2   How Climate Change Affects Extreme Weather Events

Weather Event	Climate-Related Effect
Tropical Cyclones	Increase in intensity and frequency with significant risks for coastal and inland flooding before, during and after landfall (Elsner, Kossin, and Jagger, 2008; Kossin, Olander, and Knapp 2013).
Wildfires	Increase in frequency and intensity of large wildfires due to elevated temperature, persistent and prolonged drought and changing wind patterns (USGCRP 2018). The cumulative forest area burned doubled from 1984 to 2015 with climate change.
Flooding	Coastal, inland, urban, and river floods are becoming more frequent (USGCRP 2018) because of elevated storm surges coupled with sea level rise as well as increasing heavy downpour events. (Westra, Alexander, and Zwiers 2013).
Heat waves	Heat waves continue to rise in frequency and intensity and the rate of increase has doubled since 1975 (Blunden, Arndt, and Hartfield 2018). Global surface temperatures are expected to exceed 1.5°C (2.7°F) between 2030 and 2052 (IPCC 2018).
Drought	Droughts are increasing in many areas and groundwater is being depleted at a rate that far exceeds natural cycles of replenishment (USGCRP 2018). Globally, approximately four billion people live under severe water scarcity at least one month of the year (Mekonnen and Hoekstra 2015).

hazard and experience immediate health consequences. For example, a person exposed to extreme heat may experience heatstroke, organ system failure, and death. Other examples include burns from wildfire and drowning in floodwater. Indirect impacts are mediated through proximal and distal factors such as societal impact, effect on public health systems, land use changes, disrupted ecosystems, and more (Banwell et al. 2018; USGCRP 2018). Indirect impact examples include increasing incidence of water-or vector-borne diseases from standing floodwater and prolonged power outages resulting in a disrupted cold chain required for ongoing vaccination campaigns.

Locations where health care is delivered may also suffer direct impacts from climate hazards, resulting in facility damage (e.g., flooding). Health care facilities may also suffer indirect impacts, such as service disruptions due to power loss, supply chain disruption, and loss of personnel. Disruptions in facility functioning may be compounded by worker exhaustion or absenteeism (Chowdhury et al. 2019) and concerns for family safety and childcare needs for those who are available to work (Charney, Rebmann, and Flood, 2015). The following section highlights four types of extreme weather events that significantly affected health care facilities with examples of direct and indirect effects to the health care system.

Tropical Cyclones

Tropical storms and cyclones result in direct health care infrastructure destruction that can cause facility evacuation and discontinuation of services. Hurricanes cause damage through high winds and tornados, and simultaneously cause flooding from heavy rain and storm surge. Hurricane Michael in Florida caused structural damage resulting in the closure and evacuation of at least nine hospitals, five nursing homes, and fifteen assisted-living facilities (Evans 2018). Hurricane Katrina caused the closure of 94 dialysis centers in the affected region due to direct damage of infrastructure (Kopp et al. 2007).

Indirect impacts from tropical storms occur because of damage to telecommunication networks, loss of medical records and patient health information, interruptions to clean water supply, loss of transportation and supply chains, and power outages (Irvin-Barnwell et al. 2020; Kopp et al. 2007; Norcross et al. 1993; Silverman et al. 1995). Power outages may halt use of imaging modalities used to diagnose injuries and other health conditions, make monitors and mechanical ventilators inoperable, and disrupt blood product and other medication availability due to a lack of refrigeration. Impacts to transportation may result from damage to landing zones for air medical transportation and damage to roads, which ultimately limit emergency medical services, and may result in delays in care (Crutchfield and Harkey, 2019).

Hurricanes and tropical storms also lead to indirect impacts on health care facilities due to loss of supply chains locally and globally. Hurricane Maria devastated Puerto Rico in 2017 (Figure 25.2) and disrupted critical medical device and pharmaceutical supplies for the United States for months despite never hitting the U.S. mainland. Eleven of the top twenty global pharmaceutical companies had manufacturing facilities in Puerto Rico, which supported 90,000 employees and produced thousands of essential medical products. The mainland United States experienced widespread shortages of critical medical devices and pharmaceuticals, as a result of direct damage to factories as well as loss of energy, supply chains, and critical personnel (Food and Drug Administration 2017).

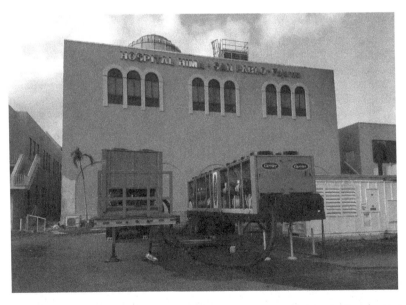

Portable generators brought in to restore power at a hospital in Fajardo, Puerto Rico after Hurricane Maria, 2017
Used with permission by Charles Little, DO.

Other indirect effects include worsening of existing challenges with water and sanitation, vaccination, primary prevention services, and access to health care, especially for the most medically and socially vulnerable populations (Isbell and Bhoojedhur, 2019). For example, in 2019 Tropical cyclones Idai and Kenneth overwhelmed Mozambique and Zimbabwe with destruction of livelihoods and properties, resultant infectious disease outbreaks and food insecurity, which drove thousands of residents into deeper poverty (Centre for Research on the Epidemiology of Disasters [CRED] 2019; U.S. Agency for International Development 2019).

Wildfires

Wildfires can result in direct damage to health care infrastructure and supporting industries. For example, 2018 was the most destructive year for wildfires in California history, with more than 1.8 million acres burned and more than 23,000 building structures lost, including health care facilities (National Interagency Coordination Center 2019). In November of 2018 alone, at least three hospitals, six intermediate care facilities, and four congregate living health facilities were evacuated due to wildfire risk (California Department of Public Health 2018). Pharmacies were also closed, resulting in scarcity of crucial respiratory medications in the face of increasing demand exacerbated by widespread smoke exposure (Thompson 2018).

Wildfires also indirectly affect health care delivery by destroying roads with downed trees and debris, ultimately hindering evacuation as well as patient access to facilities. (Cova et al. 2011). Wildfires can lead to power grid disruptions, both accidental and intentional. Following the 2019 fires in California, electric companies preemptively shut off power to 800,000 people to prevent electrical arching from above-ground power lines and thus reduce additional wildfire risk. The outcome included thousands at risk for wildfires cut off from information and the loss of power for lifesaving medical device operation (CBS 2019). Additionally, although larger health facilities were able to rely on back-up generators, smaller facilities, such as community health centers that assist the most underserved populations, were left without electricity for days. Of the community centers surveyed, 97 percent relied on refrigeration for medications like insulin and vaccinations, and less than half had backup power options at their facility (Sherer 2019). Furthermore, the aftermath of this power-shutdown revealed that many urban hospitals in California located in high fire-hazard-zones lacked plans to address fire-related risks, such as loss of power and forced evacuation (Adelaine et al. 2017).

Flooding

Extreme precipitation events, sea level rise, and tropical cyclones often result in flooding, which may directly affect health care facilities (USGCRP 2018). Extreme precipitation events, such as the unprecedented rainfall in 2019 that resulted in massive flooding in the U.S. Midwest, have become 30 percent more frequent and intense in the last sixty years (Madsen and Willcox, 2012). During the Midwest flooding, many hospitals and at least twelve long-term care facilities were forced to evacuate and close (American Hospital Association [AHA] 2019).

Indirect effects of flooding result from disruptions and damage to transportation and water treatment systems. In the 2019 Midwest floods, many roadways were inaccessible, which affected transportation for hospital employees, patients, and emergency medical services (AHA 2019). Simultaneously, farms that supplied local food were flooded, leading to food shortages that may have affected health care facilities relying upon local supply for nutrition for staff, visitors, and patients. In addition, flooding can lead to sewage overflow events and contribute to drinking water contamination, which poses grave risks to public health and increases health care utilization (Brokamp et al. 2017; Olds et al. 2018).

When severe flooding events occur in high-income countries, the results can be dramatic. However, high-income countries have relatively advanced water management systems and urban planning design, which serve to mitigate possible impact on the population. When flooding events occur in low- and middle-income countries, the risk of population-wide impact and excess mortality due to lack of infrastructure redundancy and preparedness is much higher. A recent study showed that fewer than one in five hospitals surveyed in Africa had disaster plans in place despite several prior flood events in the region. (Koka et al. 2018). Similarly, backup communication and energy sources were routinely shown to be lacking or nonexistent (Koka et al. 2018). Staff absenteeism during floods and insufficient supplies at the facilities to sustain demand during transportation interruptions have also been identified as concerns (Farley et al. 2017).

Extreme Heat

Extreme heat events directly impact health care facilities by causing power-outages ("brown-outs") and cause utilization surges for heat-related illnesses (Davis and Novicoff, 2018; Dhainaut et al. 2004; Hess, Saha, and Luber, 2014; Schmeltz, Petkova, and Gamble, 2016; Wondmagegn et al. 2019). Surges in health care treatment may quickly overwhelm underprepared or under-resourced facilities, and ultimately affect the most vulnerable patients.

Extreme heat indirectly affects facilities by driving up operating costs and energy consumption for indoor cooling, particularly in lower latitudes (Bawaneh et al. 2019). Simultaneously, power-outages may leave health care facilities without air conditioning and ventilation, ultimately exacerbating health conditions and result in poor health outcomes (Steffen, Hughes, and Perkins, 2014). Power outages have been associated with major disruptions in health care, including communication and information technology, staffing, food and nutrition, potable water, and wastewater management (Klein, Rosenthal, and Klausner, 2012). Power outages tend to preferentially affect resource limited health care facilities in all countries. For example, in 2017, after power outages from Hurricane Irma, approximately 160 nursing homes lost power, leading to at least eight heatstroke deaths and hundreds of emergency evacuations. (Reisner, Fink, and Yee, 2017). Power outages also contribute to an increase in call volume of emergency medicine services and increase health care utilization for many complaints, which may stress already poorly functioning health systems and potentially negatively impact routine emergency care (Prezant et al. 2005; Rand et al. 2005).

Natural Systems and Resources

Climate-related stressors, such as sea level rise and water scarcity, have consequences on health care facilities and surrounding communities. Coastal flooding can result in damage to health care systems and disruption in care. Drought in arid regions can also negatively affect the delivery of health care services.

Sea Level Rise

Coastal areas worldwide are increasingly being threatened by sea level rise, storm surges, and resultant flooding (Fleming et al, 2018; Hauer, Evans, and Mishra, 2016). In the United States alone, more than 133 million people live in counties along a shoreline, and this population continues to increase (Kildow et al. 2016). Worldwide, 40 percent of the global population lives within sixty miles of the coast (United Nations 2017). The most at-risk cities are those in North America, South America, Africa, and Asia with projected billions of dollars in losses by 2050 and millions of forced inland evacuations. Small island developing states are at particular risk due to their low-lying geography coupled with a lack of resources for adaptation and response

(Schnitter et al. 2018; WHO 2017). In the United States, more than 60,000 miles in roads and bridges, trillions of dollars in property, and public infrastructure are currently threatened by sea level rise (USGCRP 2018).

In the United States, states are independently recognizing the risks that sea level rise poses to health facilities. Virginia recently assessed coastal health-infrastructure vulnerability and projected reduced access to many health facilities and other critical infrastructure due to rising sea levels and storm surge (Liu, Behr, and Diaz, 2016). Similarly, North and South Carolina completed a health care vulnerability assessment as it pertains to threats to water infrastructure posed by sea level rise (Allen et al. 2019). Currently, the Charleston, South Carolina medical district routinely floods due to storm surges (Runkle et al. 2018). High exposure urban coastal cities are calling for improved community preparedness and risk assessments (Lane et al. 2013). To date, little collective significant action has been taken to mitigate the coming impact of sea level rise on coastal communities and health facilities.

Water Scarcity

Clean water is needed for all basic health care operations and climate change is likely to further strain water availability in many regions. Health care facilities require large volumes of water for sanitation, medical processing, laundry, food service, surgical and medical procedures such as dialysis, heating, and cooling (Environmental Protection Agency [EPA] 2012; Huttinger et al. 2017; U.S. Department of Energy 2011). In the United States, health care facilities use approximately seven percent of total water used in commercial facilities (EPA 2012). A single large U.S. hospital uses 43.6 million gallons of water annually at a cost of approximately $202,200 (U.S. Energy Information Administration 2012).

Clean water shortages have a negative impact on health care facilities, particularly in low- and middle-income countries (LMICs). In a recent survey of 129,000 hospitals in seventy-eight LMICs, 50 percent lack piped water, 33 percent lack improved sanitation, 39 percent lack handwashing soap, 39 percent lack adequate infectious waste disposal, and 73 percent lack sterilization equipment (Cronk and Bartram 2018). In another survey, less than two thirds of hospitals surveyed had a reliable water source (Chawla et al. 2016). A baseline lack of clean water can negatively affect efficiency and success during health emergencies and compromise the ability to deliver emergency care in a safe manner for patients and personnel (Hsia et al. 2012).

International Frameworks for Health Care System Resilience

The chapter thus far has outlined stressors to health care facilities as a result of climate-related events. In response to known risks and in preparation for future climate-scenarios, international and domestic organizations have collaborated to provide frameworks and toolkits to guide health care facilities with resilience planning and green transformation—designing, constructing, operating, and maintaining buildings in ways that conserve natural resources and reduce pollution. These initiatives are reviewed along with case studies demonstrating their successful incorporation into health care facility planning.

WHO Operational Framework for Building Climate-Resilient Health Systems

In 2015, the WHO put forth an operational framework for health system climate resilience. The six traditional health system building blocks are identified as a foundation for the development of health system elements that should be targeted to enhance climate resilience, as shown in Figure 25.2 (WHO 2015). The framework recognizes the importance of leadership and governance in addition to a strong and educated health workforce to enhance climate resilience.

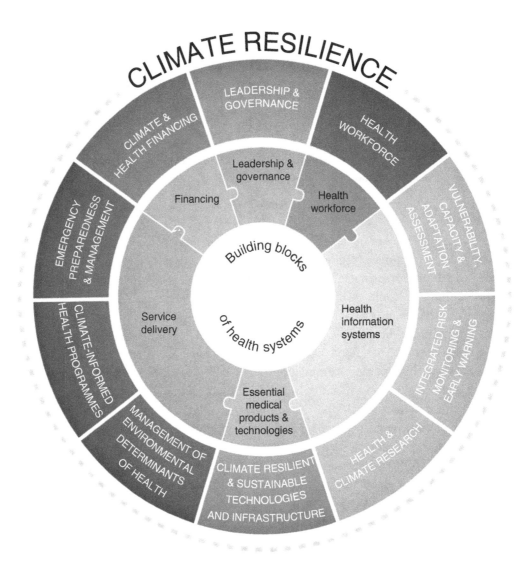

Figure 25.2   Ten components comprising the WHO Operational Framework for Building Climate-Resilient Health Systems
Source: WHO (2015). Used with permission.

Resiliency-driven health service delivery requires robust emergency preparedness for extreme weather events, climate-informed health programs (e.g., vector-borne disease), and management of the environmental determinants of health (e.g., nutrition and air quality). A climate-related approach to health information systems requires (1) assessments to guide understanding of vulnerability to climate risks, capacity of the system to respond, and identification of adaptations; (2) integrated risk monitoring and early warning systems; and (3) guidance for the utilization of climate research on health. This framework specifically recommends that health care systems invest in sustainable and resilient technologies and infrastructure, emphasizing the importance of integrating a climate lens into health facilities to maintain their functionality during and after disasters. Implementation of these recommendations improves the likelihood of crucial service delivery during a disaster and simultaneously improves efficiency and reduces daily operation costs.

Sendai Framework for Disaster Risk Reduction (SFDRR)

The United Nations Sendai Framework for Disaster Risk Reduction (SFDRR)—an international covenant adopted in 2015 to establish common goals and standards for disaster risk reduction—formalizes climate change as a disaster-risk multiplier and provides guidelines to reduce disaster risk and build resilience (United Nations 2015). The goal of the SFDRR is to provide evidence-based disaster management guidance, and actively involve adopters to "prepare, review and periodically update preparedness policies, plans and programmes with the involvement of all relevant institutions, considering climate change scenarios and their impact, and to facilitate the participation of all sectors and stakeholders" (United Nations 2015). Strong accountability is fundamental to the framework, which contains thirty-eight indicators to track progress in implementing the seven targets, which aim to reduce disaster mortality and damage to critical infrastructure and economies through increased multihazard early warning systems, improved national and local mitigation strategies, and enhanced international cooperation. The framework also incorporates the related dimensions of Sustainable Development Goals related to poverty, sustainability, and climate action.

The UNFCCC Nairobi Work Programme and National Adaptation Plans

The United Nations Framework Convention on Climate Change convenes countries to address climate change mitigation and adaptation. Adaptation initiatives in developing countries, including the least developed countries and small island developing states, have been emphasized because of the greater risks to their communities and people from climate change (Patz et al. 2007). In 2005, the Nairobi Work Programme was initiated to assist nations in understanding, assessing, and making informed decisions around climate change with specific focus on adaptation actions and enhancing knowledge (UNFCCC 2019b). National adaptation plans (NAPs) were subsequently recommended as a framework to encourage countries to identify needs and risks in the intermediate and long term and subsequently implement policy strategies to meet identified needs. Health and health care are critical components of NAPs, sometimes termed "H-NAPs" (WHO 2014). There are currently eighteen LMIC countries with NAPs (United Nations Framework Convention on Climate Change [UNFCCC] 2020) with another 80 of the more than 150 LMICs with plans underway (UNFCCC 2019a). The components of the H-NAP include groundwork, preparatory elements, implementation strategies, and reporting, monitoring, and reviewing with the overall objective of specifying priorities to minimize health risks of climate change (Ebi and Prats 2015; WHO 2014). Together the Nairobi Work Programme and NAPs serve to promote effective adaptation action for at-risk populations and nations.

Green and Resilient Health Care

Health care facility vulnerability and resilience are deeply connected to environmental and energy sustainability. Health care facilities are large consumers of energy, water, and other resources, which make them more vulnerable when disruptions occur due to climate-related events. Therefore, by increasing efficiency of resource utilization under normal operating conditions, a hospital becomes more self-sufficient and is able to stay open longer with fewer external inputs during a disaster. Toolkits that approach resilience coupled with sustainability have been developed by national and international organizations. Key features are summarized in Table 25.3.

The **Smart Hospital Initiative (SHI)** (PAHO 2017) was developed by the Pan American Health Organization (PAHO) to promote hospital resilience in the Caribbean and Latin

America. The three pillars of the SHI are resilient (safe), sustainable (smart), and environmentally sound (green) facilities. The goal of the initiative is to increase resilience of operations among the approximately 70 percent of hospitals in the Caribbean and Latin America that are located in areas designated as "at risk" of disaster impacts (PAHO 2014). The conceptual framework for health facilities centers around three objectives: (1) structural, nonstructural, and functional resilience; (2) small carbon footprint; and (3) small environmental footprint.

The Smart Hospitals Toolkit was created over several years by the PAHO Disaster Mitigation Advisory Group with input from leaders across the region. Implementation of the toolkit requires a stepwise approach (PAHO 2017). The first step is assessing the hospital safety index using preestablished metrics. The outcome of this assessment is then used to identify risk, urgency of change, and underlying vulnerability of the community. The second step is employment of a "green checklist" whereby opportunities are identified to improve energy efficiency, water conservation, air quality, food waste, and waste management. Simultaneously, the financial feasibility of each intervention is assessed. Third, baseline assessment tools allow hospitals to determine the necessary extent of work and the cost associated with it. The remaining steps involve preparation, recruitment, evaluation, and maintenance planning. More than thirty countries and four territories in the Caribbean and Latin America have adopted the hospital safety index, and at least 11,530 people have been trained as safe hospitals evaluators (PAHO 2016).

The United States Department of Health and Human Services' **Sustainable and Climate-Resilient Health Care Facilities Initiative (SCRHCFI)** (U.S. Department of Health and Human Services 2014) is another resource available to assist facilities in preparing for and responding to extreme weather events. The five steps of the framework are (1) climate risks and community vulnerability assessment; (2) land use, building design, and regulatory content; (3) infrastructure protection and resilience planning; (4) essential clinical care service delivery planning; and (5) environmental protection and ecosystem adaptations. Each element features a checklist and list of relevant resources.

Canada similarly developed the **Health Care Facility Climate Change Resiliency Toolkit** (Canadian Coalition for Green Health Care and Novia Scotia Department of Environment 2013). The toolkit includes a facilitator's guide, an assessments checklist with seventy-eight questions, and a resource guide. It addresses components of supply chain, infrastructure, and emergency management and health care services to assist facilities in identifying and addressing gaps (Paterson et al. 2014).

Table 25.3   Health Care Facility Resilience Toolkits

Overview of main features of three toolkits for health care facility resilience			
	Health Care Facility Climate Change Resiliency Toolkit (Canada)	**Sustainable and Climate Resilient Health Care Facilities Toolkit (U.S.)**	**PAHO Smart Hospitals Toolkit**
Type of facility	Hospitals	Hospitals, residential health care, ambulatory care, and home care	Small and medium-sized facilities, hospitals with 200+ beds
Focus resiliency areas	Emergency management, sustainability, infrastructure	Infrastructure, critical services, personnel, supply chain	Sustainability and infrastructure
Format	Facilitator's guide, resiliency assessment checklist, resources, case studies	Best practices document, five-element framework, checklists, case studies	Hospital Safety Index, Green Checklist, cost benefit analysis, training aids, lessons learned
Website	http://www.greenhealthcare.ca	https://toolkit.climate.gov	www.paho.org

Source: Adapted from Balbus et al. (2016).

In order to provide practical funding for such initiatives, the World Bank Group **Climate Change and Health Diagnostic** (WHO and World Bank Group 2018) supports climate-smart health care in effort to "link knowledge to investment." They identify climate-smart health care as the intersection between low-carbon health care and resilient health interventions. The framework identifies climate stresses that disrupt health care systems and contribute to poor health. It provides country-level guidance for identifying climate threats as well as engaging and educating stakeholders across multiple disciplines. The framework prioritizes interventions based on accessed barriers and opportunities and, importantly, uniquely links them to a lending portfolio to support identified prioritized actions.

Case Studies

UNIVERSITY OF TEXAS MEDICAL CENTER GETS RESILIENCE RIGHT

The University of Texas Medical Center (TMC), one of the largest medical and research facilities in the world, developed a hazard mitigation plan after Tropical Storm Allison devastated the medical center in 2001. Tropical Storm Allison caused more than $5 billion in damages to southern Louisiana and southeast Texas due to extreme precipitation and resultant flooding (National Oceanic and Atmospheric Administration [NOAA] 2001). At least twenty-two people died as a result of the direct effects from flooding and electrocution in Harris County, Texas and 45,000 buildings flooded (NOAA 2001). Three major hospitals were shut down, resulting in forced transfers and evacuations (Cocanour et al. 2002). Following the storm, transdisciplinary stakeholders from Houston met and developed a hazard mitigation plan including forty-two proactive, sustainable measures to mitigate risks of future disasters including flood infrastructure development (USGCRP 2019). Outcomes of plan included a new combined heat and power utility plant elevated above flood levels and a stormwater management system to enhance water drainage across the medical campus. Other major improvements included installation of a storm-resistant roof, relocation of communication systems, replacement of fuel storage tanks from under to above-ground units, installation of flood gates and flood walls, and enhanced flood alert systems (Fang et al. 2014). When Hurricane Harvey made landfall in 2017, there was a very different outcome. Despite more than forty inches of rainfall, TMC was able to continue operations with minimal interruption (Phillips et al.2017).

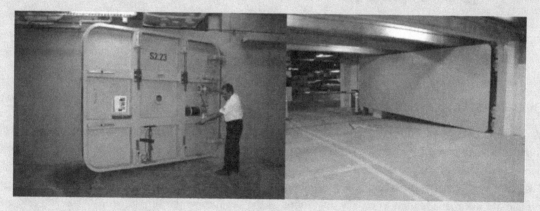

Texas Medical Center flood door and flood gate in facility parking lot
Used with permission by Nick Fang, PhD, PE.

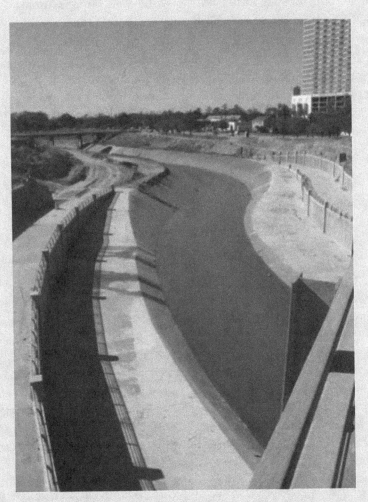

Widened channel near Texas Medical Center, created in response to damages caused by Hurricane Allison
Used with permission by Nick Fang, PhD, PE.

VANCOUVER COASTAL HEALTH ADDRESSES A WARMING CLIMATE

In 2018, Vancouver Coastal Health in conjunction with Fraser Health committed to prioritizing and incorporating plans for current and future acute and chronic climate stressors (Lower Mainland Facilities Management 2018). They partnered with diverse leaders in their community to reinforce old infrastructure and build new facilities that incorporated scientific predictions and relevant local hazards such as extreme precipitation and warming temperatures. Additionally, these hospitals are integrating climate risk management into daily operations of the facilities, while simultaneously training and engaging facility members, the general public, government leaders and health system administration teams.

APPLYING THE WORLD BANK DIAGNOSTIC IN MADAGASCAR

Madagascar is a "climate and health hotspot" because of its susceptibility to extreme weather events coupled with a high proportion of the population living in poverty. The World Bank Climate Change and Health Diagnostic was implemented to identify current and future climate-related risks and opportunities for the health sector (World Bank Group 2018). From the initial diagnostic assessment six interventions were formulated including development of a low-carbon strategy for the health sector, scaling up community small and medium enterprise programming and markets for energy efficiency, scaling up waste management programs, scaling up Green Hospital Initiatives, promoting water use efficiency, establishment of training programs, and a health system-wide cost-benefit analyses (World Bank Group 2018). These interventions also support climate-related health priorities in the areas of nutrition, water-related illness, extreme weather events, vector-borne diseases, and air pollution.

SMART HOSPITALS IN THE CARIBBEAN: STORIES OF SUCCESS

Georgetown Hospital in Saint Vincent and the Grenadines and Pogson Hospital in Saint Kitts and Nevis both underwent significant infrastructure and operational changes based on implementation of the PAHO Smart Hospitals Initiative (Bynoe and Caribbean Community Climate Change Centre 2013; Bynoe, Social Impact Unit, and Caribbean Community Climate Change Centre 2013). Georgetown Hospital underwent significant infrastructure work to improve ventilation, water management, plumbing and sanitary fixtures, and energy efficiency. One of the largest projects was installation of an emergency energy supply system (generator and solar photovoltaic) with a return on investment estimated in only four to six years (Buter 2018). Almost a 58 percent reduction in electrical consumption was seen after the improvements (Buter). Pogson Hospital similarly addressed energy efficiency through efficient lighting, safety with new doors, and water conservation.

PEEBLES HOSPITAL, BRITISH VIRGIN ISLANDS

Peebles Hospital in the British Virgin Islands is the primary public hospital for the region. In 2014, it completed comprehensive upgrades and facilities expansion utilizing Smart Hospital construction principles (Devitt 2016) and was given an "A" rating by the PAHO Safety Index Calculator. During Hurricanes Irma and Maria in 2018, the hospital remained fully operational for patient care with only minor window cracks despite widespread destruction to surrounding buildings (PAHO 2018). In fact, it hosted the National Emergency Operations Center and the Ministry of Health during disaster and recovery processes (PAHO 2018). Additionally, the building served as a temporary shelter for displaced persons for months after the event.

Economics and Equity: Closing the Gaps in Health System Resilience in Low-Income Countries

Although climate-resilient health care systems are critically important in all countries, the specific challenges and opportunities differ greatly between geographic regions as well as between high-income, middle-income and low-income countries. High- and low-income countries have varying abilities to raise capital to invest in resilience. In low-income countries, despite potential high returns on investments, financial barriers often limit action. To address these barriers, the Green Climate Fund was developed to pool financial resources from private and public sectors and provide grants, loans, and equity toward mitigation and adaptation initiatives. To date, 129 projects are underway with the potential to have a positive impact on an estimated 353 million people. Priority is given to African states, least developed countries, and small island developing states (Green Climate Fund 2020). Other funding mechanisms include the Global Environment Facility, Adaptation Fund, and Least Developed Country Fund. Further funding opportunities are available at climatefundsupdate.org.

There is a critical need to ensure available funds are being used to incorporate resilient and green principles into new construction projects and retrofitting of existing facilities within the health sector. Lending organizations can help countries implement sustainable projects by providing the necessary expertise and oversight during various stages of project development. Additionally, with organizational restructuring, climate resilient principles can become embedded within official development aid for health care systems and infrastructure in low-income countries (CRED and United Nations International Strategy for Disaster Reduction 2016; Dresser et al. 2016; Patz et al. 2007). Many success stories exist and can serve as guidance and motivation for further initiatives. As an example, a United Nations Development Programme pilot study installed photovoltaic panels in rural Zimbabwe clinics that had no electricity before the project. The initiative was cost neutral in four years with a carbon payback of less than two years (World Bank Group 2017). A similar project at Bir Hospital in Nepal, funded through the World Bank Group, installed a solar grid to power critical care areas of the public hospital (World Bank Group 2017).

Critical gaps in current health system structures in low-income countries can decrease overall resilience and substantially influence outcomes in a population's health. One such example is the lack of functional emergency care systems in LMICs, which are crucial to address everyday emergencies and disasters due to climate influenced events (Carlson et al. 2019). Currently, insufficient funding and political will are allocated to strengthen this essential portion of the health care system (Reynolds et al. 2017). In 2019, a new World Health Assembly (2019) resolution (72.16) was passed that called for comprehensive approach to ensuring timely care for the acutely ill and injured and emphasized that robust and "well-prepared everyday emergency care systems are vital for mitigating the impact of disasters and mass casualty events and for maintaining delivery of health services in fragile situations and conflict-affected areas." To begin to address this need, policymakers and funders should consider emergency care initiatives as a critical component of building climate resilience as emergency departments are often the front lines of disaster management. Simultaneously, emergency care systems can be strengthened through a government directorate dedicated to emergency care, domestic investment in dedicated emergency units, establishment of emergency care training programs, and implementation of formal evidence-based triage and treatment protocols (Reynolds et al. 2017).

Research Needs

Hospitals and health care facilities operate within complex systems, which include physical infrastructure, human infrastructure, energy and water resources, transportation and waste removal services, security services, communications, information technology, food systems, and more. During acute and chronic climate-related disasters, population health depends on the entire system being able to provide the right service in the right place in a timely manner. To achieve this, research priorities include:

- Systems-based analysis of past successes and failures of health care systems during different types of disasters to understand critical weakness and possible decision-making points influencing health care operations and service delivery

- Development of empirically based models that integrate simulated performance of critical health infrastructure and patient behavior during disasters in order to accurately project health impacts and critical points of vulnerability and intervention

Multidisciplinary research involving social and behavioral science, mathematical modeling, economics, engineering, health science, and more can improve our understanding of human behaviors and health care system functioning during disasters. Although a number of programs in the United States support research into community or urban infrastructure resilience in general, none focus on applying these concepts in a sophisticated manner to health care facility resilience specifically. A recent set of themes for research priorities for broader community resilience has been proposed that includes (1) resilient frameworks, (2) physical infrastructure systems (buildings and critical infrastructure, lifeline systems), (3) social systems, and (4) economic systems (Koliou et al. 2017). This framework provides a useful priority list for research in health care systems, which also relies upon these four domains.

Summary

Climate-related disasters not only cause injuries and traumatic deaths but set into motion a cascade of direct and indirect impacts on health care facilities and supporting sectors that ultimately may result in increased morbidity and mortality. Therefore, building resilient and sustainable health care systems is essential given the projected increasing severity of extreme events due to climate change. Multiple toolkits and guidance documents as well as case examples exist to guide a health care facility transformation. However, there are currently crucial unmet research and financial investment needs, especially in the least developed countries. Additionally, significant gaps remain in local, national, and international policy development around building health system resiliency. Informed policies and strong partnerships coupled with significant investment will be vital for ensuring proactive changes to enable health care resilience.

KEY TERMS

Climate Change and Health Diagnostic: A five-stage diagnostic by the World Bank Group to support climate-smart health care and ultimately, to improve morbidity and mortality.

Climate-resilient health system: Capable to anticipate, respond to, cope with, recover from and adapt to climate-related shocks and stress, so as to bring sustained improvements in population health, despite an unstable climate (WHO 2015).

Resilience: The ability of a system and its component parts to anticipate, absorb, accommodate, or recover from the effects of a hazardous event in a timely and efficient manner, including through ensuring the preservation, restoration, or improvement of its essential basic structures and functions (IPCC 2012).

Smart Hospital Initiative (SHI): A seven-step toolkit by the Pan American Health Organization (PAHO) focused on building safe, smart, and green facilities in the Caribbean and Latin America.

Sustainable and Climate-Resilient Health Care Facilities Initiative (SCRHCFI): U.S. Department of Health and Human Services' online resource available to assist facilities in preparing for and responding to extreme weather events using a five-step framework.

Vulnerability: Exposure, sensitivity, and adaptive capacity (USGCRP 2016).

DISCUSSION QUESTIONS

1. What are the benefits of creating climate-resilient health systems? What are potential problems from incentivizing resilience in high- and low-income countries?

2. What are examples of extreme weather effects and their impact on health care facilities?

3. What initiatives are available to assist health care facilities build resilience?

References

Adelaine, S. A., M. Sato, Y. Jin, and H. Godwin. 2017. "An Assessment of Climate Change Impacts on Los Angeles (California USA) Hospitals, Wildfires Highest Priority." *Prehospital Disaster Medicine* 32 (5):556–2. doi:10.1017/S1049023X17006586.

American Hospital Association. 2019. "Historic Flooding in Midwest Affects Hospitals." *March* 18, 2019. https://www.aha.org/news/headline/2019-03-18-historic-flooding-midwest-affects-hospitals.

Allen, T., T. Crawford, B. Montz, J. Whitehead, S. Lovelace, A. D. Hanks, A. R. Christensen, and G. D. Kearney. 2019. "Linking Water Infrastructure, Public Health, and Sea Level Rise: Integrated Assessment of Flood Resilience in Coastal Cities." *Public Works Management and Policy* 24 (1):110–39.

Balbus, J., P. Berry, M. Brettle, S. Jagnarine-Azan, A. Soares, C. Ugarte, L. Varangu, and E. Villalobos Prats. 2016. "Enhancing the Sustainability and Climate Resiliency of Health Care Facilities: A Comparison of Initiatives and Toolkits." *Revista panamericana de salud pública* 40 (3):174–80.

Banwell, N., S. Rutherford, B. Mackey, R. Street, and C. Chu. 2018. "Commonalities between Disaster and Climate Change Risks for Health: A Theoretical Framework." *International Journal of Environmental Research and Public Health* 15 (3). doi:10.3390/ijerph15030538.

Bawaneh, K., F. Ghazi Nezami, M. Rasheduzzaman, and B. Deken. 2019. "Energy Consumption Analysis and Characterization of Healthcare Facilities in the United States." *Energies* 12 (19). doi:10.3390/en12193775.

Bell, S. A., M. Abir, H. Choi, C. Cooke, and T. Iwashyna. 2018. "All-Cause Hospital Admissions among Older Adults after a Natural Disaster." *Annals of Emergency Medicine* 71 (6):746–54. doi:10.1016/j.annemergmed.2017.06.042.

Berkowitz, S., H. Seligman, J.Meigs, and S. Basu. 2018. "Food Insecurity, Healthcare Utilization, and High Cost: A Longitudinal Cohort Study." *American Journal of Managed Care* 24 (9):399–404.

Blunden, J., D. S. Arndt, and G. Hartfield. 2018. "State of the Climate in 2017." *Bulletin of the American Meteorological Society* 99 (8):Si–S310 https://journals.ametsoc.org/doi/pdf/10.1175/2018BAMSState oftheClimate.1.

Brokamp, C., A. F. Beck, L. Muglia, and P. Ryan. 2017. "Combined Sewer Overflow Events and Childhood Emergency Department Visits: A Case-Crossover Study." *Science of the Total Environment* 607–8:1180–7. doi:10.1016/j.scitotenv.2017.07.104.

Buter, C. 2018. *Health Facilities and Disaster Resilience: PAHO Smart Hospital Project.* Pan American Health Organization. https://www.apha.org/-/media/files/pdf/membergroups/phn/paho_webinar_slides .ashx?la=enandhash=B637962F0BEACAFC475181C072D9CE98CA866531.

Bynoe, M., and Caribbean Community Climate Change Centre. 2013. *An Economic Appraisal of a SMART Hospital Initiative: Pogson Medical Centre–St. Kitts Nevis.* https://www.paho.org/en/file/62022/download?token=kXOALD7u.

Bynoe, M., Social Impact Unit, and Caribbean Community Climate Change Centre. 2013. *An Economic Appraisal of a SMART Hospital.* https://www.paho.org/disasters/index.php?option=com_docman& view=download&category_slug=smart-hospitals-toolkit&alias=2181-cost-benefit-analysis-full-report-st-vincent-hospital&Itemid=1179&lang=en.

California Department of Public Health. 2018. "Health Care Facility Evacuations." *November* 19, 2018. https://www.cdph.ca.gov/Programs/CHCQ/LCP/Pages/2018-Facility-Evacuations.aspx.

Canadian Coalition for Green Health Care and Novia Scotia Department of Environment. 2013. *Health Care Facility Climate Change Resiliency Toolkit.* http://www.greenhealthcare.ca/climate resilienthealthcare/toolkit/.

Carlson, L. C., T. A. Reynolds, L. A. Wallis, and E. J. Calvello Hynes. 2019. "Reconceptualizing the Role of Emergency Care in the Context of Global Healthcare Delivery." *Health Policy Plan* 34 (1):78–82. doi:10.1093/heapol/czy111.

CBS. 2019. "Wildfires Rage in California as Residents Scramble without Power." October 10, 2019. cbsnews.com/news/wildfires-california-fires-rage-as-residents-scramble-without-power-pge/.

Centre for Research on the Epidemiology of Disasters. 2019. *Disasters in Africa: 20 Year Review (2000–2019*)*. Brussels: CRED. https://cred.be/sites/default/files/CredCrunch56.pdf.

Centre for Research on the Epidemiology of Disasters and United Nations International Strategy for Disaster Reduction. 2016. *Power and Death: Disaster Mortality 1996–2015*. https://www.unisdr.org/files/50589_creddisastermortalityallfinalpdf.pdf

Charney, R., T. Rebmann, and R. Flood. 2015. "Emergency Childcare for Hospital Workers during Disasters." *Pediatric Emergency Care* 31 (12):839–43.

Chawla, S. S., S. Gupta, F. M. Onchiri, E. B. Habermann, A. L. Kushner, and B. T. Stewart. 2016. "Water Availability at Hospitals in Low- and Middle-Income Countries: Implications for Improving Access to Safe Surgical Care." *Journal of Surgical Research* 205 (1):169–78. doi:10.1016/j.jss.2016.06.040.

Chowdhury, M. A. B., A. J. Fiore, S. A. Cohen, C. Wheatley, B. Wheatley, M. P. Balakrishnan, M. Chami et al. 2019. "Health Impact of Hurricanes Irma and Maria on St Thomas and St John, US Virgin Islands, 2017–2018." *American Journal of Public Health* 109 (12):1725–32. doi:10.2105/AJPH.2019.305310.

Cocanour, C., S. Allen, J. Mazabob, J. Sparks, C. Fischer, J. Romans, and K. Lally. 2002. "Lessons Learned from the Evacuation of an Urban Teaching Hospital." *Archives of Surgery* 137:1141–45.

Cova, T. J., D. M. Theobald, J. B. Norman, and L. K. Siebeneck. 2011. "Mapping Wildfire Evacuation Vulnerability in the Western US: The Limits of Infrastructure." *GeoJournal* 78 (2):273–85. doi:10.1007/s10708-011-9419-5.

Cronk, R., and J. Bartram. 2018. "Environmental Conditions in Health Care Facilities in Low- and Middle-Income Countries: Coverage and Inequalities." *International Journal of Hygiene and Environmental Health* 221 (3):409–22. doi:10.1016/j.ijheh.2018.01.004.

Crutchfield, A. S., and K. A. Harkey. 2019. "A Comparison of Call Volumes before, during, and after Hurricane Harvey." *American Journal of Emergency Medicine* 37 (10):1904–6. doi:10.1016/j.ajem.2019.01.007.

Davis, J., S. Wilson, A. Brock-Martin, S. Glover, and E. Svendsen. 2010. "The Impact of Disasters on Populations with Health and Health Care Disparities." *Disaster Medicine and Public Health Preparedness* 4 (1):30–38.

Davis, R. E., and W. M. Novicoff. (2018). "The Impact of Heat Waves on Emergency Department Admissions in Charlottesville, Virginia, U.S.A." *International Journal of Environmental Research and Public Health* 15 (7). doi:10.3390/ijerph15071436.

Department for International Development. 2011. *Defining Disaster Resilience: A DFID Approach Paper*. London: DFID. https://assets.publishing.service.gov.uk/government/uploads/system/uploads/attachment_data/file/186874/defining-disaster-resilience-approach-paper.pdf.

Devitt, C. K. 2016. "Department Profile: British Virgin Islands Health Services Authority Biomedical Engineering Department." *September* 30, 2016. https://1technation.com/department-profile-british-virgin-islands-health-services-authority-biomedical-engineering-department/

Dhainaut, J. F., Y. E. Claessens, C. Ginsburg, and B. Riou. 2004. "Unprecedented Heat-Related Deaths during the 2003 Heat Wave in Paris: Consequences on Emergency Departments." *Critical Care* 8 (1):1–2. doi:10.1186/cc2404.

Doran, K. M., R. P. McCormack, E. L. Johns, B. G. Carr, S. W. Smith, L. R. Goldfrank, and D. C. Lee. 2016. "Emergency Department Visits for Homelessness or Inadequate Housing in New York City before and after Hurricane Sandy." *Journal of Urban Health* 93 (2):331–44. doi:10.1007/s11524-016-0035-z.

Dresser, C., J. Allison, J. Broach, M. E. Smith, and A. Milsten. 2016. "High-Amplitude Atlantic Hurricanes Produce Disparate Mortality in Small, Low-Income Countries." *Disaster Medicine and Public Health Preparedness* 10 (6):832–37. doi:10.1017/dmp.2016.62.

Ebi, K. L., and E. V. Prats. 2015. "Health in National Climate Change Adaptation Planning." *Annals of Global Health* 81 (3):418–26. doi:10.1016/j.aogh.2015.07.001.

Elsner, J. B., J. P. Kossin, and T. H. Jagger. 2008. "The Increasing Intensity of the Strongest Tropical Cyclones." *Nature* 455 (7209):92–95. doi:10.1038/nature07234.

Environmental Protection Agency. 2012. "Saving Water in Hospitals." http://www.imusenvironmentalhealth.org/assets/38/7/saving_water_in_hospitals.pdf.

Evans, M. 2018. "Hurricane Michael Forces Florida Hospitals to Shut Down." *Wall Street Journal* *October* 12, 2018. https://www.wsj.com/articles/hurricane-michael-forces-florida-hospitals-to-shut-down-1539287788.

Fang, Z., G. Dolan, A. Sebastian, and P. B. Bedient. 2014. "Case Study of Flood Mitigation and Hazard Management at the Texas Medical Center in the Wake of Tropical Storm Allison in 2001." *Natural Hazards Review* 15 (3). doi:10.1061/(asce)nh.1527-6996.0000139.

Farley, J. M., I. Suraweera, W. Perera, J. Hess, and K. L. Ebi. 2017. "Evaluation of Flood Preparedness in Government Healthcare Facilities in Eastern Province, Sri Lanka." *Global Health Action* 10 (1):1331539. doi:10.1080/16549716.2017.1331539.

Food and Drug Administration. 2017. *Securing the Future for Puerto Rico: Restoring the Island's Robust Medical Product Manufacturing Sector.* Washington, DC: FDA. https://www.fda.gov/media/108975/download.

Fleming, E., W. Sweet, M. Craghan, J. Haines, J. F. Hart, H. Stiller, and A. Sutton-Grier. 2018. "Coastal Effects." In *Climate Science Special Report: Fourth National Climate Assessment, Vol. I*, edited by D. J. Wuebbles, D. W. Fahey, K. A. Hibbard, D. J. Dokken, B. C. Stewart, and T. K. Maycock, 322–52. Washington, DC: U.S. Global Change Research Program. https://nca2018.globalchange.gov/chapter/coastal.

Gray, B., and K. Hebert. 2006. *After Katrina: Hospitals in Hurricane Katrina.* Washington, DC: Urban Institute.https://www.urban.org/sites/default/files/publication/50896/411348-Hospitals-in-Hurricane-Katrina.PDF.

Green Climate Fund. 2020. "Projects and Programmes." https://www.greenclimate.fund/what-we-do/projects-programmes.

Hauer, M. E., J. M. Evans, and D. R. Mishra. 2016. "Millions Projected to Be at Risk from Sea-Level Rise in the Continental United States." *Nature Climate Change* 6 (7):691–95. doi:10.1038/nclimate2961.

Health Care Without Harm. 2018. *Safe Haven in the Storm.* Reston VA: HCWH. https://noharm-uscanada.org/sites/default/files/documents-files/5146/Safe_haven.pdf.

Hess, J. J., S. Saha, and G. Luber. 2014. "Summertime Acute Heat Illness in U.S. Emergency Departments from 2006 through 2010: Analysis of a Nationally Representative Sample." *Environmental Health Perspectives* 122 (11):1209–15. doi:10.1289/ehp.1306796.

Hsia, R. Y., N. A. Mbembati, S. Macfarlane, and M. E. Kruk. 2012. "Access to Emergency and Surgical Care in Sub-Saharan Africa: The Infrastructure Gap. *Health Policy Plan* 27 (3):234–44. doi:10.1093/heapol/czr023.

Hutchins, S., K. Bouye, G. Luber, L. Briseno, C. Hunter, and L. Corso. 2018. "Public Health Agency Responses and Opportunities to Protect Against Health Impacts of Climate Change among US Populations with Multiple Vulnerabilities." *Journal of Racial and Ethnic Health Disparities* 5:1159–70.

Huttinger, A., R. Dreibelbis, F. Kayigamba, F. Ngabo, L. Mfura, B. Merryweather, A. Cardon, and C. Moe. 2017. "Water, Sanitation and Hygiene Infrastructure and Quality i.n Rural Healthcare Facilities in Rwanda." *BMC Health Services Research* 17 (1): 517. doi:10.1186/s12913-017-2460-4.

Intergovernmental Panel on Climate Change. 2012. *Glossary of Terms.* Cambridge, UK and New York: Cambridge University Press. https://archive.ipcc.ch/pdf/special-reports/srex/SREX-Annex_Glossary.pdf.

Intergovernmental Panel on Climate Change. 2018. Summary for Policymakers. In *Global Warming of 1.5°C. An IPCC Special Report on the Impacts of Global Warming of 1.5°C above Pre-Industrial Levels and Related Global Greenhouse Gas Emission Pathways, in the Context of Strengthening the Global Response to the Threat of Climate Change, Sustainable Development, and Efforts to Eradicate Poverty*, edited by V. Masson-Delmotte, P. Zhai, H.-O. Pörtner, D. Roberts, J. Skea, P. R. Shukla, A. Pirani, W. Moufouma-Okia et al., 3–24. Geneva: IPCC.

Irvin-Barnwell, E. A., M. Cruz, C. Maniglier-Poulet, J. Cabrera, J. Rivera Diaz, R. De La Cruz Perez, C. Forrester et al. 2020. "Evaluating Disaster Damages and Operational Status of Health-Care Facilities during the Emergency Response Phase of Hurricane Maria in Puerto Rico." *Disaster Medicine and Public Health Preparedness* 14 (1):80–88. doi:10.1017/dmp.2019.85.

Isbell, T., and S. Bhoojedhur. 2019. "AD297: Cyclones Add to Mozambique's Public Health Challenges."AccessedJune21,2020.https://www.afrobarometer.org/publications/ad297-cyclones-add-mozambiques-public-health-challenges.

Issa, A., K. Ramadugu, P. Mulay, J. Hamilton, V. Siegel, C. Harrison, C. M. Campbell et al. 2018. "Deaths Related to Hurricane Irma—Florida, Georgia, and North Carolina, September 4–October 10, 2017." *MMWR. Morbidity and Mortality Weekly Report* 67 (30):829–32.

Kabene, S. M., C. Orchard, J. M. Howard, M. A. Soriano, and R. Leduc. 2006. "The Importance of Human Resources Management in Health Care: A Global Context." *Human Resources for Health* 4:20. doi:10.1186/1478-4491-4-20.

Kildow, J., C. Colgan, P. Johnston, J. Scorse, and M. Farnum. 2016. *State of the U.S. Ocean and Coastal Economies: 2016 Update.* Monterey CA: National Ocean Economics Program, Middlebury Institute of International Studies. http://midatlanticocean.org/wp-content/uploads/2016/03/NOEP_National_Report_2016.pdf.

Kishore, N., D. Marques, A. Mahmud, M. V. Kiang, I. Rodriguez, A. Fuller, P. Ebner et al. 2018. "Mortality in Puerto Rico after Hurricane Maria." *New England Journal of Medicine* 379 (2):162–70. doi:10.1056/NEJMsa1803972.

Klein, K. R., M. S. Rosenthal, and H. A. Klausner. 2012. "Blackout 2003: Preparedness and Lessons Learned from the Perspectives of Four Hospitals." *Prehospital and Disaster Medicine* 20 (5):343–9. doi:10.1017/s1049023x00002818.

Koka, P. M., H. R. Sawe, K. R. Mbaya, S. S. Kilindimo, J. A. Mfinanga, V. G. Mwafongo, L. A. Wallis, and T. A. Reynolds. 2018. "Disaster Preparedness and Response Capacity of Regional Hospitals in Tanzania: A Descriptive Cross-Sectional Study." *BMC Health Services Research* 18 (1):835. doi:10.1186/s12913-018-3609-5.

Koliou, M., J. W. van de Lindt, T. P. McAllister, B. R. Ellingwood, M. Dillard, and H. Cutler. 2017. "State of the Research in Community Resilience: Progress and Challenges." *Sustainable and Resilient Infrastructure* 1–21. https://doi.org/10.1080/23789689.2017.1418547.

Kopp, J. B., L. K. Ball, A. Cohen, R. J. Kenney, K. D. Lempert, P. E. Miller, P. Muntner, N. Qureshi, and S. A. Yelton. 2007. "Kidney Patient Care in Disasters: Lessons from the Hurricanes and Earthquake of 2005." *Clinical Journal of the American Society of Nephrology* 2 (4):814–24. doi:10.2215/CJN.03481006.

Kossin, J. P., T. L., Olander, and K. R. Knapp. 2013. "Trend Analysis with a New Global Record of Tropical Cyclone Intensity." *Journal of Climate* 26 (24):9960–76. doi:10.1175/jcli-d-13-00262.1.

Lane, K., K. Charles-Guzman, K. Wheeler, Z. Abid, N. Graber, and T. Matte. 2013. "Health Effects of Coastal Storms and Flooding in Urban Areas: A Review and Vulnerability Assessment." *Journal of Environmental and Public Health* 2013:913064. doi:10.1155/2013/913064.

Liu, H., J. G. Behr, and R. Diaz. 2016. "Population Vulnerability to Storm Surge Flooding in Coastal Virginia, USA." *Integrated Environmental Assessment and Management* 12 (3):500–9. doi:10.1002/ieam.1705.

Lower Mainland Facilities Management. 2018. *Moving towards Climate Resilient Health Facilities for Vancouver Coastal Health*. Vancouver, BC: LMFM. https://bcgreencare.ca/system/files/resource-files/VCH_ClimateReport%2BAppendices_Final_181025.pdf.

Madsen, T., and N. Willcox. 2012. *When It Rains It Pours: Global Warming and the Increase in Extreme Precipitation from 1948 to 2011*. Denver, CO: Environment America Research & Policy Center. https://environmentamerica.org/sites/environment/files/reports/When%20It%20Rains,%20It%20Pours%20vUS.pdf.

Mekonnen, M., and A. Hoekstra. 2015. "Four Billion People Facing Severe Water Scarcity." *Science Advances* 2:7. https://advances.sciencemag.org/content/advances/2/2/e1500323.full.pdf.

National Interagency Coordination Center. 2019. *Wildland Fire Summary and Statistics Annual Report 2018*. Boise, ID: NICC. https://www.predictiveservices.nifc.gov/intelligence/2018_statssumm/annual_report_2018.pdf.

National Oceanic and Atmospheric Administration. 2001. *Service Assessment: Tropical Storm Allison*. Silver Spring, MD: NOAA. https://www.weather.gov/media/publications/assessments/allison.pdf.

National Oceanic and Atmospheric Administration National Centers for Environmental Information. 2020. "U.S. Billion-Dollar Weather and Climate Disasters." *April* 8, 2020. https://www.ncdc.noaa.gov/billions/.

Norcross, E. D., B. M. Elliott, D. B. Adams, and F. A. Crawford. 1993. "Impact of a Major Hurricane on Surgical Services in a University Hospital." *American Surgeon* 59 (1):28–33. http://europepmc.org/abstract/MED/8480928.

Olds, H. T., S. R. Corsi, D. K. Dila, K. M. Halmo, M. J. Bootsma, and S. L. McLellan. 2018. "High Levels of Sewage Contamination Released from Urban Areas after Storm Events: A Quantitative Survey with Sewage Specific Bacterial Indicators." *PLoS Medicine* 15 (7):e1002614. doi:10.1371/journal.pmed.1002614.

Pan American Health Organization. 2014. *Strategic Plan 2013–2018*. Washington, DC: PAHO. https://reliefweb.int/report/world/paho-strategic-plan-2013-2018-disaster-risk-reduction-and-response-more-resilient.

Pan American Health Organization . 2016. *Plan of Action for Disaster Risk Reduction 2016–2021*. Washington, DC: PAHO. https://www.paho.org/hq/dmdocuments/2016/CD55-17-e.pdf.

Pan American Health Organization . 2017. *Smart Hospitals Toolkit*. Washington, DC: PAHO. https://iris.paho.org/bitstream/handle/10665.2/34977/9789275119396_eng.pdf?sequence=1.

Pan American Health Organization . 2018. *Putting SMART to the Test—Weathering Climate Change in the Caribbean*. Washington, DC: PAHO. https://www.paho.org/en/file/62011/download?token= BgEz0pWX.

Paterson, J., P. Berry, K. Ebi, and L. Varangu. 2014. "Health Care Facilities Resilient to Climate Change Impacts." *International Journal of Environmental Research and Public Health* 11 (12):13097–116. doi:10.3390/ijerph111213097.

Patz, J. A., H. K. Gibbs, J. A. Foley, J. V. Rogers, and K. R. Smith. 2007. "Climate Change and Global Health: Quantifying a Growing Ethical Crisis." *EcoHealth* 4 (4):397–405. doi:10.1007/s10393-007-0141-1.

Phillips, R., R. Schwartz, W. McKeon, and M. Boom. 2017. "Lessons in Leadership: How the World's Largest Medical Center Braced for Hurricane Harvey." October 25, 2017. https://catalyst.nejm.org/lessons-leadership-texas-medical-center-hurricane-harvey/ (webpage no longer active).

Prezant, D. J., J. Clair, S. Belyaev, D. Alleyne, G. I. Banauch, M. Davitt, K. Vandervoots et al. 2005. "Effects of the August 2003 Blackout on the New York City Healthcare Delivery System: A Lesson for Disaster Preparedness." *Critical Care Medicine* 33 (1 suppl):S96–101. doi:10.1097/01.ccm.0000150956.90030.23.

Rand, D., D. Mener, E. Lerner, and N. DeRobertis. 2005. "The Effect of an 18-Hour Electrical Power Outage on an Urban Emergency Medical Services System." *Prehospital Emergency Care* 9 (4):391–7.

Reisner, N., S. Fink, and V. Yee. 2017. "Eight Dead from Sweltering Nursing Home as Florida Struggles after Irma." *New York Times, September* 13, 2017. https://www.nytimes.com/2017/09/13/us/nursing-home-deaths-florida.html.

Reynolds, T., H. Sawe, A. Rubiano, S. D. Shin, L. Wallis, and C. N. Mock. 2017. "Strengthening Health Systems to Provide Emergency Care." In *Disease Control Priorities*. 3rd ed., edited by D. T. Jamison, H. Gelband, S. Horton, P. Jha, R. Laxminarayan, C. N. Mock, and R. Nugent, 247–65. Washington, DC: World Bank.

Runkle, J., E. R. Svendsen, M. Hamann, R. K. Kwok, and J. Pearce. 2018. "Population Health Adaptation Approaches to the Increasing Severity and Frequency of Weather-Related Disasters Resulting From our Changing Climate: A Literature Review and Application to Charleston, South Carolina." *Current Environmental Health Reports* 5 (4):439–52. doi:10.1007/s40572-018-0223-y.

Santos-Burgoa, C., A. Goldman, E. Andrade, N. Barrett, U. Colon-Ramos, M. Edberg, and S. Zeger. 2018. *Ascertainment of the Estimated Excess Mortality from Hurricane Maria in Puerto Rico: Project Report*. Washington, DC: Milken Institute School of Public Health, George Washington University. https://publichealth.gwu.edu/sites/default/files/downloads/projects/PRstudy/Acertainment%20of%20the%20Estimated%20Excess%20Mortality%20from%20Hurricane%20Maria%20in%20Puerto%20Rico.pdf.

Schmeltz, M. T., E. P. Petkova, and J. L. Gamble. 2016. "Economic Burden of Hospitalizations for Heat-Related Illnesses in the United States, 2001–2010." *International Journal of Environmental Research and Public Health* 13 (9). doi:10.3390/ijerph13090894.

Schnitter, R., M. Verret, P. Berry, T. Chung Tiam Fook, S. Hales, A. Lal, and S. Edwards. 2018. "An Assessment of Climate Change and Health Vulnerability and Adaptation in Dominica." *International Journal of Environmental Research and Public Health* 16 (1). doi:10.3390/ijerph16010070.

Sherer, P. 2019. "California Power Blackouts Reveal Widespread Vulnerability in Health Care System." *October* 17, 2019. https://www.directrelief.org/2019/10/california-power-blackouts-reveal-vulnerability-in-healthcare/.

Silverman, M. A., M. Weston, M. Llorente, C. Beber, and R. Tam. 1995. "Lessons Learned from Hurricane Andrew: Recommendations for Care of the Elderly in Long-Term Care Facilities." *Southern Medical Journal* 88 (6):603–8.

Steffen, W., L. Hughes, and S. Perkins. 2014. *Heatwaves: Hotter, Longer, More Often*. Potts Point: Climate Council of Australia. https://www.climatecouncil.org.au/uploads/9901f6614a2cac7b2b88 8f55b4dff9cc.pdf.

Sternberg, E., G. Lee, and D. Huard. 2004. "Counting Crises: US Hospital Evacuations 1971–1999." *Prehospital and Disaster Medicine* 19:150–7.

Swerdel, J. N., G. G. Rhoads, N. M. Cosgrove, J. B. Kostis, and Myocardial Infarction Data Acquisition System Study Group. 2016. "Rates of Hospitalization for Dehydration Following Hurricane Sandy in New Jersey." *Disaster Medicine and Public Health Preparedness* 10 (2):188–92. doi:10.1017/dmp.2015.169.

Texas Hospital Association. 2018. *Hurricane Harvey Analysis: Texas Hospitals' Preparation Strategies for Future Disaster Response*. Austin: THA. https://capitol.texas.gov/tlodocs/85R/handouts/C2102018051010001/7d5c2c0d-a060-4a24-8eae-4ae4b7a8bebc.PDF.

Thomas, K. S., D. Dosa, K. Hyer, L. M. Brown, S. Swaminathan, Z. Feng, and V. Mor. 2012. "Effect of Forced Transitions on the Most Functionally Impaired Nursing Home Residents." *Journal of the American Geriatric Society* 60 (10):1895–1900. doi:10.1111/j.1532-5415.2012.04146.x.

Thompson, C. A. 2018. "Hospital Pharmacies in Northern California Deal with State's Largest Wildfire." *American Journal of Health-System Pharmacy* 75 (22):1762–4. doi:10.2146/news180066.

U.S. Agency for International Development. 2019. "Southern Africa—Tropical Cyclone Idai—Fact Sheet." *April* 4, 2019. https://www.usaid.gov/cyclone-idai/fy19/fs4.

U.S. Department of Energy. 2011. *Hospitals Save Costs with Water Efficiency.* Washington, DC: Energy Efficiency Renewable Energy Information Center. https://www1.eere.energy.gov/buildings/publications/pdfs/alliances/hea_water_efficiency_fs.pdf.

U.S. Department of Health and Human Services. 2014. *Primary Protection: Enhancing Health Care Resilience for a Changing Climate.* Washington, DC: USDHHS. https://toolkit.climate.gov/sites/default/files/SCRHCFI%20Best%20Practices%20Report%20final2%202014%20Web.pdf.

U.S. Energy Information Administration. 2012. "Energy Characteristics and Energy Consumed in Large Hospitals in the United States in 2007." *August* 17, 2012. https://www.eia.gov/consumption/commercial/reports/2007/large-hospital.php.

United Nations Framework Convention on Climate Change. 2019a. "Eight Years of NAPs: Where Are We Now?" *February* 26, 2019. http://napexpo.org/napblogger/our_blog/national-adaptation-plans-eight-years-of-naps-where-are-we-now/.

United Nations Framework Convention on Climate Change. 2019b. "Nairobi Work Programme on Impacts, Vulnerability and Adaptation to Climate Change." https://unfccc.int/topics/adaptation-and-resilience/workstreams/nairobi-work-programme-on-impacts-vulnerability-and-adaptation-to-climate-change#eq-2.

United Nations Framework Convention on Climate Change. 2020. "National Adaptation Plans." https://www4.unfccc.int/sites/NAPC/Pages/national-adaptation-plans.aspx.

United Nations. 2015. *Sendai Framework for Disaster Risk Reduction 2015-2030.* Geneva: United Nations Office for Disaster Risk Reduction. https://www.unisdr.org/files/43291_sendaiframeworkfordrren.pdf.

United Nations. 2017. "Factsheet: People and Oceans." https://sustainabledevelopment.un.org/content/documents/Ocean_Factsheet_People.pdf.

U.S. Global Change Research Program. 2016. *The Impacts of Climate Change on Human Health in the United States: A Scientific Assessment.* Washington, DC: USGCRP. https://s3.amazonaws.com/climatehealth2016/high/ClimateHealth2016_FullReport.pdf.

U.S. Global Change Research Program. 2018. *Fourth National Climate Assessment Vol. II: Impacts, Risks, and Adaptation in the United States.* Washington, DC: USGCRP. https://nca2018.globalchange.gov/downloads/NCA4_2018_FullReport.pdf.

U.S. Global Change Research Program. 2019. "After Record-Breaking Rains, a Major Medical Center Improves Resilience." *U.S. Climate Resilience Toolkit. August* 12, 2019. https://toolkit.climate.gov/case-studies/after-record-breaking-rains-major-medical-centers-hazard-mitigation-plan-improves.

Westra, S., L. V. Alexander, and F. W. Zwiers. 2013. "Global Increasing Trends in Annual Maximum Daily Precipitation." *Journal of Climate* 26 (11):3904–18. doi:10.1175/jcli-d-12-00502.1.

Willoughby, M., C. Kipsaina, N. Ferrah, S. Blau, L. Bugeja, D. Ranson, and J. E. Ibrahim. 2017. "Mortality in Nursing Homes Following Emergency Evacuation: A Systematic Review." *Journal of the American Medical Directors Association* 18 (8):664–70. doi:10.1016/j.jamda.2017.02.005.

Wondmagegn, B. Y., J. Xiang, S. Williams, D. Pisaniello, and P. Bi. 2019. "What Do We Know about the Healthcare Costs of Extreme Heat Exposure? A Comprehensive Literature Review." *Science of the Total Environment* 657:608–18. doi:10.1016/j.scitotenv.2018.11.479.

World Bank Group. 2017. *Climate-Smart Healthcare: Low-Carbon and Resilience Strategies for the Health Sector.* Washington, DC: World Bank. http://documents.worldbank.org/curated/en/322251495434571418/pdf/113572-WP-PUBLIC-FINAL-WBG-Climate-smart-Healthcare-002.pdf.

World Bank Group. 2018. *Madagascar Climate Change and Health Diagnostic: Risks and Opportunities for Climate-Smart Health and Nutrition Investment.* Washington, DC: World Bank. http://documents.worldbank.org/curated/en/936661516004441146/pdf/121945-12-1-2018-11-21-5-WorldBankMadagascarClimateChangeandHealthDiagnosticJan.pdf.

World Health Assembly. 2019. *Emergency Care Systems for Universal Health Coverage: Ensuring Timely Care for the Acutely Ill and Injured. May* 28, 2019. https://apps.who.int/gb/ebwha/pdf_files/WHA72/A72_R16-en.pdf.

World Health Organization. 2014. *WHO Guidance to Protect Health from Climate Change through Health Adaptation Planning*. Geneva: WHO. https://apps.who.int/iris/bitstream/handle/10665/137383/9789241508001_eng.pdf?sequence=1.

World Health Organization. 2015. *Operational Framework for Building Climate Resilient Health Systems*. Geneva: WHO. https://www.afro.who.int/sites/default/files/2017-06/9789241565073_eng.pdf.

World Health Organization. 2017. *Small Island Developing States Health and WHO Country Presence Profile*. Geneva: WHO. https://apps.who.int/iris/bitstream/handle/10665/255804/WHO-CCU-17.08-eng.pdf;jsessionid=9DA117F2CD8E87C18C3C303F10ADF63A?sequence=1.

World Health Organization and World Bank Group. 2018. *Methodological Guidance Climate Change and Health Diagnostic: A Country-Based Approach for Assessing Risks and Investing in Climate-Smart Health Systems*. Washington, DC: World Bank. http://documents.worldbank.org/curated/en/552631515568426482/pdf/122328-WP-PUBLIC-WorldBankClimateChangeandHealthDiagnosticMethodologyJan.pdf.

CHAPTER 26

HEALTH PROFESSIONAL CLIMATE ENGAGEMENT

Amy Collins, Shanda Demorest, and Sarah Spengeman

Introduction

The health care sector is on the frontline of the climate crisis, bearing the shifting burden of disease attributable to climate change along with injuries and illnesses related to extreme weather events. Extreme weather disasters can disrupt health care infrastructure, access, and delivery. However, at the same time, health care operations contribute to climate change and the burden of disease, with the health care sector responsible for nearly 10 percent of United States greenhouse gas emissions (Eckelman and Sherman 2016). As the only sector with a healing mission, the health care sector has a historic opportunity to use its political, economic, and ethical influence to promote **climate-smart health care** and other climate solutions to protect human health.

Health professionals are **trusted messengers**, and historical **social movements** have taught us that they can be powerful advocates for systemic change. Health professionals have many opportunities to use their trusted voices and health expertise to educate patients, the public, policymakers, and health care administrators about the health impacts of climate change and the carbon footprint of the health care sector, as well as advocate for climate solutions locally, nationally, and internationally.

Social Movements

Health professionals have been instrumental in the success of many social movements that have sought to advance social justice, protect the vulnerable, and safeguard human health and our environment (McCally 2002). Social movements are collective actions in which the public is alerted, educated, and then mobilized to challenge prevailing economic and political norms to redress social problems and restore critical social values.

The Special Challenge of Climate Change

The first major challenge to addressing climate change is the absence of one single source of the problem to target—and the lack of a single solution. There are many responsible actors and many sources of emissions, which presents a challenge for organizers and activists to coalesce around a single actor and a single solution.

The second challenge is one of mobilizing support for climate action. Past social movements were primarily fought by those directly affected by the injustice. Although climate change already has adverse impacts on human health, many people still see it as a distant threat that may not affect them personally. Health professionals have an opportunity to help people understand the many ways climate

KEY CONCEPTS

- Health professionals serve on the front lines of the climate health crisis.

- Health professionals are trusted messengers.

- Other social movements have taught us that health professionals can be powerful champions for social change.

- The health care sector can leverage its political, ethical, and economic influence to advance climate solutions.

- Health professionals have many opportunities to advocate for climate-smart health care and climate policy solutions.

change is *already* harming health and how it has the potential to be disastrous for the health of future generations if we fail to act.

The third major challenge to addressing climate change is time. Never before has the window for action been so narrow. As former President Obama noted in 2014, "we are the first generation to feel the impact of climate change and the last generation that can do something about it."

Stories of Success: Historical Social Movements

Although the challenge of climate change is unprecedented, historical social movements offer lessons. We have learned that a small group of dedicated advocates who act as trusted messengers, or persons regarded as credible sources of health information, can successfully mobilize the public to support transformative leadership across society. To be successful, social movements need to shape public opinion while also persuading decision-makers to implement policy solutions (Moyer 1987).

The Nuclear Crisis

In the 1960s, Physicians for Social Responsibility (PSR) emerged as U.S. physicians organized to address the threat of nuclear weapons. PSR helped launch an international movement of physicians which was instrumental in building support for a comprehensive nuclear test ban treaty. PSR was effective in influencing public opinion because physicians were viewed by the public as highly credible and trusted messengers. By drawing attention to the health impacts of nuclear testing, physicians helped break down partisanship around the issue of nuclear arms and defense (Alexander 2013). Before the 1960s, nuclear testing and the arms race had been seen, even by the American Medical Association (AMA), as a political issue (Alexander). PSR helped reframe the debate by educating the public about how their health was *currently* being impacted. In the 1960s, by pointing to research that showed the presence of strontium-90 (a by-product of nuclear testing) in children's teeth, physicians employed a powerful public education strategy that connected with both hearts (children are a powerful subject) and minds (sound scientific research communicated by credible sources). This effort led to the signing of the Limited Test Ban Treaty, which ended above-ground nuclear tests by the United States, the USSR, and Britain in 1963 (PSR 2000).

Tobacco

In the first half of the twentieth century, public health advocates faced an uphill battle in the fight against tobacco. Smoking was widely accepted in American society and was promoted by sophisticated advertising campaigns and powerful corporate interests (Yale University Library 2018). Recognizing the deep trust people have for medical professionals, tobacco companies aggressively courted physician endorsements as a key advertising strategy (Gardner and Brandt 2006).

The tide began to shift in the 1950s when a growing number of studies linked smoking to cancer. In 1953, the *Journal of the American Medical Association* (JAMA) stopped publishing cigarette advertisements and banned cigarette companies from exhibiting at AMA conventions (Gardner and Brandt 2006). In 1964, the U.S. Surgeon General released the first report of the Surgeon General's Advisory Committee on Smoking and Health. Based on more than 7,000 articles, the report concluded that cigarette smoking is a cause of lung and laryngeal cancer (Centers for Disease Control and Prevention [CDC] 1999). Health organizations relied on medical research to persuade Congress to pass the first Federal Cigarette Labeling and

Advertising Act of 1965, which required cigarette packages to be labeled with a health warning (Association of Centers for the Study of Congress n.d.). In the 1980s and 1990s, other messaging strategies such as the negative health impacts of secondhand smoke helped to change public attitudes and beliefs about smoking and persuade policymakers to take action to reduce smoking rates. The validation of tobacco use as a significant threat to human health was key to the success of the tobacco control movement. Tobacco control efforts, including education and public policy, are estimated to be associated with avoidance of eight million premature deaths between 1964-2012 in the United States alone (Holford et al. 2014).

Mercury

The advocacy of Health Care Without Harm (HCWH), the organization that led the global campaign for mercury-free health care, provides additional lessons in successful organizing for social change. In 1997, the Environmental Protection Agency (EPA) found that medical waste incinerators were the fourth largest source of mercury emissions in the United States (EPA 1997). HCWH's strategy began with engaging a single hospital in eliminating mercury-based medical devices, starting with a Mercury Awareness Day and a thermometer swap at Beth Israel Deaconess Medical Center (BIDMC) in Boston (Karliner, Cohen, and Orris 2014). By focusing attention at the local level and creating a visible "media moment," HCWH was able to provide a model of success to persuade hospital leaders across the United States to eliminate mercury devices. This example illustrated the campaign's key message: that hospitals and health professionals have an ethical responsibility to not contribute to the diseases they are aiming to treat. By using the model of BIDMC and the "first, do no harm" message, HCWH was able to scale mercury elimination in hospitals across the United States (Karliner et al. 2014).

In July 2007, after pressure from HCWH and other European nongovernmental organizations, the European Union agreed to ban the sale of mercury thermometers for use in health care. The successful elimination of mercury in hospitals across the globe, as well as the passage of local, national, and regional policies prohibiting use of these devices, helped set the stage for a global treaty. After three years of negotiations, 140 countries agreed to the Minamata Convention, which phases out the export, import, and manufacturing of mercury-containing products, including thermometers and blood pressure devices by 2020 (United Nations Environment Programme 2019).

Lessons Learned

What are key lessons for health professional climate advocates from historical social movements?

- Health professionals are trusted sources of health information.
- A health framework supports policy action by helping to break down partisanship.
- Health professionals can accelerate global social, economic, and political change by starting at the local level and using health sector action to build the case for policy change.

Health professionals can use these lessons to guide movement-building to accelerate climate solutions. However, it is important to recognize that it is not necessary to win over every opponent. Organizing body 350.org emphasizes this with their Spectrum of Allies (Figure 26.1).

Using this model, early adopters of the idea that climate change affects health will help elevate the message and "recruit" key stakeholders to shift the trend from opposition to

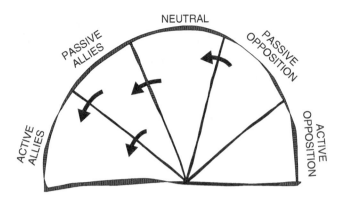

Figure 26.1   Spectrum of Allies
Source: 350.org (n.d.).

acceptance. This transition from opposition to neutrality to support has been demonstrated in recent studies around belief in global warming. Between 2009 and 2018, the percentage of Americans who are concerned or alarmed about global warming increased from 51 percent to 59 percent (Yale Program on Climate Change Communication 2019). Thus, employing a human health narrative led by health professionals shows promise as the foundation for necessary climate action by influencers and decision-makers around the world.

Why Health Professionals Should Advocate for Climate Solutions

Patient advocacy is inherent to the role of the health professional and a critical component of the provider-patient relationship. In its Declaration of Professional Responsibilities, the AMA (2017) stated that physicians should "advocate for political, economic, educational and social systemic changes that protect human health and well-being." In addition, the American Board of Internal Medicine has called for a "commitment to the promotion of public health and preventive medicine, as well as public advocacy on the part of each physician" (Brennan et al. 2002). (Figure 26.2).

Although many health professionals recognize that advocacy is important, few engage because of the demands of clinical care, competing priorities, concern about being per-

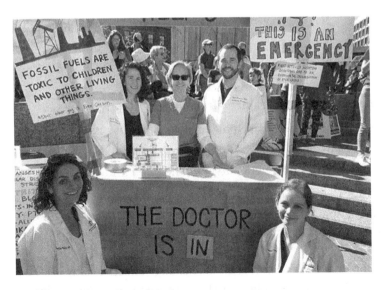

Figure 26.2   Health professional advocacy
Source: Courtesy of A. Collins.

ceived as political, and lack of awareness about how to take action. However, it is critical that health professionals actively engage in and prioritize climate advocacy for the following reasons:

- Climate change is having an adverse impact on health. Medical societies are calling on health professionals to take climate action by calling on health professionals to advocatinge for policies that reduce greenhouse gas emissions help reduce health care's carbon footprint, and educate patients and communities about climate change and health (Medical Society Consortium on Climate and Health n.d.).

- The health care sector contributes to climate change.

- Extreme weather events can disrupt health care access, delivery, and supply chains.

- Health professionals are trusted messengers. In 2019, for the eighteenth consecutive year, nurses topped the Gallup Poll as America's most trusted profession ranking number one for honesty and integrity, with doctors and pharmacists ranked third and fourth (Reinhart 2020). Research has shown that primary care providers are the most trusted source of information about climate change (Maibach et al. 2015).

- Climate advocacy is in keeping with the oath to "first, do no harm."

Advocacy within the Health Care Sector

Why Start with the Health Care Sector?

Health care leaders can use their ethical influence to drive climate solutions, use their economic power to move markets, and leverage their political influence to drive policy change. Health care can make the case—with its ethical, political, and economic clout—that promoting climate solutions is in the interest of both human and environmental health.

Health Care's Responsibility

The health care sector is responsible for almost 10 percent of U.S. greenhouse gas emissions (Eckelman and Sherman 2016). Furthermore, if the global health care sector were a country, it would be the fifth largest emitter of greenhouse gas emissions (HCWH 2019a). Hospitals are energy and water intensive, generate huge amounts of waste, and have large supply chains procuring billions of dollars of food, pharmaceuticals, supplies, and devices. In fact, the supply chain is a major contributor to health care's climate footprint, contributing to 71% of health care's emissions via the production, transport, and disposal of goods. (HCWH 2019a). In addition, hospitals generate waste anesthetic gases, serve large amounts of meat, and have a significant transportation footprint, all contributing to health care emissions. Thus, the health sector has many opportunities to align operations with its healing mission and implement climate-smart strategies to both improve health and mitigate climate change (Figure 26.3).

Climate-smart health care is defined as low-carbon, resilient health care with the following strategies: investments in renewable energy and energy efficiency, waste minimization and sustainable waste management, sustainable transportation and water policies, low-carbon procurement policies, and resilience strategies to withstand extreme weather events (World Bank 2017).

Why Is the Health Care Sector Influential?

The health care sector holds immense power in decision-making from an economic, political, and ethical perspective.

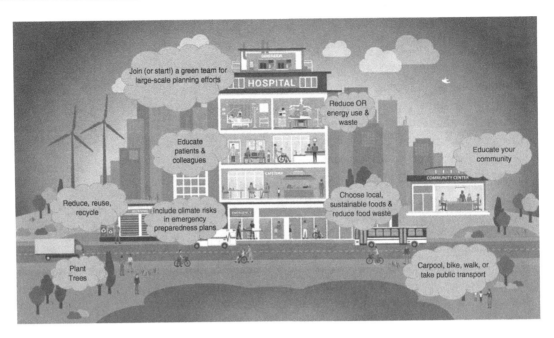

Figure 26.3   How to promote climate-smart health care within a hospital
Source: Nurses Climate Challenge (2020).

Economic Influence

As the largest industry in the United States, the health care sector has significant economic power (Thompson 2018). Health spending in the United States is 18 percent of national gross domestic product (GDP) and is projected to grow 5.5 percent annually (Cuckler et al. 2018). Hospitals are often the largest employers in their communities, and hospitals and health systems top the list of the largest employers in many states (Rege 2018). The health care sector has an enormous supply chain with the purchasing volume of the top group purchasing organizations of over $189 billion in 2017 (Gooch 2017).

Political Influence

Because hospitals are major employers, elected officials are interested in hearing from hospital leaders and other health professionals. Health professionals can influence public policy by framing environmental sustainability in terms of improving patient outcomes and reducing health care costs.

Ethical Influence

As a sector dedicated to protecting health, health care has moral credibility that can be leveraged to reframe climate change as a threat to the health of the communities they serve. As a mission-driven sector, health care can be a trusted voice at the policymaking table.

Health Care's Opportunity

The health care sector has a unique responsibility and historic opportunity to protect public health from climate change, improve community resilience and accelerate the transition to a low carbon future. Hospitals are valued "**anchor institutions**": they are rooted in place, hold significant investments in real estate and social capital, and are among the largest employers in their communities (Schwarz 2017). As anchor institutions, hospitals can leverage their influence to improve local health, economies, and resilience.

The health care sector can shift trends by implementing **climate-smart health care** strategies and leverage its purchasing power to lead the transformation to a low-carbon economy. By investing in regional clean energy projects and purchasing food from local farms, hospitals not only advance climate solutions; they also support local, sustainable jobs that promote healthy, equitable communities (Norris and Howard 2015).

How Health Professionals Can Engage within Their Health Care Facility

Clinical Champions

Health professionals working to advance sustainable health care have come to be known as **"clinical champions."** Practice Greenhealth defines clinical champions as health professionals "who advocate for change, leverage their influence within the organization, and lead their peers on sustainability issues so that it becomes a part of the culture and operating norms for the facility" (2016). An engaged clinical workforce can be a boost for a successful hospital sustainability program.

Clinical champions can educate their colleagues through grand rounds and other presentations. They can also work within the hospital settings with colleagues from operating rooms, environmental services, food services, purchasing, facilities management, pharmacy, and disaster management to advocate for climate-smart health care strategies.

Recognizing the value of health professional engagement, many leading hospitals have identified clinical champions. Practice Greenhealth (2019) reported that 71 percent of all Environmental Excellence Award winners had identified a clinical champion to lead efforts on clinical engagement and education, and 96 percent of their Top 25 performing hospitals and 100 percent of their Circle of Excellence award winners had appointed a clinical champion in 2018.

How to Get Started

Health professionals can start by becoming a champion in their department or unit. If a facility is a member of Practice Greenhealth (2020a), champions can use the engaged leadership toolkit (Practice Greenhealth 2020b) to develop a strategy for talking to hospital's leaders about sustainability.

At the Bedside

Research by Maibach and colleagues (2015) has shown that most Americans do not understand the health implications of climate change but that primary care providers and public health professionals are the most trusted professions to deliver the climate message. Health care providers have a critical opportunity to integrate climate education into routine provider–patient conversations. For example:

- While caring for patients with heat-related illnesses, a provider can educate about the health impacts of extreme heat and opportunities for patients to reduce their risk of heat-related illness.

- While treating a patient with tick-borne illness, a clinician can provide education about how rising temperatures are causing changes in the prevalence and geographical distribution of tick- and other vector-borne diseases, along with advice about how to reduce risk.

- During evaluation of a patient with an asthma exacerbation, providers can educate about local air pollution index and pollen counts.

By talking to patients about climate change and health, clinicians are communicating that climate change is a serious public health issue and that solutions exist. Such education can be provided not only during conversations with patients and families but also in discharge instructions and patient educational materials such as flyers and posters (HCWH 2020).

Clinically Sustainable Health Care

The tremendous resources required to provide clinical care significantly contribute to health care's carbon footprint. In the process of providing patient care, health professionals order many diagnostic tests and treatments, use large amounts of supplies and devices, routinely prescribe and administer many medications, and perform procedures and surgeries. Although often necessary to provide optimal patient care, these clinical interventions do not *always* add value, *can* cause harm, and contribute to both wasteful health care spending and health care pollution.

Although the attention to health care waste has been motivated by interest in reducing costs and improving patient safety, reducing wasteful health care practices can yield environmental co-benefits including emissions reduction. There are opportunities to make health care services more environmentally responsible without compromising patient safety, satisfaction, or efficiency. In addition, there are opportunities for individual health professionals to be good environmental stewards of health care resources and decrease optimize the environmental impact performance of the care they provide. These opportunities have led to the emerging concept of **clinical sustainability**.

According to Dr. Cassandra Thiel, assistant professor at New York University School of Medicine, clinical sustainability analyzes "the processes of providing clinical care and aims to identify ways to improve the environmental performance of clinical practice without compromising the quality of care. It looks closely at *how* we use health care resources and *why* we use them the way we do, in an effort to reduce clinical medicine's overall environmental footprint" (C. Theil, personal communication, April 3, 2019). Scholars engage in lifecycle assessment research to drive clinical sustainability forward and support evidence-based clinical and device use decisions by sustainability and health professionals.

In individual practice, health professionals can conserve health care resources and reduce waste by minimizing unnecessary surgeries, tests, and interventions as well as by becoming educated about the environmental impact of health care interventions and processes. One way to do that is by evaluating pharmaceutical prescribing practices. Pharmaceuticals contribute to the health care sector's carbon footprint; this contribution is estimated at 21 percent of the overall footprint of the health sector in England (Sustainable Development Unit 2013). Health professionals can take action by making evidence-based prescribing decisions, limiting medication quantities and refills, and recommending nonpharmaceutical interventions when appropriate (Qaseem et al. 2017). In viewing health care waste through an environmental lens, health professionals have an opportunity to promote clinically sustainable health care as a key strategy in advancing climate-smart health care.

Health Professional Leadership for Broader Social Change

Health professionals have tremendous opportunities to leverage their trusted voices, influence public policy, and build support for climate solutions at all levels of society.

Advocating with Policymakers

Climate change is often viewed as a partisan issue. Policymakers expect to hear from members of environmental interest groups in support of climate action, but environmental interest groups rarely focus on human health. Thus, health professionals have the opportunity to shift the climate change conversation from a political debate to a focus on protecting health. As major employers and large consumers of energy, representatives of health systems and hospitals can also make a strong business case for investing in clean energy as a way to reduce health care operating costs. Many elected leaders want to do the "right thing," but they must be able to make the case to their constituents and colleagues that investing in climate solutions is a justifiable use of limited public resources. Health professionals can equip policymakers with the information necessary to advance climate solutions.

Effective Communication with Policymakers

It is not necessary to be an expert on climate change or clean energy policy to effectively influence elected representatives. The most important expertise a health professional can bring to conversations with policymakers is their direct experience serving patients and communities affected by climate change.

The first step to being an effective policy advocate is knowing one's representatives at the city, county, state, and federal levels, as well as the policy areas they are directly responsible for. Developing a relationship with elected officials starts with an introductory meeting to explain why climate change is an important health concern. Regular communications with elected representatives help establish health professionals as a trusted source of information and ensures that representatives know they will be held accountable for their decisions. It is important to share relevant facts and data about climate change and health and to provide specific recommendations for policy solutions. Furthermore, personal stories of how climate change places patients or communities at risk helps put a human face to the data. Because stories hinge upon shared human experiences, they are more likely than facts to be remembered by policymakers.

Amplifying the Voice of the Health Professional

When it comes to policy advocacy, there is power in numbers. Elected officials need to know that the health professional community is united in declaring a climate-health emergency and calling for urgent climate action (climatehealthaction.org 2019).

Leveraging the Media to Amplify the Message

Coverage of climate change by the media does not match the scope or urgency of the crisis. For example, only twenty-two of the top fifty U.S. newspapers covered the 2018 Intergovernmental Panel on Climate Change (IPCC) Special Report citing a decade to dramatically reduce emissions to avoid catastrophic climate change (Macdonald 2018). Health professionals clearly have an opportunity to educate journalists about climate change and health and increase media coverage.

There are two primary ways to encourage journalists and news outlets to produce or print stories about climate and health. The first is through creating content with proactive outreach to the press. The second option is to make the climate and health message visible at events or as part of other stories the media may already be covering.

Traditional Media Outreach

Proactive outreach to the media involves making direct contact with media outlets, editors, and journalists, and encouraging them to cover or publish articles about climate and health by submitting opinion pieces such as op-eds or letters to the editor (LTEs). Health professionals have an advantage in publishing submissions because editors often want opinion articles to come from individuals who have credibility on the topic they are writing about.

Both op-eds and LTEs provide the strong, informed, and focused opinion of the author. Compelling op-eds include stories that demonstrate the author's direct experience with or knowledge of climate change and health. LTEs are shorter, more succinct, and are usually written in response to a published article or recent event.

For both op-eds and LTEs, timing is everything. Health professionals should watch for opportunities such as the publication of a new climate or health report, a recently introduced bill or an upcoming hearing, or an extreme weather event and then clearly connect the current event to how climate change is harming health locally. All opinion pieces should end with a focus on solutions and a clear call to action.

The more health professionals interact with journalists, provide valuable information, and serve as a trusted source, the more likely journalists are to reach out to cover climate and health stories.

Just Show Up

The second primary way to get media coverage is to show up where the media will already have a presence. For instance, by signing up to testify at a hearing, health professionals can educate policymakers and the public and may be quoted in the press. Public marches, protests, and demonstrations are also often covered by the press. Health professionals can make themselves more visible at climate events by wearing white coats or scrubs, carrying signs with messages such as "climate change is a health emergency," and marching together.

Finally, educating journalists about climate change can increase coverage. Health journalists are already covering stories about health care, and environmental journalists are already covering stories about energy and the environment. When an article is published on increasing asthma rates, for example, health professionals can contact the journalist and explain the effect climate change is having on air quality. Similarly, if an article from an environmental journalist addresses how renewable energy creates jobs, health professionals can contact the author and explain how climate solutions also benefit health. Doing so not only educates the journalist and increases the likelihood this frame will be used for their next story, but also provides them with a trusted source of information.

Social Media

Social media can be used to reframe public conversation about climate change to focus on health while also holding elected leaders accountable for their actions. Social media is an effective way to communicate with elected representatives in a public way. Health professionals can comment on representatives' pages, thank them for their position or vote, or express displeasure when they do not support policies that advance climate solutions. A survey of congressional staff showed that nearly two thirds of respondents reported that social media was a somewhat important or very important tool for understanding constituents' views and opinions (Congressional Management Foundation 2011). Social media can increase the effectiveness and amplify the impact of in-person meetings, e-mails, and phone calls.

Individual Climate Action

Given the enormity and urgency of the climate crisis, personal climate action can feel futile. However, environmental action at home and can build momentum for broader advocacy and changes at the local, institutional, and national level. Individual action communicates to others what is personally important and can ultimately start to shift social norms. Research has shown that the four most effective individual actions to reduce one's carbon footprint with the potential to drive systemic change are having one fewer child, living car free, avoiding air travel, and eating a plant-based diet (Wynes and Nicholas 2017). In this study, Wynes and Nicholas evaluated a variety of lifestyle choices and found that these four behaviors have greater potential to reduce emissions than commonly promoted strategies such as recycling and upgrading household light bulbs. By leading by example, individuals let others know that they value environmental action which can motivate others to make similar lifestyle choices and ultimately drive larger, systemic changes. For example, a survey by Westlake (2018) found that around half of respondents who knew someone who had given up flying because of climate change reported personally flying less as a result. Other powerful individual actions are described next.

Voting and Campaign Contributions

An important individual action is financially supporting candidates and political parties with climate platforms and voting for candidates at the local, state, and federal levels that prioritize aggressive climate action. Individuals can receive guidance from the League of Conservation Voters, Be a Climate Voter, and the Environmental Voter Project.

Divestment

Individuals can also divest their financial holdings from fossil fuels and invest in environmentally responsible funds and companies using guidance from Fossil Free Funds (2019) and Fossil Free USA (n.d.b) Individuals can also encourage their employers to offer fossil-free employer-sponsored retirement plans.

Join a Group

It can be empowering to join relevant climate groups that can influence public opinion or organizational and political policy. As the climate activist Bill McKibben says, "The most important thing an individual can do is not be an individual." Joining a group such as Physicians for Social Responsibility, the Nurses Climate Challenge, or Medical Students for a Sustainable Future (Figure 26.4) is a way to feel less isolated and allow an individual to work together with other climate champions and be a part of a collective advocacy effort.

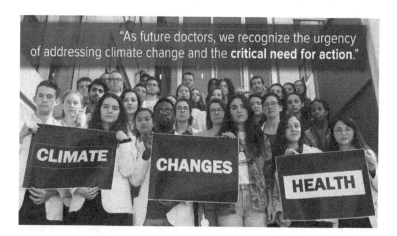

Figure 26.4   Students at Warren Alpert Medical School of Brown University
Source: Courtesy of A. Zhang.

Charitable Donations

Health professionals can align their charitable contributions with their environmental principles and consider making charitable donations to organizations that are working to promote climate solutions.

Talk about Climate

Thirty-five percent of Americans say they discuss global warming with family and friends often or occasionally, whereas 65 percent say they rarely or never talk about it (Leiserowitz et al. 2018). Because the majority of Americans are concerned about climate (Yale Program on Climate Change Communication 2019), health professionals are encouraged to use their trusted voices and talk about the health impacts of climate change and solutions with their patients, colleagues, family, and friends on a regular basis. Although individual action can be powerful and rewarding, it alone will not solve the climate crisis. Individuals must continue to demand broad political and societal changes.

Encouraging Trends

There are many positive signs that health professionals are increasingly recognizing their responsibility to address climate change and advocate for climate solutions.

Climate Change in Health Program Curricula

Medical and nursing schools are increasingly incorporating the health impacts of climate change into their curricula as the voice of students demanding its inclusion has grown louder. The 2018 Lancet Countdown on Climate Change and Health U.S. policy brief recommends that climate change and health education should be rapidly integrated into health professional curricula and continuing medical education (Salas, Knappenberger, and Hess 2018).

Leffers et al. (2017) highlight how climate curricula in nursing education is imperative, yet there are no current models or guidelines for integration. In 2020, a core cohort of nursing schools from across the United States launched a partnership with the Nurses Climate Challenge (2020) to integrate climate change into coursework and curricula. By using Nurses Climate Challenge resources, faculty leading the initiatives within their schools of nursing have the flexibility to integrate regionally and culturally relevant content into their programming.

Medical schools in the United States are starting to provide climate and health education primarily through lectures and electives, but most are not including climate education in their core curriculum (Wellbery et al. 2018). In 2019, the University of Colorado School of Medicine held its first Climate Medicine two-week elective course for fourth-year medical students (Lemery n.d.). University of California San Francisco offers a climate change course as part of its Inquiry Course in the UCSF Medical School Bridges Program (Fleischer 2017). Icahn School of Medicine at Mt. Sinai is taking a different approach and is integrating climate and health education into existing medical school courses through its Climate Change Curriculum Infusion Project (Cayon 2019).

Recognizing the need for climate education, growing numbers of medical students are inviting guest speakers and developing educational programs on their own. Overall, however, the number of medical schools providing climate and health education is small and there remains tremendous opportunity for more schools to integrate climate into their core curriculum. Recognizing this opportunity, in 2019 the AMA adopted a policy supporting climate education in undergraduate, graduate, and continuing medical education with a goal that all trainees and practicing physicians will have understanding of the health impacts of climate change and be able to counsel patients on how to protect themselves from climate risks (AMA 2019).

Climate and health curricula has gained attention at a global level as well. The International Federation of Medical Students Association (IFMSA 2016) released its Climate and Health training manual. In 2018, IFMSA launched the 2020 Vision for Climate-Health in Medical Curricula, an online advocacy platform, calling for all medical schools globally to include climate and health in their curricula by 2020 (IFMSA 2018). Finally, it is encouraging to note that many schools and programs around the world have joined a coalition launched by Columbia University's Mailman School of Public Health that supports including climate change in health education (Columbia University 2020).

Medical Society and Health Organization Leadership

Recognizing the health impacts of climate change and the power of health professional advocacy, medical societies and health organizations around the world are coming together to amplify the voice of health professionals.

In the United States, more than two dozen medical societies representing over half a million physicians have joined the Medical Society Consortium for Climate and Health, with a mission to organize, empower, and amplify the voice of the nation's doctors to convey how climate change is harming our health and how climate solutions will improve it.

By 2020, more than 160 U.S. health and medical organizations have endorsed the Call to Action on Climate, Health and Equity, which outlines a ten-point policy action agenda and calls on government officials, elected officials, businesses, civic leaders, and candidates for office to recognize climate change as a health emergency and work to implement the recommendations in the policy agenda (climatehealthaction.org 2019).

The World Medical Association (WMA 2015) has called on physicians and medical societies to keep health central to the climate debate and advocate for implementation of the Paris Agreement. In the United Kingdom, the Health Alliance on Climate Change was founded by a number of royal medical and nurse's colleges, bringing together physicians, nurses, and other health professionals to communicate the health impacts of climate change and advocate for solutions (BMJ Publishing Group 2019).

State Health Professional Climate Advocacy

In recent years, health professionals have launched state-based health professional climate action groups dedicated to educating the public and policymakers about the health threats of climate change and advocating for clean energy and investments in climate preparedness and resilience (Medical Society Consortium on Climate and Health n.d.). (Figure 26.5).

Civil Disobedience

In the era of the climate crisis, health professionals are increasingly turning toward nontraditional advocacy, including civil disobedience, to demand immediate climate solutions to protect our future. In a powerful call to action, Dr. Richard Horton, editor in chief of *The Lancet*, called on health professionals worldwide to engage in nonviolent, social protest to demand solutions to protect patients from the climate crisis (Doctors for Extinction Rebellion 2019). (Figure 26.6).

Health professionals are calling attention to the many ways climate affects health and are calling for action by participating in Extinction Rebellion, Global Climate Strikes, Fire Drill Fridays, and by forming nonviolent clinician climate action groups with support from the Civil Disobedience Center.

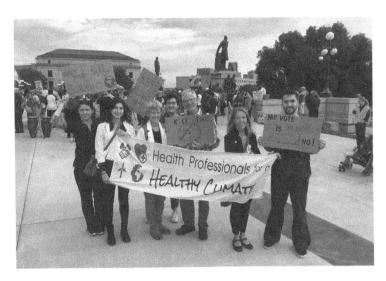

Figure 26.5   Minnesota Health Professional Climate Action Group "Health Professionals for a Healthy Climate"
Source: Courtesy of S. Demorest.

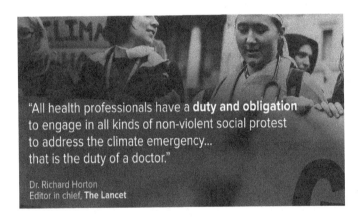

Figure 26.6   Health professionals engaging in civil disobedience
Source: Courtesy of HCWH.

Fossil Fuel Divestment

Fossil fuel divestment is a way for health care professionals to ensure that their investments uphold their environmental and health values. The World Medical Association has recommended that its national medical associations and all health organizations begin the process of divesting from fossil fuel companies (Wellbery et al. 2018). Some U.S. and international health organizations have already partially or completely divested from fossil fuels (Fossil Free USA n.d.a). In 2020, the *British Medical Journal* issued a call to action for health professionals and medical organizations worldwide to divest from fossil fuels and restore hope for the future well-being of our planet and human health (Abbasi and Godlee 2020). They also offer guidance to help individuals and organizations successfully divest (UK Health Alliance on Climate Change 2017).

Hospital and Health System Leadership

With support and guidance from HCWH, health care facilities around the world are reducing their carbon footprint, transitioning to clean, renewable energy, building climate-resilient facilities, and investing in community health and resilience.

Health care systems are increasingly setting ambitious climate and clean energy goals. For example, Kaiser Permanente, which operates thirty-nine hospitals and more than 700 medical offices, set a goal to be carbon net positive by 2025 (Kaiser Permanente 2018). Contributing approximately 5 percent of the United Kingdom's total emissions, the National Health Service has commissioned an expert panel to guide the system towards a goal of net zero emissions (NHS n.d.).

HCWH's global campaign to advance climate-smart health care, the Health Care Climate Challenge, had over 200 participants in 2020, representing the interests of more than 22,000 hospitals and health centers in thirty-three countries (HCWH 2019b). Eighteen health care institutions, representing the interests of more than 1,200 hospitals and health centers in ten countries, have also pledged to implement 100 percent renewable electricity in their facilities (HCWH 2019b).

Hospitals and health care systems are increasingly leveraging their role as anchor institutions to drive market and systems change, while also strengthening health, equity, and resilience at the local level. Many U.S. health systems and hospitals have adopted the Cool Food Pledge, committing to offer more plant-forward meals, while tracking their food-related emissions and joining with other major food distributors and servicers to shift the food system to be more sustainable. Hospitals such as Cleveland Clinic, Seattle Children's Hospital, and the Medical University of South Carolina, among many others, are investing in tree planting on their own campuses and in their communities to support cleaner air, counter the urban heat-island effect, and improve stormwater management, especially in historically disadvantaged communities (Arbor Day Foundation 2020).

Health care systems are also demonstrating leadership at the state, national, and international levels. In both the United States and Europe, health care institutions have come together to form Health Care Climate Councils: leadership bodies devoted to moving the sector toward climate-smart health care while leveraging their economic and political influence for market and policy change. In 2017 and 2019, the U.S. Health Care Climate Council traveled to Washington, D.C. to advocate for climate and health solutions with congressional representatives. In California, Massachusetts, and Washington, hospitals and health systems have formed Health Care Climate Alliances to bring health care's voice to the climate and clean energy policymaking process. Twenty-four U.S. health care systems, operating more than 800 hospitals, have also joined We Are Still In, pledging to support the goals of the historic Paris Agreement.

Summary

Climate change poses an urgent global threat to human health and health care delivery. Health professionals have led social movements in the past, yielding results that have changed public attitudes and shaped policy outcomes. Health professionals have a historic opportunity to reframe climate change as a health issue while also transforming the health care sector and advancing policy solutions. With its moral credibility, purchasing power, and political and economic influence, the health care sector is uniquely poised to accelerate the transition to a healthy and sustainable future. There are many advocacy tools and resources available to health professionals, and positive trends including new curricula in nursing and medical schools, the formation of clinician climate action groups, and the commitment of health systems to 100 percent renewable energy show that health professionals can lead climate solutions.

KEY TERMS

Anchor institutions: Enterprises such as universities and hospitals that are rooted in their local communities by mission, invested capital, or relationships to customers, employees, and vendors.

Climate-smart health care: Low carbon, resilient health care strategies.

Clinical champions: Clinicians who advocate for change, leverage their influence within the organization, and lead their peers on sustainability issues so that it becomes a part of the culture and operating norms for the facility.

Clinical sustainability: The processes of providing clinical care and identification of ways to improve the environmental performance of clinical practice without compromising the quality of care. It looks closely at how we use health care resources and why we use them the way we do, in an effort to reduce clinical medicine's overall environmental footprint.

Social movements: Collective actions in which the public is alerted, educated, and then mobilized to challenge the economic and political leaders and the whole society to redress social problems and restore critical social values.

Trusted messengers: Persons regarded as credible sources of health information.

DISCUSSION QUESTIONS

1. What lessons that can be learned from historical social movements about the role of health professionals in advancing solutions that can be applied to the climate justice movement?

2. You are a health professional committed to working on climate solutions within your facility. Your clinical supervisor has asked you why you believe health professionals should be concerned about climate change with so many competing health care priorities. What is your response? What are your three to five key messages for your clinical supervisor? Consider the same question for your hospital CEO.

3. What are your three to five key messages about why health professionals should advocate for climate solutions? How can health professionals amplify these messages? What are some examples of audiences health professionals can reach? Would you have different messages for different audiences? If so, identify several audiences and key messages for each.

4. A group of health professional students at an academic medical center has asked you how they can individually have an impact on climate change in their personal and professional lives. What do you tell them?

Online Resources

Health Care Without Harm, https://noharm-uscanada.org

Medical Students for a Sustainable Future as an online resource https://ms4sf.org

Practice Greenhealth, https://practicegreenhealth.org

Nurses Climate Challenge, https://nursesclimatechallenge.org

U.S. Call to Action on climate, health, and equity, https://climatehealthaction.org/cta/climate-health-equity-policy

Medical Society Consortium on Climate and Health, https://medsocietiesforclimatehealth.org

References

350.org. n.d.. *Spectrum of Allies.* https://trainings.350.org/resource/spectrum-of-allies/.

Abbasi, K.. and F. Godlee. 2020. "Investing in Humanity: The BMJ's Divestment Campaign." *BMJ* 368 (167). https://doi.org/10.1136/bmj.m167.

Alexander, S. 2013. "The origins of Physicians for Social Responsibility (PSR) and International Physicians for the Prevention of Nuclear War (IPPNW)." *Social Medicine* 7 (3):120–26.

American Medical Association. 2017. "A Declaration of Professional Responsibility H-140.900." https://policysearch.ama-assn.org/policyfinder/detail/medical%20ethic?uri=%2FAMADoc%2FHOD.xml-0-431.xml.

American Medical Association. 2019. "AMA Adopts New Policies at 2019 Annual Meeting." June 12, 2019. https://www.ama-assn.org/press-center/press-releases/ama-adopts-new-policies-2019-annual-meeting?mc_cid=1e1e669256&mc_eid=448c3c9a4a.

Arbor Day Foundation. 2020. "Tree Campus Healthcare." https://www.arborday.org/programs/tree-campus-healthcare/?Trackingid=404.

Association of Centers for the Study of Congress. n.d. "Federal Cigarette Labeling and Advertising Act." http://acsc.lib.udel.edu/exhibits/show/legislation/cigarette-labeling.

Brennan, T., L. Blank, J. Cohen, H. Kimball, N. Smelser, R. Copeland, R. Lavizzo-Mourey et al. 2002. Medical Professionalism in the New Millennium: A Physician Charter. *Annals of Internal Medicine* 136 (3):243–6. https://annals.org/aim/fullarticle/474090/medical-professionalism-new-millennium-physician-charter.

BMJ Publishing Group. 2019. "Climate Change." https://www.bmj.com/campaign/climate-change.

Cayon, C. 2019. "Preparing Medical Students for a Warmer World." January 3, 2019. https://www.commondreams.org/views/2019/01/03/preparing-medical-students-warmer-world.

Centers for Disease Control. 1999. "Achievements in Public Health, 1900–1999: Tobacco Use—United States, 1900–1999. *MMWR. Morbidity and Mortality Weekly Report* 48 (43):986–93.

Climatehealthaction.org. 2019. "U.S. Call to Action on Climate, Health, and Equity: A Policy Action Agenda." https://climatehealthaction.org/cta/climate-health-equity-policy/.

Columbia University. 2020. "List of GCCHE [Global Consortium on Climate and Health Education] Member Institutions." https://www.mailman.columbia.edu/research/global-consortium-climate-and-health-education/list-gcche-member-institutions.

Congressional Management Foundation. 2011. *#SocialCongress: Perceptions and Use of Social Media on Capitol Hill.* Washington, DC: CMF. http://www.congressfoundation.org/storage/documents/CMF_Pubs/cmf-social-congress-2011.pdf.

Cuckler, G. A., A. M. Sisko, J. A. Poisal, S. P. Keehan, S. D. Smith, A. J. Madison, C. J. Wolfe, and J. C. Hardesty. 2018. "National Health Expenditure Projections, 2017–26: Despite Uncertainty, Fundamentals Primarily Drive Spending Growth." *Health Affairs* 37 (3). https://doi.org/10.1377/hlthaff.2017.1655.

Doctors for Extinction Rebellion. 2019. *Lancet Editor "Doctors Obliged to Protest" about Health and Climate* [Video]. YouTube. October 24, 2019. https://www.youtube.com/watch?v=2x6sBfV64N4&feature=youtu.be.

Eckelman, M. J., and J. Sherman. 2016. "Environmental Impacts of the U.S. Health Care System and Effects on Public Health." *PLoS ONE* 11 (6):e0157014. https://doi.org/10.1371/journal.pone.0157014.

Environmental Protection Agency. 1997. *Hospital/Medical/Infectious Waste Incinerators: Background Information for Promulgated Standards and Guidelines—Regulatory Impact Analysis for New And Existing Facilities.* Report EPA-453/R-97-009B. Research Triangle Park, NC: EPA. https://www3.epa.gov/ttn/ecas/docs/ria/solid-waste_ria_final_hospital-waste-incinerators_1997-07.pdf.

Fossil Free Funds. 2019. "Are Your Savings Invested in Fossil Fuels?" https://fossilfreefunds.org/blog/2017/03/23/are-your-savings-supporting-clean-energy-or-fossil-fuels.html.

Fossil Free USA. n.d.a. "1000+ divestment commitments." https://gofossilfree.org/divestment/commitments/.

Fossil Free USA. n.d.b. "Your Roadmap to Divestment." https://gofossilfree.org/usa/your-roadmap-to-personal-divestment/.

Fleischer, D. 2017. "UCSF Medical School Inquiry Course Explores Link between Climate Change and Health." https://sustainability.ucsf.edu/1.659.

Gardner, M. N., and A. M. Brandt. 2006. "'The Doctors' Choice Is America's Choice': The Physician in US Cigarette Advertisements, 1930–1953." *American Journal of Public Health* 96 (2):222–32. doi: 10.2105/AJPH.2005.066654.

Gooch, K. 2017. "4 of the largest GPOs." February 6, 2017. https://www.beckershospitalreview.com/finance/4-of-the-largest-gpos-2017.html.

Health Care Without Harm. 2019a. *Health Care's Climate Footprint*. Brussels: HCWH. https://noharm-global.org/sites/default/files/documents-files/5961/HealthCaresClimateFootprint_092319.pdf.

Health Care Without Harm. 2019b. "The Health Care Climate Challenge." https://noharm-uscanada.org/healthcareclimatechallenge.

Health Care Without Harm. 2020. "Climate and Health Patient Education." https://noharm-uscanada.org/content/us-canada/climate-and-health-patient-education.

Holford, T. R., R. Meza, K. E. Warner, C. Meernik, J. Jeon, S. H. Moolgavkar, and D. T. Levy. 2014. Tobacco Control and the Reduction in Smoking-Related Premature Deaths in the United States, 1964–2012." *JAMA* 311 (2):164–71. doi: 10.1001/jama.2013.285112.

Intergovernmental Panel on Climate Change. 2018. *Global Warming of 1.5°C. An IPCC Special Report on the Impacts of Global Warming of 1.5°C above Pre-Industrial Levels and Related Global Greenhouse Gas Emission Pathways, in the Context of Strengthening the Global Response to the Threat of Climate Change, Sustainable Development, and Efforts to Eradicate Poverty*, edited by V. Masson-Delmotte, P. Zhai, H.-O. Pörtner, D. Roberts, J. Skea, P. R. Shukla, A. Pirani, W. Moufouma-Okia et al. Geneva: IPCC.

International Federation of Medical Students' Associations. 2016. *Training Manual: Climate and Health: Enabling Students and Young Professionals to Understand and Act upon Climate Change Using a Health Narrative*. Copenhagen: IFMSA. https://ifmsa.org/wp-content/uploads/2017/03/Final-IFMSA-Climate-and-health-training-Manual-2016.pdf.

International Federation of Medical Students' Associations. 2018. *Sixty-Fifth Session of the WHO Regional Committee for the Eastern Mediterranean Agenda Item 5 (c): Draft of WHO Global Strategy on Health, Environment, and Climate Change*. Copenhagen: IFMSA. https://ifmsa.org/wp-content/uploads/2018/10/IFMSA-Statement-5c_health_environment_climate_change.pdf.

Kaiser Permanente. 2018. "We Will Be Carbon Neutral in 2020." September 10, 2018. https://about.kaiserpermanente.org/community-health/news/kaiser-permanente-finalizes-agreement-to-enable-carbon-neutralit.

Karliner, J., G. Cohen, G., and P. Orris. 2014. "Lessons in Forging Global Change." *Stanford Social Innovation Review* Winter 2014. https://ssir.org/articles/entry/lessons_in_forging_global_change

Leffers, J., R. M. Levy, P. K. Nicholas, and C. F. Sweeney. 2017. "Mandate for the Nursing Profession to Address Climate Change through Nursing Education." *Journal of Nursing Scholarship* 49 (6):679–87. https://doi.org/10.1111/jnu.12331.

Leiserowitz, A., E. Maibach, C. Roser-Renouf, S. Rosenthal, M. Cutler, and J. Kotcher. 2018. "Climate Change in the American Mind: March 2018." April 27, 2018. http://climatecommunication.yale.edu/publications/climate-change-american-mind-march-2018/2/.

Lemery, J. n.d. "4th Year Medical Student Elective: Climate Medicine EMED 8010." https://www.coloradowm.org/courses/med-student-electives/4th-year-medical-student-elective-climate-medicine-emed-8010/.

Macdonald, T. 2018. "Majority of Top US Newspapers Fail to Mention Landmark Climate Change Report on Their Homepages." [Blog post] .October 8, 2018. https://www.mediamatters.org/new-york-times/majority-top-us-newspapers-fail-mention-landmark-climate-change-report-their?redirect_source=/blog/2018/10/08/Majority-of-top-US-newspapers-fail-to-mention-landmark-climate-change-report-on-their-home/221608.

Maibach, E. W., J. M. Kreslake, C. Roser-Renouf, S. Rosenthal, G. Feinberg, and A. A. Leiserowitz. 2015. "Do Americans Understand that Global Warming Is Harmful to Human Health? Evidence from a National Survey. *Annals of Global Health* 81 (3):396–409. https://doi.org/10.1016/j.aogh.2015.08.010.

McCally, M. 2002. "Health and the Environment." *Annals of the American Academy of Political and Social Science*, 584:145–58.

Medical Society Consortium on Climate and Health. n.d.. "About." https://medsocietiesforclimatehealth.org/about/.

Moyer, B. 1987. "The Movement Action Plan: A Strategic Framework Describing the Eight Stages of Successful Social Movements." https://www.historyisaweapon.com/defcon1/moyermap.html.

National Health Service. n.d.. "A net zero NHS." https://www.england.nhs.uk/greenernhs/a-net-zero-nhs/.

Norris, T., and T. Howard. 2015. *Can Hospitals Heal America's Communities?* Washington, DC: Democracy Collaborative. https://community-wealth.org/sites/clone.community-wealth.org/files/downloads/CanHospitalsHealAmericasCommunities.pdf.

Nurses Climate Challenge. 2020. "About Us." https://nursesclimatechallenge.org/about.

Physicians for Social Responsibility. 2000. *Physicians for Social Responsibility: A History of Accomplishments*. Washington, DC: PSR. https://secure2.convio.net/psr/documents/history.pdf.

Practice Greenhealth. 2016. *2016 Sustainability Benchmark Report.* Reston, VA: Practice Greenhealth. https://practicegreenhealth.org/sites/default/files/2019-10/2016.practice.greenhealth.sustainability.benchmark.report_0.pdf.

Practice Greenhealth. 2019. *2018 Sustainability Benchmark Data.* Reston, VA: Practice Greenhealth. https://practicegreenhealth.org/sites/default/files/2019-11/2019_sustainability_benchmark_data.pdf.

Practice Greenhealth. 2020a. "About Us." https://practicegreenhealth.org/about/about-us.

Practice Greenhealth. 2020b. *Engaged Leadership Toolkit.* Reston, VA: Practice Greenhealth. https://practicegreenhealth.org/engaged-leadership-toolkit.

Qaseem, A., T. J. Wilt, R. M. McLean, and M. A. Forciea. 2017. "Noninvasive Treatments for Acute, Subacute, and Chronic Low Back Pain: A Clinical Practice Guideline from the American College of Physicians." *Annals of Internal Medicine* 166 (7):514–30. doi: 10.7326/M16-2367.

Rege, A. 2018. "Hospitals Are the Biggest Employers in These 13 States." November 14, 2018. https://www.beckershospitalreview.com/hospital-management-administration/hospitals-are-the-biggest-employers-in-these-13-states.html.

Reinhart, R. J. 2020. "Nurses Continue to Rate Highest for Honesty, Ethics." Gallup. January 6, 2020. https://news.gallup.com/poll/274673/nurses-continue-rate-highest-honesty-ethics.aspx.

Salas, R. N., P. Knappenberger, and J. Hess. 2018. *2018 Lancet Countdown on Health and Climate Change Brief for the United States of America.* London: Lancet Countdown.

Schwarz, D. F. 2017. "What You Need to Know about Hospital Roles in Community Investment." [Blog post]. March 15, 2017. https://www.rwjf.org/en/blog/2017/03/can-hospitals-defy-tradition.html.

Sustainable Development Unit. 2013. *Carbon Footprint Update for NHS in England.* Cambridge: SDU. http://www.sduhealth.org.uk/documents/Carbon_Footprint_summary_NHS_update_2013.pdf.

Thompson, D. 2018. "Health Care Just Became the U.S.'S Largest Employer." *The Atlantic.* January 9, 2018. https://www.theatlantic.com/business/archive/2018/01/health-care-america-jobs/550079/.

UK Health Alliance on Climate Change. 2017. "Briefing: Divesting Your Health Organization from Fossil Fuels." http://www.ukhealthalliance.org/divestment/?mc_cid=f5c2dac814&mc_eid=8a77e96a25.

United Nations Environment Programme. 2019. "Minamata Convention on Mercury." http://www.mercuryconvention.org/Convention/History/tabid/3798/language/en-US/Default.aspx.

Wellbery, C., P. Sheffield, K. Timmireddy, M. Safarty, A. Teherani, and R. Fallar. 2018. "It's Time for Medical Schools to Introduce Climate Change into Their Curricula." *Academic Medicine* 93 (12):1774–7. doi: 10.1097/ACM.0000000000002368.

Westlake, S. 2018. "A Counter-Narrative to Carbon Supremacy: Do Leaders Who Give Up Flying Because of Climate Change Influence the Attitudes and Behaviour of Others?" Unpublished doctoral dissertation, Cardiff University. *SSRN.* http://dx.doi.org/10.2139/ssrn.3283157.

World Bank. 2017. *Climate-Smart Healthcare: Low-Carbon and Resilience Strategies for the Health Sector.* Washington, DC: World Bank. http://documents.worldbank.org/curated/en/322251495434571418/pdf/113572-WP-PUBLIC-FINAL-WBG-Climate-smart-Healthcare-002.pdf.

World Medical Association. 2015. "Physician Leaders Call for Health to Be Protected in Climate Change Agreement." November 15, 2015. https://www.wma.net/news-post/physician-leaders-call-for-health-to-be-protected-in-climate-change-agreement/.

Wynes, S., and K. A. Nicholas. 2017. "The Climate Mitigation Gap: Education and Government Recommendations Miss the Most Effective Individual Actions." *Environmental Research Letters* 12 (7):091001.

Yale Program on Climate Change Communication. 2019. "Global Warming's Six Americas." http://climatecommunication.yale.edu/about/projects/global-warmings-six-americas/.

Yale University Library. 2018. "Selling Smoke: Tobacco Advertising and Anti-Smoking Campaigns." http://exhibits.library.yale.edu/exhibits/show/sellingsmoke.

CHAPTER 27

SPECIFIC IMPACTS UPON HUMAN HEALTH

Caleb Dresser and Satchit Balsari

Introduction

Climate change affects every organ system in the human body. For many, these health impacts are among the most immediately visible and personally concerning aspects of climate change. The purpose of this chapter is to provide an overview of our current clinical understanding of the ways in which human diseases are impacted by climate change.

Examining the impact of climate change on each organ system of the human body reveals common themes. Environmental heat, airborne particulate matter, ecosystem changes, food insecurity, and sequalae of climate-related disasters appear again and again as principal exposures. Health impacts are unequally distributed; the burden of disease, disability, and death disproportionately affects the most vulnerable on global, national, and local levels. Extremes of age, lower socio-economic status, the presence of comorbid conditions, and social marginalization are significant mediating factors influencing individual vulnerability and the unequal disease burdens explored in this chapter. In addition, many of the most harmful impacts occur in settings with limited resilience due to weak health care systems.

Cardiovascular Disease

Coronary Artery Disease, Myocardial Infarction, and Cardiac Arrest

The impact of climate change on coronary artery disease and its sequelae is mediated via variable, warming ambient air temperatures and increased levels of airborne particulate matter.

Myocardial infarction and temperature: Extremely hot or cold weather is linked to increased rates of myocardial infarction (MI), and variability in temperature compared to local norms rather than absolute temperature appears to be a significant factor (Claeys et al. 2017). A 2013 study found a hazard ratio of 1.44 for myocardial infarction when there was extreme heat in the preceding two days, and 1.36 for extreme cold (Madrigano et al. 2013); a 2018 meta-analysis of thirty research papers showed a 1.6 percent increase in the risk of hospitalization for myocardial infarction for every degree Celsius of temperature increase, and a pooled estimate of MI mortality risk of 1.639 during heat waves (Sun al. 2018). The clinical impact of extremes of heat may be minimized by use of air conditioning in populations where this is an option (Davis et al. 2003).

Myocardial infarction and air quality: Myocardial infarction has been linked to elevated levels of ground level ozone, particulate matter, and wildfire smoke (Haikerwal et al. 2015; Mustafic et al. 2012; Reid et al. 2016), which result in a combination of systemic inflammatory response, sympathetic activation, increased blood coagulation and platelet activation, leading to the development of atherothrombosis

KEY CONCEPTS

- Patients with chronic illnesses as well as other vulnerable individuals may suffer negative health impacts because of extreme weather events, which often results in increased health care utilization.

- Clinicians practicing in temperate climates should be alert to the potential arrival of tropical and subtropical infectious diseases in their region.

- Heat-related illnesses can affect most organ systems, and impacts range from direct heat injury to an increased risk of birth anomalies.

- Mental illness, including suicide, posttraumatic stress disorder, and depression, will increase as a result of natural disasters, heat stress, social displacement, and other climate-related factors.

- Health care providers should identify and counsel vulnerable patients regarding prevention actions to consider during anticipated climate-related events such as heat waves, toxic algal blooms, wildfires, and floods. These may range from personal protective measures to health planning, sheltering or evacuation planning.

and subsequent cardiovascular pathology (Claeys et al. 2017). Particulate and ozone levels are expected to worsen in certain areas as regional heating, wildfires, desertification, and dust storms intensify. Ongoing fossil fuel use is another source of concern.

Cardiac arrest: Out of hospital cardiac arrest can be the result of innumerable possible conditions, and attribution to a primary cardiovascular cause is generally inferential rather than absolute. Within these limitations, there is evidence that extremes of environmental small-particle air pollution ($PM_{2.5}$) are associated with increased rates of out of hospital cardiac arrest, likely from cardiovascular causes. An Australian study found a 6.98 percent increase in the risk of out-of-hospital cardiac arrest, with particular risk in older adults, for every 9 mcg/m^3 increase in $PM_{2.5}$ over a two-day period (Haikerwal et al. 2015). High-risk patients should consider taking protective steps, including use of air filters or indoor sheltering or temporary evacuation from affected areas, during air quality events such as wildfires and dust storms.

Coronary artery disease: Long-term risk of coronary artery disease (CAD) and other cardiovascular injury has been linked with local air quality and cold temperatures; chronic inflammation is a hypothesized mechanism (Claeys et al. 2017). Regional warming may reduce CAD rates in cold regions, although this effect has not yet been demonstrated longitudinally.

Atrial Fibrillation

Atrial fibrillation is a common, potentially life-threatening condition. Inflammatory changes and other stresses secondary to exposure to $PM_{2.5}$ are believed to increase the rate of atrial fibrillation; a 10 mcg/m^3 increase in $PM_{2.5}$ has been associated with a 3.8 percent increase in the risk of atrial fibrillation occurrence in a large observational study (Liu et al. 2018), whereas in a study of patients with implanted pacemakers, a 26 percent increase in the odds of atrial fibrillation occurrence was observed for every 6 mcg/m^3 increase in $PM_{2.5}$ in the hours preceding the event (Link et al. 2013). Although the degree of effect is variable and likely depends on the origin of the particulate matter, the overall association appears plausible.

Heat stress also appears to contribute to the onset of atrial fibrillation. An Italian study showed the incidence of new onset atrial fibrillation increased significantly in the twenty-four hours following days with a heat index greater than 44 (Brunetti et al. 2014). In a separate study, patients with atrial fibrillation were found to have a 6 percent increase in risk of dying on extremely hot days (Zanobetti et al. 2013).

Given the anticipated increase in frequency and severity of heat waves and air quality events, elderly patients may benefit from avoiding high temperature locations or polluted air, ensuring adequate hydration, and seeking immediate medical attention for symptoms such as palpitations and lightheadedness.

Health care utilization: Health care utilization for cardiovascular disease increases with increased particulate matter, ground-level ozone, and extremes of temperature. Wildfire smoke, which contains an array of particulates and toxins and is expected to become an increasing hazard as a result of climate change, increases emergency department utilization for cardiovascular complaints, particularly in patients over age sixty-five on days with heavy smoke burden (Wettstein et al. 2018). Utilization for atrial fibrillation has also been linked to levels of particulate matter in the hemisphere, with 1.4–3 percent increases in the rate of presentation for atrial fibrillation for every 10 mcg/m^3 of particulate matter in the atmosphere (Solimini and Renzi 2017). Recent meta-analysis has also shown associations between risk of atrial fibrillation and levels of ground-level $PM_{2.5}$ and ozone (Shao et al. 2016).

Extremes of temperature have been associated with increased health care utilization and rates of cardiovascular events; whereas the impact of cold tends to be a delayed effect over several days, heat immediately increases the risk of cardiovascular events requiring hospital treatment. This effect has been replicated in multiple studies in North America, Asia, and the Middle East (Mohammadi et al. 2018). Use of emergency medical services by patients with hypertension and prior cardiovascular disease has also been found to increase on hot days (Brunetti et al. 2014). Providers who care for patients with cardiovascular disease should prepare for increased utilization by these patients during heat waves and in urban or wildfire-affected areas where levels of ozone or particulate matter are significantly elevated.

Respiratory Disease

Asthma

Asthma affects at least 339 million people globally and is responsible for more than 417,918 deaths every year (World Health Organization 2020). It is among the most common diseases of childhood in wealthy nations and disproportionately affects historically underserved populations in urban areas. Asthmatics can expect significant increases in risk of exacerbation as a result of exposure to heat, humidity, allergenic pollens, air pollution, and harmful algal blooms caused by global climate change.

Heat and Humidity: Increased temperature and humidity are important mediators of exacerbations in the asthmatic patient. Increased airway temperatures have been shown to increase activity in the vagal pulmonary C-fibers that mediate bronchoconstriction in a rat model (Lin et al. 2015), and increased pulmonary resistive indices have been found in horses with equine asthma exposed to high-temperature environments (Bullone, Murcia, and Lavoie 2016). In humans, numerous studies have shown that heat and humidity have significant clinical implications for the asthmatic patient; extremes of heat and rainfall have been associated with increased asthma-related hospitalization rates (Soneja et al. 2016), humidity has been self-reported as a trigger in patients with allergic asthma (Hayes et al. 2013), and extreme heat has been linked to hospitalizations during the hot season (Lam et al. 2016).

Pollen: Airborne pollen exposure in the temperate zone has increased in recent years as a result of climate change and is likely to increase further in the future in terms of total pollen concentrations (Katelaris and Beggs 2018), length of pollen seasons (Ziska et al. 2011), and pollen allergenicity (Ziska and Beggs 2012). Increased asthma hospitalization rates have been linked to grass and tree pollen (Guilbert et al. 2018; Heguy et al. 2008). Emergency system activations for asthma in Genoa have been associated with high levels of airborne pollen (Tosca et al. 2014), as have emergency department presentations for asthma in New York (Jariwala et al. 2014). New populations will also be affected, as the ranges for common allergen-producing plants such as ragweed shift in response to changes in the climate; an additional forty-four million people in Europe could suffer from ragweed allergies by the middle of the twenty-first century (Lake et al. 2017).

Air quality: Air pollution, including particulate matter and ground-level ozone, has a proinflammatory effect on the human respiratory tree; this can lead to asthma exacerbations and increased asthma incidence (Trasande and Thurston 2005). Elevated ozone levels have been associated with increased hospital admissions for asthma in Ontario (Burnett et al. 1994), and both ozone and $PM_{2.5}$ have been associated with increased risk of hospitalization for asthma in New York, particularly in young children (Silverman and Ito 2010). Patients with asthma and families with asthmatic children should be vigilant for climate-change-related increases in particulate matter and ozone in their communities, consider air filter use, and avoid outdoor activity during periods of poor air quality.

Harmful Algae Blooms: Residents living within 1.6 km of the coastline can experience a 44 percent increase in rates of admission for asthma during harmful algal blooms ("red tide" events), which are becoming larger and more common because of climate-related increases in ocean surface temperature (Kirkpatrick et al. 2006). Pre- and postexposure spirometry has confirmed decreases in forced expiratory volume (FEV1) and peak flow rate in asthma patients who are exposed to brevetoxins produced by harmful algae (Fleming et al. 2007). For patients with asthma living on coastlines where harmful algae blooms occur, climate change is likely to increase rates of asthma attacks and simultaneously increase health care utilization for treatment. Additionally, the geographic range of these blooms is likely to eventually extend well into temperate-zone waters such as the North Sea (Peperzak 2005).

Chronic Obstructive Pulmonary Disease

Chronic obstructive pulmonary disease (COPD) is a progressive, debilitating, and ultimately fatal lung disease caused by inhaled irritants such as those in cigarette smoke and in rare cases genetic predisposition. COPD is characterized by stepwise decline in lung function associated with exacerbation events, in which a stressor causes inflammation and abrupt decline in lung function with resulting respiratory distress. Climate change is expected to increase exposure of vulnerable COPD patients to stressors including temperature extremes, increased humidity, weather fluctuations, airborne particulate matter, and ground-level ozone to varying degrees in different geographic regions.

Airborne particulates and ground-level ozone are of particular concern. Emergency department presentation rates (Arbex et al. 2009) and hospital admission rates for COPD have been associated with increased levels of ground-level ozone and PM10 (Burnett et al. 1994; Medina-Ramon, Zanobetti, and Schwartz 2006; Schwartz 1994a). In addition, high levels of airborne particulates have been shown to increase the risk of death in patients with COPD by as much as 25 percent (Schwartz 1994b). Patients with COPD may benefit from access to air filters, clean air spaces, or opportunities to relocate to cleaner air during temporary air pollution events such as wildfires. Health care providers should discuss preventative measures with their patients and be alert to early signs of COPD exacerbation during periods of poor air quality.

Pneumonia

Pneumonia is a result of acute inflammation due to infection of the lung by a diverse array of bacteria, viruses and fungi; in the United States alone, pneumonia leads to more than 544,000 emergency department visits and 48,000 deaths per year (National Center for Health Statistics 2017). Climate change can be expected to lead to an increase in the incidence of pneumonia in a variety of settings around the world, mediated by climate-related natural disasters, harmful algal blooms, air pollution, and famines caused by regional crop failures (Mirsaeidi et al. 2016).

Climate-Related Natural Disasters: Infrastructure destruction, for example, loss of shelter after tropical cyclones, and increased exposure to pathogens in the postdisaster environment are believed to place affected persons at higher risk of developing pneumonia, a trend that is likely to be magnified by climate change. Multiple studies in Africa, South Asia, and East Asia have revealed increased incidence and rates of hospital admission for pneumonia and other respiratory infections following natural disasters including typhoons and flooding events due to heavy rainfall (Biswas and Mukhopadhyay 1999; Kondo et al. 2002; Siddique et al. 1991; van Loenhout et al. 2018). Clinicians should be particularly alert for fungal pneumonia in the postdisaster environment (Kao et al. 2005; Kawakami et al. 2012).

Harmful Algae Blooms: Harmful algae blooms, also known as red tide events, are expected to increase in frequency in coming decades as a result of climate change and have been shown to be associated with an increased risk of pneumonia. For example, a 2006 study documented an overall 19 percent increase in the rate of diagnosis of pneumonia in a Florida emergency room during a red tide event; patients living within 1.6 km of the coastline experienced a 31 percent increase in pneumonia admissions (Kirkpatrick et al. 2006).

Temperature Variability: Outdoor ambient temperatures are expected to become increasingly variable in most regions as climate change progresses, presenting a potential stressor that can lead to pneumonia in susceptible individuals, such as the young, the elderly, and those with underlying lung disease. Increases in this variability, as measured by the change in temperature between two consecutive days, have been linked with increased emergency department visits for childhood pneumonia in an Australian study (Xu, Hu, and Tong 2014).

Air Pollution and Airborne Particulate Matter: Airborne particulate matter and ground-level ozone are expected to increase in many areas under most climate-change scenarios. Evidence from studies in Asia, Europe, and North America shows that days with increased $PM_{2.5}$, PM_{10}, and ozone levels are associated with increased admission rates for pneumonia (Ion-Nedelcu et al. 2008; Schwartz 1994; Tsai and Yang 2014). There is also evidence that populations with long-term exposure to elevated $PM_{2.5}$ levels have higher rates of community-acquired pneumonia (Neupane et al. 2010).

Malnutrition and Famine: Available evidence indicates that climate change will lead to increased food insecurity, malnutrition, micronutrient deficiency, and childhood stunting, especially in low- and middle-income countries (Phalkey et al. 2015). Given the substantial amount of evidence that malnutrition contributes to increased rates of infection and mortality from pneumonia (Ginsburg et al. 2015; Schlaudecker, Steinhoff, and Moore 2011), it is plausible that pneumonia rates may rise in populations experiencing increased food insecurity and undernutrition rates as a result of climate change, although further research is needed to definitively link this this causal pathway with climate change.

Coccidiomycosis

Coccidiomycosis (valley fever) is a fungal pulmonary infection caused by inhalation of airborne spores, which can lead to severe lung injury and death. Exposure to coccidiomycosis increases in dry and windy conditions in which there are larger amounts of airborne soil and dust. Coccidiomycosis infection rates in Arizona show a seasonal pattern correlating to dry and dusty environmental conditions (Comrie 2005; Park et al. 2005). Large human outbreaks have been documented in other settings after environmental conditions led to large amounts of airborne soil dust (Williams et al. 1979). Given the vast areas of the globe that are projected to undergo desertification leading to increases in airborne dust, it is possible that coccidiomycosis will be an increasing threat in regions where this fungus is known to occur.

Pneumonic Plague

Pneumonic plague is the result of infection with *Yersinia pestis*, typically transmitted to humans by fleas who leave their typical rodent hosts; mortality can exceed 50 percent, even with treatment. Over the past 200 years, many outbreaks have occurred when environmental triggers have led to population fluctuations and displacement of rodent populations, causing increased contact with humans (McMichael 2017). Climate modeling suggests that abrupt changes in local environment, which can be expected to lead to displacement of rodent populations, are to be expected in the future with increasing frequency. Clinicians practicing in regions such as the Southwest United States, Central Asia, or Northern Madagascar where there is endemic infection of wildland rodent populations should maintain a high index of suspicion after abrupt changes in local environmental conditions.

Pulmonary Hantavirus

Hantavirus is transmitted to humans from the bodily fluids of infected rodents and can lead to severe pulmonary disease, carrying a substantial mortality risk. Previous human outbreaks have been associated with abrupt changes in environmental conditions resulting in increased contact between rodents and humans (Bayard et al. 2004; Williams et al. 1997). Thus, the increased climate variability projected to occur in coming decades may lead to increased risk of future outbreaks in humans (Engelthaler et al. 1999; Yates et al. 2002), although further research is needed to define and quantify this risk.

Renal Disease

Pathologies arising from heat stress or dehydration due to either increased ambient temperature or decreased access to potable water are the principal foreseeable threats to kidney health as a result of climate change.

Acute Kidney Injury

Acute kidney injury (AKI) occurs when renal function is abruptly decreased, typically leading to a decrease in urine output and an increase in serum blood urea nitrogen (BUN) and creatinine; the most common cause is reduced renal perfusion due to hypotension or volume depletion. Rising ambient temperatures, which are expected in most regions in summertime as a result of climate change, lead to increased metabolic demand, respiration, and perspiration, ultimately leading to total body fluid depletion. This is further exacerbated if a supply of potable water is not immediately available for thirst-triggered oral rehydration, a situation that is likely to become increasingly common in arid, semiarid, and summertime temperate settings, particularly for outdoor workers. The result is decreased intravascular volume, decreased renal perfusion, and renal cell injury; in some cases this can involve death of the renal tubule cells (acute tubular necrosis). This can be further exacerbated by use of medications that affect the cardiovascular system, including common antihypertensive and diuretic medications. Treatment is focused on replenishment of intravascular volume, avoidance of nephrotoxic substances, and avoidance of further injury; most individuals will recover renal function within three weeks. Clinicians should counsel patients on diuretics and antihypertensives about the importance of heat protection and hydration during hot weather.

Global Warming Nephropathy, Chronic Kidney Disease of Unknown Origin (CKDu), and Mesoamerican Nephropathy

CKDu is an emerging global epidemic, first observed in young, otherwise healthy agricultural workers in El Salvador and Sri Lanka, and has now been observed in a large number of settings in the semiarid tropics where average ambient temperatures are rising and rainfall is decreasing as a result of climate change. Affected individuals do not display the traditional risk factors for chronic kidney disease (CKD), yet develop progressive renal failure, usually beginning in the third decade (Roncal-Jimenez et al. 2016). In regions with poor health care infrastructure, access to hemodialysis is limited and thus this disease becomes fatal. Extensive research in South Asia and Central America has evaluated a range of possible etiologic factors, including possibly nephrotoxic well water, rehydration with sugary beverages, and concomitant infection with malaria (Madero, Garcia-Arroyo, and Sanchez-Lozada 2017; Siriwardhana et al. 2015); as of this writing the majority of evidence points to recurrent heat stress and dehydration as the primary cause of this disease (Nerbass et al. 2017). Ecological analysis strongly suggests that this disease pattern is a direct result of global climate change interacting with the socioeconomic realities of affected nations (Glaser et al. 2016); clinicians working in settings with large agricultural populations and a warming, drying local environment or who treat migrant populations should familiarize themselves with the literature surrounding CKDu and take appropriate steps such as serum creatinine measurement to screen potentially affected patients for this devastating disease.

Nephrolithiasis

Nephrolithiasis (kidney stone formation) is the result of changes in solute load and solubility in the renal pelvis. Although extremes of both alkalinity and more commonly acidity can precipitate stone formation, the most universal predisposing factor is increased proportional solute load, typically as a result of renal water reabsorption in the nephron due to dehydration or low intravascular volume. For reasons similar to those outlined regarding AKI, global climate change is likely to lead to increased risk of dehydration, resulting in increased kidney stone formation. Increased risk of emergency department visits for renal colic on hot days has already been documented; projections suggest "up to a 10 percent increase in the prevalence rate [of nephrolithiasis] in the next half century secondary to the effects of global warming, with a coinciding 25 percent increase in health-care expenditures" (Fakheri and Goldfarb 2011).

Urinary Tract Infections

Urinary tract infection (UTI) occurs when bacteria enter the urinary tract and are able to reproduce. Successful bacterial colonization is more difficult when there is increased flushing of bacteria out of the urinary tract as a result of forward urine flow during micturition. Decreased urine output, which occurs with heat stress and volume depletion, impairs this process. Environmental heating and drying associated with climate change can be expected to increase incidence of this disease. Two studies have linked UTI and pyelonephritis with ambient daily temperatures, suggesting that information on protection from heat stress and maintenance of adequate hydration should be universally taught to all residents in affected areas (Borg et al. 2017; Liu et al. 2017).

Neurologic Disease

Stroke

Risk of suffering an acute cerebrovascular accident (stroke) will increase as a result of climate change in many regions, predominantly as a result of increased heat stress and increased exposure to airborne particulate matter such as that from wildfires.

Airborne particulate matter from wildfire smoke has been consistently found to increase emergency department presentations for cerebrovascular disease, with a relative risk of 1.22 in a retrospective analysis of the 2015 wildfire season in California (Wettstein et al. 2018) and a relative risk of 1.69 during the 2011 Wallow fire in New Mexico (Resnick et al. 2015). The mechanism is likely related to inflammatory changes associated with $PM_{2.5}$ exposure, particularly to the pro-inflammatory combustion products in wildfire smoke. Patients at elevated baseline risk of cerebrovascular accident may benefit from protective measures such as air filter use or evacuation from smoke-affected regions if feasible.

Increasing environmental heat is expected to result in increased risk of stroke. Although individual study results are mixed, there is an overall trend toward increased risk of both hemorrhagic and ischemic strokes with high ambient temperatures, particularly when the temperature increase is rapid and the patients are male or elderly (Lavados, Olavarria, and Hoffmeister 2018). Modeling suggests that a 20 percent increase in hemorrhagic stroke and a 100 percent increase in ischemic stroke relative to 1980 baselines could be seen in Beijing, China by 2080, principally as a result of climate change (T. Lee et al. 2018). Similar work has shown the potential for a 150 percent increase in years of life lost as a result of strokes in Tianjen, China by 2050 due to higher ambient temperatures (G. Lee et al. 2018).

Dementia

Although there is no evidence linking development of dementia with climate change, there is substantial evidence linking climate-related environmental changes, particularly increased ambient temperatures and risk of heat waves, with increased mortality rates in patients who already carry a diagnosis of dementia. Analysis of over eleven million patients in the United States revealed an 8 percent increase in the risk of death in patients with Alzheimer's disease and 6 percent increase in the risk of death in patients with dementia on days with extreme heat (Zanobetti et al. 2013). Hospitalization rates for patients with dementia have also been found to increase during periods of exceptionally high temperatures relative to local baseline conditions. It is likely that the observed increases in hospitalization rates and mortality result from the decreased ability of patients suffering from dementia to take heat-adaptive actions such as seeking cooler environments, increasing fluid consumption, and adjusting clothing. It is of paramount importance that caregivers of these patients take proactive steps to ensure their safety during periods of extreme heat.

Konzo and Neurolathyrism

Konzo is a spastic upper motor neuron disorder caused by ingestion of cyanide and other compounds in bitter cassava, affecting populations across sub-Saharan Africa (Kashala-Abotnes et al. 2019). Neurolathyrism is similar to konzo in that it is a crippling, permanent neurologic disease resulting from ingestion of the grasspea (*Lathyrus sativus*) native to northern and eastern Africa and the Mediterranean basin. There is a well-documented relationship between drought conditions and outbreaks of both diseases, as subsistence-farming populations switch to consuming larger amounts of drought-resistant cassava or grasspea (Banea-Mayambu et al. 1997; Getahun et al. 1999, 2002). There is widespread concern that as drought frequency increases in sub-Saharan Africa, subsistence cultivation of grasspea and cassava, and resulting cases of konzo and neurolathyrism, will increase. This scenario would be particularly devastating to the long-term resilience of affected populations, as survivors are often left incapacitated, requiring lifelong assistance from family members and their community. As these diseases are incurable, interventions should likely focus on providing alternate approaches to food security during droughts (Oluwole 2015).

Ciguatera

Ciguatera is a potentially debilitating neurologic disorder resulting from ingestion of ciguatoxin in the flesh of tropical marine fish. Although many affected individuals recover fully, others are left with persistent and in some cases debilitating symptoms (Centers for Disease Control and Prevention 2019). Clinicians can expect to see a rise in ciguatera poisoning in coming decades as a result of increasing sea surface temperatures leading to increased risk of *Gambierdiscus toxicus* blooms and incorporation into the marine food chain (Gingold, Strickland, and Hess 2014; Tester et al. 2010). Steps to monitor for dinoflagellate blooms and reduce reliance on tropical marine fisheries may help reduce incidence of this disease.

Reproductive Health and Disease

Direct heat stress, disaster impacts, interpersonal violence, and health care access disruption are the principal mechanisms through which global climate change will affect reproductive health and disease.

Birth Anomalies, Preterm Delivery, and Fetal Death

There is substantial evidence linking environmental heat with adverse outcomes in pregnancy. Elevated ambient temperatures at specific timepoints in the first trimester have been linked to specific patterns of developmental abnormalities, including neural tube defects, cardiac anomalies, and hypospadias (Agay-Shay et al. 2013; Auger et al. 2017b; Kilinc et al. 2016). Extreme heat has also been linked to both increased rates of preterm delivery and increased rates of fetal death, likely as a result a maternal physiologic stress (Cox et al. 2016; Kuehn. and McCormick 2017). As global climate change leads to increased average ambient temperatures and increasingly common heat waves, women who are pregnant or trying to conceive are advised to avoid high-heat environments—an objective that their employers, families, and communities should support them in accomplishing.

Fetal death and preterm delivery also increase in the wake of climate-related natural disasters. Experience from Hurricane Charley, Hurricane Andrew, and other storms revealed an increase in fetal deaths and preterm deliveries, likely as a result of maternal stressors associated with the disaster and postdisaster environment (Antipova and Curtis 2015; Grabich et al. 2016; Zahran et al. 2014). Given anticipated increases in the average intensity of landfalling tropical cyclones around the world, it appears reasonable for affected communities to put programs in place to prioritize the early evacuation of pregnant patients to areas with appropriate access to obstetric care.

Another troubling cause of birth defects, the mosquito-borne Zika virus, has the potential to significantly expand its range as a result of climate change. Zika infection has been linked to microcephaly, premature delivery, and miscarriage when initial infection occurs during pregnancy (World Health Organization 2018). There is mounting evidence that this threat, which expanded rapidly across tropical and subtropical regions starting in 2015, could eventually expand into new, previously temperate regions as a result of climate change (Asad and Carpenter 2018). It is believed that warmer temperatures facilitate spread of the virus (Tesla et al. 2018), suggesting that long-term climate-related risks may exist even outside areas of current transmission activity.

Sexual Violence and Domestic Violence

There is a well-documented association between exposure to natural disasters and increased risk of intimate partner violence and gender-based violence. This has been seen in post hurricane environments in the United States, following disasters including earthquakes in Iran, and elsewhere (Anastario, Shehab, and Lawry 2009; Harville et al. 2011; Sohrabizadeh 2016). Sequelae include both physical and mental health outcomes (Schumacher et al. 2010). Given the anticipated increase in weather-related natural disasters as a result of climate change, disaster planners and clinicians should be alert to this risk and implement preventative measures such as gender-disaggregated shelters and emergency obstetrics/gynecology services.

Climate refugees represent a second, related population that is at significantly elevated risk of sexual and gender-based violence (Keygnaert et al. 2014). Displacement from existing social structures, absence of consistent rule of law along migration routes, and altered power structures create a situation in which many migrants are extremely vulnerable to sexual assault or coercion and in which many intact families may experience extreme levels of interpersonal stress (Freedman 2016).

Access to Women's Health Care

Availability of basic women's health care can be significantly impaired during periods of natural disaster. Evidence from recent hurricanes in the United States has been linked to decreased access to contraception (Leyser-Whalen, Rahman, and Berenson 2011), decreased access to screening for sexually transmitted diseases (Kissinger et al. 2007), and increased risk of unavailability of women's health care in general, including antenatal care (Callaghan et al. 2007). As the incidence of climate-related natural disasters increases, efforts must be made to ensure continued access to women's health services.

Ocular Disease

Retinal Detachment

Retinal detachment is an acute, vision threatening disorder of the eye in which the retina detaches from posterior tissues. A 2011 review of more than 23,000 cases of retinal detachment in Taiwan revealed a positive association with ambient temperature (Lin et al. 2011), and a 2017 study revealed that increasing ambient temperature from 15°Celsius (C) to 25°C (59°F to 77°F) resulted in an increased risk of retinal detachment, with an odds ratio of 1.98 to 2.71 depending on age (Auger et al. 2017a). These findings suggest that incidence could potentially increase across large regions of the globe in coming decades as a result of climate change.

Cataracts

Cataracts occur when any of a variety of factors lead to clouding of the lens of the eye, resulting in permanent, progressive blurring of the patient's vision, sometimes ultimately requiring surgical replacement of the lens. Research in India has shown a possible link between heatstroke and subsequent cataract formation (Minassian, Mehra, and Jones 1984). Animal studies have demonstrated heating of ocular lens up to several degrees above core body temperature when in direct sunlight in hot weather, providing a potential pathophysiologic mechanism (Al-Ghadyan and Cotlier 1986; Johnson 2004). There is also evidence that extreme heat while a fetus is in utero is associated with elevated risk of congenital cataracts (Van Zutphen et al. 2012). Although a definitive link between climate change and cataract formation has yet to be demonstrated, the environmental and pathophysiological basis for such a link is plausible based on available information.

Ocular Infectious Disease

It is very likely that the typical geographic ranges of a variety of ocular infections will change along with the climate. There are scattered reports of dilofilariasis, a parasitic infection of the eye common in tropical regions, appearing in Hungary and Romania, well outside typical ranges for this infection (Arbune and Dobre 2015; Boss, Sosne, and Tewari 2017; Doczi et al. 2015). Similarly, expert opinion anticipates that the burden of fungal keratitis in temperate regions will increase substantially as the climate warms (Johnson 2004). Clinicians treating ocular infections should increase their index of suspicion for fungal or parasitic etiologies previously uncommon in their region of practice.

Hematology and Oncology

Malignancy

Risk of cancer and hematologic malignancy in relation to climate is an incompletely explored field. The impact of climate change is likely to vary significantly across different geographies, and it is probable that many climate-related effects that raise the risk of malignancy will be local in nature, for example, weather-related damage to industrial facilities or mobilization of toxins from Superfund sites as a result of rising water tables. Clinicians, public health professionals, and community health advocates should familiarize themselves with anticipated climate change effects and assess how these may affect toxic and infectious exposure sources in their community.

Combustion of forested areas contaminated with radiologic material is of increasing concern as temperate zone and boreal forests warm and dry as a result of climate change. Numerous studies have examined the potential consequences of a forest fire in the Chernobyl exclusion zone (Bondar et al. 2014); combustion of the entire region would be expected to result in between 20 and 240 solid tumors in Europe (Evangeliou et al. 2014), and, although observational studies of actual combustion have revealed much lower radiologic emissions associated with the much smaller burning patterns seen in recent decades (Evangeliou et al. 2016), increases in magnitude of forest fires are to be expected in coming decades.

A very different set of mechanisms affect risk of skin cancer. Although the overall impact of climate change and transitioning to carbon-free energy sources on surface ultraviolet (UV) radiation levels is as yet unclear (Bais et al. 2015), duration of outdoor time will likely increase in many temperate regions due to warming, leading to increased ultraviolet light exposure and increased risk of skin cancers if appropriate preventative measures are not taken (Kaffenberger, et al. 2017). There is already some evidence that climate change may be contributing to rising rates of dermatologic malignancies in agricultural workers in the mountains of Ecuador (Harari Arjona et al. 2016). Sun protective measures should be emphasized in previously cool regions that are now rapidly warming.

Psychiatric Disease

Climate change exacerbates a range of psychiatric diseases as a result of environmental stressors and resulting social instability, livelihood instability and forced migration. There is a growing literature on psychiatric pathologies resulting directly from the presence of or impacts of climate change. For example, a 2018 study linked "shifting from monthly temperatures between 25°C and 30°C to > 30°C [with] increases [in] the probability of mental health difficulties by 0.5 percent points, [and] 1°C of 5-year warming. . . with a 2% point increase in the prevalence of mental health issues, and. . . exposure to Hurricane Katrina. . . with a 4% point increase" (Obradovich et al. 2018). There is significant concern that depression among children and teenagers is increasing in many areas as result of climate change and its effects (Majeed and Lee 2017), and there is evidence that climate-change related concerns are now a feature of obsessive-compulsive checking concerns in some populations (Jones et al. 2012). Mental health issues associated with loss of environmentally dependent livelihoods such as farming and herding are also increasingly well documented (Ellis and Albrecht 2017; Furberg, Evengard, and Nilsson 2011).

Suicide

There is significant evidence supporting climate-related stressors as important contributors to suicide risk. Drought (Hanigan et al. 2012), changes in climate affecting crop growth

(Kabir 2018), and forced migration increase risk of suicide or suicidal ideation; there is also evidence that increased summertime heat may be associated with an increased risk of suicide (Akkaya-Kalayci et al. 2017; Fountoulakis et al. 2016). Loss of social supports and social roles is another important contributor to suicide risk. There is substantial evidence that these losses play a significant role in the increased risk of suicide among migrants and refugees; as climate change drives increasing population displacement, displaced communities and their health care providers will need to aggressively screen for suicidal ideation in affected persons and address it in a culturally appropriate manner (Mandavia et al. 2017).

Schizophrenia and Antipsychotic Medication Safety

Patients with schizophrenia are at elevated risk of death during hot weather (Page et al. 2012; Schmeltz and Gamble 2017) and exhibit increased utilization of emergency medical facilities (Hansen et al. 2018; Thompson et al. 2018; Wang et al. 2014). Mechanisms may include impaired heat tolerance, less access to air conditioning, or decreased utilization of other adaptive strategies. In addition, patients on stable doses of antipsychotics have been found to have impaired heat tolerance and more rapid core temperature rise than healthy controls (Hermesh et al. 2000), and there are case reports of heatstroke in patients on antipsychotic medication (Lee, Chen, and Chang 2015). Although it is unclear to what degree medication use, underlying disease, and other factors contributed to these findings, they do emphasize the importance of protection from hot environments for this population.

Posttraumatic Stress Disorder

Posttraumatic stress disorder (PTSD) is a long-term condition characterized by persistent, intrusive thoughts, anxiety, depression, and flashbacks. PTSD develops as a result of exposure to traumatic events, ranging from natural disasters to combat to sexual assault. There is substantial evidence that natural disasters lead to increased incidence of PTSD (DeSalvo et al. 2007; Neria, Nandi, and Galea 2008; Rataj, Kunzweiler, and Garthus-Niegel 2006), in some cases affecting as much as a quarter of the exposed population (Cerda et al. 2013; Galea et al. 2008). Given the anticipated increase in weather-related natural disasters resulting from climate change, it is expected that PTSD rates in affected communities will increase substantially. Forced migration is another source of PTSD that will increase with climate change as environmental stressors drive populations from their land (Meze-Hausken 2004); both the processes of migration, which can involve abuses or exploitation, and the destinations, which include refugee camps and marginalized roles in host societies, create situations in which vulnerable migrants are exposed to traumatic events and interpersonal interactions (Shultz et al. 2019). Finally, PTSD resulting from exposure to or participation in armed conflict may increase in coming decades; although quantification and prognostication are necessarily imprecise, there is growing concern that the social disruptions and food insecurity resulting from climate change will ultimately lead to a rise in armed conflict over the course of the twenty-first century (Burke et al. 2009; Levy, Sidel, and Patz 2017; Schleussner et al. 2016).

Depression

Depression is a potentially debilitating condition characterized by decreased activity levels and self-actualization, circadian changes, and decreased sense of self-worth. Although causes of depression are multifactorial, there is substantial evidence that negative changes in the personal environment can trigger or exacerbate depressive symptoms, and there is accumulating evidence that social and environmental changes resulting from climate change including changed subsistence patterns, exposure to climate-related natural disasters, and forced migration are now contributing to the global burden of depression (Ellis and Albrecht 2017; Obradovich et al. 2018; Rataj, Kunzweiler, and Garthus-Niegel 2016). Providers are advised to familiarize themselves with locally relevant climate-related stressors that may be affecting their patients and take proactive steps to screen for clinical impacts.

Anxiety

Anxiety has been shown to increase in the aftermath of natural disasters (Rataj, Kunzweiler, and Garthus-Niegel 2016) and in response to chronic environmental stressors such as decreasing rainfall and other factors affecting crop production (Ellis and Albrecht 2017). Anxiety regarding the entity of climate change itself, and its sequelae, has also been identified as a new mental health issue, although large-scale research on this topic is as yet lacking (Glaser 2008).

Dermatologic Disease

Cutaneous Infections

As the planet warms, it is expected that functional biomes will shift northwards; the result will be increased incidence of subtropical or tropical skin conditions well north of their current geographic distribution and more northerly extension of temperate zone diseases (Balato et al. 2014). In the Americas, research shows expanding ranges for Lyme disease, leishmaniasis, and certain fungal infections (Kaffenberger et al. 2017). In Europe, warming temperatures may be contributing to wound infections with regionally unexpected bacteria (Sganga et al. 2009). There is significant concern that the transmission range of a variety of tick-borne dermatoses may be altered globally (Andersen and Davis 2017).

Skin infections resulting from exposure to climate-change-related flooding present an additional concern; according to the International Society of Dermatology Climate Change Committee, flooding increases the risk of impetigo, tinea corporis, leishmaniasis, bites and stings, scabies, and cutaneous larva migrans, all of which providers should be prepared to treat in the postflood environment (Dayrit et al. 2018).

Hand, Foot, and Mouth Disease

Hand, foot, and mouth disease (HFMD) is a common childhood enteroviral disease that results in seven to ten days of rash and other symptoms; although cases are typically self-limited, deaths do occur. Viral transmission improves with increasing humidity and warming temperatures up to approximately 20 C; recent modeling in China suggests a substantial increase in caseloads in areas that are currently cooler than this threshold, resulting in a 3–5 percent increase nationally by 2090 (Schmidt 2018; Zhao et al. 2018). These results are consistent with findings from other parts of the world (Andersen and Davis 2015), and there is now concern that rising rates of HFMD may be linked to climate change (Coates, Davis, and Andersen 2019).

Skin Cancer

Although the overall effects of climate change on the surface UV exposure levels that contribute to malignancy are unclear, there is concern that individual UV exposure may rise in temperate and subarctic regions as the population spends more time outside.

Gastrointestinal Disease

Gastroenteritis

There is substantial evidence that warmer temperatures are associated with an increase in infectious gastroenteritis (Ghazani et al. 2018). A recent meta-analysis identified an anticipated 8–11 percent increase in the relative risk of diarrheal disease worldwide by the end of the twenty-first century, albeit with a substantial margin of error because of the limited number of relevant high-quality studies (Kolstad and Johansson 2011). There is also substantial evidence that extreme weather events, particularly those involving high rainfall and flooding, lead to outbreaks of infectious gastroenteritis. Floodwaters in the aftermath of deluges and hurricanes typically carry high loads of bacteria and other pathogens, increasing risk of drinking water contamination. For example, medical records from typhoon Haiyan in the Philippines reveal increased rates of admission for gastroenteritis, particularly in children (van Loenhout et al. 2018). Similar effects have been described throughout the world (Davies et al. 2014).

Hepatitis A

Hepatitis A is a waterborne viral infection of the liver transmitted via fecal contamination of drinking water. Research in Spain shows a 24 percent increase in the relative risk of developing hepatitis A after exceptionally rainy weeks (Gullon et al. 2017), and modeling in China projects an increase in hepatitis A infections associated with flooding events in coming decades (Gao et al. 2016). Public health authorities will likely need to expand prevention efforts in regions that anticipate increased rainfall as a result of climate change.

Intestinal Schistosomiasis

Schistosomiasis is a parasitic infection caused by parasitic flatworms that can invade the gastrointestinal tract, bloodstream, and urinary tract. It is currently a significant health problem in central and eastern Africa, the Middle East, southern China, South America, and other regions with favorable ecologic conditions. Research in southern China suggests that the effective transmission range will expand northward in coming decades (Zhu, Fan, and Peterson 2017). In east Africa, however, the anticipated effect is less clear, as decreases in the snail host range may offset any expansion of the suitable niche for the flatworm parasite itself (Stensgaard et al. 2013). Whether the net global effect of climate change is overall range expansion or a shifting of ranges to new regions and out of old ones (Stensgaard et al. 2019), it is very likely that there will be communities that face schistosomiasis as a novel climate-related health threat, and public health authorities in potentially affected regions should be alert to this hazard.

Endocrine Disease

Diabetes

Diabetes mellitus represents a substantial fraction of endocrine disease throughout the world, and type II diabetes is one of the fastest-growing chronic diseases in both the developing and the developed world. Climate change will affect diabetics through both heat stress (Westphal et al. 2010) and potential disruption of health care services including insulin availability, which is of particular concern given the relatively large fraction of the population living with this condition (Ford et al. 2006).

Morbidity and mortality: Environmental heat is a substantial and potentially lethal threat to diabetic patients (Li et al. 2014; Schwartz 2005). Patients with diabetes have been found to be at particular risk of myocardial infarction during heat waves, showing greater heat sensitivity than the average population (Lam et al. 2018). Similarly, a review of over seven million deaths in the United States revealed an increased risk of death for diabetics on hot days, with an odds ratio of 1.035 on days with extreme heat (Medina-Ramon et al. 2006).

Weather-related natural disasters, which are expected to increase in frequency and severity as a result of climate change, are also particularly lethal for diabetic patients. In one study, risk of death for diabetic patients more than doubled following a major hurricane (Hendrickson and Vogt 1996). Additional concerns related to insulin availability are outlined in this section.

Health Care Utilization: Diabetic patients increase health care utilization during hot weather. Increases in diabetic patients' use of emergency departments during heat waves are well documented (Cook, Wellik, and Fowke 2011; Knowlton et al. 2009). Similarly, a review of outpatient medical consultations in England revealed a 9 percent increase in the odds of diabetic patients seeking medical consultation for every degree centigrade increase in environmental temperature above 22°C (Hajat et al. 2017). It is likely that this increase in care-seeking is at least in part caused by impaired thermoregulation (Cook, Wellik, and Fowke 2011). It is currently unclear to what degree other factors are also at play, but it appears prudent for diabetic patients to focus on sheltering in cool areas during periods of extreme heat.

Insulin Availability: Insulin-dependent diabetics who cannot access insulin are at risk of uncontrolled hyperglycemia, infection, hyperglycemic coma, and diabetic ketoacidosis. Availability of consistently refrigerated insulin is of paramount importance to this population. Climate change threatens insulin availability through both environmental heating and risk of weather-related natural disasters which disrupt healthcare access and supply chains. Insulin slowly degrades over time, and this process is accelerated at increased temperatures, though it should be noted that many preparations of insulin retain more than 90 percent of their potency after several weeks at 40°C (Gill 2000).

Insulin availability following natural disasters is likely to be an increasing problem. Large proportions of those seeking care after hurricanes need continuity of care that was disrupted by the disaster, and demand for insulin at field clinics can easily outstrip supply (Alson et al. 1993). Transitioning to alternate insulin regimens during disaster and use of insulin syringes in crowded evacuation centers present additional hazards (Cefalu et al. 2006). Patients are advised to keep their insulin supplies with them during evacuation; responders should be prepared to address the needs of diabetics without access to insulin.

Multisystem Heat-Related Illness

It is expected that cases of heat exhaustion and heatstroke will increase as a result of climate change. Clinicians, workplace supervisors, athletic coaches, and most laypersons should familiarize themselves with the symptoms of both conditions and know when to get help for these acute, life-threatening conditions.

Heat Exhaustion

The physiology of heat exhaustion is well explored in other publications; it represents a state of depleted reserves, in which the body's ability to maintain thermal homeostasis is becoming compromised but has not yet failed. Patients may have cool, clammy skin, decreased energy, and abnormal vital signs including tachypnea and tachycardia. Treatment is focused on removing the patient from the hot environment, replacing fluids and electrolytes, and ensuring return to homeostasis.

Heatstroke

The endpoint of unchecked heat stress following failure of regulatory mechanisms is heatstroke, in which a rising core body temperature leads to multisystem organ failure, coma, and death. Patients may appear confused or unconscious and will often have hot, dry skin. Treatment is focused on rapid, aggressive cooling, for example via cold water immersion or chilled bladder irrigation; supportive care will often involve intubation, sedation, and chemical paralysis to protect airway function and reduce metabolic activity. For most clinicians and laypersons, the key to patient survival will be early recognition, cooling, and activation of emergency medical services. Emergency departments and intensive care units should be prepared for an increase in the number of heatstroke patients during heat waves.

Infectious Disease, Immunology, and Toxicology

Some topics are beyond the scope of this chapter. Although a variety of organ-system-specific impacts of climate change on infectious diseases, allergens, and toxic exposures have been mentioned, these topics require in-depth exploration beyond what can be accomplished here. Other chapters in this textbook and a wide range of outside sources provide further reading on these subjects.

Summary

Climate change has the potential to affect every organ system in the human body. Effects will vary significantly by region; clinicians should familiarize themselves with the specific manifestations that can be anticipated within their practice environment. Patients with asthma, diabetes, cardiovascular disease, dementia, and psychiatric illness are at particular risk, as are patients with limited mobility, the elderly, the very young, the socially marginalized, and the economically disadvantaged.

DISCUSSION QUESTIONS

1. You are explaining why you're worried about climate change to a relative at a holiday party. Which of the potential health impacts of climate change feel most immediately concerning to you personally, based on where you currently live?

2. You run a visiting nurse (VNA) program in suburban community. A four-day heat wave is forecast for next week. Which of your patients are most at risk? What actions would you like to take?

3. As a member of the public health commission for a small town in your home state, what are some specific steps you can take to address the risk of climate-related health impacts in your community?

4. Medical problems specific to one organ system—for example, atrial fibrillation—are usually managed by a specific specialty in the traditional medical system. What are the advantages and disadvantages of this approach when it comes to the multisystem threat presented by climate change and climate-related natural disasters?

5. You are part of a church group that works with refugees as they resettle in your community. What are some impacts of climate change that you'll want to keep in mind as you partner with them to meet their needs?

References

Agay-Shay, K., M. Friger, S. Linn, A. Peled, Y. Amitai, and C. Peretz. 2013. "Ambient Temperature and Congenital Heart Defects." *Human Reproduction* 28 (8):2289–97.

Akkaya-Kalayci, T., B. Vyssoki, D. Winkler, M. Willeit, N. D. Kapusta, G. Dorffner, and Z. Özlü-Erkilic. 2017. "The Effect of Seasonal Changes and Climatic Factors on Suicide Attempts of Young People." *BMC Psychiatry* 17 (1):365.

Al-Ghadyan, A. A., and E. Cotlier. 1986. "Rise in Lens Temperature on Exposure to Sunlight or High Ambient Temperature." *British Journal of Ophthalmology* 70 (6):421–6.

Alson, R., D. Alexander, R. B. Leonard, and L. W. Stringer. 1993. "Analysis of Medical Treatment at a Field Hospital Following Hurricane Andrew, 1992." *Annals of Emergency Medicine* 22 (11):1721–8.

Anastario, M., N. Shehab, and L. Lawry. 2009. "Increased Gender-Based Violence among Women Internally Displaced in Mississippi 2 Years Post-Hurricane Katrina." *Disaster Medicine and Public Health Preparedness* 3 (1):18–26.

Andersen, L. K., and M. D. Davis. 2015. "The Effects of the El Nino Southern Oscillation on Skin and Skin-Related Diseases: A Message from the International Society of Dermatology Climate Change Task Force." *International Journal of Dermatology* 54 (12):1343–51.

Andersen, L. K., and M. D. Davis. 2017. "Climate Change and the Epidemiology of Selected Tick-Borne and Mosquito-Borne Diseases: Update from the International Society of Dermatology Climate Change Task Force." *International Journal of Dermatology* 56 (3):252–9.

Antipova, A., and A. Curtis. 2015. "The Post-Disaster Negative Health Legacy: Pregnancy Outcomes in Louisiana after Hurricane Andrew." *Disasters* 39 (4):665–86.

Arbex, M. A., G. M. de Souza Conceição, S. P. Cendon, F. F. Arbex, A. C. Lopes, E. P. Moysés, S. L. Santiago et al. 2009. "Urban Air Pollution and Chronic Obstructive Pulmonary Disease-Related Emergency Department Visits." *Journal of Epidemiology and Community Health* 63 (10):777–83.

Arbune, M., and M. Dobre. 2015. "Dirofilariasis—An Emergent Human Parasitosis in Romania." *Acta Parasitologica* 60 (3):485–7.

Asad, H., and D. O. Carpenter. 2018. "Effects of Climate Change on the Spread of Zika Virus: A Public Health Threat." *Reviews on Environmental Health* 33 (1):31–42.

Auger, N., M.-A. Rhéaume, M. Bilodeau-Bertrand, T. Tang, and T. Kosatsky. 2017a. "Climate and the Eye: Case-Crossover Analysis of Retinal Detachment after Exposure to Ambient Heat." *Environmental Research* 157:103–9.

Auger, N., W. D. Fraser, L. Arbour, M. Bilodeau-Bertrand, and T. Kosatsky. 2017b. "Elevated Ambient Temperatures and Risk of Neural Tube Defects." *Occupational and Environmental Medicine* 74 (5):315–20.

Bais, A. F., R. L. McKenzie, G. Bernhard, P. J. Aucamp, M. Ilyas, S. Madronich, and K. Tourpalia. 2015. "Ozone Depletion and Climate Change: Impacts on UV Radiation." *Photochemical & Photobiological Sciences* 14 (1):19–52.

Balato, N., M. Megna, F. Ayala, A. Balato, M. Napolitano, and C. Patruno. 2014. "Effects of Climate Changes on Skin Diseases." *Expert Review of Anti-Infective Therapy* 12 (2):171–81.

Banea-Mayambu, J. P., T. Tylleskär, N. Gitebo, N. Matadi, M. Gebre-Medhin, and H. Rosling. 1997. "Geographical and Seasonal Association between Linamarin and Cyanide Exposure from Cassava and the Upper Motor Neurone Disease Konzo in Former Zaire." *Tropical Medicine & International Health* 2 (12):1143–51.

Bayard, V., P. T. Kitsutani, E. O. Barria, L. A. Ruedas, D. S. Tinnin, C. Muñoz, I. B. de Mosca et al. 2004. "Outbreak of Hantavirus Pulmonary Syndrome, Los Santos, Panama, 1999–2000." *Emerging Infectious Diseases* 10 (9):1635–42.

Biswas, R., D. Pal, and S.P. Mukhopadhyay. 1999. "A Community Based Study on Health Impact of Flood in a Vulnerable District of West Bengal." *Indian Journal of Public Health* 43 (2):89–90.

Bondar, Y. I., A. D. Navumau, A. N. Nikitin, J.Brown, and M. Dowdall. 2014. "Model Assessment of Additional Contamination of Water Bodies as a Result of Wildfires in The Chernobyl Exclusion Zone." *Journal of Environmental Radioactivity* 138:170–6.

Borg, M., P. Bi, M. Nitschke, S. Williams, and S. McDonald. 2017. "The Impact of Daily Temperature on Renal Disease Incidence: An Ecological Study." *Environmental Health* 16 (1):114.

Boss, J. D., G. Sosne, and A. Tewari. 2017. "Ocular Dirofilariasis: Ophthalmic Implication of Climate Change on Vector-Borne Parasites." *American Journal of Ophthalmology Case Reports* 7:9–10.

Brunetti, N. D., D. Amoruso, L. De Gennaro, G. Dellegrottaglie, G. Di Giuseppe, G. Antonelli, and M. Di Biase. 2014. "Hot Spot: Impact of July 2011 Heat Wave in Southern Italy (Apulia) on Cardiovascular Disease Assessed by Emergency Medical Service and Telemedicine Support." *Telemedicine Journal and e-Health* 20 (3):272–81.

Bullone, M., R. Y. Murcia, and J. P. Lavoie. 2016. "Environmental Heat and Airborne Pollen Concentration Are Associated with Increased Asthma Severity in Horses." *Equine Veterinary Journal* 48 (4):479–84.

Burke, M. B., E. Miguel, S. Satyanath, J. A. Dykema, and D. B. Lobell. 2009. "Warming Increases the Risk of Civil War in Africa." *Proceedings of the National Academy of Sciences of the USA* 106 (49):20670–4.

Burnett, R. T., R. E. Dales, M. E. Raizenne, D. Krewski, P. W. Summers, G. R. Roberts, M. Raad-Young, T. Dann, and J. Brook. 1994. "Effects of Low Ambient Levels of Ozone and Sulfates on the Frequency of Respiratory Admissions to Ontario Hospitals." *Environmental Research* 65 (2):172–94.

Callaghan, W. M., S. A. Rasmussen, D. J. Jamieson, S. J. Ventura, S. L. Farr, P. D. Sutton, T. J Mathews et al. 2007. "Health Concerns of Women and Infants in Times of Natural Disasters: Lessons Learned from Hurricane Katrina." *Maternal and Child Health Journal* 11 (4):307–11.

Cefalu, W. T., S. R. Smith, L. Blonde, and V. Fonseca. 2006. "The Hurricane Katrina Aftermath and Its Impact on Diabetes Care: Observations from 'Ground Zero': Lessons in Disaster Preparedness of People with Diabetes." *Diabetes Care* 29 (1):158–60.

Centers for Disease Control and Prevention. 2019. "Ciguatera Fish Poisoning Fact Sheet." Accessed April 9, 2019. https://www.cdc.gov/nceh/ciguatera/.

Cerda, M., M. Paczkowski, S. Galea, K. Nemethy, C. Péan, and M. Desvarieux. 2013. "Psychopathology in the Aftermath of the Haiti Earthquake: A Population-Based Study of Posttraumatic Stress Disorder and Major Depression." *Depression and Anxiety* 30 (5):413–24.

Claeys, M. J., S. Rajagopalan, T. S. Nawrot, and R. D. Brook. 2017. "Climate and Environmental Triggers of Acute Myocardial Infarction." *European Heart Journal* 38 (13):955–60.

Coates, S. J., M. D. P. Davis, and L. K. Andersen. 2019. "Temperature and Humidity Affect the Incidence of Hand, Foot, and Mouth Disease: A Systematic Review of the Literature—A Report from the International Society of Dermatology Climate Change Committee." *International Journal of Dermatology* 58 (4):388–99.

Comrie, A. C. 2005. "Climate Factors Influencing Coccidioidomycosis Seasonality and Outbreaks." *Environmental Health Perspectives* 113 (6):688–92.

Cook, C. B., K. E. Wellik, and M. Fowke. 2011. "Geoenvironmental Diabetology." *Journal of Diabetes Science and Technology* 5 (4):834–42.

Cox, B., A. M. Vicedo-Cabrera, A. Gasparrini, H. A. Roels, E. Martens, J. Vangronsveld, B. Forsberg, and T. S. Nawrot. 2016. "Ambient Temperature as a Trigger of Preterm Delivery in a Temperate Climate." *Journal of Epidemiology and Community Health* 70 (12):1191–9.

Davies, G. I., L. McIver, Y. Kim, M. Hashizume, S. Iddings, and V. Chan. 2014. "Water-Borne Diseases and Extreme Weather Events in Cambodia: Review of Impacts and Implications of Climate Change." *International Journal of Environmental Research and Public Health* 12 (1):191–213.

Davis, R. E., P. C. Knappenberger, P. J. Michaels, and W. M. Novicoff. 2003."Changing Heat-Related Mortality in the United States." *Environmental Health Perspectives* 111 (14):1712–8.

Dayrit, J. F., L. Bintanjoyo, L. K. Andersen, M. Dennis, and P. Davis. 2018. "Impact of Climate Change on Dermatological Conditions Related to Flooding: Update from the International Society of Dermatology Climate Change Committee." *International Journal of Dermatology* 57 (8):901–10.

DeSalvo, K. B., A. D. Hyre, D. C. Ompad, A. Menke, L. L. Tynes, and P. Muntner. 2007. "Symptoms of Posttraumatic Stress Disorder in a New Orleans Workforce Following Hurricane Katrina." *Journal of Urban Health* 84 (2):142–52.

Doczi, I., L. Bereczki, T. Gyetvai, I. Fejes, Á. Skribek, Á. Szabó, S. Berkes et al. 2015. "Description of Five Dirofilariasis Cases in South Hungary and Review Epidemiology of This Disease for the Country." *Wiener klinische Wochenschrift* 127 (17–18):696–702.

Ellis, N. R., and G. A. Albrecht. 2017. "Climate Change Threats to Family Farmers' Sense of Place and Mental Wellbeing: A Case Study from the Western Australian Wheatbelt." *Social Science & Medicine* 175:161–8.

Engelthaler, D. M., D. G. Mosley, J. E. Cheek, C. E. Levy, K. K. Komatsu, P. Ettestad, T. Davis et al. 1999. "Climatic and Environmental Patterns Associated with Hantavirus Pulmonary Syndrome, Four Corners Region, United States." *Emerging Infectious Diseases* 5 (1):87–94.

Evangeliou, N., Y. Balkanski, A. Cozic, W. M. Hao, A. P. Møller 2014. "Wildfires in Chernobyl-Contaminated Forests and Risks to the Population and the Environment: A New Nuclear Disaster about to Happen?" *Environment International* 73:346–58.

Evangeliou, N., S. Zibtsev, V. Myroniuk, M. Zhurba, T. Hamburger, A. Stohl, Y. Balkanski et al. 2016. "Resuspension and Atmospheric Transport of Radionuclides due to Wildfires near the Chernobyl Nuclear Power Plant in 2015: An Impact Assessment." *Scientific Reports* 6:26062.

Fakheri, R. J., and D. S. Goldfarb, 2011. "Ambient Temperature as a Contributor to Kidney Stone Formation: Implications of Global Warming." *Kidney International* 79 (11):1178–85.

Fleming, L. E., B. Kirkpatrick, L. C. Backer, J. A. Bean, A. Wanner, A. Reich, J. Zaias et al. 2007. "Aerosolized Red-Tide Toxins (Brevetoxins) and Asthma." *Chest* 131 (1):187–94.

Ford, E. S., A. H. Mokdad, M. W. Link, W. S. Garvin, L. C. McGuire, R. B. Jiles, and L. S. Balluz. 2006. "Chronic Disease in Health Emergencies: In the Eye of the Hurricane." *Preventing Chronic Disease* 3 (2):A46.

Fountoulakis, K. N., C. Savopoulos, P. Zannis, M. Apostolopoulou, I. Fountoukidis, N. Kakaletsis, I. Kanellos et al. 2016. "Climate Change But Not Unemployment Explains the Changing Suicidality in Thessaloniki Greece (2000–2012)." *Journal of Affective Disorders* 193:331–8.

Freedman, J. 2016. "Sexual and Gender-Based Violence against Refugee Women: A Hidden Aspect of the Refugee 'Crisis.'" *Reproductive Health Matters* 24 (47):18–26.

Furberg, M., B. Evengard, and M. Nilsson. 2011. "Facing the Limit of Resilience: Perceptions of Climate Change among Reindeer Herding Sami in Sweden." *Global Health Action* 4. doi: 10.3402/gha.v4i0.8417.

Galea, S., M. Tracy, F. Norris, and S. F. Coffey. 2008. "Financial and Social Circumstances and the Incidence and Course of PTSD in Mississippi during the First Two Years after Hurricane Katrina." *Journal of Traumatic Stress* 21 (4):357–68.

Gao, L., Y. Zhang, G. Ding, Q. Liu, C. Wang, and B. Jiang. 2016. "Projections of Hepatitis A Virus Infection Associated with Flood Events by 2020 and 2030 in Anhui Province, China." *International Journal of Biometeorology* 60 (12):1873–84.

Getahun, H., A. Mekonnen, R. TekleHaimanot, and F. Lambein. 1999. "Epidemic of Neurolathyrism in Ethiopia." *Lancet* 354 (9175):306–7.

Getahun, H., F. Lambein, M. Vanhoorne, and P. Van der Stuyft. 2002. "Pattern and Associated Factors of the Neurolathyrism Epidemic in Ethiopia." *Tropical Medicine & International Health* 7 (2):118–24.

Ghazani, M., G. FitzGerald, W. Hu, G. S. Toloo, and Z. Xu. 2018. "Temperature Variability and Gastrointestinal Infections: A Review of Impacts and Future Perspectives." *International Journal of Environmental Research and Public Health* 15 (4):766.

Gill, G. V. 2000. "Viewpoint: Stability of Insulin in Tropical Countries." *Tropical Medicine & International Health* 5 (9):666–7.

Gingold, D. B., M. J. Strickland, and J. J. Hess. 2014. "Ciguatera Fish Poisoning and Climate Change: Analysis of National Poison Center Data in the United States, 2001–2011." *Environmental Health Perspectives* 122 (6):580–6.

Ginsburg, A. S., R. Izadnegahdar, J. A. Berkley, J. L. Walson, N. Rollins, and K. P. Klugman. 2015. "Undernutrition and Pneumonia Mortality." *Lancet Global Health* 3 (12):e735–6.

Glaser, G. 2008. "Anxious about Earth's Troubles? There's Treatment." *New York Times. February* 16, 2008.

Glaser, J., J. Lemery, B. Rajagopalan, H. F. Diaz, R. García-Trabanino, G. Taduri, M. Madero et al. 2016. "Climate Change and the Emergent Epidemic of CKD from Heat Stress in Rural Communities: The Case for Heat Stress Nephropathy." *Clinical Journal of the American Society of Nephrology* 11 (8):1472–83.

Grabich, S. C., W. R. Robinson, S. M. Engel, C. E. Konrad, D. B. Richardson, and J. A. Horney. 2016. "Hurricane Charley Exposure and Hazard of Preterm Delivery, Florida 2004." *Maternal and Child Health Journal* 20 (12):2474–82.

Guilbert, A., B. Cox, N. Bruffaerts, L. Hoebeke, A. Packeu, M. Hendrickx, K. De Cremer et al. 2018. "Relationships between Aeroallergen Levels and Hospital Admissions for Asthma in the Brussels-Capital Region: A Daily Time Series Analysis." *Environmental Health* 17 (1):35.

Gullon, P., C. Varela, E. V. Martínez, and D. Gómez-Barroso. 2017. "Association between Meteorological Factors and Hepatitis A in Spain 2010–2014." *Environment International* 102:230–5.

Haikerwal, A., M. Akram, A. Del Monaco, K. Smith, M. R. Sim, M. Meyer, A. M. Tonkin, M. J. Abramson, and M. Dennekamp. 2015. "Impact of Fine Particulate Matter ($PM_{2.5}$) Exposure during Wildfires on Cardiovascular Health Outcomes." *Journal of the American Heart Association* 4(7):e001653.

Hajat, S., A. Haines, C. Sarran, A. Sharma, C. Bates, and L. E. Fleming. 2017. "The Effect of Ambient Temperature on Type-2-Diabetes: Case-Crossover Analysis of 4+ Million GP Consultations across England." *Environmental Health* 16 (1):73.

Hanigan, I. C., C. D. Butler, P. N. Kokic, and M. F. Hutchinson. 2012. "Suicide and Drought in New South Wales, Australia, 1970–2007." *Proceedings of the National Academy of Sciences of the USA* 109 (35):13950–5.

Hansen, A., P. Bi, M. Nitschke, P. Ryan, D. Pisaniello, and G. Tucker. 2008. "The Effect of Heat Waves on Mental Health in a Temperate Australian City." *Environmental Health Perspectives* 116 (10):1369–75.

Harari Arjona, R., J. Piñeiros, M. Ayabaca, and F. H. Freire. 2016. "Climate Change and Agricultural Workers' Health in Ecuador: Occupational Exposure to UV Radiation and Hot Environments." *Annali dell'Istituto superiore di sanità* 52 (3):368–73.

Harville, E. W., C. A. Taylor, H. Tesfai, X. Xiong, and P. Buekens. 2011. "Experience of Hurricane Katrina and Reported Intimate Partner Violence." *Journal of Interpersonal Violence* 26 (4):833–45.

Hayes, D., Jr., M. A. Jhaveri, D. M. Mannino, H. Strawbridge, and J. Temprano. 2013. "The Effect of Mold Sensitization and Humidity upon Allergic Asthma." *Clinical Respiratory Journal* 7 (2):135–44.

Heguy, L., M. Garneau, M. S. Goldberg, M. Raphoz, F. Guay, and M.-F. Valois. 2008. "Associations between Grass and Weed Pollen and Emergency Department Visits for Asthma Among Children in Montreal." *Environmental Research* 106 (2):203–11.

Hendrickson, L. A., and R. L. Vogt. 1996. "Mortality of Kauai Residents in the 12-Month Period Following Hurricane Iniki." *American Journal of Epidemiology* 144 (2):188–91.

Hermesh, H., R. Shiloh, Y. Epstein, H. Manaim, A. Weizman, and H. Munitz. 2000. "Heat Intolerance in Patients with Chronic Schizophrenia Maintained with Antipsychotic Drugs." *American Journal of Psychiatry* 157 (8):1327–9.

Ion-Nedelcu, N., M. Niţescu, M. Caian, R. Bacruban, and E. Ceauşu. 2008. [Effect of Air Pollution upon the Hospitalization for Acute Lower Respiratory Tract Infections among the Bucharest Municipality's Residents]. *Bacteriologia, virusologia, parazitologia, epidemiologia* 53 (2):117–20.

Jariwala, S., J. Toh, M. Shum, G. de Vos, K. Zou, S. Sindher, P. Patel et al. 2014. "The Association between Asthma-Related Emergency Department Visits and Pollen and Mold Spore Concentrations in the Bronx, 2001–2008." *Journal of Asthma* 51 (1):79–83.

Johnson, G. J. 2004. "The Environment and the Eye." *Eye (London)* 18 (12):1235–50.

Jones, M. K., B. M. Wootton, L. D. Vaccaro, and R. G. Menzies. 2012. "The Impact of Climate Change on Obsessive Compulsive Checking Concerns." *Australian and New Zealand Journal of Psychiatry* 46 (3):265–70.

Kabir, S. M. S. 2018. "Psychological Health Challenges of the Hill-Tracts Region for Climate Change in Bangladesh." *Asian Journal of Psychiatry* 34:74–7.

Kaffenberger, B. H., D. Shetlar, S. A. Norton, and M. Rosenbach. 2017. "The Effect of Climate Change on Skin Disease in North America." *Journal of the American Academy of Dermatology* 76 (1):140–7.

Kao, A. Y., R. Munandar, S. L. Ferrara, D. M. Systrom, R. L. Sheridan, S. S. Cash, and E. T. Ryan. 2005. "Case Records of the Massachusetts General Hospital. Case 19-2005. A 17-Year-Old Girl with Respiratory Distress and Hemiparesis after Surviving a Tsunami." *New England Journal of Medicine* 352 (25):2628–36.

Kashala-Abotnes, E., D. Okitundu, D. Mumba, M. J. Boivin, T. Tylleskär, and D. Tshala-Katumbay. 2019. "Konzo: A Distinct Neurological Disease Associated with Food (Cassava) Cyanogenic Poisoning." *Brain Research Bulletin* 145:87–91.

Katelaris, C. H., and P. J. Beggs. 2018. "Climate Change: Allergens and Allergic Diseases." *Internal Medicine Journal* 48 (2):129–34.

Kawakami, Y., T. Tagami, T. Kusakabe, N. Kido, T. Kawaguchi, M. Omura, and R. Tosa. 2012. "Disseminated Aspergillosis Associated with Tsunami Lung." *Respiratory Care* 57 (10):1674–8.

Keygnaert, I., A. Dialmy, A. Manço, J. Keygnaert, N. Vettenburg, K. Roelens, and M. Temmerman. 2014. "Sexual Violence and Sub-Saharan Migrants in Morocco: A Community-Based Participatory Assessment Using Respondent Driven Sampling." *Globalization and Health* 10:32.

Kilinc, M. F., S. Cakmak, D. O. Demir, O. G. Doluoglu, Y. Yildiz, K. Horasanli, and A. Dalkilic. 2016. "Does Maternal Exposure During Pregnancy to Higher Ambient Temperature Increase the Risk of Hypospadias?" *Journal of Pediatric Urology* 12 (6):407.e1–407.e6.

Kirkpatrick, B., L. E. Fleming, L. C. Backer, J. A. Bean, R. Tamer, G. Kirkpatrick, T. Kane et al. 2006. "Environmental Exposures to Florida Red Tides: Effects on Emergency Room Respiratory Diagnoses Admissions." *Harmful Algae* 5 (5):526–33.

Kissinger, P., N. Schmidt, C. Sanders, and N. Liddon. 2007. "The Effect of the Hurricane Katrina Disaster on Sexual Behavior and Access to Reproductive Care for Young Women in New Orleans." *Sexually Transmitted Diseases* 34 (11):883–6.

Knowlton, K., M. Rotkin-Ellman, G. King, H. G. Margolis, D. Smith, G. Solomon, R. Trent, and P. English. 2009. "The 2006 California Heat Wave: Impacts on Hospitalizations and Emergency Department Visits." *Environmental Health Perspectives* 117 (1):61–7.

Kolstad, E. W., and K. A. Johansson. 2011. "Uncertainties Associated with Quantifying Climate Change Impacts on Human Health: A Case Study for Diarrhea." *Environmental Health Perspectives* 119 (3):299–305.

Kondo, H., N. Seo, T. Yasuda, M. Hasizume, Y. Koido, N. Ninomiya, and Y. Yamamoto. 2002. "Post-Flood--Infectious Diseases in Mozambique. *Prehospital and Disaster Medicine* 17 (3):126–33.

Kuehn, L., and S. McCormick. 2017. "Heat Exposure and Maternal Health in the Face of Climate Change." *International Journal of Environmental Research and Public Health* 14 (8).

Lake, I. R., N. R. Jones, M. Agnew, C. M. Goodess, F. Giorgi, L. Hamaoui-Laguel, M. A. Semenov, et al. 2017. "Climate Change and Future Pollen Allergy in Europe." *Environmental Health Perspectives* 125 (3):385–91.

Lam, H. C., A. M. Li, E. Y.-Y. Chan, and W. B. Goggins III. 2016. "The Short-Term Association between Asthma Hospitalisations, Ambient Temperature, Other Meteorological Factors and Air Pollutants in Hong Kong: A Time-Series Study." *Thorax* 71 (12):1097–1109.

Lam, H. C. Y., J. C. N. Chan, A. O. Y. Luk, E. Y.-Y. Chan, and W. B. Goggins. 2018. "Short-Term Association between Ambient Temperature and Acute Myocardial Infarction Hospitalizations for Diabetes Mellitus Patients: A Time Series Study." *PLoS Medicine* 15 (7):e1002612.

Lavados, P. M., V. V. Olavarria, and L. Hoffmeister. 2018. "Ambient Temperature and Stroke Risk: Evidence Supporting a Short-Term Effect at a Population Level from Acute Environmental Exposures." *Stroke* 49 (1):255-261.

Lee, C. P., P. J. Chen, and C. M. Chang. 2015. "Heat Stroke during Treatment with Olanzapine, Trihexyphenidyl, and Trazodone in a Patient with Schizophrenia." *Acta Neuropsychiatrica* 27 (6):380–5.

Levy, B. S., V. W. Sidel, and J. A. Patz. 2017. "Climate Change and Collective Violence." *Annual Review of Public Health* 38:241–57.

Leyser-Whalen, O., M. Rahman, and A. B. Berenson. 2011. "Natural and Social Disasters: Racial Inequality in Access to Contraceptives after Hurricane Ike." *Journal of Women's Health (Larchmont)* 20 (12):1861–6.

Lin, H. C., C.-S. Chen, J. J. Keller, J.-D. Ho, C.-C. Lin, and C.-C. Hu. 2011. "Seasonality of Retinal Detachment Incidence and Its Associations with Climate: An 11-Year Nationwide Population-Based Study." *Chronobiology International* 28 (10):942–8.

Lin, Y. J., R.-L. Lin, M. Khosravi, and L.-Y. Lee. 2015. "Hypersensitivity of Vagal Pulmonary C-Fibers Induced b Increasing Airway Temperature in Ovalbumin-Sensitized Rats." *American Journal of Physiology. Regulatory, Integrative and Comparative Physiology* 309 (10):R1285–91.

Link, M. S., H. Luttmann-Gibson, J. Schwartz, M. A. Mittleman, B. Wessler, D. R. Gold, D. W. Dockery, and F. Laden. 2013. "Acute Exposure to Air Pollution Triggers Atrial Fibrillation." *Journal of the American College of Cardiology* 62 (9):816–25.

Li, G., Q. Guo, Y. Liu, Y. Li, and X. Pan. 2018. "Projected Temperature-Related Years of Life Lost from Stroke due to Global Warming in a Temperate Climate City, Asia: Disease Burden Caused by Future Climate Change." *Stroke* 49 (4):828–34.

Li, T., R. M. Horton, D. A. Bader, F. Liu, Q. Sun, and P. L. Kinney. 2018. "Long-Term Projections of Temperature-Related Mortality Risks for Ischemic Stroke, Hemorrhagic Stroke, and Acute Ischemic Heart Disease under Changing Climate in Beijing, China." *Environment International* 112:1–9.

Li, Y., L. Lan, Y. Wang, C. Yang, W. Tang, G. Cui, S. Luo et al. 2014. "Extremely Cold and Hot Temperatures Increase the Risk of Diabetes Mortality in Metropolitan Areas of Two Chinese Cities." *Environmental Research* 134:91–7.

Liu, J. M., Y.-L. Chang, R.-J. Hsu, H.-Y. Su, S.-W. Teng, and F.-W. Chang. 2017. "The Climate Impact on Female Acute Pyelonephritis in Taiwan: A Population-Based Study." *Taiwanese Journal of Obstetrics & Gynecology* 56 (4):437–41.

Liu, X., D. Kong, Y. Liu, J. Fu, P. Gao, T. Chen, Q. Fang, K. Cheng, and Z. Fan. 2018. "Effects of the Short-Term Exposure to Ambient Air Pollution on Atrial Fibrillation." *Pacing and Clinical Electrophysiology* 41 (11):1441–6.

Madero, M., F. E. Garcia-Arroyo, and L. G. Sanchez-Lozada. 2017. "Pathophysiologic Insight into MesoAmerican Nephropathy." *Current Opinion in Nephrology And Hypertension* 26 (4):296–302.

Madrigano, J., M. A. Mittleman, A. Baccarelli, R. Goldberg, S. Melly, S. von Klot, and J. Schwartz. 2013. "Temperature, Myocardial Infarction, and Mortality: Effect Modification by Individual- and Area-Level Characteristics." *Epidemiology* 24 (3):439–46.

Majeed, H., and J. Lee. 2017. "The Impact of Climate Change on Youth Depression and Mental Health." *Lancet Planetary Health* 1 (3):e94–e95.

Mandavia, A., D. Huang, J. Wong, B. Ruiz, F. Crump, J. Shen, M. Martinez et al. 2017. "Violating Clan and Kinship Roles as Risk Factors for Suicide and Stigma among Lao Refugees: An Application of the Cultural Model of Suicide and 'What Matters Most' Frameworks." *Israel Journal of Psychiatry and Related Sciences* 54 (1):39–48.

McMichael, A. 2017. *Climate Change and the Health of Nations: Famines, Fevers, and the Fate of Populations*. New York: Oxford University Press.

Medina-Ramon, M., A. Zanobetti, D. P. Cavanagh, and J. Schwartz. 2006. "Extreme Temperatures and Mortality: Assessing Effect Modification by Personal Characteristics and Specific Cause of Death in a Multi-City Case-Only Analysis." *Environmental Health Perspectives* 114 (9):1331–6.

Medina-Ramon, M., A. Zanobetti, and J. Schwartz. 2006. "The Effect of Ozone and PM_{10} on Hospital Admissions for Pneumonia and Chronic Obstructive Pulmonary Disease: A National Multicity Study." *American Journal of Epidemiology* 163 (6):579–88.

Meze-Hausken, E. 2004. "Contrasting Climate Variability and Meteorological Drought with Perceived Drought and Climate Change in Northern Ethiopia." *Climate Research* 27 (1):19–31.

Minassian, D. C., V. Mehra, and B. R. Jones. 1984. "Dehydrational Crises from Severe Diarrhoea or Heatstroke and Risk of Cataract." *Lancet* 1 (8380):751–3.

Mirsaeidi, M., H. Motahari, M. T. Khamesi, A. Sharifi, M. Campos, and D. E. Schraufnagel. 2016. "Climate Change and Respiratory Infections." *Annals of the American Thoracic Society* 13 (8):1223–30.

Mohammadi, R., H. Soori, A. Alipour, E. Bitaraf, and S. Khodakarim. 2018. "The Impact of Ambient Temperature on Acute Myocardial Infarction Admissions in Tehran, Iran." *Journal of Thermal Biology* 73:24–31.

Mustafic, H., P. Jabre, C. Caussin, M. H. Murad, S. Escolano, M.Tafflet, M.-C. Périer et al. 2012. "Main Air Pollutants and Myocardial Infarction: A Systematic Review and Meta-Analysis." *JAMA* 307 (7):713–21.

National Center for Health Statistics. 2017. "*Pneumonia.*" Centers for Disease Control and Prevention. Accessed January 2, 2019. https://www.cdc.gov/nchs/fastats/pneumonia.htm.

Nerbass, F. B., R. Pecoits-Filho, W. F. Clark, J. M. Sontrop, C. W. McIntyre, and L. Moist. 2017. "Occupational Heat Stress and Kidney Health: From Farms to Factories." *Kidney International Reports* 2 (6):998-1008.

Neria, Y., A. Nandi, and S. Galea. 2008. "Post-Traumatic Stress Disorder Following Disasters: A Systematic Review." *Psychological Medicine* 38 (4):467–80.

Neupane, B., M. Jerrett, R. T. Burnett, T. Marrie, A. Arain, and M. Loeb. 2010. "Long-Term Exposure to Ambient Air Pollution and Risk of Hospitalization with Community-Acquired Pneumonia in Older Adults." *American Journal of Respiratory and Critical Care Medicine* 181 (1):47–53.

Obradovich, N., R. Migliorini, M. P. Paulus, and I. Rahwan. 2018. "Empirical Evidence of Mental Health Risks Posed by Climate Change." *Proceedings of the National Academy of Sciences of the USA* 115 (43):10953–8.

Oluwole, O. S. 2015. "Cyclical Konzo Epidemics and Climate Variability." *Annals of Neurology* 77 (3):371–80.

Page, L. A., S. Hajat, R. S. Kovats, L. M. Howard. 2002. "Temperature-Related Deaths in People with Psychosis, Dementia and Substance Misuse." *British Journal of Psychiatry* 200 (6):485–90.

Park, B. J., K. Sigel, V. Vaz, K. Komatsu, C. McRill, M. Phelan, T. Colman et al. 2005. "An Epidemic of Coccidioidomycosis in Arizona Associated with Climatic Changes, 1998–2001." *Journal of Infectious Diseases* 191 (11):1981–7.

Peperzak, L. 2005. "Future Increase in Harmful Algal Blooms in the North Sea due to Climate Change." *Water Science and Technology* 51 (5):31–6.

Phalkey, R. K., C. Aranda-Jan, S. Marx, B. Höfle, and R. Sauerborn. 2015. "Systematic Review of Current Efforts to Quantify the Impacts of Climate Change on Undernutrition." *Proceedings of the National Academy of Sciences of the USA* 112 (33):E4522–9.

Rataj, E., K. Kunzweiler, and S. Garthus-Niegel. 2016. "Extreme Weather Events in Developing Countries and Related Injuries and Mental Health Disorders—A Systematic Review." *BMC Public Health* 16 (1):1020.

Reid, C. E., M. Brauer, F. H. Johnston, M. Jerrett, J. R. Balmes, and C. T. Elliott. 2016. "Critical Review of Health Impacts of Wildfire Smoke Exposure." *Environmental Health Perspectives* 124 (9):1334–43.

Resnick, A., B. Woods, H. Krapfl, and B. Toth. 2015. "Health Outcomes Associated with Smoke Exposure in Albuquerque, New Mexico, during the 2011 Wallow Fire." *Journal of Public Health Management and Practice* 21 (suppl 2):S55–61.

Roncal-Jimenez, C. A., R. García-Trabanino, C. Wesseling, and R. J. Johnson. 2016. "Mesoamerican Nephropathy or Global Warming Nephropathy?" *Blood Purification* 41 (1–3):135–8.

Schlaudecker, E. P., M. C. Steinhoff, and S. R. Moore. 2011. "Interactions of Diarrhea, Pneumonia, and Malnutrition in Childhood: Recent Evidence from Developing Countries." *Current Opinion in Infectious Diseases* 24 (5):496–502.

Schleussner, C. F., J. F. Donges, R. V. Donner, and H. J. Schellnhuber. 2016. "Armed-Conflict Risks Enhanced by Climate-Related Disasters in Ethnically Fractionalized Countries." *Proceedings of the National Academy of Sciences of the USA* 113 (33):9216–21.

Schmeltz, M. T., and J. L. Gamble. 2017. "Risk Characterization of Hospitalizations for Mental Illness and/or Behavioral Disorders with Concurrent Heat-Related Illness." *PLoS One* 12 (10):e0186509.

Schmidt, C. W. 2018. "More Cases of Hand, Foot, and Mouth Disease in China: A Consequence of Climate Change?" *Environmental Health Perspectives* 126 (9):94002.

Schumacher, J. A., S. F Coffey, F. H. Norris, M. Tracy, K. Clements, and S. Galea. 2010. "Intimate Partner Violence and Hurricane Katrina: Predictors and Associated Mental Health Outcomes." *Violence and Victims* 25 (5):588–603.

Schwartz, J. 1994a. "Air Pollution and Hospital Admissions for the Elderly in Detroit, Michigan." *American Journal of Respiratory and Critical Care Medicine* 150 (3):648–55.

Schwartz, J. 1994b. "What Are People Dying of on High Air Pollution Days?" *Environmental Research* 64 (1):26–35.

Schwartz, J. 2005. "Who Is Sensitive to Extremes of Temperature?: A Case-Only Analysis." *Epidemiology* 16 (1):67–72.

Sganga, G., V. Cozza, T. Spanu, P. L. Spada, and G. Fadda. 2009. "Global Climate Change and Wound Care: Case Study of an Off-Season Vibrio Alginolyticus Infection in a Healthy Man." *Ostomy/Wound Management* 55 (4):60–2.

Shao, Q., T. Liu, P. Korantzopoulos, Z. Zhang, J. Zhao, and G. Li. 2016. "Association between Air Pollution and Development of Atrial Fibrillation: A Meta-Analysis of Observational Studies." *Heart & Lung* 45 (6):557–62.

Shultz, J. M., A. Rechkemmer, A. Rai, and K. T. McManus. 2019. "Public Health and Mental Health Implications of Environmentally Induced Forced Migration." *Disaster Medicine and Public Health Preparedness* 13 (2):116–22.

Siddique, A. K., A. H. Baqui, A. Eusof, and K. Zaman. 1991. "1988 Floods in Bangladesh: Pattern of Illness and Causes of Death." *Journal of Diarrhoeal Diseases Research* 9 (4):310–4.

Silverman, R. A., and K. Ito. 2010. "Age-Related Association of Fine Particles and Ozone with Severe Acute Asthma in New York City." *Journal of Allergy and Clinical Immunology* 125 (2):367–73 e5.

Siriwardhana, E. A., P. A. J. Perera, R. Sivakanesan, T. Abeysekara, D. B. Nugegoda, and J. A. A. S. Jayaweera. 2015. "Dehydration and Malaria Augment the Risk of Developing Chronic Kidney Disease in Sri Lanka." *Indian Journal of Nephrology* 25 (3):146–51.

Sohrabizadeh, S. 2016. "A Qualitative Study of Violence against Women after the Recent Disasters of Iran." *Prehospital Emergency Care* 31 (4):407–12.

Solimini, A. G., and M. Renzi. 2017. "Association between Air Pollution and Emergency Room Visits for Atrial Fibrillation." *International Journal of Environmental Research and Public Health* 14 (6).

Soneja, S., C. Jiang, J. Fisher, C. R. Upperman, C. Mitchell, and A. Sapkota. 2016. "Exposure to Extreme Heat and Precipitation Events Associated with Increased Risk of Hospitalization for Asthma in Maryland, U.S.A." *Environmental Health* 15:57.

Stensgaard, A. S., J. Utzinger, P. Vounatsou, E. Hürlimann, N. Schur, C. F. L. Saarnak, C. Simoonga et al. 2013. "Large-Scale Determinants of Intestinal Schistosomiasis and Intermediate Host Snail Distribution across Africa: Does Climate Matter?" *Acta Tropica* 128 (2):378–90.

Stensgaard, A. S., P. Vounatsou, M. E. Sengupta, and J. Utzinger. 2019. "Schistosomes, Snails and Climate Change: Current Trends and Future Expectations." *Acta Tropica* 190:257–68.

Sun, Z., C. Chen, D. Xu, and T. Li. 2018. "Effects of Ambient Temperature on Myocardial Infarction: A Systematic Review and Meta-Analysis." *Environmental Pollution* 241:1106–14.

Tesla, B., L. R. Demakovsky, E. A. Mordecai, S. J. Ryan, M. H. Bonds, C. N. Ngonghala, M. A. Brindley, and C. C. Murdock. 2018. "Temperature Drives Zika Virus Transmission: Evidence from Empirical and Mathematical Models." *Proceedings of the Royal Society of London. Series B* 285 (1884):20180795.

Tester, P. A., R. L. Feldman, A. W. Nau, S. R. Kibler, and R. W. Litakera. 2010. "Ciguatera Fish Poisoning and Sea Surface Temperatures in the Caribbean Sea and the West Indies." *Toxicon* 56 (5):698–710.

Thompson, R., R. Hornigold, L. Page, and T. Waite. 2018. "Associations between High Ambient Temperatures and Heat Waves with Mental Health Outcomes: A Systematic Review." *Public Health* 161:171–91.

Tosca, M. A., S. Ruffoni, G. W. Canonica, and G. Ciprandi. 2014. "Asthma Exacerbation in Children: Relationship among Pollens, Weather, and Air Pollution." *Allergologia et Immunopathologia (Madrid)* 42 (4):362–8.

Trasande, L., and G. D. Thurston. 2005. "The Role of Air Pollution in Asthma and Other Pediatric Morbidities." *Journal of Allergy and Clinical Immunology* 115 (4):689–99.

Tsai, S. S., and C. Y. Yang. 2014. "Fine Particulate Air Pollution and Hospital Admissions for Pneumonia in a Subtropical City: Taipei, Taiwan." *Journal of Toxicology and Environmental Health Part A* 77 (4):192–201.

van Loenhout, J. A. F., J. G. Cuesta, J. E. Abello, J. M. Isiderio, M. L. de Lara-Banquesio, and D. Guha-Sapir. 2018. "The Impact of Typhoon Haiyan on Admissions in Two Hospitals in Eastern Visayas, Philippines." *PLoS One* 13 (1):e0191516.

Van Zutphen, A. R., S. Lin, B. A. Fletcher, and S.-A. Hwang. 2012. "A Population-Based Case-Control Study of Extreme Summer Temperature and Birth Defects." *Environmental Health Perspectives* 120 (10):1443–9.

Wang, X., E. Lavigne, H. Ouellette-Kuntz, and B. E. Chen. 2014. "Acute Impacts of Extreme Temperature Exposure on Emergency Room Admissions Related to Mental and Behavior Disorders in Toronto, Canada." *Journal of Affective Disorders* 155:154–61.

Westphal, S. A., R. D. Childs, K. M. Seifert, M. E. Boyle, M. Fowke, P. Iñiguez, and C. B. Cook. 2010. "Managing Diabetes in the Heat: Potential Issues and Concerns." *Endocrine Practice* 16 (3):506–11.

Wettstein, Z. S., S. Hoshiko, J. Fahimi, R. J. Harrison, W. E. Cascio, and A. G. Rappold. 2018. "Cardiovascular and Cerebrovascular Emergency Department Visits Associated with Wildfire Smoke Exposure in California in 2015." *Journal of the American Heart Association* 7 (8).

Williams, P. L., D. L. Sable, P. Mendez, and L. T. Smyth. 1979. "Symptomatic Coccidioidomycosis Following a Severe Natural Dust Storm. An Outbreak at the Naval Air Station, Lemoore, Calif." *Chest* 76 (5):566–70.

Williams, R. J., R. T. Bryan, J. N. Mills, R. E. Palma, I. Vera, F. De Velasquez, E. Baez et al. 1997. "An Outbreak of Hantavirus Pulmonary Syndrome in Western Paraguay." *American Journal of Tropical Medicine and Hygiene* 57 (3):274–82.

World Health Organization. 2018. "Zika Virus Factsheet." https://www.who.int/news-room/fact-sheets/detail/zika-virus.

World Health Organization. 2020. "Fact Sheet: Asthma." https://www.who.int/en/news-room/fact-sheets/detail/asthma.

Xu, Z., W. Hu, and S. Tong. 2014. "Temperature Variability and Childhood Pneumonia: An Ecological Study." *Environmental Health* 13 (1):51.

Yates, T. L., J. N. Mills, C. A. Parmenter, T. G. Ksiazek, R. R. Parmenter, J. R. Vande Castle, C. H. Calisher et al. 2002. "The Ecology and Evolutionary History of an Emergent Disease: Hantavirus Pulmonary Syndrome." *BioScience* 52 (11):989.

Zahran, S., I. M. Breunig, B. G. Link, J. G. Snodgrass, S. Weiler, and H. W. Mielke. 2014. "Maternal Exposure to Hurricane Destruction and Fetal Mortality." *Journal of Epidemiology and Community Health* 68 (8):760–6.

Zanobetti, A., M. S. O'Neill, C. J. Gronlund, and J. D. Schwartz. 2013. "Susceptibility to Mortality in Weather Extremes: Effect Modification by Personal and Small-Area Characteristics." *Epidemiology* 24 (6):809–19.

Zhao, Q., S. Li, W. Cao, D.-L. Liu, Q. Qian, H. Ren, F. Ding et al. 2018. "Modeling the Present and Future Incidence of Pediatric Hand, Foot, and Mouth Disease Associated with Ambient Temperature in Mainland China." *Environmental Health Perspectives* 126 (4):047010.

Zhu, G., J. Fan, and A. T. Peterson. 2017. "Schistosoma Japonicum Transmission Risk Maps at Present and under Climate Change in Mainland China." *PLoS Neglected Tropical Diseases* 11 (10):e0006021.

Ziska, L., K. Knowlton, C. Rogers, D. Dalan, N. Tierney, M. A. Elder, W. Filley et al. 2011. "Recent Warming by Latitude Associated with Increased Length of Ragweed Pollen Season in Central North America." *Proceedings of the National Academy of Sciences of the USA* 108 (10):4248–51.

Ziska, L. H., and P. J. Beggs. 2012. "Anthropogenic Climate Change and Allergen Exposure: The Role of Plant Biology." *Journal of Allergy and Clinical Immunology* 129 (1):27–32.

CHAPTER 28

CLIMATE CHANGE AND LOSS OF BIODIVERSITY

Richard Salkowe and Mark R. Hafen

Introduction

Biodiversity is defined as the variability among all life forms that exist on Earth. These variations have evolved as a result of billions of years of competitive and cooperative relationships between interacting organisms and the physical environment in which they reside. This has led to the development of the diverse **ecosystems** that exist on our planet at the present time. Fossil evidence of biological diversity on Earth dates from 2 billion to 3.5 billion years ago. The primordial species that existed during that time frame were single-celled prokaryotic microorganisms, lacking a true nucleus, and they were capable of withstanding the extremes of a geologically unstable planet. These **prokaryotes** gradually diversified to include, in part, thermophilic bacteria that were capable of withstanding extreme heat, methane-producing archaebacteria, and eventually photosynthetic oxygen-producing cyanobacteria. The biodiversity that is evident in these varied examples of early life on Earth exemplify the adaptations and alterations in single-celled organisms that occurred over the course of more than a billion years in response to environmental challenges.

The subsequent evolution of multicellular organisms and, eventually, the diverse flora and fauna that comprise life on our planet in the twenty-first century did not occur without interruption. Our planet has succumbed to multiple species extinction events over the course of the past 500 million years associated with climate-related temperature fluctuations, sea level changes, large scale volcanic eruptions, and asteroid impacts. Five major **mass extinction** events have occurred over the past 500 million years that have been classified as such because of the magnitude of loss of biodiversity and the abundance of species that were eradicated during the extinction time frame. It is estimated that 75–99 percent of the more than five billion species that have ever existed on our planet suffered their demise during these historical mass extinction events (Kunin and Gaston 1996; Richter 2015; Stearns and Stearns 1999) and the recovery to preextinction levels of biodiversity may have taken as long as ten million years (Jablonski 1991).

Causes and Consequences of Biodiversity Loss

Approximately 8.7 million eukaryotic organisms have been estimated to inhabit our planet today, but it is believed more than 80 percent of **eukaryotes** have yet to be identified (Mora et al. 2011) and if prokaryotic microorganisms are included, planet Earth may contain nearly one trillion diverse species (Locey and Lennon 2011). However, this abundance of diversity is confronted by the stark reality that we may be on the precipice of a sixth mass extinction event and it is associated with anthropogenic climate-related influences (Ceballos, Ehrlich, and Dirzo 2017). Loss of species diversity is occurring at a rate that is 1,000 to 10,000 times

KEY CONCEPTS

- Climate change is expected to have a major effect on global biodiversity in the coming decades.

- Climate change and other human impacts are already altering worldwide ecosystems.

- Human health and well-being requires the maintenance of ecosystem biodiversity.

greater than the natural background rate of one to five species per year (Wilson 2007). Dozens of species are estimated to be going extinct every day (Center for Biological Diversity n.d.; Chivian and Bernstein 2008) and midrange climate warming scenarios from a recent study, which included 20 percent of Earth's terrestrial surface area, approximate that 15–37 percent of all species will be "committed to extinction" by 2050 (Thomas et al. 2004).

Although climate change is a significant driver with respect to biodiversity loss, it is important to note that a combination of anthropogenic influences, including agriculture, logging, ranching, overpopulation, infrastructure expansion, invasive species, and pollution, have contributed to and potentiated the adverse effects of a warming planet. The combination of habitat destruction and climate change provide limited refuge for many species that are under stress. This is exemplified by the United Nations' estimate that 7.3 million hectares of tropical forest are destroyed each year for logging and agricultural land clearing (Food and Agriculture Organization 2005). Greater than one half of all plant and animal species are found in tropical rain forests. Degradation of this essential ecosystem has far ranging consequences on human health ranging from the loss of potential lifesaving medicines to alterations in climate associated with carbon sequestration processes by forest trees and the burning of forest land (Salkowe 2016). Over one half of all tropical rain forests have been cleared and the World Wildlife Federation estimates that approximately 15 percent of all greenhouse gas emissions are attributable to deforestation (World Wildlife Federation n.d.).

The 7.7 billion human inhabitants of our planet have placed extreme demands on natural resources. Our burgeoning population has led to rapid urbanization and infrastructure development and this has compromised natural habitats and is often associated with the introduction of invasive species that threaten the native biota in their respective communities. Natural habitat corridors are fragmented by poorly planned urban development resulting in a vast array of challenges to affected species ranging from decreased access to food and water resources to limitations in genetic diversity associated with compromised nesting and breeding habitats.

Pollution is an unfortunate sequela of the production and consumption of synthetic and natural resources in the twenty-first century and extends from the burning of fossil fuels to the distribution of chemicals and waste in our water supply. Water pollution from pesticides and industrial byproducts containing polychlorinated biphenyls (PCBs), bisphenol A, and phthalates has been associated with compounds that interfere with normal endocrine hormonal functions, which may lead to developmental abnormalities and altered reproductive capacity in humans (Salkowe 2016). Herbicides and agricultural pesticides damage natural flora and reduce food supply for certain species. Air pollution from sulfur and nitrogen emissions produces "acid rain" with deleterious effects on multiple species (United Nations Economic Commission for Europe n.d.).

This combination of planetary maladies has been underway since the advent of permanent human settlements approximately 12,000 years ago. The subsequent agricultural and, more recent, industrial revolutions have exacerbated our climate change dilemma. We are now faced with a unique paradox that was not encountered during historical mass extinction events on our planet. Homo sapiens was not an inhabitant of Earth during prior mass extinction events. At the present time, human beings reside on planet Earth as a relatively nonnomadic and overabundant omnivore species and our well-being is dependent on the preservation of a significant diversity in a vast array of vulnerable species and ecosystems that filter air, purify water, protect us from hazards, and provide essential food resources. There is limited opportunity for refuge from the cascading consequences of biodiversity loss that are underway as a result of a changing climate.

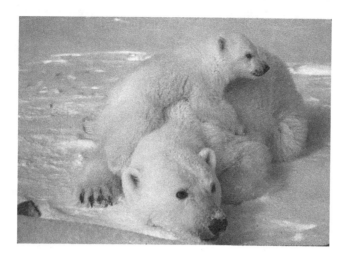

Figure 28.1 Arctic polar bear and cub
Source: Courtesy U.S. Fish and Wildlife Service, Schliebe, Scott, public domain.

In 1911, the famous naturalist and conservationist John Muir informed us that, "When we try to pick out anything by itself, we find it hitched to everything else in the universe." Muir was describing the interactions and interdependencies that exist among the physical and biologic components of our environment. These relationships result in the diverse ecosystems that are essential to our well-being. The effects of biodiversity loss are clear when we consider the well-documented climate change-related loss of habitat and the subsequent extinction risk for threatened apex predator species such as the Arctic polar bear (Figure 28.1). However, the insidious consequences of biodiversity loss become more evident when we understand that the Arctic polar bear is also an indicator species and the polar bear's compromised habitat serves as a harbinger of the adverse effects of a warming planet for the entire Arctic biome. These complex interactions are the foundation of our planet's varied ecosystems and our sustainability is dependent on the preservation of these diverse relationships. Laidre et al. (2018) provide us with a salient reminder in stating that, "we frequently fail to consider how environmental conditions and interspecies interactions molded evolution over geological timescales, or the importance of these evolutionary events to modern-day ecology. As the climate continues to warm, there are certain to be surprises."

Historical Perspective

Prior extinction events that led to a significant loss of biodiversity and compromised species abundance have been documented throughout the fossil record. Our geologic past serves as a prologue to the potential risks associated with the evidence of a rapidly changing climate on our planet in the twenty-first century. A review of the etiology and consequences of the five mass extinction events that occurred over the past 500 million years will provide a contextual basis for understanding the deleterious effects of climate change on biodiversity and species abundance.

The first of the recognized mass extinction events occurred during the geological time frame known as the "Ordovician," which ended approximately 444 million years ago with a cataclysmic combination of events associated with climate-related glaciation, tectonic plate movements, and lower sea levels (Harper, Hammarlund, and Rasmussen 2014). An estimated 86 percent of species were lost over the course of a million years during the end of this geological period (Richter 2015). Land-based animals did not exist during the Ordovician, so the extinction event specifically affected marine organisms. A cooling planet resulted in a global decrease in sea level with the resultant loss of tropical marine genera (Finnegan et al. 2012). A temperature decline of approximately 10°C (18°F) allowed continental ice to expand to tropical latitudes (Pohl, Austermann, and Donnadieu 2018). Consequently, the highest level of species loss occurred in the tropical oceans where the glaciation associated spreading ice sheet provided limited refuge for the biota that were acclimated to warm water temperatures.

The second mass extinction event occurred approximately 375 million years ago during the Late Devonian period and led to the demise of 70–80 percent of all animal species which were present on our planet at that time (Richter 2015). This mass extinction comprised a series of 8–10 smaller extinctions that occurred over twenty million years. The Devonian was known as the "Age of Fish" as there were no large land animals in existence; it was not until the latter part of this geologic time frame that land-based plants and insects emerged. During the Late Devonian, the "stony" coral species that are present on modern coral reefs first appeared. The Devonian extinction event was particularly severe with respect to the demise of reef building species such as tabulate coral and a significant number of abundant arthropod species, known as trilobites. Over 20,000 species of trilobites were present prior to the onset of the Devonian extinction, ranging from 1 mm to 72 cm in size, and these animals served essential roles in the marine ecosystem as filter feeders, scavengers and as a food source for larger marine animals.

It is hypothesized that newly developing terrestrial vascular plant species with deep root systems released an abundance of nutrients into shallow waters, which led to algal blooms that compromised available oxygen levels and suffocated the shallow water species (Algeo et al. 1995). Microorganisms that were capable of tolerating this anoxic environment fed off the algal blooms and emitted hydrogen sulfide as a waste product that contributed to the toxicity of ocean waters during this time frame (Baraniuk 2015). Asteroid impacts, plate tectonics, and climate change have also been implicated in this event, which had a cumulative devastating effect on biodiversity. It would take 260 million years after the Devonian extinction for reef building coral to reemerge on our planet (Global Reef Project 2010).

The End Permian geological period that occurred approximately 252 million years ago represents the third mass extinction event and is widely recognized as the most severe extinction event in the history of our planet. This time period has been categorized as the "Great Dying" and it is believed to represent the closest our planet has ever been to the total annihilation of all existing life forms (Solly 2018). An estimated 96 percent of marine life, 70 percent of terrestrial animals, and 90 percent of all life forms on planet Earth succumbed to the forces of climate change that occurred during this extinction. This was a catastrophic global warming event and has been reported to be the result of an asteroid impact or a breakdown in the Earth's protective ozone layer. However, recent research suggests that 300,000 years of volcanic eruptions that were occurring during the Permian culminated in the injection of massive amounts of magma beneath the Earth's surface. This led to the extensive burning of subterranean coal deposits that had accumulated during the preceding Carboniferous geologic period. The geochemical evidence supports the fact that the burning of this sedimentary rock led to the release of massive amounts of greenhouse gases including carbon dioxide, methane, and sulfur. This led to acid rain that decimated the forests and ocean acidification and deoxygenation that destroyed most of the marine life (Burger 2018; Burgess, Muirhead, and Bowring 2017; Nuccitelli 2018). It is estimated that ocean surface temperatures increased by 11°C during the Late Permian-Triassic transition with a resultant 76 percent decrease in global ocean oxygen levels. Deep sea floor environments were particularly compromised and modeling estimates indicate that 40 percent of all sea floor environments became completely anoxic (Gannon 2018). This event is believed to have occurred rapidly over the course of 100,000 years, a small amount of time in our planet's geologic history. The trilobite species that remained after the Devonian extinction met their final demise during this time period and it was the most significant extinction event in the history of insect arthropods. It would take an estimated ten million years to restore the approximate level of biodiversity that existed before the "Great Dying."

The correlation between modern anthropogenic climate forcing factors such as fossil fuel burning and the processes of global warming that occurred during the End Permian extinction reveal the risks of biodiversity loss associated with a course of unabated greenhouse gas emissions. The National Oceanic and Atmospheric Administration indicates that ocean surface temperatures have increased by 0.13°C per decade over the past century and the UN World Meteorological Organization's Provisional Statement on the State of the Global Climate in 2018, predicts that we may see atmospheric temperature increases of 3–5°C by the end of the century (World Meteorological Organization 2018). Justin Penn and Curtis Deutsch, oceanographers from the University of Washington, inform us that, "under a business-as-usual emissions scenarios, by 2100, warming in the upper ocean will have approached 20 percent of warming in the late Permian, and by the year 2300, it will reach between 35 and 50 percent" (Penn et al. 2018; University of Washington 2018). These findings highlight the potential for an extinction event arising from a warming trend associated with anthropogenic-induced climate change.

The fourth mass extinction event in Earth's history occurred approximately 201 million years ago, during the End Triassic geological period, when an estimated 80 percent of existing species were eradicated from the planet. The life forms that managed to survive the Late Permian mass extinction had gradually evolved by the time of the Triassic to reveal the first mammalian small rodent-like creatures and the earliest dinosaurs on our planet. The End Triassic extinction occurred in a relatively short geological time frame of approximately 40,000 years. All of the land masses that exist on Earth at the present time were coalesced into one supercontinent, known as Pangea, during the beginning of the Triassic geological period. Because of tectonic activity associated with shifts in the Earth's mantle layer, Pangea began to break apart during the late Triassic and large-scale volcanic activity ensued. Researchers in the Department of Earth, Atmospheric and Planetary Sciences at the Massachusetts Institute of Technology have determined that this massive volcanic activity lead to significant releases of greenhouse gases, including carbon dioxide, methane, and sulfur, which resulted in a significant loss of biodiversity among both plant and animal species (Chu 2013) This provided an opportunity for the reptilian biota that withstood the environmental challenge to gradually evolve into the first dinosaur species that inhabited Earth. Some scientists believe the late Triassic event involved a series of background extinctions and, as such, it should be not labeled as a single mass extinction event. There are also theories promoting an asteroid impact as the initiating cause of this extinction but recent evidence correlating the onset of the extinction with massive volcanic activity supports the premise that the End Triassic extinction was a result of greenhouse gas emissions associated with the fragmentation of the Pangea landmass. In this regard, the causal factors associated with planetary global warming during this event were similar to the prior Permian extinction, although on a smaller scale.

The fifth mass extinction event occurred approximately sixty-six million years ago during the End Cretaceous geologic period. Approximately 76 percent of all species on our planet succumbed to this event, which marks the end of the nonavian dinosaurs on Earth and the ascent of the mammalian species. A 10 km asteroid impact in the Yucatan peninsula has been implicated as a significant factor in this extinction occurrence although volcanic activity has been highlighted in multicausal theories pertaining to this devastating event. Climate simulations indicate that global wildfires associated with the asteroid impact led to the ejection of soot into the atmosphere, which darkened the sky for several years. The resulting absence of sunlight led to the cessation of photosynthesis and the demise of the plant species that provided essential support for the planetary food chain (Bardeen et al. 2017). The lack of sunlight and the sulfur-laden soot emissions are hypothesized to have resulted in global cooling with annual mean surface air temperatures decreasing by at least 26°C and subfreezing temperatures on a large portion of the planet lasting for three to sixteen years. Even in the tropical regions, annual mean air temperatures declined from 27°C to 5°C (Herrle et al. 2015). This rapid cooling occurred subsequent to one of the warmest periods on our planet when the polar regions were ice free and average ocean temperatures of up to 35°C (95°F) were prevalent. Julia Brugger, at the Potsdam Institute for Climate Research, suggest that dinosaurs were adapted to the preceding warm environment and were unable to tolerate this rapid cooling (Brugger, Feulner, and Petri 2017). It took an estimated thirty years for the climate to recover from the initial effects of the asteroid impact. There is ongoing debate in the scientific community regarding the ultimate cause of the End Cretaceous extinction. Although an extrinsic asteroid impact has been given primacy in the recent debate regarding the origin of the fifth mass extinction, plate tectonics and volcanic activity have also been linked to the event. This may have been a multicausal extinction, but the ultimate end result reveals that a significant change in global climate occurred. This culminated in a mass extinction event with devastating consequences for the diversity and the abundance of species that inhabited our planet during the End Cretaceous geological period.

Biodiversity Loss in the Twenty-First Century

We are now facing the prospect of a sixth mass extinction event. This has been referred to as the **anthropocene** extinction as it is attributed to human activity. The combined influences of agricultural expansion, industrialization and overpopulation have created challenges to a vast array of species ranging from single-celled eukaryotes in Arctic sea ice to the megafauna of the Serengeti plains. This episode of extinctions began over 12,000 years ago during the Late Pleistocene Epoch. More than 300 mammalian species have been eradicated since the onset of this event along with the 2.5 billion years of unique evolutionary history that accompanied the establishment of these species on our planet (Davis, Faurby, and Svenning 2018). A review of vertebrate taxa evaluated by the International Union for Conservation of Nature (IUCN) reveals that 338 vertebrate extinctions have occurred in the past 500 years (Ceballos et al. 2015). Ceballos, Ehrlich, and Dirzo (2017), in a review of 27,600 terrestrial vertebrate species that presently exist on Earth, have determined that ongoing diminished species population size and range shrinkage are indicative of a "massive erosion of biodiversity and of the ecosystem services essential to civilization," which they categorize as a "biological annihilation."

In contrast, some scientific researchers are more selective in their assessment of the present state of species extinction and avoid comparison with the five historical mass extinction events (Barnosky et al. 2011; Brannen 2017). Although these scientists acknowledge the severity of biodiversity loss that has occurred over the past 12,000 years, they indicate that aggressive intervention may prevent a cataclysm comparable to the historical mass extinction events. Smithsonian paleontologist, Doug Erwin, informs us that a mass extinction event, classified as the loss of 75 percent or more of all living organisms, would be dependent on an ecosystem's undefined **"tipping points"** (Brannen 2017). These "tipping points" would lead to the collapse of entire ecosystems and would be the cumulative result of an unmanageable combination of environmental stressors which exceeded an ecosystem's survival capacity. Faced with the myriad of environmental challenges that are present on Earth in the twenty-first century, the pertinent question is, will our present day and projected anthropogenic induced climate change be the "tipping point" for the onset of a sixth mass extinction?

Climate change is expected to become the greatest driver of change in global biodiversity in the coming decades (Molinos et al. 2016). A worldwide assessment of the effects of a warming planet on amphibian species indicates that more than one third of the 6,300 known species are threatened with extinction and that mountainous amphibian species with limited altitudinal range are the most compromised (Wake and Vredenburg 2008). Additional research suggests that climate change leading to warmer ocean temperatures will lead to major changes in the geographic range of marine biodiversity. This would result in potential extinctions of thermal intolerant species in tropical oceans and the migration of capable species from the tropics to polar regions with an unknown effect on the extant native biota in these areas (Finnegan et al. 2015). The combination of human impacts and climate change will place coastal species at increased risk in tropical regions, including the Indo-Pacific, the Caribbean, and the Gulf of Mexico. Mark Urban, from the Department of Ecology and Evolutionary Biology at the University of Connecticut, performed a review of 131 previously published studies and concluded that unabated greenhouse gas emissions will threaten 16 percent of existing species with extinction due to climate change by the end of the century (Urban 2015). Anthony Barnosky, at the University of California, Berkeley, surmises that the sixth mass extinction could occur in just a few centuries "under conditions that resemble the 'perfect storm' which coincided with past mass extinctions: multiple, atypical high-intensity ecological stressors, including rapid, unusual climate change and highly elevated atmospheric CO2" (Barnosky et al. 2011). A review of global ecosystems that are presently succumbing to the forces of climate change with respect to biodiversity loss will provide us with an opportunity to determine if existing ecological stressors are, in fact, providing the "tipping point" that may result in the sixth mass extinction event on Earth.

Marine and Coastal Ecosystems

The world's oceans comprise 71 percent of our planet's total surface area and contain 97 percent of Earth's water resources. It is estimated that 50 to 80 percent of all life forms and 99 percent of habitable space on our planet is located in the ocean. Our oceans meet the shoreline along a global path that exceeds 217,000 miles of coastal interface. A changing climate associated with greenhouse gas emissions has significant effects on marine and coastal biodiversity associated with sea level rise, ocean acidification, ocean deoxygenation, and an increase in storm intensity. The circulation of ocean currents, known as the global conveyor belt, is influenced by warming ocean temperatures. This circulation pattern influences the upwelling of nutrients that provide sustenance for the **phytoplankton** that form the foundation of the ocean food chain in our polar regions. Sea level rise provides a threat to the coastal flora and fauna that are dependent on a narrow range of physical features, ranging from salinity gradients and shoreline topography to nesting and breeding habitats. Coral reefs provide habitat for approximately one quarter of all marine species and the 2018 report by the Intergovernmental Panel on Climate Change concludes that "the majority of warmer water coral reefs that exist today (70–90 percent) will largely disappear" if ocean temperatures increase by 1.5°C (2.7°F) (Intergovernmental Panel on Climate Change 2018; Markham 2018). It is evident that our planetary well-being is dependent on the preservation of the physical and biological balances that maintain the integrity of a healthy ocean system. This balance is threatened by climate change and a more thorough investigation of ocean ecosystem biological and physical interdependencies, from algal species to marine mammals, will assist in substantiating our concerns.

Polar Ocean Ecosystems

The poles have been described as the "most sensitive regions to climate change on Earth" (National Snow and Ice Data Center 2020). In the Arctic, changes in ocean temperature have contributed to the melting of sea ice, which has had a major effect on the entire ecosystem. Key observational indicators have led scientists to conclude that, "the Arctic biophysical system is now clearly trending away from its 20th Century state and into an unprecedented state, with implications not only within but beyond the Arctic" (Box et al. 2019). Ecosystem components including sea ice biota, plankton, deep-sea benthic organisms, marine fishes, seabirds, and marine mammals are experiencing pressure from climate induced changes in their physical, chemical, and biological environment (Conservation of Arctic Flora and Fauna International Secretariat 2017). The loss of sea ice due to warmer ocean temperatures will lead to changes in the microscopic marine algae, classified as phytoplankton, that form the foundation of the Arctic food chain. Smaller algae species, yielding lower levels of carbon, may be less nutritious for the **zooplankton** that are dependent on phytoplankton as a food source (Neeley et al. 2018). Zooplankton species ranging from Arctic copepods to Antarctic krill are showing evidence of declines in number in their respective ecosystems associated with changes in sea ice distribution and native phytoplankton abundance (Figure 28.2). The primary native polar krill and copepod species are highly adapted to cold ocean temperatures and their ability to thrive in an environment with warmer temperatures compounds the concerns pertaining to this vital part of the food chain in the polar regions (Hinder et al. 2014; Pinones and Fedorov 2016). Marine fishes, seabirds, and mammals are dependent on the zooplankton for sustenance. The ability for nonnative phytoplankton species to migrate from warmer ocean waters to the polar regions and the capacity for zooplankton to adapt to, both, warmer water temperatures and an alternative food source will determine the fate of the polar ecosystems as a result of climate change.

Tropical Ocean Ecosystems

Anthropogenic-induced global warming has deceased the oxygenation of ocean waters in many areas. Warmer waters hold less oxygen and lead to changes in ocean circulation and stratification, which result in decreased levels of available oxygen. Oxygen levels in some tropical regions have decreased by 40 percent in the last fifty years with a global average loss of 2 percent (Poppick 2019; Stramma et al. 2008). Although some species such as squid and jellyfish are more tolerant of lower ocean oxygen levels, crustaceans and fish have experienced die-off events sec-

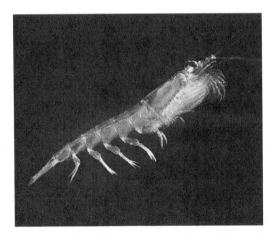

Figure 28.2 Antarctic krill
Source: Courtesy Uwe Kils, Creative Commons, Share Alike 3.0.

ondary to low oxygen levels (Grantham et al. 2004). Coastal water **dead zones** are primarily attributable to nutrient runoff, but open ocean dead zones are increasing as a result of climate change and warmer water temperatures. These areas of decreased oxygenation are known as oxygen minimum zones and they are expanding in surface area and depth with secondary loss of habitat for species that require higher oxygen levels. Recent dead zones have been found in tropical waters including the Arabian Sea and the Indian Ocean. Hypoxic areas have increased by 4.5 million km^2 at depths of 200–700 m in tropical and subtropical waters (Stramma et al. 2010).

Coral reefs are predominantly located in tropical waters and they support one of the world's most diverse ecosystems. The IUCN indicates that coral reefs support over 500 million people, worldwide, who are dependent on vibrant reef ecosystems for their daily subsistence (International Union for Conservation of Nature 2017). However, climate change has led to the recognition of coral reefs as one of the most threatened ecosystems on our planet. An increase in tropical ocean water of 1°C (1.8°F) has led to mass bleaching of coral reefs in several parts of the world. The burning of fossil fuels results in the release of greenhouse gases, which are responsible for the acidification of ocean waters. This has a harmful effect on reef building corals. Thermal stress increases susceptibility to invasive bacterial diseases and prolonged bleaching results in the death of the affected coral. These multiple environmental challenges have a devastating effect on the biodiversity of the coral reef ecosystem and the 25 percent of all marine fish species that are dependent on a healthy coral reef habitat.

Coastal Ecosystems

Coastal ecosystem biota exhibit unique adaptations to the energy, salinity, and moisture gradients that are present along our world's coastlines (Burkett et al. 2008). These ecosystems are under stress due to alterations in land use and the challenges associated with a changing climate (see Case Study: Tampa Bay, Florida, and Biodiversity Loss). Increases in freshwater and ocean temperature, ocean acidification, sea level rise, weather pattern alterations, ocean currents, and increased levels of carbon dioxide in the environment will serve as disruptive forces for the biodiversity of coastal flora and fauna (Paice and Chambers 2016). All species of sea turtles will face limitations in nesting sites associated with an increase in sea level and an increase in beach temperature. Because fish maintain the same body temperature as their surrounding environment, increased water temperatures will challenge the vitality of highly adapted shallow water coastal fish species.

Rainforest Ecosystems

Home to more than one half of all plants and wildlife on our planet, tropical rainforests provide a critical role in absorbing carbon dioxide from the atmosphere. Unfortunately, deforestation is limiting the ability for rainforests to act as carbon sinks and is, in fact, contributing to the warming of the earth's atmosphere by the release of carbon dioxide associated with forest burning. Compounding this is the estimation that increased atmospheric temperatures will lead to a 10–20 percent decrease in rainfall in rainforests in the Amazon basin, which would gradually change the forest ecosystems into savannah ecosystems. In a worst-case scenario, the decrease in forest canopy cover would perpetuate a cycle of drought and lead to what has been classified as an "Amazon dieback." Recent research has indicated that the Amazon rainforest is sufficiently resilient to withstand a major "dieback" scenario (Yale School of Forestry and Environmental Studies 2020). However, climate change associated temperature increases and resource compromise are threatening diverse rainforest species ranging from the Hawaiian honeycreeper to Australian Lemuroid ringtail possums.

Desert Ecosystems

Although a warming planet may seem to be less of a threat to desert ecosystems, many of the plant and animal species that live in the desert are already living at a physiological thermal maximum tolerance level. An increase in temperature may not be sustainable for key components of the desert ecosystem.

Research suggest that changes in temperature and precipitation will affect the desert by altering biotic components such as the soil crusts that help to maintain soil stability and carbon and nitrogen levels that serve as habitats for microorganisms (Chinese Academy of Sciences 2018). Stanley Smith, an ecologist from the University of Nevada, predicts that massive increases in carbon dioxide associated with greenhouse gas emissions will eventually transform desert ecosystems by encouraging invasive plant growth. This may disturb the delicately balanced desert ecosystems by changing the nutrient cycle, fire cycle, and distribution of water (Hill 2000).

Mountain Ecosystems

Approximately 85 percent of water that humans depend on originates from mountain ecosystems (U.S. Geologic Survey n.d.). The varied topographic, climatic, and biologic gradients in mountain ranges throughout the world make these ecosystems particularly vulnerable to changes in temperature and precipitation. Upward altitude shifting of plant species in high mountain systems will challenge the habitats of the native alpine vegetation. Mountain temperatures are rising at twice the rate of the rest of the world. The resultant decrease in snowfall will affect water availability and has allowed species, such as elk, to expand their forage range. This has had a negative effect on the ecosystem's seasonal woodsy plants and impacted the population of plant dependent songbirds (Castro 2017). A warmer planet will influence the chemistry of mountain soils by shifting the balance of nutrients. This may disrupt fragile, high-elevation grasses, flowers, and trees (Mayor et al. 2017).

CASE STUDY: TAMPA BAY, FLORIDA, AND BIODIVERSITY LOSS

Tampa Bay is an estuary along west Florida's Gulf of Mexico coast. Much of the estuary is highly urbanized, notably by the cities of Tampa and St. Petersburg and their surrounding suburbs, and pressure for additional development is putting stress on the bay's remaining natural ecosystems. Historically, Tampa Bay was surrounded by salt marshes, salterns (aka salt flats or salt barrens), mangroves, and tidal creek ecosystems. Today, however, urbanization has been responsible for heavy modification of most of the rivers and streams that empty into the bay, and many smaller creeks have been completely eliminated. The remaining tidal wetland ecosystems are sandwiched between rising water levels of the bay and the impacts created by increased urban development.

Specifically, biodiversity in the Tampa Bay region is being affected by a phenomenon known as "coastal squeeze." Coastal squeeze is a form of coastal habitat loss in which ecosystem habitats in the intertidal zone decline or disappear, because these environments are caught between rising sea levels on one side and the low-lying human-built environment on the other (Borchert et al. 2018; Pontee 2013). Often the gray infrastructure constructed to protect the built environment from the impacts of rising seas, such as sea walls and revetments, also prevents coastal ecosystems from migrating landward over time in response to sea level rise. The potential, for example, of landward migration of wetlands in the Tampa Bay region have been found to be low (Borchert et al. 2018). At the same time, the impervious surfaces of urban development impact the hydrology of coastal ecosystems, affecting sedimentation, water quality, and nutrient distribution (Torio and Chmura 2013). This can reduce the overall spatial extent of the mosaic of habitats in the wetlands that support many species and thus have a negative impact on biodiversity.

Loss of biodiversity is also occurring as the result of climate change and sea level rise. The conversion of salt marsh and saltern ecosystems to mangroves has been modeled and documented in both Tampa Bay and other coastal areas of the Gulf of Mexico (Armitage et al. 2015; Raabe, Roy, and McIvor 2012; Radabaugh et al. 2018; Sherwood and Greening 2014). The loss of the former two wetlands reduces or eliminates the habitats upon which many bay and gulf species—plant and animal—depend, particularly sea animals in their juvenile stages. And although mangroves are themselves a critical ecosystem to the bay, they cannot provide the same biotic and abiotic factors that support all of the marsh and saltern species. Both plant and animal biodiversity decline as a result. Even the mangroves are not immune to impacts from climate change and urbanization. Indeed, changes to freshwater flow and overall hydrologic connectivity can lead to the loss of these ecosystems as well (Osland et al. 2018).

The changes in all of these wetland ecosystems have potentially farther-reaching impacts to biodiversity. For example, changes to the filtration and sedimentation processes provided by salt marshes affect bay water quality (chemistry, salinity, clarity, etc.), and ultimately nearshore gulf water quality. Salt water intrusion due to sea level rise affects freshwater and upland ecosystems further inland, as well as the ability of the coastal wetlands themselves to adapt to increased inundation and higher salinities (Osland et al. 2018). All of these add up to ecological stress and threaten the ability of the Tampa Bay estuary and the environments around it to maintain their biodiversity.

Finally, the very health, welfare, and economic well-being of the human populations living in this region are affected by coastal squeeze, climate change, and impacts to Tampa Bay wetland ecosystems. Sources of food, employment, and shoreline protection are lost, threatening the urban environment itself (Borchert et al. 2018). People living in the Tampa Bay region have a vested interest in developing better land use practices and in balancing urban growth with wetland conservation measures (Lester and Matella 2016; Sherwood and Greening 2014). Both ecological and economic valuations of wetland ecosystem benefits must be conducted to understand the threats climate change, and in particular coastal squeeze, pose to biodiversity and to human populations that are dependent upon it (Russell and Greening 2015; Sherwood and Greening 2014).

Summary

Climate change is expected to become the greatest driver of change in global biodiversity in the coming decades (Molinos et al. 2016). The cumulative forces of climate change are taking a visible toll on the biodiversity of our planet and the human health consequences are evident in measures ranging from altered air quality to the loss of food and medicinal resources. From bleached coral reefs and anoxic dead zones in our oceans to habitat loss for Arctic polar bears, the damage to species and ecosystems is evident. Anthropogenic induced warming has led to decreased ocean productivity, altered food web dynamics, reduced abundance of habitat-forming species, shifting species distributions, and a greater incidence of disease (Hoegh-Guldberg and Bruno 2010). The consequences of increasing global temperatures, higher levels of atmospheric carbon dioxide, ocean acidification, and higher sea levels are particularly alarming when viewed from an ecosystem perspective. An ecosystems approach provides insight into the physical and biological characteristics of stressed environments ranging from polar oceans to our planet's deserts. Component ecosystem species ranging from the phytoplankton that form the foundation of the Arctic food chain to the soil microbes that support plant life in mountain ecosystems are under threat. Davis et al. (2018) remind us that "extinction is part of evolution, but the unnatural rapidity of current species losses forces us to address whether we are cutting off twigs or whole branches from the tree of life." The overwhelming evidence of climate change-related loss of biodiversity raises the question of how close are we to a "tipping point" where the effects of climate change lead to the insurmountable devastation of a "sixth mass extinction" event and an unmanageable challenge to human health and well-being.

DISCUSSION QUESTIONS

1. How do the five historical mass extinction events relate to climate change related loss of biodiversity in the twenty-first century?

2. How do changes in the biodiversity of single celled microbial organisms have the potential to adversely affect entire ecosystems?

3. How does climate change-related biodiversity loss affect human health?

KEY TERMS

Anthropocene: Relating to the current geologic age, characterized by the predominantly human influence on climate and the environment.

Biodiversity: The variability among all life forms that exist on Earth.

Dead zones: Areas in the ocean of such low oxygen concentration that animal life suffocates and dies.

Ecosystem: A biological community of interacting organisms and their physical environment.

Eukaryote: An organism whose cells contain a nucleus within a membrane.

Mass extinction: A loss of 75 percent of the world's species in a period defined as two million years or less.

Phytoplankton: Microscopic marine algae. Phytoplankton is the base of several aquatic food webs.

Prokaryote: Microscopic single-celled organism that lacks a distinct nucleus.

Tipping point: A scenario when an ecosystem undergoes significant changes to biodiversity.

Zooplankton: Animal-like constituent of plankton- protozoa, small crustaceans, fish eggs, and larvae.

References

Algeo, T. J., R. Berner, J. B. Maynard, and S. E. Scheckler. 1995. "Late Devonian Oceanic Anoxic Events and Biotic Crises: 'Rooted' in the Evolution of Vascular Land Plants?" *GSA Today* 5 (3):64–66.

Armitage, A. R., W. E. Highfield, S. D. Brody, and P. Louchouarn. 2015. "The Contribution of Mangrove Expansion to Salt Marsh Loss on the Texas Gulf Coast." *PLoS ONE* 10 (5):e0125404.

Baraniuk, C. 2015. "The Devonian Extinction Saw the Oceans Choke to Death." *BBC. June* 23, 2015. http://www.bbc.com/earth/story/20150624-the-day-the-oceans-died.

Bardeen, C. G., R. R. Garcia, O. B. Toon, and A. J. Conley. 2017. "On Transient Climate Change at the Cretaceous-Paleogene Boundary due to Atmospheric Soot Injections." *Proceedings of the National Academy of Sciences of the USA* 114 (36):E7415–E7424.

Barnosky. A. D., N. Matzke, S. Tomiya, G. O. U. Wogan, B. Swartz, T. B. Quental, C. Marshall et al. 2011. "Has the Earth's Sixth Mass Extinction Already Arrived?" *Nature* 471:51–57.

Borchert, S. M., M. J. Osland, N. M. Enwright, and K. T. Griffith. 2018. "Coastal Wetland Adaptation to Sea Level Rise: Quantifying Potential for Landward Migration and Coastal Squeeze." *Journal of Applied Ecology* 55:2876–87.

Box, J. E., W. T. Colgan, T. R. Christensen, W. T. Colgan, T. R. Christensen, N. M. Schmidt, M. Lund, F.-J. W. Parmentier, R. Brown et al. "Key Indicators of Arctic Climate Change: 1971–2017. *Environmental Research Letters* 14 (4):045010.

Brannen, P. 2017. "Earth Is Not in the Midst of a Sixth Mass Extinction." *The Atlantic June* 13, 2017. https://www.theatlantic.com/science/archive/2017/06/the-ends-of-the-world/529545/.

Brugger, J., G. Feulner, and S. Petri. 2017. "Baby, It's Cold Outside: Climate Model Simulations of the Effects of the Asteroid Impact at the End of the Cretaceous." *Geophysical Research Letters* 44:419–27.

Burger, B. J. 2018. "What Caused Earth's Largest Mass Extinction Event? New Evidence from the Permian-Triassic Boundary in Northeastern Utah." Pre-Print. Department of Geology, Utah State University.

Burgess, S. D, J. D. Muirhead, and S. A. Bowring. 2017. "Initial Pulse of Siberian Traps Sills as the Trigger of the End-Permian Mass Extinction." *Nature Communications* 8:2017.

Burkett, V. R., R. J. Nicholls, L. Fernandez, and C. D. Woodroffe. 2008. "Climate Change Impacts on Coastal Biodiversity." University of Wollongong Research Online. https://ro.uow.edu.au/scipapers/217/.

Castro, J. 2017. "Climate Change Ripples through Mountain Ecosystems." *LiveScience January* 12, 2017. https://www.livescience.com/17949-climate-change-cascading-effects.html.

Ceballos G., P. R. Ehrich, A. D. Barnosky, A. García, R. M. Pringle, and T. M. Palmer. 2015. "Accelerated Modern Human-Induced Species Losses: Entering the Sixth Mass Extinction." *Science Advances* 1 (5): e1400253.

Ceballos, G., P. R. Ehrlich, and R. Dirzo. 2017. "Biological Annihilation via the Ongoing Sixth Mass Extinction Signaled by Vertebrate Population Losses and Declines." *Proceedings of the National Academy of Sciences of the USA* 114:E6089–E6096.

Center for Biological Diversity. n.d. "Halting the Extinction Crisis." https://www.biologicaldiversity.org/programs/biodiversity/elements_of_biodiversity/extinction_crisis/.

Chinese Academy of Sciences. 2018. "Climate Change to Impact Desert Ecosystems: Chinese Researchers." *August* 17, 2018. http://english.cas.cn/newsroom/archive/news_archive/nu2018/201808/t20180817_196187.shtml.

Chivian, E., and A. Bernstein, eds. 2008. *Sustaining Life: How Human Health Depends on Biodiversity.* New York: Oxford University Press.

Chu, J. 2013. "Huge and Widespread Volcanic Eruptions Triggered the End-Triassic Extinction." *MIT News March* 21, 2013. http://news.mit.edu/2013/volcanic-eruptions-triggered-end-triassic-extinction-0321.

Conservation of Arctic Flora and Fauna. 2017. *State of the Arctic Marine Biodiversity: Key Findings and Advice for Monitoring.* Akureyri, Iceland: CAFF International Secretariat.

Davis, M., S. Faurby, and J. C. Svenning. 2018. "Mammal Diversity Will Take Millions of Years to Recover from the Current Biodiversity Crisis." *Proceedings of the National Academy of Sciences of the USA* 115:11262–7.

Finnegan, S., S. C. Anderson, P. G. Harnik, C. Simpson, D. P. Tittensor, J. E. Byrnes, Z. V. Finkel et al. 2015. "Paleontological Baselines for Evaluating Extinction Risk in the Modern Oceans." *Science* 348 (6234):5675.

Finnegan, S., N. A. Heim, S. E. Peters, and W. W. Fischer. 2012. "Climate Change and the Selective Signature of the Late Ordovician Mass Extinction." *Proceedings of the National Academy of Sciences of the USA* 109 (18):6829-34.

Food and Agriculture Organization. 2005. *Global Forest Resources Assessment 2005. Progress towards Sustainable Forest Management.* Rome: FAO. http://www.fao.org/3/a0400e/a0400e00.htm.

Gannon, M. 2018. "How Rising Temperatures Suffocated 96% of Sea Life in Earth's Biggest Extinction." *Live Science December* 10, 2018. https://www.livescience.com/64270-animals-suffocated-permian-extinction.html.

Global Reef Project. 2010. "Coral Reef History." http://globalreefproject.com/coral-reef-history.php.

Grantham, B. A., F. Chan, K. L. Nielsen, D. S. Fox, J. A. Barth, A. Huyer, J. Lubchenco, and B. A. Menge. 2004. "Upwelling-Driven Nearshore Hypoxia Signals Ecosystem and Oceanographic Changes in the Northeast Pacific." *Nature* 429:749–54.

Harper, D. A. T., E. Hammarlund, and C. M. O. Rasmussen. 2004. "End Ordovician Extinctions: A Coincidence of Causes." *Gondwana Research* 25:1294–1307.

Herrle, O., C. J. Schroder-Adams, W. Davis, A. T. Pugh, J. M. Galloway, and J. Fath. 2015. "Mid-Cretaceous High Arctic Stratigraphy, Climate, and Oceanic Anoxic Events." *Geology* 43 (5):403.

Hill, D. 2000. "Deserts Threatened by Climate Change." *Science November* 2, 2000. https://www.sciencemag.org/news/2000/11/deserts-threatened-climate-change.

Hinder, S. L., M. B. Gravenor, M. Edwards, et al. 2014. "Multi-Decadal Range Changes vs. Thermal Adaptation for North East Atlantic Oceanic Copepods in the Face of Climate Change." *Global Change Biology* 21 (1):140–6.

Hoegh-Guldberg, O., and J. F. Bruno. 2010. "The Impact of Climate Change on the World's Marine Ecosystems." *Science* 328:1523–8.

Intergovernmental Panel on Climate Change. 2018. *Global Warming of 1.5°C. An IPCC Special Report on the Impacts of Global Warming of 1.5°C above Pre-Industrial Levels and Related Global Greenhouse Gas Emission Pathways, in the Context of Strengthening the Global Response to the Threat of Climate Change, Sustainable Development, and Efforts to Eradicate Poverty*, edited by V. Masson-Delmotte, P. Zhai, H.-O. Pörtner, D. Roberts, J. Skea, P. R. Shukla, A. Pirani, W. Moufouma-Okia et al. Geneva: IPCC. https://www.ipcc.ch/sr15/.

International Union for Conservation of Nature. 2017. "Coral Reefs and Climate Change." https://www.iucn.org/resources/issues-briefs/coral-reefs-and-climate-change.

Jablonski, D. 1991. "Extinctions: A Paleotological Perspective." *Science* 253 (5021).

Kunin, W. E., and K. Gaston, eds. 1996. *The Biology of Rarity: Causes and Consequences of Rare–Common Differences*. New York: Springer.

Laidre, K. L., I. Stirling, J. A. Estes, A. Kochnev, and J. Roberts. 2018. "Historical and Potential Future Importance of Large Whales as Food for Polar Bears." *Frontiers in Ecology and the Environment* 16 (9):515–24.

Lester, C., and M. Matella. 2016. "Managing the Coastal Squeeze: Resilience Planning for Shoreline Residential Development." *Stanford Environmental Law Journal* 36:23–61.

Locey, K. J., and J. T. Lennon. 2011. "Scaling Laws Predict Global Microbial Diversity." *Proceedings of the National Academy of Sciences of the USA* 113:5970–5.

Markham, A. 2018. "Half a Degree of Warming Could Be the Difference between Survival and Extinction for Many Species." *Union of Concerned Scientists Blog, October* 9, 2018. https://blog.ucsusa.org/adam-markham/half-a-degree-of-warming-could-mean-species-extinction.

Mayor, J. R., N. J. Sanders, A. T. Classen, et al. 2017. "Elevation Alters Ecosystem Properties across Temperate Treelines Globally." *Nature* 542:91–95.

Molinos, J. G., B. S. Halpern, D. S. Schoeman, C. J. Brown, W. Kiessling, P. J. Moore, J. M. Pandolfi et al. 2016. "Climate Velocity and the Future Global Redistribution of Marine Biodiversity." *Nature Climate Change* 6:83–88 .

Mora, C., D. P. Tittensor, S. Adl, A. G. B. Simpson, and B. Worm. 2011. "How Many Species Are There on Earth and in the Ocean?" *PLoS Biology* 9 (8). https://doi.org/10.1371/journal.pbio.1001127.

National Snow and Ice Data Center. 2020. "Quick Facts on Arctic Sea Ice." https://nsidc.org/cryosphere/quickfacts/seaice.html.

Neeley, A. R., L. A. Harris, and K. E. Frey. 2018. "Unraveling Phytoplankton Community Dynamics in the Northern Chukchi Sea under Sea-Ice-Covered and Sea-Ice-Free Conditions." *Geophysical Research Letters* 45 (15):7663–71.

Nuccitelli, D. 2018. "Burning Coal May Have Caused Earth's Worst Mass Extinction." *Guardian March* 12, 2018. https://www.theguardian.com/environment/climate-consensus-97-per-cent/2018/mar/12/burning-coal-may-have-caused-earths-worst-mass-extinction.

Osland, M. J., L. C. Fehera, J. López-Portillo, R. H. Daya, D. O. Sumanc, J. M. Guzmán Menéndez, and V. H. Rivera-Monroye. 2018. "Mangrove Forests in a Rapidly Changing World: Global Change Impacts and Conservation Opportunities along the Gulf of Mexico Coast." *Estuarine, Coastal and Shelf Science* 214:120–40.

Paice, R., and J. Chambers. 2016. *Climate Change Impacts on Coastal Ecosystems. CoastAdapt Impact Sheet 8*. Southport, Australia: National Climate Change Adaptation Research Facility, Gold Coast. https://coastadapt.com.au/sites/default/files/factsheets/T312_9_Coastal_Ecosystems.pdf.

Penn, J. L., C. Deutsch, J. L. Payne, and E. A. Sperling. 2018. "Temperature-Dependent Hypoxia Explains Biogeography and Severity of End-Permian Marine Mass Extinction." *Science* 362 (6419):eaat1327.

Pinones, A., and A. V. Fedorov. 2016. "Projected Changes of Antarctic Krill Habitat by the End of the 21st Century." *Geophysical Research Letters* 43 (16):8580–9.

Pohl, A., J. Austermann, and Y. Donnadieu. 2018. "Modeling Ordovician Ice Sheet and the Sea-Level Fingerprint of Its Collapse: Toward a Consistent Picture of the Ordovician Glaciation." *Geophysical Research Abstracts* 20.

Pontee, N. 2013. "Defining Coastal Squeeze: A Discussion." *Ocean & Coastal Management* 84:204–7.

Poppick, L. 2019. "The Ocean Is Running Out of Breath, Scientists Warn." *Scientific American February* 25, 2019. https://www.scientificamerican.com/article/the-ocean-is-running-out-of-breath-scientists-warn/.

Raabe, E. A., L. C. Roy, and C. C. McIvor. 2012. "Tampa Bay Coastal Wetlands. Nineteenth to Twentieth Century Tidal Marsh-to-Mangrove Conversion." *Estuaries and Coasts* 35:1145–62.

Radabaugh, K. R., R. P. Moyer, A. R. Chappel, C. E. Powell, I. Bociu, B. C. Clark, and J. M. Smoak. 2018. "Coastal Blue Carbon Assessment of Mangroves, Salt Marshes, and Salt Barrens in Tampa Bay, Florida, USA." *Estuaries and Coasts* 41:1496–1510.

Richter, V. 2015. "The Big Five Mass Extinctions." *Cosmos: The Science of Everything. July* 6, 2015. https://cosmosmagazine.com/palaeontology/big-five-extinctions.

Russell, M., and H. Greening. "Estimating Benefits in a Recovering Estuary: Tampa Bay, Florida." *Estuaries and Coasts* 38 (suppl 1):S9–S18.

Salkowe, R. 2016. "Biodiversity and Human Health." In *Auerbach's Wilderness Medicine*, 7th ed., edited by P. Auerbach, T. A. Cushing, and N. S. Harris, 2535–42. Philadelphia: Elsevier.

Sherwood, E. T., and H. S. Greening. 2014. "Potential Impacts and Management Implications of Climate Change on Tampa Bay Estuary Critical Coastal Habitats." *Environmental Management* 53:401–15.

Solly, M. 2018. "How Did the 'Great Dying' Kill 96 Percent of Earth's Ocean-Dwelling Creatures?" *Smithsonian December* 11, 2018. https://www.smithsonianmag.com/smart-news/how-did-great-dying-kill-96-percent-earths-ocean-dwelling-creatures-180970992/#2bjRHwzOfLiQ5S48.99.

Stearns, B. P, and S. C. Stearns. 1999. *Watching, From the Edge of Extinction*. New Haven: Yale University Press; 1999.

Stramma, L., G. C. Johnson, J. Sprintall, and V. Mohrholz. 2008. "Expanding Oxygen-Minimum Zones in the Tropical Oceans." *Science* 320 (5876):655–8.

Stramma, L., S. Schmidtko, L. A. Levin, and G. C. Johnson. 2010. "Ocean Oxygen Minima Expansions and Their Biological Impacts." *Deep Sea Research Part 1: Oceanographic Research Papers* 57 (4):587–95.

Thomas, C. D., A. Cameron, R. E. Green, M. Bakkenes, L. J. Beaumont, Y. C. Collingham, B. F. N. Erasmus et al. 2004. "Extinction Risk from Climate Change." *Nature* 427 (6970):145–8.

Torio, D. D., and G. L. Chmura. 2013. "Assessing Coastal Squeeze of Tidal Wetlands." *Journal of Coastal Research* 29 (5):1049–61.

United Nations Economic Commission for Europe. n.d. "Air pollution, Ecosystems and Biodiversity." http://www.unece.org/environmental-policy/conventions/envlrtapwelcome/cross-sectoral-linkages/air-pollution-ecosystems-and-biodiversity.html .

University of Washington. 2018. "Biggest Mass Extinction Caused by Global Warming Leaving Ocean Animals Gasping for Breath." *AAAS EurekAlert December* 6, 2018. https://www.eurekalert.org/pub_releases/2018-12/uow-bme113018.php.

Urban, M. C. 2015. "Accelerating Extinction Risk from Climate Change." *Science* 348 (6234).

U.S. Geologic Survey. n.d. "Climate Change in Mountain Ecosystems." https://www.usgs.gov/centers/norock/science/climate-change-mountain-ecosystems-ccme?qt-science_center_objects=0#qt-science_center_objects.

Wake, D. B., and V. T. Vredenburg. 2008. "Are We in the Midst of the Sixth Mass Extinction? A View from the World of Amphibians." In *In the Light of Evolution: Vol. II: Biodiversity and Extinction*, edited by J. C. Avise, S. P. Hubbell, and F. J. Ayala, 27–44. Washington, DC: National Academies Press.

Wilson, E. O. 2007. "Biophilia and the Conservation Ethic." In *Evolutionary Perspectives on Environmental Problems*, edited by D. J. Penn and I. Mysterud. Piscataway, NJ: Transaction Publishers.

World Meteorological Organization. 2018. "WMO Climate Statement: Past 4 Years Warmest on Record." *November* 29, 2018. https://public.wmo.int/en/media/press-release/wmo-climate-statement-past-4-years-warmest-record.

World Wildlife Federation. n.d. "Deforestation and Forest Degradation." https://www.worldwildlife.org/threats/deforestation-and-forest-degradation.

Yale School of Forestry and Environmental Studies. 2020. "Climate Change and Tropical Forests." https://globalforestatlas.yale.edu/climate-change/climate-change-and-tropical-forests.

CHAPTER 29

ECOSYSTEM SERVICES

Lydia Olander, Sara Mason, Heather Tallis, Joleah Lamb,
Yuta J. Masuda, and Randall Kramer

What Are Ecosystem Services?

People living in many tropical regions collect wood and shellfish from mangrove forests. These same mangroves are fish nurseries helping to support local and global fisheries. The forests accumulate and sequester carbon helping to reduce climate change. The trunks and roots of these trees slow down storm winds and waves protecting coastal communities from storm impacts. These benefits are examples of **ecosystem services**: the benefits that nature provides to people. Mangroves can also provide dis-services, such as mosquitos that can be a nuisance to people and carry disease.

There are three types of ecosystem services: provisioning, regulating, and cultural (Millennium Ecosystem Assessment 2005; Carpenter et al. 2009; Potts et al. 2016). **Provisioning services** are the most familiar, including crops, fish, timber, and drinking water. Most **provisioning services** are bought and sold in markets and have a market value. **Regulating services** are less apparent but often immensely important to people. These include the filtration and purification of water by wetlands or shellfish and the regulation of erosion of sediments that can support and build productive coastal deltas but also fill up hydropower, irrigation, drinking, and flood control reservoirs. Ecosystems such as wetlands regulate water flows in ways that buffer and reduce flooding frequency and intensity. Coastal habitats such as marshes, mangroves, or coral reefs can reduce wave energy, protecting shorelines from erosion, which, in some cases, offers significant protection to property and people. **Regulating services** also benefit agricultural areas by providing habitat for pollinator species (such as bees) or pest control species (such as birds). **Cultural services** include the opportunity for outdoor recreational or cultural activities, such as boating, swimming, hiking, hunting, and fishing, which can provide substantial economic value in many places (U.S. Bureau of Economic Analysis 2019). Other cultural services are more difficult to quantify but can be very important to people. These include the beauty and aesthetics of natural or partly natural areas (e.g., lakes, forests, pastoral landscapes), the sense of peace and release of stress associated with being in a natural setting, the satisfaction from being able to choose a way of life that depends on natural resources (e.g., fishing, farming), and spiritual or cultural connection to a place that is important to many people including Indigenous peoples.

Although our dependence on ecosystem services may not be obvious in daily life, humans simply could not live on this planet without them. This stark reality was demonstrated in 1991 when eight scientists were sealed into a miniature earth system, called Biosphere 2. It was designed with a rainforest, a grassland, a desert, fresh and saltwater wetlands with mangrove trees, and a coral reef in a miniature ocean to inform the future of life support systems for long-term space travel

KEY CONCEPTS

- Ecosystem services are the benefits that nature provides to people.

- Many of the services that nature provides are linked either directly or indirectly to human health outcomes.

- These ecosystem services are likely to be severely affected by climate change, with multiple health consequences.

(Nelson 2018). Amazingly, the scientists were able to produce sufficient food without synthetic fertilizers or pesticides, but they faced many problems with rampant growth of cockroaches, ants, algae, and morning glories, as well as the overproduction of carbon dioxide and underproduction of oxygen from their plants. This experiment clarified how many benefits nature provides to our daily life and how much we still have to learn about how to manage them. Ecosystem services are provided by natural systems in a delicate balance, and effects of climate change have the potential to drastically alter or disrupt these services.

How Does Climate Change Affect Ecosystem Services that Have an Impact on Human Health?

In this section, we describe how various ecosystem services affect human health and then discuss how climate change might disrupt or alter the delivery of these services.

Provisioning Services

Food (Crops, Livestock and Seafood)

Nature can be directly linked to human health through provisioning services. Clearly, human food and nutrition security are tightly tied to ecosystems' provision of healthy crops and fisheries. Globally, approximately 82 percent of the calories in the human food supply are provided by terrestrial plants (mostly cultivated crops), 16 percent by terrestrial animals (mostly cultivated livestock), and 1 percent by aquatic animals and plants (Food and Agriculture Organization [FAO] 2019). Capture fisheries and aquaculture together provide 17 percent of animal protein consumed by the global population and micronutrients in seafood can lower risk of cardiovascular disease; improve maternal health and pregnancy outcomes and increase early childhood physical and cognitive development; improve immune system function; and alleviate health issues associated with micronutrient deficiencies such as anemia, rickets, childhood blindness, and stunting (Bennett, Carpenter, and Caraco 2001; Hicks et al. 2019). Undernutrition contributes to the death of roughly three million children per year (Black et al. 2013), and 29 percent of the global population faced micronutrient deficiencies in 2010 (Webb et al. 2018) and an estimated 12 percent of the global population was at risk of protein deficiency in 2017 (Medek, Schwartz, and Myers 2017).

Climate change will alter temperature, precipitation, and carbon dioxide concentrations, which may have a significant impact on crop yields, although net effects on yields are still unclear (Grassini, Eskridge, and Cassman 2013; Lin and Huybers 2012; Ray et al. 2012; Ziska and Bunce 2007). Climate model projections generally indicate less precipitation in currently arid and semiarid regions and greater precipitation in the polar latitudes (Collins et al. 2013) and regional changes in extreme temperatures and heavy precipitation (Intergovernmental Panel on Climate Change [IPCC] 2018). Rising temperatures are expected to have a negative impact on major crops with each degree Celsius increase in global mean temperature causing a reduction in yield of 6 percent for wheat, 3.2 percent for rice, 7.4 percent for maize, and 3.1 percent for soybeans (Zhao et al. 2017). Warming temperatures can also increase the survival of insect pests in the winter, increasing their number and expanding their range (Bale et al. 2002; Bebber, Ramotowski, and Gurr 2013), and the spread of invasive plants and animals spurred by climate change may do significant damage to crops (Ziska et al. 2011). Crop pathogens, fungi, and weeds may also increase (Flood 2010). Extreme weather events such as prolonged heat, drought, and excessive rainfall, which are increasingly frequent with climate change, have also been shown to decrease crop yields in some cases (Lesk, Rowhani, and Ramankutty 2016; Powell and Reinhard 2016; Mäkinen et al. 2017; IPCC 2018). However, in isolated regions and for certain crop types weather extremes have actually increased yields (Mäkinen et al. 2017). Increasing concentrations of carbon dioxide may improve crop performance by increasing rates of photosynthesis and water use efficiency (Long et al. 2006; Ziska and Bunce 2007). The expected net effect of these various elements of climate change on crop yields is less predictable.

Emerging evidence also suggests that the *CO$_2$ fertilization effect will drive reductions in crop nutrient content*. The protein content of grains and tubers, such as rice, wheat, barley, and potatoes may decline 7–15 percent, and zinc and iron concentrations in cereal grains and legumes may decrease 3–11 percent (Myers et al. 2014). Rising CO$_2$ concentrations put hundreds of millions at risk of zinc, iron, and/or protein deficiency (Myers et al. 2017).

Climate change is likely to alter access to fish populations as ocean temperatures shift, and reduce fishery production. Changes in temperature patterns in the ocean are already driving shifts in the location and average depth of fish stocks (Perry et al. 2005; Nye et al. 2009). Changing locations can change access for local fishing communities or price of seafood, which may reduce access to seafood protein especially for lower-income communities (Hicks et al. 2019). Though fish distributions are changing and expected to continue to change, it is still uncertain if net fish production and fishery productivity will be altered by climate change (Brander 2007; Free et al. 2019; Smale et al. 2019; Cheung et al. 2010). Coral reefs are the habitat type most threatened by climate change due to rising ocean temperatures and ocean acidification, with projections of significant loss of area and local extinctions of these habitats (Burke et al. 2011; Hoegh-Guldberg et al. 2007; Hughes et al. 2017; IPCC 2019), and in many tropical countries coral reefs account for a significant amount (10–12 percent) of fish caught; up to 25 percent in developing tropical nations (Garcia and de Leiva Moreno 2003). It is also possible that changes in climate may alter the nutritional composition of phytoplankton communities (the basis of many marine food chains), resulting in changes to nutritional content of fish; however, further study of these micronutrient changes is needed to determine their specific impacts on human health (Myers et al. 2017).

Naturally Sourced Medicines

Although not yet clear how, climate change may alter the distribution of medicinal resources found in nature, and their chemical compounds. Tree, plant, algal, and terrestrial and marine animal extracts contain a variety of bioactive compounds such as polyphenols (including flavonoids, phenolic acids, tannins), phytoestrogens (including lignans), stilbenes, carotenoids, and sterols (Marris 2006; Holmbom et al. 2007; Moutsatsou 2007), the properties of which can result in anticancer activity, antiatherogenic potential, and antioxidant potential (Kris-Etherton et al. 2002; Karjalainen, Sarjala, and Raitio 2010). Natural medicines are still the primary source of treatments in some countries, with up to 80 percent of the population using traditional forms of medicine (World Health Organization 2002). Pharmaceutical extracts of natural materials or synthetics designed to mimic them account for a large number of today's western medicines. For example, the precursor to today's aspirin was prepared from willow bark as early as 400 BCE (Mahdi et al. 2006). Today's leading malaria drug, artemisinin, was originally derived from leaves of the Asian wormwood plant, *Artemisia annua* (Miller and Su 2011). Climate change may drive variation in the concentration and effectiveness of medically active compounds in some plants (Gairola et al. 2010; Mishra 2016). There has been recent interest in marine bioprospecting, especially with regards to new anti-infective drugs derived from marine microbes (Xu et al. 2018), but marine microbes are also vulnerable to climate change (Webster and Hill 2007), meaning important medicinal microbes may never be discovered. It is uncertain how climate change will alter the distribution of medicinal plants and the concentration of their active compounds, but it is clear that the habitats where they grow are under stress and will be changing (Gairola et al. 2010; Khanum, Mumtaz, and Kumar 2013; Maikhuri et al. 2018; Zhao et al. 2018).

Regulating Services

Pollination

Pollination by native insects is an important regulating input to many crops that benefit human nutrition. Bees are generally the main providers of pollination services, but insects, birds, bats and other animals, also contribute (FAO 2019). Crops at least partially pollinated by animals account for 35 percent of global food production (Klein et al. 2007) and are particularly significant in the supply of micronutrients for human consumption, for example, accounting for more than 90 percent of available vitamin C and more than 70 percent of available vitamin A (Eilers et al. 2011).

Climate change may affect food production of flowering species by reducing the abundance of pollinating insects and shifting their regional distributions (Abrol 2012; Hegland et al. 2009; Memmott et al. 2007; Potts et al. 2016). Warming affects the timing of flowering and will generally cause plant communities to migrate poleward (Parmesan and Yohe 2003); however, it is less likely that pollinators and their life cycles will shift in tandem. Both pollinator and flowering plant species may be at risk of extinction because of the reduced overlap in timing of flowering and pollinator emergence (Myers et al. 2017). Modeling indicates that global pollinator declines will influence adult intake of foods that provide vitamin A and folate, increasing the risk of heart disease, stroke, diabetes, and certain cancers (Smith et al. 2015).

Inland Flood Reduction

Ecosystems can help reduce inland flood risk during moderate storms by capturing and slowing down floodwaters and helping floodwaters infiltrate into groundwater (Burek et al. 2012; Dixon et al. 2016; Watson et al. 2016). Using simulation modeling at a regional scale in Europe, Burek et al. (2012) found that natural ecosystems could reduce twenty-year peak floods by up to 15 percent locally and 4 percent regionally. Even slight flood reductions can make the difference between a small flood and a disaster if it means stream banks and levees hold. Climate change is already accelerating the frequency and intensity of storms, increasing flooding in many areas (Collins et al. 2013; Kundzewicz et al. 2008; Wobus et al. 2017). These increases amplify the value of nature's regulating role in reducing flooding and storm surge from moderate sized storm events. At the same time, more frequent large events exceed the capacity of natural systems to regulate water flows and reduce floods. Under increased CO_2 conditions plants close their stomata and transpire less water, leading to more water in streams (Fowler et al. 2019). Although this may be helpful in low water conditions, it could contribute to greater flood risk in some areas. Worsening flooding and reduced ability of natural systems to mitigate these events results in the direct health impacts of flooding on loss of life and injury, but also may result in increases in chronic respiratory illness that have been observed after floods (Jakucbicka et al. 2010). In addition, increased contamination from overwhelmed septic systems, water treatment facilities, and animal agriculture will affect water sources including groundwater, which supplies 31.5 percent of the global population with drinking water. This is likely to enhance outbreaks of enteric illness (Andrade et al. 2018; Murphy et al. 2017).

Coastal Protection

Coastal habitats can reduce impacts from storm surge, sea level rise, and coastal flooding. Numerous studies have found that coastal ecosystems (salt marshes, mangroves, bivalve reefs, seagrass, coral reefs, barrier islands etc.) can help attenuate storm surge, stabilize eroding coastlines, reduce the force of incoming waves, and reduce coastal storm damages and injury (Das and Vincent 2009; Gedan et al. 2011; Shepard et al. 2012; Bayas et al. 2011). Although these natural systems can attenuate impact to coastal communities, they cannot stop it completely. One study determined that salt marsh vegetation was responsible for 60 percent of the wave attenuation during storm events (Möller et al. 2014). In the Philippines mangroves currently reduce flooding that affects over half a million people, 23 percent of whom live below the poverty line (WAVES 2017; Beck et al. 2018). For a given twenty-five-year event (flooding level expected to occur every twenty-five years) coral reefs currently reduce flooding for more than 8700 km^2 of land and 1.7 million people; these benefits increase for larger events (Beck et al. 2018).

Climate change—through influences on ocean acidification, marine heat waves, sea level rise induced inundation, coastal erosion, and saltwater intrusion—threatens protective coral reefs, mangroves, and marshes (Scavia et al. 2002; Smale et al. 2019; Speers et al. 2016). For example, the IPCC (2018) reports a 70–99 percent predicted further decline in coral reefs, depending on the future climate scenario. In addition, climate change through sea level rise and increased storm intensity will likely result in higher high tides and larger and more frequent storm surges and coastal flooding, all of which are particularly problematic for heavily populated, low-lying areas (Knutson et al. 2010; Vitousek et al. 2017; Wahl et al. 2015).

Increases in coastal flooding are primarily driven by climate change induced sea level rise and increased storm intensity, but this is exacerbated by the loss of coastal habitats from human development. Coastal flooding leads to health impacts including immediate deaths and subacute morbidity and mortality, specifically, from related outbreaks such as hepatitis E, gastrointestinal diseases, and leptospirosis, which are associated with sewage runoff and displaced populations, as well as associated physiological distress (Alderman, Turner, and Tong 2012; Lane et al. 2013; Wright, D'Elia, and Nichols 2019).

Another factor to consider is the capacity of some coastal systems, like seagrass ecosystems, to sequester, kill, and inhibit waterborne pathogens, reducing the likelihood of human exposure. This is particularly important when there is increased sewage and wastewater runoff associated with coastal flooding or overflow of combined sewer-stormwater systems in urban centers following extreme rainfall events. Unfortunately, climate change-induced increased storm frequency combined with coastal human development is driving losses in the extent of these habitats (see Case Study 1).

CASE STUDY 1 CLIMATE CHANGE INFLUENCES THE CAPACITY FOR SEAGRASS ECOSYSTEMS TO SEQUESTER WATERBORNE PATHOGENS

Joleah Lamb

Disease outbreaks in marine environments are expected to increase in the coming years because of expanding human populations on the coast and associated heightened contaminant and pollutant runoff (Grant et al. 2012). Natural ecosystems like seagrasses may represent a mitigation mechanism. Seagrasses and their microbiome have shown chemical and biological regulation of pathogens in vivo (Kumar et al. 2008; Mani, Bharathi, and Patterson 2012). A recent study revealed that the presence of intact seagrass beds resulted in 50 percent reductions in the relative abundance of potential bacterial pathogens capable of causing disease in marine organisms and people (Lamb et al. 2017). Pathogens affected included eleven of twelve of the most critically important groups of antibiotic-resistant pathogens reported this year by the World Health Organization (WHO).

The pathogen-reducing services of seagrasses may extend to other aspects of human health through indirect pathways. Coastal communities can rely heavily on coral-reef associated fish for protein and micronutrients, with fishery productivity dropping three-fold in some cases of reef loss (Rogers, Blanchard, and Mumby 2014). Seagrasses adjacent to reefs can protect this contribution to nutritional health by keeping corals free from disease (Burke et al. 2011). Nutritional health could also be improved through aquaculture practices supported by seagrasses (Troell et al. 2014).

Climate change may have profound implications for the ability of seagrass ecosystems to mitigate waterborne pathogens by further altering their distribution, productivity, and community structure. Seagrass is found on every continental shelf except for Antarctica but has declined globally with the rate of loss on the rise since 1990 (Waycott et al. 2009). It has been suggested that seagrass may actually benefit from rising levels of carbon dioxide through increased photosynthesis and carbon acquisition that support increased growth rates or densities (Borum et al. 2016). However, predicted increases in sea level and tidal range could reduce seagrass extent. Hurricanes, cyclones, and other storms cause disturbance that has resulted in seagrass decline in many parts of the world (Orth et al. 2006), and climate change is expected to increase the intensity of extreme weather events and reduce periods between them (Hoyos et al. 2006). Finally, acidification could negatively influence microbial functional diversity, reducing some pathogen control mechanisms.

Water Quality Regulation

Natural ecosystems, such as seagrasses, forests, and riverbanks, purify water through the filtration of contaminants (heavy metals, pathogenic microorganisms, etc.) and through the sequestration of nutrients that can become pollutants in high concentrations (nitrogen and phosphorous) (Burge et al. 2016; Mitsch et al. 2001; Pizzuto 2012; Tufenkji, Ryan, and Elimelech 2002).

In many places climate change is expected to increase the quantity and intensity of rainfall, which may reduce the ability of natural habitats to capture and filter pollutants because of high-volume water flows and increased upstream erosion exacerbating pollutant and nutrient runoff (Delpla et al. 2009; Kistemann et al. 2002; Kundzewicz et al. 2008; Melillo 2014).

As a result, previously sequestered contaminants, such as mercury or arsenic, can get released into waterways and food chains, which can affect human health. For example, exposure to mercury has been associated with neurocognitive deficits, multiorgan impairment (e.g., kidney, heart, liver), and reduced immune function (Bellanger et al. 2013). High levels of nitrogen in drinking water can cause methemoglobinemia (World Health Organization 2011), reproductive problems (Kramer et al. 1994), and cancer (non-Hodgkin's lymphoma, bladder and ovarian cancer) (Weyer et al. 2001).

Nutrient pollution also commonly drives eutrophication (overfertilization of waterways), which may cascade into harmful algal blooms. Human contact of high toxin by-products from algal blooms can occur through swimming, respiration (aerosols that contain toxins), or consumption of contaminated drinking water, fish, or shellfish (Cooke and Kennedy 2009; Smith 2003; Van Dolah 2000). Around 10 percent of foodborne disease outbreaks in the United States and over 60,000 global intoxication incidents per year are from algal toxins. In coastal marine habitats, these harmful algal blooms can also lead to fishery closures that limit access to seafood for seafood dependent communities. The frequency, growth rate, and longevity of these harmful algal blooms is likely exacerbated by climate change through increased water temperatures (Gobler et al. 2017; Hallegraeff 2010) and the loss of natural filtration habitats (e.g., sea grasses and forests bordering streams).

Air Quality Regulation

Ecosystems also provide a *regulating service by helping to clean our air and reducing exposure to air pollutants that cause respiratory diseases* (including asthma), cardiovascular diseases, adverse pregnancy outcomes (such as preterm birth), and even death (Haines and Patz 2004). Certain tree species improve air quality by filtering out gases and airborne particulates such as ozone (O_3), sulfur dioxide (SO_2), nitrogen dioxide (NO_2), carbon monoxide (CO), and particulate matter smaller than 10μm (particulate matter [PM]10) (Bowler et al. 2010; Lindgren and

Elmqvist 2017). For example, trees in the contiguous United States removed 17.4 million metric tons of air pollution in 2010 (range: 9.0–23.2 million metric tons), which was calculated to avoid more than 850 incidences of human mortality and 670,000 incidences of acute respiratory symptoms (Nowak et al. 2014). Globally, street trees in urban areas are providing reductions in particulate air pollution for millions of people (McDonald et al. 2016). These benefits are concentrated in urban areas where both sources of air pollution and human populations are greatest.

Climate change is likely to inflict particular stress on urban and suburban trees through increases in pests and pathogens (Meineke et al. 2013; Tubby and Webber 2010) making it more difficult to sustain healthy urban tree cover that filters air pollution. *Climate change will also increase air pollution levels* through increases in ozone (Beggs 2004; Bloomer et al. 2009; Fiore, Naik, and Leibensperger 2015; Jacob and Winner 2009), making this air-filtration ecosystem service ever more important. Air pollution concentrations have worsened in almost 70 percent of cities around the globe between 2010 and 2016 (Watts et al. 2018).

Heat Regulation

Vegetation, especially trees, significantly help reduce local air temperatures. Loss of forests between 2000 and 2010 resulted in warming of 0.38 ± 0.02 (mean $\pm$ SE) and $0.16 \pm 0.01°C$ in tropical and temperate regions respectively. In tropical regions, where average temperatures are already near human physiological thresholds, a 50 percent reduction in forest was associated with an increased local surface temperature of $1.08 \pm 0.25°C$ ($\sim 2°F$) (Prevedello et al. 2019) (See Case Study 2). In urban areas around the world, street trees are already providing over sixty-five million people with a 0.5 to 2.0°C (0.9 to 3.6°F) reduction in maximum air temperatures (McDonald et al. 2016).

CASE STUDY 2   CLIMATE CHANGE AND DEFORESTATION INFLUENCE THE CAPACITY OF TROPICAL FORESTS TO COOL COMMUNITIES AND BENEFIT HEALTH

Yuta J. Masuda, Ike Anggraeni, Edward T. Game, June Spector, Nicholas H. Wolff

Tropical forests can provide cooling services that benefit the health of local communities. Shade from trees reduces ground level solar radiation and individual tropical trees transpire hundreds of liters of water a day for a cooling power equivalent to two household air conditioning units (Ellison et al. 2017). In rural villages in East Kalimantan, Indonesia, one study (Masuda et al. 2019) found temperatures between 2.6 and 8.3°C higher in open fields compared to nearby forests—a temperature differential so large it is equivalent to nearly a century of projected warming under high greenhouse gas emissions scenarios (Rogelj, Meinshausen, and Knutti 2012). In this same Indonesian region, a randomized control trial found significant effects of forest temperature regulation on heat stress and cognitive function (Masuda et al. 2019; Suter et al. 2019).

The cooling services provided by forests will likely become more important under climate change, especially in the tropics. Communities in low-latitude tropical countries are already exposed to thermal thresholds reaching unsafe levels (Mora et al. 2017). These communities are especially at risk of heat-related illness because many are engaged in subsistence agriculture or other manual labor, occupations that are particularly vulnerable to increases in heat exposure (United Nations Environmental Programme 2016). They also often lack access to infrastructure and alternative livelihood options. As a result, expected additional heat exposure driven by climate change could further erode their already low resilience to environmental, economic, and other shocks (Coffel, Horton, and de Sherbinin 2017), which in turn increases risks of creating and perpetuating poverty traps (Barrett, Garg, and McBride 2016). Simultaneous deforestation is likely to further heighten the loss of cooling services from forests. Additional impacts from excessive heat exposure include increased risk of injuries or accidents (Spector et al. 2016; Crowe et al. 2015), adverse mental health impacts (Berry, Bowen, and Kjellstrom 2010), kidney disease (Wesseling et al. 2013; Crowe et al. 2013), and even death (Barreca et al. 2013). In the long-term, deforestation events increase CO_2 in the atmosphere and lead to increasing incidence of extreme heat events, chronic temperature increases, and unpredictable weather patterns (Bonan 2008; Lawrence and Vandecar 2015; Lawton et al. 2001).

This can be an important factor during extreme heat events, which are becoming more frequent globally under climate change. One quarter of global landmass has experienced an intensification of heat extremes (maximum temperature in the hottest day of the year) by more than 1°C (1.8°F) over just a few decades (Schleussner, Pfleiderer, and Fischer 2017). Climate-induced changes in temperature combined with exposure show that vulnerability to extremes of heat has risen since 1990, with 157 million more people exposed to heatwave events in 2017, compared with 2000 (Watts et al. 2018). High temperatures over 39°C (102°F) have been linked to heatstroke and cardiovascular and renal disease (Watts et al. 2018; Kovats and Hajat 2008).

Fire Regulation

Natural fires produce a regulating service that reduces the risk of catastrophic wildfire. Natural small and frequent surface fire burns in grasslands and fire-associated forests maintain the habitats and associated species and reduce the fuel load, limiting the frequency of catastrophic wildfire (fires that kill a majority of trees in the canopy and can cause significant economic and ecological damage) (Pausas and Keeley 2019). Frequent fires reduce fuel load and establish a pattern of smaller, more frequent fires, which produce overall less smoke over time than catastrophic wildfires. Severe wildfires have the potential to be devastating to human communities through direct loss of life and property but also indirectly through impacts to water and air quality. Wildfires may release significant amounts of sediment (Silins et al. 2009), nutrients (Smith 2003), heavy metals (Kelly et al. 2006), and other contaminants (Crouch et al. 2006) with implications for the supply of safe drinking water (Bladon et al. 2014; Emelko et al. 2011).

Wildfires can also produce massive plumes of smoke over wide areas. Average global mortality from landscape fire smoke exposure between 1997 and 2006 was 339,000 deaths annually with the highest rates in sub-Saharan Africa and Southeast Asia (Johnston et al. 2012). Following large 1997 fires in Indonesia, an estimated twenty million people in that country suffered from respiratory problems, with 19,800–48,100 premature mortalities (Heil, Langmann, and Aldrian 2007). Peatland forest fires with dangerous levels of airborne particulate matter now occur almost every year in Indonesia (Harrison, Page, and Limin 2009). In the western United States, about forty-six million people of all ages were exposed to at least one smoke wave (two consecutive days of wildfire-related $PM_{2.5} > 20\ \mu g/m^3$) during 2004 to 2009 and experienced a 7.2 percent increase in risk of respiratory-related hospital admissions during smoke wave days (Liu et al. 2017). Levels of PM10, the most frequently studied pollutant, were 1.2 to 10 times higher due to wildfire smoke compared to nonfire periods and/or locations (Liu et al. 2015). Respiratory disease was the most frequently studied health condition and had the most consistent results, with exacerbations of asthma, chronic obstructive pulmonary disease, bronchitis, and pneumonia. Recent studies now also report an increased risk of respiratory infections and associated mortality (Reid et al. 2016) and reduced height in adulthood (Tan-Soo and Pattanayak 2019). Although the loss of natural fire regimes (fire regulation service) is a driver for increased large-scale wildfires and associated smoke events, it is not the only one.

Climate change is increasing these risks because it is leading to earlier and longer fire seasons (Intergovernmental Panel on Climate Change 2013; Pechony and Shindell 2010; Westerling et al. 2006). Future wildfire potential increases significantly with climate change in the United States, South America, central Asia, southern Europe, southern Africa, and Australia (Liu, Stanturf, and Goodrick 2010). Climate change has already increased wildfire activity across forests in the western United States, lengthened the fire season, and doubled the cumulative area that would have burned in this same region between 1984 and 2016 (Abatzoglou and Williams 2016; Harvey 2016). Much of the western United States and areas around the Great Lakes and southeastern coast are predicted to have three to six times more weeks with "very high risk" of fire by midcentury (Barbero et al. 2015).

Climate Regulation

Natural ecosystems can directly regulate the climate by drawing down greenhouse gases from the atmosphere. As plants use carbon dioxide in photosynthesis, terrestrial ecosystems absorb around three billion tons of atmospheric carbon per year through net growth, which accounts for 30 percent of anthropogenic CO_2 emissions (Canadell and Raupach 2008). Tropical forests that hold around 250 Gt of carbon have become a net source of carbon emissions due to deforestation and degradation, releasing over 400 Tg (10^{12} g) C each year (Baccini et al. 2017; Saatchi et al. 2011). The other natural system with high carbon storage is the northern permafrost. Around 1,500 billion tons of organic carbon are stored in terrestrial soils in the northern permafrost zone but *increasing temperatures from climate change are starting to thaw it, releasing methane* (a more powerful—five to twenty times, but shorter-lived greenhouse gas than carbon dioxide). Models estimate around ninety billion tons of this carbon will be released by 2100 with more than half being lost after that (Schuur et al. 2015). Oceans and the phytoplankton within them are also a significant reservoir of carbon, taking up around 1.4 Pg C per year (Landschützer et al. 2014); the ocean has absorbed between 20 and 30 percent of anthropogenic carbon dioxide emissions since the 1980s (IPCC 2018, 2019). Griscom et al. (2017) postulate that if all terrestrial and coastal habitats were managed to maximize carbon sequestration (e.g., reforestation, agricultural management) with reasonable safeguards to maintain sufficient food production and **biodiversity** support, an additional 2.3 Pg (10^{15} g) CO_2 equivalents could be captured. This could provide one third of the mitigation needed to give us a two-thirds chance of staying below a 2°C climate threshold.

As climate change alters plant distribution patterns and growth rates, it is likely to affect climate regulation. As noted previously, the climate-driven melting of permafrost will release large amounts of potent greenhouse gases, creating a reinforcing feedback loop that will accelerate climate change (Schuur et al. 2015). In terrestrial ecosystems increased carbon dioxide has a "fertilization effect" on vegetation by increasing the efficiency of photosynthesis as long as there is enough nitrogen (the most commonly limiting element) for the plants. This is likely to increase the carbon stored in terrestrial vegetation; however, rates of decomposition and carbon loss from soils is likely to increase and the net effect in non-permafrost regions is not certain (Bonan 2008). Loss of natural ecosystems' abilities to regulate the global climate connects back to human health through the myriad linkages highlighted in this book.

Infectious Disease Regulation and Biodiversity

Climate change can influence the severity, timing, and location of infectious disease outbreaks by altering host susceptibility, infectious agents, and environmental conditions including temperature, humidity, and preferred habitat for vectors. Climate change is also shifting the spatial distribution of vector-borne and zoonotic diseases like Lyme disease, malaria, dengue, Zika, and viral encephalitis into historically cooler climates that are now warming (Gage et al. 2008; Githeko et al. 2000; Patz 2018; Patz and Reisen 2001). For mosquito-borne diseases, warmer temperatures can also exacerbate risk by increasing egg production, biting rates, and shortening the disease incubation time (Patz et al. 1996). At the same time, human migrations and travel of disease naïve populations into areas newly in range for these vector-borne diseases may mean less immunity in these communities and greater disease risk (Patz and Reisen).

Another way in which climate change may affect human disease is through losses in biodiversity resulting from altered temperature, precipitation, and hydrologic systems. The so-called **"dilution effect"** posits that changes in biodiversity in some ecosystems will impact the transmission cycle of certain pathogens. Where biodiversity is higher, the presence of hosts with a low capacity to transmit disease from host to vector can dilute the effect of highly competent hosts (Ostfeld and Keesing 2012). Conversely, reductions in diversity from climate change may increase infection risk and disease prevalence in hosts. Although there is mixed evidence about the importance of the dilution effect, empirical studies often find that decreased diversity is correlated with increased disease risk (Young et al. 2017). Appropriate policy response to these risks remains unclear, in part because climate change and other forms of disturbance affect disease through additional pathways (Young et al. 2017).

Cultural Services

Nature provides aesthetic and psychological benefits that enrich human life with meaning and emotion, and have direct connections to mental health (Chiesura 2004; Yeager et al. 2018). Aesthetic benefits from green spaces have been associated with reduced stress and with increased mental health (Berg et al. 2010; Stigsdotter et al. 2010). The use of urban green space, such as urban community gardens and other activities that enhance a sense of place, social interactions, and the strengthening of neighborhood participation, has been shown to have beneficial mental health effects (Elmqvist et al. 2013; Lindgren and Elmqvist 2017). As noted previously, climate change is likely to inflict particular stress on urban and suburban trees (Tubby and Webber 2010; Meineke et al. 2013), where green spaces are likely to be most limited and most needed.

Many communities, including Indigenous and rural, have strong cultural associations with natural ecosystems; for example, plants and animals that represent deities, access to burial grounds or family places, sufficient subsistence resources like fish or clean water, and engaging in cultural fishing or harvest practices (Pascua et al. 2017). Climate change is having disproportionate effects on some such cultural services. For example, in the Arctic, weaker sea ice and reduced longevity of ice reduces travel options and speed, and sea ice-based hunting. In addition, thawing permafrost can damage roads and infrastructure reducing access to important sites for Indigenous people (Hovelsrud et al. 2011). Low-lying small island nations are at great risk from sea level rise with entire cultural heritages at risk (Barnett and Adger 2003). These changes in the provision of cultural services driven by climate change dramatically affect cultural practices, nutrition, and mental health.

Table 29.1 summarizes the ecosystem services discussed in this section.

Table 29.1 Summary of Ecosystem Services Discussed, How Climate Affects the Ecosystems Those Services Depend on, and the Human Health Impacts Related to Those Altered Services

	Ecosystem Services	Climate Change Impacts	Ecosystem Effects	Health Impacts
Provisioning	**Crops**	Changing precipitation and weather patterns (storms, droughts etc.); increased CO_2 levels; desertification	Altered crop yield, reduced crop nutritional content, decreased soil health, increased crop pests	Food and nutrition security
	Freshwater fish	Rising water temperatures; changing precipitation patterns	Fish deaths, expansion of invasive species, increased frequency of algal blooms (causing fish death or inability to harvest fish)	Food and nutrition security
	Marine fish	Ocean acidification; rising water temperatures and changing ocean currents	Exacerbates algal blooms and dead zones, fish deaths, loss of fish nursery habitat, changing fish locations	Food and nutrition security
	Natural medicines	Climate-induced stress on habitats where medicinal organisms grow/live	Habitat loss, habitat health, ecological community shifts; range distribution shifts of medicinal organisms	Availability of and access to medicinal organisms; potential to discover new medicinal substances

	Ecosystem Services	Climate Change Impacts	Ecosystem Effects	Health Impacts
Regulating	**Pollination**	Warming temperatures; changing precipitation patterns	Changes in flower phenology; shifting (and possible mismatch) of ranges of plant and pollinator species; reduced populations or local extinction of pollinator species, all leading to reduced crop yields	Food insecurity and malnutrition due to decreased production of animal pollinated crops
	Water storage (flood protection)	Increased frequency of high intensity rainfall events	Inability of what remains of natural systems to store increased climate-change-induced floodwaters	Morbidity and mortality from floods; spread of infectious disease after flood events; mental health impacts related to flood events
	Coastal storm protection	Frequency and intensity of storms that cause significant coastal flooding; sea level rise; increased water temperatures, ocean acidification	Overwhelming of natural systems that buffer against storm surge; loss of coral reefs that buffer storm surge	Morbidity and mortality from floods; spread of infectious disease after flood events; mental health (stress) related to flood events
	Water filtration	Increased frequency of high intensity rainfall events; loss of habitats from storms, temperature, and sea level rise.	Inability of natural systems to sufficiently filter increased runoff of contaminants into waterways	Humans drinking contaminated water (e.g., contaminated with diarrheal disease-causing bacteria, heavy metals, nutrients)
	Air filtration in urban areas	Climatic conditions suitable for urban tree pests and pathogens	Pest and pathogen proliferation leading to death or decreased health of urban trees	Exposure to air pollution
	Heat regulation	Increasing temperatures and increased frequency of heat wave events	Loss of trees increases local temperatures, and pest and pathogen proliferation lead to death or decreased health of urban trees	Incidence of heat related illness, for example, heatstroke
	Reducing wildfire risk	Decreased rainfall and increased temperatures	Increased forest fire risk; spread of insect pests and pathogens that weaken trees; habitat shifts that stress trees	Morbidity and mortality from fire; exposure to smoke; contaminated freshwater sources (caused by sedimentation from fire events) with effects on drinking water quality and freshwater fisheries
	Climate regulation	Temperature and precipitation changes	Loss or reduced health of habitats that sequester and store carbon	Increased release or decreased capture and storage of carbon resulting in increased climate change (which causes all the health issues this book discusses)
	Disease regulation	Changing temperatures and precipitation patterns	Shifting and expanding ranges for disease vector species; increased vector production rates and incubation time; biodiversity loss and associated dilution effect	Increased exposure to disease carrying vectors (e.g., for malaria, Lyme); increased infection prevalence in disease hosts
Cultural	**Psychological benefits of green space/ nature exposure**	Climatic conditions suitable for urban tree pests and pathogens	Pest and pathogen proliferation leading to death or decreased health of urban trees	Reduction in mental health benefits of urban greenspace
	Cultural significance	Changing temperature and precipitation	Shifting or loss of culturally relevant habitats and species	Malnutrition related to loss of traditional food sources; mental health effects of loss or degradation of culturally relevant habitats and species

Ecosystem Solutions that Reduce Climate Change Impacts on Human Health

A diverse array of management approaches has been developed to improve the provision of ecosystem services. Most of these management approaches are not designed to reduce climate change impacts on human health, but if implemented in the right places with the right design, many could do so. Here, we provide several examples of ecosystem service management approaches that could reduce climate change impacts on human health.

Healthy soil communities store carbon and contribute to climate stabilization. Investments are already being made in management approaches like cover crops or fertilizer management to improve soil health and increase climate benefits. These same soil health improvements may benefit people by increasing the nutritional value of crops. For example, a study in Ethiopia showed that wheat grown on soils with more organic carbon had higher levels of zinc and protein (Wood and Baudron 2018).

Another example where soil health investments could which improve human health is found in northwest India is currently dominated by a rice-wheat cropping system that relies on crop residue burning to clear fields (National Academy of Agricultural Sciences 2017). This residue burning reduces soil health, and the burning itself is a major health risk, as the air pollution caused by fires contributes one quarter of high particulate air pollution levels in the winter (Sarkar, Singh, and Chauhan 2018). These pollution levels are high enough to affect the population in major cities including Delhi, where the last two years have seen national health emergencies declared during the peak burning season. Interventions that reduce crop residue burning would benefit soil health, climate, and human health.

A wide range of approaches have been designed to restore and protect forests for their carbon storage and climate mitigation benefits (in addition to their natural value). Management approaches that improve or maintain forest cover in the tropics could benefit human health by reducing heat stress (see Case Study 2). There is some evidence that efforts to protect forests in South America and Asia (but not Africa) by reducing road construction that fragments forests can reduce malaria risk (Bauhoff and Busch 2020). Some forest management approaches have been designed to help reduce wildfire risk, which is increasing under climate change (Westerling et al. 2006; Abatzoglou and Williams 2016). As these approaches are meant to reduce fires near population centers, further investment in them could also reduce smoke exposure and associated respiratory health impacts.

Investments in coastal ecosystem services can have direct climate mitigation and adaptation benefits and could also aid health if designed to do so. Investments in highly structured coastal habitats like coral reefs and mangroves can lead to reductions in storm surge and associated coastal flooding, reducing floodwater health risks, and loss of life during moderate storms. Innovative financing tools are being developed to support this ecosystem service. For example, a new kind of risk management tool called parametric insurance was recently applied to a stretch of Mexican coastline near Cancún. The insurance policy is paid for by hotel taxes, and used to recover the reef and its protective services after damage by storms.

Although many ecosystem service management options exist, it will be critical for the cost effectiveness of any ecosystem service solutions be compared to traditional health interventions. Few studies have done such comparisons. There is a need for more research on ecosystem-mediated health outcomes, especially research that focuses on how public policy responses and human behavioral changes affect ecosystems and human health (Pattanayak, Kramer, and Vincent 2017). Given the rapidly increasing pace of climate change, and increasingly clear impacts of climate on both ecosystem services and health, this is an area that warrants immediate attention from health and environment communities alike.

Summary

Ecosystem services are the benefits that nature provides to people. Many of these benefits flowing from nature influence some aspects of human health. Climate change is altering natural ecosystems on earth through a myriad of pathways thus changing their ability to provide services to people, resulting in varied human health outcomes. We have discussed how various ecosystem services affect human health and described how climate change might disrupt or alter the delivery of those services. We conclude with examples of ecosystem management activities that present possible solutions for mitigating the health effects of climate change's disruption of ecosystem services.

DISCUSSION QUESTIONS

1. Describe how climate will affect one provisioning, one regulating, and one cultural ecosystem service.

2. How might those changes identified in question 1 affect human health?

3. How might climate change influence human nutrition? What ecosystem services mediate those effects?

4. Briefly describe one example of natural resource management that could help mediate the negative health outcomes of climate change.

KEY TERMS

Biodiversity: The term biodiversity (from "biological diversity") refers to the variety of life on Earth at all its levels, from genes to ecosystems, and can encompass the evolutionary, ecological, and cultural processes that sustain life. Biodiversity includes not only species we consider rare, threatened, or endangered but also every living thing—from humans to organisms we know little about, such as microbes, fungi, and invertebrates (American Museum of Natural History, Center for Biodiversity and Conservation n.d.).

Cultural ecosystem services: Ecosystem services that describe the nonmaterial benefits that ecosystems provide to people, such as recreation opportunity, aesthetic appreciation, spiritual connection, sense of place, or appreciation for the existence of a particular habitat or species.

Dilution effect: The so-called "dilution effect" posits that changes in biodiversity in some ecosystems will impact the transmission cycle of certain pathogens. Where biodiversity is higher, the presence of hosts with a low capacity to transmit disease from host to vector can dilute the effect of highly competent hosts. Conversely, reductions in diversity may increase infection risk and disease prevalence in hosts.

Ecosystem services: Benefits people receive from nature.

Provisioning ecosystem services: Ecosystem services that represent material benefits of ecosystems that people use, appreciate, or sell. Many provisioning services have market value. These services include food production, water provision, and raw material creation (e.g., wood).

Regulating ecosystem services: Ecosystem services that regulate natural systems, such as an ecosystem's ability to regulate flooding, pollinate crops, or maintain soil health.

References

Abatzoglou, J. T., and A. P. Williams. 2016. "Impact of Anthropogenic Climate Change on Wildfire across Western US Forests." *Proceedings of the National Academy of Sciences of the USA* 113 (42):11770–5.

Abrol, D. P. 2012. "Climate Change and Pollinators." In *Pollination Biology: Biodiversity Conservation and Agricultural Production*, edited by D. P. Abrol, 479–508. Dordrecht: Springer Netherlands. https://doi.org/10.1007/978-94-007-1942-2_15.

Alderman, K., L. R. Turner, and S. Tong. 2012. "Floods and Human Health: A Systematic Review." *Environment International* 47 (October):37–47. https://doi.org/10.1016/j.envint.2012.06.003.

American Museum of Natural History. n.d. "What Is Biodiversity?" https://www.amnh.org/research/center-for-biodiversity-conservation/about-the-cbc/what-is-biodiversity-why-is-it-important-amnh.

Andrade, L., J. O'Dwyer, E. O'Neill, and P. Hynds. 2018. "Surface Water Flooding, Groundwater Contamination, and Enteric Disease in Developed Countries: A Scoping Review of Connections and Consequences." *Environmental Pollution* 236 (May):540–9. https://doi.org/10.1016/j.envpol.2018.01.104.

Baccini, A., W. Walker, L. Carvalho, M. Farina, D. Sulla-Menashe, and R. A. Houghton. 2017. "Tropical Forests Are a Net Carbon Source Based on Aboveground Measurements of Gain and Loss." *Science* 358 (6360):230–4. https://doi.org/10.1126/science.aam5962.

Bale, J. S., G. J. Masters, I. D. Hodkinson, C. Awmack, T. M. Bezemer, V. K. Brown, J. Butterfield, A. Buse, J. C. Coulson, and J. Farrar. 2002. "Herbivory in Global Climate Change Research: Direct Effects of Rising Temperature on Insect Herbivores." *Global Change Biology* 8 (1):1–16.

Barbero, R., J. T. Abatzoglou, N. K. Larkin, C. A. Kolden, and B. Stocks. 2015. "Climate Change Presents Increased Potential for Very Large Fires in the Contiguous United States." *International Journal of Wildland Fire* 24 (7):892–9. https://doi.org/10.1071/WF15083.

Barnett, J., and W. N. Adger. 2003. "Climate Dangers and Atoll Countries." *Climatic Change* 61 (3):321–37. https://doi.org/10.1023/B:CLIM.0000004559.08755.88.

Barreca, A., K. Clay, O. Deschenes, M. Greenstone, and J. S. Shapiro. 2013. *Adapting to Climate Change: The Remarkable Decline in the U.S. Temperature-Mortality Relationship over the 20th Century.* Cambridge, MA: National Bureau of Economic Research.

Barrett, C. B., T. Garg, and L. McBride. 2016. "Well-Being Dynamics and Poverty Traps." *Annual Review of Resource Economics* 8 (1):303–27.

Bauhoff, S., and J. Busch. 2020. "Does Deforestation Increase Malaria Prevalence? Evidence from Satellite Data and Health Surveys." *World Development* 127:104734.

Bayas, J. C. L., C. Marohn, G. Dercon, S. Dewi, H. P. Piepho, L. Joshi, M. van Noordwijk, and G. Cadisch. 2011. "Influence of Coastal Vegetation on the 2004 Tsunami Wave Impact in West Aceh." *Proceedings of the National Academy of Sciences of the USA* 108 (46):18612–17. https://doi.org/10.1073/pnas.1013516108.

Bebber, D. P., M. A. T. Ramotowski, and S. J. Gurr. 2013. "Crop Pests and Pathogens Move Polewards in a Warming World." *Nature Climate Change* 3 (11):985.

Beck, M. W., S. Narayan, D. Trespalacios, K. Pfliegner, I. J. Losada, P. Menéndez, A. Espejo, S. Torres, P. Díaz-Simal, and F. Fernandez. 2018. *The Global Value of Mangroves for Risk Reduction; Summary Report.* Berlin: The Nature Conservancy. https://www.conservationgateway.org/ConservationPractices/Marine/crr/library/Documents/GlobalMangrovesRiskReductionSummaryReport10.7291/V9930RBC.pdf.

Beggs, P. J. 2004. "Impacts of Climate Change on Aeroallergens: Past and Future." *Clinical & Experimental Allergy* 34 (10):1507–13. https://doi.org/10.1111/j.1365-2222.2004.02061.x.

Bellanger, M., C. Pichery, D. Aerts, M. Berglund, A. Castaño, M. Čejchanová, P. Crettaz, et al. 2013. "Economic Benefits of Methylmercury Exposure Control in Europe: Monetary Value of Neurotoxicity Prevention." *Environmental Health* 12 (1):3. https://doi.org/10.1186/1476-069X-12-3.

Bennett, E. M., S. R. Carpenter, and N. F. Caraco. 2001. "Human Impact on Erodable Phosphorus and Eutrophication: A Global Perspective. Increasing Accumulation of Phosphorus in Soil Threatens Rivers, Lakes, and Coastal Oceans with Eutrophication." *BioScience* 51 (3):227–34. https://doi.org/10.1641/0006-3568(2001)051[0227:HIOEPA]2.0.CO;2.

Berg, A. E. van den, J. Maas, R. A. Verheij, and P. P. Groenewegen. 2010. "Green Space as a Buffer between Stressful Life Events and Health." *Social Science & Medicine* 70 (8):1203–10. https://doi.org/10.1016/j.socscimed.2010.01.002.

Berry, H. L., K. Bowen, and T. Kjellstrom. 2010. "Climate Change and Mental Health: A Causal Pathways Framework." *International Journal of Public Health* 55 (2):123–32. doi:10.1007/s00038-009-0112-0.

Black, R. E., C. G. Victora, S. P. Walker, Z. A. Bhutta, P. Christian, M. de Onis, M. Ezzati, et al. 2013. "Maternal and Child Undernutrition and Overweight in Low-Income and Middle-Income Countries." *Lancet* 382 (9890):427–51. https://doi.org/10.1016/S0140-6736(13)60937-X.

Bladon, K. D., M. B. Emelko, U. Silins, and M. Stone. 2014. "Wildfire and the Future of Water Supply." *Environmental Science & Technology* 48 (16):8936–43. https://doi.org/10.1021/es500130g.

Bloomer, B. J., J. W. Stehr, C. A. Piety, R. J. Salawitch, and R. R. Dickerson. 2009. "Observed Relationships of Ozone Air Pollution with Temperature and Emissions." *Geophysical Research Letters* 36 (9). https://doi.org/10.1029/2009GL037308.

Bonan, G. B. 2008. "Forests and Climate Change: Forcings, Feedbacks, and the Climate Benefits of Forests." *Science* 320 (5882):1444–9. doi:10.1126/science.1155121.

Borum, J., O. Pedersen, L. Kotula, M. W. Fraser, J. Statton, T. D. Colmer, and G. A. Kendrick. 2016. "Photosynthetic Response to Globally Increasing CO_2 of Co-Occurring Temperate Seagrass Species." *Plant, Cell & Environment* 39 (6):1240–50.

Bowler, D. E., L. Buyung-Ali, T.M. Knight, and A. S. Pullin. 2010. "Urban Greening to Cool Towns and Cities: A Systematic Review of the Empirical Evidence." *Landscape and Urban Planning* 97 (3):147–55. https://doi.org/10.1016/j.landurbplan.2010.05.006.

Brander, K. M. 2007. "Global Fish Production and Climate Change." *Proceedings of the National Academy of Sciences of the USA* 104 (50):19709–14. https://doi.org/10.1073/pnas.0702059104.

Burek, P., S. Mubareka, R. Rojas, A. de Roo, A. Bianchi, C. Baranzelli, C. Lavalle, and I. Vandecasteele. 2012. *Evaluation of the Effectiveness of Natural Water Retention Measures. JRC Scientific and Policy Reports.* Luxembourg: Publications Office of the European Union. http://ec.europa.eu/environment/water/blueprint/pdf/EUR25551EN_JRC_Blueprint_NWRM.pdf.

Burge, C. A., C. J. Closek, C. S. Friedman, M. L. Groner, C. M. Jenkins, A. Shore-Maggio, and J. E. Welsh. 2016. "The Use of Filter-Feeders to Manage Disease in a Changing World." *Integrative and Comparative Biology* 56 (4):573–87.

Burke, L., K. Reytar, M. Spalding, and A. Perry. 2011. *Reefs at Risk Revisited.* Washington, DC: World Resources Institute. https://www.wri.org/publication/reefs-risk-revisited.

Canadell, J. G., and M. R. Raupach. 2008. "Managing Forests for Climate Change Mitigation." *Science* 320 (5882):1456–7. https://doi.org/10.1126/science.1155458.

Carpenter, S. R., H. A. Mooney, J. Agard, D. Capistrano, R. S. Defries, S. Díaz, T. Dietz, et al. 2009. "Science for Managing Ecosystem Services: Beyond the Millennium Ecosystem Assessment." *Proceedings of the National Academy of Sciences of the USA* 106 (5):1305–12. https://doi.org/10.1073/pnas.0808772106.

Cheung, W. W. L., Vi. W. Y. Lam, J. L. Sarmiento, K. Kearney, R. Watson, D. Zeller, and D. Pauly. 2010. "Large-Scale Redistribution of Maximum Fisheries Catch Potential in the Global Ocean under Climate Change." *Global Change Biology* 16 (1):24–35. https://doi.org/10.1111/j.1365-2486.2009.01995.x.

Chiesura, A. 2004. "The Role of Urban Parks for the Sustainable City." *Landscape and Urban Planning* 68 (1):129–38. https://doi.org/10.1016/j.landurbplan.2003.08.003.

Coffel, E. D., R. M. Horton, and A. de Sherbinin. 2017. "Temperature and Humidity Based Projections of a Rapid Rise in Global Heat Stress Exposure during the 21st Century." *Environmental Research Letters* 13 (1). https://iopscience.iop.org/article/10.1088/1748-9326/aaa00e.

Collins, M., R. Knutti, J. Arblaster, J.-L. Dufresne, T. Fichefet, P. Friedlingstein, X. Gao et al. 2013. "Long-Term Climate Change: Projections, Commitments and Irreversibility." In *Climate Change 2013: The Physical Science Basis. Contribution of Working Group I to the Fifth Assessment Report of the Intergovernmental Panel on Climate Change,* edited by T. F. Stocker, D. Qin, G.-K. Plattner, M. Tignor, S.K. Allen, J. Boschung, A. Nauels et al. Cambridge, UK and New York: Cambridge University Press.

Cooke, G. D., and R. H. Kennedy. 2009. "Managing Drinking Water Supplies." *Journal of Lake Reservoir Management* 17:157–74.

Crouch, R. L., H. J. Timmenga, T. R. Barber, and P. C. Fuchsman. 2006. "Post-Fire Surface Water Quality: Comparison of Fire Retardant versus Wildfire-Related Effects." *Chemosphere* 62 (6):874–89. https://doi.org/10.1016/j.chemosphere.2005.05.031.

Crowe, J., C. Wesseling, B. R. Solano, M. P. Umaña, A. R. Ramírez, T. Kjellstrom, D. Morales, and M. Nilsson. 2013. "Heat Exposure in Sugarcane Harvesters in Costa Rica." *American Journal of Industrial Medicine* 56 (10):1157–64. doi:10.1002/ajim.22204.

Crowe, J., M. Nilsson, T. Kjellstrom, and C. Wesseling. 2015. "Heat-Related Symptoms in Sugarcane Harvesters." *American Journal of Industrial Medicine* 58 (5):541–8. doi:10.1002/ajim.22450.

Das, S., and J. R. Vincent. 2009. "Mangroves Protected Villages and Reduced Death Toll during Indian Super Cyclone." *Proceedings of the National Academy of Sciences of the USA* 106 (18):7357–60. https://doi.org/10.1073/pnas.0810440106.

Delpla, I., A. -V. Jung, E. Baures, M. Clement, and O. Thomas. 2009. "Impacts of Climate Change on Surface Water Quality in Relation to Drinking Water Production." *Environment International* 35 (8):1225–33. https://doi.org/10.1016/j.envint.2009.07.001.

Dixon, S. J., D. A. Sear, N. A. Odoni, T. Sykes, and S. N. Lane. 2016. "The Effects of River Restoration on Catchment Scale Flood Risk and Flood Hydrology." *Earth Surface Processes and Landforms* 41 (7):997–1008. https://doi.org/10.1002/esp.3919.

Eilers, E. J., C. Kremen, S. S. Greenleaf, A. K. Garber, and A.-M. Klein. 2011. "Contribution of Pollinator-Mediated Crops to Nutrients in the Human Food Supply." *PLoS ONE* 6 (6):1–6. https://doi.org/10.1371/journal.pone.0021363.

Ellison, D., C. E. Morris, B. Locatelli, D. Sheil, J. Cohen, D.Murdiyarso, V. Gutierrez et al. 2017. "Trees, Forests and Water: Cool Insights for a Hot World." *Global Environmental Change* 43:51–61.

Elmqvist, T., M. Fragkias, J. Goodness, B. Güneralp, P. J. Marcotullio, R. I. McDonald, Susan Parnell et al. 2013. *Urbanization, Biodiversity and Ecosystem Services: Challenges and Opportunities: A Global Assessment.* New York: Springer.

Emelko, M. B., U. Silins, K. D. Bladon, and M. Stone. 2011. "Implications of Land Disturbance on Drinking Water Treatability in a Changing Climate: Demonstrating the Need for 'Source Water Supply and Protection' Strategies." *Water Research* 45 (2):461–72. https://doi.org/10.1016/j.watres.2010.08.051.

Fiore, A. M., V. Naik, and E. M. Leibensperger. 2015. "Air Quality and Climate Connections." *Journal of the Air & Waste Management Association* 65 (6):645–85. https://doi.org/10.1080/10962247.2015.1040526.

Flood, J. 2010. "The Importance of Plant Health to Food Security." *Food Security* 2 (3):215–31.

Food and Agriculture Organization. 2019. *The State of the World's Biodiversity for Food and Agriculture 2019.* Rome: FAO Commission on Genetic Resources for Food and Agriculture Assessments. http://www.fao.org/3/CA3129EN/CA3129EN.pdf.

Fowler, M. D., G. J. Kooperman, J. T. Randerson, and M. S. Pritchard. 2019. "The Effect of Plant Physiological Responses to Rising CO 2 on Global Streamflow." *Nature Climate Change* 9 (11):873–79. https://doi.org/10.1038/s41558-019-0602-x.

Free, C. M., J. T. Thorson, M. L. Pinsky, K. L. Oken, J. Wiedenmann, and O. P. Jensen. 2019. "Impacts of Historical Warming on Marine Fisheries Production." *Science* 363 (6430):979–83. https://doi.org/10.1126/science.aau1758.

Gage, K. L., T. R. Burkot, R. J. Eisen, and E. B. Hayes. 2008. "Climate and Vectorborne Diseases." *American Journal of Preventive Medicine Theme Issue: Climate Change and the Health of the Public* 35 (5):436–50. https://doi.org/10.1016/j.amepre.2008.08.030.

Gairola, S., N. M. Shariff, A. Bhatt, and C. P. Kala. 2010. "Influence of Climate Change on Production of Secondary Chemicals in High Altitude Medicinal Plants: Issues Needs Immediate Attention." *Journal of Medicinal Plants Research* 4 (18):1825–9. doi:10.5897/JMPR10.354.

Garcia, S. M., and I. de L. Moreno. 2003. "Global Overview of Marine Fisheries." In *Responsible Fisheries in the Marine Ecosystem*, 1–24. Rome: Food and Agriculture Organization and CABI Publishing.

Gedan, K. B., M. L. Kirwan, E. Wolanski, E. B. Barbier, and B. R. Silliman. 2011. "The Present and Future Role of Coastal Wetland Vegetation in Protecting Shorelines: Answering Recent Challenges to the Paradigm." *Climatic Change* 106 (1):7–29. https://doi.org/10.1007/s10584-010-0003-7.

Githeko, A. K., S. W. Lindsay, U. E. Confalonieri, and J. A. Patz. 2000. "Climate Change and Vector-Borne Diseases: A Regional Analysis." *Bulletin of the World Health Organization* 78 (9):1136–47.

Gobler, C. J., O. M. Doherty, T. K. Hattenrath-Lehmann, A. W. Griffith, Y. Kang, and R. W. Litaker. 2017. "Ocean Warming since 1982 Has Expanded the Niche of Toxic Algal Blooms in the North Atlantic and North Pacific Oceans." *Proceedings of the National Academy of Sciences of the USA* 114 (19):4975–80.

Grant, S. B., J.-D. Saphores, D. L. Feldman, A. J. Hamilton, T. D. Fletcher, P. L. M. Cook, M. Stewardson et al. 2012. "Taking the 'Waste' Out of 'Wastewater' for Human Water Security and Ecosystem Sustainability." *Science* 337 (6095):681–6.

Grassini, P., K. M. Eskridge, and K. G. Cassman. 2013. "Distinguishing between Yield Advances and Yield Plateaus in Historical Crop Production Trends." *Nature Communications* 4:2918.

Griscom, B. W., J. Adams, P. W. Ellis, R. A. Houghton, G. Lomax, D. A. Miteva, W. H. Schlesinger et al. 2017. "Natural Climate Solutions." *Proceedings of the National Academy of Sciences of the USA* 114 (44):11645–50. https://doi.org/10.1073/pnas.1710465114.

Haines, A., and J. A. Patz. 2004. "Health Effects of Climate Change." *JAMA* 291 (1):99–103. https://doi.org/10.1001/jama.291.1.99.

Hallegraeff, G. M. 2010. "Ocean Climate Change, Phytoplankton Community Responses, and Harmful Algal Blooms: A Formidable Predictive Challenge1." *Journal of Phycology* 46 (2):220–35. https://doi.org/10.1111/j.1529-8817.2010.00815.x.

Harrison, M. E., S. E. Page, and S. H. Limin. 2009. "The Global Impact of Indonesian Forest Fires." *Biologist* 56 (3):156–63.

Harvey, B. J. 2016. "Human-Caused Climate Change Is Now a Key Driver of Forest Fire Activity in the Western United States." *Proceedings of the National Academy of Sciences of the USA* 113 (42):11649–50.

Hegland, S. J., A. Nielsen, A. Lázaro, A.-L. Bjerknes, and Ø. Totland. 2009. "How Does Climate Warming Affect Plant-Pollinator Interactions?" *Ecology Letters* 12 (2):184–95. https://doi.org/10.1111/j.1461-0248.2008.01269.x.

Heil, A., B. Langmann, and E. Aldrian. 2007. "Indonesian Peat and Vegetation Fire Emissions: Study on Factors Influencing Large-Scale Smoke Haze Pollution Using a Regional Atmospheric Chemistry Model." *Mitigation and Adaptation Strategies for Global Change* 12 (1):113–33. https://doi.org/10.1007/s11027-006-9045-6.

Hicks, C. C., P. J. Cohen, N. A. J. Graham, K. L. Nash, E. H. Allison, C. D'Lima, D. J. Mills et al. 2019. "Harnessing Global Fisheries to Tackle Micronutrient Deficiencies." *Nature* 574 (7776):95–98. https://doi.org/10.1038/s41586-019-1592-6.

Hoegh-Guldberg, O., P. J. Mumby, A. J. Hooten, R. S. Steneck, P. Greenfield, E. Gomez, C. D. Harvell et al. 2007. "Coral Reefs Under Rapid Climate Change and Ocean Acidification." *Science* 318 (5857):1737–42. https://doi.org/10.1126/science.1152509.

Holmbom, B., S. Willfoer, J. Hemming, S. Pietarinen, L. Nisula, P. Eklund, and R. Sjoeholm. 2007. "Knots in Trees: A Rich Source of Bioactive Polyphenols." *In Materials, Chemicals, and Energy from Forest Biomass, ACS Symposium Series 954:350–62.* American Chemical Society. https://doi.org/10.1021/bk-2007-0954.ch022.

Hovelsrud, G. K., B. Poppel, B. van Oort, and J. D. Reist. 2011. "Arctic Societies, Cultures, and Peoples in a Changing Cryosphere." *Ambio* 40 (suppl 1):100–10. https://doi.org/10.1007/s13280-011-0219-4.

Hoyos, C. D., P. A. Agudelo, P. J. Webster, and J. A. Curry. 2006. "Deconvolution of the Factors Contributing to the Increase in Global Hurricane Intensity." *Science* 312 (5770):94–7.

Hughes, T. P., M. L. Barnes, D. R. Bellwood, J. E. Cinner, G. S. Cumming, J. B. C. Jackson, J. Kleypas et al. 2017. "Coral Reefs in the Anthropocene." *Nature* 546 (7656):82–90. https://doi.org/10.1038/nature22901.

Intergovernmental Panel on Climate Change. 2013: *Climate Change 2013: The Physical Science Basis. Contribution of Working Group I to the Fifth Assessment Report of the Intergovernmental Panel on Climate Change*, edited by T. F. Stocker, D. Qin, G.-K. Plattner, M. Tignor, S. K. Allen, J. Boschung, A. Nauels et al. Cambridge, UK and New York: Cambridge University Press. https://www.ipcc.ch/report/ar5/wg1/.

Intergovernmental Panel on Climate Change. 2018. *Global Warming of 1.5°C. An IPCC Special Report on the Impacts of Global Warming of 1.5°C above Pre-Industrial Levels and Related Global Greenhouse Gas Emission Pathways, in the Context of Strengthening the Global Response to the Threat of Climate Change, Sustainable Development, and Efforts to Eradicate Poverty*, edited by V. Masson-Delmotte, P. Zhai, H.-O. Pörtner, D. Roberts, J. Skea, P. R. Shukla, A. Pirani, W. Moufouma-Okia et al. Geneva: IPCC. https://www.ipcc.ch/sr15/download/#full.

Intergovernmental Panel on Climate Change. 2019. *Special Report on the Ocean and Cryosphere in a Changing Climate.* Geneva: IPCC. https://www.ipcc.ch/srocc/download-report/.

Jacob, D. J., and D. A. Winner. 2009. "Effect of Climate Change on Air Quality." *Atmospheric Environment* 43 (1):51–63. https://doi.org/10.1016/j.atmosenv.2008.09.051.

Jakubicka, T., F. Vos, R. Phalkey, M. Marx, and D. Guha-Sapir. 2010. *Health Impacts of Floods in Europe: Data Gaps and Information Needs from a Spatial Perspective.* Microdis. http://lib.riskreductionafrica.org/bitstream/handle/123456789/1122/health%20impacts%20of%20floods%20in%20europe.pdf?sequence=1.

Johnston, F. H., S. B. Henderson, Y. Chen, J. T. Randerson, M. Marlier, R. S. DeFries, P. Kinney, D. M. J. S. Bowman, and M. Brauer. 2012. "Estimated Global Mortality Attributable to Smoke from Landscape Fires." *Environmental Health Perspectives* 120 (5):695–701. https://doi.org/10.1289/ehp.1104422.

Karjalainen, E., T. Sarjala, and H. Raitio. 2010. "Promoting Human Health through Forests: Overview and Major Challenges." *Environmental Health and Preventive Medicine* 15 (1):1–8. https://doi.org/10.1007/s12199-008-0069-2.

Kelly, E. N., D. W. Schindler, V. L. St. Louis, D. B. Donald, and K. E. Vladicka. 2006. "Forest Fire Increases Mercury Accumulation by Fishes via Food Web Restructuring and Increased Mercury Inputs." *Proceedings of the National Academy of Sciences of the USA* 103 (51):19380–85. https://doi.org/10.1073/pnas.0609798104.

Khanum, R., A. S. Mumtaz, and S. Kumar. 2013. "Predicting Impacts of Climate Change on Medicinal Asclepiads of Pakistan Using Maxent Modeling." *Acta Oecologica* 49 (May):23–31. https://doi.org/10.1016/j.actao.2013.02.007.

Kistemann, T., T. Classen, C. Koch, F. Dangendorf, R. Fischeder, J. Gebel, V. Vacata, and M. Exner. 2002. "Microbial Load of Drinking Water Reservoir Tributaries during Extreme Rainfall and Runoff." *Applied and Environmental Microbiology* 68 (5):2188–97.

Klein, A.-M., B. E. Vaissière, J. H. Cane, I. Steffan-Dewenter, S. A. Cunningham, C. Kremen, and T. Tscharntke. 2007. "Importance of Pollinators in Changing Landscapes for World Crops." *Proceedings of the Royal Society B: Biological Sciences* 274 (1608):303–13. https://doi.org/10.1098/rspb.2006.3721.

Knutson, T. R., J. L. McBride, J. Chan, K. Emanuel, G. Holland, C. Landsea, I. Held et al. 2010. "Tropical Cyclones and Climate Change." *Nature Geoscience* 3 (3):157–63. https://doi.org/10.1038/ngeo779.

Kovats, R. S., and S. Hajat. 2008. "Heat Stress and Public Health: A Critical Review." *Annual Review of Public Health* 29 (1):41–55. https://doi.org/10.1146/annurev.publhealth.29.020907.090843.

Kramer, M. H., B. L. Herwaldt, G. F. Craun, R. L. Calderon, and D. D. Juranek. 1994. "Surveillance for Waterborne-Disease Outbreaks—United States 1993–1994." *MMWR. Morbidity and Mortality Weekly Report* 45 (SS-1):1–33.

Kris-Etherton, P. M., K. D. Hecker, A. Bonanome, S. M. Coval, A. E. Binkoski, K. F. Hilpert, A. E. Griel, and T. D. Etherton. 2002. "Bioactive Compounds in Foods: Their Role in the Prevention of Cardiovascular Disease and Cancer." *American Journal of Medicine* 113 (Suppl 9B, December):71S–88S.

Kumar, C. S., D. V. L. Sarada, T. P. Gideon, and R. Rengasamy. 2008. "Antibacterial Activity of Three South Indian Seagrasses, *Cymodocea serrulata*, *Halophila ovalis* and *Zostera capensis*." *World Journal of Microbiology and Biotechnology* 24:1989–1992 (2008). https://doi.org/10.1007/s11274-008-9695-5.

Kundzewicz, Z. W., L. J. Mata, N. W. Arnell, P. Döll, B. Jimenez, K. Miller, T. Oki, Z. Şen, and I. Shiklomanov. 2008. "The Implications of Projected Climate Change for Freshwater Resources and Their Management." *Hydrological Sciences Journal* 53 (1):3–10. https://doi.org/10.1623/hysj.53.1.3.

Lamb, J. B. J. A. J. M. van de Water, D. G. Bourne, C. Altier, M. Y. Hein, E. A. Fiorenza, N. Abu, J. Jompa, and C. D. Harvell. 2017. "Seagrass Ecosystems Reduce Exposure to Bacterial Pathogens of Humans, Fishes, and Invertebrates." *Science* 355 (6326)731–3.

Landschützer, P., N. Gruber, D. C. E. Bakker, and U. Schuster. 2014. "Recent Variability of the Global Ocean Carbon Sink." *Global Biogeochemical Cycles* 28 (9):927–49. https://doi.org/10.1002/2014GB004853.

Lane, K., K. Charles-Guzman, K. Wheeler, Z. Abid, N. Graber, and T. Matte. 2013. "Health Effects of Coastal Storms and Flooding in Urban Areas: A Review and Vulnerability Assessment." *Journal of Environmental and Public Health* 2013:913064. https://doi.org/10.1155/2013/913064.

Lawrence, D., and K. Vandecar. 2015. "Effects of Tropical Deforestation on Climate and Agriculture." *Nature Climate Change* 5:27–36.

Lawton, R. O., U.S. Nair, R. A. Pielke Sr., and R. M. Welch. 2001. "Climatic Impact of Tropical Lowland Deforestation on Nearby Montane Cloud Forests." *Science* 294 (5542):584–7. doi:10.1126/science.1062459.

Lesk, C., P. Rowhani, and N. Ramankutty. 2016. "Influence of Extreme Weather Disasters on Global Crop Production." *Nature* 529 (7584):84–87. https://doi.org/10.1038/nature16467.

Lin, M., and P. Huybers. 2012. "Reckoning Wheat Yield Trends." *Environmental Research Letters* 7 (2):024016.

Lindgren, E., and T. Elmqvist. 2017. "Ecosystem Services and Human Health." *Oxford Research Encyclopedia of Environmental Science* https://doi.org/10.1093/acrefore/9780199389414.013.86.

Liu, J. C., G. Pereira, S. A. Uhl, M. A. Bravo, and M. L. Bell. 2015. "A Systematic Review of the Physical Health Impacts from Non-Occupational Exposure to Wildfire Smoke." *Environmental Research* 136 (January):120–32. https://doi.org/10.1016/j.envres.2014.10.015.

Liu, J. C., A. Wilson, L. J. Mickley, F. Dominici, K. Ebisu, Y. Wang, M. P. Sulprizio et al. 2017. "Wildfire-Specific Fine Particulate Matter and Risk of Hospital Admissions in Urban and Rural Counties." *Epidemiology (Cambridge, Mass.)* 28 (1):77–85. https://doi.org/10.1097/EDE.0000000000000556.

Liu, Y., J. Stanturf, and S. Goodrick. 2010. "Trends in Global Wildfire Potential in a Changing Climate." *Forest Ecology and Management* 259 (4):685–97. https://doi.org/10.1016/j.foreco.2009.09.002.

Long, S. P., E. A. Ainsworth, A. D. B. Leakey, J. Nösberger, and D. R. Ort. 2006. "Food for Thought: Lower-Than-Expected Crop Yield Stimulation with Rising CO_2 Concentrations." *Science* 312 (5782):1918–21. https://doi.org/10.1126/science.1114722.

Mahdi, J. G., A. J. Mahdi, A. J. Mahdi, and I. D. Bowen. 2006. "The Historical Analysis of Aspirin Discovery, Its Relation to the Willow Tree and Antiproliferative and Anticancer Potential." *Cell Proliferation* 39 (2):147–55. https://doi.org/10.1111/j.1365-2184.2006.00377.x.

Maikhuri, R. K., P. C. Phondani, D. Dhyani, L. S. Rawat, N. K. Jha, and L. S. Kandari. 2018. "Assessment of Climate Change Impacts and Its Implications on Medicinal Plants-Based Traditional Healthcare System in Central Himalaya, India." *Iranian Journal of Science and Technology, Transactions A: Science* 42 (4):1827–35. https://doi.org/10.1007/s40995-017-0354-2.

Mäkinen, H., J. Kaseva, P. Virkajärvi, and H. Kahiluoto. 2017. "Shifts in Soil–Climate Combination Deserve Attention." *Agricultural and Forest Meteorology* 234–235 (March):236–46. https://doi.org/10.1016/j.agrformet.2016.12.017.

Mani, A. E., V. Bharathi, and J. Patterson. 2012. "Antibacterial Activity and Preliminary Phytochemical Analysis of Seagrass *Cymodocea rotundata*." *International Journal of Microbiology Research* 3 (2):99–103.

Marris, E. 2006. "Drugs from the Deep." *News. Nature. October* 25, 2006. https://doi.org/10.1038/443904a.

Masuda, Y, J., B. Castro, I. Anggraeni, N. H. Wolff, K. Ebi, T. Garg, E. T. Game, J. Krenz, and J. Spector. 2019. "How Are Healthy, Working Populations Affected by Increasing Temperatures in the Tropics? Implications for Climate Change Adaptation Policies." *Global Environmental Change* 56:29–40.

McDonald, R., T. Kroeger, T. Boucher, W. Longzhu, and R. Salem. 2016. "Planting Healthy Air: A Global Analysis of the Role of Urban Trees in Addressing Particulate Matter Pollution and Extreme Heat." *The Nature Conservancy and C40 Cities.* https://www.nature.org/en-us/what-we-do/our-insights/perspectives/how-urban-trees-can-save-lives/.

Medek, D. E., J. Schwartz, and S. S. Myers. 2017. "Estimated Effects of Future Atmospheric CO_2 Concentrations on Protein Intake and the Risk of Protein Deficiency by Country and Region." *Environmental Health Perspectives* 125 (8). https://doi.org/10.1289/EHP41.

Meineke, E. K., R. R. Dunn, J. O. Sexton, and S. D. Frank. 2013. "Urban Warming Drives Insect Pest Abundance on Street Trees." *PLOS One* 8 (3):e59687. https://doi.org/10.1371/journal.pone.0059687.

Melillo, J. M. 2014. *Climate Change Impacts in the United States: The Third National Climate Assessment.* Washington, DC: U.S. Global Change Research Program.

Memmott, J., P. G. Craze, N. M. Waser, and M. V. Price. 2007. "Global Warming and the Disruption of Plant–Pollinator Interactions." *Ecology Letters* 10 (8):710–17. https://doi.org/10.1111/j.1461-0248.2007.01061.x.

Millennium Ecosystem Assessment. 2005. *Ecosystems and Human Well-Being: Synthesis.* Washington, DC: Island Press. https://www.millenniumassessment.org/documents/document.356.aspx.pdf.

Miller, L. H., and X. Su. 2011. "Artemisinin: Discovery from the Chinese Herbal Garden." *Cell* 146 (6):855–8. https://doi.org/10.1016/j.cell.2011.08.024.

Mishra, T. 2016. "Climate Change and Production of Secondary Metabolites in Medicinal Plants: A Review." *International Journal of Herbal Medicine* 4 (4):27–30.

Mitsch, W. J., J. W. Day, J. W. Gilliam, P. M. Groffman, D. L. Hey, G. W. Randall, and N. Wang. 2001. "Reducing Nitrogen Loading to the Gulf of Mexico from the Mississippi River Basin: Strategies to Counter a Persistent Ecological Problem. Ecotechnology—The Use of Natural Ecosystems to Solve Environmental Problems—Should Be a Part of Efforts to Shrink the Zone of Hypoxia in the Gulf of Mexico." *BioScience* 51 (5): 373–88. https://doi.org/10.1641/0006-3568(2001)051[0373:RNLTTG]2.0.CO;2.

Möller, I., M. Kudella, F. Rupprecht, T. Spencer, M. Paul, B. K. van Wesenbeeck, G. Wolters et al. 2014. "Wave Attenuation over Coastal Salt Marshes under Storm Surge Conditions." *Nature Geoscience* 7 (10):727–31. https://doi.org/10.1038/ngeo2251.

Mora, C., C. W. W. Counsell, C. R. Bielecki, and L. V. Louis. 2017. "Twenty-Seven Ways a Heat Wave Can Kill You: Deadly Heat in the Era of Climate Change." *Circulation: Cardiovascular Quality and Outcomes* 10 (11):e004233. doi: 10.1161/CIRCOUTCOMES.117.004233.

Moutsatsou, P. 2007. "The Spectrum of Phytoestrogens in Nature: Our Knowledge Is Expanding." *Hormones (Athens, Greece)* 6 (3):173–93.

Murphy, H. M., M. D. Prioleau, M. A. Borchardt, and P. D. Hynds. 2017. "Review: Epidemiological Evidence of Groundwater Contribution to Global Enteric Disease, 1948–2015." *Hydrogeology Journal* 25 (4):981–1001. https://doi.org/10.1007/s10040-017-1543-y.

Myers, S. S., M. R. Smith, S. Guth, C. D. Golden, B. Vaitla, N. D. Mueller, A. D. Dangour, and P. Huybers. 2017. "Climate Change and Global Food Systems: Potential Impacts on Food Security and

Undernutrition." *Annual Review of Public Health* 38 (1):259–77. https://doi.org/10.1146/annurev-publhealth-031816-044356.

Myers, S. S., A. Zanobetti, I. Kloog, P. Huybers, A. D. B. Leakey, A. J. Bloom, E. Carlisle et al. 2014. "Increasing CO_2 Threatens Human Nutrition." *Nature* 510 (7503):139–42. https://doi.org/10.1038/nature13179.

National Academy of Agricultural Sciences. 2017. *Innovative Viable Solution to Rice Residue Burning in Rice-Wheat Cropping System through Concurrent Use of Super Straw Management System-Fitted Combines and Turbo Happy Seeder. Policy Brief No. 2.* New Delhi: NAAS. http://naasindia.org/documents/CropBurning.pdf.

Nelson, M. 2018. "Biosphere 2: What Really Happened?" *Dartmouth Alumni Magazine* May-June 2018. https://dartmouthalumnimagazine.com/articles/biosphere-2-what-really-happened.

Nowak, D. J., S. Hirabayashi, A. Bodine, and E. Greenfield. 2014. "Tree and Forest Effects on Air Quality and Human Health in the United States." *Environmental Pollution* 193 (October):119–29. https://doi.org/10.1016/j.envpol.2014.05.028.

Nye, J. A., J. S. Link, J. A. Hare, and W. J. Overholtz. 2009. "Changing Spatial Distribution of Fish Stocks in Relation to Climate and Population Size on the Northeast United States Continental Shelf." *Marine Ecology Progress Series* 393 (October):111–29. https://doi.org/10.3354/meps08220.

Orth, R. J., T. J. B. Carruthers, W. C. Dennison, C. M. Duarte, J. W. Fourqurean, K. L. Heck et al. 2006. "A Global Crisis for Seagrass Ecosystems." *BioScience* 56 (12):987–96.

Ostfeld, R. S., and F. Keesing. 2012. "Effects of Host Diversity on Infectious Disease." *Annual Review of Ecology, Evolution, and Systematics* 43 (1):157–82. https://doi.org/10.1146/annurev-ecolsys-102710-145022.

Parmesan, C., and G. Yohe. 2003. "A Globally Coherent Fingerprint of Climate Change Impacts across Natural Systems." *Nature* 421 (6918):37. https://doi.org/10.1038/nature01286.

Pascua, P., H. McMillen, T. Ticktin, M. Vaughan, and K. B. Winter. 2017. "Beyond Services: A Process and Framework to Incorporate Cultural, Genealogical, Place-Based, and Indigenous Relationships in Ecosystem Service Assessments." *Ecosystem Services* 26 (August):465–75. https://doi.org/10.1016/j.ecoser.2017.03.012.

Pattanayak, S. K., R. A. Kramer, and J. R. Vincent. 2017. "Ecosystem Change and Human Health: Implementation Economics and Policy." *Philosophical Transactions of the Royal Society B: Biological Sciences* 372 (1722):20160130. https://doi.org/10.1098/rstb.2016.0130.

Patz, J. A. 2018. "Altered Disease Risk from Climate Change." *EcoHealth* 15 (3):693–4. https://doi.org/10.1007/s10393-018-1382-x.

Patz, J. A., P. R. Epstein, T. A. Burke, and J. M. Balbus. 1996. "Global Climate Change and Emerging Infectious Diseases." *JAMA* 275 (3):217–23. https://doi.org/10.1001/jama.1996.03530270057032.

Patz, J. A, and W. K Reisen. 2001. "Immunology, Climate Change and Vector-Borne Diseases." *Trends in Immunology* 22 (4):171–2. https://doi.org/10.1016/S1471-4906(01)01867-1.

Pausas, J. G., and J. E. Keeley. 2019. "Wildfires as an Ecosystem Service." *Frontiers in Ecology and the Environment* https://doi.org/10.1002/fee.2044.

Pechony, O., and D. T. Shindell. 2010. "Driving Forces of Global Wildfires over the Past Millennium and the Forthcoming Century." *Proceedings of the National Academy of Sciences of the USA* 107 (45):19167–70. https://doi.org/10.1073/pnas.1003669107.

Perry, A. L., P. J. Low, J. R. Ellis, and J. D. Reynolds. 2005. "Climate Change and Distribution Shifts in Marine Fishes." *Science* 308 (5730):1912–15. https://doi.org/10.1126/science.1111322.

Pizzuto, J. 2012. "Predicting the Accumulation of Mercury-Contaminated Sediment on Riverbanks—An Analytical Approach." *Water Resources Research* 48 (7). https://doi.org/10.1029/2012WR011906.

Potts, S. G., V. Imperatriz-Fonseca, H. Ngo, J. C. Biesmeijer, T. Breeze, L. Dicks, L. Garibaldi et al. 2016. "Summary for Policymakers of the Assessment Report of the Intergovernmental Science-Policy Platform on Biodiversity and Ecosystem Services (IPBES) on Pollinators, Pollination and Food Production." hal-01946814. Post-Print. HAL. https://ideas.repec.org/p/hal/journl/hal-01946814.html.

Powell, J. P., and S. Reinhard. 2016. "Measuring the Effects of Extreme Weather Events on Yields." *Weather and Climate Extremes* 12 (June):69–79. https://doi.org/10.1016/j.wace.2016.02.003.

Prevedello, J. A., G. R. Winck, M. M. Weber, E. Nichols, and B. Sinervo. 2019. "Impacts of Forestation and Deforestation on Local Temperature across the Globe." *PLOS One* 14 (3):e0213368. https://doi.org/10.1371/journal.pone.0213368.

Ray, D. K., N. Ramankutty, N. D. Mueller, P. C. West, and J. A. Foley. 2012. "Recent Patterns of Crop Yield Growth and Stagnation." *Nature Communications* 3:1293.

Reid, C. E., M. Brauer, F. H. Johnston, M. Jerrett, J. R. Balmes, and C. T. Elliott. 2016. "Critical Review of Health Impacts of Wildfire Smoke Exposure." *Environmental Health Perspectives* 124 (9):1334–43. https://doi.org/10.1289/ehp.1409277.

Rogelj, J., M. Meinshausen, and R. Knutti. 2012. "Global Warming under Old and New Scenarios Using IPCC Climate Sensitivity Range Estimates." *Nature Climate Change* 2:248–53. https://doi.org/10.1038/nclimate1385.

Rogers, A., J. L. Blanchard, and P. .J Mumby. 2014. "Vulnerability of Coral Reef Fisheries to a Loss of Structural Complexity." *Current Biology* 24 (9):1000–5. doi: 10.1016/j.cub.2014.03.026.

Saatchi, S. S., N. L. Harris, S. Brown, M. Lefsky, E. T. A. Mitchard, W. Salas, B. R. Zutta et al. 2011. "Benchmark Map of Forest Carbon Stocks in Tropical Regions across Three Continents." *Proceedings of the National Academy of Sciences of the USA* 108 (24):9899–9904. https://doi.org/10.1073/pnas.1019576108.

Sarkar, S., R. P. Singh, and A. Chauhan. 2018. "Increasing Health Threat to Greater Parts of India Due to Crop Residue Burning." *Lancet Planetary Health* 2 (8):e327–e328.

Scavia, D., J. C. Field, D. F. Boesch, R. W. Buddemeier, V. Burkett, D. R. Cayan, M. Fogarty et al. 2002. "Climate Change Impacts on U.S. Coastal and Marine Ecosystems." *Estuaries* 25 (2):149–64. https://doi.org/10.1007/BF02691304.

Schleussner, C.-F., P. Pfleiderer, and E. M. Fischer. 2017. "In the Observational Record Half a Degree Matters." *Nature Climate Change* 7 (June):460–2. https://doi.org/10.1038/nclimate3320.

Schuur, E. A. G., A. D. McGuire, C. Schädel, G. Grosse, J. W. Harden, D. J. Hayes, G. Hugelius et al. 2015. "Climate Change and the Permafrost Carbon Feedback." *Nature* 520 (7546):171–9. https://doi.org/10.1038/nature14338.

Shepard, C. C., V. N. Agostini, B. Gilmer, T. Allen, J. Stone, W. Brooks, and M. W. Beck. 2012. "Assessing Future Risk: Quantifying the Effects of Sea Level Rise on Storm Surge Risk for the Southern Shores of Long Island, New York." *Natural Hazards* 60 (2):727–45. https://doi.org/10.1007/s11069-011-0046-8.

Silins, U., M. Stone, M. B. Emelko, and K. D. Bladon. 2009. "Sediment Production Following Severe Wildfire and Post-Fire Salvage Logging in the Rocky Mountain Headwaters of the Oldman River Basin, Alberta." *CATENA* 79 (3):189–97.

Smale, D. A., T. Wernberg, E. C. J. Oliver, M. Thomsen, B. P. Harvey, S. C. Straub, M. T. Burrows et al. 2019. "Marine Heatwaves Threaten Global Biodiversity and the Provision of Ecosystem Services." *Nature Climate Change* 9 (4):306. https://doi.org/10.1038/s41558-019-0412-1.

Smith, M. R, G. M Singh, D. Mozaffarian, and S. S Myers. 2015. "Effects of Decreases of Animal Pollinators on Human Nutrition and Global Health: A Modelling Analysis." *Lancet* 386 (10007):1964–72. https://doi.org/10.1016/S0140-6736(15)61085-6.

Smith, V. H. 2003. "Eutrophication of Freshwater and Coastal Marine Ecosystems a Global Problem." *Environmental Science and Pollution Research* 10 (2):126–39. https://doi.org/10.1065/espr2002.12.142.

Spector, J. T., D. K. Bonauto, L. Sheppard, T. Busch-Isaksen, M. Calkins, D. Adams, M. Lieblich, and R. A. Fenske. 2016. "A Case-Crossover Study of Heat Exposure and Injury Risk in Outdoor Agricultural Workers." *PLoS One* 11 (10):e0164498. doi:10.1371/journal.pone.0164498.

Speers, A. E., E. Y. Besedin, J. E. Palardy, and C. Moore. 2016. "Impacts of Climate Change and Ocean Acidification on Coral Reef Fisheries: An Integrated Ecological–Economic Model." *Ecological Economics* 128 (August):33–43. https://doi.org/10.1016/j.ecolecon.2016.04.012.

Stigsdotter, U. K., O. Ekholm, J. Schipperijn, M. Toftager, F. Kamper-Jørgensen, and T. B. Randrup. 2010. "Health Promoting Outdoor Environments - Associations between Green Space, and Health, Health-Related Quality of Life and Stress Based on a Danish National Representative Survey." *Scandinavian Journal of Public Health* 38 (4):411–17. https://doi.org/10.1177/1403494810367468.

Suter, M. K., K. A. Miller, I. Anggraeni, K. L. Ebi, E. T. Game, J. Krenz, Y. J. Masuda et al. 2019. "Association between Work in Deforested, Compared to Forested, Areas and Human Heat Strain: An Experimental Study in a Rural Tropical Environment." *Environmental Research Letters* 14 (8):084012. doi: 10.1088/1748-9326/ab2b53.

Tan-Soo, J.-S., and S. K. Pattanayak. 2019. "Seeking Natural Capital Projects: Forest Fires, Haze, and Early-Life Exposure in Indonesia." *Proceedings of the National Academy of Scienced of the USA* 116 (12):5239–45. https://doi.org/10.1073/pnas.1802876116.

Troell, M., R. L. Naylor, M. Metian, M. Beveridge, P. H. Tyedmers, C. Folke, K. J Arrow et al. 2014. "Does Aquaculture Add Resilience to the Global Food System?" *Proceedings of the National Academy of Sciences of the USA* 111 (37):13257–63.

Tubby, K. V., and J. F. Webber. 2010. "Pests and Diseases Threatening Urban Trees under a Changing Climate." *Forestry: An International Journal of Forest Research* 83 (4):451–59. https://doi.org/10.1093/forestry/cpq027.

Tufenkji, N., J. N. Ryan, and M. Elimelech. 2002. "The Promise of Bank Filtration." *Environmental Science and Technology* 36 (November): 422A-428A. https://doi.org/10.1021/es022441j.

United Nations Environmental Programme. 2016. *Climate Change and Labour: Impacts of Heat in the Workplace*. Nairobi, Kenya: UNEP.U.S. Bureau of Economic Analysis. 2019. "Outdoor Recreation." *September* 20, 2019. https://www.bea.gov/data/special-topics/outdoor-recreation.

Van Dolah, F. M. 2000. "Marine Algal Toxins: Origins, Health Effects, and Their Increased Occurrence." *Environmental Health Perspectives* 108 (suppl 1):133–41.

Vitousek, S., P. L. Barnard, C. H. Fletcher, N. Frazer, L. Erikson, and C. D. Storlazzi. 2017. "Doubling of Coastal Flooding Frequency within Decades Due to Sea-Level Rise." *Scientific Reports* 7 (1):1399. https://doi.org/10.1038/s41598-017-01362-7.

Wahl, T., S. Jain, J. Bender, S. D. Meyers, and M. E. Luther. 2015. "Increasing Risk of Compound Flooding from Storm Surge and Rainfall for Major US Cities." *Nature Climate Change* 5 (12):1093–97. https://doi.org/10.1038/nclimate2736.

Watson, K. B., T. Ricketts, G. Galford, S. Polasky, and J. O'Niel-Dunne. 2016. "Quantifying Flood Mitigation Services: The Economic Value of Otter Creek Wetlands and Floodplains to Middlebury, VT." *Ecological Economics* 130 (October):16–24. https://doi.org/10.1016/j.ecolecon.2016.05.015.

Watts, N., M. Amann, S. Ayeb-Karlsson, K. Belesova, T. Bouley, M. Boykoff, P. Byass et al. 2018. "The Lancet Countdown on Health and Climate Change: From 25 Years of Inaction to a Global Transformation for Public Health." *Lancet* 391 (10120):581–630. https://doi.org/10.1016/S0140-6736(18)32594-7.

WAVES (Wealth Accounting and the Valuation of Ecosystem Services). 2017. *Valuing the Protection Services of Mangroves in the Philippines: Policy Brief*. Washington, DC: World Bank. https://www.wavespartnership.org/sites/waves/files/kc/Policy%20Brief%20Valuing%20Protective%20Services%20of%20Mangroves%20in%20the%20Philippines.compressed.pdf.

Waycott, M., C. M. Duarte, T. J. B. Carruthers, R. J. Orth, W. C. Dennison, S. Olyarnik, A. Calladine et al. 2009. "Accelerating Loss of Seagrasses across the Globe Threatens Coastal Ecosystems." *Proceedings of the National Academy of Sciences of the USA* 106 (30):12377–81.

Webb, P., G. A. Stordalen, S. Singh, R. Wijesinha-Bettoni, P. Shetty, and A. Lartey. 2018. "Hunger and Malnutrition in the 21st Century." *BMJ* 361 (June):k2238. https://doi.org/10.1136/bmj.k2238.

Webster, N., and R. Hill. 2007. "Vulnerability of Marine Microbes on the Great Barrier Reef to Climate Change." *In Climate Change and the Great Barrier Reef*. Canberra: Australian Greenhouse Office.

Wesseling, C., J. Crowe, C. Hogstedt, K. Jakobsson, R. Lucas, and D. H. Wegman. 2013. "The Epidemic of Chronic Kidney Disease of Unknown Etiology in Mesoamerica: A Call for Interdisciplinary Research and Action." *American Journal of Public Health* 103 (11):1927–30. https://doi.org/10.2105/AJPH.2013.301594.

Westerling, A. L., H. G. Hidalgo, D. R. Cayan, and T. W. Swetnam. 2006. "Warming and Earlier Spring Increase Western U.S. Forest Wildfire Activity." *Science* 313 (5789):940–3. https://doi.org/10.1126/science.1128834.

Weyer, P. J., J. R. Cerhan, B. C. Kross, G. R. Hallberg, J. Kantamneni, G. Breuer, M. P. Jones, W. Zheng, and C. F. Lynch. 2001. "Municipal Drinking Water Nitrate Level and Cancer Risk in Older Women: The Iowa Women's Health Study." *Epidemiology* 12 (3):327.

Wobus, C., E. Gutmann, R. Jones, M. Rissing, N. Mizukami, M. Lorie, H. Mahoney et al. 2017. "Climate Change Impacts on Flood Risk and Asset Damages within Mapped 100-Year Floodplains of the Contiguous United States." *Natural Hazards and Earth System Sciences* 17 (12):2199–2211. https://doi.org/10.5194/nhess-17-2199-2017.

Wood, S. A., and F. Baudron. 2018. "Soil Organic Matter Underlies Crop Nutritional Quality and Productivity in Smallholder Agriculture." *Agriculture, Ecosystems & Environment* 266:100–8.

World Health Organization. 2002. *WHO Traditional Medicine Strategy 2002–2005*. Geneva: WHO. https://www.who.int/medicines/publications/traditionalpolicy/en/.

World Health Organization. 2011. *Nitrage and Nitrite in Drinking-Water: Background Document for Development of WHO Guidelines for Drinking-Water Quality*. Geneva: WHO. https://www.who.int/water_sanitation_health/dwq/chemicals/nitratenitrite2ndadd.pdf.

Wright, L. D., C. F. D'Elia, and C. R. Nichols. 2019. "Impacts of Coastal Waters and Flooding on Human Health." In *Tomorrow's Coasts: Complex and Impermanent*, edited by L. D. Wright and C. R. Nichols, 151–66. Coastal Research Library. Cham: Springer International Publishing. https://doi.org/10.1007/978-3-319-75453-6_10.

Xu, D., L. Han, C. Li, Q. Cao, D. Zhu, N. H. Barrett, D. Harmody et al. 2018. "Bioprospecting Deep-Sea Actinobacteria for Novel Anti-Infective Natural Products." *Frontiers in Microbiology* 9.

Yeager, R., D. W. Riggs, N. DeJarnett, D. J. Tollerud, J. Wilson, D. J. Conklin, T. E. O'Toole et al. 2018. "Association between Residential Greenness and Cardiovascular Disease Risk." *Journal of the American Heart Association* 7 (24):e009117. https://doi.org/10.1161/JAHA.118.009117.

Young, H. S., C. L. Wood, A. M. Kilpatrick, K. D. Lafferty, C. L. Nunn, and J. R. Vincent. 2017. "Conservation, Biodiversity and Infectious Disease: Scientific Evidence and Policy Implications." *Philosophical Transactions of the Royal Society B: Biological Sciences* 372 (1722):20160124. https://doi.org/10.1098/rstb.2016.0124.

Zhao, C., B. Liu, S. Piao, X. Wang, D. B. Lobell, Y. Huang, M. Huang et al. 2017. "Temperature Increase Reduces Global Yields of Major Crops in Four Independent Estimates." *Proceedings of the National Academy of Sciences of the USA* 114 (35):9326–31. https://doi.org/10.1073/pnas.1701762114.

Zhao, Q., R. Li, Y. Gao, Q. Yao, X. Guo, and W. Wang. 2018. "Modeling Impacts of Climate Change on the Geographic Distribution of Medicinal Plant Fritillaria Cirrhosa D. Don." *Plant Biosystems* 152 (3):349–55. https://doi.org/10.1080/11263504.2017.1289273.

Ziska, L. H., D. M. Blumenthal, G. B. Runion, E. R. Hunt, and H. Diaz-Soltero. 2011. "Invasive Species and Climate Change: An Agronomic Perspective." *Climatic Change* 105 (1):13–42. https://doi.org/10.1007/s10584-010-9879-5.

Ziska, L. H., and J. A. Bunce. 2007. "Predicting the Impact of Changing CO_2 on Crop Yields: Some Thoughts on Food." *New Phytologist* 175 (4):607–18.

CHAPTER 30

CLIMATE CHANGE AND HEALTH IN ALASKA: HOW DO THINGS COMPARE WITH THE "LOWER 48"?

Micah Hahn

Introduction

Spanning almost 580,000 square miles, Alaska is nearly one fifth the size of the contiguous United States. This vast region includes 34,000 miles of shoreline and three million lakes and covers many different ecosystems, ranging from Arctic tundra to coastal rainforests (Alaska Department of Fish and Game 2019). With its huge variation in geography and natural features, there is also a wide range of environmental changes happening in Alaska because of climate change (Markon et al. 2018). Although there are only a handful of meteorologic stations in Alaska with historical weather information (Alaska Climate Research Center 2019), climate modeling work over the past two decades and more recent efforts to summarize meteorologic trends for the state have provided a wealth of information about the environmental changes that are occurring in Alaska.

Simultaneously, our understanding of the human health impacts of climate change in Alaska is still developing. Much of the effort in this field has centered around community-based monitoring approaches that provide a means to track changes in environmental hazards in a specific area so that communities can evaluate the potential risk of particular activities. There have been few epidemiologic assessments of adverse health outcomes from climate change in Alaska. The dearth of research in this area is in part due to the lack of readily available clinical records and epidemiologically relevant environmental data from around the state. Additionally, many of the most prevalent health impacts in Alaska are the result of complex ecological pathways that are difficulty to untangle. Further, isolated communities with small populations make it difficult to establish statistically robust quantitative assessments.

This chapter describes climate and health in the Alaskan context, highlighting some of the environmental changes and health impacts that are unique compared to the contiguous United States. It also includes examples of how Alaskan communities have started to address health concerns related to a changing climate and discusses the future role of public health in addressing these issues in the state.

Environmental Change in Alaska

Many of the environmental anomalies that have been observed in Alaska mirror the changes that are happening in the Pacific Northwest (May et al. 2018). The annual average temperature in Alaska has been increasing steadily since the late 1970s (Markon et al. 2018) and is now 3 to 4°F warmer than the long-term average between 1951 and 1980 (Thoman and Walsh 2019). The most substantial changes in temperature are occurring in winter when the recent seasonal temperatures were

KEY CONCEPTS

- Alaska is almost one fifth the size of the contiguous United States. An understanding of climate change in the state almost always requires regional assessments. Some of the health impacts of climate change in the state are similar to those observed in the Pacific Northwest and other parts of the United States, but infrastructure and access to resources, reliance on wild foods, and winter travel strategies present unique challenges to Alaskan residents that are more similar to other Arctic regions.

- There are limited epidemiologic assessments of climate-related health impacts in Alaska. Much of our understanding comes from community-based monitoring and observations.

- OneHealth, or the connection between human, animal, and environmental health, is an important framework for understanding and planning for the health impacts of climate change in the state due to lifestyles that have people living close to the land.

- Many Alaskan communities are developing climate adaptation plans that are motivated by concerns about the health impacts of climate change. Public health has an important role to play in advancing climate solutions that simultaneously mitigate climate change while improving health outcomes and health equity in Alaska.

over 5°F warmer than the historical average across most of the state (Figure 30.1). Interior Alaska, known for frigid winter temperatures, is experiencing fewer very cold days below -30°F (Thoman and Walsh), and many northern communities are observing record-setting high temperatures during the spring transition (National Oceanic and Atmospheric Administration National Climatic Data Center 2019).

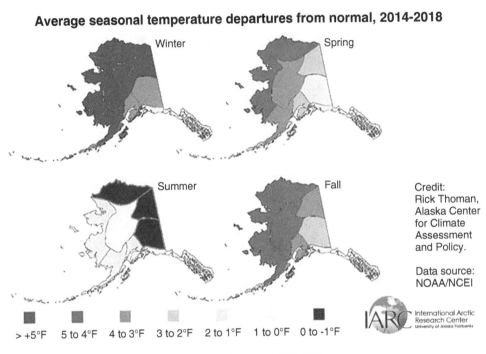

Average seasonal temperature departures from normal, 2014-2018

Figure 30.1 Average seasonal temperature departures from normal, 2014–2018
Source: Reprinted with permission from Thoman and Walsh (2019).

Average annual precipitation across Alaska has increased over the last fifty years, but year-to-year variability is large (Bieniek et al. 2014; Thoman and Walsh 2019). Regional droughts, or periods of lower than average precipitation, have occurred in parts of Alaska in the past, but new tools have allowed us to compare recent Alaskan conditions to the contiguous United States. For example, Alaska experienced a period of drought between July 2018 and October 2019. In the last week of August 2019, 1.5 percent of the state (land area roughly equivalent to the size of New Hampshire) was in "extreme drought" (National Drought Mitigation Center 2019). Many rural communities that depend on snowmelt to fill drinking water reservoirs and hydroelectric power implemented short-term water conservation strategies to deal with the shortage (Leffler 2019; City of Cordova Alaska 2019; Jenkins 2019).

Like much of the western United States, the wildfire season in Alaska is beginning earlier, and the frequency of large wildfire seasons (> 1 million acres burned) has increased 50 percent since 1990, compared to the prior four decades (Markon et al. 2018; Thoman and Walsh 2019). In 2019, Alaska's interagency fire management organization extended the wildfire season an additional month (through September 30) due to the warm, dry conditions and ongoing fires (Alaska Department of Natural Resources 2019).

Warm anomalies in the North Pacific ocean have affected Alaskan and Pacific Northwest waters in similar ways, leading to substantial impacts on a number of fisheries across the region (Bond et al. 2015; Barbeaux et al. 2018). Similarly, increasing river temperatures and declining flows to key spawning grounds have resulted in massive salmon dieoff events in both the Northwest and Alaska in recent years (Martin 2019; Sherwood 2015).

Although the trends in warming temperatures, wildfire risk, and changing ocean and river ecosystems are similar to the changes observed elsewhere in the continental United States, Alaska faces environmental challenges that are unique to high latitude regions of the world. Alaska is warming twice as fast as the global average, and recent statewide average temperatures have been exceptionally warm (Markon et al. 2018). Four of the past five years (2014–2016, 2018) were the warmest on record for the state (Thoman and Walsh 2019). Although the annual average temperature has increased across the state compared to the historical average (1951–1980), this ranges from 2.3°F of warming in the southeast to almost 6°F in the northernmost region of Alaska (Thoman and Walsh).

One of the starkest indicators of climate change in Alaska is changing sea ice. Sea ice plays an important role in regional climate, human activities, and ecosystem functions in the northern part of the state. Recent maps of the Chuckchi and Beaufort Seas demonstrate the substantial decline in sea ice that has occurred in the waters around Alaska (Figure 30.2). Because of this loss of sea ice, there is open water off the northern coast of Alaska for three to four months per year compared to a few days or weeks per year in the 1980s (Thoman and Walsh 2019).

Sea ice concentration off Alaska, 1988 vs. 2018

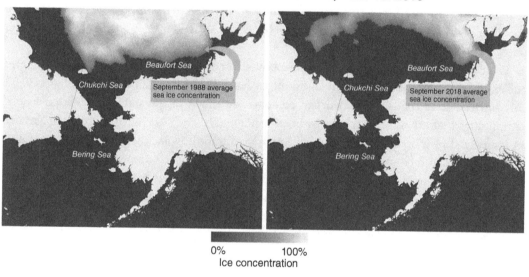

Credit: Rick Thoman, Alaska Center for Climate Assessment and Policy.
Data source: NSIDC

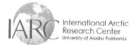

International Arctic
Research Center
University of Alaska Fairbanks

Figure 30.2   Sea ice concentration off Alaska, 1988 vs. 2018
Reprinted with permission from Thoman and Walsh (2019).

Permafrost, or ground that remains frozen for two or more years, is found beneath about half of Alaska (Markon et al. 2018). Permafrost has been thawing in Arctic regions of Alaska since the 1970s (Markon et al.), and the highest rates of near-surface warming are occurring on the North Slope (Thoman and Walsh 2019).

More than 90 percent of Alaska's glaciers are receding (Thoman and Walsh 2019). The rate of thaw between 1994 and 2013 is nearly double the 1962–2006 rate, and recent modeling studies suggest that this rate will likely continue to increase (Markon et al. 2018).

If Alaska were overlaid on the contiguous United States, it would reach from California to Florida and stretch from northern Minnesota down to Texas. The state contains a wide variety of ecosystems, including Arctic tundra in communities like Utqiagvik and Kaktovik, coastal rainforests in Ketchikan, and maritime meadows on volcanic islands in the Aleutians (Nowacki et al. 2001). Given the size and ecological diversity in the state, it is not surprising that there is enormous variation in the climate-related environmental changes that are happening throughout Alaska. Indeed, as we begin to think about the impact of these changes on the health of Alaskans, a key starting point is that your **exposure** to climate-related health threats depends on where you live in the state. In northern Alaska, the retreat of sea ice has left coastal communities vulnerable to storm surge and coastal erosion. In interior Alaska, thawing permafrost increasingly challenges roads and infrastructure. Warming oceans and changes to the marine ecosystem are putting pressure on fisheries that are the economic engine of many coastal communities. In southcentral and southeast Alaska, warming temperatures support a more rapid spruce bark beetle reproduction cycle, making Alaskan forests more susceptible to wildfires (Bentz et al. 2010; Werner et al. 2006). Mapping out the climate and health links in Alaska necessitates a regional approach to account for the diversity of environmental changes happening through the state.

How Is Alaska Different from the Contiguous United States?

In order to understand how climate change is affecting the health of Alaskans, it is important to understand three unique characteristics of life in Alaska: infrastructure and access to resources in urban and rural communities, reliance on **subsistence** foods, and winter travel strategies.

Over half of Alaskans live in the major population centers of Anchorage, Fairbanks, and Juneau, but the majority of Alaskan communities have fewer than 1,500 people (Figure 30.3). Only thirteen state roads connect urban centers, and much of the state's population live in communities that are only accessible by boat or plane (Driscoll 2015). Most rural villages are not connected to a major power grid, and many communities lack indoor piped water and sewer and instead rely on hauling water from a community water treatment facility, using a communal "washeteria" for showers, laundry, and flush toilets, or bucket toilets inside their home (Thomas et al. 2013). Communities with a majority Alaska Native population are largely located in northern, western, and interior Alaska, whereas communities with a predominantly nonnative population are located along the road system (Figure 30.3). The lack of road access and geographic spread of Alaska's rural communities severely limits the availability of health care and emergency response resources and defines the distribution system for food and household goods. Although there is usually a grocery or general store in each community, the availability of goods varies, and many people supplement their households with trips to commercial centers by plane or ferry.

Many Alaskans rely on subsistence hunting, fishing, and gathering as part of their household food supply and livelihood. This reliance on customary and traditional uses of wild, renewable resources for direct personal or family use as food, shelter, fuel, clothing, tools, or transportation means that changes in the distribution of key animal or plant species could significantly change dietary patterns or affect a household's main source of income.

Finally, the lack of a paved road system connecting much of the state means that Alaskans often use unique forms of transportation. In particular, during the winter, many frozen rivers transform to highways connecting communities that are normally separated by wilderness. For example, a team of people construct an ice road each winter across nearly 200 miles of the Kuskokwim River in Southwest Alaska. This temporary highway means that trucks can bring supplies into communities, and the 13,000 people in the region have the ability to drive to Bethel, the biggest town in the region, for medical appointments and shopping (O'Malley 2019).

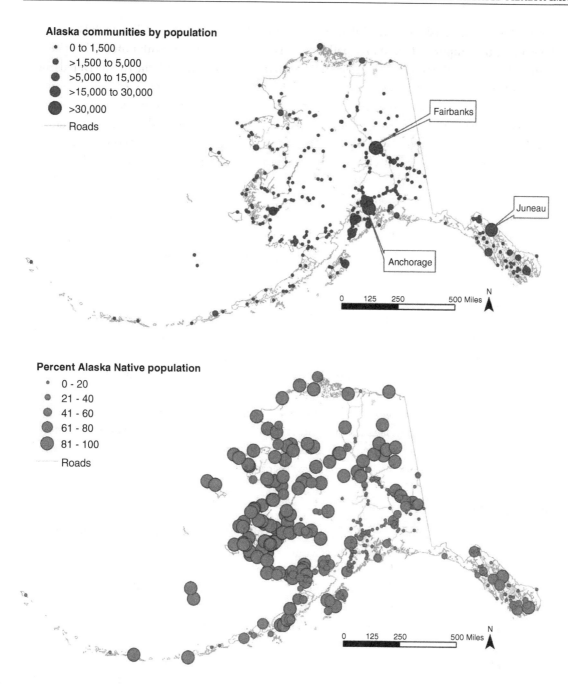

Figure 30.3 Map of the distribution and population size of Alaskan communities (top). Map of the distribution of the Alaska Native population in Alaska (bottom

Climate-Related Health Impacts in Alaska

Despite limited epidemiologic assessments of climate-related health outcomes in Alaska, community observations and to some extent, a broader look at the health impacts in other parts of the country, have helped identify the most likely health impacts of climate change in the state. One of the longest-running resources for community observations on environmental change is the Local Environmental Observer (LEO) Network where the public can submit observations of unusual environmental events and receive a response from a subject matter expert who can provide more context (Alaska Native Tribal Health Consortium 2019b). In addition, several rural communities have initiated qualitative community climate change health assessments supported by the Alaska Native Tribal Health Consortium's Center for Climate & Health that have identified important **exposure** pathways linking climate drivers with potential impacts to human health (Alaska Native Tribal Health Consortium 2019a). In 2018, the Alaska Department of Health and Social Services published a comprehensive health impact assessment of climate change in the state, which provides a broad overview of many of the potential health concerns in Alaska as well as a system for ranking health impacts to help with adaptation planning (Yoder et al. 2018). Although much of the climate and health research in the contiguous United States focuses on exposures like increased temperatures and rising sea levels that have direct health impacts, many climate-related health issues in Alaska are the result of complex ecological webs linking environmental change, culture and traditional lifestyles, and wildlife health. Some of the most pressing climate-related health concerns in Alaska are summarized next.

Accidents and Injuries due to Changing Winter Conditions

The rapid warming of winter in Alaska poses several challenges to human health, although these hazards vary in rural and urban communities. In rural communities, winter travel and hunting or fishing is often by snowmobile and depends on consistently frozen ice roads, described previously. As winters are becoming shorter and warmer, thinning ice has made travel conditions more hazardous. An epidemiologic assessment of 307 "falling through ice" events in Alaska between 1990 and 2010 showed that over a third of the events ended in a fatality and over half involved travel by snowmobile (Fleischer et al. 2014). In contrast, warmer winters in Alaska's urban centers have led to a higher frequency of "rain on snow" events that have challenged road maintenance crews to keep roads ice free and safe for automobile travel in order to prevent injuries and deaths from road accidents (Hao 2018; Richardson 2014). Across Alaska, avalanches may become more common as freeze-thaw cycles create unstable snow pack (Berwyn 2019).

Air Quality Impacts

Many of the air quality impacts of climate change in Alaska are similar to those seen in other parts of the United States. The wildfire season in Alaska is beginning earlier, and the frequency of large wildfire seasons (> one million acres burned) has increased 50 percent since 1990, compared to the prior four decades (Markon et al. 2018; Thoman and Walsh 2019). In parallel, the number of smoky days in Alaska's largest cities has also increased (Figure 30.4), exposing residents to a variety of pollutants of public health concern, including carbon monoxide (CO), nitrogen oxides (NO_x), ozone (O_3), volatile organic compounds (VOCs), as well as particulate matter (PM) (Phuleria et al. 2005). There is evidence that recent Alaskan wildfires have caused substantial asthma exacerbations in major population centers in the state (Hahn, in review).

Pollen and mold are other important climate-related environmental exposures in Alaska. People with allergies or asthma are particularly affected by these irritants. There are pollen and mold counting programs in Anchorage and Fairbanks, the two largest urban areas in the state. The counts in these cities occur two to five times per week during the allergy season and provide information on the seasonal timing and abundance of their release (Alaska Department of Health and Social Services 2017). These data show that in recent years, pollen counts in these areas were an order of magnitude above levels considered high by allergists (Alaska Department of Health and Social Services). The main source of pollen in Alaska is birch trees. Vegetation projections for Alaska show that vegetation succession after wildfires is a substantial driver of land cover in the state (Johnstone et al. 2011). The relative composition of coniferous and deciduous trees will determine the severity of pollen concentrations in the future.

Finally, dust from vehicles on dirt roads and wind-blown dust from dry river beds and glaciers is another source of air quality concerns in Alaska (Alaska Department of Environmental

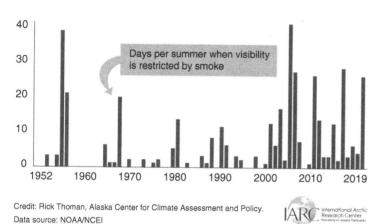

Figure 30.4 Smoky days in Alaska, 1952–2019
Source: Reprinted with permission from Thoman and Walsh (2019).

Conservation 2019b). Dry and warm conditions can exacerbate dust events and cause respiratory problems for nearby communities.

Food Safety, Nutrition, and Distribution

Many of the stressors around food and nutrition in Alaska stem from the substantial role of subsistence foods in an Alaskan diet and the climate-mediated ecological changes that are negatively affecting these animal and plant species. In 2012, Alaskans harvested almost 50 million lbs of wild fish, land and sea mammals, and wild plants for personal use (Fall 2016). On average, people living in rural areas harvested 295 lbs of wild resources (usable weight after filleting or field dressing animals) per capita. By weight, over half of the harvest was fish and shellfish, followed by land mammals (22.7 percent), marine mammals (14.0 percent), bird/eggs (2.7 percent), and wild plants (3.9 percent). Urban residents tend to gather comparatively fewer wild resources (22 lbs per person), and they predominantly harvest fish and land mammals. The rural subsistence harvest provides about 26 percent (554 kcal/per person/per day) of the average daily caloric needs in a typical 2100 kcal/day diet (Fall 2016) so a poor salmon return or lack of solid sea or river ice for transportation can have a significant impact on the available food resources in a household.

Ice cellars are vertical shafts built into the permafrost and used as frozen food storage (typically subsistence meat harvests) in many northern rural communities in Alaska. Anecdotally, residents have reported that ice cellars are failing more frequently. A decade-long monitoring program in a handful of cellars found that although the temperature inside the cellars did not increase substantially, the condition of many of the cellars deteriorated over the course of the study (Nyland et al. 2017). In addition to disturbance from nearby construction activity, flooding, and changes in the thaw depth of permafrost and salinity of the soil were noted as threats to the structural integrity of the cellars (Nyland et al.). Without safe food storage, harvested wild meats could spoil and leave households without a consistent protein source (Yoder et al. 2018).

Another important link between a changing climate and food resources in Alaska are harmful algal blooms (HABs) that produce a toxin that accumulates in shellfish and can cause paralytic shellfish poisoning (PSP), a potentially fatal neuroparalytic condition, when affected shellfish are eaten. Butter clams, mussels, razor clams, and cockles are some of the most commonly harvested by Alaskan residents (Southeast Alaska Tribal Toxins Network 2019a).

Warmer ocean temperatures off the coast of Alaska can support the growth of HABs associated with PSP (Southeast Alaska Tribal Toxins Network 2019b). Between 1993 and 2014, 117 PSP cases were reported to the Alaska state health department (Alaska Department of Health and Social Services 2015). Consumption of butter clams or mussels was associated with over half of these cases, and all cases were caused by toxin produced by *Alexandrium* algae. Another algae species that produces domoic acid has not caused any human cases in Alaska to date, but a 2015 bloom that stretched from southern California to Southeast Alaska closed commercial shellfish harvest areas along the coast (National Oceanic and Atmospheric Administration 2016). The Alaska Department of Environmental Conservation tests commercially harvested shellfish. There is currently no state-based testing program for recreational or subsistence shellfish harvest, but regional community-based monitoring has started to address this need and is discussed further in the section *Surveillance for climate-related exposures and health outcomes in Alaska*). There is also evidence that marine mammals, another important food source for Alaskans, are also being exposed to these toxins (Lefebvre et al. 2016).

A large outbreak of *Vibro parahaemolyticus* in Alaskan oysters on a cruise ship in 2004 was the northernmost documentation of *V. parahaemolyticus* illness (McLaughlin et al. 2005). Warmer than normal ocean temperatures at the farm where the oysters were harvested may have played a role in the outbreak (McLaughlin et al. 2005). This pathogen may become more of a concern in the state, particularly in coastal communities.

Vector-Borne Disease

There have been no reported locally acquired human cases of tick-borne disease in Alaska. Tularemia is a bacterial disease present in the state, but most cases of tularemia in domestic animals and humans in Alaska have been the result of handling infected wildlife rather than a tick bite (Alaska Department of Environmental Conservation (2021)). Despite the lack of clinical cases of tick-borne disease, trends in milder winters and other ecological changes have raised the concern that vector-borne diseases could emerge as a public health threat in the state (Yoder et al. 2018).

Although there are records of six tick species in Alaska from the early to mid-20th century, little is known about their distribution, abundance, or role as vectors of tick-borne pathogens. There is evidence that several species of nonnative ticks that are known vectors in the Lower 48 are being imported into the state (Durden, Beckmen, and Gerlach 2016). Most of the ticks reported to date have arrived on people and pets traveling outside of the state (Hahn et al. 2020a). Current work on ticks and tick-borne diseases in Alaska focuses on developing systematic surveillance in order to track trends in tick distribution and the establishment of nonnative species in the state (Hahn et al. 2020a).

CLINICAL CORRELATES 30.1 WHY TICK SURVEILLANCE IS AN IMPORTANT CLINICAL TOOL

Ticks transmit a remarkable diversity of viral, bacterial, nematode, and protozoan pathogens (Jongejan and Uilenberg 2004; Otranto et al. 2012), and the distribution of many ticks and tick-borne diseases continues to expand across the United States (Eisen et al. 2017; Sonenshine 2018). In clinical settings, clinicians rely on patient history to guide their differential diagnosis. Many tick-borne diseases present with nonspecific symptoms—fever, chills, muscle and joint aches—that are easily mistaken for other diseases. Without accurate information on the distribution of tick species and tick-borne pathogens, we run the risk of misdiagnosis, incorrect treatment, and undiagnosed severe, chronic disease.

There exists an imperative to monitor tick and tick-borne pathogens in our changing climate to ensure accurate diagnoses and appropriate prevention strategies.

Emerging Zoonotic Diseases

In May 2019, the Centers for Disease Control and Prevention Arctic Investigation Branch led a zoonotic disease prioritization workshop (Salyer et al. 2017) that included representatives from the state public health, veterinary, and wildlife agencies, tribal organizations, the University of Alaska, and several federal agencies. The goal of the workshop was to identify the most pressing zoonotic threats in the state based on clinical outcomes, prevalence, food safety and security concerns, potential social and economic impacts, response capacity, and the impact of changing environmental conditions. The top-priority zoonotic diseases identified during the workshop were amnesic and paralytic shellfish poisoning, zoonotic influenza, rabies, cryptosporidiosis, giardiasis, toxoplasmosis, brucellosis, and Q fever. The next step is to assess laboratory and surveillance capabilities and outbreak response and preparedness and identify gaps where additional development and capacity is needed.

CLINICAL CORRELATES 30.2 FOX AND RABIES TRANSMISSION

Rabies is a viral disease transmitted to humans through bites and scratches of infected animals. The disease is almost universally fatal with infection spread to the brain and central nervous system. It is prevented through vaccination of pets and avoiding contact with wild animals that most commonly carry the disease (bats, foxes, skunks, raccoons). Postexposure prophylaxis is available as a series given as human rabies immune globulin and through a vaccine. In Alaska, geographic information system and modeling have been used to compare human rabies cases with areas of urbanization to better inform public health decisions (Huettmann, Magnuson, and Hueffer 2017). Both arctic and red foxes in the northern regions are known reservoirs for the disease, yet climactic changes are expected to shift transmission patterns increasingly toward rabid red foxes rather than arctic foxes (Kim et al. 2014).

Shifting patterns of rabies disease transmission from animal reservoirs affected by warming temperatures and urbanization serve as important areas of interest for public health.

Mental Health and Well-Being

Climate change affects mental and behavioral health through a variety of causal pathways in Alaska. Acute events such as wildfire and extreme coastal storms and the associated destruction and loss of property, stress from traveling in unusual conditions such as unstable ice, and loss of cultural sites such as graveyards and traditional burial grounds creates stressors that can cause anxiety and depression as well as exacerbate existing mental health issues. In 2018, 21.2 percent of Alaskans reported that they been diagnosed with depression at some point in their lives (Alaska Department of Health and Social Services 2019). Several Alaska Native communities have already or are making plans to relocate because of threats from flooding and erosion. This huge shift in livelihoods and sense of place, concerns about safety, and the disruption caused in social and cultural activities are likely a substantial source of stress and depression (Bell et al. 2010).

The impacts of climate change on wild food resources is likely another important concern for mental health in Alaska. The unpredictable nature of wild foods and changes to the environment that make hunting or fishing more difficult can be an added stressor for families. Commercial fishing is an important livelihood in Alaska; In 2018 fishing employment brought in nearly $600 million in gross earnings for state residents (Warren 2019).

As in many places, the most pervasive impacts of climate change on mental in Alaska are likely through ecological grief, or "the grief felt in relation to experienced or anticipated ecological losses, including the loss of species, ecosystems and meaningful landscapes due to acute or chronic environmental change" (Cunsolo and Ellis 2018). Alaskans may be particularly affected by this sense of grief because of the deep connection of many people to the land, historically, through a reliance on natural resources, recreationally, and as a part of their cultural identity. Preliminary results from an ongoing study on the mental health impacts of wildfires in south-central Alaska show that residents report experiencing grief and feelings of loss associated with changes to the landscape after recent wildfires (M. Hahn, personal communication).

Temperature-Related Death and Illness

Although heat-related illness and death have not historically been a concern in Alaska, recent record-breaking summer temperatures (Di Liberto 2019) have opened the conversation within the public health community. Extreme heat exposures are defined in comparison to the average temperature in a given location (Sarofim et al. 2016). This means that an 29°C (85°F) day in Anchorage, Alaska may have a different health impact than an 29°C (85°F) day in Florida or Texas. Epidemiologic evidence shows that increases in temperature have a bigger impact on heat-related deaths and hospitalizations in areas where temperatures are typically cooler (Sarofim et al. 2016; Lee et al. 2014; Medina-Ramón and Schwartz 2007). This may be due to acclimatization as well as lack of air conditioning or other strategies to escape the heat in places that have historically had more moderate summer temperatures (Medina-Ramón and Schwartz 2007). In Alaska, buildings are designed to keep heat in and air conditioners are uncommon. Additionally, the dual exposures of smoke from wildfires coupled with warmer than normal temperatures means that residents are torn between staying inside and closing their windows and opening up their home to cool down.

Water-Related Shortages and Illnesses

Water and sanitation infrastructure in many rural Alaskan communities is threatened by thawing permafrost, extreme storms, and erosion. Lack of solid ground means that pipes bend and break. Damage to sewage lagoons can cause contamination of water sources for drinking, washing, and laundry (Brubaker et al. 2011; Thomas et al. 2013), and thawing permafrost can increase the turbidity of surface water. Erosion and shifting ground can cause local lakes and reservoirs to drain. Adequate water and sanitation when communities are relocating is another persistent challenge. The Alaska Native Tribal Health Consortium is developing and testing a portable sanitation system water called PASS with the intent of increasing access for homes without piped systems due to environmental conditions or pending relocation (Alaska Native Tribal Health Consortium 2016, 2019c).

OneHealth: An Alaskan Framework for Addressing the Health Impacts of Climate Change

Many of the adverse health impacts of climate change in Alaska fall at the intersection of human, animal, and environmental health. For example, changing environmental conditions that have a negative impact on salmon runs challenge an important cultural, food, and livelihood resource for Alaskans (The Salmon Project 2019). Similarly, the establishment of nonnative ticks in Alaska could pose a threat to human, domestic animal, and wildlife health. Perhaps because of the degree to which the natural world is intertwined into daily life in Alaska through food, recreation, and income, the **OneHealth** framework that acknowledges this overlap has been a foundational concept for much of the Alaskan climate and health work to date (Ruscio et al. 2015).

For several years, the Centers for Disease Control and Prevention Arctic Investigation Program and Alaska Native Tribal Health Consortium (ANTHC) have hosted quarterly OneHealth meetings to share recent climate-related environmental or outbreak events and to discuss emerging OneHealth issues. Dozens of researchers join these meetings, creating an informal network of epidemiologists, veterinarians, clinicians, and biologists across Alaska who are familiar with investigations and recent findings from human and animal agencies and intuitions in the state.

The University of Alaska Fairbanks Center for OneHealth Research has recently formed to improve research capacity and more effectively promote holistic well-being in the circumpolar North. The mission of this hub is to be a coordination center for interdisciplinary teams to design research, education, and outreach programs around OneHealth in the state (University of Alaska Fairbanks 2019).

At the state level, coordination between the Department of Health and Social Services (DHSS), the Office of the State Veterinarian (OSV), and the Alaska Department of Fish and Game (ADFG) (i.e., human, domestic animal, and wildlife health agencies, respectively) on emerging threats related to climate change are common. For example, DHSS monitors human cases of shellfish poisoning, OSV conducts testing for the commercial shellfish industry, and ADFG regulates subsistence and recreational harvest of shellfish. Similarly, with regard to ticks and tick-borne disease, DHSS monitors human cases of tick-borne disease, OSV receives tick samples from the state surveillance program (See the next section), and ADFG offices across the state are drop sites for tick specimens from the public.

Surveillance for Climate-Related Exposures and Health Outcomes in Alaska

Perhaps due to the strong OneHealth community in the state, much of the early epidemiologic work on climate and health in Alaska has focused on emerging threats at the intersection of human and animal health. Within this broad field of research, there have been several efforts to develop surveillance programs to collect ongoing information to quantify human health risk. Many of these programs have focused on environmental or wildlife monitoring rather than relying on human case reports of disease. The reason for this is threefold. First, these early surveillance programs are assessing emerging threats to human health that have caused few or no cases of human illness in the state. Second, because of the small human population in Alaska compared to other states, environmental or wildlife monitoring may be a more sensitive indicator of emerging threats. Finally, monitoring environmental data can help define the exposure pathway of these hazards and provide a target for intervention in a way that assessing human cases cannot.

Although the State of Alaska monitors harmful algal bloom toxins in the commercial shellfish industry, there is not a state program for phytoplankton monitoring or testing shellfish for subsistence or recreational harvest. As a result, regional monitoring programs have started to address this gap (Alaska Harmful Algal Bloom Network 2019). For example, Southeast Alaska Tribal Ocean Research (SEATOR) was formed in September 2013 to unify sixteen southeast Alaska tribes to collect weekly phytoplankton and water samples and biweekly shellfish samples for toxin testing (Southeast Alaska Tribal Toxins Network 2013). Shellfish samples are analyzed within forty-eight hours and posted to the online data portal so that communities can use this information to make decisions about when and where they can safely harvest shellfish.

The population living in Northwest Alaska is highly dependent on a traditional subsistence diet, which includes marine and terrestrial wildlife. The emergence of zoonotic pathogens, previously unknown in Alaskan wildlife and the release of mercury (Hg) from thawing permafrost threaten a culturally and nutritionally important food source. Additionally, the lack of strong health surveillance infrastructure in rural Alaska means that communities have limited information to monitor their risk to these emerging threats. The Alaska Native Tribal Health Consortium worked with the University of Alaska Fairbanks to develop laboratory methods and field test a blood paper test strip that communities could use to detect emerging zoonotic pathogens and contaminants (Berner 2014). Through the Rural Alaska Monitoring Program (RAMP), hunters were provided filter paper kits that they could use to take a blood sample of hunted animals (Figure 30.5). After the blood dried, they mailed the samples in for testing. This pilot community-based surveillance program empowered Alaska Native communities to monitor their risk of exposure and in order to develop appropriate adaptation strategies so they can maintain consumption of culturally important and healthy subsistence foods while reducing risk of exposure to zoonotic pathogens.

Veterinarians and the public have started finding ticks on people and pets more often than in the past. Many of the recently identified ticks are non-native, meaning that they are not known to be established in the state (Hahn et al. 2020a). In 2019, the University of

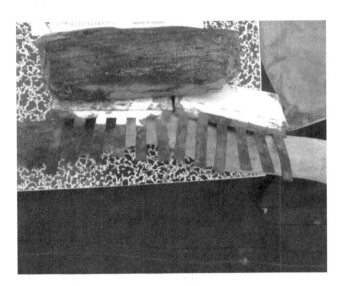

Figure 30.5   Filter paper strips properly soaked, air drying on a piece of driftwood, before being put in a prelabeled envelope and mailed to the laboratory as part of the biomonitoring program
Source: Photo courtesy of Jim Berner, Photo credit: Mike Brubaker.

Alaska-Anchorage, the Alaska Office of the State Veterinarian, and the Alaska Department of Fish and Game established the Alaska Submit-A-Tick Program (Hahn et al. 2020a). Through this surveillance program, the public, biologists, or clinicians can turn in ticks they find on themselves, pets, wildlife, or in the environment for species identification and testing. The information collected through this surveillance system will be used to monitor how many nonnative ticks are being imported through human and pet travel outside of the state and to identify areas of Alaska where nonnative ticks may become established. Additionally, these data will be used to assess the risk of tick-borne pathogen transmission from native tick species in Alaska.

The air quality monitoring network in Alaska is run by the Alaska Department of Environmental Conservation (Alaska Department of Environmental Conservation 2019a). Air quality monitors are located in large population centers based on the requirements for Environmental Protection Agency monitoring. As a result of the wildfires and long-term poor air quality in many parts of the state in 2019, many individuals and organizations installed

PurpleAir monitors to track local air quality conditions (Ellis 2019). Data are centralized on the PurpleAir network website, but it is yet to be seen how this or other similar air monitoring technology can be utilized to support public health.

A common theme of the surveillance systems discussed here is the reliance on community-based data collection and reporting. Despite limitations of citizen science, these community-based surveillance methods allow continuous data collection over a huge area of the state with relatively low human and financial resources. In the Alaskan context, this data collection strategy is particularly useful for monitoring emerging threats and identifying sentinel events as part of an early warning system. In addition, working with shellfish harvesters, hunters, or pet owners for each of these data collection efforts has the dual benefit of providing the people who are most affected with tools and information to protect the health of themselves and their families.

Climate Adaptation Planning in Alaska

Another central focus of climate and health work in Alaska has been the development of community climate adaptation plans (Figure 30.6). Generally considered a "road map" for preparing for and adapting to the local impacts of climate change, these community-driven plans were generally developed through a collaborative process between community members, Alaskan scientists, and nonprofit or science organizations in the state. In most of the plans, health and safety or community well-being are identified as overarching goals or important values. In many cases, public health concerns are cited as key motivations for action. For example, the Oscarville, Nome, and Shaktoolik Adaptation Plans refer to many of the climate-related health impacts described earlier in this chapter such as concerns related to subsistence food availability and safety, hazardous winter travel conditions, water and sanitation issues related

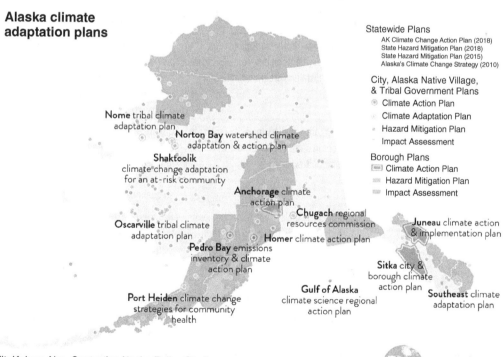

Credit: Kelsey Aho, Center for Alaska Policy Studies.

Data source: DEECD; Meeker and Kettle, 2017

Figure 30.6   Alaska climate adaptation plans
Source: Reprinted with permission from Thoman and Walsh (2019).

to thawing permafrost, or decreased air quality due to dust from dry river sloughs (Kettle, Martin, and Sloan 2017; Johnson and Gray 2014; Schaeffer et al. 2019).

One of the most recent climate planning efforts in Alaska took place in Anchorage (Hahn et al. 2019; Hahn et al. 2020b). Almost half of Alaska's population lives in Anchorage, which serves as the commercial hub for the state. Much of Alaska's supply chain infrastructure including the Port of Alaska and the largest airport are in Anchorage.

The Anchorage Climate Action Plan incorporated human health at several different points in the planning process. The Anchorage plan includes mitigation and adaptation actions in seven different sectors: Buildings and Energy, Consumption and Solid Waste, Land Use and Transportation, Health and Emergency Preparedness, Urban Forests and Watersheds, Food Systems, and Outreach and Education. The Health and Emergency Preparedness chapter includes strategies to (1) reduce health and safety impacts of climate change, (2) increase household and community resilience, (3) engage diverse communities in climate resilience planning, and (4) develop research and monitoring programs to support our understanding of and planning for the health and health impacts of climate change in Anchorage.

In addition to strategies directly connected to health in the Health and Emergency Preparedness chapter, many actions in other sectors are linked with potential **co-benefits** for health as well as potential benefits for economic development, equity, and environmental sustainability (Table 30.1). For example, one of the actions in the Anchorage plan supports lowering barriers for farmers markets to accept payment through food assistance programs including the Supplemental Nutrition Assistance Program (SNAP) and Special Supplemental Nutrition Program for Women, Infants, and Children (WIC). Realization of this action decreases carbon emissions from the Alaskan food system by encouraging consumption of locally produced

Table 30.1 Actions from the Anchorage Climate Action Plan and Their Associated Health Co-Benefits

Sector	Action	Health co-benefit
Buildings and Energy	With a focus on low-income households and renters, engage residents on low-cost ways to save money, such as installing programmable thermostats.	Supporting energy efficient housing can prevent a number of cardiorespiratory diseases through reduced exposure to extreme heat and cold, mold, dampness, and improved indoor air quality when ventilation is addressed.
Land Use and Transportation	Amend zoning codes to allow mini city centers in neighborhoods in order to create more walkable/ bikeable communities.	Urban design that supports active transportation can decrease obesity and encourage social interactions within the community. Reducing single occupancy vehicles can also improve urban air quality.
Consumption and Solid Waste	Deploy alternatively fueled vehicles—biodiesel/ electric vehicles used in solid waste collection and disposal.	Reducing the number of fossil fuel Municipal vehicles on the road can improve urban air quality.
Food Systems	Encourage and incentivize farmers' markets to accept payment through food assistance programs, including SNAP, WIC, WIC Farmers' Market Nutrition Program (FMNP), and Seniors FMNP.	Decreasing barriers for purchasing fresh, healthy produce can improve household nutrition. Shopping at neighborhood markets can also encourage social interactions within the community.
Urban Forests and Watersheds	Preserve existing forested areas through practices that repurpose already developed areas, such as establishing codes that retain minimum canopy cover on new developments and minimize removal of native soil, groundcover, and shrubs.	Preservation of greenspaces in the community can encourage residents to spend time outdoors, either recreationally or engaging in active transportation (e.g., biking and walking).

foods. At the same time, it increases access to healthy, culturally relevant foods that could improve nutrition in low-income households. On a broader scale, increased sales at farmers' markets support Alaska producers, strengthen the local food system, and improve Alaskan resilience by decreasing reliance on foods imported from out of state.

The final connection to health in the Anchorage Climate Action Plan is that, like many of the adaptation plans in rural communities, protecting public health was one of the primary values driving the development of the plan. Healthy and resilient communities have universal appeal. Regardless of political stance, it is easy to support policies and infrastructure that ensure that people can get to work after a heavy rain event or that a community has consistent piped water during a drought. In fact, there is evidence to suggest that framing climate change as a public health issue and identifying the health benefits of taking action to mitigate climate change has been compelling to a broad cross-section of Americans (Maibach et al. 2010; Myers et al. 2012; Weathers and Kendall 2016). In a place like Alaska where residents tend to be divided on politics, personal health is an important unifying value for discussing climate change.

Next Steps in Addressing Climate and Health in Alaska

One of the early proponents of addressing climate change within the field of public health, Anthony McMichael (2001) enumerated the challenges of integrating climate change impacts as risk factors using traditional epidemiologic research methods. Vast geographic scale, dynamism, and complex causal pathways are inherent characteristics of climate change that necessitate creative approaches to risk assessment. A small, dispersed population and limited clinical and environmental data augment these challenges in Alaska. Despite these limitations, there are several ways that the public health and clinical community can support climate adaptation in Alaska.

A commonly used framework for public health practice around climate change (Building Resilience Against Climate Effects, or BRACE) has five steps that lead to successful adaptation: (1) quantifying risk and assessing vulnerability, (2) projecting the disease burden, (3) assessing public health interventions, (4) development and implementation of adaptation strategies, and (5) impact evaluation (Marinucci et al. 2014). In Alaska, state, regional, and community surveillance activities described in this chapter support risk and vulnerability assessments (Table 30.2). Data collected through these programs can support epidemiologic assessments of climate-related exposures that characterize populations that are sensitive to particular environmental hazards and help identify thresholds for public health intervention. However, many of these monitoring programs are chronically under-resourced and rely on Alaskan residents to report their observations. Development of state and regional capacity to support surveillance activities, process and manage data, and report results back to the public in a timely and culturally relevant format would enhance the effectiveness of these programs.

In many small, Alaskan communities, the impacts of climate change on health are very apparent, and a highly detailed, quantitative assessment of health outcomes may not always be necessary before starting to devise adaptation solutions. This approach is reflected in many of the community climate adaptation plans that utilize community discussions and prioritization activities to define high priority issues they would like to address. However, after communities have identified their priority actions, there is often lack of support for implementation of adaptation programs and evaluation of adaptation strategies.

Finally, a major gap in climate and health research and planning in Alaska are scenario-based health risk assessments (aka climate change health impact projections) (Hess 2015). These projections are based on quantitative epidemiologic relationships between environmental change and health outcomes in the present applied to models of expected climatic changes in the coming decades. Most assessments to date have focused on direct health outcomes such as heat illness and mortality (Huang et al. 2011) that are not currently a major concern in Alaska; however, respiratory health outcomes, waterborne illness, and injury associated with extreme storms are Alaska-relevant health concerns that could be modeled using these methods (Hsu et al. 2018; Kintziger et al. 2017; Conlon et al. 2016). Downscaled projections of expected climatic changes are available for Alaska (Scenario Network of Alaska and Arctic Planning–University of Alaska Fairbanks 2019) and are a key resource for these epidemiologic investigations in Alaska.

Table 30.2   Representative Examples of Climate and Health Activities in Alaska within the BRACE Framework and Classified by Geographic Scope

Climate and health adaptation activities	Geographic scope		
	Statewide	**Group of communities**	**Community**
Quantifying risk and assessing vulnerability	State of Alaska Climate and Health Impact Assessment; Alaska-Submit-A-Tick surveillance program; Local Environmental Observer (LEO) Network	Harmful algal bloom monitoring; biofilter paper monitoring for emerging zoonoses; pollen monitoring; epidemiologic assessment of falling through ice	Community climate adaptation plans; ANTHC Community Climate Change and Health Assessments; epidemiologic assessment of exposure to particulate matter from wildfire smoke and cardiorespiratory outcomes
Projecting the disease burden	*Lack of research in this area*		
Assessing public health interventions	*Lack of research in this area*		
Development and implementation of adaptation strategies		Development of portable water/sanitation system for relocating communities (Alaska Native Tribal Health Consortium 2019c)	Community adaptation plans; Anchorage Climate Action Plan
Impact evaluation	*Lack of research in this area*		

Conclusion

Alaska faces enormous challenges with regard to changing environmental conditions and impacts on infrastructure, food and water resources, and cultural and recreational activities that have implications for the physical and mental health of residents. Additionally, direct impacts of climate change on health including smoke exposures from wildfire, increasing summer temperatures, and accidents and injuries during unpredictable winter travel conditions will add additional stress to Alaska's public health and clinical services. Although some of the health impacts of climate change that have been observed in the state are similar to other regions of the United States, many aspects of Alaskan life create challenges that are unique within our national context.

We have gained considerable insight into the impacts of the changing environment on the health of communities through conversations and community observations over the past decade. Moving forward, more quantitative information about the health burden of environmental exposures in Alaskan communities could support adaptation planning by characterizing populations that are sensitive to particular environmental hazards, identifying thresholds for public health intervention, projecting expected future health impacts, and supporting evaluation of adaptation strategies.

In addition to the traditional epidemiologic and programmatic role of public health, collaboration in climate action planning can be a key opportunity to infuse health considerations across sectors of a municipal or community government. In order to take advantage of this moment in time when communities in Alaska and elsewhere are dramatically shifting their energy, transportation, food, and waste management systems, it is essential that the public health community advocates for climate mitigation strategies that simultaneously improve public health and health equity.

DISCUSSION QUESTIONS

1. What are some unique characteristics of life in Alaska that influence people's exposure to climate-mediated environmental changes?

2. How does changing sea ice extent affect the health of Alaskan communities?

3. Explain how a failed salmon run could affect the physical and mental health of an Alaskan community.

4. What is the role of community-based monitoring in understanding the impact of climate change on health in Alaska?

5. Why is ecological surveillance relevant to clinical patient care?

6. How would you design a surveillance system to collect information on climate-related health outcomes in Alaska?

7. What is the relevance of the OneHealth framework to climate change in Alaska?

8. Explain how the development of climate adaptation plans relate to protecting public health.

KEY TERMS

Co-benefits: Ancillary benefits (to health in this context) of policies and actions to decrease greenhouse gas emissions (Haines 2017).

Exposure: Contact between a person and one or more biological, chemical, or physical stressors, including stressors affected by climate change (e.g., extreme heat, extreme weather) (Gamble et al. 2016). In Alaska, many exposures are the result of complex ecological processes such as changes to salmon runs that affect nutrition as well as anxiety and mental health around food resources.

OneHealth: A collaborative, multisectoral, and transdisciplinary approach—working at the local, regional, national, and global levels—with the goal of achieving optimal health outcomes recognizing the interconnection between people, animals, plants, and their shared environment (Centers for Disease Control and Prevention 2019).

Subsistence: Alaska state law defines subsistence use as "the noncommercial, customary and traditional uses of wild, renewable resources by a resident domiciled in a rural area of the state for direct personal or family consumption as food, shelter, fuel, clothing, tools, or transportation, for the making and selling of handicraft articles out of nonedible by-products of fish and wildlife resources taken for personal or family consumption, and for the customary trade, barter, or sharing for personal or family consumption" (State of Alaska 2016). The Alaska Federation of Natives describes subsistence as "the hunting, fishing, and gathering activities which traditionally constituted the economic base of life for Alaska's Native peoples and which continue to flourish in many areas of the state today" (Alaska Federation of Natives 2012).

Acknowledgment

Thank you to Sarah Yoder, Mike Brubaker, John Walsh, and Rick Thoman for reviewing this chapter and providing valuable comments.

References

Alaska Climate Research Center. 2019. "Climate Station Map." http://climate.gi.alaska.edu/station-map.

Alaska Department of Environmental Conservation. 2019a. "Alaska Air Quality Index." https://dec.alaska.gov/Applications/Air/airtoolsweb/Aq/.

Alaska Department of Environmental Conservation. 2019b. "Dust in Alaska." https://dec.alaska.gov/air/anpms/dust/.

Alaska Department of Environmental Conservation (2020). "Tickborne Diseases." https://dec.alaska.gov/eh/vet/ticks/tickborne-diseases/.

Alaska Department of Fish and Game. 2019. "Ecosystems." https://www.adfg.alaska.gov/index.cfm?adfg=ecosystems.list.

Alaska Department of Health and Social Services. 2015. "Paralytic Shellfish Poisoning—Alaska, 1993–2014." *Epidemiologic Bulletin* 1.

Alaska Department of Health and Social Services. 2017. "Pollen and Outdoor Mold Season Update." *State of Alaska, Epidemiology Bulletin* 10. http://www.epi.alaska.gov/bulletins/docs/b2017_10.pdf.

Alaska Department of Health and Social Services. 2019. "Alaska Behavioral Risk Factor Surveillance System (BRFSS)." http://ibis.dhss.alaska.gov/query/selection/brfss23/BRFSSSelection.html.

Alaska Department of Natural Resources. 2019. "Extreme Conditions Extend Alaska Wildfire Season to Sept. 30." Press Release, August 26. 2019. http://dnr.alaska.gov/commis/pic/releases/82619 Extreme conditions extend Alaska wildfire season to Sept 30.pdf.

Alaska Federation of Natives. 2012. "The Right to Subsist: Federal Protection of Subsistence in Alaska." https://www.nativefederation.org/wp-content/uploads/2018/07/2010-april8-the-right-to-subsistence.pdf.

Alaska Harmful Algal Bloom Network. 2019. "National, Regional and Statewide HABs Programs." https://aoos.org/alaska-hab-network/regional-and-state-habs-programs/.

Alaska Native Tribal Health Consortium. 2016. "Portable Alternative Sanitation System (PASS), Final Report–Kivalina." https://anthc.org/clean-water-and-sanitation/portable-alternative-sanitation-system-final-report-kivalina-alaska/.

Alaska Native Tribal Health Consortium. 2019a. "Community Climate Assessment Reports." https://anthc.org/what-we-do/community-environment-and-health/center-for-climate-and-health/climate-health-3/.

Alaska Native Tribal Health Consortium. 2019b. "LEO Network." https://anthc.org/what-we-do/community-environment-and-health/leo-network/.

Alaska Native Tribal Health Consortium. 2019c. "Portable Alternative Sanitation System Connects In-Home Sanitation Systems Where It Was Impossible Before." https://anthc.org/news/portable-alternative-sanitation-system-connects-in-home-sanitation-systems-where-it-was-impossible-before/.

Barbeaux, S., K. Aydin, B. Fissel, K. Holsman, B. Laurel, W. Palsson, K. Shotwell, Q. Yang, and S. Zador. 2018. "Chapter 2: Assessment of the Pacific Cod Stock in the Gulf of Alaska Executive Summary." *In Stock Assessment and Fishery Evaluation Report for the Groundfish Resources of the Gulf of Alaska.* Anchorage, AK: North Pacific Fishery Management Council. https://archive.afsc.noaa.gov/refm/docs/2019/GOApcod.pdf.

Bell, J., M. Brubaker, K. Graves, and J. Berner. 2010. "Climate Change and Mental Health: Uncertainty and Vulnerability for Alaska Natives." *Center for Climate and Health Bulletin* (3):1–10.

Bentz, B. J., J. Régnière, C. J. Fettig, E. M. Hansen, J. L. Hayes, J. A. Hicke, R. G. Kelsey, J. F. Negrón, and S. J. Seybold. 2010. "Climate Change and Bark Beetles of the Western United States and Canada: Direct and Indirect Effects." *BioScience* 60 (8):602–13. https://doi.org/10.1525/bio.2010.60.8.6.

Berner, J. 2014. "The Rural Alaska Monitoring Program." https://vimeo.com/125515030.

Berwyn, B. 2019. "Avalanches Menace Colorado as Climate Range Raises the Risk." *Inside Climate News, March* 9, 2019. https://insideclimatenews.org/news/08032019/avalanche-climate-change-risk-snow-storm-forecast-colorado-switzerland.

Bieniek, P. A, J. E Walsh, R. L. Thoman, and U. S. Bhatt. 2014. "Using Climate Divisions to Analyze Variations and Trends in Alaska Temperature and Precipitation." *Journal of Climate* 27 (8):2800–18. https://doi.org/10.1175/JCLI-D-13-00342.1.

Bond, N. A., M. F. Cronin, H. Freeland, and N. Mantua. 2015. "Causes and Impacts of the 2014 Warm Anomaly in the NE Pacific." *Geophysical Research Letters* 42 (9):3414–20.

Brubaker, M., J. Berner, R. Chavan, and J. Warren. 2011. "Climate Change and Health Effects in Northwest Alaska." *Global Health Action* 4 (1):8445. https://doi.org/10.3402/gha.v4i0.8445.

Centers for Disease Control and Prevention. 2019. "One Health Basics." https://www.cdc.gov/onehealth/basics/index.html.

City of Cordova Alaska. 2019. "Water Conservation 08/29/19." https://www.cityofcordova.net/residents/services/water-status/1194-water-conservation-08-29-19.

Conlon, K., K. Kintziger, M. Jagger, L. Stefanova, C. Uejio, and C. Konrad. 2016. "Working with Climate Projections to Estimate Disease Burden: Perspectives from Public Health." *International Journal of Environmental Research and Public Health* 13 (8): 804. https://doi.org/10.3390/ijerph13080804.

Cunsolo, A., and N. R. Ellis. 2018. "Ecological Grief as a Mental Health Response to Climate Change-Related Loss." *Nature Climate Change* 8 (4):275–81. https://doi.org/10.1038/s41558-018-0092-2.

Di Liberto, T. 2019. "High Temperatures Smash All-Time Records in Alaska in Early July 2019." NOAA climate.gov. 2019. https://www.climate.gov/news-features/event-tacker/high-temperatures-smash-all-time-records-alaska-early-july-2019.

Driscoll, D. 2015. "Community-Based Sentinel Surveillance as an Innovative Tool to Measure the Health Effects of Climate Change in Remote Alaska." In *Global Climate Change and Human Health, edited by George Luber and Jay Lemery*, 407–29. San Francisco, CA: Jossey-Bass.

Durden, L. A., K. B. Beckmen, and R. F. Gerlach. 2016. "New Records of Ticks (Acari: Ixodidae) from Dogs, Cats, Humans, and Some Wild Vertebrates in Alaska: Invasion Potential." *Journal of Medical Entomology* 53 (6):1391–95. https://doi.org/10.1093/jme/tjw128.

Eisen, R. J., K. J. Kugeler, L. Eisen, C. B. Beard, and C. D. Paddock. 2017. "Tick-Borne Zoonoses in the United States: Persistent and Emerging Threats to Human Health." *ILAR Journal*, March, 1–17. https://doi.org/10.1093/ilar/ilx005.

Ellis, T. 2019. "UAF Project Seeks to Provide Air Quality Data for Rural, Remote Alaska Areas." Alaska Public Media. https://www.alaskapublic.org/2019/07/25/uaf-project-seeks-to-provide-air-quality-data-for-rural-remote-alaska-areas/.

Fall, J. A. 2016. "Regional Patterns of Fish and Wildlife Harvests in Contemporary Alaska." *Arctic* 69 (1):47–64.

Fleischer, N. L., P. Melstrom, E. Yard, M. Brubaker, and T. Thomas. 2014. "The Epidemiology of Falling-through-the-Ice in Alaska, 1990-2010." *Journal of Public Health* 36 (2):235–42. https://doi.org/10.1093/pubmed/fdt081.

Gamble, J. L., J. Balbus, M. Berger, K. Bouye, V. Campbell, K. Chief, K. Conlon et al. 2016. "Chapter 9: Populations of Concern." In *The Impacts of Climate Change on Human Health in the United States: A Scientific Assessment*, 247–86. Washington, DC: U.S. Global Change Research Program. doi:10.7930/J0Q81B0T.

Hahn MB, Disler G, Durden L, Coburn S, Witmer F, George W, Beckmen K, and R Gerlach. (2020a). Establishing a baseline for tick surveillance in Alaska: Tick collection records from 1909-2019. *Ticks and Tick-borne Disease*. 11(5): 101495.

Hahn MB, Kemp C, Ward-Waller C, Donovan S, Schmidt JI, and S Bauer (2020b). Collaborative climate mitigation and adaptation planning with university, community, and municipal partners: A case study in Anchorage Alaska. *Local Environment*. 25(9): 648–665.

Hahn MB, Kuiper G, O'Dell K, Fischer EV, and S Magzamen (In review). Wildfire smoke is associated with an increased risk of cardiorespiratory emergency room visits in Alaska.

Hahn, M., S. Kilcoyne, C. Kemp, C. Ward-Waller, A. Long, S. Donovan, B. Brettschneider, and L. Roderick (Eds). 2019. "Anchorage Climate Action Plan." http://www.muni.org/Departments/Mayor/AWARE/ResilientAnchorage/pages/climateactionplan.aspx.

Haines, A. 2017. "Health Co-Benefits of Climate Action." *Lancet Planetary Health* 1 (1):e4–e5. doi:10.1016/S2542-5196(17)30003-7.

Hao, K. 2018. "Microsoft Is Enabling Alaska to Reduce Car Deaths on Icy Roads." *Quartz February* 27, 2018. https://qz.com/1216050/microsoft-is-working-with-alaska-to-reduce-car-deaths-on-icy-roads/.

Hess, J. 2015. "Climate Change Health Impact Projections." In *Global Climate Change and Human Health, edited by George Luber and Jay Lemery*, 385–406. San Francisco, CA: Jossey-Bass.

Hsu, W.-H., S.-A. Hwang, S. Saha, P. J. Schramm, A. R. Van Zutphen, K. Conlon, and S. Lin. 2018. *Projecting Climate-Related Disease Burden: A Case Study on Methods for Projecting Respiratory Health Impacts*. Atlanta: National Center for Environmental Health, Centers for Disease Control and Prevention. https://www.cdc.gov/climateandhealth/docs/ProjectingDiseaseRespiratoryCaseStudy_508.pdf.

Huang, C., A. G. Barnett, X. Wang, P. Vaneckova, G. Fitzgerald, and S. Tong. 2011. "Projecting Future Heat-Related Mortality under Climate Change Scenarios: A Systematic Review." *Environmental Health Perspectives*. Washington, DC: Public Health Service, U.S. Department of Health and Human Services. https://doi.org/10.1289/ehp.1103456.

Huettmann, F., E. E. Magnuson, and K. Hueffer. 2017. "Ecological Niche Modeling of Rabies in the Changing Arctic of Alaska." *Acta Veterinaria Scandinavica* 59 (1):18. doi:10.1186/s13028-017-0285-0.

Jenkins, E. 2019. "Metlakatla, Which Depends on Water, Has Moved Quickly to Accommodate the Realities of Drought." Alaska Public Media. https://www.alaskapublic.org/2019/11/20/metlakatla-which-depends-on-water-has-moved-quickly-to-accommodate-the-realities-of-drought/.

Johnson, T., and G. Gray. 2014. "Shaktoolik, Alaska: Climate Change Adaptation for an At-Risk Community Adaptation Plan." U.S. Climate Resilience Toolkit.

Johnstone, J. F., T. S. Rupp, M. Olson, and D. Verbyla. 2011. "Modeling Impacts of Fire Severity on Successional Trajectories and Future Fire Behavior in Alaskan Boreal Forests." *Landscape Ecology* 26 (4):487–500. https://doi.org/10.1007/s10980-011-9574-6.

Jongejan, F., and G. Uilenberg. 2004. "The Global Importance of Ticks." *Parasitology* 129:S3–14. https://doi.org/10.1017/S0031182004005967.

Kettle, N., J. Martin, and M. Sloan. 2017. *Nome Tribal Climate Nome Tribal Climate Adaptation Plan*. Fairbanks, AK: Nome Tribal Climate Center for Climate Assessment and Policy.

Kim, B. I., J. D. Blanton, A. Gilbert, L. Castrodale, K. Hueffer, D. Slate, and C. E. Rupprecht. 2014. "A Conceptual Model for the Impact of Climate Change on Fox Rabies in Alaska, 1980–2010." *Zoonoses Public Health* 61 (1):72–80. doi:10.1111/zph.12044.

Kintziger, K. W., M. A. Jagger, K. C. Conlon, K. F. Bush, B. Haggerty, L. H. Morano, K. Lane et al. 2017. "Technical Documentation on Exposure-Response Functions for Climate-Sensitive Health Outcomes." http://www.cdc.gov/climateandhealth/BRACE.htm.

Lee, M., F. Nordio, A. Zanobetti, P. Kinney, R. Vautard, and J. Schwartz. 2014. "Acclimatization across Space and Time in the Effects of Temperature on Mortality: A Time-Series Analysis." *Environmental Health* 13 (1):89. https://doi.org/10.1186/1476-069X-13-89.

Lefebvre, K. A., L. Quakenbush, E. Frame, K. B. Huntington, G. Sheffield, R. Stimmelmayr, A. Bryan, et al. 2016. "Prevalence of Algal Toxins in Alaskan Marine Mammals Foraging in a Changing Arctic and Subarctic Environment." *Harmful Algae* 55 (May):13–24. https://doi.org/10.1016/j.hal.2016.01.007.

Leffler, J. 2019. "Rain a Respite for Southeast Water Conservation Measures." Alaska Public Media. https://www.alaskapublic.org/2019/06/20/rain-a-respite-for-southeast-water-conservation-measures/.

Maibach, E. W., M. Nisbet, P. Baldwin, K. Akerlof, and G. Diao. 2010. "Reframing Climate Change as a Public Health Issue: An Exploratory Study of Public Reactions." *BMC Public Health* 10 (1):299. https://doi.org/10.1186/1471-2458-10-299.

Marinucci, G. D, G. Luber, C. K Uejio, and S. Saha. 2014. "Building Resilience against Climate Effects—A Novel Framework to Facilitate Climate Readiness in Public Health Agencies." *International Journal of Environmental Research and Public Health* 11:6433–58. https://doi.org/10.3390/ijerph110606433.

Markon, C., S. Gray, M. Berman, L. Eerkes-Medrano, T. Hennessy, H. P. Huntington, J. Littell et al. 2018. "Chapter 26 : Alaska." In *Impacts, Risks, and Adaptation in the United States: The Fourth National Climate Assessment, Vol. II*, edited by D. R. Reidmiller, C. W. Avery, D. R. Easterling, K. E. Kunkel, K. L. M. Lewis, T. K. Maycock, and B. C. Stewart, 1185–1241. Washington, DC: U.S. Global Change Research Program. https://doi.org/10.7930/NCA4.2018.CH26.

Martin, M. C.. 2019. "Warm Waters across Alaska Cause Salmon Die-Offs." Juneau Empire. https://www.juneauempire.com/news/warm-waters-across-alaska-cause-salmon-die-offs/.

May, C., C. H. Luce, J. H. Casola, M. Chang, J. Cuhaciyan, M. Dalton, S. E. Lowe et al. 2018. "Chapter 24 : Northwest. In *Impacts, Risks, and Adaptation in the United States: The Fourth National Climate Assessment, Vol. II*, edited by D. R. Reidmiller, C. W. Avery, D. R. Easterling, K. E. Kunkel, K. L. M. Lewis, T. K. Maycock, and B. C. Stewart, 1036–1100. Washington, DC: U.S. Global Change Research Program. https://doi.org/10.7930/NCA4.2018.CH24.

McLaughlin, J. B, A. DePaola, C. A. Bopp, K. A. Martinek, N. P. Napolilli, C. G. Allison, S. L. Murray et al. 2005. "Outbreak of Vibrio Parahaemolyticus Gastroenteritis Associated with Alaskan Oysters." *New England Journal of Medicine* 353 (14):1463–70. http://www.ncbi.nlm.nih.gov/pubmed/16207848.

McMichael, A. J. 2001. "Global Environmental Change as 'Risk Factor': Can Epidemiology Cope?" *American Journal of Public Health* 91 (8):1172–74.

Medina-Ramón, M., and J. Schwartz. 2007. "Temperature, Temperature Extremes, and Mortality: A Study of Acclimatisation and Effect Modification in 50 US Cities." *Occupational and Environmental Medicine* 64 (12):827–33. https://doi.org/10.1136/oem.2007.033175.

Myers, T. A., M. C. Nisbet, E. W. Maibach, and A. A. Leiserowitz. 2012. "A Public Health Frame Arouses Hopeful Emotions about Climate Change." *Climatic Change* 113 (3–4):1105–12. https://doi.org/10.1007/s10584-012-0513-6.

National Drought Mitigation Center. 2019. "Drought in Alaska." https://www.drought.gov/drought/states/alaska.

National Oceanic and Atmospheric Administration. 2016. "West Coast Harmful Algal Bloom." *NOAA News. September* 15, 2016. https://oceanservice.noaa.gov/news/sep15/westcoast-habs.html.

National Oceanic and Atmospheric Administration National Climatic Data Center. 2019. "U.S. Selected Significant Climate Anomalies and Events–May and Spring 2019." 2019. https://www.ncdc.noaa.gov/sotc/national/201905.

Nowacki, G., P. Spencer, T. Brock, M. Fleming, and T. Jorgenson. 2001. "Ecoregions of Alaska and Neighboring Territory." Reston, VA: U.S. Geological Survey. https://databasin.org/datasets/6a792aa584344d3ca98745b201b64223.

Nyland, K. E., A. E. Klene, J. Brown, N. I. Shiklomanov, F. E. Nelson, D. A. Streletskiy, and K. Yoshikawa. 2017. "Traditional Inupiat Ice Cellars in Barrow, Alaska - Characteristics, Temperature Monitoring, and Distribution." *Geographical Review* 107 (1):143–58. https://doi.org/10.1111/j.1931-0846.2016.12204.x.

O'Malley, J. 2019. "Alaska Relies on Ice. What Happens When It Can't Be Trusted?" *New York Times, April* 10, 2019. https://www.nytimes.com/2019/04/10/us/alaska-ice-melting.html.

Otranto, D., E. Brianti, M. Latrofa, G. Annoscia, S. Weigl, R. Lia, G. Gaglio, et al. 2012. "On a Cercopithifilaria Sp. Transmitted by Rhipicephalus Sanguineus: A Neglected, but Widespread Filarioid of Dogs." *Parasites & Vectors* 5 (1):1. https://doi.org/10.1186/1756-3305-5-1.

Phuleria, H. C., P. M. Fine, Y. Zhu, and C. Sioutas. 2005. "Air Quality Impacts of the October 2003 Southern California Wildfires." *Journal of Geophysical Research Atmospheres* 110 (7):1–11. https://doi.org/10.1029/2004JD004626.

Richardson, J. 2014. "Fairbanks DOT Increasing Use of Brine for Slick Roads." *Fairbanks Daily News-Miner November* 14, 2014. http://www.newsminer.com/news/local_news/fairbanks-dot-increasing-use-of-brine-for-slick-roads/article_0aa6291e-6c9c-11e4-b355-bfb480125f0c.html.

Ruscio, B. A., M. Brubaker, J. Glasser, W. Hueston, and T. W. Hennessy. 2015. "One Health—a Strategy for Resilience in a Changing Arctic." *International Journal of Circumpolar Health* 74:27913. https://doi.org/10.3402/ijch.v74.27913.

Salyer, S. J., R. Silver, K. Simone, and C. B. Behravesh. 2017. "Prioritizing Zoonoses for Global Health Capacity Building—Themes from One Health Zoonotic Disease Workshops in 7 Countries, 2014–2016." *Emerging Infectious Diseases* 23 (December):S57–64. https://doi.org/10.3201/eid2313.170418.

Sarofim, M. C., S. Saha, M. D. Hawkins, D. M. Mills, J. Hess, R. Horton, P. Kinney, J. Schwartz, and A. St. Juliana. 2016. "Chapter 2: Temperature-Related Death and Illness." In *The Impacts of Climate Change on Human Health in the United States: A Scientific Assessment*, 43–68. Washington, DC: U.S. Global Change Research Program. https://doi.org/10.7930/J0MG7MDX.

Scenario Network of Alaska and Arctic Planning (SNAP). 2019. "SNAP Data Portal." University of Alaska Fairbanks. https://www.snap.uaf.edu/tools-data/data-downloads.

Schaeffer, J. Q., A. Rittgers, P. Johnson, A. Davis, B. Grunau, J. Hebert, and M. Doyle. 2019. *Pektayiinata = We Are Resilient, Oscarville Tribal Climate Adaptation Plan*. Oscarville, AK: Oscarville Traditional Village. http://cchrc.org/media/Oscarville_Adaptation_Plan.pdf.

Sherwood, C. 2015. "Thousands of Salmon Die in Hotter-than-Usual Northwest Rivers." *Reuters July* 27, 2015. https://www.reuters.com/article/us-usa-oregon-salmon/thousands-of-salmon-die-in-hotter-than-usual-northwest-rivers-idUSKCN0Q203P20150728.

Sonenshine, D. E. 2018. "Range Expansion of Tick Disease Vectors in North America: Implications for Spread of Tick-Borne Disease." *International Journal of Environmental Research and Public Health* 15 (3):478. doi:10.3390/ijerph15030478.

Southeast Alaska Tribal Toxins Network. 2013. "Paralytic Shellfish Poisoning Monitoring Program." *May* 20, 2019. http://www.seator.org/resources.

Southeast Alaska Tribal Toxins Network. 2019a. "Alaska Shellfish ID Chart." http://www.seator.org/PDF_Documents/AK%20Shellfish%20ID%20Chart.pdf.

Southeast Alaska Tribal Toxins Network. 2019b. "Harmful Algal Blooms and Climate Change." http://www.seator.org/PDF_Documents/HABS%20and%20Global%20Warming.pdf.

State of Alaska. 2016. "Alaska Statutes." 2016. http://www.akleg.gov/basis/statutes.asp#16.05.940%0D.

The Salmon Project. 2019. "Archive." https://salmonproject.org/research/.

Thoman, R., and J. E. Walsh. 2019. *Alaska's Changing Environment: Documenting Alaska's Physcial and Biological Changes through Observations*, edited by H. R. McFarland. Fairbanks: International Arctic Research Center, University of Alaska-Fairbanks.

Thomas, T. K., J. Bell, D. Bruden, M. Hawley, and M. Brubaker. 2013. "Washeteria Closures, Infectious Disease and Community Health in Rural Alaska: A Review of Clinical Data in Kivalina, Alaska." *International Journal of Circumpolar Health* 72 (1):21233. https://doi.org/10.3402/ijch.v72i0.21233.

University of Alaska Fairbanks. 2019. "Center for One Health Research." https://www.uaf.edu/onehealth/index.php.

Warren, J. 2019. "Fishing Jobs Decline 4.9 Percent in 2018." *Alaska Economic Trends* (November):4–6, 15.

Weathers, M. R., and B. E. Kendall. 2016. "Developments in the Framing of Climate Change as a Public Health Issue in US Newspapers." *Environmental Communication* 10 (5):593–611. https://doi.org/10.1080/17524032.2015.1050436.

Werner, R. A., E. H. Holsten, S. M. Matsuoka, and R. E. Burnside. 2006. "Spruce Beetles and Forest Ecosystems in South-Central Alaska: A Review of 30 Years of Research." *Forest Ecology and Management* 227:195–206. https://doi.org/10.1016/j.foreco.2006.02.050.

Yoder, S., S. Deglin, M. Pachoe, A. Hamade, P. Anderson, Y. Springer, J. Mclaughlin, and L. Castrodale. 2018. "Assessment of the Potential Health Impacts of Climate Change in Alaska." *State of Alaska, Epidemiology Bulletin* 20 (1). http://dhss.alaska.gov/dph/Epi.

CHAPTER 31

THE GLOBAL ENERGY TRANSITION AND PUBLIC HEALTH IN A CHANGING CLIMATE

Hanna Linstadt, Cecilia J. Sorensen and Morgan D. Bazilian

Introduction

The energy sector is currently the dominant contributor to climate change, accounting for 60 percent of total greenhouse gas (GHG) emissions globally (United Nations 2020). The transition of the global energy landscape toward a low-carbon system should serve to protect human health and limit the effects of climate change. In this chapter we discuss how climate change and access to energy are both closely tied to health and how pursuing zero-carbon and accessible energy will help improve health by both mitigating climate change and improving access to reliable energy. We see that energy and health are tied closely in two ways that are discussed in this chapter. First, mitigating emissions and air pollution—at least in part with zero carbon energy sources—will likely decrease respiratory and cardiovascular disease and prevent millions of premature deaths. Second, increasing access to energy—especially clean energy—is also needed to improve the health and socio-economic well-being of vulnerable populations.

The future effects of climate change on health are acknowledged in the Intergovernmental Panel on Climate Change's Special Report on Global Warming of 1.5°C, which recommends limiting warming to 1.5°C (2.7°F) above preindustrial levels in order to protect human and planetary health (IPCC 2018). Our ability to limit warming to 1.5°C largely depends on the global energy transition away from fossil fuels. Minimizing emissions will be important in minimizing the multitude of health risks associated with climate change.

The transition to affordable and clean energy is also important to address public health. The United Nations Sustainable Development Goals, a blueprint to pursue prosperity of all people and our planet, recognizes the importance of clean energy for health and prosperity. Sustainable Development Goal 7 (SDG7), "Affordable and Clean Energy," strives to reach three main goals by 2030: to provide universal access to "affordable, reliable, sustainable and modern energy"; to increase production and use of renewable energy; and to improve energy efficiency (International Energy Agency [IEA] et al. 2020). These goals can be reached by transitioning the global energy landscape from a fossil fuel-based system to clean energy (Gielen et al. 2019; IEA et al. 2020). Access to clean, reliable, and affordable energy services will improve human well-being, especially within impoverished communities, as it allows for improved health care delivery, hygiene, education, and employment.

The global energy transition is the process through which the energy sector transforms from fossil fuel-based toward zero-carbon. Climate experts have advised that this transition must occur by the middle of the century to limit extreme harms

KEY CONCEPTS

- Transitioning to a low-carbon energy economy serves to protect human health in the short and long term by reducing air pollution and mitigating the pervasive effects of climate change.

- Access to clean, reliable, and affordable energy services will improve human well-being, especially within impoverished communities, as it allows for improved health care delivery, hygiene, education, and employment.

- Although there has been improvement in international financial support to aid the least-developed countries in transitioning to clean energy, sustained investment is still greatly needed to ensure an equitable transition and simultaneous achievement of global goals laid out by the Paris Agreement.

to human health and societal well-being (International Renewable Energy Agency 2020). This chapter briefly discusses the current trends in the global energy supply, followed by the relationship between the global energy transition and how it can mitigate climate change. We then discuss the state of access to clean energy and electricity and how the global energy transition can address this issue. The two matters of climate change and access to reliable and affordable electricity each affect health, and there are opportunities in the global energy transition to improve both issues.

Current Trends in Global Energy Supply

The global energy landscape is currently undergoing dramatic transformation. Although the energy sector has historically relied almost exclusively on carbon-based fuel, the proportion of production and use of renewable energy has increased over the past few decades as the cost of renewables drops and battery storage improves (Center for Climate and Energy Solutions 2020; Watts et al. 2019). The power generation sector accounts for 38 percent of total energy-related CO_2 emissions, and the replacement of fossil fuels with clean energy sources would decrease these emissions (Watts et al. 2019). Over the past decade, renewable energy consumption has grown faster than total energy consumption, increasing renewable energy's share in the global energy mix. These trends are most heavily noted within electricity generation (IEA et al. 2020). As of 2018, renewable energy accounted for 45 percent of the growth in electricity generation, with wind and solar representing over half of this growth (Watts et al. 2019).

Recent energy trends could lead to a larger share of renewable energy in the global market. The trend began before this decade, as renewable energy production in 2019 increased more than demand, and electricity from fossil fuel-based sources decreased despite an overall increase in energy consumption (Kåberger 2020). The following year, coal, oil, and nuclear power demand began to decrease, and renewable energy demand increased (IEA 2020). These changes equate to an increase in the renewable energy sector's global share of fuel and power sectors (IEA 2020). Overall, renewable energy's contribution to electricity generation is expected to continue to grow (IEA 2020).

Although there have been significant gains in renewable energy among the power sector, the heating and transport sectors have not seen such robust growth. Projections anticipate the share of heat consumption from renewable sources will increase from only 10 percent to 12 percent between 2019 and 2024 (IEA 2019). Increasing the use of renewable energy sources in the heating and transport sectors could help transition away from fossil fuels to a zero-carbon energy sector.

Carbon dioxide emissions related to energy have steadily increased by roughly one per cent per year in the 2010s (International Renewable Energy Agency 2020); however, with the decrease in energy demand in 2020 came a significant decline in global CO_2 emissions (IEA 2020). The future, however, is unclear—economic recovery efforts from COVID-19 could lead to a rebound in fossil fuel use and GHG emissions, which has been seen in prior times of economic recovery (Hepburn, O'Callaghan, Stern, Stiglitz, and Zenghelis 2020).

The Energy Transition and Climate Change

International negotiations and collaborations to meet these goals are currently structured through the United Nations Framework Convention on Climate Change, under which the Paris Agreement was nearly universally adopted in 2015. The goal of the Paris Agreement is to reduce GHG emissions to limit temperature increase in this century to 2°C (3.6°F) above the preindustrial levels and to actively pursue a limit of 1.5°C.

The Paris Agreement provides a mechanism for developed nations to help developing nations in their efforts to decrease GHG emissions by providing financial resources to mitigate climate change. By signing the Paris Agreement, nations set their own national climate action plans and publicly assess their progress every five years, and developed countries agree to support developing countries in their own climate action plans.

The sum of nations' commitments and progress are currently insufficient to meet the goal of lowering emissions to limit warming to 2°C. Carbon dioxide emissions must decrease by at least 45 percent compared to 2010 levels by 2030 and net-zero emissions by the year 2050 to reach this goal (IPCC 2018). It is currently estimated that 2030 emissions will be lowered only by half of what is needed to limit warming to 2°C and only one fifth of what is necessary to achieve a limit of 1.5°C (Watts et al. 2019). There are multiple reasons why the global community is falling short, including insufficient commitments by developed nations who produce the vast majority of GHG emissions, and insufficient assistance to developing countries that are trying to transition to use of more renewable energy. Though there has been improvement in financial support—international flows doubled to $21.4 billion between 2010 and 2017—only 12 percent of these funds reached the least-developed countries who need the support the most (IEA et al. 2020).

Reducing CO_2 emissions to reach the Paris Agreement goal requires transformation of the global energy system. Electrification with clean power has the ability to mitigate 60 percent of the needed decrease in emissions (IEA et al. 2020). An analysis from International Renewable Energy Agency (2020) shows that increasing deployment renewable energy sources with electrification and improved energy efficiency can contribute to as much as 90 percent of the CO_2 emission reductions needed by the year 2050.

Global Energy Poverty and the SDGs

Despite the recent changes in the global energy landscape, hundreds of millions of people still lack access to basic electricity and clean energy options (IEA et al. 2020)—both of which are needed to meet the Sustainable Development Goals. There has been progress over the past two decades (Energy Information Administration 2017), as fewer people today lack access to electricity than ever before. Between 2010 and 2018, the number of people without access to electricity declined from 1.2 billion to 789 million, and this number is expected to reach 620 million by 2030 (IEA et al. 2020). This decline is largely attributed to the increase in affordable electrification solutions like off-grid solar technologies (IEA et al. 2020), as well as the decreasing cost of renewables (Energy Information Administration 2017). Though renewables would be beneficial in many regions—especially developing nations—new renewable generation capacity varies significantly by region. Of new renewable energy capacity additions in 2019, 54 percent were added in Asia, whereas Africa accounted for only 4.3 percent of the total (United Nations Environment Programme 2020).

Despite modest average improvements in access to clean and reliable energy, there has been unequal progress across global regions and urban versus rural environments. Latin America, eastern Asia, and southeastern Asia are all approaching universal access, and central Asia and southern Asia reached greater than 92 percent access as of 2018 (IEA et al. 2020). Sub-Saharan Africa, however, has 47 percent access as of 2018, which, although increased from 34 percent in 2010, still accounts for 70 percent of the current global deficit in electricity (IEA et al. 2020). By 2030, 85 percent of the population lacking access to electricity is expected to be in sub-Saharan Africa (IEA et al. 2020).

Disparities in access are also seen between urban and rural populations. As of 2018, 97 percent of urban populations had electricity access versus only 80% of rural populations

(IEA et al. 2020). Electricity availability in rural populations has increased from 70 percent in 2010, largely in part because of off-grid solutions (IEA et al. 2020). Over the past decade, approximately 135 million people gained access to electricity via home systems or solar lighting with off-grid or mini-grid access (IEA et al. 2020).

There is also a large difference between high-, middle- and low-income countries in terms of energy—specifically regarding the types of fuel used for cooking. The Lancet Countdown 2019 reports that only 7.5 percent of households in low-income countries and only 40 percent of households in middle-income countries have access to clean fuels and technologies for cooking (Watts et al. 2019). Lack of access to clean fuel increases exposure to indoor air pollution, which is very harmful to human health, accounting for approximately three million premature deaths each year (IEA et al. 2020).

Many leaders in global politics have recognized the importance of universal electrification within the next decade, specifically via the United Nations' Sustainable Development Goals. SDG7, "Access to Sustainable and Reliable Energy," underpins achievement of several other related SDGs. As noted earlier, reaching the goal of Good Health and Well-being (SDG3) depends heavily upon access to modern reliable energy by underserved populations, as energy access allows for adequate hygiene, functioning health care systems, and other essential public health services (International Renewable Energy Agency 2018).

SDG1 aims to eliminate poverty in all of its forms (United Nations Department of Economic and Social Affairs 2020). Energy access is key to this goal, as access to energy and electricity can help lift people out of poverty by allowing individuals and communities to start and maintain businesses, pursue education (United Nations Department of Economic and Social Affairs 2014), and improve health and sanitation. SDG1 also calls for improved resilience of those vulnerable to climate-related extreme events and other social or economic disasters. Renewable energy in particular helps improve resiliency of communities (Bouley et al. 2017), since independent grids can help communities maintain power access when they would otherwise be cut off from a grid. SDG3, "Good Health and Well-being," also depends on access to clean and reliable energy, for reasons including minimizing exposure to air pollution, increasing access to safe and reliable drinking water, and improving access to health care and education, among other reasons that are discussed in the following section.

Clean Water and Sanitation (SDG6) also ties in closely with energy, as access to safe and clean water is often dependent on energy for treatment and transportation of clean water and the elimination of wastewater. Decent Work and Economic Growth (SDG8) also benefits from the economic growth and jobs provided by the renewable energy sector (Gielen et al. 2019). For example, between 2012 and 2018, jobs in the renewable energy sector increased from 7.3 million to 11 million and is expected to triple by 2030 (IEA et al. 2020).

Unfortunately, reports show that we are not on track to meet the goals of SDG7 by 2030. We are currently increasing access to electricity at a rate of 0.82 percent per year as of 2018 but would need to increase this number to 0.87 percent per year in order to reach universal access to electricity by 2030 (IEA et al. 2020). The global share of renewable energy in the total global energy mix is unlikely to reach 36 percent in time (IEA et al. 2020), as we are currently at approximately 19 percent (IEA and International Renewable Energy Agency 2017) and are on track to reach only 21% by 2030 (World Bank 2017). We are also slated to fall short on the energy efficiency goal. We are currently reducing energy intensity by 2.1 percent per year and are projected to maintain this level to 2030; however, the goal is to decrease by 2.6 percent per year by 2030 (World Bank 2017). Thus, though significant strides have been made in improving access to electricity, producing and deploying renewable energy sources, and increasing energy efficiency, more is needed to reach the SDG7 goal by 2030.

Clean Energy Transitions and Health

Moving forward, it is clear that the success of both the Paris Agreement and the Sustainable Development Goals related to protecting human health will depend heavily on the transition to renewable energy as the basis for universal access to this energy. There are myriad benefits of the energy transition on health, which are discussed next.

Shifting away from carbon-based energy sources will likely improve health by decreasing harmful air pollution (Watts et al. 2021). According to the World Health Organization (WHO), air pollution leads to seven million premature deaths every year (WHO 2014). Most of these deaths are from stroke, heart disease, respiratory diseases and infections, and lung cancer (WHO 2014). Projections estimate that if we are able to decrease emissions enough to limit warming to 2°C, we could decrease the number of premature deaths from air pollution by up to 346,000 annually by 2030 and up to 1.5 million annually by 2050 (Vandyck et al. 2018). Some progress has been seen already, as Europe and the Western Pacific regions have seen small decreases in the number of premature deaths, mainly from closing of coal power plants (Watts et al. 2019).

Approximately one billion people today rely on health facilities without electricity supply, especially in rural areas (International Renewable Energy Agency 2018). Health care facilities need reliable energy for medical devices, sanitation and disinfection methods, refrigeration for medications and vaccines, and lighting (WHO and World Bank 2014). Resource-poor populations that lack energy access in homes or health care facilities therefore would benefit in a variety of ways from the establishment of renewable electricity in their communities.

Renewable energy, such as solar and wind power, increase the resilience of health care facilities. Disasters cut off supplies for energy and electricity and have rendered resource-poor health care facilities unable to function in times of extreme weather events or other significant disruptions (Kishore et al. 2018). The adoption of local renewable and sustainable energy, however, buffers against this and allows continuation of health care services during disaster scenarios or other stressors on energy and social system (WHO and World Bank 2014).

Access to clean and renewable energy is especially important in low-resource settings by providing clean energy for cooking, heating, and hygiene (Puliti 2020; United Nations Environment Programme 2020b). There are currently three billion people—mostly in Asia and sub-Saharan Africa—without access to clean fuels and technologies who instead must use wood, charcoal, dung, and coal as fuel for cooking (IEA et al. 2020; Watts et al. 2019). These fuels emit harmful indoor air pollution, which results in increased incidence of health problems like respiratory disease and infections, cardiovascular disease, and death (Fullerton, Bruce, and Gordon 2008). Indoor air pollution results in approximately four million premature deaths globally every year, and women and children account for 60 percent of these premature deaths (United Nations n.d.). Access to clean energy for cooking will improve health by decreasing the indoor pollutants, thereby decreasing the avoidable respiratory diseases and premature deaths (Health and Environment Linkages Initiative. n.d.; Watts et al. 2021). Clean cooking and heating technologies will also prevent further GHG emissions that would otherwise be produced by traditional cooking and heating methods (Anenberg 2012).

Not only will clean cooking technology avoid premature deaths linked to indoor air pollution, it will also help improve gender equity (U.S. Agency for International Development 2019). Women and girls spend significantly more time cooking and collecting water and fuel to cook with (Cecelski 2006), which could be spent pursuing education or other beneficial activities. Therefore, improving access to clean cooking technology will improve health by decreasing harmful indoor air pollution as well as help improve gender equity.

Reliable energy also contributes to better health as it aids in access to clean water and proper sanitation of waste, which minimizes the transmission water-borne disease and allows for handwashing and other aspects of good hygiene (United Nations Environment Programme 2020a). Access to safe water for drinking, sanitation, and hygiene has the potential to prevent over 9 percent of the entire global disease burden and 6.3 percent of all deaths (Prüss-Üstün, Bos, Gore, and Bartram 2008).

Not only does access to modern energy improve the health of resource-poor populations, it also expands access to education, which in turn leads to improved well-being. Education is a fundamental social determinant of health (Hahn and Truman 2015), and reliable and sustainable energy will allow for more access to schools and online educational resources.

Job security and job creation are another benefit of the global transition to renewable energy (IEA and International Renewable Energy Agency 2017; Ram, Aghahosseini, and Breyer 2020). Access to clean and reliable electricity allows people and communities to pursue financial security and economic growth. Not only does renewable energy provide affordable and reliably available electricity for businesses, but it also provides growing opportunities for employment in itself. In the United States alone, the clean energy sector currently employs over three million people, which is fourteen times what the coal, gas, oil, and other fossil fuel industries employ (Ettenson 2017). It will likely employ a great deal more in the future as well, as we move toward more investments in the renewable energy and replace coal-powered infrastructure.

Conclusion

The global energy landscape appears to be transitioning toward a low-carbon system; however, gains are unevenly distributed across the globe, and the transition is not occurring fast enough to meet targets designed to limit warming this century. Transitioning to clean energy imparts a multitude of benefits to health and well-being, including reducing respiratory and cardiovascular diseases and premature deaths resulting from air pollution. Improving access to modern energy will also improve health by allowing access to health care itself, as well as improving cooking and heating technology, gender equity, education, job security, and economic growth. It is possible, though difficult, to address these two significant challenges, and multinational cooperation will be essential to success.

References

Anenberg, S. 2012. "Clean Stoves Benefit Climate and Health." *Nature* 490 (7420):343.

Bouley, T., S. Roschnik, J. Karliner, S. Wilburn, S. Slotterback, R. Guenther, P. Orris, T. Kasper, B. L. Platzer, and K. Torgeson. 2017. *Climate-Smart Healthcare: Low-Carbon and Resilience Strategies for the Health Sector.* Washington, DC: World Bank Group.

Cecelski, E. 2006. *From the Millenium Development Goals towards a Gender-Sensitive Energy Policy Research and Practice: Empirical Evidence and Case Studies.* The Hague: ENERGIA/DfID Collaborative Research Group on Gender and Energy.

Center for Climate and Energy Solutions. 2020. *Renewable Energy.* https://www.c2es.org/content/renewable-energy/. Accessed July 23, 2020.

Energy Information Administration. 2017. *Global Access to Electricity Has Increased over the Past Two Decades.* https://www.eia.gov/todayinenergy/detail.php?id=31552.

Ettenson, L. 2017. *US Clean Energy Jobs Surpass Fossil Fuel Employment.* February 1. https://www.nrdc.org/experts/lara-ettenson/us-clean-energy-jobs-surpass-fossil-fuel-employment.

Fullerton, D. G., N. Bruce, and S. B. Gordon. 2008. "Indoor Air Pollution from Biomass Fuel Smoke Is a Major Health Concern in the Developing World." *Transactions of the Royal Society of Tropical Medicine and Hygiene* 102 (9):843–851.

Gielen, D., F. Boshell, D. Saygin, M. D. Bazilian, N. Wagner, and R. Gorini. 2019. "The Role of Renewable Energy in the Global Energy Transformation." *Energy Strategy Reviews* 24:38–50.

Hahn, R. A., and B. I. Truman. 2015. "Education Improves Public Health and Promotes Health Equity." *International Journal of Health Services: Planning, Administration, Evaluation* 45 (4):657–678.

Health and Environment Linkages Initiative. 2020. *Indoor air pollution and household energy.* https://www.who.int/heli/risks/indoorair/indoorair/en/. Accessed July 23, 2020.

Hepburn, C., B. O'Callaghan, N. Stern, J. Stiglitz, and D. Zenghelis. 2020. "Will COVID-19 Fiscal Recovery Packages Accelerate or Retard Progress on Climate Change?" *Oxford Review of Economic Policy.* Published online 8 May 2020. https://doi.org/10.1093/oxrep/graa015.

Intergovernmental Panel on Climate Change. 2018. *Global Warming of 1.5°C. An IPCC Special Report on the Impacts of Global Warming of 1.5°C above Pre-Industrial Levels and Related Global Greenhouse Gas Emission Pathways, in the Context of Strengthening the Global Response to the Threat of Climate Change, Sustainable Development, and Efforts to Eradicate Poverty,* edited by V. Masson-Delmotte, P. Zhai, H.-O. Pörtner, D. Roberts, J. Skea, P. R. Shukla, A. Pirani, W. Moufouma-Okia et al. Geneva: IPCC.

International Energy Agency. 2019. *Renewables 2019.* Paris: IEA. https://www.iea.org/reports/renewables-2019.

International Energy Agency. 2020. *Global Energy Review 2020.* Paris: IEA. https://www.iea.org/reports/global-energy-review-2020.

International Energy Agency, and International Renewable Energy Agency. 2017. *Perspectives for the Energy Transition—Investment Needs for a Low-Carbon Energy System.* Paris and Abu Dhabi: IRENA and IEA.

International Energy Agency, International Renewable Energy Agency, United Nations Statistics Division, World Bank, World Health Organization. 2020. *Tracking SDG 7: The Energy Progress Report 2020.* Washington, DC: World Bank. https://openknowledge.worldbank.org/handle/10986/33822.

International Renewable Energy Agency. 2016. *The Power to Change: Solar and Wind Cost Reduction Potential to 2025.* Abu Dhabi: IRENA.

International Renewable Energy Agency. 2018. *Healthcare.* https://www.irena.org/offgrid/Healthcare.

International Renewable Energy Agency. 2020. *Global Renewables Outlook: Energy Transformation 2050.* Abu Dhabi: IRENA.

International Renewable Energy Agency. 2020. *Energy Transition.* https://irena.org/energytransition. Accessed August 18, 2020.

Kåberger, T. 2020. "Global Power Sector Developments: RE Finally Dominated Growth." Renewable Energy Institute. https://www.renewable-ei.org/en/activities/column/REupdate/20200302.php.

Kishore, N., N. Kishore, D. Marqués, A. Mahmud, M. V. Kiang, I. Rodriguez, A. Fuller, P. Ebner et al. 2018. "Mortality in Puerto Rico after Hurricane Maria." *New England Journal of Medicine* 379 (2):162–170.

Prüss-Üstün, A., R. Bos, F. Gore, and J. Bartram. 2008. *Safer Water, Better Health: Costs, Benefits and Sustainability of Interventions to Protect and Promote Health.* Geneva: World Health Organization.

Puliti, R. 2020. *Energy Access Takes Center Stage in Fighting COVID-19 (Coronavirus) and Powering Recovery in Africa.* April 22. https://www.worldbank.org/en/news/opinion/2020/04/22/energy-access-critical-to-overcoming-covid-19-in-africa.

Ram, M., A. Aghahosseini, and C. Breyer. 2020. "Job Creation during the Global Energy Transition Towards 100% Renewable Power System by 2050." *Technological Forecasting and Social Change* 151:119682.

United Nations. 2020. *Ensure Access to Affordable, Reliable, Sustainable and Modern Energy.* Sustainable Development Goals. https://www.un.org/sustainabledevelopment/energy/. Accessed August 18, 2020.

United Nations Department of Economic and Social Affairs. 2014. *Electricity and Education: The Benefits, Barriers, and Recommendations for Achieving the Electrification of Primary and Secondary Schools.* New York: UNDESA.

United Nations Department of Economic and Social Affairs. 2020. *Goal 1: End Poverty in All Its Forms Everywhere.* https://sdgs.un.org/goals/goal1.

United Nations Environment Programme. 2020. *Uptick for Renewable Electricity Generation in 2019.* April 20. https://www.unenvironment.org/news-and-stories/story/uptick-renewable-electricity-generation-2019.

United Nations Environment Programme. 2020a. *Goal 6: Ensure Access to Water and Sanitation for All.* Sustainable Development Goals 2020. https://www.un.org/sustainabledevelopment/water-and-sanitation/. Accessed July 23, 2020.

United Nations Environment Programme. 2020b. *Goal 7: Affordable and Clean Energy.* Sustainable Development Goals 2020. https://www.unenvironment.org/explore-topics/sustainable-development-goals/why-do-sustainable-development-goals-matter/goal-7. Accessed July 23, 2020.

U.S. Agency for International Development. 2019. *Empowering Women and Girls. Updated February* 28, 2019. https://www.usaid.gov/energy/gender. Accessed July 23, 2020.

Vandyck, T., K. Keramidas, A. Kitous, J. V. Spadaro, R. Van Dingenen, M. Holland, and B. Saveyn. 2018. "Air Quality Co-Benefits for Human Health and Agriculture Counterbalance Costs to Meet Paris Agreement Pledges." *Nature Communications* 9 (1):4939.

Watts, N., M. Amann, N. Arnell, S. Ayeb-Kaisson, K. Belesova, M. Boykoff, P. Byass et al. 2019. "The 2019 Report of the Lancet Countdown on Health and Climate Change: Ensuring that the Health of a Child Born Today Is Not Defined by a Changing Climate." *Lancet* 394 (10211):1836–78.

Watts, N., et al. (2021). "The 2020 report of The Lancet Countdown on health and climate change: responding to converging crises." *Lancet* 397 (10269):129–170.

World Bank. 2017. *Sustainable Energy for All Global Tracking Framework: Progress toward Sustainability*. Washington, DC: World Bank.

World Health Organization. 2014. "7 Million Premature Deaths Annually Linked to Air Pollution." news release, March 25. https://www.who.int/mediacentre/news/releases/2014/air-pollution/en/.

World Health Organization and World Bank. 2014. *Access to Modern Energy Services for Health Facilities in Resource-Constrained Settings: A Review of Status, Significance, Challenges and Measurement*. Geneva: WHO.

LOSS OF THE WORLD'S CORAL REEFS AND WHAT IT MEANS FOR HUMAN HEALTH AND WELL-BEING: THREATS TO SEAFOOD SECURITY, NUTRITION, DISEASE RISK, PHYSICAL HAZARDS, AND LIVELIHOODS

Carolyn Sotka

Key Concepts

- Warm-water coral reefs are considered to be the marine ecosystem most threatened by climate-related ocean change, especially ocean warming and acidification. If trends continue, all the reefs in the world could be gone by 2070.

- Loss of coral reefs has serious implications for human health and can compromise seafood security and associated nutritional benefits, increase risks of disease, and increase exposure to new physical hazards including flooding.

- Illnesses associated with loss of healthy coral ecosystems include micronutrient deficiencies and suboptimal neurodevelopmental in children, adult obesity, diabetes, seafood poisoning, cardiovascular disease, and cancer. In some cases, a return to traditional seafood-based diets can slow these harms and improve nutritional outcomes and human health.

- Loss of coral reefs jeopardizes coastal economies, livelihoods, property, and cultural services that are supportive of social cohesion and well-being.

- High in diversity, reefs have sedentary animals that protect or defend themselves through chemical means, which can yield marine-based pharmaceuticals.

Introduction

Healthy coral reefs are one of the most beautiful, biologically diverse, culturally significant, and economically vital ecosystems on earth. Tropical or **warm-water reefs** provide food security and livelihoods for more than 275 million people worldwide and in over 100 countries (Pendleton et al. 2016; Burke et al. 2011). Reefs are the first line of defense for coastal shorelines and reduce risk from wave-induced or sea level rise flooding; protecting life and property for those living within 100-year flood zones (Díaz et al. 2019). Reefs also attract tourism and recreational activities with an estimated combined global value of at least $2.7 trillion per year including food and other ecosystem goods and services (International Year of the Reef [IYOR] 2018). Coral reefs are considered the "rainforests of the ocean," hosting 25 percent of all marine life and 4,000 species of fish alone (IYOR 2018; Burke et al. 2011).

Yet tropical coral reefs are delicate, cover less than 1 percent of the ocean floor, and are extremely vulnerable to a variety of stressors (see Figure B.2.1). In fact, coral reefs are considered to be the marine ecosystem most threatened by climate-related ocean change, especially ocean warming and acidification (Intergovernmental Panel on Climate Change [IPCC] 2019).

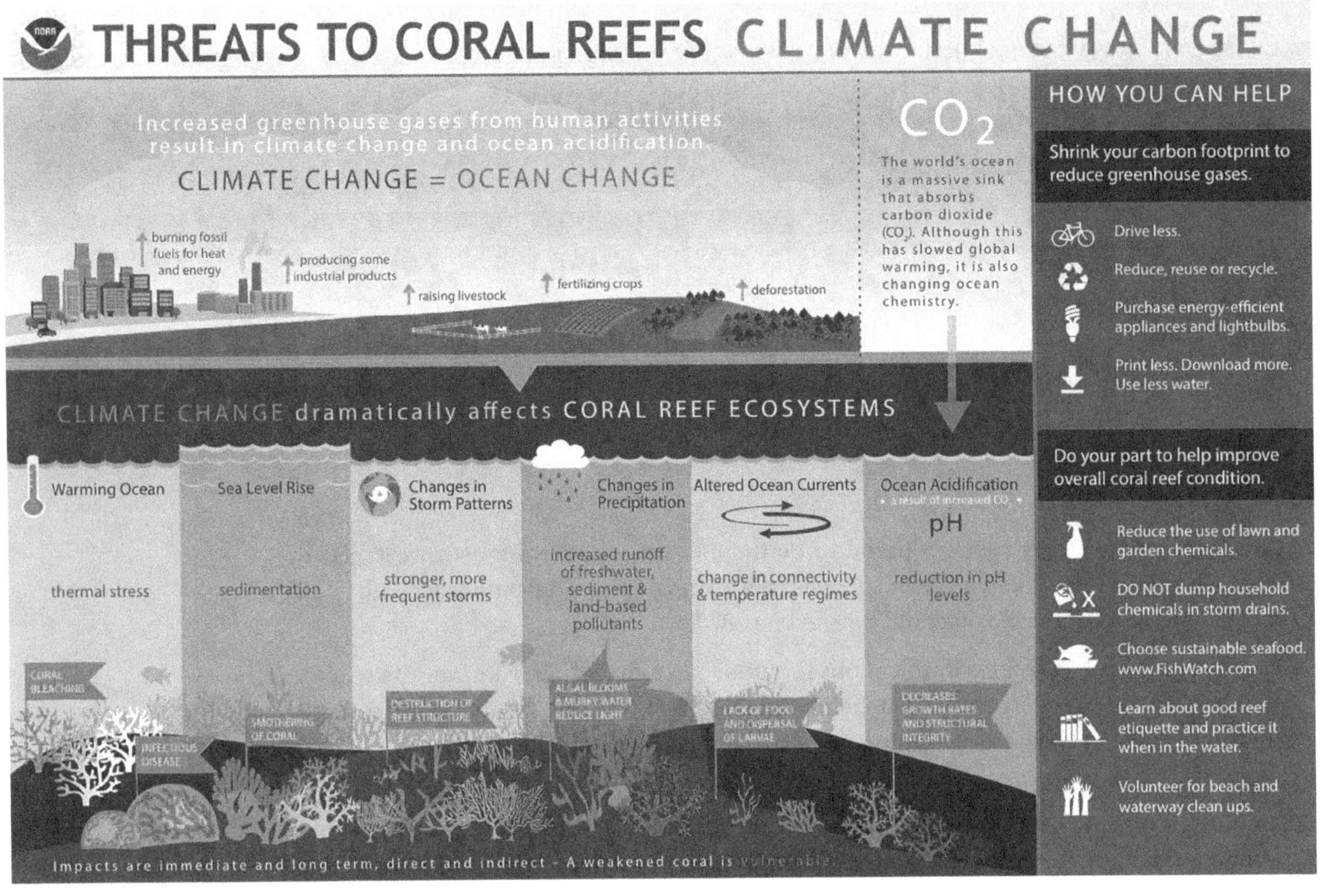

Figure B.2.1 The varied effects of climate change are changing the ocean; these changes dramatically affect coral reef ecosystems

Source: National Ocean Service (NOS, 2019b), courtesy of National Oceanic and Atmospheric Administration (NOAA)'s National Ocean Service, https://oceanservice.noaa.gov/facts/coralreef-climate.html#transcript.

Other drivers interact with and further exacerbate coral extinction including poor water quality due to sediment and nutrient runoff, frequency of extreme storms events, increased incidence of disease, overexploited fishing, and sea level rise (see Figure B.2.2).

Over the last thirty to forty years, the average cover of living coral on tropical reefs has declined by approximately 50–75 percent in nearly all regions of their range (Bruno et al. 2019). If global warming trends continue, all the reefs in the world could be gone by 2070 (Morrison et al. 2019; Hoegh-Guldberg et al. 2018; Heron et al. 2018). Since 1998, heat waves have bleached or killed corals in more than 90 percent of reefs listed as World Heritage sites worldwide, including in the Galapagos Islands, Hawaii, and Australia (Morrison et al. 2019; Heron et al. 2018).

For example, in the Great Barrier Reef, the world's largest reef system, half of the corals died in 2016 and 2017 because of mass bleaching caused by rising seawater temperatures (Hughes et al. 2019). When corals are stressed under this condition, they expel the beneficial microscopic algae (zooxanthellae) living in their tissues, causing the coral to turn completely white (NOS 2019a). These events were very rare, once every few decades before the 1980s but in the years since, the frequency of coral bleaching has increased such that reefs no longer have sufficient time to recover between severe episodes (Hughes et al. 2018; Pierre-Louis and Plumer 2018). **Ocean acidification** presents an additional challenge and can inhibit coral reef recovery. The increase in CO_2 in the atmosphere absorbed by the ocean reduces calcification rates in reef-building and reef-associated organisms by altering seawater chemistry through decreases in pH. This affects the growth and structural integrity of coral reefs (IYOR 2018; IPCC 2019).

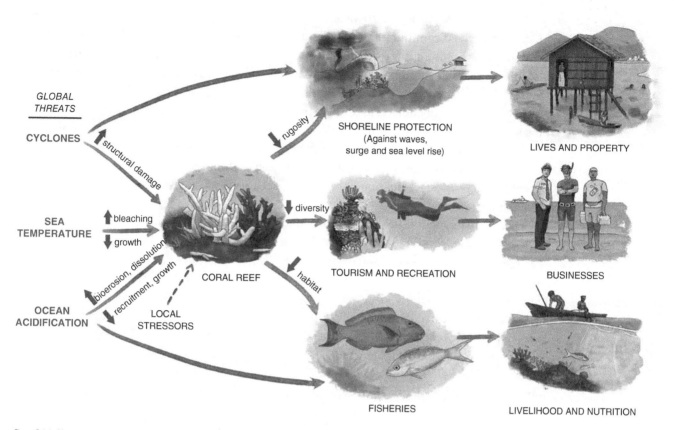

Figure B.2.2 Main actors and relationships in the effect of local and global factors along typical tropical coastal areas involving coral reefs and other ecosystems

Source: Reproduced from Hoegh-Guldberg, Pendleton, and Kaup (2019), with permission from Adrien Comte and Linwood Pendleton, updated from Pendleton et al. (2016), reproduced with permission of Vanessa González Ortiz .

Healthy reef ecosystem functioning is connected to the well-being of people who directly or indirectly benefit from tropical corals reefs (Woodhead et al. 2019; Moberg and Folke 1999). When coral cover declines, so does habitat complexity (Bruno et al. 2019; Alvarez-Filip et al. 2009, 2011) and diversity of reef inhabitants, including fishes and invertebrates (Bruno et. al. 2019; Idjadi and Edmunds 2006; Jones et al. 2004; Pratchett et al. 2008). Increasing water temperatures can shift where fish live and travel in search of their preferred prey and habitat. Rising water temperatures can kill off both the fish and food sources they depend on (Pierre-Louis 2019).

The loss of warm-water reefs greatly compromises the ecosystem services they provide to society such as provisioning services including livelihood, seafood security, and associated health impacts or other goods (Woodhead et al. 2019; Grafeld et al. 2017); cultural services like recreation, tourism, and well-being (Brander, Van Beukering, and Cesar 2007), and regulating services such as coastal protection (Ferrario et al. 2014).

Reef ecosystems protect coastal communities, businesses, and residents from wave action and storms, providing risk reduction benefits to an estimated 100 to 197 million people that live below 10-meter elevation and within 50 kilometers of reefs (Woodhead et al. 2019; Ferrario et al. 2014). These same communities are on the frontline of extreme weather events and potential exposure to increased risk of infectious disease (Food and Agriculture Organization [FAO] 2015).

Climate change predictions paint a bleak picture for corals and the human communities who rely upon them. Achieving the ambitious emissions reduction targets of limiting global warming to 1.5°C (2.7°F) above the preindustrial period by 2030–2052, could still cause a loss of 70–90 percent of reefs. Even just a half degree higher—hitting 2.0°C (3.6°F)—would be catastrophic and result in a 99 percent loss (Hoegh-Guldberg et al. 2018; IPCC 2019)

Seafood insecurity has led to an acceleration of a "nutrition transition" toward processed foods, and affected communities face a double burden of disease from childhood micronutrient deficiencies plus an increase in adult obesity, diabetes, and metabolic and heart disease. Diminished seafood consumption during pregnancy also increases the risk of child suboptimal neurodevelopmental outcomes, including compromised cognition and fine motor skills (see Case Study 1). Loss of coral reefs can also increase foodborne illness risks, such ciguatera fish poisoning, which is on the rise and has no cure, for communities that rely on local supplies and for travelers (see Case Study 2). High in diversity, reefs have sedentary animals like sponges, corals, and tunicates that protect or defend themselves through chemical means and can yield potential discoveries for marine-based pharmaceuticals to meet public health needs (see Case Study 3).

Healthy reefs support healthy coastal economies, and coral reef tourism is a critical, undervalued ecosystem service (Spalding et al. 2017). Tourism in the 30 percent of the world's reefs that are travel destinations, annually generates $US 36 billion dollars globally from international and domestic visitors. This includes on-reef tourism such as diving, snorkeling, and glass bottom-boat tours, and indirect contributions from calm waters, beaches, views, and seafood. Economic benefits go beyond tourism: in the Caribbean, the Mesoamerican Reef system supports an economic value across tourism, commercial fisheries, and coastal development of $6.2 billion annually. In the Coral Triangle in Southeast Asia, the number is even higher at $13.9 billion (United Nations Environment Programme 2018). In the U.S. Florida Keys, coral reefs have an asset value of $8.5 billion and generate $4.4 billion in local sales, $2 billion in local income, and 70,400 full and part-time jobs (NOAA 2019).

Conversely, economic disruption from loss of fisheries and reef ecosystem stability has been associated with physical and mental health harms including fear, anger, exhaustion, and depression. Repeated and sustained stress releases cortisol, lowers production of dopamine and serotonin levels, and can have long-term physical impacts such as disease (Nichols 2014). In addition to disrupting provisioning services (e.g., fisheries, food security), climate change can undermine cultural services, such as cognitive and experiential benefits (Woodhead et al. 2019). The gathering and sharing of fish encompasses a range of cultural values including subsistence and knowledge values and social cohesion (Grafeld et al. 2017). Other wellbeing metrics for reef fishers are enjoyment, a sense of identity, tradition, prestige, and lifestyle (Cinner 2014; Woodhead et al. 2019).

CASE STUDY 1: FOOD SECURITY, NUTRITION, DISEASE, AND EXPOSURE TO PHYSICAL HAZARDS: LOSS OF SMALL-SCALE FISHERIES IN PACIFIC ISLAND COUNTRIES AND TERRITORIES AND HEALTH IMPACTS

Coral loss leads to reduced fisheries production, both commercially and for subsistence, which jeopardizes livelihoods and food security and increases poverty throughout the world's tropics. This highlights a key issue of equity for millions of people who depend on these valuable ecosystems (Hoegh-Guldberg et al. 2018; Spalding et al. 2014; Halpern et al. 2015). For many, fish are the primary source of animal protein, making up to 70 percent of diet in coastal and island countries (Pierre-Louis 2019; FAO 2014)

Loss of coral reefs has serious implications for human nutrition. Nine of the ten most obese nations on Earth are found in the South Pacific (Golden, C. Harvard Chan 2019 podcast). The collapse of local fisheries has led to an acceleration of a "nutrition transition" toward processed foods such as canned meats, instant noodles, cereals, rice, and sugar-sweetened beverages (Charlton et al. 2016). Also, food imports to countries such as Samoa and Tonga now exceed total exports (Morrison et al. 2019; Savage, McIver, and Schubert 2019).

Pacific Island countries and territories face a double burden of disease, with a high prevalence of food insecurity and childhood micronutrient deficiencies, accompanied by an increase in adult obesity, diabetes, and metabolic and heart disease. In these remote areas, there are very limited options to replace micronutrients lost, such as iron, zinc, vitamin A, vitamin B12, and fatty acids (Charlton et al. 2016).

Fish intake (consumption of 60 g fish/day) is associated with a 36 percent reduced mortality risk from heart disease and a 12 percent reduction in mortality from all causes (FAO 2017; Thilsted et al. 2016). Fish are a rich source of B12, zinc, and iron—essential for growth, brain function, and nervous system maintenance. Bioavailable calcium in small fish are particularly important in the diets of the poor, which are often low in milk products (FAO 2017; Thilsted et al. 2016).

Fish provide a unique source of long chain omega-3 fatty acids, intake of which, during pregnancy, is associated with reduced risk of early preterm delivery (and a modest increase in birth weight). Lower seafood consumption during pregnancy increases the risk of the child's suboptimal neurodevelopmental outcomes, including cognition and fine motor skills. In addition, fish enhance the uptake of micronutrients from plant-sources (FAO 2017; Thilsted et al. 2016).

Researchers are developing nutritional biomarkers such as hemoglobin to look at anemia, diabetes, and fatty acid profiles. In most cases, a return to traditional seafood-based diets can slow these epidemics and community-supported reef conservation can improve nutritional outcomes and human health (Golden, C. Harvard Chan 2019).

Investigating fish-food security and nutrition linkages is challenging given the complexities and interrelated factors including fish prices, wages, social security, household diet diversity, intrahousehold allocation of food, and child growth (FAO 2017). In 2017, cause of deaths in the Pacific from preventable diseases like diabetes, cardiovascular disease, and cancer has risen to 86 percent, compared to 80 percent just six years before, in part due to people's increased reliance on imports (Morrison et al. 2019; World Health Organization 2018).

Additional factors to consider are impacts to small-scale and subsistence fishers, who rely on the healthy and diverse ecosystems as the fundamental basis for their livelihoods. Twenty-five percent of small-scale fisheries fish primarily on coral reef (Woodhead et al. 2019; Teh, Teh, and Sumaila 2013) and degradation of coral reefs extends to products from a range of taxa used for subsistence and cash income (Woodhead et al. 2019; Albert et al. 2015). The lack of available resources can increase competition, restrict access to fisheries, shift fishing efforts to further locations, and increase exposure to new physical risks (FAO 2017; Weeratunge et al. 2011). Shifts in gender roles, physical demands and exposure to more dangerous occupational hazards are important factors to consider and can affect the entire community (FAO 2017).

CASE STUDY 2: CIGUATERA FISH POISONING IN THE GULF OF MEXICO AND THE CARIBBEAN

Climate-change-induced reef loss or damage can increase risk of seafood poisoning in communities that rely on local supplies but also pose a serious and underrecognized hazard for travelers. Ciguatera fish poisoning is an illness that is on the rise and occurs after eating reef fish contaminated with toxins produced by the dinoflagellate, *Gambierdiscus toxicus* (Ansdell 2019).

Dead coral reefs can provide a hospitable surface for colonization of filamentous and calcareous macroalgae, a substrate preferred by *G. toxicus* (Hallegraeff, Anderson, and Cembella 1995). Dinoflagellates are ingested by herbivorous fish. The toxins produced by *G. toxicus* are then biomodified and concentrated by intermediate species as they pass up the marine food chain to carnivorous fish, such as barracuda and finally to humans. Ciguatoxins are concentrated in fish liver, intestines, roe, and heads (Ansdell 2019).

Up to 50,000 cases of ciguatera poisoning are reported annually worldwide. Because the disease is underrecognized and underreported, this is likely a significant underestimate. The incidence in travelers to highly endemic areas (the tropical and subtropical waters between the latitudes of 35°N and 35°S) has been estimated as high as three cases per one hundred people (Ansdell 2019).

The incidence and geographic distribution of ciguatera poisoning are increasing because of warming oceans and tropicalization of species. Newly recognized areas of risk include the Canary Islands, the eastern Mediterranean, and the western Gulf of Mexico. Also, cases of ciguatera poisoning are seen with increasing frequency in nonendemic areas because of increased global trade in seafood products. Today, ciguatera has become a more visible human health threat due to increased global travel and appearance in nonendemic areas from increased global trade in seafood products (Ansdell 2019; FAO 2018).

People who have ciguatera may experience nausea, vomiting, and neurologic symptoms such as tingling fingers or toes. They also may find that cold things feel hot and hot things feel cold. Ciguatera has no cure. Symptoms usually go away in days or weeks but can last for years. There is no readily available test for ciguatera toxins in humans and no specific antidote; only symptoms can be treated (Ansdell 2019; FAO 2018).

Fish that are most likely to cause ciguatera poisoning are large carnivorous reef fish, such as barracuda, grouper, moray eel, amberjack, sea bass, or sturgeon. Omnivorous and herbivorous fish such as parrot fish, surgeonfish, and red snapper can also be a risk (Ansdell 2019).

For years, ciguatera had been an issue for developing countries but typically with very limited resources to support local research. Researchers are looking for detection methods for a quick and easy field test, like a dipstick method or biosensor technologies (FAO 2018). Communities directly affected by ciguatera use different ways to lower risk of exposure, sometimes with cats and small dogs to test fish before consumption. Elderly people are sometimes willing to take the risk of eating the fish for the community (FAO 2018).

CASE STUDY 3: MARINE PHARMACEUTICALS AND LOSS OF LIFESAVING DRUGS FROM THE SEA

Healthy coral reefs provide a virtually untapped source of marine-based pharmaceuticals and natural products that can greatly enhance quality of life and combat human illnesses (Sandifer et al. 2007). High in diversity, reefs have sedentary animals like sponges, corals, and tunicates that protect or defend themselves through chemical means, which can yield potential discoveries to meet human health needs and cures (Katona 2015).

For example, coral reef sponges contain bioactive chemical compounds used in anti-viral and anti-cancer drugs, including the HIV drug AZT, a breakthrough in AIDS treatment in the late 1980s. An antileukemia drug was the first marine drug approved for cancer treatment in 1969 (Smithsonian Institution 2019). The National Cancer Institute has invested in the discovery and development of anticancer drugs from the ocean, with over thirty in preclinical and clinical trials to treat a variety of cancers (Sandifer et al. 2007).

Other coral reef products on the market include a pain medication derived from the cone snail (Sandifer et al. 2007). The list of chemotherapy agents, antibiotics, antivirals, anesthetics, adhesives, and marine genetic products being used or developed to treat cancer, leukemia, cystic fibrosis, heart disease, wounds, and infections includes at least 18,000 products derived from 4,800 marine species (Arrieta, Arnaud-Haond, and Duarte 2010).

Summary

Coral reefs are the marine ecosystem most threatened from anthropogenic climate change and are projected to be lost unless global carbon emissions are slashed to 45 percent of 2010 levels by 2030 (IPCC 2019). The related human health consequences are unprecedented and need to be considered in disaster planning and as potential health benefits in marine resource planning (Sutton-Grier and Sandifer 2018). Experts suggest the plight of coral reefs could push nations past societal and political tipping points (Morrison et al. 2019). Engineered solutions to combat further loss or strengthen resiliency and rebuilding of some reefs show promise, including restoration, assisted species relocation, use of marine protected areas, and coral gardening. Such actions are most successful when they are community supported and science based, using local and Indigenous knowledge, with long-term reduction or removal of nonclimatic stressors, and under the lowest levels of warming humanly achievable (IPCC 2019).

Key Terms

Ocean acidification: Presents an additional challenge and can inhibit coral reef recovery. The increase in CO_2 in the atmosphere absorbed by the ocean reduces calcification rates in reef-building and reef-associated organisms by altering seawater chemistry through decreases in pH. This affects the growth and structural integrity of coral reefs.

Warm-water reefs: Warm-water coral reefs occupying habitats that are close to the surface (0–100 meters) where they secrete calcium carbonate skeletons that accumulate over time, creating a complex reef matrix that provides habitat for hundreds of thousands of marine species.

References

Albert, J. A., S. Albert, A. Olds, A. Cruz-Trinidad, and A.-M. Schwarz. 2015. "Reaping the Reef: Provisioning Services from Coral Reefs in Solomon Islands." *Marine Policy* 62:244–51.

Alvarez-Filip, L., N. K. Dulvy, J. A. Gill, I. M. Cote, and A. R. Watkinson. 2009. "Flattening of Caribbean Coral Reefs: Region-Wide Declines in Architectural Complexity." *Proceedings of the Royal Society of London. Series B* 276:3019–25.

Alvarez-Filip, L., J. A. Gill, N. K. Dulvy, A. L. Perry, A. R. Watkinson, and I. M. Coté. 2011. "Drivers of Region-Wide Declines in Architectural Complexity on Caribbean Reefs." *Coral Reefs* 30:1051–60.

Ansdell, V. E. 2019. "Chapter 2: Preparing International Travelers." In *Yellow Book—Travelers' Health. CDC Food Poisoning from Marine Toxins*. Atlanta, GA: Centers for Disease Control and Prevention. https://wwwnc.cdc.gov/travel/yellowbook/2020/preparing-international-travelers/food-poisoning-from-marine-toxins.

Arrieta, J. M., S. Arnaud-Haond, and C. M. Duarte. 2010. "What Lies Underneath: Conserving the Oceans' Genetic Resources." *Proceedings of the National Academy of Sciences of the USA* 107 (43):18318–24. doi:10.1073/pnas.0911897107.

Brander, L. M., P. Van Beukering, and H. S. J. Cesar. 2007. "The Recreational Value of Coral Reefs: A Meta-Analysis." *Ecological Economics* 63 (1):209–18. https://doi.org/10.1016/j.ecolecon.2006.11.002.

Bruno, J. F., I. M. Côté, L. T. Toth. 2019. "Climate Change, Coral Loss, and the Curious Case of the Parrotfish Paradigm: Why Don't Marine Protected Areas Improve Reef Resilience." *Annual Review of Marine Science* 11:307–34.

Burke, L., K. Reytar, M. Spalding, and A. Perry. *2011. Reefs at Risk Revisited.* Washington, DC: World Resources Institute. http://pdf.wri.org/reefs_at_risk_revisited.pdf. Calculated at WRI based on data from LandScan High Resolution Global Population Data Set, Oak Ridge National Laboratory, 2007.

Charlton, K. E., J. Russell, E. Gorman, Q. Hanich, A. Delisle, B. Campbell, and J. Bell. 2016. "Fish, Food Security and Health in Pacific Island Countries and Territories: A Systematic Literature Review." *BMC Public Health* 16:285. doi: 10.1186/s12889-016-2953-9.

Cinner, J. 2014. "Coral Reef Livelihoods." *Current Opinion in Environmental Sustainability* 7:65–71. https://doi.org/10.1016/j.cosust.2013.11.025.

Díaz, S., J. Settele, E. S. Brondízio, H. T. Ngo, M. Guèze, J. Agard, A. Arneth et al. 2019. *Summary for Policymakers of the Global Assessment Report on Biodiversity and Ecosystem Services of the Intergovernmental Science-Policy Platform on Biodiversity and Ecosystem Services*. Bonn, Germany: Intergovernmental Science-Policy Platform on Biodiversity and Ecosystem Services .https://ipbes.net/global-assessment-report-biodiversity-ecosystem-services.

Ferrario, F., M. W. Beck, C. D. Storlazzi, F. Micheli, C. C. Shepard, and L. Airoldi. 2014. "The Effectiveness of Coral Reefs for Coastal Hazard Risk Reduction and Adaptation." *Nature Communications* 5:3794, https://doi.org/10.1038/ncomms4794.

Food and Agriculture Organization. 2014. *The State of World Fisheries and Aquaculture: Opportunities and Challenges*. Rome: FAO. http://www.fao.org/3/a-i3720e.pdf.

Food and Agriculture Organization. 2015. *Voluntary Guidelines for Securing Sustainable Small-Scale Fisheries in the Context of Food Security and Poverty Eradication.* Rome: FAO. http://www.fao.org/3/a-i4356en.pdf.

Food and Agriculture Organization. 2017. *Strengthening Sector Policies for Better Food Security and Nutrition Results: Fisheries and Aquaculture. Policy Guidance Note 1.* Rome: FAO. http://www.fao.org/3/a-i6227e.pdf.

Food and Agriculture Organization. 2018. "Experts Meet for Deep Dive on Ciguatera Fish Poisoning." *November* 30, 2018. http://www.fao.org/fao-who-codexalimentarius/news-and-events/news-details/en/c/1173604.

Golden, C. Harvard Chan Podcast. 2019. "The Connection between Coral Reefs and Human Health." *February* 21, 2019. https://www.hsph.harvard.edu/news/multimedia-article/coral-reefs-health-nutrition/.

Grafeld, S., K. L. L. Oleson, L. Teneva, and J. N. Kittinger. 2017. "Follow That Fish: Uncovering the Hidden Blue Economy in Coral Reef Fisheries." *PLoS One* 12 (8):e0182104. https://doi.org/10.1371/journal. pone.0182104.

Hallegraeff, G. M., D. M. Anderson, and A. D. Cembella, eds. 1995. *Manual on Harmful Marine Microalgae.* New York: UNESCO.

Halpern, B. S., M. Frazier, J. Potapenko, K. S. Casey, K. Koenig, C. Longo, J. S. Lowndes et al. 2015. "Spatial and Temporal Changes in Cumulative Human Impacts on the World's Ocean." *Nature Communications* 6 (1):7615. doi:10.1038/ncomms8615.

Heron, S. F., R. van Hooidonk, J. Maynard, K. Anderson, J. C. Day, E. Geiger, O. Hoegh-Guldberg et al. 2018. *Impacts of Climate Change on World Heritage Coral Reefs: Update to the First Global Scientific Assessment.* Paris: UNESCO World Heritage Centre.

Hoegh-Guldberg, O., D. Jacob, M. Taylor, M. Bindi, S. Brown, I. Camilloni, A. Diedhiou et al. 2018. "Impacts of 1.5°C Global Warming on Natural and Human Systems." In *Global Warming of 1.5°C. An IPCC Special Report on the Impacts of Global Warming of 1.5°C above Pre-Industrial Levels and Related Global Greenhouse Gas Emission Pathways, in the Context of Strengthening the Global Response to the Threat of Climate Change, Sustainable Development, and Efforts to Eradicate Poverty*, edited by V. Masson-Delmotte, P. Zhai, H.-O. Pörtner, D. Roberts, J. Skea, P. R. Shukla, A. Pirani, W. Moufouma-Okia et al., 175–311. Geneva: Intergovernmental Panel on Climate Change. https://www.ipcc.ch/sr15/chapter/chapter-3/.

Hoegh-Guldberg, O., L. Pendleton, and A. Kaup. 2019. "People and the Changing Nature of Coral Reefs." *Regional Studies in Marine Science* 30 (July 2019). https://www.sciencedirect.com/science/article/pii/S2352485518306637.

Hughes, T. P., J. T. Kerry, S. R. Connolly, A. H. Baird, C. M. Eakin, S. F. Heron, A. S. Hoey et al. 2019. "Ecological Memory Modifies The Cumulative Impact Of Recurrent Climate Extremes." *Nature Climate Change* 9:40–43.

Hughes, T. P., K. D Anderson, S. R. Connolly, S. F. Heron, J. T. Kerry, J. M. Lough, A. H. Baird et al. 2018. "Spatial and Temporal Patterns of Mass Bleaching of Corals in the Anthropocene." *Science* 359 (6371):80–83.

Idjadi, J. A., and P. J. Edmunds. 2006. "Scleractinian Corals as Facilitators for Other Invertebrates on a Caribbean Reef." *Marine Ecology Progress Series* 319:117–27.

International Year of the Reef. 2018. "Benefits of Coral Reefs." https://www.iyor2018.org/about-coral-reefs/benefits-of-coral-reefs/.

Intergovernmental Panel on Climate Change. 2019. "Summary for Policymakers." In *IPCC Special Report on the Ocean and Cryosphere in a Changing Climate*, edited by H.-O. Pörtner, D. C. Roberts, V. Masson-Delmotte, P. Zhai, M. Tignor, E. Poloczanska, K. Mintenbeck et al. Geneva: IPCC.

Jones, G. P., M. I. McCormick, M. Srinivasan, and J. V. Eagle. 2004. "Coral Decline Threatens Fish Biodiversity in Marine Reserves." *Proceedings of the National Academy of Sciences of the USA* 101:8251–3.

Katona, S. 2015. "Marine Animals in Human Medicine: Will a Sponge Save Your Life?" Ocean Health Index. *January* 22, 2015. http://www.oceanhealthindex.org/news/Marine_Animals_Human_Medicine.

Moberg, F., and C. Folke. 1999. "Ecological Goods and Services of Coral Reef Ecosystems." *Ecological Economics* 29 (2):215–33. https://doi.org/10.1016/S0921-8009(99)00009-9.

Morrison, T. H., T. P. Hughes, W. N. Adger. K. Brown, J. Barnett, M. C. Lemos, D. Huitema et al. 2019. "Comment: Save Reefs to Rescue All Ecosystems: An Approach that Tackles the Underlying Causes of Coral-Reef Decline Could Be Applied to Other Habitats." *Nature* 573:333–6.

National Oceanic and Atmospheric Administration. 2019. Florida Keys National Marine Sanctuary website. Accessed June 21, 2020. https://floridakeys.noaa.gov/.

Nichols, J. 2014. *Blue Mind: The Surprising Science that Shows How Being Near, In, On, or Under Water Can Make You Happier, Healthier, More Connected and Better at What You Do.* New York: Little Brown Spark Publishing.

National Ocean Service. 2019a. "Ocean Facts—What Is Coral Bleaching?" National Ocean Service. Accessed February 17, 2020. https://oceanservice.noaa.gov/facts/coral_bleach.html.

National Ocean Service. 2019b. "Threats To Coral Reefs: How Does Climate Change Affect Coral Reefs?" National Ocean Service. Accessed February 17, 2020. https://oceanservice.noaa.gov/facts/coralreef-climate.html.

Pendleton, L. H., O. Hoegh-Huldberg, C. Langdon, and A. Comte. 2016. "Multiple Stressors and Ecological Complexity Require a New Approach to Coral Reef Research." *Frontiers in Marine Science* 3:1–5. doi: 10.3389/fmars.2016.00036.

Pierre-Louis, K. 2019. "The World Is Losing Fish to Eat as Oceans Warm, Study Finds." *New York Times,* February 28, 2019.

Pierre-Louis, K., and B. Plumer. 2018. "Global Warming's Toll on Coral Reefs: As If They're 'Ravaged by War.'" *New York Times,* January 4, 2018. https://www.nytimes.com/2018/01/04/climate/coral-reefs-bleaching.html?module=inline.

Pratchett, M. S., P. L. Munday, S. K. Wilson, N. A. J. Graham, J. E. Cinner, D. R. Bellwood, G. P. Jones, N. V. C. Polunin, and T. R. McClanahan. 2008. "Effects of Climate-Induced Coral Bleaching on Coral-Reef Fishes: Ecological and Economic Consequences." *Oceanography and Marine Biology* 46 (46): 251–96. doi: 10.1201/9781420065756.ch6.

Sandifer, P., C. Sotka, D. Garrison, and V. Fay. 2007. *Interagency Oceans and Human Health Research Implementation Plan: A Prescription for the Future.* Washington, DC: Interagency Working Group on Harmful Algal Blooms, Hypoxia, and Human Health of the Joint Subcommittee on Ocean Science and Technology.

Savage, A., L. McIver, and L. Schubert. 2019. "Review: The Nexus of Climate Change, Food and Nutrition Security and Diet-Related Non-Communicable Diseases in Pacific Island Countries and Territories." *Climate and Developmen* 12 (2):120–33.

Smithsonian Website. 2019. "From Sea Sponge to HIV Medicine." https://ocean.si.edu/ocean-life/invertebrates/sea-sponge-hiv-medicine.

Spalding, M. D., S. Ruffo, C. Lacambra, I. Meliane, L. Z. Hale, C. C.Shepard, and M. W. Beck. 2014. "The Role of Ecosystems in Coastal Protection: Adapting to Climate Change and Coastal Hazards." *Ocean and Coastal Management* 90:50–57. doi:10.1016/j.ocecoaman.2013.09.007.

Spalding, M. D., L. Burke, S. A.Wood, J. Ashpole, J. Hutchison, and P. zu Ermgassene. 2017. "Mapping the Global Value and Distribution of Coral Reef Tourism." *Marine Policy* 82:104–13. doi:10.1016/j.marpol.2017.05.014.

Sutton-Grier, A. E., and P. A. Sandifer. 2018. "Conservation of Wetlands and Other Coastal Ecosystems: a Commentary on their Value to Protect Biodiversity, Reduce Disaster Impacts, and Promote Human Health and Well-Being." *Wetlands* 39:1295–1302.

Teh, L. S., L. C. Teh, and U. R. Sumaila. 2013. "A Global Estimate of the Number of Coral Reef Fishers." *PLoS One* 8:e65397.

Thilsted, S. H., A. Thorne-Lyman, P. Webb, J. R. Bogard, R. Subasingh, M. J. Phillips, and E. H. Allison. 2016. "Sustaining Healthy Diets: The Role of Capture Fisheries and Aquaculture for Improving Nutrition in the Post-2015 Era." *Food Policy* 61:126–31.

United Nations Environment Programme. 2018. *The Coral Reef Economy: The Business Case for Investment in the Protection, Preservation and Enhancement of Coral Reef Health.* Nairobi, Kenya: UNEP. https://wedocs.unep.org/bitstream/handle/20.500.11822/26694/Coral_Reef_Economy.pdf?sequence=1&isAllowed=y.

Weeratunge, N., D. Pemsl, P. Rodriguez, O. L. Chen, M. C. Badjeck, A. M. Schwarz, C. Paul, J. Prange, and J. Kelling. 2011. *Planning the Use of Fish for Food Security in Solomon Islands.* Manado, Indonesia: Coral Triangle Support Partnership.

World Health Organization. 2018. *Progress on the Prevention and Control of Noncommunicable Diseases in the Western Pacific Region: Country Capacity Survey 2017.* Manila: Regional Office for the Western Pacific, WHO.

Woodhead, A. J., C. C. Hicks, A. V. Norström, G. J. Williams, and N. A. J. Graham. (2019). "Coral Reef Ecosystem Services in the Anthropocene." *Functional Ecology* 2019:1–12.

THE *NURSES CLIMATE CHALLENGE*: A MODEL FOR HEALTH PROFESSIONAL CLIMATE ACTION

Shanda Demorest

Key Concepts

- Nurses as holistic and trusted professionals have immense potential to lead action on climate change.

- The diverse range of nursing practice gives nurses the opportunity to leverage their knowledge and position to influence climate action at the bedside, through education, and action at a public policy level.

- The *Nurses Climate Challenge* is one approach to educating health professionals about the health impacts of climate change that could be adapted and applied to other disciplines.

Americans consistently rate nurses as the most highly trusted professionals (Brenan 2018). Nurses care for and connect with people during the most meaningful and difficult times of their lives. They are specially trained to strike a balance between cutting-edge science and the art of human connection, and they work with people across all ages in all settings. Furthermore, the American Nurses Association (2015) advocates that "the registered nurse practices in an environmentally safe and healthy manner," which broadens the profession to one that exists far beyond the bedside and into the world.

Climate Affects Health

Leading health organizations and experts have deemed climate change to be a grave global public health threat (American Public Health Association [APHA] 2018; Centers for Disease Control and Prevention [CDC] 2018; Watts et al. 2018; World Health Organization [WHO] 2018). Specifically, climate change has health impacts from air pollution, extreme heat, vector-borne diseases, food- and waterborne illness, mental health issues, and many others (U.S. Global Change Research Program [USGCRP] 2018). These health impacts disproportionately affect vulnerable and marginalized populations. Although this issue naturally fits within the nursing scope of practice, the nursing profession does not yet have consistent or streamlined protocols for incorporating content into nursing schools or practice settings.

Despite the lack of widespread nursing engagement, some organizations have successfully led in integrating climate change into the profession (Cook, Demorest, and Schenk 2019). For example, Alliance of Nurses for Healthy Environments (ANHE 2018) is a national organization aimed at empowering nurses to act on environmental challenges that include water security, workplace and environmental chemical exposures, and climate change via engagement strategies in education and policy work. In addition, the interdisciplinary nonprofit organization Health Care Without Harm (HCWH 2018) supports the health care industry in implementing environmental sustainability initiatives around energy use and waste across entire health care systems. It was through the partnership of ANHE and HCWH that the Nurses Climate Challenge was born.

The Nurses Climate Challenge

The Nurses Climate Challenge (2019) was the nation's first nurse-led campaign to educate health professionals about the human health impacts of climate change. When the challenge was launched in May 2018 at the Alliance of Nurses for Healthy Environments Summit and the CleanMed conference (the joint conference of Health Care Without Harm and Practice Greenhealth), the team aspired toward a goal of educating 5,000 health professionals.

Online registration for the challenge was free and open to all nurses, nursing students, and former nurses of all educational backgrounds. Nurses who registered to participate in the Nurses Climate Challenge became "Nurse Climate Champions" and gained access to a comprehensive toolkit with evidence-based, regional resources to share in their own settings.

Resources for the Nurses Climate Challenge:

- Outline of steps and timeline for planning, promoting, and hosting successful education sessions

- Sample e-mail for engaging leadership

- Short (ten-minute) PowerPoint presentation on the health impacts of climate change

- Long (twenty- to thirty-minute) PowerPoint presentation on the health impacts of climate change

- Talking points and strategies for having challenging conversations about climate change

- Guide to how nurses can be hospitals' climate champions

- Guide for acting in the health care setting and in one's personal life

After hosting a session, Nurse Climate Champions were asked to report (via the website) the number of people they had educated on climate and health issues and to answer questions on some basic metrics regarding their audience's reception of the content. The original goal of educating 5,000 health professionals on climate and health was met within ten months of the project launch. In May 2019, the Nurses Climate Challenge team increased the goal to educating 50,000 health professionals on climate and health issues by 2022.

Diversity, Breadth, and Depth

Within twenty months of launching, nearly 1,000 nurses from forty-seven U.S. states and twenty countries registered to become Nurse Climate Champions. Participants' roles and settings varied widely. Approximately one third of champions served in staff nursing roles, one fifth in nurse educator roles, with the rest of the champions being nurse leaders, advanced practice nurses, researchers, community nurses, and student nurses (Demorest et al. 2019). In addition, Nurse Climate Champions who practiced in health systems that were members of Practice Greenhealth (2017)—a national organization which aims to implement environmental sustainability initiatives within health systems—were introduced by the Nurses Climate Challenge team to leaders within the health systems' sustainability departments to deepen climate and sustainability work within those settings.

Nurse Climate Champions reported educating in a variety of settings such as hospital staff meetings, grand rounds, conferences, community events, classrooms, student clinical sites, and break rooms. Across all educational sessions, champions reported very high levels of audience engagement, strong interest in implementing environmental sustainability initiatives, and very little dissent from participants (Demorest et al. 2019).

Lessons Learned and Growing the Challenge

Although engagement in the Nurses Climate Challenge has been robust and the outcomes surpassed early goals, the national campaign alone is not a comprehensive model for other health professional education on climate change. The Nurses Climate Challenge as an educational campaign was based on the premise that nurses must *understand* about climate and health impacts before they *care* about them—and nurses must *care* about climate and health impacts before they *act* on them. However, with bold global goals of reducing carbon emissions, climate change education is insufficient. To further tackle emissions, the team developed a repertoire of action-oriented climate advocacy resources for champions to use in the workplace and at home such as:

- Resources for nurses to participate in Energy Star Treasure Hunts, an Environmental Protection Agency (2019) program supporting efforts to find energy saving opportunities on nursing units within their health care setting

- Guidance for champions to recommend clean energy to their hospital administration

- Meeting script for elected officials about climate change policy issues

The Nurses Climate Challenge engaged hundreds of nurses across the country and around the world in climate change by offering resources to those who registered to become Nurse Climate Champions. Furthermore, the challenge facilitated the education of thousands of others by empowering the registered champions to educate their peers about the health impacts of climate change. Given nurses' roles as holistic and trusted professionals, it follows that issues of climate change and health care are a necessary area of expansion to the profession not only for individual nurses serving as Nurse Climate Champions but also broadly in bedside care, formalized nursing education, and in public policy. The holistic, systems-wide approach of nursing can better prepare entire interdisciplinary clinical teams to take climate change into account when assessing, diagnosing, caring for, and discharging patients within the clinical care setting. In addition, educating nursing students *before* they enter practice settings will better prepare them to care for patients who will continue to exhibit signs of climate-related health effects. Finally, climate-educated nurses advocating for climate-smart legislation with their local policymakers will influence policy that not only addresses human health but also the health of the ecosystems in which we live. Early success suggests that the framework of the Nurses Climate Challenge could serve as a model for climate education and action not only in the nursing profession but in other health care disciplines as well.

References

Alliance of Nurses for Healthy Environments. 2018. "Climate Change and Health." https://envirn.org/climate-change/.

American Nurses Association. 2015. "Environmental Health." https://www.nursingworld.org/practice-policy/work-environment/health-safety/environmental-health/.

American Public Health Association. 2018. "Climate Change." https://www.apha.org/topics-and-issues/climate-change.

Brenan, M. 2018. "Nurses Again Outpace Other Professions for Honesty, Ethics." Gallup. December 20, 2018. https://news.gallup.com/poll/245597/nurses-again-outpace-professions-honesty-ethics.aspx.

Centers for Disease Control and Prevention. 2018. "Climate and Health." https://www.cdc.gov/climate-andhealth/default.htm.

Cook, C., S. Demorest, and E. Schenk. 2019. "Nurses and Climate Action." *American Journal of Nursing* 119 (4):54–60.

Demorest, S., S. Spengeman, E, Schenk, C. Cook, and H. Levey Weston. 2019. "The Nurses Climate Challenge: A National Campaign to Engage 5,000 Health Professionals Around Climate Change." *Creative Nursing* 25 (3):208–15.

Environmental Protection Agency. 2019. *Energy Star Treasure Hunts.* https://www.energystar.gov/buildings/about-us/campaigns/treasure_hunt.

Health Care Without Harm. 2018. "Climate and Health." https://noharm-uscanada.org/issues/us-canada/climate-and-health/#initiatives.

Nurses Climate Challenge. 2019. *Nurses Climate Challenge.* https://nursesclimatechallenge.org/.

Practice Greenhealth. 2017. "About." https://practicegreenhealth.org/about.

U.S. Global Change Research Program. 2018. *Impacts of Climate Change on Human Health in the United States: A Scientific Assessment.* Washington, DC: USGCRP.

Watts, N., M. Amann, S. Ayeb-Karlsson, K. Belesova, T. Bouley, M. Boykoff, P. Byass et al. 2018. "The Lancet Countdown on Health and Climate Change: From 25 Years of Inaction to a Global Transformation for Public Health." *Lancet* 391 (10120):581–630.

World Health Organization. 2018. "Climate Change and Health." https://www.who.int/news-room/fact-sheets/detail/climate-change-and-health.

Abiotic factor: Nonliving chemical or physical factor that can affect an ecosystem.

Active transport: The use of nonmotorized transportation forms, such as walking, cycling, or public transit.

Adaptation: According to the Intergovernmental Panel on Climate Change, the process of adjustment to new conditions. In human systems, climate adaptation seeks to moderate harm and/or exploit beneficial opportunities. In some natural systems, human intervention may facilitate adjustment to expected climate and its effects. Also, efforts to lessen the impacts of climate change through measures to prepare populations for a changing climate, such as disaster preparedness and flood control.

Adaptive management: A framework that uses regularly updated models to facilitate iterative management of complex systems subjects with multiple stakeholders (Holling 1978; National Research Council 2004).

Aeroallergen: Any airborne substance, such as pollen or spores, that triggers an allergic reaction.

Aerobiology: A subset of biology that studies the dynamics of organic particles and small organisms that can be passively transported by air. Aerobiologists are associated with the measuring and reporting of airborne pollen and fungal spores as a public health service.

Aerosol: A suspension of fine solid particles or liquid droplets, in air or another gas.

Air toxins: Airborne pollutants that cause or may cause cancer or other serious health effects, such as reproductive effects or birth defects, or adverse environmental and ecological effects.

Ambient air: Regulatory term within the Environmental Protection Agency's (EPA's) National Ambient Air Quality Standards that refers to "the atmosphere, external to buildings, to which the general public has access."

Amnesic shellfish poisoning: Poisoning syndrome occurring from the consumption of shellfish contaminated with domoic acid.

AMPA: α-amino-3-hydroxy-5-methyl-4-isoxazolepropionic acid, a neurotransmitter that has an action like that of glutamate.

Anchor institutions: Enterprises such as universities and hospitals that are rooted in their local communities through mission, invested capital, or relationships to customers, employees, and vendors.

Anthropocene: Relating to the current geologic age, characterized by the predominantly human influence on climate and the environment.

Anthropogenic: Originating from human activity.

Arboviruses: Viruses transmitted by mosquitoes, ticks, and midges. They include the important human pathogens yellow fever virus, dengue virus, chikungunya virus, and Zika virus.

Atmosphere: The gaseous envelope of a planet such as Earth.

Attainment area: A location with concentrations of criteria pollutants that are below the levels established by the EPA's National Ambient Air Quality Standards.

Attribution: The process of proving that a response is actually a direct result of a forcing, beyond simply observing a correlation between cause and effect. For example, see **Attribution experiment**.

Attribution experiment: In the context of climate modeling, an attribution experiment is one in which a known forcing agent is withheld to determine the degree to which the result is a direct result of that forcing agent. For example, using a global climate model to simulate the twentieth century with and without the observed increase in CO_2 concentration—the latter experiment not resulting in global warming attributes global warming to the CO_2 increase.

Benefit-Cost Analysis (BCA): An analysis that compares the costs and benefits of an action in monetary terms.

Bias: In the context of global climate models (GCMs), a bias is a discrepancy between today's climate as simulated by the GCM and that observed in real data (in situ measurements, satellite observations, etc.). A typical GCM bias might be that India does not receive enough rainfall or that the eastern Pacific Ocean is too cold. Some GCM biases are systemic (i.e., common across most of the GCMs from around the world) or vary enough from GCM to GCM that they effectively cancel out in the ensemble average of GCMs.

Biodiversity: From "biological diversity"; the variability among all life forms that exist on Earth.

Biogenic: Originating from natural sources. Often used in the climate literature to describe emissions including volatile organic compounds released from trees and vegetation, such as monoterpenes and iso-prenes, as well as emissions of nitrogen compounds from soil.

Biological hazards: Communicable disease pathogens that when exposed to populations may cause loss of life, injury, or other health impacts.

Biosphere: The regions of a planet in which life can exist.

Biotic factor: A living factor that can affect an ecosystem.

Boundary value problem: A model experiment in which the results will be strongly influenced by factors external to (or literally at the boundaries of) the system being modeled. This is the case in future climate change experiments (see **Future experiment**).

Capacity: The measure of all the strengths, attributes, and resources available to a community, society, or organization (e.g., people) that can be used to achieve agreed goals.

Chlorofluorocarbon: Fluorinated gas (F-gas)—a potent greenhouse gas; a synthetic chemical capable of destroying the earth's atmosphere more quickly than it can naturally restore itself. These migrate into the upper atmosphere and break down and release chlorine and bromine ions, which catalyze the breakdown of the ozone molecules, and each ion can destroy thousands of ozone molecules. The Montreal Protocol success-fully phased cholorfluorocarbons out of production and consumption.

Clean Air Act: A U.S. federal law that regulates air emissions from stationary and mobile sources. Among other things, this law authorizes the Environmental Protection Agency to establish National Ambient Air Quality Standards to protect public health and public welfare and to regulate emissions of hazardous air pollutants.

Climate-altering pollutants: Pollutants that contribute to global warming.

Climate change: The systematic change in the long-term state of the atmosphere over multiple decades (or longer); a combination of human-induced and natural climatic changes or human-induced changes alone.

Climate Change and Health Diagnostic: Five-stage diagnostic created by the World Bank Group to support climate-smart health care and ultimately, to improve morbidity and mortality.

Climate change communication: Material designed to inform, persuade, or engage with climate change. Material may be delivered face to face or using a variety of media.

Climate change impact: Any number of effects of the long-term variation in average weather conditions occurring across the globe.

Climate crisis: The anthropogenic impacts that have accelerated the earth's warming and environmental destruction to near-catastrophic levels.

Climate feedback: Forcing in the climate system that is both a cause and effect of itself and either acts to amplify (positive feedback) or dampen the initial forcing (negative feedback).

Climate mitigation: Efforts to reduce climate-altering pollutant concentrations through reductions in emissions and/or increases in carbon capture.

Climate models: Multifaceted tools that complement observations and theory. (also see **Global climate model**).

Climate penalty: Increase in air pollutants (eg. surface ozone, $PM_{2.5}$) resulting from regional climate warming in the absence of precursor emission changes.

Climate-related disaster: Serious disruption influenced by long-term meteorologic conditions caused by changes in long-term weather patterns.

Climate resiliency: The capacity of communities to prepare for, protect, and recover from the impacts associated with climate-related events.

Climate-resilient health system: Health system that can anticipate, respond to, cope with, recover from, and adapt to climate-related shocks and stress, in order to bring sustained improvements in population health (World Health Organization 2015).

Climate sensitivity: How strongly the global climate system responds to a given amount of forcing (see **Radiative forcing**).

Climate-smart health care: Low carbon, resilient health care strategies.

Climate variability: Regular patterns in the Earth system that occur over periods of months to decades. (also see **Internal variability**)

Climatologic hazards: Weather conditions that, when they occur over a period of time, may cause loss of life, injury, or other health impacts.

Clinical champions: Clinicians who advocate for change, leverage their influence within the organization, and lead their peers on sustainability issues

Clinical sustainability: The processes of providing clinical care and identification of ways to improve the environmental performance of clinical practice without compromising the quality of care. It looks closely at how we use health care resources and why we use them the way we do, in order to reduce clinical medicine's overall environmental footprint.

Coarse particles: A type of particulate matter found near roadways and dusty industries, with an aerodynamic diameter larger than 2.5 micrometers and smaller than 10 micrometers in diameter (PM_{10}).

Co-benefits: Positive benefits (air quality, health, economic, aesthetic, ecosystem) related to the reduction of greenhouse gases.

Co-harms: Adverse health impacts of climate mitigation strategies.

Combined sewer overflow: The untreated and partially treated human and industrial waste, toxic materials, stormwater, and debris that exceed the holding capacity of the sewer system. Resulting runoff pollutes nearby and downstream rivers, streams, and other bodies of water.

Common but differentiated responsibilities: A foundational principle of environmental law aimed at facilitating fairness and cooperation between developed and developing nations. This principle is based on the premise that although all nations have the same responsibility to protect the environment and encourage sustainable development, their obligations to meet such responsibilities are nonetheless proportionate with their commensurate level of resources, capabilities, and advantages/disadvantages.

Concentration: The amount of a substance present in the medium, for example, carbon dioxide or methane in the atmosphere, usually expressed as parts per million.

Concentration Response Function: see **Dose-, Exposure-,** or **Concentration Response Function**

Conflict hazards: Conditions of human conflict that when exposed to a population may cause loss of life, injury, or other health impacts.

Consumerism: A preoccupation with and inclination toward the purchase of consumer goods.

Control experiment: A "long" global change model (GCM) simulation (typically simulating a time period of 1,000 years or more) in which greenhouse gas concentrations (and other facts such as solar output) are held constant. Control experiments can be used to determine how large an externally (such as human-) forced trend (in a different experiment) should be in order to be "detectable" amid the background, natural climate variability.

Cost-effectiveness analysis (CEA): An analysis that determines which alternative most efficiently uses available resources (monetary or not) to achieve a given goal.

Cost-of-illness (COI): A measure of the costs resulting from a disease or condition (or the monetary expression of total burden of disease), including the direct medical and nonmedical costs, lost productivity, and other costs to society.

Counterfactual: Hypothetical exploration of what might have happened if initial conditions had been as stipulated.

Cryosphere: The frozen water parts of a planet such as Earth.

Cryptobiotic crusts: Communities of living organisms, often containing fungi and cyanobacteria that form crusts on soils in arid regions such as deserts.

Cultural ecosystem services: Ecosystem services that describe the nonmaterial benefits that ecosystems provide to people, such as recreation opportunity, aesthetic appreciation, spiritual connection, sense of place, or appreciation for the existence of a particular habitat or species (see **Ecosystem services**).

Cultural worldview: A preference for a particular type of social control and organization; for example, egalitarians emphasize equal status and collective problem-solving whereas individualists emphasize personal autonomy and economic freedom.

Cumulative impacts: The health risks and impacts caused by multiple pollutants, usually emitted by multiple sources of pollution in a community, and their interactions with each other and any social vulnerabilities that exist in the community.

Cyclone: Weather phenomenon featuring a central region of low pressure surrounded by air flowing in an inward spiral and generating maximum sustained winds speeds of 74 mph or greater.

Dead zones: Areas of oceans and lakes that contain little or no oxygen because of nutrient inputs.

Dehydration: A significant loss of body fluid that impairs normal body function.

Delta method: A commonly used method to create a temperature projection time series that relies on mean climate warming applied to the observed present-day climate.

Demography: The statistical study of living populations with regard to dynamic changes in their size, structure, and distribution in time and space.

Dengue: Term used to refer both to a virus and to the disease caused when this virus infects humans. Dengue is an arbovirus primarily transmitted to humans by *Aedes* species. Dengue infection typically manifests as a self-limited acute febrile illness; however, a range of symptoms are possible, including life-threatening hemorrhagic shock. No specific treatment exists beyond supportive care.

Diarrhetic shellfish poisoning: Poisoning syndrome that occurs from the consumption of shellfish contaminated with okadaic acid.

Diazotrophic: Refers to atmospheric N_2 and the organisms able to use this atmospheric gas to make more complex forms of nitrogen such as ammonia.

Dilution effect: The so-called "dilution effect" posits that changes in biodiversity in some ecosystems will affect the transmission cycle of certain pathogens. Where biodiversity is higher, the presence of hosts with a low capacity to transmit disease from host to vector can dilute the effect of highly competent hosts. Conversely, reductions in diversity may increase infection risk and disease prevalence in hosts.

Disability adjusted life year (DALY): A measure of disease burden that incorporates both years of life lost due to premature mortality and years lost due to disability (World Health Organization n.d.).

Disaster: A serious disruption involving widespread human morbidity and mortality, which exceeds the ability of the affected community or society to cope using its own resources.

Disaster risk management: The systematic process of lessening the adverse impacts of hazards and the possibility of disaster.

Disaster risk reduction: The concept and practice of lowering disaster risks through systematic efforts to analyze and manage the causal factors of disasters, including through reduced exposure to hazards, lessened vulnerability of people, wise management of land and the environment, and improved preparedness for adverse events.

Dispersion: Distribution of air pollution into the atmosphere.

Diurnal temperature range (DTR): The difference between daily maximum and minimum temperatures.

Dose-, Exposure-, or **Concentration Response Function:** The **relative risk** of adverse health outcomes at various dose, exposure, or concentration levels.

Drought: A period of deficiency of moisture in the soil such that there is inadequate water required for plants, animals, and human beings.

Early warning system: A predictive modeling tool used by epidemiologists, meteorologists, and others to anticipate environmental hazards such as heat waves and hurricanes.

Eclampsia: See **Preeclampsia**.

Ecosystem: A biological community of interacting organisms and their physical environment.

Ecosystem services: Benefits people receive from nature.

eHealth: The use of distance-spanning technology for health care and the use of electronic documentation of health services, including telemedicine, activities such as home monitoring of vital signs using mobile technology, and electronic health surveillance systems.

El Niño: Natural climate phenomenon in which the temperature of the surface of the eastern equatorial Pacific Ocean warms by a few degrees Celsius.

Emissions: The amount of a substance added to the medium in a given time period. In the context of climate change, **emissions** refers to the amount of greenhouse gases added to the atmosphere per year (e.g., ~19 Gt of C per year). The relationship with concentration in terms of climate change mitigation strategies is important; for example, reduction of emissions does not necessarily lead to a decline in concentration.

End point approach: An approach in which vulnerability is viewed as the impacts that result from the added effects of climate change influences, using projections from climate modeling. From these projections, impacts on individuals with existing health predispositions and vulnerabilities are estimated; community vulnerabilities are understood as the aggregate of individual vulnerabilities.

Energy balance: The ability of greenhouse gases to trap heat in the atmosphere.

Energy efficiency: Reducing energy consumption by using less energy to perform the same task or attain the same level of output. This is distinguished from energy conservation, the concept of reducing energy consumption through minimizing energy-consuming activities, which requires changes in individual behavior.

Ensemble: In the context of climate modeling, an ensemble is a group of different global climate models (GCMs) that have conducted an otherwise identical experiment. Their results can be averaged to produce a multimodel ensemble mean; their spread or variance is a measure of the scientific uncertainty associated with that prediction. An ensemble may also be composed of an experiment conducted several times by a *single* GCM conducting an experiment several times, identical in every way except for the weather on the first day of the experiment (i.e., the initial conditions). In that case, the ensemble mean can be used to isolate the true forced response (according to that GCM) whereas the variance likely represents internal variability.

Environmental exposure pathways: The physical course taken by hazardous substances from point of origin through human contact.

Environmental justice: The fair treatment and meaningful involvement of all people regardless of race, color, national origin, or income, with respect to the development, implementation, and enforcement of environmental laws, regulations, and policies (EPA: https://www.epa.gov/environmentaljustice).

Eukaryote: An organism whose cells contain a nucleus within a membrane.

Exposure: Contact between a person and one or more biological, chemical, or physical stressors, including stressors affected by climate change.

Exposure Response Function: see **Dose-, Exposure-,** or **Concentration Response Function**

Extraterrestrial hazards: Extraterrestrial objects that, when exposed to populations, may cause loss of life, injury, or other health impacts.

Extreme climate events: Occur when the exacerbation of extreme weather events lasts for a prolonged period of time, for example, a season.

Extreme heat event: A period with notably greater than-normal surface temperatures and moisture for a specific geographic location and time of year.

Extreme weather events: Cyclones, hurricanes, drought, or flooding of a frequency, duration, or intensity that would not normally be predicted by past observations.

Extrinsic incubation period: The time required for the pathogen to (1) establish an infection in a blood-feeding vector and (2) multiply or develop to the point where it can be further transmitted during subsequent vector feedings.

Feedback Loops: Feedback loops are a "cyclical process triggered by environmental change that leads back to more change," such as melting ice caps that in turn expose darker land mass absorbing more solar heat and triggering greater warming. Another example is ozone depletion, which increases ultraviolet radiation, which in turn suppresses the human immune system (Lenton et al. 2019).

Flood: A significant rise of water level in a stream, lake, reservoir, or coastal region

Forced migration: The involuntary movements of refugees and internally displaced people (those displaced by conflict or persecution within their country of origin) as well as people displaced by natural or environmental disasters, famine, chemical or nuclear disasters, or development projects.

Forcing: A factor, either actual or hypothetical, which drives change in the climatic system (see **Climate sensitivity** and **Radiative forcing**).

Fossil fuel: A natural fuel such as coal or gas, formed in the geological past from the remains of living organisms.

Frames, framing: The selection and emphasis of particular meanings in communication, for example, a "public health frame" in climate change communication stresses the relevance of public health to climate change.

Future experiment: Global climate model experiments that simulate a future period of time (say, out to the year 2100) given a prescribed scenario of future greenhouse gas scenarios (see **Representative concentration pathways**).

Gender mainstreaming: The concept of integrating a gendered perspective into policy design, process, planning, implementation, and evaluation to promote equality between women and men.

General Comment 14:   Drafted by the Committee on Economic, Social and Cultural Rights to explain the meaning of the **right to health**; adopted by UN members in 2000.

Global circulation model: Complex mathematical models of the Earth's atmosphere and oceans that are used to study the likely environmental impacts of shifts in greenhouse gas emissions, such as changes in temperature, precipitation, and sea level.

Global climate change: The long-term variation in average weather conditions that occur across the globe.

Global climate model (GCM):   Computerized representation of the laws of physics that govern how the atmosphere, ocean, and other features of the climate system operate and interact.

Global warming potential (GWP):   A particular potential to absorb energy emitted from the Earth's surface and atmosphere.

Governance: The totality of "political, organizational and administrative processes through which stakeholders, including governments, civil society and private-sector interest groups, articulate their interests, exercise their legal rights, make decisions, meet their obligations, and mediate their differences" (Swinburn et al. 2019)

Greenhouse effect: A naturally occurring phenomenon that, through its capture of the sun's energy, raises the Earth's baseline average temperature by 33°C (91°F).

Greenhouse gases: Atmospheric constituents whose molecular geometry render them particularly effective at intercepting thermal radiation (emitted by the surface of Earth) and reemitting it to the atmosphere rather than allowing it to escape to space. Examples include carbon dioxide, water vapor, ozone, and methane. Rising concentrations of greenhouse gases lead to a net energy imbalance in Earth's climate, requiring an increase in global average temperature (hence the widely used term *greenhouse effect*).

Grid cell: The basic unit of space in a global climate model (GCM). GCMs divide the global climate system into a large number of discrete cells, and the governing equations of the atmosphere, ocean, etc. are all solved for within each of these grid cells. The size of a grid cell is a function of the GCMs resolution, and can vary from GCM to GCM depending on scientific objective and/or computer resources available.

Harvesting effects: Also referred to as mortality displacement, a short-term increase in mortality followed by reduced mortality, especially among susceptible people who may have died regardless of heat exposure within the next few days.

Hazard: A dangerous phenomenon, substance, human activity, or condition that may cause loss of life, injury, or other health impacts.

Hazard avoidance: The category of risk treatment that seeks to avoid the incidence and prevalence of hazards.

Health–climate nexus: The impact of the climate crisis on human health and the intersection of the health and climate fields.

Health impact assessment: A combination of procedures, methods, and tools by which a policy, project, or hazard may be judged as to its potential effects on the health of a population and the distribution of those effects within the population (WHO 1999).

Health impact function: Equation used to estimate the number of health outcomes (e.g., mortality or morbidity events) in a population associated with a given exposure.

Health system: According to the World Health Organization, a health system consists of all the activities whose primary purpose is to promote, restore or maintain health. This includes efforts to influence determinants of health as well as more direct health-improving activities (WHO 2000).

Health system stress testing: Focusing on climate-related hypothetical scenarios, the effective operations of the health system is assessed and approaches for managing acute and chronic climate events are developed. Such exercises increase the capacity of health systems and related sectors to adapt and respond to climate-related shocks and challenges.

Health vulnerability and adaptation assessments: These allow local, regional, and national levels of government to understand climate change-related health risks, identify populations that are most at risk, recognize vulnerabilities in the health system, and inform effective and inclusive adaptation actions and response measures.

Heat syncope: Fainting or dizziness as a result of overheating (*syncope* is the medical term for fainting). It is a type of *heat* illness. The basic symptom of heat syncope is fainting, with or without mental confusion.

Heat wave: A period of time when daily temperatures rise above a specified threshold high-end temperature (e.g., the 95th or 99th percentile of X-year seasonal or monthly averages) for at least two consecutive days in a given location. Temperature thresholds usually factor in both absolute temperature and humidity, with specific units varying by monitoring jurisdiction.

Historical trauma: Cumulative trauma across both one person's lifespan and across generations, resulting from political, economic, and environmental stressors.

Human rights: The entitlements everyone has, by virtue of being born, to live a life of equality and dignity.

Human rights–based approaches: Explicitly assist governments to meet their internationally and nationally binding human rights obligations and empower people to know and claim their rights.

Hydrofluorocarbons (HFCs): Potent short-lived climate pollutants (SLCP) used in air conditioning, refrigeration, solvents, some foams such as fire extinguishing systems, and aerosols. HFCs are orders of magnitude more potent than carbon dioxide and have a much shorter atmospheric lifetime. The Kigali Amendment to the Montreal Protocol, agreed to in 2016, specifically added HFCs to the list of gases to phase down.

Hydrologic cycle: The sequence of conditions through which water passes from vapor to precipitation in the form of liquids and solids then back to vapor through the process of evaporation and transpiration.

Hydrologic hazards: Movement of water that, when exposed to populations, may cause loss of life, injury, or other health impacts.

Hydrosphere: The solid, liquid, and gaseous water parts of a planet such as Earth.

Hypotension: Low blood pressure, which can cause fainting or dizziness when the brain does not receive enough blood.

Incremental adaptation: Occurs when information on the risks of climate change is integrated into policies and measures, without changing underlying assumptions. This includes improving public health and health care services for climate-relevant health outcomes, without necessarily considering the possible impacts of climate change.

Incubation period: Time between exposure to the hazard and biological onset of disease.

Indigenous: There is no universally recognized definition of Indigenous peoples; however, key features include self-identification as Indigenous; historical continuity with precolonial and/or presettler societies; links to territories and surrounding natural resources; distinct social, economic, or political systems; and distinct language, culture, and beliefs (United Nations 2015).

Information deficit model: A uni-directional communication model which assumes the audience requires education, information, or facts in order to be engaged with a topic.

Integrated assessment model: Computer modeling frameworks that link human behaviors (e.g., population characteristics, economic development, emissions of greenhouse gases, etc.) with physical earth dynamics (e.g., atmosphere-ocean interactions, carbon storage in the biosphere, etc.) in order to inform environmental policy.

Initial conditions: In the context of climate modeling, the particular state of the climate system at the first time step of a GCM simulation. In other words, the weather. In weather forecasting, initial conditions are crucially important; in general, the better we know the state of the atmosphere *now*, the better our forecast of the weather in forty-eight hours will be. In climate modeling, the initial conditions are long forgotten before the time period attempting to be predicted (decades in the future). In fact, it is becoming commonplace for GCM experiments to be run many times with extremely slight random noise added to the initial conditions to *ensure* that the initial conditions are not influencing the long–range climate change projection.

Intergovernmental Panel on Climate Change (IPCC): Expert panel established in 1988 by the World Meteorological Organization (WMO) and the United Nations Environment Programme (UNEP) to summarize the state of the science on climate change, impacts, and policy response strategies. The group consists of over 2,500 international voluntary scientists who curate periodic "assessment reports" that are later reviewed by representatives of the member states of the United Nations, which in turn will either reject or accept them.

Internal variability: Loosely synonymous with *natural* climate variability, internal variability refers to the fluctuations in climate that are not driven by changes in *external* forcing agents such as greenhouse gases, volcanic eruptions, and solar output.

Internally displaced persons: Migrants forced from their homes who have not crossed an international border and remain under the jurisdiction of their own national governments.

Kampala Convention: A legally binding instrument, restricted for use within the African Union, designed to protect internally displaced persons

Kigali Amendment: The Kigali Amendment to the Montreal Protocol was adopted in 2016 to phase down the use of hydrofluorocarbons (HFCs) by cutting consumption and production.

Landslides: All types of gravity-induced ground movements, ranging from rock falls through slides/slumps, avalanches, and flows, triggered mainly by precipitation, seismic activity, and volcanic eruptions.

Land-use planning: The process undertaken by public authorities to identify, evaluate, and decide on different options for the use of land.

Lithosphere: The rocky, outer part of the Earth.

Low-emission vehicles: Gas-alternative or gas-hybrid vehicles that lower climate altering pollutant emissions per passenger mile traveled, with concurrent reductions in air pollutant emissions.

Lyme disease: Tick-borne illness primarily caused by one of three species of the *Borreliella* bacteria. Infection is typically divided into three clinical phases—early localized, early disseminated, and late—based on time from the primary tick bite. Rash is the most typical finding of early localized disease, whereas early disseminated disease can manifest with cardiac and/or neurologic symptoms anywhere from weeks to months after the initial bite. If left untreated, late disease can develop months to years after initial exposure and most typically manifests as a relapsing polyarticular arthritis, though chronic fatigue and neurologic symptoms can also occur. Early localized infections are easily treated with antibiotics, whereas treatment for later stages is more nuanced.

Major depressive disorder: A mood disorder characterized by a pervasive and persistent sense of hopelessness and despair.

Malaria: Febrile illness caused by the *Plasmodium* parasites *P. falciparum, P. vivax, P. malariae, P. ovalae,* and *P. knowelsi.* The uncomplicated illness typically manifests as fever in addition to a range of nonspecific symptoms. Complicated infections may affect any or a number of organ system(s), Anti-parasitic treatment varies according to the causative species. Inadequately or untreated infections can recur after apparent cure.

Malnutrition: A broad term that refers to all forms of poor nutrition, including **undernutrition,** overweight, and obesity. Malnutrition is caused by a complex array of factors, including dietary inadequacy (deficiencies, excesses, or imbalances in energy, protein, and micronutrients), infections, and sociocultural factors (Global Nutrition Report 2018).

Mass extinction: A loss of 75 percent of the world's species in a period defined as two million years or less.

Mental health: A state of well-being in which every individual realizes their own potential, can cope with the normal stresses of life, can work productively and fruitfully, and is able to contribute to the community.

Meteorologic hazards: Acute weather conditions that, when exposed to populations, may cause loss of life, injury, or other health impacts.

Mitigation: The process of reducing the severity or seriousness of something; used in the climate literature in reference to the reduction of climate-altering pollutant concentrations either through reductions in emissions or increases in gas capture processes.

Model: A representation that mimics relevant features of the situation being studied.

Mobile source: Sources of air pollution including on-road vehicles and nonroad vehicles and engines.

Montreal Protocol: A multilateral environmental agreement that focuses on the reduction of ozone depleting substances.

Multilateral: A policy, proposal, or act that has been agreed upon by three or more parties. From a climate perspective, multilateral agreements are key to affecting temperature increases and greenhouse gas accumulation.

Narratives: Stories and meaning-making in communication, for example, through relating climate change to people's real-life experiences.

National Adaptation Programmes of Action (NAPAs):   Drafted by least developed countries to identify their most "urgent and immediate adaptation needs"—those for which further delay in implementation would increase vulnerability to climate change or increase adaptation costs at a later stage—and submitted to the United Nations Framework Convention on Climate Change for possible funding from the Least Developed Country Fund.

National Ambient Air Quality Standards (NAAQS):   Clean Air Act-mandated ambient air limits for air pollutants considered harmful to public health and to the environment.

Nationally Determined Contributions (NDCs):   The Paris Agreement requires that each country communicate the explicit ways in which they will reduce emissions and by how much; NDCs are a country's stated targets and timelines.

Natural hazard: Natural process or phenomenon that may cause loss of life, injury, or other health impacts, property damage, loss of livelihoods and services, social and economic disruption, or environmental damage.

Nitrogen oxides (NO_x):   A class of precursor compounds that, when combined in the atmosphere in the presence of sunlight along with **volatile organic compounds,** can form ground-level ozone, a major component of smog.

Nonstructural mitigation: Any measure that uses knowledge, practice, or agreement to reduce risks and impacts, in particular through policies and laws, public awareness raising, training, and education.

Ocean acidification: The decrease in the pH values of Earth's oceans primarily due to chemical reactions between seawater and carbon dioxide as it is absorbed from the atmosphere. The increase in CO_2 in the atmosphere absorbed by the ocean reduces calcification rates in reef-building and reef-associated organisms by altering seawater chemistry through decreases in pH.

Occupational hazard: Hazard experienced specifically in the workplace because of the worksite or the nature of the work.

Occupational illness: Chronic ailment or disease caused by work-related exposures.

Occupational injury: Physical—and potentially mental— harm resulting from work-related activities.

OneHealth: A collaborative, multisectoral, and transdisciplinary approach—working at the local, regional, national, and global levels—with the goal of achieving optimal health outcomes recognizing the interconnection between people, animals, plants, and their shared environment (CDC 2019).

Ozone (O_3):   A major air pollutant and colorless, unstable gas with a pungent odor. Ozone is a powerful lung irritant that is harmful in the lower atmosphere (**troposphere**) but a beneficial component of the upper atmosphere (**stratosphere**).

Ozone layer: Blanket of diffuse gases encircling the earth as part of the upper atmosphere, at a distance of 12 to 50 kilometers above the surface; also refers to three oxygen atoms (ozone, or O3) that concentrate there.

Parallel processing: The computation strategy often employed in climate modeling wherein the world is split into a number of tiles (each tile containing many grid cells), and the equation solving within those tiles is distributed across a number of individual computer processors. Parallel processing significantly speeds up a global climate model experiment that needs to simulate a long time period (say, 2006 through 2100) at a reasonable spatial resolution.

Paralytic shellfish poisoning: Poisoning syndrome that occurs from the consumption of shellfish contaminated with saxitoxin.

Parameterization: The implementation of a real physical process in the climate system into a global climate model (GCM) without directly simulating that physical process. Rather, the process is implemented by way of its relationship with other *parameters* that are more confidently solved for by the GCM.

Paris Agreement Carbon Budget: The amount of CO_2 the globe can emit and still meet goals set by the Paris Agreement.

Paris Climate Agreement: An international treaty created among attendees of the 2015 United Nations Climate Change conference in Paris, France, aimed at reducing the emission of gases responsible for global warming

Particulate matter (PM):   A major air pollutant comprising a complex mixture of extremely small particles and liquid droplets. Particle pollution is made up of a number of components, including acids (such as nitrates and sulfates), organic chemicals, metals, and soil or dust particles. Fine particles, such as those found in smoke and haze, are 2.5 micrometers in diameter and smaller ($PM_{2.5}$).

Peaker plants: Power plants that generally run only when there is a high demand, known as peak demand, for electricity.

Phenology: The study of periodic plant and animal lifecycle events and how these are influenced by seasonal and interannual variations in climate.

Photochemical: A chemical reaction initiated by the absorption of energy in the form of light.

Photodermatitis: A form of allergic contact dermatitis whereby the allergen is activated by light in order to induce an allergic response.

Phytoplankton: Microscopic marine algae at the base of several aquatic food webs.

PM$_{2.5}$: Fine particulate matter that can remain suspended in the air for long periods of time. It has been linked with increased risk of pulmonary and cardiovascular disease.

Policymakers: Governmental actors who directly promulgate policies in public spaces, private actors who promulgate policies within their governance structures and influence public policy, and other nongovernmental actors that influence public policy through advocacy, research, activism, and lending subject matter expertise in formal and informal ways, such as advising multilateral negotiations.

Polluter pays principle: The principle that polluters and users of natural resources bear the full environmental and social costs of their actions, ensuring that a more complete picture of the cost is reflected in the ultimate market price for a good or service.

Polyether: Polymeric, often chain-like, organic compounds containing ether linkages.

Posttraumatic stress disorder (PTSD): A mental health condition triggered by a terrifying event—war, disaster, or physical or emotional trauma.

Precautionary principle: States that political, social, and economic responses to environmental threats should move forward with all deliberate speed rather than embrace inertia until definite scientific answers are found.

Precursor: An air pollutant emitted directly from a source. Often used in describing the pollutant building blocks that drive formation of secondary pollutants.

Preeclampsia/Eclampsia: Complications of pregnancy including high blood pressure and protein loss in urine that may eventually lead to seizures and death for both mother and baby without prompt intervention.

Preparedness: The knowledge and capacities developed by people to effectively anticipate, respond to, and recover from, the impacts of likely, imminent, or current hazard events or conditions.

Prevention: The outright avoidance of adverse impacts of hazards and related disasters.

Primary pollutant: An air pollutant emitted directly from a source.

Primary prevention: Avoidance of adverse outcomes before they occur at the population level, by reducing risk factors for specific hazards within groups of healthy individuals. Distinct from *primordial prevention*.

Primordial prevention: Prevention of health hazards from occurring. Distinct from *primary prevention*.

Pro-environmental behavior: Personal action that addresses climate change, such as reducing energy usage in the home.

Progressive realization of the right to health: A specific and continuing state obligation to move as expeditiously and effectively as possible toward the full realization of the **right to health**. Retrogressive measures are not permissible (health rights must not deteriorate), and states must prove any such measures were introduced only after the most careful consideration of all alternatives.

Projection: Defined by the Intergovernmental Panel on Climate Change as the "response of the climate system to emission or concentration scenarios of greenhouse gases and aerosols, or radiative forcing scenarios, often based upon simulations by climate models."

Prokaryote: Microscopic single-celled organism that lacks a distinct nucleus.

Provisioning ecosystem services: Ecosystem services that represent material benefits of ecosystems that people use, appreciate, or sell. Many provisioning services have market value. These services include food production, water provision, and raw material creation (e.g., wood).

Psychological distance: The perception of being disconnected from an issue such as climate change; psychological distance has four dimensions: temporal (distance in time), social (distance between oneself and others), spatial (geographical distance), and uncertainty (how certain it is that an event will happen).

Public engagement: The extent to which people are cognitively, affectively (emotionally), and behaviorally connected with a problem such as climate change.

Quality-Adjusted Life Year (QALY) and Disability-Adjusted Life Year (DALY): Metrics used for measuring morbidity benefits or costs; see Chapter 24 for detailed explanations

Radiative forcing: The planetary energy imbalance (incoming minus outgoing) due to a particular forcing agent. Some anthropogenic forcings can result in a negative radiative forcing, such as aerosols (as they reflect incoming solar radiation). Anthropogenic greenhouse gas forcing currently amounts to a net 1–2 W/m^2 of radiative forcing.

Ratification: In the context of the United Nations, ratification of treaties refers to the agreement by a country or state to be bound by a treaty. Ratification usually requires time for a country to gain domestic approval for the treaty and enact legislation that follows the treaties requirements.

Recovery: The restoration, and improvement where appropriate, of facilities, livelihoods, and living conditions (and health status), including efforts to reduce disaster risk factors.

Red tides: Common term for blooms of microalgae and cyanobacteria that contain red pigments, causing an appearance of "red paint" on the surface of the water.

Redfield ratio: Molar ratio of carbon:nitrogen:phosphorous of 106:16:1 as found in seawater and phytoplankton.

Refugees: Migrants forced from their homes who have crossed an international border. They are legally defined and protected by the 1951 United Nations Convention Relating to the Status of Refugees and the related 1967 Protocol.

Regulating ecosystem services: Ecosystem services that regulate natural systems, such as an ecosystem's ability to regulate flooding, pollinate crops, or maintain soil health.

Relative risk: The probability of an exposed group of people experiencing an adverse health outcome in relation to the probability of that outcome in an unexposed group.

Relocation: The action of moving a community to another place, often organized and carried out by the national government.

Renewable energy: Cleaner energy sources that include solar photovoltaic (PV) cells, wind turbines, and hydroelectric power.

Representative concentration pathways (RCPs):   Scenarios that take into account different levels of emissions and concentrations of greenhouse gases. Each scenario considers a trajectory over time that would lead to potential future climate conditions. Four RCPs are widely used in climate modeling for global change science; RCP2.6, RCP4.5, RCP6.0, and RCP8.5. The number following RCP indicates the radiative forcing (in W/m^2) at 2100.

Residence time: Relative measure of the average amount of time that a water molecule would be expected to be present within a waterbody before being lost or removed.

Resilience: The ability of a system and its component parts to anticipate, absorb, accommodate, or recover from a given insult (eg. environmental hazard) in a timely and efficient manner, including through ensuring the preservation, restoration, or improvement of its essential basic structures and functions (IPCC 2012).

Resolution: In the context of global climate models (GCMs), the size of a grid cell. A "higher resolution" GCM has smaller grid cells and, consequently, more of them (so as to completely cover the planet). Higher resolution requires exponentially greater computer resources but may enable smaller–scale (and potentially important) physical processes to be directly simulated rather than relying heavily on parameterizations.

Response: The provision of emergency services and public assistance during or immediately after a disaster in order to save lives, reduce health impacts, ensure public safety, and meet the basic subsistence needs of the people affected.

Right to health: Arising from the International Covenant on Economic, Social and Cultural Rights (Article 12) and spelled out in UN **General Comment 14** that all people are entitled to the highest attainable standard of mental and physical health. This extends to timely and appropriate health care as well as access to the underlying determinants of health, such as access to safe and potable water and adequate sanitation, safe food, nutrition and housing, healthy occupational, and environmental conditions and health information.

Risk: The potential for consequences where something of value is at stake and where outcomes are uncertain. The probability of harmful consequences, (e.g., morbidity and mortality) resulting from interactions between natural or human-induced hazards and vulnerable conditions.

Risk avoidance: Methods that avoid risk altogether (e.g., hazard avoidance and exposure avoidance).

Risk management: The systematic approach and practice of managing uncertainty to minimize potential harm and loss.

Risk multiplier: A multiplier is an economic factor that when increased/changed causes increases/changes in many other variables. A cumulatively reinforcing induced interaction between one factor and multiple variables. Climate change is a risk multiplier to health—it is multiplying the risks not only associated with climate change-induced disasters and catastrophic effects, but also those associated with health risks affected on multiple levels by climate change. For example, global warming causes water evaporation and extreme, unpredictable temperatures that affect food and water supplies, which can lead to malnutrition, diarrhea, heart and respiratory diseases, and waterborne or insect-transmitted diseases.

Risk reduction: Methods that reduce the likelihood or impact of a hazard.

Risk retention: Methods that accept the risk (also known as risk acceptance).

Risk transfer: The process of formally or informally shifting the financial consequences of particular risks from one party to another.

Risk treatment: The process of selecting and implementing of measures to modify risk. Risk treatment measures can include avoiding, optimizing, transferring, or retaining risk.

Scenarios: Alternate images or storylines for future states that include details relevant to the processes being projected.

Scientific uncertainty: In the context of global climate models (GCMs), the uncertainty due to imperfect scientific knowledge of the physics of the climate system (manifest as imperfect GCMs). The scientific uncertainty associated with future experiments is generally characterized by the *spread* among an ensemble of GCM results. Each GCM may be subject to the same assumptions about future greenhouse gas forcing, yet each GCM yielded slightly different results.

Sea inundation: An acute-onset, coastal flood event, not associated with low pressure weather systems, tides, or top-overs/breaches of barriers.

Sea level rise: The increase in the average level of all of Earth's oceans, mainly because of the melting of sea ice and expansion of saltwater as temperatures warm.

Secondary pollutant: An air pollutant that forms when other (primary) pollutants react in the atmosphere.

Secondary prevention: Once the exposure/hazard has occurred, secondary prevention aims to avoid adverse outcomes through early detection of disease among high-risk individuals.

Segmentation: The use of statistical techniques to group a population according to common characteristics.

Sendai Framework for Disaster Risk Reduction: An international covenant adopted in 2015 to establish common goals and standards for disaster risk reduction.

Senescing: In the case of algae, refers to the aging and break down of a bloom, and the associated release of pigments (and toxins) into water.

Shared socioeconomic pathways (SSPs):   A set of future scenarios that capture plausible trends in socioeconomic and environmental conditions over the twenty-first century.

Short-lived climate pollutants (SLCPs):   Pollutants that have shorter atmospheric lifetimes but are hundreds or thousands of times more potent than carbon dioxide in warming effects. The four key SLCPs are methane, hydrofluorocarbons, black carbon, and tropospheric ozone.

Skepticism (with regard to climate change):   The holding of doubts about the physical reality, human causation, or importance of climate change, and/or concerning the ability of human action to effectively address it.

Smart Hospital Initiative (SHI):   A seven-step toolkit by the Pan American Health Organization focused on building safe, smart, and green facilities in the Caribbean and Latin America.

Social cost of carbon (SCC):   A measure of the net present value to the global society of emitting one additional unit of CO_2.

Social marketing: The application of principles from commercial marketing for socially desirable ends.

Social movements: Collective actions in which the public is alerted, educated, and then mobilized to challenge the economic and political leaders and the whole society to redress social problems and restore critical social values.

Societal uncertainty: In the context of future experiments, the uncertainty due to the fact that we cannot predict exactly how much greenhouse gases will continue to increase over the course of this century. Even if there was no scientific uncertainty, societal uncertainty would be inevitable. Societal uncertainty is built into the enterprise of climate modeling for global change by simulating four different RCPs—to account for a wide range of possible futures in terms of population, economics, technology, policy, etc.

Soot: A black, carbonaceous substance produced during incomplete combustion of fossil fuels.

Starting point approach: A second vulnerability framework in which environmental and social processes are included, more easily incorporating environmental justice concerns; social and economic processes of marginalization and inequalities are diagnosed as the causes of climate vulnerability.

Stationary sources: Place-bound emitters of air pollution including factories, refineries, boilers, and power plants.

Storm: Any disturbed state of an astronomical body's atmosphere, especially affecting its surface, and strongly implying severe weather.

Storm runoff: Rainfall and snowmelt that flows across impervious surfaces.

Stratosphere/Stratospheric ozone layer: The layer of the earth's atmosphere that extends between 12 and 50 km above the earth, as distinguished from the troposphere, which resides within the first 12 km above earth. The stratosphere contains the highest concentration of ozone, known as the "ozone layer." Its function is to protect the earth from harmful ultraviolet (UV-B) radiation, which in high concentrations has dire effects on human health

Structural mitigation: Any physical construction aimed to reduce or avoid possible impacts of hazards, or application of engineering techniques to achieve hazard-resistance and resilience in structures or systems

Subsistence: Alaska state law defines subsistence use as "the noncommercial, customary and traditional uses of wild, renewable resources by a resident domiciled in a rural area of the state for direct personal or family consumption as food, shelter, fuel, clothing, tools, or transportation, for the making and selling of handicraft articles out of nonedible by-products of fish and wildlife resources taken for personal or family consumption, and for the customary trade, barter, or sharing for personal or family consumption" (State of Alaska 2019). The Alaska Federation of Natives (AFN) describes subsistence as "the hunting, fishing, and gathering activities which traditionally constituted the economic base of life for Alaska's Native peoples and which continue to flourish in many areas of the state today" (Alaska Federation of Natives 2012).

Sustainable and Climate-Resilient Health Care Facilities Initiative (SCRHCFI): U.S. Department of Health and Human Services' online resource available to assist facilities in preparing for and responding to extreme weather events using a five-step framework

Sustainable development: Development that meets the needs of the present without compromising the ability of future generations to meet their own needs.

Sustainable Development Goals (SDGs): Seventeen aspirational goals for global well-being, created by the United Nations in 2015. Example targets include ending poverty and protecting the planet from climate change.

Synergistic reaction: A reaction where the combination of one or more factors leads to result much greater than the sole effect of individual factors, such as human exposure to multiple harmful chemicals that produce unforeseen health effects, as in the case of DDT.

Technological hazards: Human-made technologies that when exposed to populations may cause loss of life, injury, or other health impacts.

Tertiary prevention: Once exposure/hazard has occurred, involves treatment of established conditions in order to avoid further deterioration (which may include permanent disability and/or death).

Thermoregulation: A process to maintain a relatively constant core body temperature, which is critical to the survival of the creature, even when the surrounding temperature is different.

Tipping point: A scenario when an ecosystem undergoes significant changes to biodiversity. A threshold beyond which the impact may be many times greater than expected, such as the irreversible loss of ice sheets once the temperature and melting rate has reached a particular level that in turn triggers greater warming.

Total committed emissions from the energy sector: An estimate of future CO_2 emissions, considering business-as-usual operations of existing and proposed energy infrastructure. Usually described in the context of a particular carbon budget. See Paris Agreement Carbon Budget.

Transactional sex: A sexual relationship formed as a response to forced migration and food shortages based on the need for resources such as food, fuel wood, and transportation.

Transformation: Changes in social and other structures that mediate the construction of risk.

Transitional adaptation: Can occur with changes in underlying assumptions, including shifts in attitudes and perceptions. This includes vulnerability mapping, early warning systems, and other measures when they explicitly incorporate climate change.

Triple-policy energy mitigation strategy: Avoidance of **tipping points** and **negative synergistic reactions** requires simultaneously (1) ending reliance on fossil fuels, (2) creation of net-zero emissions energy systems, and (3) development of aggressive carbon-removal strategies.

Troposphere: The lowest layer of the atmosphere, in which the air temperature decreases with height. The depth of the troposphere is roughly 11 km on average, but with considerable geographical and seasonal variation. The boundary between the troposphere and the next layer above, the stratosphere, is called the tropopause; above this altitude, temperature begins to increase with height.

Trusted messengers: Persons regarded as credible sources of health information.

Ultrafine particles: Particulate matter of nanoscale size (less than 0.1 μm or 100 nm in diameter), which are not distinctly regulated by the National Ambient Air Quality Standards.

Uncertainty: The probability that a statement is (in)valid; the IPCC uses shorthand statements (such as "very likely") to equate to numerical probabilities (e.g., "very likely" corresponds to ">90 percent probability").

Undernutrition: Exists when a combination of insufficient food intake, health, and care conditions results in one or more of the following: underweight for age, short for age (stunted), thin for height (wasted), or functionally deficient in vitamins and/or minerals (micronutrient malnutrition).

Undernourishment: The condition in which an individual's habitual food consumption is insufficient to provide the amount of dietary energy required to maintain a normal, active, healthy life (Global Nutrition Report 2018). Prevalence of undernourishment (PoU) is a complex, aggregated measure of undernourishment at the national level.

UN Environment Programme (UNEP or UNE):   UNEP is the leading global environmental authority that sets the global environmental agenda, advocates for the environment, and promotes the coherent implementation of the environmental dimension of sustainable development. A United Nations program under the General Assembly organ, UNEP has historically been one of the least funded of the funds or programs.

Urban heat island (UHI):   An urban or metropolitan area that is significantly warmer than its surrounding rural areas (see **Urban heat island effect.**)

Urban heat island effect: A phenomenon where the higher thermal storage capacity of the urban environment combines with a relatively high concentration of local heat sources to increase temperatures relative to surrounding areas. The UHI effect results in both elevated surface and air temperatures; built environment materials re-radiate heat at night, raising nighttime temperatures.

Value: In the psychology literature, a guiding principle in the life of a person.

Value of a statistical life (VSL):   A calculation of the value of a small change in the risk of death, better termed "value of mortality risk."

Vasodilation: The dilation of blood vessels, which decreases blood pressure.

Vernalization: The biological requirement of cold temperature exposure required by some plants prior to spring flowering.

Vector-borne diseases (VBD):   Infectious diseases transmitted by arthropod vectors (e.g., mosquitoes and ticks).

Volatile organic compounds (VOCs):   Along with nitrogen oxides, precursor compounds of ozone, a major component of smog.

Voltage-gated sodium channels: Transmembrane proteins that allow sodium ions to travel across membranes and cause depolarization of neurons, resulting in an action potential.

Voluntary migration: The voluntary movement of persons who are able to choose the timing and destination of their migrant journey, usually in search of improved economic opportunities.

Vulnerability: Susceptibility to harms and risks, which includes inequality of social, economic, and environmental conditions, in addition to individual health factors; the propensity or predisposition to be adversely affected. The Intergovernmental Panel on Climate Change defines vulnerability as the degree to which a system is susceptible to, or unable to cope with, adverse effects of climate change, including climate variability and extremes. Vulnerability is a function of the character, magnitude, and rate of climate variation to which a system is exposed, its sensitivity, and its adaptive capacity.

Warm-water reefs: Warm-water coral reefs occupying habitats that are close to the surface (0–100 meters) where they secrete calcium carbonate skeletons that accumulate over time, creating a complex reef matrix that provides habitat for hundreds of thousands of marine species.

Wildfire: Fires in forest or brush grasslands that cover extensive areas and usually do extensive damage.

Willingness-to-pay (WTP) or Willingness-to-accept (WTA):   WTP is what an individual would pay to avoid a health impact; WTA is the least amount of payment an individual would accept to experience the health impact.

World Health Organization (WHO): A specialized agency under the United Nations System, under the umbrella of the United Nations Economic and Social Council. Its primary role is to direct and coordinate international health within the UN system. Its main areas of work are in health systems, health through the lifecycle, noncommunicable and communicable diseases; preparedness, surveillance, and response; and corporate services. They mostly work on climate adaptation, not mitigation.

World Meteorological Organization (WMO): An international body with 193 member states that falls under the umbrella of the United Nations. It provides international cooperation on weather, climate, hydrological services, and other geophysical sciences among its member countries.

Zooplankton: Animal-like constituent of plankton- protozoa, small crustaceans, fish eggs, and larvae.

References

Alaska Federation of Natives. 2012. "The Right to Subsist: Federal Protection of Subsistence in Alaska." https://www.nativefederation.org/wp-content/uploads/2018/07/2010-april8-the-right-to-subsistence.pdf.

Centers for Disease Control and Prevention. 2019. "One Health Basics." https://www.cdc.gov/onehealth/basics/index.html.

Environmental Pretection Agency. 2020. "Environmentaj Justice." Accessed April 30, 2020. https://www.epa.gov/environmentaljustice.

Global Nutrition Report. 2018. *Global Nutrition Report: Shining a Light to Spur Action on Nutrition.* Bristol, UK: Development Initiatives.

Holling, C. S. 1978. *Adaptive Environmental Assessment and Management.* Chichester, UK: John Wiley & Sons.

Intergovernmental Panel on Climate Change. 2012. "Glossary of Terms." In *Managing the Risks of Extreme Events and Disasters to Advance Climate Change Adaptation. A Special Report of Working Groups I and II of the Intergovernmental Panel on Climate Change*, edited by C. B. Field, V. Barros, T. F. Stocker, D. Qin, D. J. Dokken, K. L. Ebi, M. D. Mastrandrea et al., 555–64. Cambridge, UK, and New York: Cambridge University Press.

Lenton, T., J. Rockström, O. Gaffney, S. Rahmstorf, K. Richardson, W. Steffen, and H. J. Schellnhuber. 2019. "Climate Tipping Points—Too Risky to Bet Against." *Nature* November 27, 2019. https://www.nature.com/articles/d41586-019-03595-0.

National Research Council, Division on Earth and Life Studies, Ocean Studies Board, Water Science and Technology Board, Committee to Assess the U.S. Army Corps of Engineers Methods of Analysis and Peer Review for Water Resources Project Planning, Panel on Adaptive Management for Resource Stewardship. 2004. *Adaptive Management for Water Resources Project Planning.* Washington, DC: National Academies Press.

State of Alaska. 2019. "Alaska Statutes." http://www.akleg.gov/basis/statutes.asp#16.05.940.

Swinburn, B. A., V. I. Kraak, S. Allender, V. J. Atkins, P. I. Baker, J. R. Bogard, H. Brinsden et al. 2019. "The Global Syndemic of Obesity, Undernutrition, and Climate Change: *The Lancet* Commission Report." *Lancet* 393:791–846.

United Nations Permanent Forum on Indigenous Issues. 2015. *Who Are Indigenous Peoples? 5th Session. Fact Sheet 1.* New York, United Nations.

World Health Organization. 1999. *Health Impact Assessment as a Tool for Intersectoral Health Policy.* Bonn, Germany: WHO European Centre for Environment and Health/European Centre for Health Policy.

World Health Organization. 2000. *Health Systems: Improving Performance.* Geneva, Switzerland: WHO. https://www.who.int/whr/2000/en/whr00_en.pdf?ua=1.

World Health Organization. 2015. *Operational Framework for Building Climate Resilient Health Systems.* Geneva, Switzerland: WHO. https://www.afro.who.int/sites/default/files/2017-06/9789241565073_eng.pdf.

World Health Organization. 2020. "Metrics: Disability-Adjusted Life Year (DALY)." Accessed June 26, 2020. https://www.who.int/healthinfo/global_burden_disease/metrics_daly/en/.

World Health Organization. n.d. "Metrics: Disability-Adjusted Life Year (DALY)." https://www.who.int/healthinfo/global_burden_disease/metrics_daly/en/.